NURSING DIAGNOSIS MANUAL

Planning, Individualizing, and Documenting Client Care

6TH EDITION

Marilynn E. Doenges, APN, BC—Retired

Clinical Specialist—Adult Psychiatric/Mental Health Nursing,
Adjunct Faculty (Ret)
Beth-El College of Nursing and Health Sciences, CU–Springs
Colorado Springs, Colorado

Mary Frances Moorhouse, RN, MSN, CRRN

Adjunct Nursing Faculty/Clinical Instructor
Pikes Peak Community College
Colorado Springs, Colorado
Nurse Consultant
TNT-RN Enterprises

Alice C. Murr, BSN, RN—Retired

Retired Legal Nurse Consultant, certified Rehabilitation Case
Manager, and certified practitioner in Critical Care Nursing
Parkville, Missouri

F.A. DAVIS

Philadelphia

F. A. Davis Company
1915 Arch Street
Philadelphia, PA 19103
www.fadavis.com

Printed in the United States of America

Last digit indicates print number: 10 9 8 7 6 5 4 3 2 1

Acquisitions Editor: Jacalyn Sharp
Senior Content Project Manager: Amy M. Romano
Design and Illustrations Manager: Carolyn O'Brien

As new scientific information becomes available through basic and clinical research, recommended treatments and drug therapies undergo changes. The author(s) and publisher have done everything possible to make this book accurate, up to date, and in accord with accepted standards at the time of publication. The author(s), editors, and publisher are not responsible for errors or omissions or for consequences from application of the book and make no warranty, expressed or implied, in regard to the contents of the book. Any practice described in this book should be applied by the reader in accordance with professional standards of care used in regard to the unique circumstances that may apply in each situation. The reader is advised always to check product information (package inserts) for changes and new information regarding dose and contraindications before administering any drug. Caution is especially urged when using new or infrequently ordered drugs.

Library of Congress Cataloging-in-Publication Data

Names: Doenges, Marilynn E., 1922–, author. | Moorhouse, Mary Frances, 1947–, author. | Murr, Alice C., 1946–, author.
Title: Nursing diagnosis manual: planning, individualizing, and documenting client care / Marilynn E. Doenges, Mary Frances Moorhouse, Alice C. Murr.
Description: Sixth edition. | Philadelphia, PA : F.A. Davis Company, [2019] | Includes bibliographical references and indexes.
Identifiers: LCCN 2018042458 (print) | LCCN 2018043379 (ebook) | ISBN 9780803694965 | ISBN 9780803676770 (pbk.)
Subjects: | MESH: Nursing Diagnosis. | Patient Care Planning | Nursing Records
Classification: LCC RT48.6 (ebook) | LCC RT48.6 (print) | NLM WY 100.4 | DDC 616.07/5—dc23
LC record available at http://lccn.loc.gov/2018042458

To our families and friends, who much of the time have had to manage without us while we work and dream, as well as cope with our struggles and frustrations.

The Doenges families: the late Dean, Jim; Barbara and Bob Lanza; David, Monita, Matthew, and Tyler; and John, Holly, Nicole, and Kelsey; and the Daigle families: Nancy, Jim; Jennifer, Brandon, Annabelle, Will, and Henry Smith-Daigle; and Jonathan, Kim, and Mandalyn JoAn.

The Moorhouse family: the late Jan; sons Paul, Jason, and Thenderlyn Moorhouse; granddaughters Alexa and Tanner Plant; Mary Isabella Moorhouse; and the perfect great-grandchild, Quinton Russell Plant.

To my children: Kevin and Tammy Carroll and Darin and Ck Carroll; the best grandchildren ever: Chelsea-Jane, Matthew, Joseph, Nathan, and Ben Carroll; and my perfect great-grandchildren: Maxwell Carroll Bockerstette and Eisley Jo Bockerstette. You are my joy. Mom/Grammy Murr.

To our FAD family, especially Jacalyn Sharp and Amy Romano, our production team who assisted us in meeting deadlines and completing this new edition, and Robert Allen for teaching old nurses new technology.

To the nurses we are writing for, who daily face the challenge of meeting the needs of clients in varied settings and are looking for a practical way to organize and document this care. We believe that nursing diagnosis and these guides will help.

And to NANDA-I and the international nurses who are facilitating the development and dissemination of nursing diagnoses—we continue to champion your efforts and the work of promoting standardized languages.

The American Nurses Association (ANA) *Social Policy Statement* of 1980 was the first to define nursing as the diagnosis and treatment of human responses to actual and potential health problems. This definition, when combined with the ANA *Scope and Standards of Practice,* has provided impetus and support for the use of nursing diagnosis. Defining *nursing* and its effect on client care supports the growing awareness that nursing care is a key factor in client survival and in the maintenance, rehabilitative, and preventive aspects of healthcare. Changes and new developments in healthcare delivery in the past decades have given rise to the need for a common framework of communication to ensure continuity of care for the client moving between multiple healthcare settings and providers.

This book is designed to aid the student nurse and the practitioner in identifying interventions commonly associated with specific nursing diagnoses as disseminated by NANDA International. These interventions are the activities needed to implement and document care provided to the individual client and can be used in varied settings from acute to community/home care.

Chapter 1 presents a brief discussion of the nursing process and introduces the concept of evidence-based practice. Standardized nursing languages (SNLs) are discussed in Chapter 2, with a focus on NANDA-I (nursing diagnoses), NIC (interventions), and NOC (outcomes). NANDA-I has 244 diagnosis labels with definitions, defining characteristics, and related or risk factors used to define a client need or problem. NIC is a comprehensive standardized language providing more than 550 direct and indirect intervention labels with definitions and a list of activities a nurse might choose to carry out for each intervention. NOC language provides more than 540 outcome labels with definitions; a set of indicators describing specific client, caregiver, family, or community states related to the outcome; and a 5-point Likert-type measurement scale that can demonstrate client progress even when outcomes are not fully met. Chapter 3 addresses the assessment process using a nursing framework for data collection, such as the Diagnostic Divisions Assessment Tool.

A creative approach for developing and documenting the planning of care is demonstrated in Chapter 4. Mind or Concept Mapping is a technique or learning tool provided to assist you in achieving a holistic view of your client, enhance your critical-thinking skills, and facilitate the creative process of planning client care. For more in-depth information and inclusive plans of care related to specific medical/psychiatric/obstetrical and newborn conditions (with rationale and the application of the diagnoses), refer to the larger work also published by the F. A. Davis Company: *Nursing Care Plans: Guidelines for Individualizing Client Care Across the Life Span,* 10th ed. (Doenges, Moorhouse, & Murr, 2019). Psychiatric/mental health and maternal/newborn plans of care are available on the Davis Plus Web site.

Chapter 6 contains 850 disorders and health conditions reflecting all specialty areas with associated nursing diagnoses written as client problem/need statements to aid you in validating the assessment and diagnosis steps of the nursing process.

In Chapter 5, the heart of the book, all the nursing diagnoses are listed alphabetically for ease of reference and include the diagnoses accepted for use by NANDA-I 2018–2020. The alphabetization of diagnoses follows NANDA-I's own sequencing, whereby diagnoses are alphabetized first by their key term, which is capitalized. Subordinate terminology or descriptors of the diagnosis are presented in lowercase words and are alphabetized secondarily to the key term (for example, chronic Pain is alphabetized under P, following acute Pain). Each approved diagnosis includes its location in NANDA-I's Taxonomy II (see Appendix A), definition, and information divided into the NANDA-I categories of Related or Risk Factors and Defining Characteristics. Related/Risk Factors information reflects causative or contributing factors that can be useful for determining whether the diagnosis is applicable to a particular client. Defining Characteristics (signs and symptoms or cues) are listed as subjective and/or objective and are used to confirm problem diagnoses, aid in formulating outcomes, and provide additional data for choosing appropriate interventions. We have not deleted or altered NANDA-I's listings; however, on occasion, we have added to their definitions and suggested additional criteria to provide clarification and direction. These additions are denoted with brackets [ ].

NANDA-I nursing diagnosis labels are designed to be multiaxial with seven axes or descriptors. An *axis* is defined as a dimension of the human response that is considered in the diagnostic process (see Appendix B). Sometimes an axis may be included in the diagnostic concept, such as ineffective community Coping, in which the unit of care (i.e., community) is named. Some are implicit, such as Activity Intolerance, in which the individual is the unit of care. At times, an axis may not be pertinent to a particular diagnosis and will not be a part of the nursing diagnosis label. For example, the time frame (e.g., acute, intermittent) or body part (e.g., cerebral, oral, skin) may not be relevant to each diagnostic situation.

Desired Outcomes/Evaluation Criteria are identified to assist you in formulating individual client outcomes and to support the evaluation process. Sample NOC linkages to the nursing diagnosis are provided.

Nursing priorities are used to group the suggested interventions, which are primarily directed to adult care, although interventions designated as across the lifespan do include pediatric and geriatric considerations and are designated by an icon. In general, the interventions can be used in multiple settings—acute care, rehabilitation, community clinics, home care, or private practice. Most interventions are independent or nursing originated; however, some interventions are collaborative orders (e.g., medical, psychiatric), and you will need to determine when this is necessary and take the appropriate action. Icons are also used to differentiate collaborative interventions, diagnostic studies, and medications, as well as transcultural considerations. All of these "specialized" interventions are presented with icons, rather than being broken out under separate headings, to maintain their sequence within the prioritization of all nursing interventions for the diagnosis. Additionally, in support of evidence-based practice, rationales are provided for the interventions and references for these rationales are cited.

The inclusion of Documentation Focus suggestions is to remind you of the importance and necessity of recording the steps of the nursing process.

As noted, with few exceptions, we have presented NANDA-I's recommendations as formulated. We support the belief that practicing nurses and researchers need to study, use, and evaluate the diagnoses as presented. Nurses can be creative as they use the standardized language, redefining and sharing information as the diagnoses are used with individual clients. As new nursing diagnoses are developed, it is important that the data they encompass are added to assessment tools and current databases. As part of the process by clinicians, educators, and researchers across practice specialties and academic settings to define, test, and refine nursing diagnosis, nurses are encouraged to share insights and ideas with NANDA-I at the following address: NANDA International, PO Box 72, Mountain, WI 54149; e-mail: info@nandainternational.com

Marilynn E. Doenges
Mary Frances Moorhouse
Alice C. Murr

CONTENTS

CHAPTER 1

The Nursing Process:
The Foundation of Quality Client Care

DEFINING THE PROFESSION

In the world of healthcare, nursing has long struggled to establish itself as a profession. Dictionary terms describe nursing as "a calling requiring specialized knowledge and often long and intensive academic preparation; a principal calling, vocation, or employment; the whole body of persons engaged in a calling."[1] Throughout the history of nursing, unfavorable stereotypes (based on the view of nursing as subservient and dependent on the medical profession) have negatively affected the view of nursing as an independent entity. In its early developmental years, nursing did not seek or have the means to control its own practice. Florence Nightingale, in discussing the nature of nursing in 1859, observed that "nursing has been limited to signify little more than the administration of medicines and the application of poultices."[2] Although this attitude may persist in some small degree, the nursing profession has defined what makes nursing unique and has identified a body of professional knowledge. As early as 1896, nurses in the United States banded together to seek standardization of educational programs and laws governing their practice. The task of nursing since that time has been to create descriptive terminology reflecting specific nursing functions and levels of competency.[3] Erickson, Tomlin, and Swain stated the belief that "nursing will thrive as a unique and valued profession when nurses present a theory and rationalistic model for their practice, correct misleading stereotypes, locate control with clients, and actively participate in processes for change."[4]

In the past several decades, more than a dozen prominent nursing scholars (e.g., Rogers, Parse, and Henderson) have developed conceptualizations to define the nature of nursing. Because much of nursing is nonphenomenological or nonobservable, the nature of nursing cannot be explained using the usual parameters of scientific investigation. Kikuchi proposes that conceptualizations about nursing are philosophic in nature and as such are still testable.[5] As nursing research continues the work of establishing the profession as independent in its own right, the value of nursing goals is being understood and the difference between nursing and other professions is being delineated. Nursing is now recognized as both a science and an art concerned with the physical, psychological, sociological, cultural, and spiritual concerns of the individual. The science of nursing is based on a broad theoretical framework; its art depends on the caring skills and abilities of the individual nurse. The importance of the nurse within the healthcare system is noted in many positive ways, and the profession of nursing is acknowledging the need for its practitioners to act professionally and be accountable for the care they provide.

Barely a century after Florence Nightingale noted that "the very elements of nursing are all but unknown," the American Nurses Association (ANA) developed its first Social Policy Statement in 1980, defining nursing as "the diagnosis and treatment of *human responses* to actual or potential health problems."[6] Human responses (defined as people's experiences with and responses to health, illness, and life events) are nursing's phenomena of concern. In 1995, this statement was revisited, updated, and titled "Nursing's Social Policy Statement." This policy statement acknowledged that since the release of the original statement, "nursing has been influenced by many social and professional changes, as well as by the science of caring."[7]

The statement delineated four essential features of today's contemporary nursing practice:

1. Attention to the full range of human experiences and responses to health and illness without restriction to a problem-focused orientation
2. Integration of objective data with knowledge gained from an understanding of the client's or group's subjective experience
3. Application of scientific knowledge to the processes of diagnosis and treatment
4. Provision of a caring relationship that facilitates health and healing[7]

Thus, nursing's role includes the promotion of health as well as the performance of activities that contribute to recovery from or adjustment to illness. This is reflected in ANA's 2003 *Nursing's Social Policy Statement*, which recognized nursing's full scope of care by defining nursing as "the protection, promotion, and optimization of health and abilities, prevention of illness and injury, alleviation of suffering through the diagnosis and treatment of human response, and advocacy in the care of individuals, families, communities, and populations."[8] Also, nurses support the right of clients to define their own health-related goals and to engage in care that reflects their personal values. Emphasis is placed on the mind-body-spirit connection with a holistic view of the individual as nurses facilitate the client's efforts in striving for growth and development.

In your readings, you will likely encounter other definitions of nursing. As your knowledge and experience develop, your definition of nursing may change to reflect your personal nursing philosophy, your focus on a particular care setting or population, or your specific role. For example, although the definition of nursing developed by Erickson, Tomlin, and Swain is more than 30 years old, it remains viable and timely because it incorporates the concepts noted previously with today's holistic approach to care. Their definition includes what nursing is, how it is accomplished, and the goals of nursing: "Nursing is the holistic helping of persons with their self-care activities in relation to their health. This is an interactive, interpersonal process that nurtures strengths to enable development, release, and channeling of resources for coping with one's circumstances and environment. The goal is to achieve a state of perceived optimum health and contentment."[4]

An understanding of human nature is certainly important in the development of a philosophy of nursing. Understanding that "needs motivate behavior" helps the nurse to determine the client's needs at a particular moment in time. Maslow's hierarchy of needs[9] provides a basis for understanding that unmet needs can interfere with an individual's holistic growth and may even result in physical or mental distress and illness. Other theorists have also studied how people are similar, providing the nurse with more information to help understand the client. For example, Erik Erikson's observations on the stages of psychological development suggest that the individual is a "work in progress" accomplishing age-specific maturational tasks throughout the life span. Piaget's cognitive stages address how thinking develops and how individuals adapt to and organize their environment intellectually.[4] However, in the end, the individual is the primary source of information about himself/herself. The nurse needs to listen with an open mind and empathic, unconditional acceptance to what the client is relating. Knowing how people are alike provides a basis to understanding human nature. However, each person is unique, and the nurse needs to look for the client's model of the world and how it relates to the client's own situation.

The nursing profession is further defined by fundamental philosophical beliefs that have been identified over time as essential to the practice of nursing. These values and assumptions offer guidance to the nurse and need to be kept in mind to enhance the quality of nursing care provided:

- The client is a human being who has worth and dignity.
- Humans manifest an essential unity of mind/body/spirit.[7]
- There are basic human needs that must be met (Maslow's hierarchy of needs).
- When these needs are not met, problems arise that may require intervention by another person until the individuals can resume responsibility for themselves.
- Human experience is contextually and culturally defined.[7]
- Health and illness are human experiences.[7]
- Clients have a right to quality health and nursing care delivered with interest, compassion, and competence with a focus on wellness and prevention.

- The presence of illness does not preclude health, nor does optimal health preclude illness.[7]
- The therapeutic nurse-client relationship is important in the nursing process and provision of individualized care.

Finally, the ANA Code of Ethics for Nurses[10] addresses the need for nurses to respect human dignity, acknowledge the uniqueness of each client, and honor the client's right to privacy. The Code (which has been updated on several occasions, the latest in 2015) states (in part) "Nursing encompasses the protection, promotion, and restoration of health and well-being, the prevention of illness and injury; and the alleviation of suffering in the care of individuals, families, groups, communities, and populations . . . ", revealing the broadening of understanding of nursing's civic professionalism. The Code calls on nurses to assume responsibility for individual nursing judgments and actions and for the delegation of nursing activities to others. Nurses are encouraged to maintain competence in nursing, contribute to the ongoing development of the profession, and participate in the implementation and improvement of standards. This last goal can be accomplished by using the results of nursing research to engage in evidence-based nursing practice.

The roots of evidence-based practice lie in the efforts of many in the past. Hippocrates described the symptoms and course of illnesses and related them to the seasons, geographical area, and types of people associated with each. These hypotheses founded the rational approach to the understanding of disease. As knowledge grew and the germ theory of disease was accepted, epidemiology began to count disease events, leading to the establishment of a central government agency to collect and record data. This led to the posing of questions in the form of testable hypotheses, the collection of data to support or refute hypotheses,

and the development of statistical tools to summarize numerical data.[11] The work of Pasteur and Koch expanded the understanding of causal relationships between bacterial causes of many diseases, leading to reducing illness and mortality.

Florence Nightingale used statistics to measure health, identify causes of mortality, evaluate health services, and reform institutions. After the Crimean War, she began organizing committees, assembling data, and preparing reports and hearings on how administrative inadequacies affected clients' health. Her work resulted in British Army Hospital and government reforms in the interest of preventing death and disease. She became an honorary member of the American Statistical Association in 1874, and her papers were read at a National Social Science Congress in 1863 and at the nurses' congress of the Chicago World's Fair in 1893. The efforts of these pioneers laid the groundwork for the development of evidence-based practice.

Barnsteiner and Provost note that "the current definition [of evidence-based practice] is the integration of best research evidence with clinical expertise and patient values"[12]—that is, both research and nonresearch components are combined to create evidence-based practice. Quantitative research is invaluable in measuring the effectiveness of nursing interventions, while qualitative studies capture the preferences, attitudes, and values of healthcare consumers. However, the nurses' clinical judgment and individual client needs and perspectives must also be included. Research supports that evidence-based practice includes "enhancing the quality and reliability of health care, improving health outcomes, and reducing variations in care and costs." As nurses work to provide cost-effective care in the best setting for the client, "the most important [and challenging] requirement for practicing nurses in the 21st century will be to utilize [appropriate] evidence available to improve practice."[13]

ADMINISTERING NURSING CARE

Nursing leaders have identified a process that "combines the most desirable elements of the art of nursing with the most relevant elements of systems theory, using the scientific method."[14] This *nursing process* incorporates an interactive and interpersonal approach with a problem-solving and decision-making process that serves as a framework for the delivery of nursing care.[15–17]

The concept of a nursing process was first introduced in the 1950s as a three-step process of assessment, planning, and evaluation based on the scientific method of observing, measuring, gathering data, and analyzing the findings. Years of study, use, and refinement have led nurses to expand the nursing process to five distinct steps that provide an efficient method of organizing thought processes for clinical decision making, problem solving, and the delivery of higher-quality, individualized client care. The nursing process now consists of the following:

- *Assessment* or the systematic collection of data relating to clients;
- *Diagnosis or need identification* involving the analysis of collected data to identify the client's needs;
- *Planning,* which is a two-part process of identifying goals and the client's desired outcomes to address the assessed health and wellness needs along with the selection of appropriate nursing interventions to assist the client in attaining the outcomes;
- *Implementation* or putting the plan of care into action; and
- *Evaluation* by determining the client's progress toward attaining the identified outcomes and the client's response to and the effectiveness of the selected nursing interventions for the purpose of altering the plan as indicated.

Because these five steps are central to nursing actions in any setting, the nursing process is now included in the conceptual framework of nursing curricula and is accepted as part of the legal definition of nursing in the Nurse Practice Acts of most states.

When a client enters the healthcare system, whether as an inpatient, a clinic outpatient, or a home-care client, the nursing process steps are set into motion. The nurse collects data, identifies client needs (nursing diagnoses), establishes goals, creates measurable outcomes, and selects nursing interventions to assist the client in achieving these outcomes and goals. Finally, after the interventions have been implemented, the nurse evaluates the client's responses and the effectiveness of the plan of care in reaching the desired outcomes and goals to determine whether or not the needs or problems have been resolved and the client is ready to be discharged from the care setting. If the identified needs or problems remain unresolved, further assessment, additional nursing diagnoses, alteration of outcomes and goals, or changes of interventions are required.

Although we use the terms *assessment, diagnosis, planning, implementation,* and *evaluation* as separate, progressive steps, in reality they are interrelated. Together these steps form a continuous circle of thought and action that recycles throughout the client's contact with the healthcare system. Figure 1.1 depicts a model for visualizing this process. You can see that the nursing process uses the nursing diagnosis, which is the clinical judgment product of critical thinking. Based on this judgment, nursing interventions are selected and implemented. Figure 1.1 also shows how the progressive steps of the nursing process create an understandable model of both the products and the processes of critical thinking contained within the nursing process. The model graphically emphasizes both the dynamic and cyclic characteristics of the nursing process.

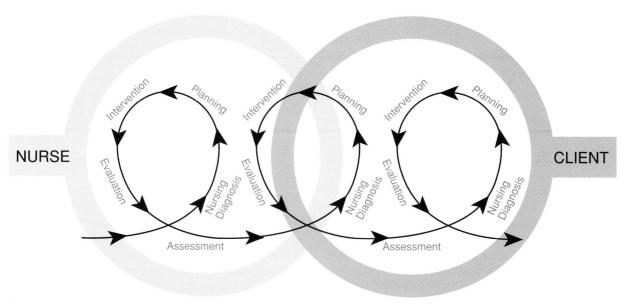

Figure 1.1 Diagram of the nursing process. The steps of the nursing process are interrelated, forming a continuous circle of thought and action that is both dynamic and cyclical.

The scientific method of problem solving introduced in the previous section is used almost instinctively by most people, without conscious awareness.

FOR EXAMPLE   While studying for your semester finals, you snack on pepperoni pizza. After going to bed, you are awakened by a burning sensation in the center of your chest. You are young and in good health and note no other symptoms (assessment). You decide that your pain is the result of the spicy food you have eaten (diagnosis). You then determine that before you can return to sleep, you need to relieve the discomfort with an over-the-counter preparation (planning). You take a liquid antacid for your discomfort (implementation). Within a few minutes, you note the burning sensation is relieved, and you return to bed without further concern (evaluation).

As you see, this is a process you routinely use to solve problems in your life that can be readily applied to client-care situations. You need only to learn the new terms describing the nursing process rather than having to think about each step (assessment, diagnosis/need identification, planning, implementation, and evaluation) in an entirely new way.

To effectively use the nursing process, the nurse needs to possess and apply some basic abilities. Particularly important is a thorough knowledge of science and theory, not only as applied in nursing but also in other related disciplines such as medicine and psychology. Creativity is needed in the application of nursing knowledge, as is adaptability in handling change and the many unexpected happenings that occur. As a nurse, you must make a commitment to practice your profession in the best possible way, trusting in yourself and your ability to do your job well and displaying the necessary leadership to organize and supervise as your position requires. In addition, intelligence, well-developed interpersonal skills, and competent technical skills are essential.

FOR EXAMPLE   A diabetic client's irritable behavior could be the result of low serum glucose or the effects of excessive caffeine intake. However, it could also arise from a sense of helplessness regarding life events. A single behavior may have varied causes. It is important that your nursing assessment skills identify the underlying etiology to provide appropriate care.

The practice responsibilities presented in the definitions of nursing and the nursing process are explained in detail in the publication *Nursing: Scope & Standards of Practice*.[18] The standards provide workable guidelines to ensure that the practice of nursing can be carried out by each nurse. Table 1.1 presents an abbreviated description of the standards of clinical practice. With the ultimate goal of quality healthcare, the effective use of the nursing process will result in a viable nursing care system that is recognized and accepted as nursing's body of knowledge and that can be shared with other healthcare professionals.

ADVANTAGES OF USING THE NURSING PROCESS

There are many advantages to using the nursing process:

- The nursing process provides an organizing framework for meeting the individual needs of the client, the client's family/significant other(s), and the community.
- The steps of the nursing process focus the nurse's attention on the "individual" human responses of a client/family or group to a given health situation, resulting in a holistic plan of care addressing the specific needs of the client/family or group.
- The nursing process provides an organized, systematic method of problem solving (while still allowing for creative solutions) that may minimize dangerous errors or omissions in caregiving and avoid time-consuming repetition in care and documentation.
- The use of the nursing process promotes the active involvement of clients in their healthcare, enhancing

TABLE 1.1	**ANA Standards of Nursing Practice**

Standards of Practice

Describe a competent level of nursing care as demonstrated by the nursing process that encompasses all significant actions taken by the nurse in providing care and forms the foundation of clinical decision making.

1. Assessment: The registered nurse (RN) collects comprehensive data pertinent to the healthcare consumer's health and/or situation.
2. Diagnosis: The RN analyzes the assessment data to determine the diagnoses or the issues.
3. Outcome Identification: The RN identifies expected outcomes for a plan individualized to the healthcare consumer or the situation.
4. Planning: The RN develops a plan that prescribes strategies and alternatives to attain expected outcomes.
5. Implementation: The RN implements the identified plan.
   a. Coordination of Care: The RN coordinates care delivery.
   b. Health Teaching and Health Promotion: The RN employs strategies to promote health and a safe environment.
   c. Consultation: The graduate-level specialty nurse or advanced-practice RN provides consultation to influence the identified plan, enhance the abilities of others, and effect change.
   d. Prescriptive Authority and Treatment: The advanced-practice RN uses prescriptive authority, procedures, referrals, treatments, and therapies in accordance with state and federal laws and regulations.
6. Evaluation: The RN evaluates progress toward attainment of outcomes.

Standards of Professional Performance

Describe roles expected of all professional nurses appropriate to their education, position, and practice setting.

7. Ethics: The RN integrates practices ethically.
8. Culturally Congruent Practice: The RN practices in a manner that is congruent with cultural diversity and inclusion principles.
9. Communication: The RN communicates effectively in a variety of formats in all areas of practice.
10. Collaboration: The RN collaborates with the healthcare consumer, family, and others in the conduct of nursing practice.
11. Leadership: The RN demonstrates leadership in the professional practice setting and the profession.
12. Education: The RN attains knowledge and competence that reflects current nursing practice.
13. Evidence-Based Practice and Research: The RN integrates evidence and research findings into practice.
14. Quality of Practice: The RN contributes to quality nursing practice.
15. Professional Practice Evaluation: The RN evaluates her or his own nursing practice in relation to professional practice standards and guidelines, relevant statutes, rules, and regulations.
16. Resource Utilization: The RN utilizes appropriate resources to plan and provide nursing services that are safe, effective, and financially responsible.
17. Collegiality/Environmental Health: The RN practices in an environmentally safe and healthy manner.

Source: American Nurses Association. (2010). *Nursing: Scope & Standards of Practice.* 2nd ed. Silver Spring, MD: Nursesbooks.org.

consumer satisfaction. Such participation increases clients' sense of control over what is happening to them, stimulates problem solving, and promotes personal responsibility, all of which strengthen the client's commitment to achieving the identified goals.

- The use of the nursing process enables you as a nurse to have more control over your practice. This enhances the opportunity for you to use your knowledge, expertise, and intuition constructively and dynamically to increase the likelihood of a successful client outcome. This, in turn, promotes greater job satisfaction and your professional growth.
- The use of the nursing process provides a common language (nursing diagnosis) for practice, unifying the nursing profession. Using a system that clearly communicates the plan of care to coworkers and clients enhances continuity of care, promotes achievement of client goals, provides a vehicle for evaluation, and aids in the development of nursing standards. In addition, the structure of the process provides a format for documenting the client's response to all aspects of the planned care.
- The use of the nursing process provides a means of assessing nursing's economic contribution to client care. The nursing process supplies a vehicle for the quantitative and qualitative measurement of nursing care that meets the goal of cost-effectiveness and still promotes holistic care.

Nursing is continuing to evolve into a well-defined profession with a more clearly delineated definition and phenomena of concern. Fundamental philosophical beliefs and qualities have been identified that are important for the nurse to possess in order to provide quality care.

The nursing profession has developed a body of knowledge that contributes to the growth and well-being of the individual and the community, the prevention of illness, the maintenance and/or restoration of health, and the relief of pain and provision of support when a return to health is not possible. The nursing process is the basis of all nursing actions and is the essence of nursing, providing a flexible, orderly, and logical problem-solving approach for administering nursing care so that client (whether individual, community, or population) needs for such care are met comprehensively and effectively. It can be applied in any healthcare or educational setting, in any theoretical or conceptual framework, and within the context of any nursing philosophy.

Each step of the nursing process builds on and interacts with the other steps, ensuring an effective practice model. Inclusion of the standards of clinical nursing practice provides additional information to reinforce understanding and opportunities to apply knowledge.

Please note, the term *client* rather than *patient* is used in this book to reflect the philosophy that the individuals or groups you work with are legitimate members of the decision-making process with some degree of control over the planned regimen and are able, active participants in the planning and implementation of their care.[4]

Next, we introduce the language described in the nursing process. This includes NANDA International's classification of nursing diagnoses,[19] the Iowa Intervention and Outcome Projects: Nursing Interventions Classification (NIC),[20] and the Nursing Outcomes Classification (NOC).[21] NANDA-I, NIC, and NOC have combined their classification systems (NNN Alliance) to provide a comprehensive nursing language.

References

1. Merriam-Webster Online Dictionary. Retrieved May 2018, from https://www.merriam-webster.com/dictionary/profession.
2. Nightingale, F. (1859). *Notes on Nursing: What It Is and What It Is Not*. Facsimile edition. Philadelphia: J. B. Lippincott, 1946.
3. Jacobi, E. M. (1976). Foreword. In Flanigan, L. (ed.) *One Strong Voice: The Story of the American Nurses' Association*. Kansas City, MO: American Nurses Association.
4. Erickson, H. C., Tomlin, E. M., Swain, M. A. (1983). *Modeling and Role-Modeling: A Theory and Paradigm for Nursing*. Englewood Cliffs, NJ: Prentice Hall.
5. Kikuchi, J. F. (1999). Clarifying the nature of conceptualizations about nursing. *Can J Nurs Res*, 30(4), 115–128.
6. American Nurses Association. (1980). *Nursing: A Social Policy Statement*. Kansas City, MO: American Nurses Publishing.
7. American Nurses Association. (1995). *Nursing's Social Policy Statement*. Washington, DC: American Nurses Publishing.
8. American Nurses Association. (2003). *Nursing's Social Policy Statement*. Washington, DC: Nursesbooks.org.
9. Maslow, A. H. (1970). *Motivation and Personality*. 2nd ed. New York, NY: Harper & Row.
10. Fowler, M. D. M. (ed.). (2015). *Guide to the Code of Ethics for Nurses with Interpretive Statements*. Silver Spring, MD: Nursesbooks.org.
11. Stolley, P. D., Lasky, T. (1995). *Investigating Disease Patterns: The Science of Epidemiology*. Scientific American Library, no. 57. New York, NY: WH Freeman.
12. Barnsteiner, J., Provost, S. (2002). How to implement evidence-based practice: Some tried and true pointers. *Reflect Nurs Leadersh*, 28(2), 18.
13. Mazurik Melnyk, B., Gallagher-Ford, L., Fineout-Overholt, E. (2014). The establishment of evidence-based practice competencies for practicing registered nurses and advanced practice nurses in real-world clinical settings: Proficiencies to improve healthcare quality, reliability, patient outcomes, and costs. *Worldviews Evid Based Nurs*, 11(1), 5–15.
14. Shore, L. S. (1988). *Nursing Diagnosis: What It Is and How to Do It, a Programmed Text*. Richmond, VA: Medical College of Virginia Hospitals.
15. Peplau, H. E. (1952). *Interpersonal Relations in Nursing: A Conceptual Frame of Reference for Psychodynamic Nursing*. New York, NY: Putnam.
16. King, L. (1971). *Toward a Theory for Nursing: General Concepts of Human Behavior*. New York, NY: Wiley.
17. Yura, H., Walsh, M. B. (1988). *The Nursing Process: Assessing, Planning, Implementing, Evaluating*. 5th ed. Norwalk, CT: Appleton & Lange.
18. American Nurses Association. (2015). *Nursing: Scope & Standards of Practice*. 3rd ed. Silver Spring, MD: Nursesbooks.org.
19. NANDA International Inc. (2018). *Nursing Diagnoses: Definitions & Classification 2018–2020*. 11th ed. New York, NY: Thieme.
20. Butcher, H. K., et al (eds). (2018). *Nursing Interventions Classification (NIC)*. 7th ed. St. Louis, MO: Mosby.
21. Moorhead, S., Johnson, M., Maas, M., et al. (eds). (2018). *Nursing Outcomes Classification (NOC)*. 6th ed. St. Louis, MO: Mosby.

CHAPTER 2

The Language of Nursing: NANDA, NIC, NOC, and Other Standardized Nursing Languages

In this chapter, we look at the process and progress of describing the work of nursing because, as Lang has stated, "If we cannot name it, we cannot control it, practice it, teach it, finance it, or put it into public policy."[1] At first glance, nursing seems to be a simple task. However, over many years, the profession has struggled, in part as a result of changes in healthcare delivery and financing, the expansion of nursing's role, and the dawning of the computer age. Gordon reminded us that classification system development parallels knowledge development in a discipline.[2] As theory development and research have begun to define nursing, it has become necessary for nursing to find a common language to describe what nursing is, what nursing does, and how to codify it. Thus, the terms "classification systems" and "standardized language" have been embraced, and the work continues.

Changes in the healthcare system occur at an ever-increasing rate. One of these changes is the movement to a paperless (computerized or electronic) client record. The use of electronic healthcare information systems is rapidly expanding, and the focus has shifted from its original uses—financial and personnel management functions—to the efficient documentation of the client encounter, whether a single office visit or a lengthy hospitalization. The move to electronic documentation is being fueled by changes in healthcare delivery and reimbursement as well as the growth of alternative healthcare settings (outpatient surgeries, home health, rehabilitation or subacute units, extended or long-term care facilities, etc.), all of which increase the need for a commonality of communication to ensure continuity of care for the client who moves from one setting or level of care to another.

These changes in the business and documentation of healthcare require the industry to generate data about its operations and outcomes. Evaluation and improvement of provided services are important to the delivery of cost-effective client care. Therefore, providers and consumers interested in outcomes of care benefit from accurate documentation of the care provided and the client's response. With the use of language or terminology that can be coded, healthcare information can be recorded in terms that are universal and easily entered into an electronic database and that can generate meaningful reporting data about its operation and outcomes. In short, standardized language is required.

A standardized language contains formalized terms that have definitions and guidelines for use. For example, if the impact of nursing care on financial and clinical outcomes is to be analyzed, coding of this information is essential. While it has been relatively easy to code medical procedures, nursing is more of an enigma because its work has not been so clearly defined.

Since the 1970s, nursing leaders have been working to define the profession of nursing and to develop a commonality of words describing practice (a framework of communication and documentation) so that nursing's contribution to healthcare is captured, is visible in healthcare databases, and is thereby recognized as essential. Therefore, the focus of the profession has been on the effort to classify tasks and to develop standardized nursing languages (SNLs) to better demonstrate what nursing is and what nursing does.

Around the world, nursing researchers continue their efforts to identify and label people's experiences with (and responses to) health, illness, and life processes as they relate to the scope of nursing practice.

The use of universal nursing terminology directs our focus to the central content and process of nursing care by identifying, naming, and standardizing the "what" and "how" of the work of nursing—including both direct and indirect activities. This wider application for a standardized language has spurred its development.

A recognized pioneer in SNL is NANDA International's "nursing diagnosis."[3] Simply stated, a nursing diagnosis is defined as a clinical judgment about individual, family, or community responses to actual or potential health problems and life processes. Nursing diagnoses provide the basis for selecting nursing interventions to achieve outcomes for which the nurse is accountable.[4] NANDA-I nursing diagnoses currently include 244 labels with definitions, defining characteristics, and related or risk factors used to define a client need or problem. Once the client's need is defined, outcomes can be developed and nursing interventions chosen to achieve the desired outcomes.

The linkage of client problems or nursing diagnoses to specific nursing interventions and client outcomes has led to the development of several other SNLs, including Clinical Care Classification (originally Home Health Care Classification),[5,6] Nursing Interventions Classification (NIC),[7] Nursing Outcomes Classification (NOC),[8] Omaha System-Community Health Classification System (OS),[9] Patient Care Data Set (now retired),[10] and Perioperative Nursing Data Set (PNDS).[11]

Whereas some of these languages (e.g., OS and PNDS) are designed for a specific client population, the NANDA-I, NIC, and NOC languages are comprehensively designed for use across systems and settings and at individual, family, and community or population levels.[12]

NIC is a comprehensive standardized language providing 565 direct and indirect intervention labels with definitions. A list of activities a nurse might choose to carry out for each intervention is also provided and can be modified as necessary to meet the specific needs of the client. These research-based interventions encompass a broad range of nursing practices, addressing both general practice and specialty areas, including direct care as well as support or administrative activities.

NOC is also a comprehensive standardized language providing 540 outcome labels with definitions; a set of indicators describing specific client, caregiver, family, or community states related to the outcome; and a five-point Likert-type scale that facilitates tracking clients across care settings and that can demonstrate client progress even when outcomes are not fully met. The outcomes are research based and are applicable in all care settings, clinical specialties, and across the life span.

In addition, NIC and NOC have been linked to the Omaha System problems, to resident assessment protocols used in extended/long-term care settings, and to NANDA-I. This last linkage created the NANDA, NIC, NOC (NNN) Taxonomy of Nursing Practice. The combination of NANDA-I nursing diagnoses, NOC outcomes, and NIC interventions in a common unifying structure provides a comprehensive nursing language recognized by the American Nurses Association (ANA) that is coded in the Systematized Nomenclature of Medicine (SNOMED), a multidisciplinary terminology supporting the electronic client record.

Having an SNL entered into international-coded terminology allows nurses to describe the care received by the client and to document the effects of that care on client outcomes, and it facilitates the comparison of nursing care across worldwide settings and diverse databases. In addition, it supports research by comparing client care delivered by nurses with that delivered by other providers, which is essential if nursing's contribution is to be recognized and nurses are to be reimbursed for the care they provide.

The current 12 versions of SNLs (consisting of two data element sets and 10 terminologies) recognized by the ANA have been submitted to the National Library of Medicine for inclusion in the Unified Medical Language System Metathesaurus. The Metathesaurus provides a uniform, integrated distribution format from over 100 biomedical vocabularies and classifications (the majority in English and some in multiple languages), and it links many different names for the same concepts, establishing new relationships among terms from different source vocabularies.

Indexing of the entire medical record supports disease management activities (including decision support systems), research, and analysis of outcomes for quality improvement for all healthcare disciplines. Coding also supports telehealth (the use of telecommunications technology to provide medical information and healthcare services over distance) and facilitates access to healthcare data across care settings and different computer systems.

So, to those who stated "Nursing will thrive as a unique and valued profession when nurses present a theory and rationalistic model for their practice . . . and actively participate in processes for change,"[13] we answer, "We are actively participating in processes for change, and as a profession, we will continue to grow."

References

1. Clark, J., Lang, N. (1992). Nursing's next advance: An internal classification for nursing practice. *Int Nurs Rev*, 39, 109–111, 128.
2. Gordon, M. (1998). Nursing nomenclature and classification system development (archived independent study module). *Online J Issues Nurs*. Retrieved May 2018 from http://ana.nursingworld.org/mods/archive/mod30/cec2full.htm.
3. NANDA International. (2003). *Nursing Diagnoses: Definitions & Classifications 2003–2004*. Philadelphia, PA: NANDA International.
4. Herdman, T. H., Kamitsuru, S. (eds). (2018). *NANDA, International Inc. Nursing Diagnoses: Definitions and Classification, 2018–2020*. 11th ed. New York, NY: Thieme.
5. Saba, V. K. (1994). *Home Health Care Classification (HHCC) of Nursing Diagnoses and Interventions*. (Revised). Washington, DC: Author.
6. Saba, V. K. (2012). *Clinical Care Classification (CCC) System*. 2nd ed. New York, NY: Springer.
7. Butcher, H. K., Bulechek, G. M., et al. (eds). (2018). *Nursing Interventions Classification (NIC)*. 7th ed. St. Louis, MO: Elsevier.
8. Moorhead, S., et al. (eds). (2018). *Nursing Outcomes Classification (NOC): Measurement of Health Outcomes*. 6th ed. St. Louis, MO: Elsevier.
9. Martin, K. S., et al. (2005). *The Omaha System: A Key to Practice, Documentation, and Information Management*. 2nd ed. Omaha, NE: Health Connections Press.
10. Ozboldt, J. G. (1996). From minimum data to maximum impact: Using clinical data to strengthen patient care. *Adv Pract Nurs Q*, 1, 62–69.
11. Association of periOperative Registered Nurses (AORN). (2010). *Perioperative Nursing Data Set [PNDS] The Perioperative Nursing Vocabulary*. 3rd ed. Denver, CO: AORN.
12. Johnson, M., et al. (eds). (2011). *NOC and NIC Linkages to NANDA-I and Clinical Conditions: Supporting Critical Reasoning and Quality Care (NANDA, NOC, and NIC Linkages)*. 3rd ed. St. Louis, MO: Mosby.
13. Erickson, H. C., Tomlin, E. M., Swain, M. A. P. (1983). *Modeling and Role-Modeling*. Englewood Cliffs, NJ: Prentice Hall.

CHAPTER 3

The Assessment Process: Developing the Client Database

*N*ursing: Scope & Standards of Practice[1] addresses the assessment process. The standard stipulates that the data-collection process is systematic and ongoing, with the registered nurse collecting comprehensive data pertinent to the healthcare consumer's health and/ or situation involving the healthcare consumer, family, and healthcare providers as appropriate, in holistic data collection. The priority of the data collection is based on the healthcare consumer's immediate condition or the anticipated needs of the healthcare consumer or situation. Data are collected using appropriate evidence-based assessment techniques, instruments, and tools with the relevant data documented in a retrievable format.

THE CLIENT DATABASE

The assessment step of the nursing process is focused on eliciting a profile of the client that allows the nurse to identify client problems or needs and corresponding nursing diagnoses, to plan care, to implement interventions, and to evaluate outcomes. This profile, or *client database,* supplies a sense of the client's overall health status, providing a picture of the client's physical, psychosocial, emotional, sexual, cultural, spiritual/ transpersonal, cognitive, age-related, and developmental levels; economic status; functional abilities; and lifestyle. It is a combination of data gathered from the history-taking interview (a method of obtaining SUBJECTIVE information by talking with the client or significant others and listening to their responses), from the physical examination (a "hands-on" means of obtaining OBJECTIVE information), and from the results of laboratory tests and diagnostic studies. To be more specific, subjective data are what the client/ significant others perceive and report, and objective data are what the nurse observes and gathers from other sources.

Assessment involves three basic activities:

- Systematically gathering data
- Organizing or clustering the data collected
- Documenting the data in a retrievable format

GATHERING DATA—THE INTERVIEW

Information in the client database is obtained primarily from the client (who is the most important or primary source) and then from family members/significant others (secondary sources), as appropriate, through conversation and by observation during a structured interview. Clearly, the interview involves more than simply exchanging and processing data. Nonverbal communication is as important as the client's choice of words in providing the data. The ability to collect data that are meaningful to the client's health concerns depends heavily on the nurse's knowledge base; on the choice and sequence of questions; and on the ability to give meaning to the client's responses, integrate the data gathered, and prioritize the resulting information.

Insight into the nature and behavior of the client is essential as well.

The nurse's initial responsibility is to observe, collect, and record data without drawing conclusions or making judgments or assumptions. Self-awareness is a crucial factor in the interaction because perceptions, judgments, and assumptions can easily color the assessment findings unless they are recognized.

The quality of a history improves with experience with the interviewing process. Tips for obtaining a meaningful history include the following:

- Be a good listener.
- Listen carefully and attentively for whole thoughts and ideas, not merely isolated facts.
- Use the skills of active listening, silence, and acceptance to provide ample time for the person to respond. Be as objective as possible.
- Identify only the client's or significant others' contributions to the history.

The interview question is the major tool used to acquire information. How the question is phrased is an important skill for obtaining the desired results and getting the information necessary to make accurate nursing diagnoses. *Note:* Some questioning strategies to avoid include closed-ended and leading questions, probing, and agreeing or disagreeing that implies that the client is "right" or "wrong." It is important to remember, too, that the client has the right to refuse to answer any question, no matter how reasonably phrased.

The following are nine effective data-collection questioning techniques:

1. Open-ended questions allow clients maximum freedom to respond in their own way, impose no limitations on how the question may be answered, and can produce considerable information.
2. Hypothetical questions pose a situation and ask the client how it might be handled.
3. Reflecting or "mirroring" responses is a useful technique in getting at underlying meanings that might not be verbalized clearly.
4. Focusing consists of eye contact (within cultural limits), body posture, and verbal responses.
5. Giving broad openings encourages the client to take the initiative in what is to be discussed.
6. Offering general leads encourages the client to continue.
7. Exploring pursues a topic in more depth.
8. Verbalizing the implied gives voice to what has been suggested.
9. Encouraging evaluation helps clients to consider the quality of their own experiences.

The client's medical diagnosis can provide a starting point for gathering data. Knowledge of the anatomy and physiology of the specific disease process and severity of the condition also helps in choosing and prioritizing precise portions of the assessment. For example, when examining a client with severe chest pain, it may be wise to evaluate the pain and the cardiovascular system in a focused assessment before addressing other areas, possibly at a later time. Likewise, the duration and length of any assessment depend on circumstances such as the client's condition and the situation's urgency.

The data collected from the client or significant others contain a vast amount of information, some of which may be repetitious. However, some of the data will be valuable for eliciting information that was not recalled or volunteered previously. Enough material needs to be noted in the history so that a complete picture is presented and yet not so much that the information will not be read or used.

GATHERING DATA—THE PHYSICAL EXAMINATION

The physical examination is performed to gather objective information and serves as a screening device. Four common methods used during the physical examination are inspection, palpation, percussion, and auscultation. These techniques incorporate the senses of sight, hearing, touch, and smell. For the data collected during the physical examination to be meaningful, it is vital to know the normal physical and emotional characteristics of humans well enough to be able to recognize deviations. To gain as much information as possible from the assessment procedure, the same format should be used each time a physical examination is performed to lessen the possibility of omissions.

Laboratory and other diagnostic studies are a part of the information-gathering stage providing supportive evidence. These studies aid in the management, maintenance, and restoration of health. In reviewing and interpreting laboratory tests, it is important to remember that the origin of the test material does not always correlate to an organ or body system (e.g., a urine test to detect the presence of bilirubin and urobilinogen could indicate liver disease, biliary obstruction, or hemolytic disease). In some cases, the results of a test are *nonspecific* because they indicate only a disorder or abnormality and not the location of the cause of the problem (e.g., an elevated erythrocyte sedimentation rate [ESR] suggests the presence but not the location of an inflammatory process).

In evaluating laboratory tests, it is advisable to consider which medications (e.g., heparin, promethazine) are being administered to the client, including over-the-counter and herbal supplements (e.g., vitamin E), because these have the potential to alter, blur, or falsify results, creating a misleading diagnostic picture.

DOCUMENTING AND CLUSTERING THE DATA

Data gathered during the interview and physical examination, as well as from other records/sources, are organized and recorded in a concise, systematic way and clustered into similar categories. Various formats have been used to accomplish this, including a review of body systems. This approach has been utilized by both medicine and nursing for many years but was initially developed to aid the physician in making medical diagnoses. Currently, nursing is developing and fine-tuning its own tools for recording and clustering data. Several nursing models available to guide data collection include Doenges and Moorhouse's Diagnostic Divisions (Table 3.1),[2,3] Gordon's Functional Health Patterns,[4] and the Nursing Assessment Tool for Data Collection (NATDC).[5]

The use of a nursing model as a framework for data collection (rather than a body systems approach [assessing the heart, moving on to the lungs, etc.] or the commonly known head-to-toe approach) has the advantage of focusing data collection on the nurse's phenomena of concern—the human responses to health, illness, and life processes.[6] This facilitates the identification and validation of *nursing* diagnosis labels to describe the data accurately.

REVIEWING AND VALIDATING FINDINGS

The nurse's initial responsibility is to observe, collect, and record data without drawing conclusions or making judgments or assumptions. Self-awareness is a crucial factor in this interaction because perceptions, judgments, and assumptions can easily color the assessment findings.

Validation is an ongoing process that occurs during the data-collection phase and upon its completion, which is when the data are reviewed and compared. The nurse should review the data to be sure that the recordings are factual, to identify errors of omission, and to compare the objective and subjective data for incongruencies or inconsistencies that require additional investigation or a more focused assessment. Data that are grossly abnormal are rechecked, and any temporary factors that may affect the data are identified and noted. Validation is particularly important when the data are conflicting, when the data sources may be unreliable, or when serious harm to the client could result from any inaccuracies. Validating the information reduces the possibility of drawing wrong inferences or conclusions that could result in inaccurate nursing diagnoses, incorrect outcomes, or inappropriate nursing actions. This can be done by sharing the assumptions with the individuals involved (e.g., client, significant other/family) and having them verify the accuracy of those conclusions. Sharing pertinent data with other healthcare professionals, such as the physician, dietitian, or physical therapist, can aid in collaborative planning of care. Data given in confidence should not be shared with other individuals (unless withholding that information would hinder appropriate evaluation or care of the client).

TABLE 3.1	General Assessment Tool

This is a suggested guideline/tool applicable in most care settings for creating a client database. It provides a nursing focus (Doenges & Moorhouse's Diagnostic Divisions of Nursing Diagnoses) that will facilitate planning client care. Although the sections are alphabetized here for ease of presentation, they can be prioritized or rearranged to meet individual needs. (Sample excerpts from psychiatric and obstetrical assessment tools are available on Davis Plus.)

Adult Medical/Surgical Assessment Tool

General Information

Name: _____ Age: _____ DOB: _____ Gender: _____ Race: _____
Admission Date: _____ Time: _____ From: _____
Reason for this visit/admission (primary concern): _____
Source of information: _____ Reliability (1–4, with 4 = very reliable): _____

Activity/Rest

Subjective (Reports)

Occupation: _____ Able to participate in usual activities/hobbies: _ Leisure time/diversional activities: _____
Ambulatory: _____ Gait (describe): _____ Activity level (sedentary to very active; use scale if available): _____
Regular exercise (type): _____
Changes in muscle mass/tone/strength: _____
History of problems/limitations imposed by condition (e.g., immobility, transfer difficulties, weakness, breathlessness):
_____
Feelings (e.g., exhaustion, restlessness, boredom, dissatisfaction): _____
Developmental factors (e.g., delayed/age appropriate): _____
Sleep: Hours: _____ Naps: _____ Aids: _____ Insomnia: _____ Related to: _____
  Difficulty falling asleep: _____ Difficulty staying asleep: _____
  Rested on awakening: _____ Excessive grogginess: _____ Bedtime rituals: _____
  Relaxation techniques: _____ Sleeps on more than one pillow: _____
Use of oxygen (type): _____ When used: _____
Medications or herbals for/affecting sleep: _____

Objective (Exhibits)

Observed response to activity: Heart rate: _____ Rhythm (reg/irreg): _____ Blood pressure: _____ Respiratory rate: _____
  Pulse oximetry: _____
Mental status (e.g., cognitive impairment, withdrawn/lethargic): _____
Neuromuscular assessment: Muscle mass/tone: _____ Posture (e.g., normal, stooped, curved spine): _____
  Tremors (location): _____ ROM: _____
  Strength: _____ Deformity: _____
Mobility aids (list): _____

Circulation

Subjective (Reports)

History of/treatment date: High blood pressure: _____ Brain injury: _____ Stroke: _____ Heart condition/surgery: _____
Rheumatic fever: _____ Palpitations: _____ Syncope: _____ Pain in legs: _____ Ankle/leg edema: _____ Blood clots: _____
Bleeding tendencies: _____ Spinal cord injury/dysreflexia episodes (describe): _____
Slow/delayed healing (describe): _____
Extremities: Numbness (location): _____ Tingling (location): _____
Cough (describe)/hemoptysis: _____
Change in frequency/amount of urine: _____
Medications/herbals: _____

Objective (Exhibits)

Color (e.g., pale, cyanotic, jaundiced, mottled, ruddy): Skin: _____ Mucous membranes: _____ Lips: _____ Nailbeds: _____
  Conjunctiva: _____ Sclera: _____
Skin moisture (e.g., dry, diaphoretic): _____
BP (R & L): Lying: _____ Sitting: _____ Standing: _____ Pulse pressure: _____ Auscultatory gap: _____
Pulses (palpated 1–4 strength): Carotid: _____ Temporal: _____ Jugular: _____ Radial: _____ Femoral: _____ Popliteal: _____
  Posttibial: _____ Dorsalis pedis: _____
Cardiac (palpation): Thrill: _____ Heaves: _____

TABLE 3.1 **continued**

Heart sounds (auscultation): Rate: _____ Rhythm: _____ Quality: _____ Friction rub: _____
  Murmur (describe location/sounds): _____
Vascular bruit (location): _ Jugular vein distention: _____
Breath sounds (describe location & sounds): _____
Extremities: Temperature: _____ Color: _____ Capillary refill (1-3 sec): _____ Edema (+1 to +4): _____ Varicosities
(location): _____ Nail abnormalities: _____ Distribution/quality of hair: _____ Trophic skin changes: _____

Ego Integrity

Subjective (Reports)

Relationship status: _____
Expressed concerns (e.g., financial, relationships, recent or anticipated lifestyle/role changes, recent tour(s) of combat duty): __
Stress factors: _____ Usual ways of handling stress: _____
Expression of feelings of: Anger: _____ Anxiety: _____ Fear: _____ Grief: _____ Helplessness: _____ Hopelessness: _____
  Powerlessness: _____
Cultural factors/ethnic ties: _____
Religious affiliation: _____ Active/practicing: _____ Practices prayer/meditation: _____
  Religious/spiritual concerns: _____ Desires clergy visit: _____
Expression of sense of connectedness/harmony with self and others: _____
Medications/herbals: _____

Objective (Exhibits)

Emotional status (check those that apply):
  Calm: _____ Anxious: _____ Angry: _____ Withdrawn: _____ Fearful: _____ Irritable: _____ Restive: _____ Euphoric: _____
Observed body language: _____ Observed physiological responses (e.g., crying, change in voice quality/volume): _____
Changes in energy field: Temperature: _____ Color: _____ Distribution: _____ Movement: _____ Sounds: _____

Elimination

Subjective (Reports)

Usual bowel elimination pattern: _____ Character of stool (e.g., hard, soft, liquid): _____ Stool color (e.g., brown, black,
yellow, clay colored, tarry): _____ Last BM/character of stool: _____ Constipation (acute/chronic): _____ Diarrhea
(acute/chronic): _____ Bowel incontinence: _____ History of bleeding: _____ Hemorrhoids/fistula: _____
  Laxative use: _____ How often: _____ Enema/suppository: _____ How often: _____
Usual voiding pattern and character of urine: _____
  Difficulty voiding: _____ Urgency: _____ Frequency: _____ Retention: _____ Bladder spasms: _____
  Pain/burning: _____
Urinary incontinence (type & time of day usually occurs): _____
History of kidney/bladder disease or stones: _____
Diuretic use: _ Other medications/herbals: _____

Objective (Exhibits)

Abdomen (auscultation): Bowel sounds (location/type): _____ Abdomen (palpation): Soft/firm: _____ Tenderness/
pain (quadrant location): _____ Distention: _____ Palpable mass: _____ Size/girth: _____

Bladder palpable: _____ Residual (per scan): _____ Overflow voiding: _____
Rectal sphincter tone (describe): _____ Hemorrhoids/fistulas: _____
  Stool in rectum: _____ Impaction: _____ Occult blood: (+ or −): _____
Presence/use of catheter or continence devices: _____ Ostomy appliances (describe appliance and location): _____

Food/Fluid

Subjective (Reports)

Usual diet (type): _____ Calorie/carbohydrate/protein/fat (g/day): _____ # of meals daily: _____
Snacks (# daily, time consumed, type): _____
Last meal consumed/content: _____
Food preferences: _____ Food allergies/intolerances: _____
Cultural or religious food preparation concerns/prohibitions: _____
Usual appetite: _____ Change in appetite: _____
Usual weight: _____ Unexpected/undesired weight loss or gain: _____
Nausea/vomiting: _____ Related to? _____ Heartburn/indigestion: _____ Related to? _____ Relieved by? _____

(table continues on page 16)

TABLE 3.1 **General Assessment Tool** (continued)

Chewing/swallowing problems: _____ Gag/swallow reflex (present): _____
  Facial injury/surgery: _____ Stroke/other neurologic deficit: _____
Teeth: Normal: _____ Dentures (full/partial): _____ Loose/absent teeth: _____ Sore mouth/gums: _____
Dental hygiene practices: _____ Professional dental care/frequency: _____
Diabetes/type: _____ Controlled with diet/pills/insulin: _____
Vitamin/food supplement use: _____ Medications/herbals: _____

Objective (Exhibits)

Current weight: _____ Height: _____ Body build: _____ Body fat %: _____
Skin turgor (e.g., firm, supple, dehydrated): _____ Mucous membranes (moist/dry): _____
Edema (describe): Generalized: _____ Dependent: _____ Feet/ankles: _____ Periorbital: _____ Abdominal/ascites: _____
Jugular vein distention: _____
Breath sounds (auscultation)/location: Normal: _____ Diminished: _____ Crackles: _____ Wheezes: _____
Condition of teeth/gums: _____ Appearance of tongue: _____ Mucous membranes: _____
Bowel sounds (quadrant location/type): _____ Hernia/masses: _____
Urine S/A or Chemstix: _____ Serum glucose (Glucometer): _____

Hygiene

Subjective (Reports)

Ability to carry out activities of daily living: Independent/dependent (levels 1–4, with 1 = *no assistance needed* to 4 = *completely dependent*):
  Mobility: _____ Needs assistance (describe): _____ Assistance provided by: _____
    Equipment/prosthetic devices required: _____
  Feeding: _____ Needs assistance preparing/eating (describe): _____ Assistive devices: _____
  Bathing: _____ Needs assistance setup/regulating water temperature/washing body parts (describe): _____
  Preferred time of personal care/bath: _____
  Dressing: _____ Needs assistance selecting clothing/dressing self (describe): _____
  Toileting: _____ Needs assistance transferring/cleaning self (describe): _____

Objective (Exhibits)

General appearance: Manner of dress: _____ Grooming/personal habits: _____
  Condition of hair/scalp: _____
Body odor: _____ Presence of vermin (e.g., lice, scabies): _____

Neurosensory

Subjective (Reports)

History of brain injury, trauma, stroke (residual effects): _____
Fainting spells/dizziness: _____ Headaches (location/type/frequency): _____
Tingling/numbness/weakness (location): _____
Seizures: _____ History/onset: _____ Type (e.g., generalized, partial): _____ Frequency: _____ Aura (describe): _____
  Postical state: _____ How controlled: _____
Vision loss/changes: ____ Glasses/contacts: ____ Last exam: ___ Glaucoma: ___ Cataract: ___ Eye surgery (type/date): ____
Hearing loss: _____ Sudden/gradual: _____ Hearing aids: _____ Last exam: _____
Sense of smell (changes): _____ Epistaxis: _____
Sense of taste (changes): _____
Other: _____

Objective (Exhibits)

Mental status (note duration of change):
  Oriented: Person: _____ Place: _____ Time: _____ Situation: _____
  Check all that apply: Alert: _____ Drowsy: _____ Lethargic: _____ Stuporous: _____ Comatose: _____
  Cooperative: _____ Follows commands: _____ Agitated/restless: _____ Combative: _____
  Delusions (describe): _____ Hallucinations (describe): _____
  Affect (describe): _____ Speech: _____
  Memory: Recent: _____ Remote: _____
  Pupil shape: _____ Size/reaction: R/L: _____ Accommodation: _____
  Facial droop: _____ Swallowing: _____
  Hand grasp/release, R: _____ L: _____

TABLE 3.1 **continued**

Coordination: _____ Balance: _____ Walking: _____ Sitting: _____ Standing: _____
Deep tendon reflexes (present/absent/location): _____ Tremors: _____ Posturing: _____ Paralysis (L/R): _____

Pain/Discomfort

Subjective (Reports)

Primary focus: Location: _____ Intensity (use pain scale/pictures): _____
 Quality (e.g., stabbing, aching, burning): _____ Radiation: _____
 Frequency: _____ Duration: _____
Precipitating/aggravating factors: _____
How relieved: OTC/prescription: _____ Nonpharmaceuticals/therapies: _____
Associated symptoms (e.g., nausea, sleep problems, photosensitivity): _____
Effect on daily activities: _____ Relationships: _____ Job: _____ Enjoyment of life: _____
Additional pain focus/describe: _____
Cultural expectations regarding pain perception and expression: _____

Objective (Exhibits)

Facial grimacing: _____ Guarding affected area: _____ Posturing: _____ Behaviors: _____ Narrowed focus: _____
Emotional response (e.g., crying, withdrawal, anger): _____
Vital sign changes (acute pain): BP: _____ Pulse: _____ Respirations: _____

Respiration

Subjective (Reports)

Dyspnea/related to: _____ Precipitating factors: _____ Relieving factors: _____
Airway clearance (e.g., spontaneous/device): _____
Cough (e.g., hard, persistent, croupy): _____ Sputum color/character: _____ Requires suctioning: _____
History of/date: Bronchitis: _____ Emphysema: _____ Tuberculosis: _____ Recurrent pneumonia: _____
Exposure to noxious fumes/allergens, infectious agents/diseases, poisons: _____
Smoker: _____ packs/day: _____ # of pack years: _____ Cigar use: _____ Smokeless: _____ Vapes: _____
Use of respiratory aids: _____ Oxygen (type, frequency, rate): _____
Medications/herbals: _____

Objective (Exhibits)

Respirations (spontaneous/assisted): _____ Rate: _____ Depth: _____ Chest excursion (e.g., equal/symmetrical): _____ Use of
 accessory muscles: _____ Nasal flaring: _____ Fremitus: _____
Breath sounds (describe): _____ Egophony: _____
Skin/mucous membrane color (e.g., pale, cyanotic): _____ Clubbing of fingers: _____
Sputum characteristics: _____
Mentation (e.g., calm, anxious, restless): _____
Pulse oximetry: _____

Safety

Subjective (Reports)

Allergies/sensitivity (medications, foods, environment, iodine, latex): _____
 Type of reaction: _____
Blood transfusion/number: _____ Date: _____ Reaction (describe): _____
Exposure to infectious diseases (e.g., measles, influenza, pink eye, whooping cough): _____
Exposure to pollution, toxins, poisons/pesticides, radiation (describe reactions): _____
Geographic areas lived in/recent travel: _____
Immunization history/date: Tetanus: _____ MMR: _____ Polio: _____ Hepatitis: _____ Pneumonia: _____ Influenza: _____ HPV: _____
Altered/suppressed immune system (list cause): _____
History of sexually transmitted infection (date/type): _____ Testing: _____
High-risk behaviors (specify): _____
Uses seat belt regularly: _____ Uses bike helmet: _____ Other safety devices: _____
Workplace safety/health issues (describe): _____ Occupation: _____ Currently working: _____ Rate working
conditions (e.g., safety, noise, heating, water, ventilation): _____
History of injuries (e.g., fall, vehicle crash, blast, gunshot, electrical, chemical): _____ Fractures/dislocations: _____
Arthritis/unstable joints: _ Joint replacement surgeries (type and date): _____ Back problems: _____
Skin problems (e.g., rashes, lesions, moles, breast lumps, enlarged nodes)/describe: _____

(table continues on page 18)

| TABLE 3.1 | General Assessment Tool (continued) |

Delayed healing (describe): _____
Cognitive limitations (e.g., disorientation, confusion): _____
Sensory limitations (e.g., impaired vision/hearing, detecting heat/cold, taste, smell, touch): _____
Prosthesis (type and date received): _____ Ambulatory devices: _____
Violence (episodes or tendencies): _____

Objective (Exhibits)

Body temperature/method (e.g., oral, rectal, temporal, tympanic): _____
Skin integrity (mark location on diagram): Scars: _____ Rashes: _____ Lacerations: _____ Ulcerations: _____ Bruises: _____
Blisters: _____ Drainage: _____ Burns (degree/% of body surface): _____

Musculoskeletal: General strength: _____ Muscle tone: _____ Gait: _____ ROM: _____ Paresthesia/paralysis: _____
Results of testing (e.g., cultures, immune function, TB, hepatitis): _____

Sexuality (Component of Social Interaction)

Subjective (Reports)

Sexually active: _____ Monogamous/committed relationship: _____ Use of condoms: _____
Birth control method: _____
Sexual concerns/difficulties: _____ Recent change in frequency/interest: _____ Pain/discomfort: _____

Objective (Exhibits)

Comfort level with subject matter: _____

Female: Subjective (Reports)

Menstruation: Age at menarche: _____ Length of cycle: _____ Duration: _____ Number of pads/tampons used/day: _____
Last menstrual period: _____ Bleeding between periods: _____ Menopausal: _____ Last period: _____ Hysterectomy (type/
date): _____ Problems with: Hot flashes: _____ Night sweats: _____ Vaginal lubrication: _____ Vaginal discharge: _____
Gynecological/breast surgery (type and date): _____
Infertility concerns: _____ Type of therapy: _____
Pregnant now: _____ Para: _____ Gravida: _____ Due date: _____
Practices breast self-examination: _____ Last mammogram: _____ Last Pap smear: _____
Hormonal therapy: _____ Supplemental calcium: _____ Other medications/herbals: _____

Female: Objective (Exhibits)

Breast examination: _____
Genitalia: _____ Warts/lesions: _____ Vaginal bleeding/discharge: _____
Test results: _____ Pap: _____ Mammogram: _____ STI: _____

Male: Subjective (Reports)

Penis: Circumcised: _____ Lesions/discharge: _____ Vasectomy: _____
Prostate disorder/voiding difficulties: _____

TABLE 3.1 **continued**

Practices self-examination: Breast: _____ Testicles: _____
Last proctoscopic/prostate examination: _____ Last PSA: _____
Medications/herbals: _____

Male: Objective (Exhibits)

Genitalia: Penis: _____ Warts/lesions: _____ Bleeding/discharge: _____ Testicles (e.g., descended, lumps): _____
Prostate: _____
Breast examination: _____
Test results: _____ STI: _____ PSA: _____

Social Interactions

Subjective (Reports)

Relationship status: Single: _____ Married: _____ Living with partner: _____ Divorced: _____ Widowed: _____
  Years in relationship: _____ Perception of relationship: _____ Concerns/stresses: _____
Role within family structure: _____ Number/age of children: _____
  Individuals living in home: _____ Caregiver (to whom & how long): _____
Extended family/availability: _____ Other support person(s): _____
Perception of relationship with family members: _____
Ethnic/cultural affiliation: _____ Strength of ethnic identity: _____ Lives in ethnic community: _____
Feelings of (describe): Mistrust: _____ Rejection: _____ Unhappiness: _____ Loneliness/isolation: _____
Problems related to illness/condition: _____
Difficulties with communication (e.g., speech, another language, brain injury): _____
  Use of communication aids (list): _____ Requires interpreter: _____
Genogram: (complete on separate form)

Objective (Exhibits)

Communication/speech: Clear: _____ Slurred: _____ Unintelligible: _____ Aphasic: _____
  Unusual speech pattern/impairment: _____ Laryngectomy present: _____
  Use of speech/communication aids: _____
Verbal/nonverbal communication with family/significant other(s): _____
  Family interaction (behavioral) pattern: _____

Teaching/Learning

Subjective (Reports)

Communication: Dominant language (specify): _____ Second language: _____
  Literate (reading/writing): _____
Education level: _____ Learning disabilities (specify): _____ Cognitive limitations: _____
Culture/ethnicity: _____ Where born: _____ If immigrant, how long in this country: _____
Health and illness beliefs/practices/customs: _____
  Which family member makes healthcare decisions/is spokesperson for client: _____
Presence of Advance Directives: _____ Code status: _____ Durable Medical Power of Attorney: _____ Designee: _____
Organ Donor status: _____ Health goals: _____
Current health problem/need: _____ Client understanding of problem: _____
Special healthcare concerns (e.g., impact of religious/cultural practices, healthcare decisions, family involvement): _____
Familial risk factors (indicate relationship): Diabetes: _____ Thyroid (specify): _____ Tuberculosis: _____
Heart disease: _____ Stroke: _____ High BP: _____
  Epilepsy/seizures: _____ Kidney disease: _____ Cancer: _____ Mental illness/depression: _____ Other: _____
Prescribed medications (list each separately):
  Drug: _____ Dose: _____ Times (circle last dose): _____
  Take regularly: _____ Purpose: _____ Side effects/problems: _____
Nonprescription drugs/frequency:
  OTC drugs: _____ Vitamins: _____ Herbals: _____ Street drugs: _____
Alcohol (amount/frequency): _____ Tobacco: _____ Smokeless tobacco: _____
Admitting diagnosis per provider: _____
Reason for hospitalization/visit per client: _____
  History of current problem/concern: _____
  Client expectations of this hospitalization/visit: _____
Will admission cause any lifestyle changes (describe): _____

(table continues on page 20)

TABLE 3.1	General Assessment Tool (continued)

Previous illnesses and/or hospitalizations/surgeries: _____

Evidence of failure to improve: _____

Last complete physical examination: _____

Discharge Plan Considerations

Projected length of stay (hours/days): _____ Anticipated date of discharge: _____

  Date information obtained: _____ Source: _____

Resources available: Persons: _____ Financial: _____ Community supports: _____ Groups: _____

Areas that may require alteration/assistance: Food preparation: _____ Shopping: _____ Transportation: _____

Ambulation: _____ Self-care (specify): _____ Socialization: _____

  Medication/IV therapy: _____ Treatments: _____ Wound care: _____ Supplies: _____

  Homemaker/maintenance (specify): _____ Physical layout of home (specify): _____

Anticipated changes in living situation after discharge: _____ Living facility other than home (specify): _____

Referrals (date/source/services): Social services: _____ Rehabilitation: _____

  Dietary: _____ Home care: _____ Resp/O_2: _____ Equipment: _____ Supplies: _____ Other: _____

SUMMARY

The assessment step of the nursing process emphasizes and should provide a holistic view of the client. The generalized assessment done during the overall data-gathering process creates a profile of the client. A focused, or more detailed, assessment may be warranted given the client's condition or emergent time constraints, or it may be done to obtain more information about a specific issue that needs expansion or clarification. Both types of assessments provide important data that complement each other. A successfully completed assessment creates a picture of clients' states of wellness, their response to health concerns or problems, and individual risk factors—this is the foundation for identifying appropriate nursing diagnoses, developing client outcomes, and choosing relevant interventions necessary for providing individualized care.

References

1. American Nurses Association. (2010). *Nursing: Scope & Standards of Practice*. 2nd ed. Silver Spring, MD: Nursesbooks.org.
2. Doenges, M. E., Moorhouse, M. F., Murr, A. C. (2016). *Nurse's Pocket Guide: Diagnoses, Interventions, and Rationales*. 14th ed. Philadelphia, PA: F. A. Davis.
3. Doenges, M. E., Moorhouse, M. F., Murr, A. C. (2019). *Nursing Care Plans: Guidelines for Individualizing Client Care Across the Lifespan*. 10th ed. Philadelphia, PA: F. A. Davis.
4. Gordon, M. (2008). *Assess Notes: Nursing Assessment and Diagnostic Reasoning*. Philadelphia, PA: F. A. Davis.
5. Souza Carneiro, C. E., et al. (2014). Construction and validation of a data collection tool for the clinical assessment of human responses of outpatients with chronic cardiovascular diseases. *Int J Nurs Knowl*, 25(3), 161–167.
6. American Nurses Association. (1995). *Nursing's Social Policy Statement*. Washington, DC: American Nurses Association.

CHAPTER 4

Concept or Mind Mapping to Create and Document the Plan of Care

The plan of care may be recorded on a single page or in a multiple-page format, with one page for each nursing diagnosis or client diagnostic statement. The format for documenting the plan of care is determined by agency policy. As a practicing professional, you might use a computer with a plan-of-care database, preprinted standardized care plan forms, or clinical pathways. Whichever form you use, the plan of care enables visualization of the nursing process and must reflect the basic nursing standards of care; personal client data; nonroutine care; and qualifiers for interventions and outcomes, such as time, frequency, and amount.

As students, you are asked to develop plans of care that often contain more detail than what you see in the hospital plans of care. This is to help you learn how to apply the nursing process and create individualized client care plans. However, even though much time and energy may be spent focusing on filling in the columns of traditional clinical care plan forms, some students never develop a holistic view of their clients and fail to visualize how each client need interacts with other identified needs. A new technique, or *megacognitive* learning tool, has been developed to assist you in visualizing the linkages and understanding the interrelationships among a client's health concerns, to enhance and evaluate your critical thinking skills, and to facilitate the creative process of planning client care.[1,2]

CONCEPT OR MIND MAPPING CLIENT CARE

Have you ever asked yourself whether you are more right-brained or left-brained? Those who naturally use their left brains are more linear in their thinking. Right-brain thinkers see more in pictures and illustrations. It is best for nurses to use the whole brain (right and left) when thinking about providing the broad scope of nursing care to clients.

No More Columns!

Traditional nursing care plans are linear—that is, they are designed in columns. They speak almost exclusively to the left brain. The traditional nursing care plan is organized according to the nursing process, which guides us in problem-solving the nursing care we give. However, the linear nature of the traditional plan does not facilitate interconnecting data from one "row" to another or between parts in a column. Concept mapping allows us to show the interconnections among various client symptoms, interventions, and problems as they impact each other.

You can keep the parts that are great about traditional care plans (problem-solving and categorizing), but change the linear or columnar nature of the plan to a design that uses the whole brain—bringing left-brained, linear problem-solving together with the free-wheeling, interconnected, creative right brain. Joining concept mapping and care planning enables you to create a whole picture of a client with all the interconnections identified.

There are several diverse and innovative ways to mind map or to concept map nursing care plans.[3] The examples in this chapter use mind mapping and require placing the client at the center, with all ideas on one page (for a whole picture); the examples also use color coding and creative energy.[4,5] When doing a large mapped plan of care, a light poster board is often used so that all ideas fit on one page.

Components of a Concept Map

Tony Buzan developed the idea of mind mapping as a way to depict how ideas about a main subject are related. Mapping represents graphically the relationships and interrelationships of ideas and concepts.[6] It fosters and encourages critical thinking through brainstorming about a particular subject. Mueller, Johnston, and Bligh took the process of mind mapping and combined it with care planning to enhance nursing students' critical thinking and provision of holistic nursing care.[3] This process has also been referred to as concept mapping.

Instead of starting at the top of the page, concept mapping starts at the page's center. The main concept of our thinking goes in this center stage place.

From that central thought, simply begin thinking of other main ideas that relate to the central topic.

These ideas radiate out from the central idea like spokes of a wheel (see subsequent discussion); however, they do not have to be added in a balanced manner. The "wheel" does not have to be round.

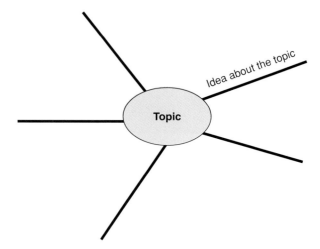

You will generate further ideas related to each spoke (see subsequent discussion), and your mind will race with even more ideas from those thoughts, which can be represented through pictures or words.

As you think of new ideas, write them down immediately. This may require going back and forth from one area of the page to another. Writing your concept map by hand allows you to move faster. Avoid

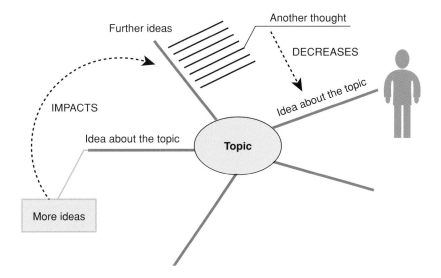

using a computer to generate a map because it hinders the fast-paced process. You can group different concepts together by color coding or by placement on the page (see subsequent discussion).

As you see connections and interconnections among groups of ideas, use arrows or lines to connect those concepts (refer to the dotted lines). You can also add defining phrases that explain how the interconnected thoughts relate to one another, as in the figure above.

Some left-brain thinkers find it very difficult to start their ideas in the middle of a page. If you are this type of thinker, try starting at the top of the page (see subsequent discussion), but you must still represent your ideas in illustration form, not in paragraphs.

Concept maps created by different people look different. They are unique to the mind's eye picture, so do not expect your map to be the same as someone else's.

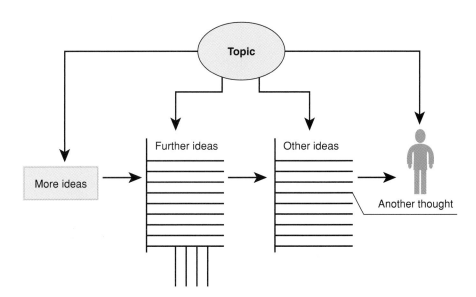

Concept mapping is an exciting alternative format for illustrating a written plan of care. A mapped care plan will look very different from traditional plans of care, which are usually completed on linear forms.

To begin mapping a client plan of care, you must begin with the central topic—the client. Now you are thinking like a nurse. Create a shape that signifies "client" to you and place it at your map's center. If your hand just cannot start at the center, then put the shape at the top. This will help you remember that the client, not the medical diagnosis or condition, is the focus of your plan. All other pieces of the map will be connected in some manner to the client. Many different pieces of information about the client can be connected directly to the client. For example, each of the following pieces of critical client data could stem from the center:

- 78-year-old widower
- No family in the state
- Obese
- Medical diagnosis of recurrent community-acquired pneumonia

Now, you must do a bit of thinking about how you think. To create the rest of your map, ask yourself how *you* plan client care. For example, which of these items do you see first or think of first as the basis for your plan: the clustered assessment data, nursing diagnoses, or outcomes? Whichever piece you choose becomes your first layer of connections. Suppose when thinking about a plan of care for a female client with heart failure, you think first in terms of all the nursing diagnoses about that woman and her condition. Your map would start with the diagnoses featured as the first "branches," with each one listed separately in some way on the map.

Completing the map then becomes a matter of adding the rest of the pieces of the plan using the nursing process and your own way of thinking or planning as your guide. If you began your map using nursing diagnoses, you might think, "What signs and symptoms or data support these diagnoses?" Then, you would connect clusters of supporting data to the related nursing diagnosis. Or you might think, "What client outcomes am I trying to achieve when I address this nursing diagnosis?" In that case, you would next connect client outcomes (or NOC labels) to the nursing diagnoses.

To keep your map clear, as suggested previously, use different colors and maybe a different shape, spoke, or line for each piece of the care plan that you add. For example:

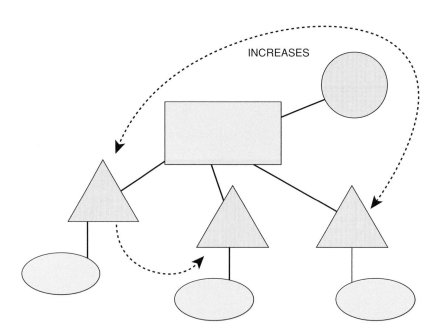

INCREASES

- Red for signs and symptoms (to signify danger)
- Yellow for nursing diagnoses (for "stop and think what this is")
- Green for nursing interventions or NIC labels (for "go")
- Blue (or some other color) for outcomes or NOC labels

When all the pieces of the nursing process are represented, each branch of the map is complete. There should be a nursing diagnosis (supported by subjective and objective assessment data), nursing interventions, desired client outcome(s), and any evaluation data, all connected in a manner that shows there is a relationship among them.

It is critical to understand that there is no preset order for the pieces because one cluster is not more or less important than another (or one is not "subsumed" under another). It is important, however, that those pieces within a branch be in the same order in each branch.

So, you might ask, how is this different from writing out information in a linear manner? What makes mapping so special? One of the things you may have discovered about caring for clients is that the care you deliver is very interconnected. Taking care of one problem often results in the simultaneous correction of another. For example, if you resolve a fluid volume problem in a client with heart failure, you will also positively impact the client's gas exchange and decrease his or her anxiety. These kinds of interconnections cannot be shown on linear plans of care, yet they are what practicing nurses see in their mind's eye all the time. These interconnections can be represented on a map with arrows or dotted or dashed lines that tie related ideas together. Then, defining phrases that explain the nature of the interconnection can be added to further clarify the relationship, as shown in Figure 4.1.

In addition to the pieces of the nursing process, other components of care can be illustrated on a map. Nurses have certain responsibilities when clients have diagnostic tests (such as an angiography or a bronchoscopy). These tests can be connected to the appropriate piece of your map, along with the correct nursing interventions related to those tests. Another item to be added is potential complications or collaborative problems.

Taking your clients' needs one step further, try asking every client you have (medical, surgical, or otherwise), "What is the most important thing to you now in relation to why you are here?" Obtaining this information builds an alliance between you and your client, and together you can work toward that desired outcome. Add it to your map and see how your plan of care becomes more client centered (refer to Fig. 4.2).

SUMMARY

Concept maps allow you to do something that is different and creative. They require you to think (and learn), make connections, and use colors and shapes. They help you to focus on the client, and having the map on one page helps you to understand the "whole picture" better. Concept maps also help you become better organized and develop your own unique approach to "thinking like a nurse" much sooner.

A student who had written many traditional plans of care in her previous nursing program wrote the following about concept-mapped care plans:

Concept mapping is painting a picture using colors of the rainbow on blank paper to tell the story of your client using "NANDA" nursing diagnoses and the nursing process. Previously, I was a student in prison (my mind) who hated the words "CARE PLAN," writing page after page in narrative form. It was laborious to do and boring to read. There was no life or heartbeat.

Concept mapping opened the prison doors, and my care plan took on human form with a VOICE, a beating HEART, and COLOR while still incorporating the nursing process and standardized nursing language. My mind now took on the professional thought process for which NANDA, NIC, and NOC were created to facilitate nursing; however, the magic was in concept mapping, which removed all my fears, and the client became a beautiful painting with a heartbeat.[3]

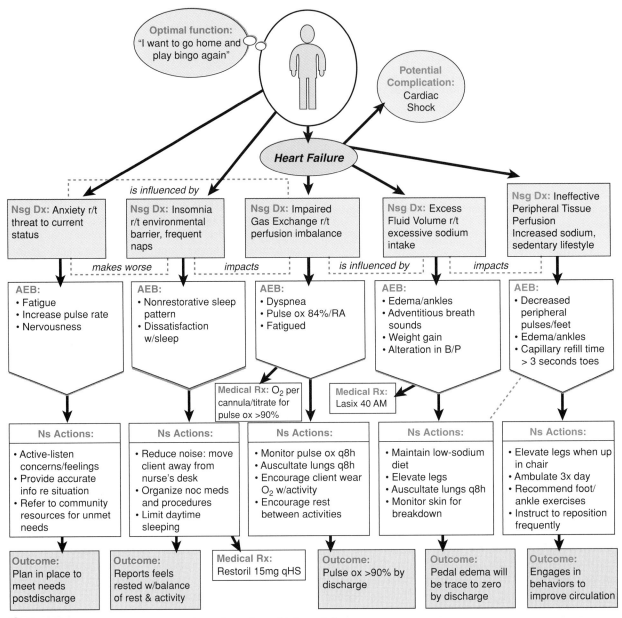

Figure 4.1 Concept map of a plan of care for a client with heart failure.

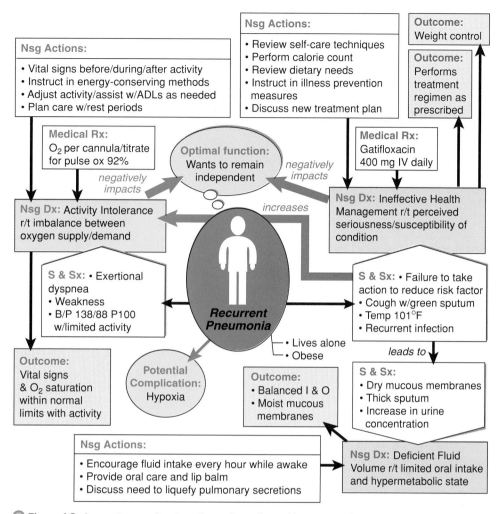

Nsg Actions:
- Vital signs before/during/after activity
- Instruct in energy-conserving methods
- Adjust activity/assist w/ADLs as needed
- Plan care w/rest periods

Nsg Actions:
- Review self-care techniques
- Perform calorie count
- Review dietary needs
- Instruct in illness prevention measures
- Discuss new treatment plan

Outcome: Weight control

Outcome: Performs treatment regimen as prescribed

Medical Rx: O_2 per cannula/titrate for pulse ox 92%

Optimal function: Wants to remain independent

negatively impacts

negatively impacts

Medical Rx: Gatifloxacin 400 mg IV daily

Nsg Dx: Activity Intolerance r/t imbalance between oxygen supply/demand

increases

Nsg Dx: Ineffective Health Management r/t perceived seriousness/susceptibility of condition

Recurrent Pneumonia

S & Sx:
- Exertional dyspnea
- Weakness
- B/P 138/88 P100 w/limited activity

S & Sx:
- Failure to take action to reduce risk factor
- Cough w/green sputum
- Temp 101°F
- Recurrent infection

- Lives alone
- Obese

leads to

Outcome: Vital signs & O_2 saturation within normal limits with activity

Potential Complication: Hypoxia

Outcome:
- Balanced I & O
- Moist mucous membranes

S & Sx:
- Dry mucous membranes
- Thick sputum
- Increase in urine concentration

Nsg Actions:
- Encourage fluid intake every hour while awake
- Provide oral care and lip balm
- Discuss need to liquefy pulmonary secretions

Nsg Dx: Deficient Fluid Volume r/t limited oral intake and hypermetabolic state

Figure 4.2 Concept map of a plan of care for a client with pneumonia.

References

1. Gull, B., Bowman, J. (2006). Concept mapping: A strategy for teaching and evaluating critical thinking in nursing education. *Nurse Educ Pract*, 6(4), 199–206.
2. Senita, J. (2008). The use of concept maps to evaluate critical thinking in the clinical setting. *Teaching and Learning in Nursing*, 3(1), 6–10.
3. Schuster, P. (2015). *Concept Mapping: A Critical-Thinking Approach to Care Planning*. 4th ed. Philadelphia: F. A. Davis.
4. Mueller, A., Johnston, M., Bligh, D. (2001). Mind-mapped care plans, a remarkable alternative to traditional nursing care plans. *Nurse Educ*, 26(2), 75–80.
5. Mueller, A., Johnston, M., Bligh, D. (2002). Viewpoint: Joining mind mapping and care planning to enhance student critical thinking and achieve holistic nursing care. *Int J Nurs Terminol Classif*, 13(1), 24–27.
6. Buzan, T. (1995). *The Mind Map Book*. 2nd ed. London: BBC Books.

CHAPTER 5

Nursing Diagnoses in Alphabetical Order

Activity Intolerance [Specify Level]

Taxonomy II: Activity/Rest—Class 4 Cardiovascular/Pulmonary Responses (00092) [**Diagnostic Division:** Activity/Rest], Submitted 1982, revised 2017

DEFINITION: Insufficient physiological or psychological energy to endure or complete required or desired daily activities.

RELATED FACTORS
Physical deconditioning
Sedentary lifestyle
Immobility
Imbalance between oxygen supply and demand

DEFINING CHARACTERISTICS

Subjective
Fatigue, generalized weakness
Exertional discomfort, dyspnea

Objective
Abnormal heart rate or blood pressure response to activity
ECG change [e.g., arrhythmia, conduction abnormality, ischemia]

FUNCTIONAL LEVEL CLASSIFICATION[3]
Level I: Walk, regular pace, on level indefinitely; climb one flight or more, but more short of breath than normal
Level II: Walk one city block [or] 500 ft on level; climb one flight slowly without stopping
Level III: Walk no more than 50 ft on level without stopping; unable to climb one flight of stairs without stopping
Level IV: Dyspnea and fatigue at rest
Sample Clinical Applications: Anemias, angina, aortic stenosis, bronchitis, emphysema, cancers, diabetes mellitus, dysmenorrhea, heart failure, HIV/AIDS, labor/preterm labor, leukemias, mitral stenosis, obesity, pain, pericarditis, peripheral vascular disease, rheumatic fever, thrombocytopenia, tuberculosis, uterine bleeding

Information that appears in brackets has been added by the authors to clarify and enhance the use of the nursing diagnoses.

DESIRED OUTCOMES/EVALUATION CRITERIA

Sample **NOC** linkages:

Activity Tolerance: Physiological response to energy-consuming movements with daily activities
Energy Conservation: Personal actions to manage energy for initiating and sustaining activity
Endurance: Capacity to sustain activity
Psychomotor Energy: Personal drive and energy to maintain activities of daily living, nutrition, and personal safety

Client Will (Include Specific Time Frame)

- Identify negative factors affecting activity tolerance and eliminate or reduce their effects when possible.
- Use identified techniques to enhance activity tolerance.
- Participate in necessary/desired activities.
- Report measurable increase in activity tolerance.
- Demonstrate a decrease in physiological signs of intolerance (e.g., pulse, respirations, and blood pressure remain within client's usual range).

ACTIONS/INTERVENTIONS

Sample **NIC** linkages:

Activity Therapy: Prescription of and assistance with specific physical, cognitive, social, and spiritual activities to increase the range, frequency, or duration of an individual's (or group's) activity
Energy Management: Regulating energy use to treat or prevent fatigue and optimize function
Exercise Promotion: Facilitation of regular physical activity to maintain or advance to a higher level of fitness and health

NURSING PRIORITY NO. 1   To identify causative/precipitating factors:

- Note presence of acute or chronic illness, such as heart failure, pulmonary disorders, hypothyroidism, diabetes mellitus, AIDS, anemias, cancers, acute and chronic pain, etc. *Many factors cause or contribute to fatigue, but the term "activity intolerance" implies that the client cannot endure or adapt to increased energy or oxygen demands caused by an activity.*[1,8,9]
- Assess cardiopulmonary response to physical activity by measuring vital signs, noting heart rate and regularity, respiratory rate and work of breathing, and blood pressure before, during, and after activity. Note progression or accelerating degree of fatigue. *Dramatic changes in heart rate and rhythm, changes in usual blood pressure, and progressively worsening fatigue result from imbalance of oxygen supply and demand. These changes are potentially greater in the frail, elderly population.*[1,3,10,11]
- Note treatment-related factors such as side effects and interactions of medications. *Can affect nature and degree of activity intolerance.*
- Determine if client is receiving medications such as vasodilators, diuretics, or beta blockers. *Orthostatic hypotension can occur with activity because of medication effects (vasodilation), fluid shifts (diuresis), or compromised cardiac pumping function.*[15]
- Note client reports of difficulty accomplishing tasks or desired activities. Evaluate current limitations or degree of deficit in light of usual status and what the client perceives causes, exacerbates, and helps the problem. *Provides comparative baseline, influences choice of interventions, and may reveal causes that the client is unaware of affecting energy, such as sleep deprivation, smoking, poor diet, depression, or lack of support.*[2,10,11]

 Diagnostic Studies   Evidence Based Practice   Medications   Pediatric/Geriatric/Lifespan

- Ascertain ability to sit, stand, and move about as desired. Note degree of assistance necessary and/or use of assistive equipment. *Helps to differentiate between problems relating to movement and problems with oxygen supply and demand characterized by fatigue and weakness.*[2,8,9,11]
- Identify activity needs versus desires (e.g., client barely able to walk up stairs but states would like to play racquetball). *Assists caregiver in dealing with reality of situation as well as the feasibility of goals client wants to achieve when developing activity plan.*
- Assess emotional or psychological factors affecting the current situation. *Stress and/or depression may be exacerbating the effects of an illness, or depression may be the result of therapy and/or limitations.*

NURSING PRIORITY NO. 2   To assist client to deal with contributing factors and manage activities within individual limits:

- Monitor vital signs before and during activity, watching for changes in blood pressure, heart and respiratory rate, and post-activity vital sign response. *Vital signs may change during activity (including higher or lower pulse or blood pressure) and should return to baseline within 5 to 7 min after activity if response to activity is normal.*[1]
- Observe respiratory rate, noting breathing pattern, breath sounds, skin color, and mental status. *Pallor and/or cyanosis, presence of respiratory distress, or confusion may be indicative of need for oxygen during activities, especially if respiratory infection or compromise is present.*
- Plan care with rest periods between activities *to reduce fatigue.*
- Assist with self-care activities. Adjust activities or reduce intensity level, or discontinue activities that cause undesired physiological changes. *Prevents overexertion.*
- Increase exercise/activity levels gradually; encourage stopping to rest for 3 minutes during a 10-minute walk, or sitting down instead of standing to brush hair. *Methods of conserving energy.*
- Encourage expression of feelings contributing to or resulting from condition. Provide positive atmosphere while acknowledging difficulty of the situation for the client. *Helps to minimize frustration, rechannel energy.*
- Involve client/significant others (SOs) in planning of activities as much as possible. *May give client opportunity to perform desired or essential activities during periods of peak energy.*
- Assist with activities and provide and monitor client's use of assistive devices. *Enables client to maintain mobility while protecting from injury.*
- Promote comfort measures and provide for relief of pain *to enhance client's ability and desire to participate in activities.*[9,11] (Refer to NDs acute Pain, chronic Pain.)
- Provide referral to collaborative disciplines, such as an exercise physiologist, psychological counseling/therapy, occupational/physical therapy, and recreation/leisure specialists. *May be needed to develop individually appropriate therapeutic regimens.*
- Prepare for/assist with and monitor effects of exercise-capacity testing. *May be performed to determine degree of oxygen desaturation and/or hypoxemia that occurs with exertion or to optimize titration of supplemental oxygen when used.*[5,8]
- Implement graded exercise or rehabilitation program under direct medical supervision. *Gradual increase in activity avoids excessive myocardial workload and associated oxygen demand and has been shown to exert positive health benefits, even in those with chronic diseases. One intervention review found that for people with mild to moderate systolic heart failure, there was neither a reduction nor an increase in the risk of death with exercise. However, following exercise training, there was a reduction in hospital admissions due to systolic heart failure.*[4]
- Administer supplemental oxygen, medications, prepare for surgery, and other treatments, as indicated. *Type of therapy or medication is dependent on the underlying condition and might include medications (e.g., antiarryhthmics, bronchodilators) or surgery (e.g., stents or coronary artery bypass graft) to improve myocardial perfusion and systemic circulation. Other treatments might include iron preparations or blood transfusion to treat severe anemia or use of oxygen and bronchodilators to improve respiratory function.*[6,7,12,14]

➕ Acute Care   Collaborative   🏠 Community/ Home Care   🌐 Cultural

NURSING PRIORITY NO. 3 To promote wellness (Teaching/Discharge Considerations):

- Review expectations of client/SOs/providers and explore conflicts or differences. *Help to establish goals and to reach agreement for the most effective plan.*
- Assist or direct client/SOs to plan for progressive increase of activity level, aiming for maximal activity within the client's ability. *Promote improved or more normal activity level, stamina, and conditioning.*
- Instruct client/SOs in monitoring response to activity and in recognizing signs/symptoms that indicate need to alter activity level. *Assist in self-management of condition and in understanding of reportable problems. Research studies continue to confirm that regular physical activity not only reduces the risk of many adverse outcomes, but it also provides health benefits.*[8,9,13,16]
- Give client information that provides evidence of daily or weekly progress *to sustain motivation.*
- Assist client to learn and demonstrate appropriate safety measures, such as using assistive devices correctly, wearing glasses, and having a companion when walking *to prevent injuries.*
- Provide information about proper nutrition to meet metabolic and energy needs, obtaining or maintaining normal body weight. *Energy is improved when nutrients are sufficient to meet metabolic demands.*[1,16]
- Encourage client to use relaxation techniques, such as visualization or guided imagery, as appropriate. *Useful in maintaining positive attitude and enhancing sense of well-being.*
- Encourage participation in self-care, recreation, or social activities and hobbies appropriate for situation. (Refer to ND decreased Diversional Activity Engagement.)
- Monitor laboratory values (such as for anemia) and pulse oximetry *to identify areas of concern that may require further assessment or intervention.*

DOCUMENTATION FOCUS

Assessment/Reassessment
- Level of activity as noted in Functional Level Classification.
- Causative or precipitating factors.
- Client reports of difficulty or change.

Planning
- Plan of care and who is involved in planning.
- Teaching plan.

Implementation/Evaluation
- Response to interventions, teaching, and actions performed.
- Modifications to plan of care.
- Attainment or progress toward desired outcome(s).

Discharge Planning
- Referrals to other resources.
- Long-term needs and who is responsible for actions.

References

1. Newfield, S. A., et al. (2007). *Cox's Clinical Applications of Nursing Diagnosis: Adult, Child, Women's, Psychiatric, Gerontic, and Home Health Considerations.* 5th ed. Philadelphia, PA: F. A. Davis.
2. Stanley, M. (2005). In Blair, K. A., Beare, P. G. (eds). *Gerontological Nursing: Promoting Successful Aging with Older Adults.* 3rd ed. Philadelphia: F. A. Davis.
3. Gordon, M. (2014). *Manual of Nursing Diagnosis.* 13th ed. St. Louis, MO: Mosby.
4. Taylor, R. S., et al. (Updated 2014). Exercise-based rehabilitation for heart failure. *Cochrane Library.* Retrieved February 2018 from http://onlinelibrary.wiley.com/doi/10.1002/14651858.CD003331.pub4/full.
5. Foss, C. M., et al. (2001). Exercise testing for evaluation of hypoxemia and/or desaturation: Revision & update. *Resp Care,* 46(5), 514–522.
6. Finn, S. D., et al. (2014). 2014 ACC/AHA/AATS/PCNA/SCAI/STS focused update of the guideline for the diagnosis and management of patients with stable ischemic heart disease: A report of the American College of Cardiology/American Heart Association Task Force on Practice Guidelines and the American Association for Thoracic Surgery, Preventive

Cardiovascular Nurses Association, Society for Cardiovascular Angiography and Interventions, and Society of Thoracic Surgeons. *J Am Coll Cardiol*, 64(18), 1929.

7. *Congestive Heart Failure in Adults*. (2002). Bloomington, MN: Institute for Clinical Systems Improvement.

8. Michael, K. M., Allen, J. K., Macko, R. E. (2006). Fatigue after stroke: Relationship to mobility, fitness, ambulatory activity, social support, and falls efficacy. *Rehabil Nurs*, 31(5), 210–217.

9. Graf, C. (2006). Functional decline in hospitalized older adults. *Am J Nurs*, 106(1), 58–67.

10. Winkelman, C., Chlan, L. (2009). Bed rest in health and critical illness: A body systems approach. *AACN Adv Crit Care*, 20(3), 254–266.

11. Hurr, H. K., et al. (2005). Activity intolerance and impaired physical mobility in elders. *Int J Nurs Terminol Classif*, 16(3–4), 47–53.

12. Exercise-induced bronchoconstriction and asthma: EPC Evidence Reports. (2010). *Agency for Healthcare Research and Quality (AJRQ)*. Retrieved February 2018 from https://archive .ahrq.gov/research/findings/evidence-based-reports/er189-abstract.html.

13. 2008 Physical Guidelines for Americans, Summary. (Update 2018). *Office of Disease Prevention and Health Promotion*. Retrieved February 2018 from https://health.gov/paguidelines/ guidelines/summary.aspx.

14. Koh, H. K., et al. (2007). Inhaled corticosteroids compared to placebo for prevention of exercise-induced bronchoconstriction. *Cochrane Library*. Retrieved February 2018 from http:// onlinelibrary.wiley.com/doi/10.1002/14651858.CD002739 .pub3/full.

15. Mussi, C., et al. (2009). Orthostatic hypotension as cause of syncope in patients older than 65 years admitted to emergency departments for transient loss of consciousness. *J Gerontol A Biol Sci Med Sci*, 64(7), 801–806.

16. Kitzman, D. W., et al. (2016). Effect of caloric restriction or aerobic exercise training on peak oxygen consumption and quality of life in obese older patients with heart failure and preserved ejection fraction: A randomized, controlled trial. *JAMA*, 315(1), 36–46.

risk for Activity Intolerance

Taxonomy II: Activity/Rest—Class 4 Cardiovascular/Pulmonary Response (00094) [**Diagnostic Division:** Activity/Rest], Submitted 1982, revised 2013, 2017

DEFINITION: Susceptible to experiencing insufficient physiological or psychological energy to endure or complete required or desired daily activities, which may compromise health.

RISK FACTORS

Imbalance between oxygen supply/demand

Immobility, physical deconditioning; sedentary lifestyle

Inexperience with an activity

At Risk Population: History of previous activity intolerance

Associated Condition: Circulatory or respiratory condition

Sample Clinical Applications: Anemias, angina, aortic stenosis, bronchitis, emphysema, dysmenorrhea, heart failure, HIV/AIDS, labor/preterm labor, leukemias, mitral stenosis, obesity, pain, pericarditis, peripheral vascular disease, rheumatic fever, thrombocytopenia, tuberculosis, uterine bleeding

DESIRED OUTCOMES/EVALUATION CRITERIA

Sample NOC linkages:

Endurance: Capacity to sustain activity

Energy Conservation: Personal actions to manage energy for initiating and sustaining activity

Psychomotor Energy: Personal drive and energy to maintain activities of daily living, nutrition, and personal safety

Client Will (Include Specific Time Frame)

• Verbalize understanding of potential loss of ability in relation to existing condition.

• Participate in conditioning or rehabilitation program to enhance ability to perform.

• Identify alternative ways to maintain desired activity level (e.g., if weather is bad, walking in a shopping mall could be an option).

• Identify conditions or symptoms that require medical reevaluation.

 Acute Care   Collaborative   Community/ Home Care   Cultural

ACTIONS/INTERVENTIONS

Energy Management: Regulating energy use to treat or prevent fatigue and optimize function

Exercise Promotion: Facilitation of regular physical activity to maintain or advance to a higher level of fitness and health

NURSING PRIORITY NO. 1   To assess factors affecting current situation:

- Note presence of medical diagnosis and/or therapeutic regimens (e.g., AIDS, chronic obstructive pulmonary disease, cancer, heart failure or other cardiac problems, anemia, multiple medications or treatment modalities, extensive surgical interventions, musculoskeletal trauma, neurological disorders). *These have potential for interfering with client's ability to perform at a desired level of activity. Note: Many factors cause or contribute to fatigue, but activity intolerance implies that the individual cannot endure or adapt to increased energy or oxygen demands caused by an activity.*[1]
- Ask client/significant other (SO) about usual level of energy *to identify potential problems and/or client's/SO's perception of client's energy and ability to perform needed or desired activities.*
- Identify factors (e.g., age, functional decline, malnutrition, painful conditions, breathing problems, vision or hearing impairments; need for mobility assistance; client resistive to efforts; unsuitable climate or weather conditions; unsafe areas to exercise) *that could block or affect desired level of activity.*
- Determine current activity level and physical condition with observation, exercise capacity testing, use of functional level classification system (e.g., Gordon's), as appropriate. *Provides baseline for comparison and opportunity to track changes.*

NURSING PRIORITY NO. 2   To develop/investigate alternative ways to remain active within the limits of the disabling condition/situation:

- Implement physical therapy or exercise program in conjunction with the client and other team members, such as a physical and/or occupational therapist, exercise or rehabilitation physiologist. *Collaborative program with short- and long-term achievable goals enhances likelihood of success and may motivate client to adopt a lifestyle of physical exercise for enhancement of health.*[2]
- Promote or implement progressive conditioning program and support inclusion in exercise or activity groups *to prevent or limit effects of deconditioning. Instruct client in energy-conserving activities and benefits of alternating activity and rest periods while continuing activities. Note: studies continue to support the positive effects of exercise training on exercise [activity] tolerance.*[6,7]
- Instruct client in proper performance of unfamiliar activities and/or alternate ways of doing familiar activities *to learn methods of conserving energy and promote safety in performing activities.*

NURSING PRIORITY NO. 3   To promote wellness (Teaching/Discharge Considerations):

- Discuss with client/SO relationship of illness or debilitating condition to inability to perform desired activity(ies). *Understanding these relationships can help with acceptance of limitations or reveal opportunity for changes of practical value.*[1,5]
- Provide information regarding factors such as smoking when one has cardiac or respiratory problems, weight management issues, or lack of motivation or interest in exercise. *Education is essential in promoting client awareness of lifestyle behaviors that can negatively affect health and may encourage client to address issues impacting ability to be active and healthy.*[3,4]
- Assist client/SO with planning for changes that may become necessary (e.g., shifting of family responsibilities, use of supplemental oxygen or medications to improve client's ability to participate in desired activities). *Anticipatory guidance facilitates adaptation if symptoms occur.*[3,4] (Refer to ND Activity Intolerance.)

• Identify and discuss symptoms for which client needs to seek medical assistance or evaluation, *providing for timely intervention.*[3]
• Refer to appropriate sources for assistance (e.g., medical specialists, smoking cessation, dietary counseling, psychological counseling) and/or assistive equipment, as needed, *to sustain or improve activity level and to promote client safety.*

DOCUMENTATION FOCUS

Assessment/Reassessment
• Identified and potential risk factors for individual.
• Current level of activity tolerance and blocks to activity.

Planning
• Treatment options, including physical therapy or exercise program, other assistive therapies and devices.
• Lifestyle changes that are planned, who is to be responsible for each action, monitoring methods.

Implementation/Evaluation
• Responses to interventions, teaching, and actions performed.
• Attainment or progress toward desired outcome(s).
• Modification of plan of care.

Discharge Planning
• Referrals for medical assistance and evaluation.

References

1. Cox, H. C., et al. (2002). *Clinical Applications of Nursing Diagnosis: Adult, Child, Women's, Psychiatric, Gerontic, and Home Health Considerations.* 4th ed. Philadelphia, PA: F. A. Davis.
2. Stanley, M. (2004). In Blair, K. A., Beare, P. G. (eds). *Gerontological Nursing: Promoting Successful Aging in the Older Adult.* 3rd ed. Philadelphia, PA: F. A. Davis.
3. American Heart Association. (Updated 2017). Lifestyle changes for heart failure. Retrieved March 2015 from http://www.heart.org/HEARTORG/Conditions/HeartFailure/Prevention TreatmentofHeartFailure/Lifestyle-Changes-for-Heart-Failure_UCM_306341_Article.jsp#.WoydKExFz4g.
4. King, L. (2012). Developing a progressive mobility activity protocol. *Orthop Nurs*, 31(5), 253–262.
5. Borroso, J., et al. (2010). Physiological and psychosocial factors that predict HIV-related fatigue. *AIDS Behav*, 14(6), 1415–1427.
6. 2008 Physical Guidelines for Americans, Summary. (Updated 2018). *Office of Disease Prevention and Health Promotion.* Retrieved February 2018 from https://health.gov/paguidelines/guidelines/summary.aspx.
7. Taylor, R. S., et al. (Updated 2014). Exercise-based rehabilitation for heart failure. *Cochrane Database of Systematic Reviews.* Retrieved February 2018 from http://www.cochrane.org/CD003331/VASC_exercise-based-rehabilitation-for-heart-failure.

 Acute Care   Collaborative   Community/Home Care   Cultural

ineffective Activity Planning

Taxonomy II: Coping/Stress Tolerance—Class 2 Coping Responses (00199) **[Diagnostic Division:** Activity/Rest**]**, Submitted 2008, revised 2017

DEFINITION: Inability to prepare for a set of actions fixed in time and under certain conditions.

RELATED FACTORS

Unrealistic perception of event [or] personal abilities
Insufficient social support
Insufficient information-processing ability
Pattern of procrastination; flight behavior when faced with proposed solution
Hedonism

DEFINING CHARACTERISTICS

Subjective
Worried/excessive anxiety/fear about a task to be undertaken

Objective
Pattern of failure, or procrastination
Insufficient resources (e.g., financial, social, knowledge)
Absence of plan; insufficient organizational skills
Unmet goals for chosen activity
Sample Clinical Applications: Depression, bipolar disorder, learning disabilities or dyslexia, chronic conditions (e.g., fibromyalgia, fatigue syndrome)

DESIRED OUTCOMES/EVALUATION CRITERIA

Sample NOC linkages:
Motivation: Inner urge that moves or promotes an individual to positive action(s)
Social Support: Reliable assistance from others

Client Will (Include Specific Time Frame)
• Acknowledge difficulty with follow-through of activity plan.
• Identify negative factors affecting ability to plan activities.
• Willingly prepare to develop own plan for activity.
• Report lessened anxiety and fear toward planning.
• Be aware of and make plan to deal with procrastination.

ACTIONS/INTERVENTIONS

Sample NIC linkages:
Self-Awareness Enhancement: Assisting a patient to explore and understand his/her thoughts, feelings, motivations, and behaviors
Values Clarification: Assisting another to clarify her/his own values in order to facilitate effective decision making
Support System Enhancement: Facilitation of support to patient by family, friends, and community

 Diagnostic Studies   Evidence Based Practice   Medications 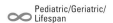 Pediatric/Geriatric/Lifespan

NURSING PRIORITY NO. 1   To identify causative/precipitating factors:

- Determine individual problems with planning and follow through with activity plan. *Identifies individual difficulties, such as anxiety regarding what kind of activity to choose, lack of resources, lack of confidence in own ability.*[1]
- Perform complete physical examination. *May have underlying problems, such as allergies, hypertension, asthma, chronic pain, that contribute to fatigue and difficulty undertaking task.*[2]
- Review medication regimen. *Side effects may contribute to fatigue, affecting client's desire to get involved in any activity.*[2]
- Assess mental status; use Beck's Depression Scale as indicated. *Anxieties and depression can interfere with client's ability and desire to be active.*[5]
- Identify client's personal values and perception of self, including strengths and weaknesses. *Provides information that will be helpful in planning care and choosing goals for this individual.*[1]
- Determine client's need to be in control, fear of dependency on others (although may need assistance from others), belief he or she cannot do the task. *Indicative of external locus of control, where client sees others as having the control and ability.*[1]
- Identify cultural or religious issues that may affect how individual deals with issues of life. *Often person learns strict ideas in family of origin, such as rituals of Catholicism or the demands of prayers for Muslims, that affect how they see their ability to make choices or manage own life.*[1]
- Discuss awareness of procrastination, need for perfection, fear of failure. *Although client may not acknowledge it as a problem, this may be a factor in difficulty in planning for, choosing, and following through with activities that might be enjoyed.*[3,8,9]
- Assess client's ability to process information. *Low self-esteem, anxiety, and possibly difficulty with thinking may interfere with perceptions.*[4]
- Discuss possibility that client is motivated by pleasure to avoid pain (hedonism). *Individual may seek activities that bring pleasure to avoid painful experiences and not realize he or she is using this to keep from completing tasks.*[4,7]
- Note availability and use of resources. *Client may have difficulty if family and friends are not supportive and other resources are not readily available.*[1]

NURSING PRIORITY NO. 2   To assist client to recognize and deal with individual factors that do or could interfere with activities and begin to plan appropriate activities:

- Encourage expression of feelings contributing to or resulting from situation. Maintain a positive atmosphere without seeming overly cheerful. *Helps client to begin to be aware of frustration and redirect energy into productive actions.*[5]
- Discuss client's perception of self as worthless and not deserving of success and happiness. *This belief is common among individuals who struggle with feelings of low self-esteem/self-confidence. They believe that anything they do is bound to fail, and feelings of anxiety and worry contribute to failure. Procrastinating and postponing the task results in failure. Sometimes the underlying feelings are those of wanting to be perfect, and the task may not be perfect if it is finished.*[4,8]
- Gently confront ambivalent, angry, or depressed feelings. *Client may react negatively and withdraw if these feelings are not dealt with in a sensitive manner.*[1]
- Help client learn how to reframe negative thoughts about self into a positive view of what is happening. *Reframing turns a negative thought into something positive to change how it affects the individual.*[1]
- Involve client/significant others (SOs) in planning an activity. *Having the support of the family and nurse will help promote success.*[1]
- Direct client to start with one desired or needed activity and to break it down into specific steps. *Makes activity more manageable, and as each step is accomplished, individual feels more confident about ability to finish the task.*[1]

 Acute Care   Collaborative   Community/ Home Care   Cultural

- Encourage client to recognize procrastinating behaviors and make a decision to change. *Procrastination is a learned behavior, possibly in the family of origin, and serves many purposes for the individual. It can be changed but requires motivation and strong desire.*[3,8,9]
- Accompany client to activity of own choosing, encouraging participation together, if appropriate. *Support from caregiver may enable client to begin participating and gain confidence.*[1,9]
- Assist client to develop skills of relaxation, imagery or visualization, and mindfulness. *Using these techniques can help the client learn to overcome stress and be able to manage life's difficulties more effectively.*[2,6]
- Assist client to investigate the idea that seeking pleasure (hedonism) is interfering with motivation to accomplish goals. *Some philosophers believe that pleasure is the only good for a person, and the individual does not see other aspects of life, interfering with accomplishments.*[7]

NURSING PRIORITY NO. 3 To promote wellness (Teaching/Discharge Criteria):

- 🏠 Assist client to identify life goals and priorities. *Often individual has not thought about the possibility of these ideas and, when asked to do this, begins to think he or she can accomplish some goals.*[1]
- Review treatment goals and expectations of client and SOs. *Helps to clarify what has been discussed and decisions that have been made and provides an opportunity to change goals as needed.*[1]
- Discuss progress in learning to relax and deal productively with anxieties and fears. *As client sees that progress is being made, feelings of worthwhileness will be enhanced and individual will be encouraged to continue working toward goals.*[2,3]
- ⊕ Identify community resources such as social services, senior center, or classes *to provide support and options for activities and change.*
- ⊕ Refer for cognitive therapy. *This structured therapy can help the individuals identify, evaluate, and modify underlying assumptions and dysfunctional beliefs they may have and begin the process of change. Learning to set own schedule with reminders can also help client to get tasks done in a timely manner.*[5]

DOCUMENTATION FOCUS

Assessment/Reassessment
- Specific problems exhibited by client.
- Causative or precipitating factors.
- Client reports of difficulty making and following through with plans.

Planning
- Plan of care and who is involved in planning.
- Teaching plan.

Implementation/Evaluation
- Response to interventions, teaching, and actions performed.
- Attainment or progress toward desired outcome(s).

Discharge Planning
- Referrals to other resources.
- Long-term needs and who is responsible for actions.

References

1. Schuyler, D. (2003). Cognitive therapy for depression. *Prim Psychiatry*, 10(5), 33–36.
2. Berczi, I. (1994). Stress and disease: The contributions of Hans Selye to neuroimmunology. In Berczi, I., Szélenyi, J. (eds). *Advances in Psychoneuroimmunology*. New York: Plenum Press, 1–15.
3. Marano, H. E. (2009, latest review 2016). Ending procrastination. Retrieved February 2018 from http://www.psychologytoday.com/articles/200310/ending-procrastination.
4. Ellis, A. (1994). Showing people they are not worthless individuals. *Voices: The Art and Science of Psychotherapy*, 1(2), 74–77.

 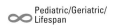

5. Beck, A. C., Beck, A. T. (1995). Cognitive therapy for depression. *Clin Psychol*, 48(3), 3–5.
6. Hopper, J. (2009, revised 2015). Cultivating mindfulness. Retrieved February 2018 from https://www.jimhopper.com/mindfulness-and-meditation/cultivating-mindfulness.
7. Moore, A. (2004, revised 2013). Hedonism. *The Stanford Encyclopedia of Philosophy*. Retrieved February 2018 http://plato.stanford.edu/entries/hedonism/.
8. California Polytechnic State University. (2012). Procrastination. Retrieved February 2018 from https://asc.calpoly.edu/ssl/procrastination.
9. Gura, T. (2009). I'll do it tomorrow. *Scientific American Mind*, 19, 32–39.

risk for ineffective Activity Planning

Taxonomy II: Coping/Stress Tolerance—Class 2 Coping Responses (0026) [**Diagnostic Division:** Activity/Rest], Submitted 2010; Revised 2013

DEFINITION: Susceptible to an inability to prepare for a set of actions fixed in time and under certain conditions, which may compromise health.

RISK FACTORS
Unrealistic perception of event or personal abilities
Insufficient social support
Insufficient information-processing ability
Flight behavior when faced with proposed solution
Pattern of procrastination
Hedonism
Sample Clinical Applications: Depression, bipolar disorder, learning disabilities/dyslexia, chronic conditions (e.g., fibromyalgia, fatigue, multiple sclerosis)

DESIRED OUTCOMES/EVALUATION CRITERIA

Sample **NOC** linkages:
Motivation: Inner urge that motivates or prompts an individual to positive action(s)
Decision-Making: Ability to make judgments and choose between two or more alternatives
Social Support: Reliable assistance from others

Client Will (Include Specific Time Frame)
• Express awareness of negative factors or actions that can interfere with planning.
• Establish mindfulness and relaxation activities to lessen anxiety.
• Develop a plan, including the time frame, for a task to be completed.

ACTIONS/INTERVENTIONS

Sample **NIC** linkages:
Self-Responsibility Facilitation: Encourage a patient to assume more responsibility for own behavior
Self-Modification Assistance: Reinforce self-directed change initiated by the patient to achieve personally important goals
Mutual Goal Setting: Collaborate with patient to identify and prioritize care goals, then develop a plan for achieving those goals

 Acute Care   Collaborative   Community/Home Care   Cultural

NURSING PRIORITY NO. 1   To identify causative/precipitating factors related to risk:

- Determine circumstances of client's situation that may impact participating in selective activities. *Identifies areas for client to begin to change behavior.*
- Note client's ability to process information. *Compromised mental ability, low self-esteem, and anxiety can interfere with dealing with planning of activities of life.*[15]
- Review health history and medications. *Underlying physical or emotional factors, such as fatigue, stress, or medication side effects, can affect ability to engage in tasks.*[3,11,18]
- Evaluate mental status, using Beck's Depression Scale or other inventories as indicated. *Depression, anxiety, and/or mental illness can potentially interfere with client's ability to plan desired activities.*[16]
- Discuss religious/cultural and personal values and perception of self, including view of strengths and weaknesses. *These factors affect every aspect of client's life, including how he/she views ability to make choices or manage life.*[9,15]
- Ascertain need for control, fear of dependency on others, or belief they will not be able to do the task. *Although client may need assistance, he/she may have external locus of control and see others as having control and the ability to do things the client is not able to do.*[17]
- Investigate client's awareness of procrastination, need for perfection, or fear of failure. *These issues may be interfering with client's choosing to manage planning of life activities.*[8]
- Discuss issue of avoiding pain by seeking pleasure (hedonism). *People sometimes avoid pain by choosing activities that provide pleasure but don't get needed tasks accomplished.*[7,8,9]
- Note availability and use of resources and social support. *Lack of resources or insufficient support limit client's ability to engage in activities.*

NURSING PRIORITY NO. 2   To assist client to recognize and deal with risk factors that interfere with appropriate activities:

- Encourage recognition of feelings associated with issues that prevent client from planning desired activities. *Awareness of frustration and/or anxiety will help client redirect energy into productive activities.*[5,10]
- Help client to reframe negative thoughts about self into a positive view of what he/she is able to achieve. *The belief that individuals are worthless and not deserving of success and happiness is prevalent among many people who are anxious, leading to the belief that anything tried is doomed to failure.*[2,5,6,14]
- Encourage client to recognize procrastinating behaviors and make a decision to change. *Often this learned behavior comes from the family of origin. A decision to change may require therapy to change the ingrained habit.*[5,11,13]
- Develop a plan with the client to deal with activities in small steps. *Learning to do this will help client to feel more organized and successful in completing the desired task.*[4,5,12]
- Encourage client to engage in activity of choice with a friend, family member. *Support may encourage client to pursue activity and be successful at completion.*[1]
- Investigate with the client the possibility that seeking pleasure (hedonism) may interfere with achieving life goals. *Individual may believe that pleasure is the only good and avoid tasks or activities viewed as not fun or pleasurable, thereby interfering with accomplishments.*[7]

NURSING PRIORITY NO. 3   To promote wellness (Teaching/Discharge Criteria):

- Identify life goals and priorities. *If the individual has never thought about setting goals, he or she may begin to think about the possibility of being successful.*[12]
- Discuss use of relaxation techniques and mindfulness to deal with anxieties and stressors. *Enables client to deal with life's difficulties more effectively, helping client to view self as worthwhile and encouraging continued work toward goals.*[3,6]

 Diagnostic Studies   Evidence Based Practice   Medications   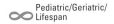 Pediatric/Geriatric/Lifespan

- Identify community resources, such as social services, senior center, or classes. *Provides an opportunity to be involved in different activities and be successful in trying new activities.*
- Refer for cognitive therapy as indicated. *May help client to deal with basic assumptions and dysfunctional beliefs in order to become successful.*[5,13]

DOCUMENTATION FOCUS

Assessment/Reassessment
- Individual risk factors identified.
- Client concerns or difficulty making and following through with plan.

Planning
- Plan of care and who is involved in planning.
- Teaching plan.

Implementation/Evaluation
- Response to interventions, teaching, and actions performed.
- Attainment or progress toward outcomes.
- Client's plan for the future.

Discharge Planning
- Referrals to other resources.
- Long-term need and who is responsible for actions.

References

1. Davis, J. L. (2005, reviewed 2009). *Coping With Anxiety.* Retrieved February 2018 from http://www.webmd.com/anxiety-panic/guide/coping-with-anxiety.
2. Blanicka, P. (2002). Reframing: The essence of mediation. Retrieved February 2018 from http://www.mediate.com/articles//blanciak.cfm.
3. Stress relievers: Tips to tame stress. (2016). Mayo Clinic Staff. Retrieved February 2018 from http://www.mayoclinic.com/health/stress-relievers/MY01373.
4. Marano, H. E. (2003, revised 2009, last reviewed 2016). Ending procrastination. *Psychol Today.* Retrieved February 2018 from http://www.psychologytoday.com/articles/200310/ending-procrastination.
5. Butler, A. C., Beck, A. T. (1995). Cognitive therapy for depression. *Clin Psychol,* 48(3), 3–5.
6. Hopper, J. (2009, revised 2015). Cultivating mindfulness. Retrieved February 2018 from https://www.jimhopper.com/mindfulness-and-meditation/cultivating-mindfulness/.
7. Moore, A. (2004, revised 2013). Hedonism. *The Stanford Encyclopedia of Philosophy.* Retrieved February 2018 from http://plato.stanford.edu/entries/hedonism/.
8. Gura, T. (2009). I'll do it tomorrow. *Scientific American Mind,* December/January, 32–39.
9. The Arizona Direct Care Curriculum Project. (2011). Activity planning. *Principles of Caregiving: Aging and Physical Disabilities, Chapter 7.* Retrieved February 2018 from http://www.azdirectcare.org/uploads/APDChap7-ActivityPlanningJan11.pdf.
10. Reblin, M., Uchino, B. N. (2008). Social and emotional support and its implication for health. *Curr Opin Psychiatry,* 21(2), 201–205.
11. Marano, H. E. (2003, revised 2010, last review 2016). Procrastination: Ten things to know. *Psychol Today.* Retrieved February 2018 from http://www.psychologytoday.com/articles/200308/procrastination-ten-things-know.
12. No author listed. (1996–2018). Personal goal setting—Planning to live your life your way. *MindTools.* Retrieved February 2018 from http://www.mindtools.com/page6.html.
13. Pucci, A. R. (2010). *The Client's Guide to Cognitive-Behavioral Therapy.* Weirton, WV: National Association of Cognitive-Behavioral Therapists.
14. Townsend, M. T. (2010). *Essentials of Psychiatric Mental Health Nursing: Concepts of Care in Evidence-Based Practice.* 5th ed. Philadelphia, PA: F. A. Davis, 143–146.
15. Das, J. P., Naglieri, J. A., Murphy, D. B. (n.d.). Individual differences in cognitive processes of planning: A personality variable? *The Psychological Record.* Digital book. Retrieved February 2018 from http://www.thefreelibrary.com/Individual+differences+in+cognitive+processes+of+planning%3A+a.-a017150075.
16. Beck Institute for Cognitive Behavior Therapy. (2016). Unbeatable assessment tools to help patients heal. Retrieved February 2018 from https://beckinstitute.org/get-informed/tools-and-resources/professionals/patient-assessment-tools/.
17. Mills, H., Reiss, N., Dombeck, M. Stress reduction and management. Retrieved May 2018 from https://www.gulfbend.org/poc/view_doc.php?type=doc&id;=1229&cn;=117.
18. Scott, E. (2012, updated 2017). Top 10 things to know about the effects of stress. *About.com.* Retrieved February 2018 from http://stress.about.com/od/understandingstress/tp/effects_stress.htm.

 Acute Care   Collaborative   Community/Home Care   Cultural

Acute Substance Withdrawal Syndrome

Taxonomy II: Coping/Stress Tolerance—Class 3 Neurobehavioral Stress (00258) [**Diagnostic Division:** Safety], Approved 2016

DEFINITION: Serious multifactorial sequalae following abrupt cessation of an addictive compound

RELATED FACTORS

Developed dependence to alcohol or other addictive substances
Heavy use of an addictive substance over time
Sudden cessation of an addictive substance
Malnutrition

DEFINING CHARACTERISTICS

Subjective

Nausea

Objective

Acute confusion
Anxiety
Disturbed sleep pattern
Risk for electrolyte imbalance
Risk for injury
At Risk Population: History of previous withdrawal symptoms
Older adults
Associated Condition: Comorbid mental disorder
Comorbid serious physical illness
Sample Clinical Applications: Alcohol intoxication, drug overdose

DESIRED OUTCOMES/EVALUATION CRITERIA

Sample NOC linkages:

Substance Withdrawal Severity: Severity of signs and symptoms of withdrawal from addictive drugs, tobacco, alcohol
Alcohol [or] Drug Abuse Cessation Behavior: Personal actions to eliminate alcohol [or] drug use that poses a threat to health
Substance Addiction Consequences: Severity in change in health status and social functioning due to substance addiction

Client Will (Include Specific Time Frame)

- Be free of adverse reactions to withdrawal, e.g., stable vital signs, alert and oriented, no cardiac dysrhythmias, electrolyte imbalance, hallucinations, or seizures.
- Commit to cessation of substance(s) used.
- Engage in behaviors/lifestyle changes to eliminate substance use.
- Use available personal, professional, and community resources.
- Manage own activities of daily living including work/school schedule.
- Engage in appropriate social interactions.

(continues on page 42)

 Diagnostic Studies   Evidence Based Practice   Medications   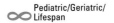 Pediatric/Geriatric/ Lifespan

Acute Substance Withdrawal Syndrome (continued)

ACTIONS/INTERVENTIONS

Sample NIC linkages:

Substance Use Treatment: Alcohol Withdrawal: Care of patient experiencing sudden cessation of alcohol consumption

Substance Use Treatment: Drug Withdrawal: Care of patient experiencing drug detoxification

Substance Use Treatment: Care of patient and family members demonstrating dysfunction as a result of substance abuse or dependence

---

NURSING PRIORITY NO. 1   To determine degree of impairment/compromise:

- Identify comorbidities—medical conditions/psychiatric disorders and currently prescribed medications. *Underlying cardiovascular disease is compounded by withdrawal; chronic lung diseases are common, affecting oxygenation, chronic infections may be present as well as traumatic injuries, suggesting additional testing, monitoring, and potential treatment needs.*
- Determine if naloxone (Narcan) administered, how many doses, and time of last dose. *Used to reverse opioid overdose but duration of action of some opioids may exceed that of Narcan, requiring repeat doses.*
- Review toxicology results of urine and blood. *To determine substances used, necessary interventions, and potential complications. Note: Symptoms and timing of occurrence depend on type of substance(s) used and last dose.*
- Assess level of consciousness, ability to speak, and response to commands. *Speech may be garbled, confused, or slurred. Response to commands may reveal inability to concentrate, impaired judgment, or muscle coordination deficits.*
- Determine stage of alcohol withdrawal syndrome (AWS) using Clinical Institute Withdrawal Assessment for Alcohol-Revised (CIWA-AR) tool. *AWS usually begins 3 to 36 hours after last drink. Helps determine appropriate care setting and specific interventions.*[1] *Note: In presence of substantial language barrier, absence of reliable history, an alternate tool such as Prediction of Alcohol Withdrawal Severity Scale (PAWSS) may be more appropriate.*[2]
- Observe for behavioral responses such as hyperactivity, disorientation, confusion, sleeplessness, irritability. *Hyperactivity related to CNS disturbances may escalate rapidly. Sleep deprivation may aggravate disorientation or confusion. Progression of symptoms may indicate impending hallucinations or delirium tremens (DTs) in alcohol withdrawal.*[4]
- Auscultate breath sounds noting adventitious sounds such as rhonchi, wheezes, crackles. *Client is at risk for atelectasis related to hypoventilation and pneumonia.*
- Review chest x-ray, arterial blood gas (ABG), or pulse oximetry. *Respiratory compromise common, e.g., right lower lobe pneumonia common in alcohol-debilitated clients and is often due to chronic aspiration.*
- Measure weight and compare to usual weight and norms for age and body size. Note skin turgor, status of mucous membranes, muscle tone/wasting, presence of edema. *Substance abuse is often associated with malnutrition.*
- Review serum nutritional studies, e.g., albumin, transferrin, prealbumin, iron, liver function, electrolytes, hemoglobin, hematocrit. *Substance users are often malnourished, impacting organ function, energy/endurance level, immune status, general well-being.*

NURSING PRIORITY NO. 2   To facilitate safe withdrawal from substance:

- Consult with medical toxicologist or regional poison control center as needed. *Useful resources for diagnosis and management of acute/critically ill clients, especially those with multi-substance use.*[3]

 Acute Care   Collaborative   Community/ Home Care   Cultural

- Provide environmental safety as indicated, e.g., bed in low position, call device within reach, doors full open or closed position, padded side rails, family member or sitter at bedside as appropriate. *Reduces risk of injury in presence of distorted sense of reality.*
- Monitor vital signs (VS) and level of consciousness (LOC) frequently during acute withdrawal. *VS and LOC can be labile based on specific substance(s) and length of time since last used. For example, hypertension frequently occurs in acute withdrawal phase but may quickly progress to hypotension.*
- Elevate head of bed. *Decreases potential for aspiration and lowers diaphragm, enhancing lung expansion.*
- Monitor respiratory rate, depth, and pattern. Note periods of apnea or Cheyne-Stokes respirations. *Toxicity levels may change rapidly, e.g., hyperventilation common during acute alcohol withdrawal phase, or marked respiratory depression can occur because of central nervous system depressant effects of substance used.*
- 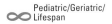 Administer supplemental oxygen, as needed. *Hypoxia may occur with respiratory depression and chronic anemia.*
- Monitor body temperature. *Elevation may occur because of sympathetic stimulation, dehydration, and/or infection, causing vasodilation and compromising venous return and cardiac output.*
- Record intake/output, 24-hour fluid balance; skin turgor, status of mucous membranes. *Preexisting dehydration, nausea/vomiting, diuresis, and diaphoresis may compromise cardiovascular function as well as renal perfusion, impacting drug clearance.*
- Administer fluid/electrolytes as indicated. *Depending on substances used, client is susceptible to excessive fluid losses and electrolyte imbalances, especially potassium and magnesium that can result in life-threatening dysrhythmias. Magnesium sulfate also beneficial in reducing tremors and seizure activity.*[3,5]
- Reorient frequently to person, place, time, and surrounding environment. *May have calming effect and limit misinterpretation of external stimuli.*
- Encourage client to verbalize anxiety. Explain substance withdrawal increases anxiety and uneasiness. *Anxiety may be physiologically or environmentally caused, and client may be unable to identify and/or accept what is happening. Note: Individuals with alcohol use disorders often also have posttraumatic stress disorder (PTSD).*[6]
- Monitor for suicidal tendencies. *May need to use emergency commitments or legal hold for client's safety once medically stable.*
- Provide symptom management as indicated. *Medications for nausea/vomiting, anxiety, trembling/"shakes," insomnia, seizure activity promote comfort and facilitate recovery.*[3]
- 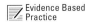 Administer medications treating specific substance(s) used. *For example, beta-adrenergic blockers may speed up the alcohol withdrawal process but are not useful in preventing seizures or DTs,*[3,4] *and methadone is used to assist opioid withdrawal.*[7] *Note: There are no Food and Drug Administration (FDA)–approved medications for treating cannabis, cocaine, or methamphetamine substance use disorders (SUDs), and medication-assisted treatments (MATs) are rarely used to treat adolescent alcohol use.*[9]
- Administer thiamine, vitamins C and B complex as indicated. *Vitamin deficiency, especially thiamine, is associated with ataxia, loss of eye movement and pupillary response, palpitations, postural hypotension, and exertional dyspnea.*[3]

NURSING PRIORITY NO. 3   To promote long-term sobriety:

- Develop trusting relationship, project an accepting attitude about substance use. *Provides client a sense of humanness, helping to decrease paranoia and distrust. (Client will be able to detect biased or condescending attitude of caregivers, negatively impacting relationship.)*
- Determine understanding of current situation. *Provides information about degree of denial, acceptance of personal responsibility, and commitment to change.*
- Arrange "intervention" or confrontation in controlled setting when client sufficiently recovered from withdrawal to address addiction issues. *Client more likely to contract for treatment while still hurting and experiencing fear and anxiety from last substance use episode.*
- Confront use of defensive behaviors—denial, projection, and rationalization. *Helps client accept the reality of the problems as they exist.*

Diagnostic Studies   Evidence Based Practice   Medications   Pediatric/Geriatric/Lifespan

- Identify individual triggers for substance use (e.g., exhaustion, loneliness/isolation, depression) and client's plans for living without drugs/alcohol. *Provides opportunity to discuss substance tension-reducing strategies and to develop and refine plan.*
- Use crisis intervention techniques to initiate behavior changes. *Calming effect enables client to be receptive to care and therapeutic interventions.*
- Instruct in use of relaxation skills, guided imagery, and visualization techniques. *Helps client relax and develop new ways to deal with stress and to problem-solve.*
- Facilitate visit by a group member/possible sponsor as appropriate, such as Alcoholics Anonymous (AA), Narcotics Anonymous (NA), Crystal Methamphetamine Anonymous (CMA), Smart Recovery. *Puts client in direct contact with support system necessary for managing sobriety and drug-free life.*
- Administer antipsychotic medications as necessary. *May be indicated for prolonged or profound psychosis following lysergic acid diethylamide (LSD) or phencyclidine (PCP) intoxication.*
- Engage entire family in multidimensional family therapy as indicated. *Program developed for adolescents with SUDs and their families to address the various influences on client's substance use by improving family functioning and collaboration with other systems, such as school and juvenile justice.*[8]

NURSING PRIORITY NO. 4   To promote optimal wellness (Teaching/Discharge Considerations):

- Review effects of substance(s) used—physical, psychological, social. *Information needed for client to make informed decisions and commit to therapeutic regimen.*
- Discuss potential for reemergence of withdrawal symptoms in stimulant abuse as early as 3 months or as late as 9 to 12 months after discontinuing use. *Early recognition of recurrence of withdrawal symptoms provides for timely intervention.*
- Review specific aftercare needs, e.g., PCP user should drink cranberry juice and continue use of ascorbic acid; alcohol abuser with liver damage should refrain from medications, anesthetics, or use household cleaning products that are detoxified in the liver. *Promotes individualized care related to specific situation.*
- Encourage balanced diet, adequate rest, exercise such as walking, biofeedback, deep meditative techniques. *These activities help restore natural biochemical balance, aid detoxification, and manage stress, anxiety.*
- Review long-term therapeutic regimen/medication-assisted treatment (MAT). *Medications such as methadone for opioid use, and Antabuse for alcohol use, may be prescribed to help maintain sobriety and reduce risk of relapse.*
- Identify community/social assistance resources, e.g., housing, food pantry, senior center/feeding station, transportation, medical care. *Provides for basic human needs, enhances coping abilities, reduces sense of isolation, and decreases risk of relapse.*
- Refer for vocational counseling/alternative schooling program as appropriate. *Provides opportunity to learn skills and obtain employment to promote independence and enhance self-esteem.*
- Encourage continued involvement in peer group therapy, individual/family counseling, drug recovery education programs. *Provides follow-up support to maintain sobriety.*
- Monitor results of periodic drug screening as appropriate. *Important to identify return to substance use or change to another drug.*

DOCUMENTATION FOCUS

Assessment/Reassessment
- Individual findings including general health status, comorbidities, signs/stage of withdrawal.
- Substance(s) used, dose, frequency, last dose.
- Results of laboratory tests/diagnostic studies.
- Effects of substance use life and relationships.

Planning
- Plan of care and who is involved in planning.
- Teaching plan.
- Plan for sobriety.

 Acute Care   Collaborative   Community/ Home Care   Cultural

Implementation/Evaluation
• Response to interventions, teaching, and actions performed.
• Attainment or progress toward desired outcomes.
• Modifications to plan.

Discharge Planning
• Long-term needs and who is responsible for actions to be taken.
• Specific referrals made.
• Plan for monitoring sobriety.

References

1. Eloma, A. S., et al. (2017). Evaluation of the appropriate use of a CIWA-Ar alcohol withdrawal protocol in the general hospital setting. *Am J Drug Alcohol Abuse*, 44(4), 418–425.
2. Moldonado, J. R., et al. (2015). Prospective validation study of the Prediction of Alcohol Withdrawal Severity Scale (PAWSS) in medically ill inpatients: A new scale for the prediction of complicated alcohol withdrawal syndrome. *Alcohol Alcohol*, 50(5), 509–518.
3. Hoffman, R. S., Weinhouse, G. L. (Updated 2017). Management of moderate and severe alcohol withdrawal syndrome. *UpTo-Date Inc*. Retrieved October 2017 from https://www.uptodate.com/contents/management-of-moderate-and-severe-alcohol-withdrawal-syndromes.
4. Burns, M. J., Lekawa, M. E., Price, J. B. (Updated 2018). Delirium tremens (DTs). *Medscape*. Retrieved June 2017 from https://emedicine.medscape.com/article/166032-overview.
5. Burton, J. (2010). Alcohol withdrawal syndrome. *Nurses Nurturing Nurses*, 19(5), 7–12.
6. U.S. Department of Veterans Affairs. (Updated 2018). PTSD and problems with alcohol use. *PTSD: National Center for PTSD*. Retrieved June 2017 from https://www.ptsd.va.gov/public/problems/ptsd-alcohol-use.asp.
7. Tetrault, J. M., Fiellin, D. A. (2012). Current and potential pharmacological treatment options for maintenance therapy in opioid-dependent individuals. *Drugs*, 72(2), 217–228.
8. Hedden, S. L., et al. (2015). Behavioral health trends in the United States: Results from 2014 national survey on drug use and health. *Substance Abuse and Mental Health Services Administration (SAMHSA)*. Retrieved January 2018 from https://www.samhsa.gov/data/sites/default/files/NSDUH-FRR1-2014/NSDUH-FRR1-2014.pdf.
9. NIDA. (2014). Principles of adolescent substance use disorder treatment: A research-based guide. *National Institute on Drug Abuse (NIDA)*. Retrieved May 2018 from https://d14rmgtrwzf5a.cloudfront.net/sites/default/files/podata_1_17_14.pdf.

Acute Substance Withdrawal Syndrome, risk for

Taxonomy II: Coping/Stress Tolerance—Class 3 Neurobehavioral Stress (00259) [**Diagnostic Division:** Safety], Approved 2016

DEFINITION: Susceptible to serious multifactorial sequalae following abrupt cessation of an addictive compound, which may compromise health

RISK FACTORS
Developed dependence to alcohol or other addictive substance
Heavy use of an addictive substance over time
Sudden cessation of an addictive substance
Malnutrition
At Risk Population: History of previous withdrawal symptoms; older adults
Associated Condition: Comorbid mental disorder or serious physical illness
Sample Clinical Applications:

DESIRED OUTCOMES/EVALUATION CRITERIA

Sample NOC linkages:
Substance Withdrawal Severity: Severity of signs and symptoms of withdrawal from addictive drugs, tobacco, alcohol

(continues on page 46)

 Diagnostic Studies   Evidence Based Practice   Medications   Pediatric/Geriatric/Lifespan

Acute Substance Withdrawal Syndrome, risk for (continued)

Alcohol [or] Drug Abuse Cessation Behavior: Personal actions to eliminate alcohol [or] drug use that poses a threat to health

Substance Addiction Consequences: Severity in change in health status and social functioning due to substance addiction

---

Client Will (Include Specific Time Frame)

- Be free of adverse reactions to withdrawal, e.g., stable vital signs, alert and oriented, no cardiac dysrhythmias, electrolyte imbalance, hallucinations, or seizures.
- Commit to cessation of substance(s) used.
- Engage in behaviors/lifestyle changes to eliminate substance use.
- Use available personal, professional, and community resources.
- Manage own activities of daily living including work/school schedule.
- Engage in appropriate social interactions.

ACTIONS/INTERVENTIONS

Sample NIC linkages:

Substance Use Treatment: Alcohol Withdrawal: Care of patient experiencing sudden cessation of alcohol consumption

Substance Use Treatment: Drug Withdrawal: Care of patient experiencing drug detoxification

Substance Use Treatment: Care of patient and family members demonstrating dysfunction as a result of substance abuse or dependence

---

NURSING PRIORITY NO. 1 To determine degree of impairment/compromise:

- Identify comorbidities—medical conditions/psychiatric disorders and currently prescribed medications. *Underlying cardiovascular disease is compounded by withdrawal; chronic lung diseases are common, affecting oxygenation; chronic infections may be present, as well as traumatic injuries, suggesting additional testing, monitoring, and potential treatment needs.*
- Determine if naloxone (Narcan) administered, how many doses, and time of last dose. *Used to reverse opioid overdose but duration of action of some opioids may exceed that of Narcan, requiring repeat doses.*
- Review toxicology results of urine and blood. *To determine substances used, necessary interventions, and potential complications. Note: Symptoms and timing of occurrence depend on type of substance(s) used and last dose.*
- Monitor for signs relative to other substances used. *Symptoms and timing of withdrawal depend on type of substance used and last dose, e.g., flu-like symptoms for heroin within 12 hours, opiates within 8–12 hours; anxiety and/or seizures for benzodiazepines within 1–4 days.*[7]
- Observe for behavioral responses such as hyperactivity, disorientation, confusion, sleeplessness, irritability. *Hyperactivity related to CNS disturbances may escalate rapidly. Sleep deprivation may aggravate disorientation or confusion. Progression of symptoms may indicate impending hallucinations or delirium tremens (DTs) in alcohol withdrawal.*[2]
- Auscultate breathe sounds noting adventitious sounds such as rhonchi, wheezes, crackles. *Client is at risk for atelectasis related to hypoventilation and pneumonia.*
- Measure weight and compare to usual weight and norms for age and body size. Note skin turgor, status of mucous membranes, muscle tone/wasting, presence of edema. *Substance abuse is often associated with malnutrition.*

 Acute Care   Collaborative   Community/Home Care   Cultural

NURSING PRIORITY NO. 2   To facilitate safe withdrawal from substance:

- Provide environmental safety as indicated, e.g., bed in low position, call device within reach, doors full open or closed position, situated close to nursing station as appropriate. *Reduces risk of injury in presence of distorted sense of reality.*
- Monitor vital signs (VS) and level of consciousness (LOC) frequently during acute withdrawal. *VS and LOC can be labile based on specific substance(s) and length of time since last used. For example, hypertension frequently occurs in acute withdrawal phase but may quickly progress to hypotension.*
- Monitor respiratory rate, depth, and pattern. *Toxicity levels may change rapidly, e.g., hyperventilation common during acute alcohol withdrawal phase or marked respiratory depression can occur because of central nervous system depressant effects of substance used.*
- Encouraging client to verbalize anxiety. *Anxiety may be physiologically or environmentally caused, and client may be unable to identify and/or accept what is happening. Note: Individuals with alcohol use disorders often also have posttraumatic stress disorder (PTSD).*[3]
- 🔍 Provide symptom management as indicated. *Medications for nausea/vomiting, anxiety, trembling/"shakes," insomnia, seizure activity promote comfort and facilitate recovery.*[1]
- 🔍∞ Administer medications treating specific substance(s) used. *For example, beta-adrenergic blockers may speed up the alcohol withdrawal process but are not useful in preventing seizures or DTs,*[1,2] *and methadone is used to assist opioid withdrawal.*[4] *Note: There are no FDA-approved medications for treating cannabis, cocaine, or methamphetamine SUDs, and medication-assisted treatments (MAT) are rarely used to treat adolescent alcohol use.*[6]
- 🔍 Administer thiamine, vitamins C and B complex as indicated. *Vitamin deficiency, especially thiamine, is associated with ataxia, loss of eye movement and pupillary response, palpitations, postural hypotension, and exertional dyspnea.*[1]

NURSING PRIORITY NO. 3   To promote long-term sobriety:

- Develop trusting relationship, project an accepting attitude about substance use. *Provides client a sense of humanness, helping to decrease paranoia and distrust.*
- Arrange "intervention" or confrontation in controlled setting when client sufficiently recovered from withdrawal to address addiction issues. *Client more likely to contract for treatment while still hurting and experiencing fear and anxiety from last substance use episode.*
- Confront use of defensive behaviors—denial, projection, and rationalization. *Helps client accept the reality of the problems as they exist.*
- Identify individual triggers for substance use (e.g., loneliness/isolation, depression) and client's plans for living without drugs/alcohol. *Provides opportunity to discuss substance tension-reducing strategies and to develop and refine plan.*
- Instruct in use of relaxation skills, guided imagery, and visualization techniques. *Helps client relax and develop new ways to deal with stress and to problem-solve.*
- Facilitate visit by a group member/possible sponsor as appropriate, such as Alcoholics Anonymous (AA), Narcotics Anonymous (NA), Crystal Methamphetamine Anonymous (CMA), Smart Recovery. *Puts client in direct contact with support system necessary for managing sobriety and drug-free life.*
- 🔍 Administer antipsychotic medications as necessary. *May be indicated for prolonged or profound psychosis following lysergic acid diethylamide (LSD) or phencyclidine (PCP) intoxication.*
- ∞ Engage entire family in multidimensional family therapy as indicated. *Program developed for adolescents with SUDs and their families to address the various influences on client's substance use by improving family functioning and collaboration with other systems, such as school and juvenile justice.*[5]

NURSING PRIORITY NO. 4   To promote optimal wellness (Teaching/Discharge Considerations):

- Review effects of substance(s) used—physical, psychological, social. *Information needed for client to make informed decisions and commit to therapeutic regimen.*

 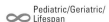

- Discuss potential for reemergence of withdrawal symptoms in stimulant abuse as early as 3 months or as late as 9 to 12 months after discontinuing use. *Early recognition of recurrence of withdrawal symptoms provides for timely intervention.*
- Review specific aftercare needs, e.g., alcohol abuser with liver damage should refrain from medications, anesthetics, or using household cleaning products that are detoxified in the liver. *Promotes individualized care related to specific situation.*
- Encourage balanced diet, adequate rest, exercise such as walking, biofeedback, deep meditative techniques. *These activities help restore natural biochemical balance, aid detoxification, and manage stress, anxiety.*
- Review long-term therapeutic regimen/medication-assisted treatment (MAT). *Medications such as methadone for opioid use, and Antabuse for alcohol use, may be prescribed to help maintain sobriety and reduce risk of relapse.*
- Identify community/social assistance resources, e.g., housing, food pantry, senior center/feeding station, transportation, medical care. *Provides for basic human needs, enhances coping abilities, reduces sense of isolation, and decreases risk of relapse.*
- Refer for vocational counseling/alternative schooling program as appropriate. *Provides opportunity to learn skills and obtain employment to promote independence and enhance self-esteem.*
- Encourage continued involvement in peer group therapy, individual/family counseling, drug recovery education programs. *Provides follow-up support to maintain sobriety.*
- Monitor results of periodic drug screening as appropriate. *Important to identify return to substance use or change to another drug.*

DOCUMENTATION FOCUS

Assessment/Reassessment
- Individual findings including general health status, comorbidities, signs/stage of withdrawal.
- Substance(s) used, dose, frequency, last dose.
- Results of laboratory tests/diagnostic studies.
- Effects of substance use life and relationships.

Planning
- Plan of care and who is involved in planning.
- Teaching plan.
- Plan for sobriety.

Implementation/Evaluation
- Response to interventions, teaching, and actions performed.
- Attainment or progress toward desired outcomes.
- Modifications to plan.

Discharge Planning
- Long-term needs and who is responsible for actions to be taken.
- Specific referrals made.
- Plan for monitoring sobriety.

References

1. Hoffman, R. S., Weinhouse, G. L. (Updated 2017). Management of moderate and severe alcohol withdrawal syndrome. *UpToDate Inc.* Retrieved October 2017 from https://www.uptodate.com/contents/management-of-moderate-and-severe-alcohol-withdrawal-syndromes.
2. Burns, M. J., Lekawa, M. E., Price, J. B. (Updated 2018). Delirium tremens (DTs). *Medscape.* Retrieved June 2017 from https://emedicine.medscape.com/article/166032-overview.
3. U.S. Department of Veterans Affairs. (Updated 2018). PTSD and problems with alcohol use. *PTSD: National Center for PTSD.* Retrieved June 2017 from https://www.ptsd.va.gov/public/problems/ptsd-alcohol-use.asp.
4. Tetrault, J. M., Fiellin, D. A. (2012). Current and potential pharmacological treatment options for maintenance therapy in opioid-dependent individuals. *Drugs, 72*(2), 217–228.

 Acute Care Collaborative Community/ Home Care Cultural

5. Hedden, S. L., et al. (2015). Behavioral health trends in the United States: Results from 2014 national survey on drug use and health. *Substance Abuse and Mental Health Services Administration (SAMHSA)*. Retrieved January 2018 from https://www.samhsa.gov/data/sites/default/files/NSDUH-FRR1-2014/NSDUH-FRR1-2014.pdf.

6. NIDA. (2014). Principles of adolescent substance use disorder treatment: A research-based guide. *National Institute on Drug Abuse (NIDA)*. Retrieved May 2018 from https://d14rmgtrwzf5a.cloudfront.net/sites/default/files/podata_1_17_14.pdf.

7. Drug withdrawal symptoms, timelines and treatment. (2018). *American Addiction Centers*. Retrieved May 2018 from https://americanaddictioncenters.org/withdrawal-timelines-treatments/.

decreased intracranial Adaptive Capacity

Taxonomy II: Coping/Stress Tolerance—Class 3 Neurobehavioral Stress (00049) [**Diagnostic Division:** Circulation], Submitted 1994

DEFINITION: Compromise in intracranial fluid dynamic mechanisms that normally compensate for increases in intracranial volumes, resulting in repeated disproportionate increases in intracranial pressure (ICP) in response to a variety of noxious and non-noxious stimuli.

RELATED FACTORS
To Be Developed

DEFINING CHARACTERISTICS

Objective
Baseline intracranial pressure (ICP) ≥10 mmHg
Disproportionate increase in intracranial pressure (ICP) following stimulus
Elevated tidal wave intracranial pressure (P_2 ICP) waveform
Repeated increase in intracranial pressure (ICP) of ≥10 mmHg for ≥5 min following external stimuli
Volume-pressure response test variation (volume: pressure ratio 2, pressure-volume index <10)
Wide-amplitude ICP waveform
Associated Condition: Brain injury; decrease in cerebral perfusion ≤50–60 mmHg; sustained increase in intracranial pressure (ICP) of 10–15 mmHg; systemic hypotension with intracranial hypertension
Sample Clinical Applications: Traumatic brain injury (TBI), cerebral edema, stroke, cranial tumors/hematomas, hydrocephalus

DESIRED OUTCOMES/EVALUATION CRITERIA

Sample NOC linkages:
Tissue Perfusion: Cerebral: Adequacy of blood flow through the cerebral vasculature to maintain brain function
Neurological Status: Ability of the peripheral and central nervous system to receive, process, and respond to internal and external stimuli

Client Will (Include Specific Time Frame)
• Demonstrate stable ICP as evidenced by normalization of pressure waveforms and response to stimuli.
• Display improved neurological signs.

ACTIONS/INTERVENTIONS

Sample NIC linkages:
Cerebral Edema Management: Limitation of secondary cerebral injury resulting from swelling of brain tissue
Cerebral Perfusion Promotion: Promotion of adequate perfusion and limitation of complications for a patient experiencing or at risk for inadequate cerebral perfusion
Intracranial Pressure (ICP) Monitoring: Measurement and interpretation of patient data to regulate intracranial pressure

 Diagnostic Studies   Evidence Based Practice   Medications   Pediatric/Geriatric/Lifespan

NURSING PRIORITY NO. 1 To assess causative/contributing factors:

- Determine factors related to individual situation (e.g., trauma such as fall, motor vehicle crash, gunshot wound, infection such as meningitis or encephalitis; brain tumor) and potential for increased ICP. *Deterioration in neurological signs/symptoms or failure to improve after initial insult may reflect decreased adaptive capacity.*

- Review results of diagnostic imaging (e.g., cerebral computed tomography [CT] scans) *to note location, type, and severity of intracranial injury. CT scan is sensitive to acute hemorrhage or skull fractures and aids in evaluating mass effect and midline shift, obliteration of the basal cisterns, or evidence of herniation.*[6]

- Monitor for change in ICP (e.g., worsening neurological signs or variations in ICP monitor waveform and pressure) and corresponding event (e.g., coughing, suctioning, position change, noise such as monitor alarms, family visit). *ICP monitoring may be done in a critically ill client with a Glasgow Coma Scale (GCS) score of 8 or less. The ICP offers data that supplement the neurological examination, and can be crucial in a client whose examination findings are affected by sedatives, paralytics, or other factors. Elevated pressure can be caused by the injury, environmental stimuli, or treatment modalities. Note: More advanced technologies are being used in some neurotrauma intensive care units to monitor electroencephalograph and bispectral index readings at the bedside to evaluate brain function while the client is in induced coma sedation with agents such as pentobarbital or propofol (Diprivan).*[2,3,6,14]

NURSING PRIORITY NO. 2 To note degree of impairment:

- Evaluate level of consciousness using GCS. *GCS remains the gold standard for objectively assessing individuals with TBIs. It assesses eye opening (e.g., awake, opens only to painful movement, keeps eyes closed), position or movement (e.g., spontaneous, purposeful, posturing), pupils (size, shape, equality, light reactivity), and consciousness or mental status (e.g., comatose, responds to pain, awake or confused). Low numbers (e.g., <8) are typically seen in clients with severe head injury and impaired cerebral perfusion requiring critical care interventions.*[2,3,6,9]

- Note purposeful and nonpurposeful motor response (e.g., posturing), comparing right and left sides. *Posturing and abnormal flexion of extremities usually indicate diffuse cortical damage. Absence of spontaneous movement on one side indicates damage to the motor tracts in the opposite cerebral hemisphere.*[1]

- Test for presence or absence of reflexes (e.g., blink, cough, gag, Babinski's reflex) and nuchal rigidity. *Helps identify location of injury (e.g., loss of blink reflex suggests damage to the pons and medulla, absence of cough and gag reflexes reflects damage to medulla, presence of Babinski's reflex indicates injury along pyramidal pathways in the brain).*[1]

- Monitor vital signs and cardiac rhythm before, during, and after activity. *Helps determine parameters for "safe" activity. Mean arterial blood pressure should be maintained above 90 mmHg to maintain cerebral perfusion pressure (CCP) greater than 70 mmHg, which reflects adequate blood supply to the brain. Fever in brain injury can be associated with injury to the hypothalamus or bleeding, systemic infection (e.g., pneumonia), or drugs. Hyperthermia exacerbates cerebral ischemia. Irregular respiration patterns can suggest location of cerebral insult. Cardiac dysrhythmias can be due to brainstem injury and stimulation of the sympathetic nervous system. Bradycardia may occur with high ICP.*[2,3,6]

- Monitor pulse oximetry or arterial blood gases, particularly pH, CO_2, and PaO_2. *A $PaCO_2$ level of 30 to 35 mmHg maintains cerebral blood flow and adequate cerebral oxygenation, while a PaO_2 of less than 65 mmHg may cause cerebral vascular dilation and further tissue damage.*[2,3,12]

- Monitor urine output and serum sodium. *Posttraumatic neuroendocrine dysfunction can result in a hyponatremic or hypernatremic state. When hyponatremia exists, cerebral edema or syndrome of inappropriate antidiuretic hormone can occur, requiring correction with fluid restriction and hypertonic IV solution. Hypernatremia can occur because of injury to the hypothalamus or pituitary stalk, causing diabetes insipidus, resulting in huge urine losses, or can be the result of excessive diuresis due to use of mannitol or furosemide administered to reduce cerebral edema.*[3]

 Acute Care   Collaborative   Community/ Home Care   Cultural

NURSING PRIORITY NO. 3   To minimize/correct causative factors/maximize perfusion:

- ✚ Perform periodic assessments of the client's level of consciousness and/or neurological status, blood pressure, breath sounds, temperature, amount of respiratory secretions, central venous pressure, heart rate and rhythm, fluid balance, nutritional status, and serial laboratory values, as with any critically ill client.
- Perform interventions specific to client with increased ICP:

  ▨ Elevate head of bed as individually appropriate. *Optimal head of bed position is determined by both ICP and coronary perfusion pressure measurements—that is, which degree of elevation lowers ICP while maintaining adequate cerebral blood flow. Studies show that in most cases, an elevation of 30 degrees significantly decreases ICP while maintaining cerebral blood flow.*[6,7]

  Maintain head and neck in neutral position, supporting with small towel rolls or pillows *to maximize venous return. Note: Lateral and rotational neck flexion has been shown to be the most consistent trigger of sustained increases in ICP.*[3,4]

  Avoid causing hip flexion of 90 degrees or more. *Hip flexion may trap venous blood in the intra-abdominal space, increasing abdominal and intrathoracic pressure and reducing venous outflow from the head, increasing cerebral pressure.*[5]

  Limit or prevent activities such as coughing, vomiting, and straining at stool and avoid or restrict use of restraints. *These factors often increase intrathoracic/abdominal pressures or agitation and markedly increase ICP.*[1]

  ⊘▨ Suction with caution and only when needed. Pass catheter just beyond end of endotracheal tube without touching tracheal wall or carina. Administer lidocaine intratracheally if indicated *to reduce cough reflex. Note: Studies have reported significant increase in ICP and decrease in CCP during suctioning in ventilated clients with brain injury, especially if they are not well sedated.*[3,15]

  ⊘▨ Hyperoxygenate before suctioning as appropriate *to minimize hypoxia. Note: Studies show that in most clients, hyperventilation is not necessary; however, therapeutic hyperventilation ($PaCO_2$ of 30 to 35 mm) may be used for a short period of time in acute neurological deterioration to reduce intracranial hypertension while other methods of ICP control are initiated.*[3,7,8,11]

- Investigate increased restlessness *to determine causative factors and initiate corrective measures as indicated:*

  Decrease extraneous stimuli and provide comfort measures (e.g., quiet environment, soft voice, tapes of familiar voices played through earphones, back massage, gentle touch as tolerated) *to reduce central nervous system stimulation and promote relaxation.*[4]

  Limit painful procedures (e.g., venipunctures, redundant neurological evaluations) to those that are absolutely necessary *in order to minimize preventable elevations in ICP.*[3]

  Provide rest periods between care activities and limit duration of procedures. Lower lighting and noise levels and schedule and limit activities *to provide a restful environment and limit spikes in ICP associated with noxious stimuli.*[3]

  Encourage family/significant others to talk to client. *Familiar voices appear to have a relaxing effect on many comatose individuals (thereby reducing ICP).*[1]

- ⊘ Administer and restrict fluid intake as necessary, and administer IV fluids via pump or control device *to maintain intravascular volume sufficient to maintain cerebral perfusion while preventing inadvertent vascular overload, cerebral edema, and increased ICP.*[6]
- Weigh as indicated. Calculate fluid balance every shift/daily *to determine fluid needs, maintain hydration, and prevent fluid overload.*[1]
- ⊘▨ Monitor and manage body temperature. Regulate environmental temperature and bed linens and use cooling blanket as indicated *to decrease metabolic and oxygen needs when fever is present or when therapeutic hypothermia therapy is used. Lowering the body temperature has been shown to lower ICP and improve outcomes for recovery.*[3,6,13]
- Provide appropriate safety measures/initiate treatment for seizures *to prevent injury and increase of ICP or hypoxia.*
- ⊘ Administer supplemental oxygen as indicated *to prevent cerebral ischemia.*

 Diagnostic Studies   Evidence Based Practice   Medications   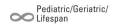 Pediatric/Geriatric/ Lifespan

- Administer medications (e.g., antihypertensives, diuretics, analgesics, sedatives, antipyretics, vasopressors, antiseizure drugs, neuromuscular blocking agents, corticosteroids) as appropriate *to maintain cerebral homeostasis and manage symptoms associated with neurological injury. Note: Controversy continues concerning the use of steroids in the setting of TBI as a neuroprotective strategy. Review of five key randomized control trials (RCTs) consistently showed that corticosteroids do not confer significant benefit in the TBI population.*[12]
- Administer enteral or parenteral nutrition *to achieve positive nitrogen balance, reducing effects of post–brain injury metabolic and catabolic states, which can lead to complications such as immunosuppression, infection, poor wound healing, loss of body mass, and multiple organ dysfunction. Studies have shown that parenteral nutritional support can be given to these clients without worsening cerebral edema.*[10]
- Prepare client for surgery as indicated (e.g., evacuation of hematoma or space-occupying lesion) *to reduce ICP and enhance circulation.*

NURSING PRIORITY NO. 4   To promote wellness (Teaching/Discharge Considerations):

- Discuss with caregivers specific situations (e.g., if client choking or experiencing pain, needing to be repositioned, constipated, blocked urinary flow) and review appropriate interventions *to prevent or limit episodic increases in ICP.*
- Identify signs/symptoms suggesting increased ICP (in client at risk without an ICP monitor), such as restlessness and deterioration in neurological responses. Review appropriate interventions.

DOCUMENTATION FOCUS

Assessment/Reassessment
- Neurological findings, noting right and left sides separately (e.g., pupils, motor response, reflexes, restlessness, nuchal rigidity); GCS.
- Response to activities and events (e.g., changes in pressure waveforms or vital signs).
- Presence and characteristics of seizure activity.

Planning
- Plan of care and who is involved in planning.
- Teaching plan.

Implementation/Evaluation
- Response to interventions and actions performed.
- Attainment or progress toward desired outcome(s).
- Modifications to plan of care.

Discharge Planning
- Future needs, plan for meeting them, and determining who is responsible for actions.
- Referrals as identified.

References

1. Doenges, M. E., Moorhouse, M. F., Murr, A. C. (2014). Craniocerebral trauma (acute rehabilitative phase). *Nursing Care Plans: Guidelines for Individualizing Client Care Across the Life Span.* 9th ed. Philadelphia, PA: F. A. Davis.
2. Brain Trauma Foundation Team (2007). Indications for intracranial monitoring: Guidelines for the management of severe traumatic brain injury. *J Neurotrauma,* 24(1 Suppl), S37–S44.
3. McNett, M. M., Gianakis, A. (2011). Nursing interventions for critically ill traumatic brain injury patients. *J Neurosci Nurs,* 42(2), 71–77.
4. Mitchell, P. H., Habermann, B. (1999). Rethinking physiological stability: Touch and intracranial pressure. *Biol Res Nurs,* 1(1), 12–19.
5. Vos, H. R. (1993). Making headway with intracranial hypertension. *Am J Nurs,* 93(2), 28–35.
6. Rangel-Castilla, L., et al. (2014). *Closed head trauma.* Retrieved February 2018 from http://emedicine.medscape.com/article/251834-overview.
7. Reddy, L. (2006). Heads up on cerebral bleeds. *Nursing,* 3(5), 4–9. Suppl, ED Insider.

 Acute Care   Collaborative   Community/Home Care   Cultural

8. Zink, E. K., McQuillan, K. (2005). Managing traumatic brain injury. *Nursing*, 35(9), 36–43.

9. Teasdale, G., Jennett, B. (1974). Assessment of coma and impaired consciousness: A practical scale. *Lancet*, 2(7872), 81–84.

10. Lump, D. (2014). Managing patients with severe traumatic brain injury. *Nursing*, 44(3), 30–37.

11. Rangel-Castillo, L., Gopinath, S., Robertson, C. S. (2008). Management of intracranial hypertension. *Neurol Clin*, 26(2), 521–541.

12. Horshide, R., et al. (2016). Do corticosteroids play a role in the management of traumatic brain injury? *Surg Neurol Int*, 7, 84.

13. Sahuquillo, J., Vilalta, A. (2007). Cooling the injured brain: How does moderate hypothermia influence the patho-physiology of traumatic brain injury? *Curr Pharm Des*, 13, 2310–2322.

14. Littlejohns, L., Bader, M. (2009). *Monitoring Technologies in Critically Ill Neuroscience Patients*. Boston: Jones and Bartlett.

15. Gholamzadeh, S., Javadi, M. (2009). Effect of endotracheal suctioning on intracranial pressure in severe head-injured patients. *Crit Care*, 13(1 Suppl), P80.

risk for Adverse Reaction to Iodinated Contrast Media

Taxonomy II: Safety/Protection—Class 5 Defensive Processes (00218) **[Diagnostic Division:** Safety], Approved 2010, revised 2013; 2017

DEFINITION: Susceptible to noxious or unintended reaction associated with the use of iodinated contrast media that can occur within seven days after contrast agent injection, which may compromise health.

RISK FACTORS

Dehydration

Generalized weakness

Anxiety

At Risk Population: Extremes of age

History of allergy; history of previous adverse effect from iodinated contrast media

Associated Condition: Chronic illness, unconsciousness

Contrast media precipitates adverse event; concurrent use of pharmaceutical agents

Fragile vein

Sample Clinical Applications: Any condition requiring the use of contrast media for diagnosis or treatment

DESIRED OUTCOMES/EVALUATION CRITERIA

Sample NOC linkages:

Allergic Response: Systemic: Severity of systemic hypersensitive immune response to a specific environmental (exogenous) antigen

Risk Control: Personal actions to understand, prevent, eliminate, or reduce modifiable health threats

Client Will (Include Specific Time Frame)

• Experience no adverse reaction from iodinated contrast media.

• Verbalize understanding of individual risks and responsibilities to avoid exposure.

• Recognize need for/seek assistance to limit allergic response/complications.

ACTIONS/INTERVENTIONS

Sample NIC linkages:

Allergy Management: Identification, treatment, and prevention of allergic responses to food, medications, insect bites, contrast material, blood, and other substances

NURSING PRIORITY NO. 1 To identify causative/precipitating factors related to risk:

- Identify the client at risk for adverse reaction prior to procedures. *A history of allergies; asthma; diabetes; renal insufficiency, including solitary kidney with elevated creatinine; thyroid dysfunction; hypertension; heart failure; current or recent use of nephrotoxic medications; or reaction to previous iodinated contrast media (ICM) administration places individual at increased risk.*[1,2]
- Ascertain type of reaction client experienced when there is a history of past reaction. *There are two types of reactions, both of which could change decisions about using ICM for diagnostic purposes. (1) Idiosyncratic reaction typically begins within 20 minutes of ICM injection. The symptoms are similar to anaphylactic reactions and can be mild (e.g., cough, itching, nasal congestion), moderate (e.g., dyspnea, wheezing), or severe (e.g., respiratory distress, arrhythmias such as bradycardia, seizures, shock, cardiopulmonary arrest). (2) Nonidiosyncratic reaction includes bradycardia, hypotension, and vasovagal reactions; neuropathy; extravasation; sensations of warmth; a metallic taste in the mouth; nausea and vomiting; and delayed reactions.*[1,3]

NURSING PRIORITY NO. 2 To assist client/caregiver to reduce or correct individual risk factors:

- Administer infusions using the "6 rights" system (right client, right medication, right route, right dose, right time, right documentation) *to prevent client from receiving improper contrast agent or dosage. Note: Clients undergoing more than one procedure at a time (such as cardiac angiography and angioplasty) receive a higher dose and are at greater risk for renal insufficiency reactions.*
- Perform imaging tests that do not require contrast media where possible *when client is at high risk for reaction.*
- Administer intravenous fluids as appropriate *to reduce incidence of contrast-induced nephropathy by supporting intravascular volume, diluting contrast media, and promoting its elimination.*[4,5]
- Administer medications (e.g., methylprednisilone [Deltasone], Benadryl) before, during, and after injection or procedures *to reduce risk or severity of reaction.*[3]
- Observe intravenous injection site frequently *to ascertain that no extravasation of contrast solution is occurring.*
- Halt infusion immediately to prevent tissue damage from contrast agent if client reports site discomfort or *redness or swelling is noted.*
- Monitor results of lab studies (e.g., creatinine clearance) *to ascertain status of kidney function.*

NURSING PRIORITY NO. 3 To promote wellness (Teaching/Discharge Criteria):

- Instruct client regarding signs and symptoms that should be reported to physician after procedures. *Weight gain, shortness of breath, decreased urination, or new or worsening edema could indicate renal insufficiency. Any delayed signs of reaction should be reported to physician immediately for possible intervention.*
- Instruct client/care provider about puncture sites and to report redness, soreness, or pain *to reduce risk of complications associated with extravasation.*
- Encourage client use of medical alert bracelet/necklace where indicated *to alert healthcare providers of prior reaction to contrast media.*

DOCUMENTATION FOCUS

Assessment/Reassessment
- Individual risk factors identified.
- Client concerns or difficulty making and following through with plan.

Planning
- Plan of care and who is involved in planning.
- Teaching plan.

 Acute Care   Collaborative   Community/ Home Care   Cultural

Implementation/Evaluation
- Response to interventions, teaching, and actions performed.
- Attainment or progress toward outcomes.

Discharge Planning
- Referrals to other resources.
- Long-term need and who is responsible for actions.

References

1. Siddiqi, N. H. (Updated 2017). Contrast medium reactions. Retrieved April 2018 from http://emedicine.medscape.com/article/422855-overview#a1.
2. Keller, D. M. (2011). Iodinated contrast media raises risk for thyroid dysfunction. *Ann Intern Med*, 172, 153–159.
3. Ilaslan, H. (Last reviewed 2015). Radiation and imaging. *Monograph from the online Merck Manual for Health Care Professionals*. Retrieved April 2018 from https://www.merckmanuals.com/home/special-subjects/common-imaging-tests/overview-of-imaging-tests.
4. Kohtz, C., Thompson, M. (2007). Preventing contrast medium-induced nephropathy. *Am J Nurs*, 107(9), 40–49.
5. Bashmore, T. M., et al. (2001). American College of Cardiology/Society for Cardiac Angiography and Interventions Clinical Expert Consensus Document on cardiac characterizations laboratory standards. A report of the American Cardiology Task Force on Clinical Expert Consensus Documents. *Am Coll Cardiol*, 37(8), 2170–2214.

---

ineffective Airway Clearance

Taxonomy II: Safety—Class 2 Physical Injury (00031) [**Diagnostic Division:** Respiration], Submitted 1980; Revised 1996, 1998, 2017

DEFINITION: Inability to clear secretions or obstructions from the respiratory tract to maintain a clear airway.

RELATED FACTORS
Excessive mucus, retained secretions
Foreign body in airway
Smoking, exposure to smoke; secondhand smoking

DEFINING CHARACTERISTICS

Subjective

Dyspnea

Objective

Diminished breath sounds; adventitious breath sounds [rales, crackles, rhonchi, wheezes]
Ineffective or absence of cough; excessive sputum
Alteration in respiratory rate or pattern
Difficulty verbalizing
Wide-eyed look; restlessness
Orthopnea
Cyanosis
Associated Condition: Airway spasm, allergic airway, asthma, chronic obstructive pulmonary disease, exudate in alveoli; hyperplasia of bronchial walls; infection; neuromuscular impairment; presence of artificial airway
Sample Clinical Applications: COPD, pneumonia, influenza, acute respiratory distress syndrome (ARDS), cancer of lung, cancer of head and neck, congestive heart failure (CHF), cystic fibrosis, neuromuscular diseases such as cerebral palsy; spinal cord injury, inhalation injuries

(continues on page 56)

 Diagnostic Studies   Evidence Based Practice   Medications   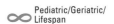 Pediatric/Geriatric/Lifespan

ineffective Airway Clearance (continued)

DESIRED OUTCOMES/EVALUATION CRITERIA

Sample NOC linkages:

Respiratory Status: Airway Patency: Open, clear tracheobronchial passages for air exchange
Risk Control: Aspiration: Personal actions to understand and prevent the passage of fluid and solid particles into the lung
Cognition: Ability to execute complex mental processes

Client Will (Include Specific Time Frame)

• Maintain airway patency.
• Expectorate or clear secretions readily.
• Demonstrate absence or reduction of congestion with breath sounds clear, respirations noiseless, and improved oxygen exchange (e.g., absence of cyanosis, arterial blood gas [ABG] results within client norms).
• Verbalize understanding of cause(s) and therapeutic management regimen.
• Demonstrate behaviors to improve or maintain clear airway.
• Identify potential complications and how to initiate appropriate preventive or corrective actions.

ACTIONS/INTERVENTIONS

Sample NIC linkages:

Airway Management: Facilitation of patency of air passages
Respiratory Monitoring: Collection and analysis of patient data to ensure airway patency and adequate gas exchange
Cough Enhancement: Promotion of deep inhalation by the patient with subsequent generation of high intrathoracic pressures and compression of underlying lung parenchyma for the forceful expulsion of air

NURSING PRIORITY NO. 1   To maintain adequate, patent airway:

• Identify client populations at risk. *Persons with impaired ciliary function (e.g., cystic fibrosis, lung transplant recipients); those with excessive or abnormal mucus production (e.g., asthma, emphysema, pneumonia, dehydration, bronchiectasis, mechanical ventilation); those with impaired cough function (e.g., neuromuscular diseases, such as muscular dystrophy, multiple sclerosis and other neuromotor conditions, such as cerebral palsy, spinal cord injury); those with swallowing abnormalities (e.g., poststroke, seizures, head/neck cancer, coma/sedation, tracheostomy, facial burns/trauma/surgery); those who are immobile (e.g., sedated individual, frail elderly, developmentally delayed, institutionalized client with multiple high-risk conditions); and infants/children (e.g., feeding intolerance, abdominal distention, emotional stressors that may compromise airway) are all at risk for problems with maintenance of open airways.*[1,2]
• Assess level of consciousness/cognition and ability to protect own airway. *This information is essential for identifying potential for airway problems, providing baseline level of care needed, and influencing choice of interventions.*
• Evaluate respiratory rate/depth and breath sounds. *Tachypnea is usually present to some degree and may be pronounced during respiratory stress. Respirations may be shallow. Some degree of bronchospasm is present with obstruction in airways and may/may not be manifested in adventitious breath sounds, such as scattered moist crackles (bronchitis), faint sounds with expiratory wheezes (emphysema), or absent breath sounds (severe asthma).*[2]

 Acute Care   Collaborative   Community/Home Care   Cultural

- Position head appropriate for age and condition/disorder. *Repositioning head may, at times, be all that is needed to open or maintain open airway in at-rest or compromised individual, such as one with sleep apnea.*
- ∞ Insert oral airway, using correct size for adult or child, when indicated. Have appropriate emergency equipment at bedside (such as tracheostomy equipment, ambu-bag, suction apparatus) *to restore or maintain an effective airway.*[3,4]
- Evaluate amount and type of secretions being produced. *Excessive and/or sticky mucus can completely obstruct or make it difficult to maintain effective airways, especially if client has impaired cough function, is very young or elderly, is developmentally delayed, has restrictive or obstructive lung disease, or is mechanically ventilated.*[2,5]
- Note ability to, and effectiveness of, cough. *Cough function may be absent, weak, or ineffective in diseases and conditions such as extremes in age (e.g., premature infant or elderly), cerebral palsy, muscular dystrophy, spinal cord injury, brain injury, postsurgery, and/or mechanical ventilation due to mechanisms affecting muscles of throat, chest, and lungs.*[5,6]
- ∞ ▱ Suction (nasal, tracheal, oral), when indicated, using correct-size catheter and suction timing for child or adult *to clear airway when secretions are blocking airways, client is unable to clear airway by coughing, cough is ineffective, infant is unable to take oral feedings because of secretions, or ventilated client is showing desaturation of oxygen by oximetry or ABGs.*[2,5,7]
- ▰ Assist with or prepare for appropriate testing (e.g., pulmonary function test or sleep studies) *to identify causative or precipitating factors.*
- ⊛ Assist with procedures (e.g., bronchoscopy, tracheostomy) *to clear or maintain open airway.*
- Keep environment free of smoke, dust, and feather pillows according to individual situation. *Remove precipitators of allergic types of respiratory reactions that can trigger/exacerbate acute episode.*[3]

NURSING PRIORITY NO. 2   To mobilize secretions:

- Elevate head of the bed or change position, as needed. *Elevation or upright position facilitates respiratory function by use of gravity; however, the client in severe distress will seek position of comfort.*[3]
- Position appropriately (e.g., head of bed elevated, client on side, rather than supine) and discourage use of oil-based products around nose *to prevent vomiting with aspiration into lungs.* (Refer to NDs risk for Aspiration, impaired Swallowing.)
- ▱ Exercise diligence in providing oral hygiene, removing substances, and keeping oral mucosa hydrated. *Airways can be obstructed by substances such as blood or thickened secretions. These can be managed by strict attention to good oral hygiene, especially in the client who is unable to provide that for self. Note: Instances of inspissated (thickened, dense, dehydrated) secretions as the cause of death have been reported.*[2]
- Encourage and instruct in deep-breathing and directed-coughing exercises; teach (presurgically) and reinforce (postsurgically) breathing and coughing while splinting incision *to maximize cough effort, lung expansion, and drainage and to reduce impairment associated with pain.*
- Mobilize client as soon as possible. *Reduces risk or effects of atelectasis, enhancing lung expansion and drainage of different lung segments.*[5]
- ▱ Administer analgesics, as indicated. *Analgesics may be needed to improve cough effort when pain is inhibiting. Note: Overmedication, especially with opioids, can depress respirations and cough effort.*
- ▱ Administer medications (e.g., expectorants, anti-inflammatory agents, bronchodilators, mucolytic agents), as indicated, *to relax smooth respiratory musculature, reduce airway edema, and mobilize secretions.*[8]
- Increase fluid intake to at least 2,000 mL/day within cardiac tolerance (may require IV in acutely ill, hospitalized client). Encourage or provide warm versus cold liquids, as appropriate. *Warm hydration can help liquefy viscous secretions and improve secretion clearance. Note: Individuals with compromised cardiac function may develop symptoms of CHF (crackles, edema, weight gain).*[4,5]
- Provide ultrasonic nebulizer or room humidifier, as needed, *to deliver supplemental humidification, helping to reduce viscosity of secretions.*

 Diagnostic Studies   Evidence Based Practice   Medications   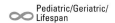 Pediatric/Geriatric/Lifespan

- 🚭📝 Assist with use of respiratory devices and treatments (e.g., intermittent positive-pressure breathing [IPPB], incentive spirometer [IS], positive expiratory pressure mask, mechanical ventilation, airway clearance vest/oscillatory airway device [flutter], assisted and directed cough techniques). *Various therapies/modalities may be required to maintain adequate airways and improve respiratory function and gas exchange depending on the cause for airway impairment. For example, an evidence-based review supports the notion that in individuals with neuromuscular conditions, cough may be made more effective by using manual assistance or positive-pressure insufflation devices. However, in clients with COPD, these same devices can be detrimental, causing decreased peak expiratory flow.* (Refer to NDs ineffective Breathing Pattern, impaired Gas Exchange, impaired spontaneous Ventilation.)[3,12]
- 🚭📝 Perform or assist client in learning airway clearance techniques, particularly when airway congestion is a chronic or long-term condition. *Numerous techniques may be used, including (but not limited to) postural drainage and percussion, flutter devices, high-frequency chest compression with an inflatable vest, intrapulmonary percussive ventilation (IVP), and active cycle of breathing technique, as indicated. Many of these techniques are the result of research in treatments of cystic fibrosis and muscular dystrophy as well as other chronic lung diseases. NOTE: Studies show that while these modalities yield short-term improvements in airway clearance, more studies are needed to measure long-term and clinically important endpoints like quality of life or rates of exacerbations.*[1,12,13]

NURSING PRIORITY NO. 3   To assess changes, note complications:

- Auscultate breath sounds, noting changes in air movement *to ascertain current status and effects of treatments to clear airways.*
- Monitor vital signs, noting blood pressure or pulse changes. Observe for increased respiratory rate, restlessness or anxiety, and use of accessory muscles for breathing, *suggesting advancing respiratory distress.*
- 🖋 Monitor and document serial chest radiographs, ABGs, pulse oximetry readings. *Identifies baseline status, influences interventions, and monitors progress of condition and/or treatment response.*
- Evaluate changes in sleep pattern, noting insomnia or daytime somnolence. *May be evidence of nighttime airway incompetence or sleep apnea.* (Refer to NDs Insomnia, Sleep Deprivation)
- 💊 Document response to drug therapy and/or development of adverse reactions or side effects with antimicrobial agents, steroids, expectorants, and bronchodilators. *Pharmacological therapy is used to prevent and control symptoms, reduce severity of exacerbations, and improve health status. The choice of medications depends on availability of the medication, the client's decision making about medication regimen, and response to any given medication.*[10]
- Observe for signs/symptoms of infection (e.g., increased dyspnea, onset of fever, increase in sputum volume, change in color or character) *to identify infectious process and promote timely intervention.*[10]
- 🖋 Obtain sputum specimen, preferably before antimicrobial therapy is initiated, *to point to effective antimicrobial agent. Note: The presence of purulent sputum during an exacerbation of symptoms is a sufficient indication for starting antibiotic therapy, but a sputum culture and antibiogram (antibiotic sensitivity) may be done if the illness is not responding to the initial antibiotic.*[10]

NURSING PRIORITY NO. 4   To promote wellness (Teaching/Discharge Considerations):

- 🏠 Assess client's/caregiver's knowledge of contributing causes, treatment plan, specific medications, and therapeutic procedures *to determine educational needs.*
- Provide information about the necessity of raising and expectorating secretions versus swallowing them *to note changes in color and amount in the event that medical intervention may be needed to prevent or treat infection.*
- Identify signs/symptoms to be reported to primary care provider. *Prompt evaluation and intervention are required to prevent/treat infection.*
- Demonstrate or assist client/significant other (SO) in performing specific airway clearance techniques (e.g., forced expiratory breathing [also called "huffing"] or respiratory muscle strength training, use of vest, chest percussion), if indicated.[1,9,11]

 Acute Care   Collaborative   Community/ Home Care   Cultural

- Review breathing exercises, effective coughing techniques, and use of adjunct devices (e.g., IPPB or IS) in pre-operative teaching *to facilitate postoperative recovery and reduce risk of pneumonia.*
- Instruct client/SO/caregiver in use of inhalers and other respiratory drugs. Include expected effects and information regarding possible side effects and interactions of respiratory drugs with other medications, over-the-counter medications, and herbals. Discuss symptoms requiring medical follow-up. *Client is often taking multiple medications that have similar side effects and potential for interactions. It is important to understand the difference between nuisance side effects (e.g., fast heartbeat after albuterol inhaler) and adverse effects (e.g., chest pain, hallucinations, or uncontrolled cardiac arrhythmia).*[8]
- Encourage and provide opportunities for rest; limit activities to level of respiratory tolerance. *Prevents or diminishes fatigue associated with underlying condition or efforts to clear airways.*
- Urge reduction or cessation of smoking. *Smoking is known to increase production of mucus and to paralyze (or cause loss of) cilia needed to move secretions to clear airway and improve lung function.*[10]
- Refer to appropriate support groups (e.g., smoking-cessation clinic, COPD exercise group, weight reduction, American Lung Association, Cystic Fibrosis Foundation, Muscular Dystrophy Association).
- Refer for/instruct in use of nocturnal continuous positive airway pressure (CPAP) therapy for treatment of sleep apnea. (Refer to NDs Insomnia, Sleep Deprivation.)

DOCUMENTATION FOCUS

Assessment/Reassessment
- Related factors for individual client.
- Breath sounds, presence and character of secretions, use of accessory muscles for breathing.
- Character of cough and sputum.

Planning
- Plan of care and who is involved in planning.
- Teaching plan.

Implementation/Evaluation
- Client's response to interventions, teaching, and actions performed.
- Attainment or progress toward desired outcome(s).
- Modifications to plan of care.

Discharge Planning
- Long-term needs and who is responsible for actions to be taken.
- Specific referrals made.

References

1. Clinical policy bulletin: Chest physiotherapy and airway clearance devices. (1995, updated 2010; last review 2017). *Aetna's Clinical Policy Bulletin.* Retrieved February 2018 from http://www.aetna.com/cpb/medical/data/1_99/0067.html.
2. Prahlow, J. A., Prahlow, T. J., Rakow, R. J. (2009). Case study: Asphyxia caused by inspissated oral and nasopharyngeal secretions. *Am J Nurs,* 109(6), 38–43.
3. McCool, F. D., Rosen, M. J. (2006). Nonpharmacologic airway clearance therapies: ACCP evidence-based clinical practice guidelines. *Chest,* 129(1 Suppl), 250S–259S.
4. Cox, H. C., et al. (2002). *Clinical Applications of Nursing Diagnosis: Adult, Child, Psychiatric, Gerontic, and Home Health Considerations.* 4th ed. Philadelphia, PA: F. A. Davis, 244–249.
5. Fink, J. B., Hunt, G. E. (eds). (1999). *Clinical Practice in Respiratory Care.* Baltimore, MD: Lippincott, Williams & Wilkins.
6. Blair, K. A. (1999). The aging pulmonary system. In Stanley, M., Beare, P. G. (eds). *Gerontological Nursing.* 2nd ed. Philadelphia, PA: F. A. Davis.
7. American Association for Respiratory Care. (2010). AARC Clinical Practice Guidelines. Endotracheal suctioning of mechanically ventilated patients with artificial airways 2010. *Respir Care,* 55(6), 758–768.
8. Vallerand, A. H., Sanoski, C. A. (2016). Bronchodilators. *Davis's Drug Guide for Nurses.* 15th ed. Philadelphia, PA: F. A. Davis.

9. Henderson, W. 7 airway clearance techniques. Retrieved February 2018 from https://lungdiseasenews.com/2017/11/20/7-airway-clearance-techniques/.

10. Global Initiative for Chronic Obstructive Lung Disease (GOLD). (2017). Global strategy for the diagnosis, management, and prevention of chronic obstructive pulmonary disease. Retrieved February 2018 from Retrieved http://www.ajmc.com/compendium/copd/global-initiative-for-chronic-obstructive-lung-disease-gold-guidelines-2017-update?p=1.

11. AHRQ Evidence Report Summaries. Treatment of disease following spinal cord injury: Summary. (2001). Retrieved February 2018 from https://archive.ahrq.gov/clinic/epcsums/spinalsum.htm.

12. Auger, A., Hernando, V., Galmache, H. (2017). Use of mechanical insufflation-exsufflation devices for airway clearance in subjects with neuromuscular disease. *Resp Care*, 62(2), 236–245.

13. Cystic Fibrosis Foundation. (No date). Global strategy for the diagnosis, management, and prevention of chronic obstructive pulmonary. https://www.cff.org/Life-With-CF/Treatments-and-Therapies/Airway-Clearance/Active-Cycle-of-Breathing-Technique/.

risk for Allergy Reaction

Taxonomy II: Safety/Protection—Class 5 Defensive Processes (00217) [Diagnostic Division: Safety], Submitted 1988; revised 2013, 2017

DEFINITION: Susceptible to an exaggerated immune response or reaction to substances, which may compromise health.

RISK FACTORS

Exposure to allergen
Exposure to environmental allergen
Exposure to toxic chemical

At Risk Population: History of food allergy; history of insect sting allergy; repeated exposure to allergen-producing environmental substance

Sample Clinical Applications: Asthma, conjunctivitis; eczema and other allergic skin rashes; food allergies and intolerances; hay fever; hives; insect stings

DESIRED OUTCOMES/EVALUATION CRITERIA

Sample **NOC** linkages:

Allergic Response: Localized: Severity of localized hypersensitive immune response to a specific environmental (exogenous) antigen

Allergic Response: Systemic: Severity of systemic hypersensitive immune response to a specific environmental (exogenous) antigen

Risk Control: Personal actions to understand, prevent, eliminate, or reduce modifiable health threats

Client Will (Include Specific Time Frame)

• Be free of signs of hypersensitive response.
• Verbalize understanding of individual risks and responsibilities in avoiding exposure.
• Identify signs/symptoms requiring prompt response.

ACTIONS/INTERVENTIONS

Sample **NIC** linkages:

Allergy Management: Identification, treatment, and prevention of allergic responses to food, medications, insect bites, contrast material, blood, and other substances

 Acute Care Collaborative Community/Home Care Cultural

NURSING PRIORITY NO. 1   To identify causative/precipitating factors related to risk:

- 🟦🏠 Question client regarding known allergies upon admission to healthcare facility. *Basic safety information to help healthcare providers prevent/prepare for safe environment for client while providing care.*
- Ascertain type of allergy and usual symptoms if client reports history of allergies (e.g., seasonal rhinitis ["hayfever"], allergic dermatitis, conjunctivitis, environmental asthma, environmental substances [e.g., mold, dust, pet dander], insect sting reactions, food intolerance, immunodeficiency such as Addison's disease, drug or transfusion reaction. *Allergies can manifest as local reactions (as may occur in skin rashes) or be systemic. Responses are many and variable. Client/caregiver may be aware of some allergies, but not all of them. It is also possible that client is having a first time allergic reaction to a substance and not know what substance caused the reaction.*[5]
- Obtain written list of drug allergies upon first contact with client. *Helps prevent adverse drug events (ADEs) while client is in facility care and aids in differentiating side effects from allergic responses. May also help improve client's understanding of reportable symptoms.*[1]
- Discuss possibility of latex allergy when entering facility care, especially when procedures are anticipated (e.g., laboratory, emergency department, operating room, wound care management, one-day surgery, dental) *so that proper precautions can be taken by healthcare providers. Note: The most severe reactions tend to occur with latex proteins contacting internal tissues during invasive procedures and when they touch mucous membranes of the mouth, vagina, urethra, or rectum.*[2] (Refer to NDs Latex Allergy Reaction and risk for Latex Reaction for related interventions.)
- ∞📋 Note client's age. *Although allergies can occur at any time in client's lifespan, there are some that can start early in life. These include food allergies (e.g., peanuts) and respiratory ailments (e.g., asthma). Note: In 2015, 8.4% of young children in the United States had asthma. Higher numbers were listed for adolescents and young adults (9.8% in persons aged 11 to 21). In 2015, it was reported that allergies affect as many as 30% percent of adults and 40% of children in the United States.*[3,5]
- ✎ Perform challenge or patch test, if appropriate, *to identify specific allergens in client with known type IV hypersensitivity. Note: Emergency department diagnosis and management depend on the history and physical examination.*
- ✎ Note response to allergen-specific IgE antibody tests where available. *Performed to measure the quantity of IgE antibodies in serum after exposure to specific antigens and has generally replaced skin tests and provocation tests, which are inconvenient, often painful, and/or hazardous to the client. Note: These tests are useful in nonemergent evaluations.*[4]

NURSING PRIORITY NO. 2   To take measures to avoid exposure and reduce/limit allergic response:

- Discuss client's current symptoms, noting reports of rash, hives, itching; teary eyes, localized swelling (e.g., of lips) or diarrhea, nausea, and feeling of faintness. Try to ascertain if client/care provider associates these symptoms with certain food, substances, or environmental factors (triggers). *May help isolate cause for a reaction. Baseline for determining where the client is along a continuum of symptoms, so that appropriate treatments can be initiated.*[5]
- Provide allergen-free environment (e.g., clean, dust-free room, use of air filters to reduce mold and pollens in air, etc.) *to reduce client exposure to allergens.*
- 💊 Collaborate with all healthcare providers to administer medications and perform procedures with client's allergies in mind. Perform challenge or patch test, if appropriate.
- Encourage client to wear medical ID bracelet/necklace *to alert providers to condition if client is unresponsive or unable to relay information for any reason.*
- 💊 Refer to physician/allergy specialists as indicated *for interventions related to specific allergy conditions.*

NURSING PRIORITY NO. 3   To promote wellness (Teaching/Discharge Criteria):

- 🏠 Instruct in/review with client and care provider(s) ways to prevent or limit client exposures. *May need or desire information regarding ways to reduce allergens at home, school, or work; may desire information regarding potential exposures when traveling, or how to manage food allergies when eating in restaurants.*[5]

 Diagnostic Studies   Evidence Based Practice   Medications   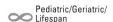 Pediatric/Geriatric/Lifespan

- Instruct in signs of reaction and emergency treatment needs. *Allergic reactions range from skin irritation to anaphylaxis. Reaction may be gradual but progressive, affecting multiple body systems, or may be sudden, requiring lifesaving treatment. Allergy can result in chronic illness, disability, career loss, hardship, and death.*
- Emphasize the critical importance of taking immediate action for moderate to severe hypersensitivity reactions *to limit life-threatening symptoms.*
- Demonstrate equipment and injection procedure, and recommend client carry auto-injectable epinephrine *to provide timely emergency treatment, as needed.*
- Emphasize necessity of informing all new care providers of allergies *to reduce preventable exposures.*
- Provide audiovisual resources and assistance numbers for emergencies. *When allergy is suspected or the potential for allergy exists, protection must begin with identification and removal of possible sources.*

DOCUMENTATION FOCUS

Assessment/Reassessment
- Individual risk factors identified.
- Client concerns or difficulty making and following through with plan.

Planning
- Plan of care and who is involved in planning.
- Teaching plan.

Implementation/Evaluation
- Response to interventions, teaching, and actions performed.
- Attainment or progress toward outcomes.

Discharge Planning
- Referrals to other resources.
- Long-term need and who is responsible for actions.

References

1. Vallente, S., Murray, L. P. (2011). Creative strategies to improve patient safety: Allergies and adverse drug reactions. *J Nurses Staff Dev*, 27(1), E1–E5.
2. Mecurio, J. (2011). Creating a latex-safe perioperative environment. *OR Nurse*, 5(6), 18–25.
3. Centers for Disease Control and Prevention (CDC). (2015). National current asthma prevalence. Retrieved February 2018 http://www.cdc.gov/asthma/asthmadata.htm.
4. No author listed. (Update 2018). Article for Lab Tests Online. Various pages. Retrieved February 2018 from https://labtestsonline.org/tests/allergy-blood-testing.
5. Asthma and Allergy Foundation of America. (2015). Allergy overview: Various pages. Retrieved February 2018 from http://www.aafa.org/page/allergies.aspx.

 Acute Care Collaborative Community/Home Care Cultural

Anxiety [Specify Level]

mild, moderate, severe, panic **Taxonomy II:** Coping/Stress Tolerance—Class 2 Coping Responses (00146) **[Diagnostic Division:** Ego Integrity], Submitted 1973; Revised 1982, 1998, 2017

DEFINITION: Vague uneasy feeling of discomfort or dread accompanied by an autonomic response (the source is often nonspecific or unknown to the individual); a feeling of apprehension caused by anticipation of danger. It is an alerting sign that warns of impending danger and enables the individual to take measures to deal with that threat.

RELATED FACTORS
Conflict about life goals; value conflict
Interpersonal transmission or contagion
Stressors
Substance misuse/[abuse]
Threat of death [perceived or actual]
Threat to current status
Unmet needs
At Risk Population: Exposure to toxin; family history of anxiety, heredity; major change; maturational or situational crisis

DEFINING CHARACTERISTICS

Subjective
Behavioral: Worried about change in life event; insomnia
Affective: Regretful; rattled; distress; apprehensiveness; nervousness, uncertainy; fear; feeling of inadequacy; worried; helplessness
Cognitive: Fear; forgetfulness; awareness of physiological symptoms
Sympathetic: Dry mouth; heart palpitations; weakness; anorexia; diarrhea
Parasympathetic: Tingling in extremities; nausea; abdominal pain; diarrhea; urinary frequency, hesitancy, urgency; faintness; fatigue; alteration in sleep pattern

Objective
Behavioral: Poor eye contact; glancing about; scanning behavior; hypervigilance; extraneous movement; fidgeting; restlessness; decrease in productivity
Affective: Increase in wariness; self-focus; irritability; jitteriness; overexcitement; anguish
Cognitive: Preoccupation; alteration in attention, concentration; diminished ability to learn or problem solve; rumination; tendency to blame others; blocking of thoughts; confusion; decrease in perceptual field
Physiological: Voice quivering; trembling; tremor; increase in tension; facial tension; increase in perspiration
Sympathetic: Cardiovascular excitation; facial flushing; superficial vasoconstriction; increase in heart or respiratory rate; increase in blood pressure; alteration in respiratory pattern; pupil dilation; twitching; brisk reflexes
Parasympathetic: Decrease in blood pressure or heart rate
Sample Clinical Applications: Major life changes or events, hospital admissions, surgery, cancer, hyperthyroidism, drug intoxication or abuse, mental health disorders

(continues on page 64)

 Diagnostic Studies Evidence Based Practice Medications Pediatric/Geriatric/ Lifespan

Anxiety [Specify Level] (continued)

DESIRED OUTCOMES/EVALUATION CRITERIA

Sample NOC linkages:

Anxiety Level: Severity of manifested apprehension, tension, or uneasiness arising from an unidentifiable source

Anxiety Self-Control: Personal actions to eliminate or reduce feelings of apprehension, tension, or uneasiness from an unidentifiable source

Coping: Personal actions to manage stressors that tax an individual's resources

Client Will (Include Specific Time Frame)

- Verbalize awareness of feelings of anxiety.
- Appear relaxed and report anxiety is reduced to a manageable level.
- Identify healthy ways to deal with and express anxiety.
- Demonstrate problem-solving skills.
- Use resources and support systems effectively.

ACTIONS/INTERVENTIONS

Sample NIC linkages:

Anxiety Reduction: Minimizing apprehension, dread, foreboding, or uneasiness related to an unidentified source or anticipated danger

Calming Technique: Reducing anxiety in patient experiencing acute distress

Dementia Management: Provision of a modified environment for the patient who is experiencing a chronic confusional state

NURSING PRIORITY NO. 1   To assess level of anxiety:

- Review familial and physiological factors, such as genetic depressive factors and psychiatric illness, active medical conditions (e.g., thyroid problems, metabolic imbalances, cardiopulmonary disease, anemia, dysrhythmias), and recent or ongoing stressors (e.g., family member illness or death, spousal conflict or abuse, loss of job). *These factors can cause or exacerbate anxiety and anxiety disorders.*[6,12,13]
- Determine current prescribed medication regimen and recent drug history of prescribed or over-the-counter (OTC) medications (e.g., steroids, thyroid preparations, weight-loss pills, caffeine). *Can heighten feelings or sense of anxiety.*[12,13]
- Identify client's perception of the threat represented by the situation. *Distorted perceptions of the situation may magnify feelings. Understanding client's point of view promotes a more accurate plan of care.*[1]
- Note cultural factors that may influence anxiety. *Individual responses are influenced by the cultural values and beliefs and culturally learned patterns of family of origin.*[3]
- Monitor physical responses (e.g., palpitations, rapid pulse, repetitive movements, pacing). *Changes in vital signs may suggest degree of anxiety client is experiencing or reflect the impact of physiological factors such as endocrine imbalances and medication effect.*[6]
- Observe behavior indicative of anxiety, *which can be a clue to the client's level of anxiety:*
- **Mild**
  Alert, more aware of environment, attention focused on environment and immediate events.
  Restless, irritable, wakeful, reports of insomnia.
  Motivated to deal with existing problems in this state.

 Acute Care   Collaborative   Community/Home Care   Cultural

- **Moderate**

  Perception narrower, concentration increased, able to ignore distractions in dealing with problem(s).

  Voice quivers or changes pitch.

  Trembling, increased pulse or respirations.
- **Severe**

  Range of perception is reduced, anxiety interferes with effective functioning.

  Preoccupied with feelings of discomfort or sense of impending doom.

  Increased pulse or respirations with reports of dizziness, tingling sensations, headache, etc.
- **Panic**

  Ability to concentrate is disrupted, behavior is disintegrated, client distorts the situation and does not have realistic perceptions of what is happening.

  May be experiencing terror or confusion or be unable to speak or move (paralyzed with fear).
- Note own feelings of anxiety or uneasiness. *Feelings of anxiety are circular, and those in contact with the client may find themselves feeling more anxious.*[2]
- Note use of drugs (including alcohol and other drugs), insomnia or excessive sleeping, and limited or avoidance of interactions with others, *which may be behavioral indicators of use of drugs to deal with problems or may indicate withdrawal from drugs or substances.*[4]
- Review results of diagnostic tests (e.g., drug screens, cardiac testing, complete blood count, chemistry panel), *which can point to physiological sources of anxiety.*
- Review coping skills used in past. *Can determine those that might be helpful in current circumstances.*[5]

NURSING PRIORITY NO. 2 To assist client to identify feelings and begin to deal with problems:

- Establish a therapeutic relationship, conveying empathy and unconditional positive regard. *Enables client to become comfortable and to begin looking at feelings and dealing with situation.*[2]
- Be available to client for listening and talking. *Establishes rapport, promotes expression of feelings, and helps client/significant other look at realities of the illness or treatment without confronting issues they are not ready to deal with.*[2]
- Encourage client to acknowledge and to express feelings—for example, crying (sadness), laughing (fear, denial), or swearing (fear, anger)—using active-listening, reflection techniques. *Often, acknowledging feelings enables client to accept and deal more appropriately with situation, thus relieving anxiety.*[7]
- Assist client to develop self-awareness of verbal and nonverbal behaviors. *Becoming aware helps client to control these behaviors and begin to deal with issues that are causing anxiety.*[8]
- Clarify meaning of feelings or actions by providing feedback and checking meaning with the client. *Validates meaning and ensures accuracy of communication.*[9]
- Acknowledge anxiety or fear. Do not deny or reassure client that everything will be all right. *Validates reality of feelings. False reassurances may be interpreted as lack of understanding or dishonesty, further isolating client.*[2]
- Be aware of defense mechanisms being used (e.g., denial, regression). *Use of defense mechanisms may be a helpful coping mechanism initially. However, continued use of such mechanisms diverts the energy that the client needs for healing, thus delaying the client from focusing and dealing with the actual problem.*[5]
- Identify coping skills the individual is using currently, such as anger, daydreaming, forgetfulness, eating, smoking, or lack of problem solving. *These may be useful for the moment but may eventually interfere with resolution of current situation.*[5]
- Provide accurate information about the situation. *Helps client to identify what is reality based and provides opportunity for client to feel reassured.*[13]
- Respond truthfully, avoid bribing, and provide physical contact (e.g., hugging, rocking) when client is a child. *Soothes fears and provides assurance. Children need to recognize that their feelings are not different from those of others.*[4]

NURSING PRIORITY NO. 3 To provide measures to comfort and aid client to handle problematic situations:

- Provide comfort measures (e.g., calm or quiet environment, soft music, warm bath, back rub, Therapeutic Touch). *Aids in meeting basic human need, decreasing sense of isolation, and assisting client to feel less anxious. Therapeutic Touch requires the nurse to have specific knowledge and experience to use the hands to correct energy field disturbances by redirecting human energies to help or heal.*[2,10]
- ∞ Modify procedures as necessary (e.g., substitute oral for intramuscular medications, combine blood draws or use fingerstick method). *Limits degree of stress and avoids overwhelming child or anxious adult.*[1]
- ∞ Manage environmental factors, such as harsh lighting, high traffic flow, excessive noise. *May be confusing or stressful to older individuals. Managing these factors can lessen anxiety, especially when client is in strange and unusual circumstances.*[1]
- Discuss the use of music and accommodate client's preferences. *Promotes calming atmosphere, helping to alleviate anxiety.*[2]
- Accept client as is. *The client may need to be where he or she is at this point in time, such as in denial after receiving the diagnosis of a terminal illness.*[2]
- Allow the behavior to belong to the client; do not respond personally. *Reacting personally can escalate the situation, promoting a nontherapeutic situation and increasing anxiety.*
- Assist client to use anxiety for coping with the situation if helpful. *Moderate anxiety heightens awareness and can help client to focus on dealing with problems.*[8]
- Encourage awareness of negative self-talk and discuss replacing with positive statements, such as using "can" instead of "can't," etc. *Negative self-talk promotes feelings of anxiety and self-doubt. Becoming aware and replacing these thoughts can enhance sense of self-worth and reduce anxiety.*[8]

PANIC STATE

- Stay with client, maintaining a calm, confident manner. *Presence communicates caring and helps client to regain control and sense of calm.*
- Speak in brief statements using simple words. *Client is not able to comprehend complex information at this time.*
- Provide for nonthreatening, consistent environment or atmosphere. Minimize stimuli and monitor visitors and interactions with others. *Lessens effect of transmission of anxious feelings.*
- Set limits on inappropriate behavior and help client to develop acceptable ways of dealing with anxiety.
- Provide safe controls and environment until client regains control. *Behavior may result in damage or injury that client will regret when control is regained, diminishing sense of self-worth.*
- Gradually increase activities and involvement with others as anxiety is decreased. *Promotes sense of normalcy, helps control feelings of anxiety.*
- Use cognitive therapy to focus on and correct faulty catastrophic interpretations of physical symptoms. *For example, thoughts of dying increase anxiety and feelings of panic. Controlling these thoughts allows client to look at situation more realistically and begin to deal appropriately with what is happening.*
- Administer anti-anxiety agents or sedatives, as ordered. *Appropriate medication can be helpful in enabling the client to regain control.*[13]

NURSING PRIORITY NO. 4 To promote wellness (Teaching/Discharge Considerations):

- Assist client to identify and deal with precipitating factors and learn new methods of coping with disabling anxiety. *Lessens possibility of repeat episodes.*[8]
- Review happenings, thoughts, and feelings preceding the anxiety attack. *Identifies factors that led to onset of attack, promoting opportunity to prevent recurrences.*[1]

 Acute Care   Collaborative   Community/ Home Care Cultural

- Identify actions and activities the client has previously used to cope successfully when feeling nervous or anxious. *Realizing that individual already has coping skills that can be applied in current and future situations can empower client.*[1]
- List helpful resources and people, including available hotline or crisis managers. *Provides ongoing and timely support.*[1]
- Encourage client to develop a regular exercise or activity program. *May be helpful in reducing level of anxiety by relieving tension and has been shown to raise endorphin levels to enhance sense of well-being.*[1]
- Assist in developing skills (e.g., awareness of negative thoughts, saying "Stop" and substituting a positive thought). *Eliminating negative self-talk can lead to feelings of positive self-esteem. (Note: Mild phobias seem to respond better to behavioral therapy.)*[9]
- Review such strategies as role-playing, use of visualizations to practice anticipated events, and prayer or meditation. *These activities can help the client practice behaviors in a safe and supportive environment, enabling individual to manage anxiety-provoking situations.*[9]
- Review medication regimen and possible interactions, especially with OTC drugs, alcohol, and herbal products. *Enhances understanding of reason for medication and can avoid untoward or harmful reactions from incompatible drugs.*[11,13]
- 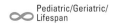 Discuss appropriate drug substitutions or changes in dosage or time of dose. *Ensures proper dosage and avoids untoward side effects. This is especially important in the elderly, who are particularly susceptible to multidrug complications.*[11]
- Refer to physician for drug management program or alteration of prescription regimen. *Drugs that often cause symptoms of anxiety include aminophylline, anticholinergics, dopamine, levodopa, salicylates, and steroids. Monitoring provides opportunity to correct possible undesirable effects of these drugs.*[11]
- Refer to individual and/or group therapy, as appropriate. *May be useful to help client deal with chronic anxiety states.*[1]

DOCUMENTATION FOCUS

Assessment/Reassessment
- Level of anxiety and precipitating or aggravating factors.
- Description of feelings (expressed and displayed).
- Awareness or ability to recognize and express feelings.
- Related substance use, if present.

Planning
- Treatment plan and individual responsibility for specific activities.
- Teaching plan.

Implementation/Evaluation
- Client involvement and response to interventions, teaching, and actions performed.
- Attainment or progress toward desired outcome(s).
- Modifications to plan of care.

Discharge Planning
- Referrals and follow-up plan.
- Specific referrals made.

References
1. Andrews, G., et al. (2002). *The Treatment of Anxiety Disorders: Clinician Guides and Patient Manuals.* 2nd ed. Cambridge, UK: Cambridge University Press.

2. Brantley, P. J., et al. (1999). Minor stressors and generalized anxiety disorder among low-income patients attending primary care clinics. *J Nerv Ment Dis*, 87, 435–440.

 Diagnostic Studies   Evidence Based Practice   Medications 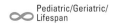 Pediatric/Geriatric/Lifespan

3. Lipson, J. G., Dibble, S. L. (2005). *Culture & Clinical Care*. 2nd ed. San Francisco, CA: UCSF Nursing Press.

4. The National Institute of Mental Health. (2005, revised 2016). *Anxiety Disorders*. Retrieved February 2018 from http://www.nimh.nih.gov/health/publications/anxiety-disorders/complete-index.shtml.

5. Wittchen, H. U., Hoyer, J. (2001). Generalized anxiety disorder: Nature and course. *J Clin Psychiatry*, 62(11 Suppl), S15–S19.

6. Kunert, P. K. (2002). Stress and adaptation. In Porth, C. M. (ed). *Pathophysiology: Concepts of Altered Health States*. Philadelphia, PA: Lippincott.

7. Moller, M. D., Murphy, M. F. (2002). *Recovering from Psychosis: A Wellness Approach*. Nine Mile Falls, WA: Psychiatric Rehabilitation Nurses Inc.

8. Bohrer, G. J. (2002). Anxiety, emotional and physical discomfort. *NurseWeek*, 3(1), 21–22. (Mountain West edition).

9. Burns, D. D. (1999, reprint 2008). *Feeling Good: The New Mood Therapy*. New York: Harper.

10. Swengros, D., et al. (2014). Promoting caring-healing relationships: Bringing Healing Touch to the bedside in a multihospital health system. *Holist Nurs Pract*, 28(6), 370–375.

11. Hayes, P. E., Dommisse, C. S. (1987). Current concepts in clinical therapeutics: Anxiety disorders, part 1. *Clin Pharm*, 6(21), 140–147.

12. Murphy, K. (2005). Anxiety: When is it too much? *Nursing Made Incredibly Easy!*, 3(5), 22–31.

13. Bhatt, N. V., Baker, M. J. (Updated 2017). *Anxiety Disorders*. Retrieved February 2018 from http://emedicine.medscape.com/article/286227-overview.

risk for Aspiration

Taxonomy II: Safety/Protection—Class 2 Physical Injury (00039) [**Diagnostic Division:** Respiration], Submitted 1988; Revised 2013, 2017

DEFINITION: Susceptible to entry of gastrointestinal secretions, oropharyngeal secretions, solids or fluids into the tracheobronchial passages, which may compromise health.

RISK FACTORS

Barrier to elevating upper body

Decrease in gastrointestinal motility

Ineffective cough

Insufficient knowledge of modifiable factors

Associated Condition: Decrease in level of consciousness; oral, facial, or neck surgery or trauma; treatment regimen

Depressed gag reflex; impaired ability to swallow; incompetent lower esophageal sphincter; increase in gastric residual or intragastric pressure; delayed gastric emptying

Presence of oral/nasal tube; enteral feedings

Sample Clinical Applications: Facial, jaw, neck surgery; vomiting, bulimia nervosa, presence of nasogastric tube, enteral feedings; brain injury, spinal cord injury

DESIRED OUTCOMES/EVALUATION CRITERIA

Sample **NOC** linkages:

Risk Control: Aspiration: Personal actions to understand and prevent the passage of fluid and solid particles into the lung

Neurological Status: Ability of the peripheral and central nervous system to receive, process, and respond to internal and external stimuli

Respiratory Status: Airway Patency: Open, clear tracheobronchial passages for air exchange

Client/Caregiver Will (Include Specific Time Frame)

• Experience no aspiration as evidenced by noiseless respirations; clear breath sounds; clear, odorless secretions.

• Identify causative or risk factors.

• Demonstrate techniques to prevent and/or correct aspiration.

 Acute Care Collaborative Community/ Home Care Cultural

ACTIONS/INTERVENTIONS

Sample NIC linkages:

Aspiration Precautions: Prevention or minimization of risk factors in the patient at risk for aspiration

Artificial Airway Management: Maintenance of endotracheal and tracheostomy tubes and prevention of complications associated with their use

Postanesthesia Care: Monitoring and management of the patient who has recently undergone general or regional anesthesia

NURSING PRIORITY NO. 1   To assess causative/contributing factors:

- Identify at-risk client according to condition/disease process as listed in Risk Factors *to determine when more active observation and/or interventions may be required.*
- ∞ ⧉ Assess for age-related risk factors potentiating risk of aspiration (e.g., premature infant, elderly infirm). *Aspiration pneumonia is more common in extremely young or old individuals, and it commonly occurs in those with chronically impaired airway defense mechanisms, including gag reflex, coughing, ciliary movement, and immune mechanisms that aid in removing material from the lower airways.*[4,13]
- ⧉ Note level of consciousness or awareness of surroundings and cognitive impairment. *Aspiration is common in comatose clients owing to inability to cough or swallow adequately and/or presence of artificial airway, mechanical ventilation, and tube feedings.*[1,13]
- ⧉ Evaluate neuromuscular dysfunction, if present, noting muscle groups involved, degree of impairment, and whether acute or of a progressive nature (e.g., stroke, cerebral palsy, Parkinson's disease, progressive supranuclear palsy, similar disabling brain diseases; Guillain-Barré syndrome, amyotrophic lateral sclerosis, psychiatric client following electric shock therapy). *May result in temporary or chronic, progressive impairment of protective muscle functions.*[7,11]
- Assess client's ability to swallow and cough; note quality of voice. *Although aspiration during swallowing is best detected by procedures such as video fluoroscopy, clinical observations are important. Sudden respiratory symptoms (such as severe coughing and cyanosis or wet phlegmy voice quality) are indicative of potential aspiration. Also, individuals with impaired or absent cough reflexes (such as may occur after a stroke, in Parkinson's disease, or during sedation) are at high risk for "silent" aspiration.*[4,9]
- Observe for neck and facial edema; e.g., client with head or neck surgery or a tracheal or bronchial injury (upper torso burns, inhalation or chemical injury). *Problems with swallowing and maintenance of airways can be expected in this client, and the potential is high for aspiration and aspiration pneumonia.*
- ⧉ Assess amount and consistency of respiratory secretions and rate and depth of respirations. *Helps differentiate the potential cause for risk of aspiration. The major pathophysiological dysfunction is the inability of the epiglottis and true vocal cords to move to close the trachea (e.g., changes in the structures themselves or because messages to the brain are absent, decreased, or impaired). Problems with coughing (clearing airways) and swallowing (pooling of saliva, liquids) increase risk of aspiration and respiratory complications.*[2–4]
- Auscultate lung sounds periodically (especially in client who is coughing frequently or not coughing at all; client with artificial airways, endotracheal and tracheostomy tubes; ventilator client being tube-fed, immediately following extubation), and observe chest radiographs *to determine decreased breath sounds, rales, or dullness to percussion that could indicate presence of aspirated food or secretions and "silent aspiration" leading to aspiration pneumonia. Note: Aspiration is the most common route of entry for both community- and hospital-acquired pneumonia.*[5]
- ⧉ Evaluate for/note presence of gastrointenstinal (GI) pathology and motility disorders. *Nausea with vomiting (associated with metabolic disorders, following surgery, or with certain medications) and gastroesophageal reflux disease can cause inhalation of gastric contents.*[3,6]

 Diagnostic Studies   Evidence Based Practice   Medications   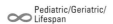 Pediatric/Geriatric/Lifespan

- Note administration of enteral feedings, which may be initiated when oral nutrition is not possible, such as in head injury, stroke, or other neurological disorders, head and neck surgery, esophageal obstruction, and discontinuous GI tract. *Potential exists for regurgitation and aspiration with the use of small or larger bore nasogastric feeding tubes, even with proper tube placement, necessitating the need for clients at high risk for aspiration associated with nasogastroenteral feedings to be evaluated for enteral feedings into the jejunum.*[7]
- Ascertain lifestyle habits (e.g., chronic use of alcohol and drugs, alcohol intoxication, tobacco, other central nervous system–suppressant drugs). *Can affect awareness as well as impair gag and swallow mechanisms.*[5]
- Assist with and review diagnostic studies (e.g., video-fluoroscopy, fiber-optic endoscopy) *that may be done to assess for presence and degree of impairment. Note: One recent retrospective study of 2,000 clients evaluated by video-fluoroscopy revealed that of those who aspirated, 55% had no protective cough reflex (silent aspiration).*[9,11]

NURSING PRIORITY NO. 2   To assist in correcting factors that can lead to aspiration:

- Place client in proper position for age and condition or disease affecting airways. *Adult and child should be upright for meals to decrease likelihood of drainage into trachea and to reduce reflux and improve gastric emptying.*[2,4] *Prone position may provide shorter gastric emptying time and decreased incidence of regurgitation and subsequent aspiration in premature infants.*[8]
- Encourage client to cough, as able, to clear secretions. *May simply need to be reminded or encouraged to cough (such as might occur in elderly person with delayed gag reflex or in postoperative, sedated client).*[2]
- Provide close monitoring for use of oxygen masks in clients at risk for vomiting. Refrain from using oxygen mask for comatose individuals.
- Keep wire cutters or scissors with client at all times when jaws are wired or banded *to facilitate clearing airway in emergencies.*
- Assist with oral care, postural drainage, and other respiratory therapies *to remove or mobilize thickened secretions that may interfere with swallowing and block airway.*[6]
- In client requiring suctioning to manage secretions:[6,9,10]
  Maintain operational suction equipment at bedside or chairside.
  Suction (oral cavity, nose, and endotracheal/tracheostomy tube) as needed, using correct size of catheter and timing for adult or child *to clear secretions in client with more frequent or congested-sounding cough; presence of coarse rhonchi and expiratory wheezing (audible with or without auscultation); visible secretions; increased peak pressures during volume-cycled ventilation; indication from client that suctioning is necessary; suspected aspiration of gastric or upper airway secretions; or otherwise unexplained increases in shortness of breath, respiratory rate, or heart rate.*
  Avoid triggering gag mechanism when performing suction or mouth care.
  Avoid keeping client supine or flat when on mechanical ventilation (especially when also receiving enteral feedings). *Supine positioning and enteral feeding have been shown to be independent risk factors for the development of aspiration pneumonia.*
- For a verified swallowing problem:[3–5,11]
  Provide a rest period prior to feeding time. *Rested person may have less difficulty with swallowing.*
  Elevate client to highest or best possible position for eating and drinking.
  Feed slowly and instruct client to take small bites and to chew thoroughly.
  Vary placement of food in client's mouth according to type of deficit (e.g., place food in right side of mouth if facial weakness present on left side). Use semisolid or soft foods that stick together and form a bolus (e.g., casseroles, puddings, stews), *which aids swallowing effort by improving client's ability to manipulate food with the tongue.*
  Avoid pureed foods and mucus-producing foods (milk).
  Determine food and liquid viscosity best tolerated by client. Add thickening agent to liquids, as appropriate. *Some individuals may swallow thickened liquids better than thin liquids.*

 Acute Care   Collaborative   Community/ Home Care   Cultural

Offer very warm or very cold liquids *to activate temperature receptors in the mouth that help to stimulate swallowing.*

Avoid washing solids down with liquids *to prevent bolus of food pushing down too rapidly, increasing risk of aspiration.*

- Provide oral medications in elixir form or crushed, if appropriate. Have client self-medicate when possible. Time medications to coincide with meals when possible.
- Refer to physician and/or speech language pathologist, as appropriate, *for medical and surgical interventions or for specific exercises to strengthen muscles and techniques to enhance swallowing.*
- When feeding tube is in place:[4,12,13]

Note radiograph and/or measurement of aspirate pH following placement of feeding tube *to verify correct position.*

Ask client about feeling of fullness and/or measure residuals just prior to feeding and several hours after feeding, when appropriate, *to prevent overfeeding.*

Elevate head of bed 30 degrees during and for at least 30 minutes after bolus feedings.

- Determine best position for infant/child (e.g., with the head of bed elevated 30 degrees and infant propped on right side after feeding). *Upper airway patency is facilitated by upright position, and turning to right side decreases likelihood of drainage into trachea.*
- Provide oral medications in elixir form or crushed, if appropriate.
- Minimize use of sedatives/hypnotics when possible. *Agents can impair coughing and swallowing.*

NURSING PRIORITY NO. 3 To promote wellness (Teaching/Discharge Considerations):

- Review individual risk or potentiating factors with client/care provider.
- Provide information about the effects of aspiration on the lungs. *Severe coughing and cyanosis (associated with eating or drinking) and voice change after swallowing indicate onset of respiratory symptoms associated with aspiration and require intervention for actual presence of aspiration.*[4,12]
- Instruct in safety concerns when feeding orally or tube feeding. (Refer to ND impaired Swallowing.)
- Train client to suction self or train family members in suction techniques (especially if client has constant or copious oral secretions) *to enhance safety/self-sufficiency.*
- Instruct individual/family member to avoid or limit activities after eating that increase intra-abdominal pressure (straining, strenuous exercise, tight or constrictive clothing). *May slow digestion or increase risk of regurgitation.*

DOCUMENTATION FOCUS

Assessment/Reassessment
- Assessment findings and conditions that could lead to problems of aspiration.
- Verification of tube placement, observations of physical findings.

Planning
- Interventions to prevent aspiration or reduce risk factors and who is involved in the planning.
- Teaching plan.

Implementation/Evaluation
- Client's responses to interventions, teaching, and actions performed.
- Foods and fluids client handles with ease or difficulty.
- Amount and frequency of intake.
- Attainment or progress toward desired outcome(s).
- Modifications to plan of care.

Discharge Planning
- Long-term needs and who is responsible for actions to be taken.

  Diagnostic Studies   Evidence Based Practice   Medications   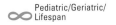 Pediatric/Geriatric/Lifespan

References

1. Swaminathan, A., Stearns, D. A., Varkey, S. B. (Updated 2017). Aspiration pneumonitis and pneumonia. Retrieved February 2018 from http://emedicine.medscape.com/article/296198-overview.

2. Newfield, S. A., et al. (2007). *Cox's Clinical Applications of Nursing Diagnosis: Adult, Child, Women's, Psychiatric, Gerontic, and Home Health Considerations.* 5th ed. Philadelphia, PA: F. A. Davis.

3. Richardson, B. (2014). Current Best Practice: Standards for Nutrition in Long Term Care. Retrieved February 2018 from http://eo2.commpartners.com/users/AHCA/downloads/140218_Slidesv2.pdf.

4. Metheny, N. A., Boltz, M., Greenberg, S. A. (2008). Preventing aspiration in older adults with dysphagia. *Am J Nurs*, 108(2), 45–46.

5. Galvan, T. J. (2001). Dysphagia: Going down and staying down. *Am J Nurs*, 101(1), 37.

6. Prahlow, J. A., Prahlow, T. J., Rakow, R. J. (2009). Case study: Asphyxia caused by inspissated oral and nasopharyngeal secretions. *Am J Nurs*, 109(38), 43.

7. Goodwin, R. S. (1996). Prevention of aspiration pneumonia: A research-based protocol. *Dimens Crit Care Nurs*, 15(2), 58–71.

8. Eichenwald, C. S. (2015). Apnea of Prematurity. Retrieved October 2018 from http://pediatrics.aappublications.org/content/pediatrics/early/2015/11/30/peds.2015-3757.full.pdf.

9. Garon, B. R., Sierzant, T., Ormiston, C. (2009). Silent aspiration: Results of 2,000 video fluoroscopic evaluations. *J Neurosci Nurs*, 41(4), 178–185.

10. American Association for Respiratory Care. (2010). AARC Clinical Practice Guidelines: Endotracheal suctioning of mechanically ventilated patients with artificial airways 2010. *Respir Care*, 55(6), 758–764.

11. Bowman, A., et al. (2005). Implementation of an evidence-based feeding protocol and aspiration risk reduction algorithm. *Crit Care Nurs Q*, 28(4), 324–333.

12. Smith Hammond, C. A., Goldstein, L. B. (2006). Cough and aspiration of food and liquids due to oral-pharyngeal dysphagia: ACCP evidence-based clinical practice guidelines, EBP compendium. *Chest*, 129(1 Suppl), 154S–168S.

13. McClave, S. A., et al. (2005). Poor validity of residual volumes as a marker for risk of aspiration in critically ill patients. *Crit Care Med*, 33(2), 324–330.

risk for impaired Attachment

Taxonomy II: Role Relationships—Class 2 Family Relationships (00058) **[Diagnostic Division:** Social Interaction], Submitted as Risk for Impaired Parent/Infant/Child Attachment 1994; Revised 2008, 2013, 2017

DEFINITION: Susceptible to disruption of the interactive process between parent/significant other and child that fosters the development of a protective and nurturing reciprocal relationship.

RISK FACTORS
Inability of parent to meet personal needs
Anxiety
Child's illness prevents effective initiation of parental contact
Disorganized infant behavior; parental conflict resulting from disorganized infant behavior
Parent-child separation; [physical barrier (e.g., infant in isolette); insufficient privacy]
Substance misuse/[abuse]
At Risk Population: Premature infant
[Difficult pregnancy and/or birth]
[Uncertainty of paternity; conception as a result of rape/sexual abuse]
[Parents who themselves experienced impaired attachment]
Sample Clinical Applications: Prematurity, genetic or congenital conditions, autism, attention deficit disorder, developmental delay (parent or child), substance abuse (parent), bipolar disorder (parent)

DESIRED OUTCOMES/EVALUATION CRITERIA

Sample NOC linkages:
Parent-Infant Attachment: Parent and infant behaviors that demonstrate an enduring affectionate bond
Parenting Performance: Parental actions to provide a child a nurturing and constructive physical, emotional, and social environment

 Acute Care   Collaborative   Community/Home Care   Cultural

Child Development: [specify age group]: Milestones of physical, cognitive, and psychosocial progression by [specify] months/years of age

---

Parent Will (Include Specific Time Frame)
- Identify and prioritize family strengths and needs.
- Exhibit nurturing and protective behaviors toward child.
- Identify and use resources to meet needs of family members.
- Demonstrate techniques to enhance behavioral organization of the infant/child.
- Engage in mutually satisfying interactions with child.

ACTIONS/INTERVENTIONS

Sample NIC linkages:

Attachment Promotion: Facilitating the development of an affective, enduring relationship between infant and parent

Family Integration Promotion: Facilitation or the growth of individuals or families who are adding an infant to the family unit

Parenting Promotion: Providing parenting information, support, and coordination of comprehensive services to high-risk families

NURSING PRIORITY NO. 1   To identify causative/contributing factors:

- Interview parents, noting their perception of situation and individual concerns. *Identifies problem areas and strengths to formulate appropriate plans to change situation that is currently creating problems for the parents.*[8]
- Assess parent/child interactions. *Identifies relationships, communication skills, and feelings about one another. The way in which a parent responds to a child and how the child responds to the parent largely determines how the child develops. Identifying the way in which the family responds to one another is crucial in determining the need for and type of interventions required.*[8]
- Ascertain availability and use of resources to include extended family, support groups, and finances. *Lack of support from or presence of extended family, lack of involvement in groups (e.g., church) or specific resources (e.g., La Leche League), and financial stresses can affect family negatively, interfering with ability to deal effectively with parenting responsibilities. Parents need support from both inside and outside the family.*[9,12]
- Determine emotional and behavioral problems of the child. *Attachment-disordered children are unable to give and receive love and affection, defy parental rules and authority, and are physically and emotionally abusive, creating ongoing stress and turmoil in the family and in future relationships.*[12]
- Evaluate parents' ability to provide protective environment and to participate in reciprocal relationship. *Parents may be immature, may be substance abusers, or may be mentally ill and unable or unwilling to assume the task of parenting. The ways in which the parent responds to the child are critical to the child's development, and interventions need to be directed at helping the parents to deal with their own issues and learn positive parenting skills.*[1,7]
- Note attachment behaviors between parent and child(ren), recognizing cultural background. *For example, lack of eye contact and touching may indicate bonding problems. Behaviors such as eye-to-eye contact, use of en face position, and talking to the infant in a high-pitched voice are indicative of attachment behaviors in American culture but may not be practiced in another culture. Failure to bond effectively is thought to affect subsequent parent-child interaction.*[4,5]

 Diagnostic Studies   Evidence Based Practice   Medications   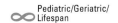 Pediatric/Geriatric/ Lifespan

• Assess parenting skill level, considering intellectual, emotional, and physical strengths and limitations. *Identifies areas of need for further education, skill training, and factors that might interfere with ability to assimilate new information.*[1,2]

NURSING PRIORITY NO. 2   To enhance behavioral organization of infant/child:

• Identify infant's strengths and vulnerabilities. *Each child is born with his or her own temperament that affects interactions with caregivers, and when these are known, actions can be taken to assist parents/caregivers to parent appropriately.*[2,7,11]
• Educate parents regarding child growth and development, where indicated, addressing parental perceptions. *Parents often have misconceptions about the abilities of their children, and providing correct information clarifies expectations and is more realistic.*[6]
• Assist parents in modifying the environment. *The environment can be changed to provide appropriate stimulation (e.g., to diminish stimulation before bedtime, to simplify when the environment is too complex to handle, to provide life space where the child can play unrestricted, resulting in freedom for the child to meet his or her needs).*[2,7] (Refer to ND readiness for enhanced organized Infant Behavior.)
• ▨ Model caregiving techniques that best support behavioral organization, such as attachment parenting. *Recognizing that the child deserves to have his or her needs taken seriously and responding to those needs in a loving fashion promotes trust, and children learn to model their behavior after what they have seen the parents do.*[9,11]
• Respond consistently with nurturance to infant/child. *Babies come wired with an ability to signal their needs by crying, and when parents respond to these signals, they develop a sensitivity that in turn develops parental intuition, providing infants with gratification of their needs and trust in their environment.*[10]

NURSING PRIORITY NO. 3   To enhance best functioning of parents:

• Develop a therapeutic nurse-client relationship. Provide a consistently warm, nurturant, and nonjudgmental environment. *Parents are often surprised to find that a tiny infant can cause so many changes in their lives and need help to adjust to this new experience. The warm, caring relationship of the nurse can help with this adjustment and provide the information and empathy they need at this time.*[1]
• Assist parents in identifying and prioritizing family strengths and needs. *Promotes positive attitude by looking at what they already do well and using those skills to address needs.*[2]
• Support and guide parents in process of assessing resources. *Outside support is important at this time, and making sure that parents receive the help they need will help them in this adjustment period.*[12]
• Involve parents in activities with the infant/child that they can accomplish successfully. *Parent participation (mentoring and modeling) in activities such as those recommended in Baby Gymboree Play and Music® creative play, and baby yoga can enable the parents to get to know their child and themselves, enhancing their confidence and self-concept.*[12]
• Recognize and provide positive feedback for nurturant and protective parenting behaviors. *Using "I" messages to let parents know their behaviors are effective reinforces continuation of desired behaviors and promotes feelings of confidence in their abilities.*[2,12]

NURSING PRIORITY NO. 4   To support parent/child attachment during separation:

• Provide parents with telephone contact as appropriate. *Knowing there is someone they can call if they have problems provides a sense of security.*[3]
• ✚ Establish a routine time for daily phone calls or initiate calls as indicated when child is hospitalized. *Provides sense of consistency and control; allows for planning of other activities so parents can maintain contact and get information on a regular basis.*[1]
• 🌐 Minimize number of professionals on team with whom parents must have contact. *Parents begin to know the individuals they are dealing with on a regular basis, fostering trust in these relationships and providing opportunities for modeling and learning.*[3]

 Acute Care   Collaborative   Community/ Home Care   Cultural

- Invite parents to use resources, such as the Ronald McDonald House, or provide a listing of a variety of local accommodations and restaurants. *When child is hospitalized out of town, parents need to have a place to stay so they can have ready access to the hospital and be able to rest and refresh from time to time.*[3]
- Arrange for parents to receive photos and progress reports from the child. *Provides information and comfort as the child progresses, allowing the parents to continue to have hope for a positive resolution.*[3]
- Suggest parents use cell phone with FaceTime, if available, or provide a photo and/or audiotape of themselves when separated for the child. *Provides a connection during the separation, sustaining attachment between parent and child.*[1]
- Consider use of a contract with parents. *Clearly communicating expectations of both family and staff serves as a reminder of what each person has committed to and serves as a tool to evaluate whether expectations are being maintained.*[3]
- Suggest parents keep a journal of infant/child progress. *Serves as a reminder of the progress that is being made, especially when they become discouraged and believe infant/child is "never" going to be better.*[3]
- 🏠 Provide "homelike" environment for situations requiring supervision of visits. *An environment that is comfortable supports the family as they work toward resolving conflicts and promotes a sense of hopefulness, enabling them to experience success when family is involved with a legal situation.*[12]

NURSING PRIORITY NO. 5   To promote wellness (Teaching/Discharge Considerations):

- 🏠 ⚕ Refer to addiction counseling or treatment, individual counseling, or family therapies as indicated. *May need additional assistance when situation is complicated by drug abuse (including alcohol), mental illness, disruptions in caregiving, or parents who are burned out with caring for child with attachment or other difficulties.*[12,13]
- Identify services for transportation, financial resources, housing, etc. *Assistance with these needs can help families focus on therapeutic regimen and on issues of parenting to improve family dynamics.*[9]
- ⚕ Develop support systems appropriate to situation (e.g., extended family, friends, social worker). *Depending on individual situation, support from extended family, friends, social worker, or therapist can assist family to deal with attachment disorders.*[10]
- Explore community resources (e.g., church affiliations, volunteer groups, day/respite care). *Church affiliations, volunteer groups, day or respite care can help parents who are overwhelmed with care of a child with attachment or other disorder.*[12]

DOCUMENTATION FOCUS

Assessment/Reassessment
- Identified behaviors of both parents and child.
- Specific risk factors, individual perceptions and concerns.
- Interactions between parent and child.

Planning
- Plan of care and who is involved in planning.
- Teaching plan.

Implementation/Evaluation
- Parents'/child's responses to interventions, teaching, and actions performed.
- Attainment or progress toward desired outcomes.
- Modifications to plan of care.

Discharge Planning
- Long-term needs and who is responsible.
- Plan for home visits to support parents and to ensure infant/child safety and well-being.
- Specific referrals made.

 Diagnostic Studies   Evidence Based Practice   Medications   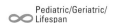 Pediatric/Geriatric/ Lifespan

References

1. Linwood, A. S. (2004). Parent-child relationships. *Encyclopedia of Children's Health*. Retrieved February 2018 from http://www.healthofchildren.com/P/Parent-Child-Relationships.html.
2. Gordon, T. How children really react to control. Retrieved February 2018 from http://www.naturalchild.org/guest/thomas_gordon.html.
3. Melnyk, B. M. (2000). Intervention studies involving parents of hospitalized young children: An analysis of the past and future recommendations. *J Ped Nurs*, 15(1), 4–13.
4. Lipson, J. G., Dibble, S. L., Minarik, P. A. (1996). *Culture & Nursing Care. A Pocket Guide*. San Francisco, CA: UCSF Nursing Press.
5. Martin, J. (1993). The gentle truth about infant bonding. *Parenting*. (December).
6. Dowshen, S. (Updated 2017). Your child's growth. Retrieved February 2018 from http://kidshealth.org/parent/growth/growing/childs_growth.html#.
7. New, M. (Updated 2016). Developing your child's self-esteem. Retrieved February 2018 from http://kidshealth.org/parent/emotions/feelings/self_esteem.html#.
8. Gordon, T. (2010). What every parent should know. Retrieved February 2018 from http://www.gordontraining.com/wp-content/uploads/What%20Every%20Parent%20Should%20Know.pdf.
9. Henningsen, M. (1996). *Attachment Disorder: Theory, Parenting and Therapy*. Evergreen, CO: Evergreen Family Counseling Center.
10. Sears, W. (1999). *Attachment Parenting: A Style That Works. Nighttime Parenting: How to Get Your Baby and Child to Sleep*. (La Leche International Book, revised edition). New York: Plume.
11. Benaroch, R. (Reviewer). (Updated 2016). What is attachment parenting? *WebMD Health and Parenting*. Retrieved February 2018 from http://www.webmd.com/parenting/what-is-attachment-parenting.
12. Adventures in parenting. (2001). *U.S. Department of Health and Human Services*. Retrieved February 2018 from https://www1.nichd.nih.gov/publications/pubs/documents/adventures_in_parenting_rev.pdf.
13. Treatment approaches for drug addiction. (2009, revised 2018). *National Institute on Drug Abuse (NIDA)*. Retrieved February 2018 from http://www.drugabuse.gov/publications/drugfacts/treatment-approaches-drug-addiction.

Autonomic Dysreflexia

Taxonomy II: Coping/Stress Tolerance—Class 3 Neurobehavioral Stress (00009) [**Diagnostic Division:** Circulation], Submitted 1988, 2017

DEFINITION: Life-threatening, uninhibited sympathetic response of the nervous system to a noxious stimulus after a spinal cord injury (SCI) at the 7th vertebra (T7) or above.

RELATED FACTORS
Gastrointestinal Stimuli:
Constipation, difficult passage of feces, fecal impaction
Digital stimulation, suppositories, enemas
Integumentary Stimuli:
Cutaneous stimulation, skin irritation
Musculoskeletal-Neurological Stimuli:
Irritating or painful stimuli below level of injury
Pressure over bony prominence or genitalia
Range of motion exercises
Spasm
Regulatory-Situational Stimuli:
Constricting clothing
Environmental temperature fluctuations
Positioning
Reproductive-Urological Stimuli:
Bladder spasm or distention
Sexual intercourse [/excitation]
Instrumentation [e.g., catheter insertion, obstruction; irrigation]
Other:
Insufficient [client] or caregiver knowledge of disease process
At Risk Population: Ejaculation; menstruation; extremes of temperature

 Acute Care Collaborative Community/Home Care Cultural

DEFINING CHARACTERISTICS

Subjective

Diffuse pain in different areas of the head

Paresthesia, chilling, blurred vision, chest pain, metallic taste in mouth, nasal congestion

Objective

Paroxysmal hypertension [sudden periodic elevated blood pressure with systolic pressure >140 mmHg and diastolic >90 mmHg]

Bradycardia or tachycardia

Diaphoresis above the injury, red blotches on skin above injury, pallor below injury

Horner's syndrome [contraction of the pupil, partial ptosis of the eyelid, enophthalmos, and sometimes loss of sweating over the affected side of the face]; conjunctival congestion

Pilomotor reflex

Associated Condition:

Bowel distention; esophageal reflux disease; gastric ulcer; gastrointestinal system pathology; gallstones; hemorrhoids

Deep vein thrombosis; pulmonary emboli

Fractures; heterotopic bone

Ovarian cyst; pregnancy; labor and delivery period

Pharmaceutical agent; substance withdrawal

Renal calculi, urinary catheterization; cystitis, urinary tract infection, detrusor sphincter dyssynergia; epididymitis

Surgical procedure; wound; sunburn

Sample Clinical Applications: Spinal cord injury

DESIRED OUTCOMES/EVALUATION CRITERIA

Sample NOC linkages:

Neurological Status: Autonomic: Ability of the autonomic nervous system to coordinate visceral and homeostatic function

Knowledge: Disease Process: Extent of understanding conveyed about a specific disease process and potential complications

Client/Caregiver Will (Include Specific Time Frame)

- Identify specific precipitating factors.
- Recognize signs and symptoms of syndrome.
- Demonstrate corrective techniques.

Client Will

Experience no episodes of dysreflexia or seek medical intervention in a timely manner.

ACTIONS/INTERVENTIONS

Sample NIC linkages:

Dysreflexia Management: Prevention and elimination of stimuli that cause hyperactive reflexes and inappropriate autonomic responses in a patient with a cervical or high thoracic cord lesion

Urinary Elimination Management [or] Bowel Management: Maintenance of an optimum urinary elimination pattern/establishment and maintenance of a regular pattern of bowel elimination

Anxiety Reduction: Minimizing apprehension, dread, foreboding, or uneasiness related to an unidentified source or anticipated danger

 Diagnostic Studies   Evidence Based Practice   Medications 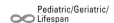 Pediatric/Geriatric/ Lifespan

NURSING PRIORITY NO. 1 To assess for precipitating factors:

- Note phase and specifics of injury. *Autonomic dysreflexia (AD) occurs in about 29% of persons with complete tetraplegia (quadraplegia). AD does not occur in the acute phase of SPI. However, some studies have identified factors that may point toward a client's likelihood of developing AD, and perhaps early in recovery. These include higher level of injury (cervical versus thoracic involvement) and more complete lesions.[1–3,6–9]*
- Assess for bladder distention, presence of bladder spasms or stones, or acute urinary tract infection. *The most common stimulus for AD is bladder irritation or overstretch associated with urinary retention or infection, blocked catheter, overfilled collection bag, or noncompliance with intermittent catheterization.*
- Evaluate for bowel distention, fecal impaction, or problems with bowel management program. *Bowel irritation or overstretch is associated with constipation or impaction; digital stimulation, suppository, or enema use during bowel program; hemorrhoids or fissures; and/or infection of gastrointestinal tract, such as might occur with ulcers or appendicitis.*
- Observe skin and tissue pressure areas, especially following prolonged sitting. *Skin and tissue irritants include direct pressure (e.g., object in chair or shoe, leg straps, abdominal support, orthotics), wounds (e.g., bruise, abrasion, lacerations, pressure ulcer), ingrown toenail, tight clothing, or sunburn or other burn.*
- Inquire about sexual activity and/or determine if reproductive issues are involved. *Overstimulation or vibration, sexual intercourse and ejaculation, scrotal compression, menstrual cramps, and/or pregnancy (especially labor and delivery) are known precipitants.*
- Inform client/care providers of additional precipitators during course of care. *Client is prone to physical conditions or treatments (e.g., intolerance to temperature extremes; deep vein thrombosis; kidney stones; fractures or other trauma; surgical, dental, diagnostic procedures), any of which can precipitate AD.*
- Note environmental temperature for extremes/drafts, *which can precipitate episode.*

NURSING PRIORITY NO. 2 To provide for early detection and immediate intervention:

- Investigate associated complaints/syndrome of symptoms (e.g., severe pounding headache, [blood pressure may be >200/100 mmHg], chest pain, irregular heart rate or dysrhythmias, blurred vision, nausea, facial flushing, metallic taste, severe anxiety; minimal symptoms or expressed complaints in presence of significantly elevated blood pressure—silent AD]). *Body's reaction to misinterpreted sensations from below the injury site, resulting in an autonomic reflex, can cause blood vessels to constrict and increase blood pressure. This is a potentially life-threatening condition, requiring immediate and correct action.[1–3,5]*
- Note onset of crying, irritability, or somnolence in infant or child *who may present with nonspecific symptoms and may not be able to verbalize discomfort.[1,6]*
- Locate and attempt to eliminate causative stimulus, moving in a stepwise fashion: *Cause can be anything that would normally cause pain or discomfort below level of injury.[1–5]*

  Assess for bladder distention: *Note: The two most common inciting stimuli are bladder and bowel distention, respectively, commonly a blocked urinary catheter.[3]*

  Empty bladder by voiding or catheterization, applying local anesthetic ointment (if indicated/per facility procedure *to prevent exacerbation of AD by procedure*).

  Ascertain that urine is free-flowing if Foley or suprapubic catheter is in place, empty drainage bag, straighten tubing if kinked, and lower drainage bag if it is higher than bladder.

  Irrigate gently or change catheter, if it is not draining freely.
- Note color, character, and odor of urine; obtain specimen for culture as indicated *(acute urinary infection can cause AD).[3]*
- Check for distended bowel *(if urinary problem is not causing AD).* Note: Fecal impaction is the second most common cause of AD.[3]

  Perform digital stimulation, checking for constipation or impacted stool. (If symptoms first appear while performing digital stimulation, stop procedure.)

 Acute Care   Collaborative   Community/ Home Care   Cultural

Apply local anesthetic ointment to rectum; remove impaction after symptoms subside *to remove causative problem without causing additional symptoms.*

- Check for skin pressure or irritation *(if bowel problem is not causing AD)*:
Perform a pressure release if sitting.
Check for tight clothing, straps, and belts.
Note whether pressure sore has developed or changed.
Observe for bruising and signs of infection.
Check for ingrown toenail, other injury to skin or tissue (e.g., burns, sunburn), or fractured bones.
- Check for other possible causes *(if skin pressure is not causing AD)*:
Menstrual cramps, sexual activity, or labor and delivery.
Abdominal conditions (e.g., colitis, ulcer).
Environmental temperature extremes.
- Take steps to reduce blood pressure, thereby *reducing potential for stroke (primary concern)*:[1–6]
Elevate head of bed immediately or place in sitting position with legs hanging down. *Lowers blood pressure by pooling of blood in legs and decreases intracranial pressure caused by vasodilation in the brain, thus reducing headache.*[3]
Loosen any clothing or restrictive devices. *Lowers blood pressure by pooling of blood in abdomen and lower extremities.*
Monitor vital signs frequently during acute episode. *Blood pressure may fluctuate quickly due to impaired autonomic regulation.* Continue to monitor blood pressure at intervals during procedures to remove cause of AD and after acute episodic symptoms subside *to evaluate effectiveness of interventions and antihypertensives.*
- Administer medications, as indicated. *If an episode is particularly severe, or persists after removal of suspected cause, antihypertensive medications with rapid onset and short duration (e.g., nifedipine, nitrates, mecamylamine diazoxide, phenoxybenzamine) may be used to block excessive autonomic nerve transmission, normalize heart rate, and reduce hypertension.*[1,4]
- 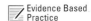 Know contraindications and cautions associated with antihypertensive medications; adjust dosage of antihypertensive medications carefully for child, elderly person, individual with known heart disease, male client using sildenafil for sexual activity, and pregnant woman. *Prevents complications, including unknown reactions in a child or systemic hypotension or seizure activity.*[4] *Note: Use of nitrate-containing medications is an absolute contraindication to sildenafil use because of the possibility of a fatal response.*[1,3]

NURSING PRIORITY NO. 3   To promote wellness (Teaching/Discharge Considerations):

- 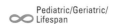 Discuss with client/caregivers warning signs of AD, as listed previously. Be aware of client's communication abilities. *AD can occur at any age from infant to very old, and the individual may not be able to verbalize a pounding headache, which is often the first symptom during onset of AD. Note: abnormal blood pressure readings may be more difficult to identify in child, unless baseline readings are known. AD management is typically initiated when the systolic BP is elevated 15 mmHg over baseline in a child and 15 to 20 mmHg over baseline for an adolescent.*[1,7]
- Ascertain that client/caregivers understand ways to avoid onset or treat syndrome as noted previously. Provide information card and instruct and periodically reinforce teaching, as needed, regarding:[1,2,5,6]
Maintaining indwelling catheter by keeping tubing free of kinks, keeping bag empty and situated below bladder level, and checking daily for deposits (bladder grit) inside catheter.
Performing intermittent catheterization as often as necessary *to prevent overfilling or distention.*
Monitoring for adequate spontaneous voiding, noting frequency and amount.
Maintaining a regular and effective bowel evacuation program.
Performing routine skin assessments.
Monitoring all systems for signs of infection and reporting promptly *for timely medical treatment.*
Scheduling routine medical evaluations.

- ∞ ✎ Instruct family member/caregiver in client's "normal" blood pressure range and proper blood pressure monitoring and plan for monitoring hypertension during acute episodes. *A spinal cord–injured client's (both adult and child) baseline blood pressure is lower than that of a noninjured person. Blood pressure 20 to 40 mmHg higher than reference range may be a sign of AD in an adult.*[6]
- 💊 Review proper use and administration of medications, when used. *Client may have medication(s) both for emergent situations and/or prevention of AD, and if so, he or she should receive medication instructions, as well as symptoms to report for immediate or emergent care, when blood pressure is not responsive.*[1,6]
- 🐾 Refer for or advise treatment of sexual and reproductive concerns, as indicated. *Client requires information and monitoring regarding sexual issues that can precipitate AD, including vibration to achieve orgasm, use of erectile dysfunction medication, and labor and delivery.*[3,7]
- Recommend wearing medical alert bracelet or necklace and carrying information card about signs/symptoms of AD and usual methods of treatment. *Provides vital information in emergency.*
- 🐾 Assist client/family in identifying emergency referrals (e.g., physician, rehabilitation nurse/home-care supervisor). Place telephone number(s) in prominent place or program numbers into client's/caregiver's cell phone.

DOCUMENTATION FOCUS

Assessment/Reassessment
- Individual findings, noting previous episodes, precipitating factors, and individual signs/symptoms.

Planning
- Plan of care and who is involved in planning.
- Teaching plan.

Implementation/Evaluation
- Client's responses to interventions and actions performed, understanding of teaching.
- Attainment or progress toward desired outcome(s).
- Modifications to plan of care.

Discharge Planning
- Long-term needs and who is responsible for actions to be taken.

References

1. Consortium for Spinal Cord Medicine, Paralyzed Veterans of America. (2001). *Acute Management of Autonomic Dysreflexia: Individuals with Spinal Cord Injury Presenting to Health-Care Facilities: Clinical Practice Guidelines. 2nd ed.* Retrieved February 2018 from http://www.pva.org/media/pdf/cpg_autonomic%20dysreflexia.pdf.
2. Acuff, M. (2005). Autonomic dysreflexia: What it is, what it does, and what to do if you experience it. *The Missouri Model Spinal Cord Injury System.* Columbia, MO: University of Missouri-Columbia, School of Health Professions.
3. Saulino, M. F. (Updated 2017). Rehabilitation of persons with spinal cord injuries. Retrieved February 2018 from https://emedicine.medscape.com/article/1265209-overview#a4.
4. Vallerand, A. H., Sanoski, C. A. (2016). *Davis's Drug Guide for Nurses.* 15th ed. Philadelphia, PA: F. A. Davis.
5. Stephenson, R. O., Berliner, J. (Updated 2018). Autonomic dysreflexia in spinal cord injury. Retrieved February 2018 from http://emedicine.medscape.com/article/322809-overview.
6. Osorio, M., Reyes, M. R., Masagli, T. L. (2014). Pediatric spinal cord injury. *Curr Phys Med Rehabil Rep*, 2(3), 158–168.
7. Ducharme, S. (2000). Sexuality and spinal cord injury. *Paraplegia News.* Retrieved February 2018 from www.stanleyducharme.com/resources/sex_spinalcord_injury.htm.
8. Krassioukov, A. V., Furlan, J. C., Fehlings, M. G. (2003). Autonomic dysreflexia in acute spinal cord injury: An under-recognized clinical entity. *J Neurotrauma*, 20(8), 707–716.
9. Widerstrom-Noga, E., Cruz-Almeida, Y., Krassioukov, A. (2004). Is there a relationship between chronic pain and autonomic dysreflexia in persons with cervical spinal cord injury? *J Neurotrauma*, 21(2), 195–204.

 Acute Care   Collaborative   Community/Home Care   Cultural

risk for Autonomic Dysreflexia

Taxonomy II: Coping/Stress Tolerance—Class 3 Neurobehavioral Stress (00010) [**Diagnostic Division:** Circulation], Submitted 1988; Revised 2000, 2013, 2017

DEFINITION: Susceptible to life-threatening, uninhibited response of the sympathetic nervous system post-spinal shock, in an individual with a spinal cord injury or lesion at T6 or above (has been demonstrated in clients with injuries at T7 and T8), which may compromise health.

RISK FACTORS
Gastrointestinal Stimuli
Constipation, difficult passage of feces, fecal impaction
Digital stimulation, suppositories, enemas
Integumentary Stimuli
Cutaneous stimulation, skin irritation
Musculoskeletal-Neurological Stimuli
Irritating or painful stimuli below level of injury
Pressure over bony prominence or genitalia
Range of motion exercises
Spasm
Regulatory-Situational Stimuli
Constricting clothing
Environmental temperature fluctuations
Positioning
Reproductive-Urological Stimuli
Bladder spasm or distention
Sexual intercourse [excitation]
Instrumentation [e.g., catheter insertion, obstruction; irrigation
Other
Insufficient [client] or caregiver knowledge of disease process
At Risk Population: Ejaculation; menstruation; extremes of temperature
Associated Condition:
Bowel distention; esophageal reflux disease; gastric ulcer; gastrointestinal system pathology; gallstones; hemorrhoids
Deep vein thrombosis; pulmonary emboli
Fractures; heterotopic bone
Ovarian cyst; pregnancy; labor and delivery period
Pharmaceutical agent; substance withdrawal
Renal calculi, urinary catheterization; cystitis, urinary tract infection, detrusor sphincter dyssynergia; epidiymitis
Surgical procedure; wound; sunburn
Sample Clinical Applications: Spinal cord injury

DESIRED OUTCOMES/EVALUATION CRITERIA

Sample NOC linkages:
Risk Control: Personal actions to understand, prevent, eliminate, or reduce modifiable health threats
Knowledge: Disease Process: Extent of understanding conveyed about a specific disease process and potential complications

(continues on page 82)

 Diagnostic Studies   Evidence Based Practice   Medications 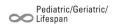 Pediatric/Geriatric/Lifespan

risk for AUTONOMIC DYSREFLEXIA (continued)

Caregiver Home Care Readiness: Preparedness of a caregiver to assume responsibility for the health care of a family member in the home

Client/Caregiver Will (Include Specific Time Frame)
- Identify risk factors present.
- Demonstrate preventive or corrective techniques.
- Be free of episodes of dysreflexia.

ACTIONS/INTERVENTIONS

Sample NIC linkages:

Dysreflexia Management: Prevention and elimination of stimuli that cause hyperactive reflexes and inappropriate autonomic responses in a patient with a cervical or high thoracic cord lesion

Surveillance: Purposeful and ongoing acquisition, interpretation, and synthesis of patient data for clinical decision making

Medication Management: Facilitation of safe and effective use of prescription and over-the-counter drugs

NURSING PRIORITY NO. 1   To assess risk factors present:

- Monitor for potential precipitating factors, including urological (e.g., bladder distention, acute urinary tract infection, kidney stones), gastrointestinal (e.g., bowel overdistention, hemorrhoids, digital stimulation), cutaneous (e.g., pressure ulcers, extreme external temperatures, dressing changes), reproductive (e.g., sexual activity, menstruation, pregnancy/delivery), and miscellaneous (e.g., pulmonary emboli, drug reaction, deep vein thrombosis). (Refer to ND Autonomic Dysreflexia for a more complete listing of precipitating factors, if indicated.)[1,2,5,6]

NURSING PRIORITY NO. 2   To prevent occurrence:

- ∞ ⬚ Monitor vital signs routinely, noting changes in blood pressure, heart rate, and temperature, especially during times of physical stress *to identify trends and intervene in a timely manner.*[1,2] *Note: The baseline blood pressure in spinal cord–injured clients (adult and child) is lower than in the general population; therefore, an elevation of 20 to 40 mmHg above baseline may be indicative of autonomic dysreflexia (AD).*[5,6]
- ⬚ Instruct all caregivers in regularly timed elimination and safe bowel and bladder or catheter care, as well as in interventions for long-term prevention of skin stress or breakdown (e.g., appropriate padding for skin and tissues, proper positioning with frequent pressure-relief actions, routine foot and toenail care) *to reduce risk of AD episode. Note: The two most common inciting stimuli are bladder and bowel distention, respectively; commonly a blocked urinary catheter.*[1,3,4,6]
- Instruct client/caregivers in additional preventive interventions (e.g., temperature control; preventing pressure ulcers, blisters, ingrown toenails; checking frequently for tight clothes or leg straps; sunburn and other burn prevention).[1,4–6]
- ⬚ Administer antihypertensive medications, as indicated. *At-risk client may be placed on routine "maintenance dose," such as when noxious stimuli cannot be removed (e.g., presence of chronic sacral pressure ulcer, fracture, acute postoperative pain).*[1]
- Refer to ND Autonomic Dysreflexia.

NURSING PRIORITY NO. 3   To promote wellness (Teaching/Discharge Considerations):

- ⬚ Review warning signs of AD with client/caregiver (e.g., sudden, severe pounding headache; flushed, red face; increased blood pressure/acute hypertension; nasal congestion; anxiety; blurred vision; metallic taste in mouth; sweating and/or flushing above the level of SCI; goose bumps; bradycardia, cardiac irregularities). *AD can develop rapidly (in minutes), thus requires quick intervention.*

 Acute Care   Collaborative   Community/ Home Care   Cultural

- Be aware of client's communication abilities. *AD can occur at any age, from infant to very old, and the individual may not be able to verbalize a pounding headache, which is often the first symptom during onset of AD.*[1]
- Ascertain that client/caregiver understands ways to avoid onset of syndrome. Provide information card and instruct and periodically reinforce teaching, as needed, regarding the following:[1–6]

    Keeping indwelling catheter free of kinks, keeping bag empty and situated below bladder level, and checking daily for deposits (bladder grit) inside catheter,

    Catheterizing as often as necessary *to prevent overfilling,*

    Monitoring voiding patterns for adequate frequency and amount,

    Performing regular bowel evacuation program,

    Performing routine skin assessments, and

    Monitoring all systems for signs/symptoms of infection and reporting promptly *for timely medical treatment.*

- Instruct family member/caregiver in proper blood pressure monitoring.
- Review use and administration of medications, when used. *Some clients are on medications routinely, and if so, they should receive instructions for routine administration, as well as symptoms to report for immediate or emergent care, when blood pressure is not responsive.*[1,5]
- Emphasize importance of regularly scheduled medical evaluations *to monitor status and identify developing problems.*
- Recommend wearing a medical alert bracelet or necklace with information card about signs/symptoms of AD and usual methods of treatment. *Provides vital information in emergencies.*
- Assist client/family in identifying emergency referrals (e.g., physician, rehabilitation nurse, or home-care supervisor). Place telephone number(s) in prominent place or program into client's/caregiver's cell phone.

DOCUMENTATION FOCUS

Assessment/Reassessment
- Individual risk factors.
- Previous episodes, precipitating factors, and individual signs/symptoms.

Planning
- Plan of care and who is involved in planning.
- Teaching plan.

Implementation/Evaluation
- Client's responses to interventions and actions performed, understanding of teaching.
- Attainment or progress toward desired outcome(s).
- Modifications to plan of care.

Discharge Planning
- Long-term needs and who is responsible for actions to be taken.

References

1. Consortium for Spinal Cord Medicine, Paralyzed Veterans of America. (2001). *Acute Management of Autonomic Dysreflexia: Individuals with Spinal Cord Injury Presenting to Health-Care Facilities: Clinical Practice Guidelines.* 2nd ed. Retrieved February 2018 from http://www.pva.org/media/pdf/cpg_autonomic%20 dysreflexia.pdf.
2. Acuff, M. (2005). Autonomic Dysreflexia: What It Is, What It Does, and What to Do If You Experience It. *The Missouri Model Spinal Cord Injury System.* Columbia, MO: University of Missouri-Columbia, School of Health Professions.
3. Saulino, M. F. (Updated 2017). Rehabilitation of persons with spinal cord injuries. Retrieved February 2018 from https:// emedicine.medscape.com/article/1265209-overview#a4.

4. National Spinal Cord Injury Association (NSCIA). (n.d.). SCI complications resource: Autonomic dysreflexia. Retrieved February 2018 http://www.spinalcord.org/contact/.
5. Stephenson, R. O., Berliner, J. (Updated 2018). Autonomic dysreflexia in spinal cord injury. Retrieved February 2018 from http://emedicine.medscape.com/article/322809-overview.
6. No author listed. (2002–2018). Autonomic dysreflexia. *SCI-Info-Pages.* Retrieved February 2018 from http://www.sci-info-pages .com/ad.html.

 Diagnostic Studies   Evidence Based Practice   Medications 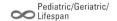 Pediatric/Geriatric/ Lifespan

disorganized infant Behavior

Taxonomy II: Coping/Stress Tolerance—Class 3 Neurobehavioral Stress (00116) [**Diagnostic Division:** Neurosensory], Submitted 1994; Revised 1998, 2017

DEFINITION: Disintegration of the physiological and neurobehavioral systems of functioning.

RELATED FACTORS
Caregiver cue misreading
Environmental overstimulation; inadequate physical environment
Feeding intolerance

DEFINING CHARACTERISTICS

Objective

Attention-interaction system: Impaired response to sensory stimuli [e.g., difficult to soothe, unable to sustain alert status]
Motor system:
Alteration in primitive reflexes; exaggerated startle response; fidgeting
Finger splay; fisting; hands to face; hyperextension of extremities
Impaired motor tone; tremor, twitching; uncoordinated movements
Physiological:
Abnormal skin color [e.g., pale, dusky]; oxygen desaturation
Arrhythmia; bradycardia; tachycardia
Feeding intolerances
Time-out signals [e.g., gaze, hiccup, sigh, slack jaw, tongue thrust]
Regulatory problems: Inability to inhibit startle reflex; irritability
State-organization system:
Active-awake; quiet-awake
Diffuse alpha electroencephalogram (EEG) activity with eyes closed; state-oscillation
Irritable crying
At Risk Population: Low postconceptual age; prematurity; prenatal exposure to teratogen
Associated Condition: Congenital or genetic disorders; infant illness; immature neurological functioning; impaired infant motor functioning; invasive procedure; infant oral impairment
Sample Clinical Applications: Prematurity, congenital or genetic disorders, meconium aspiration, respiratory distress syndrome, small for gestational age

DESIRED OUTCOMES/EVALUATION CRITERIA

Sample NOC linkages:
Neurological Status: Ability of the peripheral and central nervous system to receive, process, and respond to internal and external stimuli
Preterm Infant Organization: Extrauterine integration of physiological and behavioral function by the infant born 24 to 37 (term) weeks gestation

Infant Will (Include Specific Time Frame)
• Exhibit organized behaviors promoting achievement of optimal potential for growth and development as evidenced by modulation of physiological, motor, state, and attentional-interactive functioning.

 Acute Care Collaborative Community/ Home Care Cultural

Sample **NOC** linkages:

Child Development [specify age 1, 2 months]: Milestones of physical, cognitive, and psychosocial progression by [specify] months of age

Parent/Caregiver Will

- Recognize cues reflecting infant's stress threshold and current status.
- Identify appropriate responses (including environmental modifications) to infant's cues.
- Engage in responses to promote infant adaptation and development.
- Verbalize readiness to assume caregiving independently.

ACTIONS/INTERVENTIONS

Sample **NIC** linkages:

Environmental Management: Manipulation of the patient's surroundings for therapeutic benefit, sensory appeal, and psychological well-being

Developmental Enhancement: Infant: Facilitating optimal physical, cognitive, social, and emotional growth of child under 1 year of age

Infant Care: Newborn: Provision of care to the infant during the transition from birth to extrauterine life and subsequent period of stabilization

NURSING PRIORITY NO. 1   To assess causative/contributing factors:

- Determine infant's chronological and developmental age; note length of gestation. *These factors (prematurity, infant maturity, and stages of development) help to determine plan of care.*[1,2]
- Observe for cues suggesting presence of situations that may result in pain or discomfort. *Some behavior that appears to be disorganized may be caused by a pain source that, once identified, may be alleviated.*[1]
- Determine adequacy of physiological support. *Identifies areas of additional need.*[1]
- Evaluate level and appropriateness of environmental stimuli. *Infant behavior is affected by a wide range of stimuli. Careful assessment narrows focus of concerns.*[2]
- Ascertain parents' understanding of infant's needs and abilities. *Identifies knowledge base and areas of learning needed.*[2–4]
- Listen to parents' concerns about their capabilities to meet infant's needs. *Active listening can reassure parents, pinpoint areas to be addressed, and provide an opportunity to correct misconceptions.*[2,3]

NURSING PRIORITY NO. 2   To assist parents in providing coregulation to the infant:

- Provide a calm, nurturant, physical, and emotional environment. *Provides optimal infant comfort. Models behavior for parent(s) and optimizes learning.*[2,3]
- Encourage parents to hold infant, including skin-to-skin contact as appropriate. *Touch enhances parent-infant bonding and provides means of calming.*[3] *Research suggests skin-to-skin contact or kangaroo care may have a positive effect on infant development by enhancing neurophysiological organization and an indirect effect by improving parental mood, perceptions, and interactive behavior.*[6]
- Model gentle handling of baby and appropriate responses to infant behavior. *Provides cues to parent.*[3]
- Support and encourage parents to be with infant and participate actively in all aspects of care. *Situation may seem overwhelming to new parents. Emotional and physical support enhances coping. Parents who are able to help in the care of their infant express lower levels of helplessness and powerlessness.*[1,2]
- Encourage parents to refrain from social interaction during feedings as appropriate. *Infant may have difficulty/lack necessary energy to manage feeding and social stimulation simultaneously.*[5]

 Diagnostic Studies   Evidence Based Practice   Medications   Pediatric/Geriatric/Lifespan

- Provide positive feedback for progressive parental involvement in caregiving process. *Transfer of care from staff to parents progresses along a continuum as parents' confidence level increases and they are able to take on more complex care activities.*[7]
- Discuss infant growth and development, pointing out current status and progressive expectations as appropriate. *Augments parent knowledge of coregulation.*[2]
- Incorporate the parents' observations and suggestions into plan of care. *Demonstrates valuing of parents' input and encourages continued involvement.*[2,4]

NURSING PRIORITY NO. 3   To deliver care within the infant's stress threshold:

- ✚ Provide a consistent caregiver. *Facilitates recognition of infant cues or changes in behavior. Communication is optimized if family is familiar with caregiver.*[2]
- Identify infant's individual self-regulatory behaviors (e.g., sucking, mouthing; grasp, hand-to-mouth, face behaviors; foot clasp, brace; limb flexion, trunk tuck; boundary seeking).
- Support hands to mouth and face; offer pacifier or nonnutritive sucking at the breast with gavage feedings. *Provides opportunities for infant to self-regulate.*[2,5]
- Avoid aversive oral stimulation, such as routine oral suctioning; suction endotracheal tube only when clinically indicated. *Maximizes infant comfort, preventing undue/noxious stimulation.*[1,2]
- Use Oxyhood large enough to cover the infant's chest so arms will be inside the hood. *Allows for hand-to-mouth self-calming activities during this therapy.*[2]
- Provide opportunities for infant to grasp. *Helps with development of motor function skills and can have a calming effect.*[2,5]
- Provide boundaries or containment during all activities. Use swaddling, nesting, bunting, and caregiver's hands as indicated. *Enhances infant's feelings of security and safeness. Avoids startle reflex and accompanying distress.*[2,3]
- Allow adequate time and opportunities to hold infant. Handle infant very gently; move infant smoothly, slowly, and keep contained, avoiding sudden or abrupt movements. *Provides comfort to infant and models behavior to parent(s).*[3]
- Maintain normal alignment, position infant with limbs softly flexed and shoulders and hips adducted slightly. Use appropriate-sized diapers. *Avoids unnecessary discomfort.*[2]
- Evaluate chest for adequate expansion, placing rolls under trunk if prone position is indicated. *Provides for ease of respirations.*[2]
- Avoid restraints, including at IV sites. If an IV board is necessary, secure to limb positioned in normal alignment. *Optimizes comfort and movement.*[1,2]
- Provide a pressure-eliminating mattress, water bed, or gel pillow for infant who does not tolerate frequent position changes. *Minimizes tissue pressure and risk of tissue injury.*[2]
- Visually assess color, respirations, activity, and invasive lines without disturbing infant. Assess with "hands on" every 4 hr as indicated and prn. *Allows for undisturbed rest and quiet periods.*[2,3]
- Group care activities, schedule time for rest, and organize sleep and wake states to maximize tolerance of infant. Defer routine care when infant is in quiet sleep. *Gives infant a sense of routine and also provides for undisturbed rest and longer periods of quiet.*[2,3,5]
- Provide care with baby in side-lying position. Begin by talking softly to the baby and then placing hands in a containing hold on baby, allowing baby to prepare. Proceed with least invasive manipulations first. *Gradual build from comforting touch, to nursing care, to invasive interventions decreases overall stress of infant. Shortens perception of "being bothered" time and facilitates a more rapid calming phase.*[3]
- Respond promptly to infant's agitation or restlessness. Provide "time-out" when infant shows early cues of overstimulation. Comfort and support the infant after stressful interventions. *Decreases stress for both infant and family. Facilitates calming phase.*[3]
- Remain at infant's bedside for several minutes after procedures and caregiving to monitor infant's response and provide necessary support. *Allows for more rapid intervention(s) if infant becomes overstressed.*[3]
- 💊 Administer analgesics as individually appropriate. *Maintains optimal comfort.*[1–4]

 Acute Care   Collaborative   Community/ Home Care   Cultural

NURSING PRIORITY NO. 4 To modify the environment to provide appropriate stimulation:

- Introduce stimulation as a single mode and assess individual tolerance.

Light/Vision

- Reduce lighting perceived by infant; introduce diurnal lighting (and activity) when infant achieves physiological stability. (Daylight levels of 20 to 30 candles and night-light levels of less than 10 candles are suggested.) Change light levels gradually to allow infant time to adjust. *Lowering light levels reduces visual stimulation and provides a comforting environment. Diurnal lighting allows the stable infant to begin perception of day and night cycles and to establish circadian rhythms.*[1]
- Protect the infant's eyes from bright illumination during examinations and procedures, as well as from indirect sources, such as neighboring phototherapy treatments. *Prevents retinal damage and reduces visual stressors.*[2]
- Deliver phototherapy (when required) with Biliblanket devices if available. *Alleviates need for eye patches to protect vision.*[2]
- Provide a caregiver's face (preferably a parent's) as visual stimulus when infant shows readiness (awake, attentive). *Begins process of visual recognition.*[1]
- Evaluate/readjust placement of pictures, stuffed animal, etc., within infant's immediate environment. *Promotes state maintenance and smooth transition, allowing infant to look away easily when visual stimuli become stressful.*[5]

Sound

- Identify sources of noise in environment and eliminate/reduce *to minimize auditory stimulus, reduce startle response in infant, and provide a comforting environment:*[2]
  Speak in a low voice.
  Reduce volume on alarms and telephones to safe but not excessive volume.
  Pad metal trash can lids.
  Open paper packages such as IV tubing and suction catheters slowly and at a distance from bedside.
  Conduct rounds or report away from bedside.
  Place soft, thick fabric such as blanket rolls and toys near infant's head *to absorb sound.*
  Keep all incubator portholes closed, closing with two hands *to avoid loud snap with closure and associated startle response.*
- Refrain from playing musical toys or tape players inside incubator. *Even very soft sounds echo in an enclosed space. What an adult may find soothing is likely to overstimulate an infant.*[2,3]
- Avoid placing items on top of incubator; if necessary to do so, pad surface well. *Contact with the external parts of the incubator causes reverberation inside the chamber.*
- Conduct regular decibel (dB) checks of interior noise level in incubator (recommended not to exceed 60 dB). *Verifies that decibel levels are within acceptable range.*[2]
- Provide auditory stimulation to console and support infant before and through handling or to reinforce restfulness. *Provides modeling of behavior for family and increased comfort for infant.*[3]

Olfactory

- Be cautious in exposing infant to strong odors (e.g., alcohol, Betadine, perfumes). *Olfactory capability of the infant is very sensitive.*[1]
- Place a cloth or gauze pad scented with milk near the infant's face during gavage feeding. *Enhances association of milk with act of feeding and gastric fullness.*[2]
- Invite parents to leave near infant a handkerchief that they have scented by wearing close to their body. *Strengthens infant recognition of parents.*[2]

Vestibular

- Move and handle the infant slowly and gently. Do not restrict spontaneous movement. *Maintains comfort while encouraging motor function skill.*[2]
- Provide vestibular stimulation *to console, stabilize breathing/heart rate, or enhance growth.* Use a water bed (with or without oscillation); a motorized, moving bed or cradle; or rocking in the arms of a caregiver.

 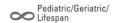

Gustatory

• Dip pacifier in milk and offer to infant for sucking and tasting during gavage feeding. *Further enhances feeding recognition with touch and taste cues.*[2]

Tactile

• Maintain skin integrity and monitor closely. Limit frequency of invasive procedures. *Decreases chance of infections. Decreases infant discomfort.*[1]
• Minimize use of chemicals on skin (e.g., alcohol, povidone-iodine, solvents) and remove afterward with warm water. *Chemical compounds remove the natural protective mechanisms of skin, and infants are often very sensitive to integumentary injury.*[1]
• Limit use of tape and adhesives directly on skin. Use DuoDerm under tape. *Helps prevent dermal injury and allergic reactions.*[1]
• Touch infant with a firm, containing touch; avoid light stroking. Provide a sheepskin or soft linen. *Note: Tactile experience is the primary sensory mode of the infant. Light stroking can cause tickle sensations that are irritating rather than pleasurable. Firm touch is reassuring.*[2]
• Encourage frequent parental holding of infant (including skin-to-skin). Supplement activity with extended family, staff, volunteers. *For family members, touch enhances bonding. If family is not readily available, infant needs regular skin-to-skin contact from caregivers for comfort and reassurance.*[3]

NURSING PRIORITY NO. 5 To promote wellness (Teaching/Discharge Considerations):

• Evaluate home environment to identify appropriate modifications. *Helps the family identify needs and begin to mentally prepare for infant homecoming.*[3]
• Identify community resources (e.g., early stimulation program, qualified childcare facilities or respite care, visiting nurse, home-care support, specialty organizations). *Begins process of resource utilization.*[2–4]
• Determine sources for equipment and therapy needs. *Facilitates transition to at-home care.*[3]
• Refer to support or therapy groups as indicated. *Provides role models, facilitates adjustment to new roles and responsibilities, and enhances coping.*[2,3]
• Provide contact number, as appropriate (e.g., primary nurse). *Supports adjustment to home setting and enhances problem solving.*[3]
• Refer to additional NDs such as risk for impaired Attachment, risk for caregiver Role Strain, compromised/disabled/readiness for enhanced family Coping, risk for delayed Development.

DOCUMENTATION FOCUS

Assessment/Reassessment

• Findings, including infant's cues of stress, self-regulation, and readiness for stimulation; chronological and developmental age.
• Parent's concerns, level of knowledge.

Planning

• Plan of care and who is involved in the planning.
• Teaching plan.

Implementation/Evaluation

• Infant's responses to interventions and actions performed.
• Parents' participation and response to interactions and teaching.
• Attainment or progress toward desired outcome(s).
• Modifications of plan of care.

Discharge Planning

• Long-term needs and who is responsible for actions to be taken.
• Specific referrals made.

 Acute Care   Collaborative   Community/Home Care   Cultural

References

1. Greene, M. F., et al. (2008). *Creasy & Resnik's Maternal-Fetal Medicine*. 6th ed. Philadelphia: W. B. Saunders.
2. London, M. L., et al. (2006). *Maternal & Child Nursing Care*. 2nd ed. Upper Saddle River, NJ: Prentice Hall.
3. Ladewig, P., London, M. L., Davidson, M. W. (2009). *Contemporary Maternal-Newborn Nursing Care*. 7th ed. Upper Saddle River, NJ: Prentice Hall.
4. Lowdermilk, D., Perry, S. (2009). *Maternity & Women's Health Care*. 7th ed. St. Louis, MO: Mosby.
5. LaRossa, M. M. (No date). Understanding preterm infant behavior in the NICU. Retrieved February 2018 from http://www.pediatrics.emory.edu/divisions/neonatology/dpc/nicubeh.html.
6. Feldman, R., et al. (2002). Comparison of skin-to-skin (kangaroo) and traditional care: Parenting outcomes and preterm infant development. *Pediatrics*, 110(1), 16–26.
7. Scharer, K., Brooks, G. (1994). Mothers of chronically ill neonates and primary nurses in the NICU: Transfer of care. *Neonatal Netw*, 13(5), 37–46.

readiness for enhanced organized infant Behavior

Taxonomy II: Coping/Stress Tolerance—Class 3 Neurobehavioral Stress (00117) [**Diagnostic Division:** Neurosensory], Submitted 1994; Revised 2013

DEFINITION: A pattern of modulation of the physiological and behavioral systems of functioning, which can be strengthened.

DEFINING CHARACTERISTICS

Objective

Parent expresses desire to enhance cue recognition

Parent expresses desire to enhance recognition of infant's self-regulatory behaviors

Parent expresses desire to enhance environmental conditions

Sample Clinical Applications: Prematurity, congenital or genetic disorders, meconium aspiration, respiratory distress syndrome, small for gestational age

DESIRED OUTCOMES/EVALUATION CRITERIA

Sample NOC linkages:

Preterm Infant Organization: Extrauterine integration of physiological and behavioral function by the infant born 24 to 37 (term) weeks gestation

Neurological Status: Ability of the peripheral and central nervous system to receive, process, and respond to internal and external stimuli

Infant Will (Include Specific Time Frame)

• Modulate physiological and behavioral systems of functioning.
• Achieve higher levels of integration in response to environmental stimuli.

Sample NOC linkages:

Child Development: [specify age group 1 or 2 months]: Milestones of physical, cognitive, and psychosocial progression by [specify] months of age

Knowledge: Infant Care: Extent of understanding conveyed about caring for a baby from birth to first birthday

Parent/Caregiver Will (Include Specific Time Frame)

• Identify cues reflecting infant's stress threshold and current status.
• Develop or modify responses (including environment) to promote infant adaptation and development.

(continues on page 90)

 Diagnostic Studies   Evidence Based Practice   Medications 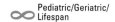 Pediatric/Geriatric/Lifespan

readiness for enhanced organized infant Behavior (continued)

ACTIONS/INTERVENTIONS

Sample NIC linkages:

Developmental Enhancement: Infant: Facilitating optimal physical, cognitive, social, and emotional growth of child under 1 year of age

Environmental Management: Manipulation of the patient's surroundings for therapeutic benefit, sensory appeal, and psychological well-being

NURSING PRIORITY NO. 1   To assess infant status and parental skill level:

- Determine infant's chronological and developmental age; note length of gestation. *These factors (prematurity, infant maturity, and stages of development) help to determine plan of care.*[1,2,5]
- Identify infant's individual self-regulatory behaviors: suck, mouth; grasp, hand-to-mouth, face behaviors; foot clasp, brace; limb flexion, trunk tuck; boundary seeking. *Assessing the infant's own regulatory coping tools alerts family and caregiver when infant is entering a stress cycle and helps determine if the infant needs assistance coping. This knowledge also helps in development of a care plan if situation warrants.*[1,2,4]
- Observe for cues suggesting presence of situations that may result in pain/discomfort. *Some behavior that appears to be disorganized may be caused by a pain source that, once identified, may be alleviated.*[1]
- Evaluate level and appropriateness of environmental stimuli. *Infant behavior is affected by a wide range of stimuli. Careful assessment narrows focus of concerns.*[2]
- Ascertain parents' understanding of infant's needs and abilities. *Identifies knowledge base and areas of additional learning need.*[2–4]
- Listen, or Active-listen, to parents' perceptions of their capabilities to promote infant's development. *When parents feel their thoughts and concerns are heard, they will feel reassured that they will be able to handle the situation.*[2,3]

NURSING PRIORITY NO. 2   To assist parents to enhance infant's integration:

- Provide positive feedback for parental involvement in caregiving process. Transfer of care from staff to parents progresses along a continuum as parents' confidence level increases and they are able to take on more responsibility.[7]
- Discuss use of skin-to-skin contact (kangaroo care [KC]) as appropriate. *Research suggests KC may have a positive effect on infant development by enhancing neurophysiological organization and an indirect effect by improving parental mood, perceptions, and interactive behavior.*[6]
- Review infant growth and development, pointing out current status and progressive expectations. *Increases parental knowledge base and level of confidence.*[2–4]
- Identify cues reflecting infant stress. *Attention to cues allows for early intervention in case of problem development.*[2–4]
- Discuss possible modifications of environmental stimuli, handling, activity schedule, sleep, and pain control needs based on infant's behavioral cues. *Stimulation that is properly timed and appropriate in complexity and intensity allows the infant to maintain a stable balance of his/her subsystems and enhances development.*[5]
- 🏠 Discuss parents' perceptions of needs and provide recommendations for modifications of environmental stimuli, activity schedule, sleep, and pain control needs. *While care provided is satisfactory, some modifications may enhance infant's integration and development.*[1,4]

 Acute Care   Collaborative   Community/Home Care   Cultural

- 🏠 Incorporate parents' observations and suggestions into plan of care. *Demonstrates value of and regard for parents' input and enhances sense of ability to deal with situation.*[2,4]

NURSING PRIORITY NO. 3 To promote wellness (Teaching/Learning Considerations):

- 🏠 Identify community resources (e.g., visiting nurse, home-care support, childcare). *Begins process of resource utilization.*[2–4]
- Refer to support group or individual role model *to facilitate ongoing adjustment to new roles and responsibilities and problem solving.*[2,3]
- Refer to additional NDs, for example, readiness for enhanced family Coping.

DOCUMENTATION FOCUS

Assessment/Reassessment

- Findings, including infant's self-regulation and readiness for stimulation; chronological and developmental age.
- Parents' concerns, level of knowledge.

Planning

- Plan of care and who is involved in the planning.
- Teaching plan.

Implementation/Evaluation

- Infant's responses to interventions and actions performed.
- Parents' participation and response to interactions/teaching.
- Attainment or progress toward desired outcome(s).
- Modifications of plan of care.

Discharge Planning

- Long-term needs and who is responsible for actions to be taken.
- Specific referrals made.

References

1. Greene, M. F., et al. (2008). *Creasy & Resnik's Maternal-Fetal Medicine*. 6th ed. Philadelphia, PA: W. B. Saunders.
2. London, M., et al. (2006). *Maternal & Child Nursing Care*. 2nd ed. Upper Saddle River, NJ: Prentice Hall.
3. Ladewig, P., London, M. L., Davidson, M. W. (2009). *Contemporary Maternal-Newborn Nursing Care*. 7th ed. Upper Saddle River, NJ: Prentice Hall.
4. Lowdermilk, D., Perry, S. (2009). *Maternity & Women's Health Care*. 7th ed. St. Louis, MO: Mosby.
5. LaRossa, M. M. (No date). Understanding preterm infant behavior in the NICU. Retrieved February 2018 from http://www.pediatrics.emory.edu/divisions/neonatology/dpc/nicubeh.html.
6. Feldman, R., et al. (2002). Comparison of skin-to-skin (kangaroo) and traditional care: Parenting outcomes and preterm infant development. *Pediatrics*, 110(1), 16–26.
7. Scharer, K., Brooks, G. (1994). Mothers of chronically ill neonates and primary nurses in the NICU: Transfer of care. *Neonatal Netw*, 13(5), 37–46.

 Diagnostic Studies   Evidence Based Practice   Medications   Pediatric/Geriatric/Lifespan

risk for disorganized infant Behavior

Taxonomy II: Coping/Stress Tolerance—Class 3 Neurobehavioral Stress (00115) [**Diagnostic Division:** Neurosensory], Submitted 1994; Revised 2013, 2017

DEFINITION: Susceptible to disintegration in the pattern of modulation of the physiological and behavioral systems of functioning, which may compromise health.

RISK FACTORS
Caregiver cue misreading; insufficient caregiver knowledge of behavioral cues
Environmental overstimulation, or insufficient environmental sensory stimulation; sensory deprivation
Feeding intolerance; infant malnutrition
Inadequate physical environment; insufficient containment within environment
Pain
At Risk Population: Low postconceptual age; prematurity; prenatal exposure to teratogen
Associated Condition: Congenital or genetic disorders; infant illness; immature neurological functioning; impaired infant motor functioning; invasive procedure; infant oral impairment
Sample Clinical Applications: Prematurity, congenital or genetic disorders, meconium aspiration, respiratory distress syndrome, small for gestational age

DESIRED OUTCOMES/EVALUATION CRITERIA

Sample NOC linkages:
Preterm Infant Organization: Extrauterine integration of physiological and behavioral function by the infant born 24 to 37 (term) weeks gestation
Neurological Status: Ability of the peripheral and central nervous system to receive, process, and respond to internal and external stimuli

Infant Will (Include specific time frame)
• Exhibit organized behaviors promoting achievement of optimal potential for growth and development as evidenced by modulation of physiological, motor, state, and attentional-interactive functioning.

Sample NOC linkages:
Child Development: [specify age group 1 or 2 months]: Milestones of physical, cognitive, and psychosocial progression by [specify] months of age
Knowledge: Infant Care: Extent of understanding conveyed about caring for a baby from birth to first birthday

Parent/Caregiver Will (Include specific time frame)
• Identify cues reflecting infant's stress threshold and current status.
• Develop or modify responses (including environment) to promote infant adaptation and development.

ACTIONS/INTERVENTIONS AND DOCUMENTATION FOCUS
Refer to ND disorganized infant Behavior for Actions/Interventions and Documentation Focus.

 Acute Care   Collaborative   Community/Home Care   Cultural

risk for Bleeding

Taxonomy II: Safety/Protection—Class 2 Physical Injury (00206) [**Diagnostic Division:** Circulation],
Submitted 2008; Revised 2013, 2017

DEFINITION: Susceptible to a decrease in blood volume, which may compromise health.

RISK FACTORS

Insufficient knowledge of bleeding precautions
At Risk Population: History of falls
Associated Condition: Aneurysm; disseminated intravascular coagulopathy; inherent coagulopathy
Gastrointestinal condition [e.g., ulcer, polyps, varices]; impaired liver function [e.g., cirrhosis]
Postpartum complications [e.g., uterine atony, retained placenta]; pregnancy complication [e.g., placenta previa/abruption]
Treatment regimen [e.g., surgery, medications, administration of platelet-deficient blood products, chemotherapy]; circumcision
Sample Clinical Applications: Trauma, brain injury, femur fracture, aortic aneurysm, esophageal varices, pancreatitis, sickle cell anemia, surgery; use of anticoagulants

DESIRED OUTCOMES/EVALUATION CRITERIA

Sample NOC linkages:
Blood Loss Severity: Severity of signs and symptoms of internal or external hemorrhage
Blood Coagulation: Extent to which blood clots within normal period of time
Risk Control: Personal actions to understand, prevent, eliminate, or reduce modifiable health threats

Client Will (Include Specific Time Frame)
- Be free of signs of active bleeding, such as hemoptysis, hematuria, or hematemesis, or excessive blood loss as evidenced by stable vital signs, skin and mucous membranes free of pallor, usual mentation, and urinary output.
- Display laboratory results for clotting times and factors within normal range for individual.
- Identify individual risks and engage in appropriate behaviors or lifestyle changes to prevent or reduce frequency of bleeding episodes.

ACTIONS/INTERVENTIONS

Sample NIC linkages:
Bleeding Precautions: Reduction of stimuli that may induce bleeding or hemorrhage in at-risk patients
Bleeding Reduction: Limitation of the loss of blood volume during an episode of bleeding

NURSING PRIORITY NO. 1   To assess risk factors:

- Assess client risk. Note possible medical diagnoses or disease processes that may lead to bleeding such as known or suspected major trauma, coagulopathies, gastric ulcers, liver disorders, pregnancy-related complications, malignancies, gram-negative sepsis, etc.
- Note type of injury(ies) present when client presents with trauma. *The pattern and extent of injury and bleeding may or may not be readily determined. For example, unbroken skin can hide a significant injury where a large amount of blood is lost within soft tissues or a crush injury resulting in interruption of the integrity of the pelvic ring can cause life-threatening bleeding from three sources (arterial, venous, and bone edge).*[1,10,11]

 Diagnostic Studies   Evidence Based Practice   Medications   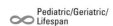 Pediatric/Geriatric/Lifespan

- Determine presence of hereditary factors, such as hereditary hemorrhagic telangiectasia, hemophilia, or other factor deficiencies; thrombocytopenia. *Hereditary bleeding or clotting disorders predispose client to bleeding complications, either spontaneous bleeding, such as nosebleeds and acute and chronic digestive tract bleeding,[2] or failure to clot in a timely manner.[1]*
- Obtain detailed history if a familial bleeding disorder is suspected. *Specialized testing may be needed and/or referral to hematologist.[1]*
- ∞ Note client's gender. *While bleeding disorders are common in both men and women, women are affected more due to the increased risk of blood loss related to menstrual cycle and child delivery procedures.[1,3]*
- Note pregnancy-related factors, as indicated. *Many factors can occur, including overdistention of the uterus—pregnant with multiples, prolonged or rapid labor, lacerations occurring during vaginal delivery, or retained placenta that can place mother at risk for postpartum bleeding.*
- Evaluate client's medication regimen. *Use of medications, such as NSAIDs, anticoagulants, corticosteroids, and certain herbals (e.g., gingko biloba), predispose client to bleeding.[4]*

NURSING PRIORITY NO. 2   To evaluate for potential bleeding:

- Monitor perineum and fundal height in postpartum client and wounds, dressings, and tubes in client with trauma, surgery, or other invasive procedures *to identify active blood loss. Note: Hemorrhage may occur because of inability to achieve hemostasis in the setting of injury or may result from the development of a coagulopathy.[2] Excessive bleeding may be defined by the individual client's physician or the facility's written policy—such as saturating two perineal pads per hour or more than 200 mL/chest tube drainage in 4 hr.[5]*
- Evaluate and mark boundaries of soft tissues in enclosed structures such as a leg or abdomen *to document expanding bruise or hematomas. Helps in identifying bleeding that may be occurring in a closed space, which renders client susceptible to complications, such as compartment syndrome or hypovolemia; permits earlier intervention.*
- Assess vital signs, including blood pressure, pulse (may be elevated initially), and respirations. Measure blood pressure lying, sitting, and standing as indicated *to evaluate for orthostatic hypotension. Note: Vital signs do not necessarily reflect the quantity of hemorrhage accurately! Fit, young patients may lose 40% of their blood volume before the systolic blood pressure drops below 100 mmHg, whereas the elderly may become hypotensive with volume loss of as little as 10%.* Monitor invasive hemodynamic parameters when present (e.g., central venous pressure) *to determine if intravascular fluid deficit exists. Note: Client could lose up to 2 L of blood into chest, abdomen, or pelvis before hypotension signals the presence of a problem.[6] The American College of Surgeons Advanced Trauma Life Support lists four classes of hemorrhage, with class I involving up to 15% blood volume loss and little change in vital signs and class IV involving blood loss greater than 40% of circulating volume and requiring aggressive resuscitation to prevent death.[7]*
- Hematest all secretions and excretions for occult blood *to more accurately determine possible source of bleeding when blood loss is occurring.*
- Note client report of pain in specific areas and whether pain is increasing, diffuse, or localized. *Can help identify bleeding into tissues, organs, or body cavities.*
- Assess skin color and moisture, urinary output, and level of consciousness or mentation. *Changes in these signs may be indicative of blood loss affecting systemic circulation or local organ function such as kidneys or brain.*
- Review laboratory data (e.g., complete blood count, including hemoglobin [Hb], platelet numbers, and function; and other coagulation factors, which may be known by number—factor I, factor II, etc., or by name—prothrombin time, partial thromboplastin time, fibrinogen, etc.) *to evaluate bleeding risk. Note: Generally, laboratory values are not helpful in acute hemorrhage because values do not change from normal until redistribution of interstitial fluid into the blood plasma occurs after 8 to 12 hours. The common problem in life-threatening acute anemia is a sudden reduction in the oxygen-carrying capacity of the blood. Depending on the etiology, this may occur with or without reduction in the intravascular volume. It is generally accepted that an acute drop in hemoglobin to a level of 7 to 8 g/dL is symptomatic.[8,12,13] Note: When one or more clotting factors are missing, produced in too small a quantity, or not functioning correctly, excessive bleeding can*

 Acute Care   Collaborative   Community/ Home Care   Cultural

occur. Loss of factors may be due to acute blood loss, transfusion of factor-deficient blood, presence of inherited bleeding disorders, drugs that alter factors (e.g., warfarin, steroids, contraceptives, NSAIDs), or medical conditions affecting organs, such as cirrhosis of the liver.[9]

- Prepare client for, or assist with, diagnostic studies, such as x-rays, computed tomography or magnetic resonance imaging scans, ultrasound, or colonoscopy, *to determine presence of injuries or disorders that could cause internal bleeding (e.g., ectopic pregnancy, damaged spleen following vehicle crash, epidural hemorrhage 2 days after a fall, reports of rectal bleeding).*

NURSING PRIORITY NO. 3 To prevent bleeding/correct potential causes of excessive blood loss:

- ⊞ Apply direct pressure and ice to bleeding site, insert nasal packing, or perform fundal massage as appropriate.
- Restrict activity and encourage bedrest or chairrest until bleeding abates.
- Maintain patency of vascular access *for fluid administration or blood replacement as indicated.*
- ∞ Assist with treatment of underlying conditions causing or contributing to blood loss, such as medical treatment of systemic infections or balloon tamponade of esophageal varices prior to sclerotherapy; proton pump inhibitor medications or antibiotics for gastric ulcer; and surgery for internal abdominal trauma or retained placenta. *Treatment of underlying conditions may prevent or halt bleeding complications.*
- Provide special intervention for an at-risk client (e.g., individual with bone marrow suppression, chemotherapy, uremia) *to prevent bleeding associated with tissue injury:*
Monitor closely for overt bleeding.
Observe for diffuse oozing from tubes, wounds, and orifices with no observable clotting *to identify excessive bleeding and/or possible coagulopathy. Note: Client with certain conditions, such as obstetric complications, gram-negative sepsis, or massive trauma, may be predisposed to develop consumptive coagulopathy or disseminated intravascular coagulation, a potentially lethal phenomenon characterized by simultaneous clotting and continual bleeding.*[2]
Maintain pressure or pressure dressings as indicated for a longer period of time. *May be required to stop bleeding, such as pressure dressings over arterial puncture site or surgical dressings.*
 Hematest secretions and excretions for occult blood *for early identification of internal bleeding.*
Protect client from trauma such as falls, accidental or intentional blows, or lacerations *that could cause bleeding.*
Use soft toothbrush or toothettes for oral care *to reduce risk of injury to oral mucosa.*
- ∞ Collaborate in evaluating need for replacing blood loss or specific components and be prepared for emergency interventions. *Institution or physician may have specific guidelines for transfusion, such as platelet count less than 20,000/mcL or Hg less than 7 g/dL, in addition to the client's clinical status.*
- ✐ Be prepared to administer hemostatic agents, such as desmopressin, *which promotes clotting and may stop bleeding by increasing coagulation factor VIII and the von Willebrand factor,* or medications to prevent bleeding, such as proton pump inhibitors *to reduce the risk of gastrointestinal bleeding and need for replacement transfusion.*

NURSING PRIORITY NO. 4 To promote wellness (Teaching/Discharge Considerations):

- 🏠 Provide information to client/family about hereditary or familial problems that predispose to bleeding complications.
- Instruct at-risk client and family regarding:
Specific signs of bleeding requiring healthcare provider notification, such as active bright bleeding anywhere, prolonged epistaxis or trauma in client with known factor bleeding tendencies, black tarry stools, weakness, vertigo, syncope, etc.
✐ The need to inform healthcare providers when taking aspirin and other anticoagulants (e.g., Lovenox, Coumadin, Plavix, Xeralto, Eliquis), especially when elective surgery or other invasive procedure is planned. *These agents will most likely be withheld for a period of time prior to elective procedures to reduce potential for excessive blood loss.*

 Diagnostic Studies   Evidence Based Practice   Medications 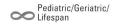 Pediatric/Geriatric/Lifespan

🖊 Importance of periodic review of client's medication regimen *to identify medications that might cause or exacerbate bleeding problems. Note: Some prescriptions, over-the-counter medications, and herbals (e.g., vitamin E, ginkgo, ginger, garlic, fish oils) promote bleeding.*[5]

🔵 Necessity of regular medical and laboratory follow-up when on Coumadin (warfarin), *to determine needed dosage changes or client management issues requiring monitoring and/or modification.*

Dietary measures to improve blood clotting, such as foods rich in vitamin K.

The need to avoid alcohol in diagnosed liver disorders or seek treatment for alcoholism in presence of alcoholic varices.

Techniques for postpartum client to check her own fundus and perform fundal massage as indicated and to contact physician for postdischarge bleeding that is bright red or dark red with large clots. *May prevent blood loss complications, especially if client is discharged early from hospital.*

DOCUMENTATION FOCUS

Assessment/Reassessment
- Individual factors that may potentiate blood loss—type of injuries, obstetrical complications, etc.
- Baseline vital signs, mentation, urinary output, and subsequent assessments.
- Results of laboratory tests or diagnostic procedures.

Planning
- Plan of care and who is involved in the planning.
- Teaching plan.

Implementation/Evaluation
- Responses to interventions, teaching, and actions performed.
- Attainment or progress toward desired outcome(s).
- Modifications to plan of care.

Discharge Planning
- Long-term needs, identifying who is responsible for actions to be taken.
- Community resources or support for chronic problems.
- Specific referrals made.

References

1. Lambing, A. (2007). Bleeding disorders: Patient history key to diagnosis. *Nurs Pract*, 32(12), 16–24.
2. Ragsdale, J. A. (2007). Hereditary hemorrhagic telangiectasia from epistaxis to life-threatening GI bleeding. *Gastroenterol Nurs*, 30(4), 293–299.
3. Sommers, M. S., Johnson, S. A., Beery, T. A. (2007). *Diseases and Disorders: A Nursing Therapeutics Manual.* 3rd ed. Philadelphia: F. A. Davis.
4. Ayers, D. M., Montgomery, M. (2009). Putting a stop to dysfunctional uterine bleeding. *Nursing*, 39(1), 44–50.
5. Beattie, S. (2007). Bedside emergency: Hemorrhage. *RN*, 70(8), 30–34.
6. Dutton, R. P. (2007). Current concepts in hemorrhagic shock. *Anesthesiol Clin North Am*, 25(1), 23–34.
7. Cabañas, J. G., Manning, J. E., Cairns, C. B. (2011). Fluid and blood resuscitation. *Tintinalli's Emergency Medicine: A Comprehensive Study Guide.* 7th ed. New York: McGraw-Hill.
8. Spahn, D. R., et al. (2006). Management of bleeding following major trauma: A European guideline. *Crit Care*, 11(1), 414.
9. Leeuwen, A. M., Kranpitz, T. R., Smith, L. (2006). *Davis Comprehensive Handbook of Diagnostic Tests with Nursing Implications.* 2nd ed. Philadelphia: F. A. Davis.
10. Smeltzer, M. D. (2010). Making a point about open fractures. *Nursing*, 40(2), 24–30.
11. Bodden, J. (2009). Treatment options in the hemodynamically unstable patient with a pelvic fracture. *Orthop Nurs*, 28(3), 109–114.
12. Kahsai, D. (2015). Acute anemia. Retrieved February 2018 from https://emedicine.medscape.com/article/780334-overview#a2.
13. Udeani, J. (2015). Hemorrhagic shock workup. Retrieved February 2018 from https://emedicine.medscape.com/article/432650-workup.

 Acute Care   Collaborative   Community/ Home Care   Cultural

risk for unstable Blood Glucose Level

Taxonomy II: Nutrition—Class 4 Metabolism (00179) [**Diagnostic Division:** Food/Fluid], Approved 2006; Revised 2013, 2017

DEFINITION: Susceptible to variation in serum levels of glucose from the normal range, which may compromise health.

RISK FACTORS
Average daily physical activity is less than recommended for gender and age
Does not accept diagnosis; insufficient knowledge of diabetes management
Excessive stress
Insufficient diabetes management or nonadherence to diabetes management plan; inadequate blood glucose monitoring; ineffective medication management
Insufficient dietary intake; excessive weight gain or loss
At Risk Population: Alteration in metal status; compromised health status; delay in cognitive development; rapid growth period
Associated Condition: Pregnancy
Sample Clinical Applications: Diabetes mellitus, diabetic ketoacidosis, hypoglycemia, gestational diabetes, corticosteroid use, total parenteral nutrition (TPN)

DESIRED OUTCOMES/EVALUATION CRITERIA

Sample **NOC** linkages:
Knowledge: Diabetes Management: Extent of understanding conveyed about diabetes, its treatment, and the prevention of complications
Diabetes Self-Management: Personal actions to manage diabetes mellitus, its treatment, and to prevent complications
Blood Glucose Level: Extent to which glucose levels in plasma and urine are maintained in normal range

Client/caregiver Will (Include Specific Time Frame)
• Acknowledge factors that may lead to unstable glucose.
• Verbalize understanding of body and energy needs.
• Verbalize plan for modifying factors to prevent or minimize shifts in glucose level.
• Maintain glucose in satisfactory range.

ACTIONS/INTERVENTIONS

Sample **NIC** linkages:
Hyperglycemia Management: Preventing and treating above-normal blood glucose levels
Teaching: Disease Process: Assisting the patient to understand information related to a specific disease process
Teaching: Prescribed Medication: Preparing a patient to safely take prescribed medications and monitor for their effects

 Diagnostic Studies   Evidence Based Practice   Medications   Pediatric/Geriatric/Lifespan

NURSING PRIORITY NO. 1   To assess risk/contributing factors:

- Determine individual factors as listed in Risk Factors. *Client or family history of diabetes, known diabetic with poor glucose control, eating disorders (e.g., morbid obesity), poor exercise habits, and failure to recognize changes in glucose needs or control due to adolescent growth spurts or pregnancy can result in problems with glucose stability.*
- Ascertain client's/significant other's (SO's) knowledge and understanding of condition and treatment needs.
- Identify individual perceptions and expectations of treatment regimen.
- Note influence of cultural, ethnic origin, socioeconomic, or religious factors impacting diabetes recognition and care, including how person with diabetes is viewed by family and community; the seeking and receiving of health care, management of factors such as dietary practices, weight, blood pressure, and lipids; and expectations of outcomes. *These factors influence client's ability to manage condition and must be considered when planning care. Numerous U.S. studies in recent years have not shown consensus on whether or not diabetes manifestations and complications disproportionately affect African Americans and Hispanics compared with non-Hispanic white adults. Some studies show differences in individuals receiving treatment for hyperlipidemia or albuminuria, control of glucose and hypertension, and preventive self-care. Some ethnic groups use folk medicine and popular remedies such as bitter food and herbs to reduce blood sugar; others may practice fasting or prayer. However, because food patterns are learned in family context and have highly symbolic associations, food choices and preparation may be the most difficult aspects of diabetes management.*[9–11]
- Determine client's awareness and ability to be responsible for dealing with situation. *Age, developmental level, and current health status affect client's ability to provide for own safety.*
- Assess client family/SO support of client. *Client may need assistance with lifestyle changes (e.g., food preparation, consumption, timing of intake and/or exercise, administration of medications).*
- Note availability and use of resources.

NURSING PRIORITY NO. 2   To assist client to develop preventative strategies to avoid glucose instability:

- Ascertain whether client and SO(s) are certain they are obtaining accurate readings on glucose-monitoring device and are adept at using device. *In addition to checking blood glucose more frequently when it is unstable, it is wise to ascertain that equipment is functioning properly and being used correctly. All available devices will provide accurate readings if properly used and maintained and routinely calibrated. However, there are many other factors that may affect the accuracy of numbers, such as size of blood drop with finger-sticking, forgetting a bolus from insulin pump, and injecting insulin into lumpy subcutaneous site. Note: Although expensive and not yet widely used because of lagging FDA approval (as of 2015), technology advances include a real-time continuous blood glucose monitoring system for detecting blood glucose trends, as well as a warning system for extreme highs and lows.*[1,13,14]
- Provide information on balancing food intake, antidiabetic agents, and energy expenditure.
- Review medical necessity for regularly scheduled lab screening and monitoring tests for diabetes. *Screening tests may include fasting plasma glucose or oral glucose tolerance tests. In the known or sick diabetic, tests can include fasting, daily (or numerous times in a day) finger-stick glucose levels. Also, in diabetics, regular testing of hemoglobin (Hgb)A_1C and the estimated average glucose help determine glucose control over time (few months). At present, there is no consensus for a hard and fast number; some guidelines state that "HgbA$_1$C level of 6.5%" is diagnostic for a diabetes diagnosis, while others indicate that a level of "less than 7%" is a reasonable goal for many, but not all patients and should be based on individualized assessment of risk for complications.*[12,13]
- Discuss home glucose monitoring according to individual parameters (e.g., six times per day for normal day and more frequently during times of stress) *to identify and manage glucose fluctuations.*

 Acute Care   Collaborative   Community/ Home Care   Cultural

- Identify common situations that could contribute to client's glucose instability on daily, occasional, or crisis basis. *Multiple factors can be in play at any time, such as missing meals, an adolescent growth spurt, or infection or other illness.*
- Review client's diet, especially carbohydrate intake. *Glucose balance is determined by the amount of carbohydrates consumed, which should be determined in needed grams/day.*[2]
- 🏠 Encourage client to read labels and choose carbohydrates described as having a low glycemic index (GI) and foods with adequate protein, higher fiber, and low fat content. *These foods produce a slower rise in blood glucose and more stable release of insulin. Note: For most people with diabetes, the first tool for managing blood glucose is some form of carbohydrate counting. Because the type of carbohydrate also affects glucose, using the GI may be helpful in "fine-tuning" blood glucose management.*[3]
- 💊 Discuss how client's antidiabetic medication(s) work. *Drugs and combinations of drugs work in varying ways with different blood glucose control and side effects. Understanding drug actions can help client avoid or reduce risk of potential for hypoglycemic reactions.*[4]

  For client receiving insulin:
- 💊 Emphasize importance of checking expiration dates of medication, inspecting insulin for cloudiness if it is normally clear, and monitoring proper storage and preparation (when mixing is required). *Affects insulin absorbability and effectiveness.*[1]
- Review type(s) of insulin used (e.g., rapid, short, intermediate, long-acting, combinations, premixed) and delivery method (e.g., subcutaneous, intramuscular injection; prefilled pen; pump). Note time when short-acting and long-acting insulins are administered. Remind client that only short-acting insulin is used in pump. *Affects timing of effects and provides clues to potential timing of glucose instability.*[1,5]
- Check injection sites periodically. *Insulin absorption can vary from day to day in healthy sites and is less absorbable in lumpy sites.*
- ∞ Ascertain that all injections are being given. *Children, teenagers, and elderly clients may forget injections or be unable to self-inject; they may need reminders and supervision.*[1]

NURSING PRIORITY NO. 3 To promote wellness (Teaching/Discharge Considerations):

- 🏠📝 Review individual risk factors and provide information *to assist client in efforts to avoid complications, such as caused by chronic hyperglycemia and acute hypoglycemia. Note: Hyperglycemia is most commonly caused by alterations in nutrition needs, inactivity, or inadequate use of antidiabetic medications. Hypoglycemia is the most common complication of antidiabetic therapy, stress, and exercise.*[1,6–8]
- Emphasize consequences of actions and choices—both immediate and long term.
- Engage client/family/caregiver in formulating a plan *to manage blood glucose level, incorporating lifestyle, age, developmental level, physical and psychological ability to manage condition.*
- 🍎 Consult with dietitian about specific dietary needs based on individual situation (e.g., growth spurt, pregnancy, change in activity level following injury).
- Encourage client to develop a system for self-monitoring *to provide a sense of control and enable client to follow own progress and assist with making choices.*
- 🍎 Refer to appropriate community resources, diabetic educator, and/or support groups as needed *for lifestyle modification, medical management, referral for insulin pump or glucose monitor, financial assistance for supplies, etc.*

DOCUMENTATION FOCUS

Assessment/Reassessment
- Findings related to individual situation, risk factors, current caloric intake, and dietary pattern; prescription medication use; monitoring of condition.
- Client's/caregiver's understanding of individual risks and potential complications.
- Results of laboratory tests and finger-stick testing.

 Diagnostic Studies   Evidence Based Practice   Medications   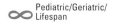 Pediatric/Geriatric/Lifespan

Planning
- Plan of care and who is involved in planning.
- Teaching plan.

Implementation/Evaluation
- Individual responses to interventions, teaching, and actions performed.
- Specific actions and changes that are made.
- Attainment or progress toward desired outcomes.
- Modifications to plan of care.

Discharge Planning
- Long-term plans for ongoing needs, monitoring and management of condition, and who is responsible for actions to be taken.
- Sources for equipment and supplies.
- Specific referrals made.

References

1. Ambler, G. R. (2010). Monitoring diabetes control (Chapter 7). In Cameron, F. J. (ed) *Caring for Diabetes in Children and Adolescents*. 3rd ed. Homebush, NSW: Blue Star Print Group.
2. Moshang, J. (2005). The growing problem of type 2 diabetes. *LPN*, 1(3), 26–34.
3. American Diabetes Association. (Updated 2014). Glycemic index and diabetes. Retrieved February 2018 from http://www.diabetes.org/food-and-fitness/food/what-can-i-eat/understanding-carbohydrates/glycemic-index-and-diabetes.html.
4. Dansinger, M. (reviewer) (2016). New type 2 diabetes treatment options. Retrieved February 2018 from https://www.webmd.com/diabetes/features/new-diabetes-medications#1.
5. Mathur, R. (2011). Insulin therapy for diabetes: Past, present and future. Retrieved February 2018 from http://www.medicinenet.com/script/main/art.asp?articlekey=11441.
6. Iscoe, K. E., et al. (2006). Efficacy of continuous real-time blood glucose monitoring during and after prolonged high-intensity cycling exercise: Spinning with a continuous glucose monitoring system. *Diabetes Technol Ther*, 8(6), 627–635.
7. McLeod, M. E. (2006). Interventions for clients with diabetes mellitus. In Ignativicius, D. D., Workman, M. L. (eds). *Medical-Surgical Nursing: Critical Thinking for Collaborative Care*. 5th ed. Philadelphia: Elsevier Saunders.
8. Asp, A. A. (2005). Diabetes mellitus. In Copstead, L. C., Banasik, J. L. (eds). *Pathophysiology*. 3rd ed. Philadelphia: Elsevier Saunders.
9. Bonds, D. E., et al. (2004). Ethnic and racial differences in diabetes care: The insulin resistance atherosclerosis study. *Diabetes Care*, 26(4), 1040–1046.
10. Kirk, J. K., et al. (2008). Disparities in A_1C levels between Hispanic and non-Hispanic white adults with diabetes: A meta-analysis. *Diabetes Care*, 31(2), 240–246.
11. Nwasuruba, C., et al. (2009). Racial differences in diabetes self-management and quality of care in Texas. *J Diabetes Complications*, 23(2), 112–118.
12. Quaseem, A., et al. (2007). Glycemic control and type 2 diabetes mellitus: The optimal hemoblogin A_1 C targets: A guidance statement from the American College of Physicians. *Ann Intern Med*, 147(6), 417–422.
13. Ramchandani, N., Saadon, Y., Jornsay, D. (2010). Diabetes under control: Real-time glucose monitoring. *Am J Nurs*, 110(4), 60–63.
14. Tucker, M. E. (2011). Continuous glucose monitors: In real time. Retrieved February 2018 from http://www.diabetesforecast.org/2015/mar-apr/continuous-glucose-monitors-in-real-time.html.
15. Khardori, R. (2018). Type 2 diabetes mellitus workup. Retrieved February 2018 from https://emedicine.medscape.com/article/117853-workup.

 Acute Care   Collaborative Community/Home Care   Cultural

risk for unstable Blood Pressure

Taxonomy II: Activity/Rest—Class 4 Cardiovascular/pulmonary Responses Physical Injury (00267) [Diagnostic Division: Circulation], Approved 2016

DEFINITION: Susceptible to fluctuating forces of blood flowing through arterial vessels, which may compromise health.

RISK FACTORS

Inconsistency with medication regimen

Orthostasis

Associated Condition: Adverse effects of cocaine, or nonsteroidal anti-inflammatory drugs (NSAIDS), or steroids

Cardiac dysrhythmia; rapid absorption and distribution of antiarrhythmia agent or vasodilator agents

Cushing syndrome; hormonal change; hyperparathyroidism; hyper- or hypothyroidism

Electrolyte imbalance; fluid retention; fluid shifts; hyperosmolar solutions

Increased intracranial pressure

Sympathetic responses

Use of antidepressant agents

This nursing diagnosis encompasses assessments and nursing interventions found in many other nursing diagnoses. For specific related information, refer to NDs, decreased intracranial Adaptive Capacity; risk for Allergy Reaction; Autonomic Dysreflexia, risk for Bleeding; risk for decreased Cardiac Output; risk for Electrolyte Imbalance; deficient Knowledge; risk for Electrolyte Imbalance; deficient Fluid Volume; excess Fluid Volume; Hyperthermia; risk for Infection; risk for Shock

Sample Clinical Applications: Adrenal crisis, primary aldosteronism, anemia; brain injury; burns; cardiogenic shock; cerebrovascular accident (CVA/stroke); pregnancy; childbirth/delivery; diabetic ketoacidosis; dialysis; drug overdose; acute kidney injury; eating disorders (anorexia/bulimia); sepsis/septicemia; shock (various types); spinal cord injury; surgery; trauma

DESIRED OUTCOMES/EVALUATION CRITERIA

Sample NOC linkages:

Cardiac Pump Effectiveness: Adequacy of blood volume ejected from the left ventricle to support systemic perfusion pressure

Symptom Control: Personal actions to minimize perceived adverse changes in physical and emotional functioning

Client/Caregiver Will

• Maintain blood pressure within acceptable limits
• Experience no cardiovascular or systemic complications
• Verbalize understanding of condition, therapeutic regimen, and preventive measures
• Initiate necessary lifestyle/behavioral changes

ACTIONS/INTERVENTIONS

Sample NIC linkages:

Hypertension Management: Preventing and treating blood pressure levels higher than normal

Hypotension Management: Preventing and treating blood pressure levels lower than normal

Medication Management: Facilitating safe and effective use of prescription and over-the-counter drugs

 Diagnostic Studies   Evidence Based Practice   Medications   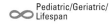 Pediatric/Geriatric/Lifespan

NURSING PRIORITY NO. 1   To identify contributing risk factors:

- Identify presence of associated conditions, for example, (1) cardiac dysfunction [including myocardial infarction, dysrhythmias, heart failure, cardiomyopathy]; (2) brain injury [including traumatic injury, stroke]; (3) fluid imbalances [either deficit or excess] and electrolyte imbalances; (4) endocrine disorders [e.g., primary aldosteronism, adrenal gland tumors, thyroid issues]; (5) acute or chronic renal disease; (6) trauma [causing damage to central and autonomic systems, including spinal cord injury]; (7) fever [such as accompanies infections/sepsis]; (8) substance use/abuse/overdose [e.g., caffeine, cocaine, other drugs of abuse]; (9) great physical/emotional stress [e.g., traumas causing anxiety, fear/panic]; (10) pregnancy; and (11) allergic reactions *that can cause or exacerbate blood pressure instability.*[1,3]
- Review current medication regimen. *Use of certain medications such as dysrrhythmia agents, vasodilators, antihypertensives, diuretics, tricyclic antidepressants, medications for Parkinson's disease can have direct effect on blood pressure.*[1,3]
- ∞ Determine how client takes medications, whether assistance is provided and by whom. *Blood pressure fluctuations can occur (1) in client who is not taking blood pressure medications as prescribed (e.g., older client living alone who doesn't understand or chooses not to follow directions and takes less or more than prescribed dose); or (2) client is taking medications as prescribed, but failing to report adverse side effects (e.g., blood pressure too low on current dose of amlodipine); (3) caregiver not involved with client medications, does not understand dosing instructions, inadvertently gives incorrect doses, or makes decisions for client (e.g., "my husband doesn't like the way that medication makes him feel, so we stopped the blood pressure medication"); (4) client/caregiver receives inadequate teaching.*[4]
- ∞ Note client age, general health, developmental and cognitive status. *These factors affect client's abilities to manage own symptoms, or respond to emergent conditions affecting blood pressure.*
- ▨ Ascertain client's current and ongoing blood pressure measurements, noting trends and sudden changes. *Note: A recent (2015) systematic review and meta-analysis of multiple studies suggest that greater systolic blood pressure variance measured early from ischemic stroke or intracerebral hemorrhage onset is associated with poor longer-term functional outcome.*[2]
- Measure blood pressure to determine risk for hypertension or hypotension, using the appropriate size and type of equipment, proper position (e.g., seated, legs uncrossed, feet flat on floor), and free of contributing factors such as consumption of caffeine, recent administration of influential medications, agitation). Be aware of numbers that are currently used to identify normal ranges of blood pressure. *Incorrect readings may result in inappropriate or lack of needed treatment.*
- Note client reports of headaches, blurred vision, chest pain, weakness or numbness in arms, legs, or face *which may indicate that blood pressure is elevated (although high blood pressure often fails to produce any noticeable symptoms until damage to the blood vessels result in serious conditions, or blood pressure rise is sudden.*[1]
- Observe for (or assess client/SO reports) sudden high blood pressure. *This condition usually occurs in a small percentage of people with high blood pressure. This can include young adults, including a high number of African American men, and individuals experiencing collagen vascular disorders, kidney issues, or pregnancy.*[3]
- Note client reports of dizziness or fainting, blurred vision, nausea, shortness of breath, thirst *which may indicate that blood pressure is fluctuating downward.*[3]
- Note whether client has potential causes for low blood pressure or hypotension. *The reason (1) may not be pathological (e.g., client reports typical blood pressure lower depending on time of day, or with medication effect; chronic kidney disease) or (2) may be indicative of pathological associated conditions (e.g., heart attack, blood loss, allergic response).*

NURSING PRIORITY NO. 2   To assist client/caregiver to reduce risk:

- Refer for and collaborate in treatment/management of underlying condition(s) *that can restore hemodynamic stability or reduce risk of blood pressure fluctuations.*
- Monitor blood pressure as indicated and evaluate trends. Correlate client's symptoms with potential or identified cause for blood pressure instability.

 Acute Care   Collaborative   Community/ Home Care   Cultural

- Address personal factors (e.g., age and developmental level, social and cultural influences, life experiences, cognitive/emotional/psychological impairment *that require modifications in healthcare management, teaching, and follow-up.*
- Discuss with client/SO those risk factors that are modifiable (e.g., taking medications as prescribed, avoiding substance misuse/[abuse]).
- Recommend changing position from supine to standing slowly and in stages, avoiding standing motionless or for long periods of time, or sitting with legs crossed *to enhance safety and reduce gravitational blood pooling in the lower extremities.*
- Identify available support systems, as needed. *Client or caregiver may need community resources (e.g., home healthcare services, assistance with medication setup/administration, supervision or day care for frail elderly or child).*
- Emphasize importance of regular and long-term medical follow-up appointments *for monitoring blood pressure and disease/condition trends and to provide for early intervention to reduce risk of complications.*
- Refer to appropriate NDs (as listed above) for related interventions.

NURSING PRIORITY NO. 3 To promote wellness (Teaching/Discharge Considerations):

- Determine most urgent need from client's/caregiver's and healthcare provider's viewpoints, *which may differ and require adjustments in teaching plan.*
- Teach home monitoring of blood pressure, where indicated, and obtain return demonstration of ability to take blood pressure (and medications) accurately.
- Recommend client keep diary of pressure readings taken at different times of the day and noting any associated symptoms. *Provides opportunity to follow trends and identify contributing factors such as medication effect.*
- Instruct client/SO in healthy eating and adequate fluid intake. *For example, obesity is a risk factor for hypertension and dehydration is a risk for hypotension. Furthermore, sodium intake can influence blood pressure in hyper- and hypotension.*
- Instruct client/SO in lifestyle modifications based on identified risks. *Exercise program, smoking cessation, stress management techniques, substance use programs not only reduce risk of blood pressure issues but also enhance general well-being.*
- Elicit client's knowledge of reportable blood pressure measurements and symptoms and who to report to. *Provides opportunity for timely intervention.*
- Review specifics and rationale for components of treatment plan. Ask client/SO if he or she has questions and/ or if he or she is willing to adhere to plan. *Helps to identify areas of concern and need for further instruction/ interventions.*
- Refer to specific NDs (as listed above) for related Teaching/Discharge considerations.

DOCUMENTATION FOCUS

Assessment/Reassessment
- Baseline and subsequent blood pressure measurements
- Medications
- Individual risk factors

Planning
- Plan of care and who is involved in planning
- Teaching plan

Implementation/Evaluation
- Client's response to interventions, teaching, and actions performed
- Status and disposition at discharge
- Attainment or progress toward desired outcome(s)
- Modifications to plan of care

 Diagnostic Studies   Evidence Based Practice   Medications   Pediatric/Geriatric/ Lifespan

Discharge Planning
• Discharge considerations and who will be responsible for carrying out individual actions
• Long-term needs and available resources
• Specific referrals made

References

1. Chandler, S. (2017). High & low blood pressure fluctuations. Retrieved May 2018 from https://www.livestrong.com/article/288427-high-low-blood-pressure-fluctuations/.
2. Manning, L. S., et al. (2015). Prognostic significance of short-term blood pressure variability in acute stroke. *Stroke*, 46, 2482–2490.
3. Lockhart, T. (2017). Sudden high blood pressure: Causes, symptoms and prevention tips. Retrieved May 2018 from https://www.livestrong.com/article/288427-high-low-blood-pressure-fluctuations/.
4. Manias, E. (2013). Communication relating to family members' involvement and understandings about patients' medication management in hospital. *Health Expect*, 18, 850–866.

---

disturbed Body Image

Taxonomy II: Self-Perception—Class 3 Body Image (00118) [**Diagnostic Division:** Ego Integrity], Approved 1973; Revised 1998, 2017

DEFINITION: Confusion in [and/or dissatisfaction with] mental picture of one's physical self.

RELATED FACTORS
Alteration in self-perception
Cultural or spiritual incongruence
[Significance of body part or functioning with regard to age, gender, developmental level, or basic human needs]

DEFINING CHARACTERISTICS

Subjective
Alteration in view of one's body; perceptions that reflect an altered view of one's body appearance
Depersonalization of body part or loss by use of impersonal pronouns
Emphasis on remaining strengths
Fear of reaction by others
Focus on past strength, function, or appearance
Negative feeling about body
Personalization of body part/loss by name

Objective
Absence of body part; alteration in body structure or function
Avoids looking at or touching one's body
Behavior of acknowledging or monitoring one's body
Change in ability to estimate spatial relationship of body to environment
Change in lifestyle, social involvement
Extension of body boundary [e.g., includes external object]
Heightened achievement
Hiding or overexposure of body part
Nonverbal response to actual or perceived change in body
Preoccupation with change or loss; refusal to verify change
At Risk Population: Developmental transition

 Acute Care   Collaborative   Community/Home Care   Cultural

Associated Condition: Alteration in body or cognitive functioning; illness; impaired psychosocial functioning; injury; surgical procedure; trauma, treatment regimen

Trauma to nonfunctioning body part

Sample Clinical Applications: Eating disorders (anorexia/bulimia nervosa), traumatic injuries, amputation, ostomies, aging process, arthritis, pregnancy, chronic renal failure, renal dialysis, burns

DESIRED OUTCOMES/EVALUATION CRITERIA

Sample **NOC** linkages:

Body Image: Perception of own appearance and body functions

Self-Esteem: Personal judgment of self-worth

Adaptation to Physical Disability: Personal actions to adapt to a significant functional challenge due to a physical disability

Client Will (Include Specific Time Frames)

- Verbalize acceptance of self in situation (e.g., chronic progressive disease, amputee, decreased independence, weight as is, effects of therapeutic regimen).
- Verbalize relief of anxiety and adaptation to altered body image.
- Verbalize understanding of body changes.
- Recognize and incorporate body image change into self-concept in accurate manner without negating self-esteem.
- Seek information and actively pursue growth.
- Acknowledge self as an individual who has responsibility for self.
- Use adaptive devices or prosthesis appropriately.

ACTIONS/INTERVENTIONS

Sample **NIC** linkages:

Body Image Enhancement: Improving a patient's conscious and unconscious perceptions and attitudes toward his/her body

Developmental Enhancement: Adolescent: Facilitating optimal physical, cognitive, social, and emotional growth of individuals during the transition from childhood to adulthood

Self-Esteem Enhancement: Assisting a patient to increase his or her personal judgment of self-worth

NURSING PRIORITY NO. 1   To assess causative/contributing factors:

- Discuss pathophysiology present or situation affecting the individual and refer to additional NDs, as appropriate. For example, when alteration in body image is related to neurological deficit (e.g., stroke), refer to ND Unilateral Neglect; for presence of severe, ongoing pain, refer to ND chronic Pain; or for loss of sexual desire/ability, refer to ND Sexual Dysfunction.
- Determine whether condition is permanent with no hope for resolution. (May be associated with other NDs such as Self-Esteem [specify] or risk for impaired Attachment when child is affected.) *Identifies appropriate interventions based on reality of situation and need to plan for long- or short-term prognosis. Note: There is always something that can be done to enhance acceptance, and it is important to hold out the possibility of living a good life with the disability.*[1]
- Assess the mental and physical influence of illness or condition on the client's emotional state (e.g., diseases of the endocrine system, use of steroid therapy). *Some diseases or conditions can have a profound effect on one's emotions and need to be considered in the evaluation and treatment of the individual's behavior and reaction to the current situation.*[1,9]

 Diagnostic Studies   Evidence Based Practice   Medications   Pediatric/Geriatric/Lifespan

- Evaluate level of client's knowledge of and anxiety related to situation. Observe emotional changes. *Provides information about starting point for providing information about illness. Emotional changes may indicate level of anxiety and need for intervention to lower anxiety before learning can take place.*[1]
- Recognize behavior indicative of overt preoccupation with body and its processes. *May interfere with ability to engage in therapy and indicate need to provide interventions to deal with concern before beginning therapy.*[2,3]
- Assume all individuals are sensitive to changes in appearance, but avoid stereotyping. *Not all individuals react to body changes in the same way, and it is important to determine how this person is reacting to changes.*[2,3]
- Have client describe self, noting what is positive and what is negative. Be aware of how client believes others see self. *Identifies self-image and whether there is a discrepancy between own view, how client's view is affected by social media, or how client believes others see him or her, which may have an effect on how client perceives changes that have occurred.*[3,4]
- ∞ Discuss meaning of loss or change to client. *A small (seemingly trivial) loss may have a big impact (such as the use of a urinary catheter or enema for bowel continence). A change in function (such as immobility) may be more difficult for some to deal with than a change in appearance. Permanent facial scarring of child may be difficult for parents to accept.*[1]
- ∞ Use developmentally appropriate communication techniques for determining exact expression of body image in child (e.g., puppet play or constructive dialogue for toddler). *Developmental capacity must guide interaction to gain accurate information.*
- Note signs of grieving or indicators of severe or prolonged depression. *May require evaluation of need for counseling or medications.*[3]
- ⊕ Determine ethnic background and cultural or religious perceptions and considerations. *Understanding how these factors affect the individual in this situation and how they may influence how individual deals with what has happened is necessary to develop appropriate interventions.*[5]
- Identify social aspects of illness or disease. *Sexually transmitted infections, sterility, or chronic conditions (e.g., vitiligo, multiple sclerosis) may affect how client views self and functions in social settings and how others view the client.*[2,8]
- Observe interaction of client with significant others (SOs). *Distortions in body image may be unconsciously reinforced by family members, or secondary gain issues may interfere with progress.*[2,8]

NURSING PRIORITY NO. 2. To determine coping abilities and skills:

- Assess client's current level of adaptation and progress. *Client may have already adapted somewhat, and information provides starting point for developing plan of care.*[2]
- Listen to client's comments and note responses to the situation. *Different situations are upsetting to different people, depending on individual coping skills, severity of the perceived changes in body image, and past experiences with similar illnesses/conditions.*[2–4,8]
- ▨ Note withdrawn behavior and the use of denial. *May be normal response to situation or may be indicative of mental illness (e.g., depression, schizophrenia).*[6] (Refer to ND ineffective Denial.)
- ⚕ Note dependence on prescription medications or use of addictive substances/alcohol. *May reflect dysfunctional coping as client turns to use of these substances to avoid dealing with changes that are occurring to body or ability to function in his or her accustomed manner.*[6]
- Identify previously used coping strategies and effectiveness. *Familiar coping strategies can be used to begin adaptation to current situation.*[2]
- ⊕ Determine individual/family/community resources. *Can provide efficient assistance and support to enable the client to adapt to changing circumstances.*

NURSING PRIORITY NO. 3 To assist client and SO(s) to deal with/accept issues of self-concept related to body image:

- Establish a therapeutic nurse-client relationship. *Conveys an attitude of caring and develops a sense of trust in which client can discuss concerns and find answers to issues confronting him or her in new situation.*[4,8]

 Acute Care   Collaborative   Community/ Home Care   Cultural

- Visit client frequently and acknowledge the individual as someone who is worthwhile. *Provides opportunities for listening to concerns and questions to promote dealing positively with individual situation and change in body image.*[1]
- Assist in correcting underlying problems when possible. *Promotes optimal healing and adaptation to individual situation (i.e., amputation, presence of colostomy, mastectomy, impotence).*[1]
- Provide assistance with self-care needs or measures, as necessary, while promoting individual abilities and independence. *Client may need support to achieve the goal of independence and positive return to managing own life.*
- Work with client's self-concept without moral judgments regarding client's efforts or progress (e.g., "You should be progressing faster; you're weak, lazy, not trying hard enough"). *Such statements diminish self-esteem and are counterproductive to progress. Positive reinforcement encourages client to continue efforts and strive for improvement.*[2,8]
- Discuss concerns about fear of mutilation, prognosis, and rejection when client is facing surgery or potentially poor outcome of procedure or illness. *Addresses realities and provides emotional support to enable client to be ready to deal with whatever the outcome may be.*[1]
- Acknowledge and accept feelings of dependency, grief, and hostility. *Conveys a message of understanding.*[1]
- Encourage verbalization of and role-play anticipated conflicts *to enhance handling of potential situations. Provides an opportunity to imagine and practice how different situations can be dealt with, thus promoting confidence.*[4]
- Encourage client and SO(s) to communicate feelings to each other and discuss situation openly. *Enhances relationship, improving sense of self-worth and sense of support.*[2]
- Alert staff to be cognizant of own facial expressions and other nonverbal behaviors. *Important to convey acceptance and not revulsion, especially when the client's appearance is affected. Clients are very sensitive to reactions of those around them, and negative reactions will affect self-esteem and may retard adaptation to situation.*[1]
- Encourage family members to treat client normally and not as an invalid. *Helps client return to own routine and begin to gain confidence in ability to manage own life.*[1]
- Encourage client to look at and touch affected body part *to begin to incorporate changes into body image. Acceptance will enhance self-esteem and enable client to move forward in a positive manner.*[1,7]
- Allow client to use denial without participating (e.g., client may at first refuse to look at a colostomy; the nurse says, "I am going to change your colostomy now" and proceeds with the task). *Provides individual time to adapt to situation.*[4]
- Set limits on maladaptive behavior; assist client to identify positive behaviors. *Self-esteem will be damaged if client is allowed to continue behaviors that are destructive or not helpful, and adaptation to new image will be delayed.*[4,10]
- Provide accurate information, as desired or requested. Reinforce previously given information. *Accurate knowledge helps client make better decisions for the future.*[4]
- Discuss the availability of prosthetics, reconstructive surgery, and physical and occupational therapy or other referrals, as dictated by individual situation. *Provides hope that situation is not impossible and the future does not look so bleak.*[1,7,8]
- Help client to select and creatively use clothing or makeup *to minimize body changes and enhance appearance.*[1]
- Discuss reasons for infectious isolation and procedures when used, and make time to sit down and talk or listen to client while in the room. *Promotes understanding and decreases sense of isolation and loneliness.*[1]

NURSING PRIORITY NO. 4 To promote wellness (Teaching/Discharge Considerations):

- Begin counseling or other therapies (e.g., biofeedback or relaxation techniques) as soon as possible. *Provides early and ongoing sources of support to promote rehabilitation in a timely manner.*[1]
- Provide information at client's level of acceptance and in small segments. *Allows for easier assimilation.*[1,2,7]

 Diagnostic Studies   Evidence Based Practice   Medications   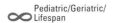 Pediatric/Geriatric/Lifespan

- Clarify misconceptions and reinforce explanations given by other health team members. *Ensures client is hearing factual information to make the best decisions for own situation.*[1,2,7]
- Include client in decision-making process and problem-solving activities. *Promotes adherence to decisions and plans that are made.*[1]
- Assist client to incorporate therapeutic regimen into activities of daily living (e.g., specific exercises, housework activities). *Promotes continuation of program by helping client see that progress can be made within own daily activities.*[1]
- Identify and plan for alterations to home and work environment or activities when necessary. *Accommodates individual needs and supports independence.*[1]
- Assist client in learning strategies for dealing with feelings and venting emotions. *Helps individual move toward healing and optimal recuperation.*[1,2]
- Offer positive reinforcement for efforts made (e.g., wearing makeup, using prosthetic device). *Client needs to hear that what he or she is doing is helping.*[1,9]
- Refer to appropriate support groups. *May need additional help to adjust to new situation and life changes.*[1]

DOCUMENTATION FOCUS

Assessment/Reassessment
- Observations, presence of maladaptive behaviors, emotional changes, stage of grieving, level of independence.
- Physical wounds, dressings; use of life support–type machine (e.g., ventilator, dialysis machine).
- Meaning of loss or change to client.
- Support systems available (e.g., SOs, friends, groups).

Planning
- Plan of care and who is involved in planning.
- Teaching plan.

Implementation/Evaluation
- Client's response to interventions, teaching, and actions performed.
- Attainment or progress toward desired outcome(s).
- Modifications of plan of care.

Discharge Planning
- Long-term needs and who is responsible for actions.
- Specific referrals made (e.g., rehabilitation center, community resources).

References

1. Tagkalakis, P., Demiri, E. (2009). A fear avoidance model in facial burn body image disturbance. *Ann Burns Fire Disasters*, 22(4), 203–207.
2. No author listed. (2009). Body image. *Women's Health*. Retrieved March 2018 fromhttp://www.womenshealth.gov/body-image/.
3. Kilic, E., et al. (2007). The effect of permanent ostomy on body image, self-esteem, marital adjustment, and sexual functioning. *Turk Psikiyatri Derg*, 18(4), 302–310.
4. Simmons, R. (2016). How social media is a toxic mirror. *Time.com*. Retrieved March 2018 from http://time.com/4459153/social-media-body-image/.
5. George, J. B., Franko, D. L. (2010). Cultural issues in eating pathology and body image among children and adolescents. *J Pediatr Psychol*, 35(3), 231–242.
6. Pimenta, A. M., et al. (2009). Relationship between body image disturbance and incidence of depression: The SUN prospective cohort. *BMC Public Health*, 9(1), 1471–2458.
7. Aacovou, I. (2005). The role of the nurse in the rehabilitation of patients with radical changes in body image due to burn injuries. *Ann Burns Fire Disasters*, 18(2), 89–94.
8. Breakey, J. W. (1997). Body image: The inner mirror. *J Prosthet Orthot*, 9(3), 107–112.
9. Kater, K. (Updated 2012). Body image health (various pages). Retrieved March 2018 from http://bodyimagehealth.org/model-for-healthy-body-image/.
10. Brandon, N. (2016). What self-esteem is and is not. *National Association for Self-Esteem*. Retrieved March 2018 from http://healthyselfesteem.org/what-self-esteem-is-and-is-not/.

 Acute Care   Collaborative   Community/Home Care   Cultural

ineffective Breastfeeding

Taxonomy II: Nutrition—Class 1 Ingestion (00104) **[Diagnostic Division:** Food/Fluid], Approved 1988; Revised 2010, 2013, 2017

DEFINITION: Difficulty feeding milk from the breasts, which may compromise nutritional status of the infant/child.

RELATED FACTORS
Insufficient parental knowledge regarding importance of breastfeeding or breastfeeding techniques
Insufficient opportunity for suckling at the breast; inadequate milk supply; delayed stage II lactogenesis
Poor infant sucking reflex
Supplemental feedings with artificial nipple; pacifier use
Maternal anxiety or ambivalence, fatigue, pain, obesity
Interrupted breastfeeding
Maternal breast anomaly
Insufficient family support

DEFINING CHARACTERISTICS

Subjective
Sore nipples persisting beyond the first week of breastfeeding
Insufficient emptying of each breast per feeding
Perceived inadequate milk supply

Objective
Infant inability to latch on to maternal breast correctly; unsustained suckling at the breast
Infant arching or crying at the breast; resisting latching on to breast
Infant crying within the first hour after breastfeeding; fussing within 1 hour of breastfeeding; unresponsive to other comfort measures
Insufficient signs of oxytocin release
Inadequate infant stooling
Insufficient infant weight gain; sustained infant weight loss
At Risk Population: Prematurity; previous breast surgery; previous history of breastfeeding failure; short maternity leave
Associated Condition: Oropharyngeal defect [e.g., cleft palate/lip; ankyloglossia (tongue-tied)]
Sample Clinical Applications: Prematurity, cleft lip/palate, ankyloglossia, Down's syndrome, child abuse or neglect, failure to thrive, diseases/infections of the breast

DESIRED OUTCOMES/EVALUATION CRITERIA

Sample **NOC** linkages:
Knowledge: Breastfeeding: Extent of understanding conveyed about lactation and nourishment of infant through breastfeeding
Breastfeeding Establishment: Maternal [or] Infant: Maternal establishment of proper attachment of an infant to and sucking from the breast for nourishment during the first 3 weeks of breastfeeding/infant attachment to and sucking from the mother's breast for nourishment during the first 3 weeks of breastfeeding
Breastfeeding Maintenance: Continuation of breastfeeding from establishment to weaning for nourishment of an infant/toddler

(continues on page 110)

 Diagnostic Studies
 Evidence Based Practice
 Medications
 Pediatric/Geriatric/ Lifespan

ineffective Breastfeeding (continued)

Client Will (Include Specific Time Frame)
• Verbalize understanding of causative or contributing factors.
• Demonstrate techniques to enhance breastfeeding experience.
• Assume responsibility for effective breastfeeding.
• Achieve mutually satisfactory breastfeeding regimen with infant content after feedings, gaining weight appropriately, and output within normal range.

ACTIONS/INTERVENTIONS

Sample NIC linkages:
Lactation Counseling: Assisting in the establishment and maintenance of successful breastfeeding
Support Group: Use of a group environment to provide emotional support and health-related information for members

NURSING PRIORITY NO. 1 To identify maternal causative/contributing factors:

• Assess client knowledge about breastfeeding and extent of instruction previously received. *Provides baseline information for identifying needs and developing plan of care.*[1,7]
• Identify cultural expectations and conflicts about breastfeeding and beliefs or practices *Various differences are possible regarding lactation, let-down techniques, and maternal food preferences.*
• ∞ Note incorrect myths/misunderstandings especially in teenage mothers, *who are more likely to have limited knowledge and more concerns about body image issues.*
• Encourage discussion of current and previous breastfeeding experience(s). *Identifies current needs and problems encountered to develop a plan of care.*[5]
• Note previous unsatisfactory experience (including self or others). *Often unsolved problems and stories told by others may cause doubt about chance for success.*[1]
• Perform physical assessment, noting appearance of breasts and nipples, marked asymmetry of breasts, obvious inverted or flat nipples, and minimal or no breast enlargement during pregnancy. *Identifies existing problems that may interfere with successful breastfeeding experience and provides opportunity to correct them when possible.*[1,7]
• Determine whether lactation failure is <u>primary</u> (i.e., maternal prolactin deficiency/serum prolactin levels, inadequate mammary gland tissue, breast surgery that has damaged the nipple, areola enervation, pituitary disorders) or <u>secondary</u> (i.e., sore nipples, severe engorgement, plugged milk ducts, mastitis, inhibition of letdown reflex, maternal/infant separation with disruption of feedings). *Primary failure may be irremediable, and alternate plans may need to be made. Secondary failure can be remedied so breastfeeding efforts can be successful.*[5] *Note: Overweight women and obese women are 2.5 times and 3.6 times, respectively, less successful in initiating breastfeeding than the general population.*[9]
• Note history of pregnancy, labor, and delivery (vaginal or cesarean section); other recent or current surgery; preexisting medical problems (e.g., diabetes mellitus, seizure disorder, cardiac diseases, presence of disabilities); or if client is adoptive mother. *While some conditions may preclude breastfeeding and alternate plans need to be made, others will need specific plans for monitoring and treatment to ensure successful breastfeeding.*[5]
• Identify maternal support systems and presence and response of significant other (SO), extended family, and friends. *Infant's father and maternal grandmother (in addition to caring healthcare providers) are important factors in whether breastfeeding is successful.*[8] *Having sufficient support enhances opportunity for a successful breastfeeding experience. Negative attitudes and comments interfere with efforts and may cause client to abandon attempt to breastfeed.*[5]

 Acute Care   Collaborative   Community/ Home Care   Cultural

- Ascertain mother's age, number of children at home, and need to return to work or school. *These factors may have a detrimental effect on desire to breastfeed. Immaturity may influence mother to avoid breastfeeding, believing that it will be inconvenient, or may cause her to be insensitive to the infant's needs. The stress of the responsibility of other children or the need to return to work can affect the ability to manage effective breastfeeding; mother will need support and information to be successful.*[6]
- Determine maternal feelings (e.g., fear, anxiety, ambivalence, depression). *Indicators of underlying emotional state that may suggest need for intervention and referral.*[1]
- Ascertain cultural expectations or conflicts about breastfeeding and beliefs and practices regarding lactation, letdown techniques, and maternal food preferences. *Understanding impact of culture and idiosyncrasies of specific feeding practices is important to determine the effect on infant feeding. The practice may be different but not inferior. For example, in many cultures, such as Mexican American, Navajo, and Vietnamese, colostrum is not offered to the newborn. Intervention is only necessary if the practice/belief is harmful to the infant.*[1,3,8]
- ∞ Note incorrect myths or misunderstandings, especially in teenage mothers *who are more likely to have limited knowledge and more concerns about body image issues.*[8]

NURSING PRIORITY NO. 2 To assess infant causative/contributing factors:

- Determine suckling problems or infant anomaly (e.g., cleft lip/palate). *These factors indicate need for interventions directed at correcting individual situation. Conditions such as cleft palate need evaluation for correction and individualized instruction in holding infant upright and using special nipple or feeding device, such as a Haberman feeder.*[1,2] *Note: One study indicated that about one-half of mothers in the study were unable to breastfeed infants with cleft lip and/or palate.*[14]
- Note prematurity. *Degree of prematurity will dictate type of interventions needed to deal with situation. Infant may be put to breast if sufficiently developed or mother may pump breast and the breast milk given via gavage. If infant breastfeeds, mother should pump afterward because the premature infant's suck cannot empty breast.*[2]
- Encourage mother to keep a log of intake and output. Review feeding schedule to note increased demand for feeding (at least eight times/day, taking both breasts at each feeding for more than 15 min on each side) or use of supplements with artificial nipple. *Provides opportunity to evaluate infant's growth, determine whether sufficient nourishment is provided, and make adjustments as needed.*[2]
- Evaluate baby latching and note observable signs of inadequate infant intake. *Inadequate latching, baby latching onto mother's nipples with sustained suckling but minimal audible swallowing noted, infant arching and crying at the breasts with resistance to latching on, decreased urinary output/frequency of stools, and inadequate weight gain all indicate need for evaluation and intervention.*[1,7]
- Determine whether baby is content after feeding or exhibits fussiness and crying within the first hour after breastfeeding. *Suggests unsatisfactory breastfeeding process.*[1]
- Note any correlation between maternal ingestion of certain foods and "colicky" response of infant. *Some foods may seem to result in reaction by the infant, and identification and elimination may correct the problem.*[2]

NURSING PRIORITY NO. 3 To assist mother to develop skills of successful breastfeeding:

- Provide emotional support to mother. Use one-to-one instruction with each feeding during hospital stay/clinic visit. *New mothers say they would like more support, encouragement, and practical information, especially when they are discharged early. Contact during each feeding provides the opportunity to develop nurse-client relationship in which these goals can be attained.*[1] *Note: Adoptive mothers choosing to breastfeed will require more supportive instruction from a lactation consultant to assist with induced lactation techniques.*[8]
- Encourage skin-to-skin or kangaroo care, especially for the premature infant. *Studies show that early skin-to-skin mother-infant contact is correlated with exclusive breastfeeding while in the hospital.*[16,21]
- Inform mother how to assess and correct a latch if needed. Demonstrate asymmetric latch by aiming infant's lower lip as far from base of the nipple as possible and then bringing infant's chin and lower jaw in contact with breast while mouth is wide open and before upper lip touches breast. *This position allows infant to use both tongue and jaw more effectively to obtain milk from the breast.*[17,21]

- Discuss early infant feeding cues (e.g., rooting, lip smacking, sucking fingers or hand) versus the late cue of crying. *New mothers may not be aware that these behaviors indicate hunger and may not respond appropriately. Early recognition of infant hunger promotes timely and more rewarding feeding experience for infant and mother.*[1,8]
- Recommend avoidance or overuse of supplemental bottle feedings and pacifiers (unless specifically indicated). *These can lessen infant's desire to breastfeed. The shape of the mouth and lips and the sucking mechanism are different for breast and bottle, and the infant may be confused by the difference, causing interference in the breastfeeding process and increasing risk of early weaning. Note: Adoptive mothers may not develop a full breast milk supply, necessitating supplemental feedings.*[1,8]
- Restrict use of nipple shields (i.e., only temporarily to help draw the nipple out) and then place baby directly on nipple. *These have been found to contribute to lactation failures. Shields prevent the infant's mouth from coming into contact with the mother's nipple, which is necessary for continued release of prolactin (promoting milk production) and can interfere with or prevent establishment of adequate milk supply. However, temporary use of shield may be beneficial in the presence of severe nipple cracking. Hand pumps can also help draw a flat nipple out before latching.*[6]
- Discuss and demonstrate breastfeeding aids (e.g., infant sling, nursing footstool, or pillows) and suggest using a variety of nursing positions *to find the most comfortable ones for mother and infant. Positions particularly helpful for "plus-sized" women or those with large breasts include the "football" hold, with infant's head to mother's breast and body curved around behind her, or lying down to nurse.*[10]
- ▧ Encourage frequent rest periods, sharing household and childcare duties. *The new mother may feel overwhelmed with taking care of infant and carrying out other household duties; having assistance can limit fatigue and facilitate relaxation at feeding times.*[6] *Note: Research suggests a correlation between psychological stress and development of breast disease (e.g., breast pain, milk stasis, mastitis) leading to early weaning.*[19]
- Suggest abstinence or restriction of tobacco, caffeine, alcohol, drugs, and excess sugar, as appropriate. *May affect milk production/letdown reflex and can be passed on to the infant.*[1]
- Promote early management of breastfeeding problems. *Dealing with problems in a timely manner will promote successful breastfeeding.*[1,7]

  For example:

Engorgement: Wear supportive bra; apply heat or cool applications to the breasts and massage from chest wall down to nipple; soothe "fussy baby" before latching on the breast and properly position baby on breast/nipple; alternate the side on which baby starts nursing; nurse round the clock or pump with piston-type electric breast pump with bilateral collection chambers at least 8 to 12 times/day; and avoid using bottle, pacifier, or supplements.[13]

Sore nipples: Wear 100% cotton fabrics, do not use soap/alcohol/drying agents on nipples, and avoid use of nipple shields or nursing pads that contain plastic; cleanse and pat dry with a clean cloth; apply thin layer of highly purified anhydrous (HPA) lanolin on nipple. *Note:* This cream is edible and does not need to be removed before breastfeeding.[12,18] Administer a mild pain reliever as appropriate. Infant should latch on least sore side or begin with hand expression to establish letdown reflex, properly position infant on breast and nipple, and use a variety of nursing positions. Break suction after breastfeeding is complete.

Clogged ducts: Use larger bra or extender to avoid pressure on site; use moist or dry heat and gently massage from above plug down to nipple; nurse infant, hand express, or pump after massage; and nurse more often on affected side.

Inhibited letdown: Use relaxation techniques before nursing (e.g., maintain quiet atmosphere, massage, apply heat to breasts, have beverage available, assume position of comfort, place infant on mother's chest, skin-to-skin). Encourage mother to relax and enjoy her baby.

Mastitis: Promote bedrest (with infant) for several days; administer antibiotics; provide warm, moist heat before and during nursing; and empty breasts completely, continuing to nurse baby at least 8 to 12 times/day, or pumping breasts for 24 hours, and then resuming breastfeeding as appropriate.

- ▧ Demonstrate use of hand expression, hand pump, and electric piston-type breast pump with bilateral collection chamber when necessary to maintain or increase milk supply. *Note: Studies indicate that mothers taught*

 Acute Care   Collaborative   Community/ Home Care   Cultural

hands-on pumping increased the mean daily volume of milk by 48%.[20] *The need to use a pump to store milk for feedings while the mother is away (i.e., going back to work or simply to allow time away from the infant) demands some degree of proficiency in the use of the pump.*[1]

NURSING PRIORITY NO. 4 To condition infant to breastfeed:

- Scent breast pad with breast milk and leave in bed with infant along with mother's photograph when separated from mother for medical purposes (e.g., prematurity).
- Increase skin-to-skin contact (kangaroo care).
- Provide practice times at breast for infant to "lick and learn."
- Express small amounts of milk into baby's mouth.
- Have mother pump breast after feeding to enhance milk production.
- Use supplemental nutrition system cautiously when necessary.
- Identify special interventions for feeding in presence of cleft lip/palate.
  These measures promote optimal interaction between mother and infant and provide adequate nourishment for the infant, enhancing successful breastfeeding.[1,21]

NURSING PRIORITY NO. 5 To promote wellness (Teaching/Discharge Considerations):

- Schedule follow-up visits with healthcare provider 24 to 48 hours after hospital discharge and 2 weeks after birth. *Provides opportunity to evaluate milk intake and breastfeeding process and adequacy of home situation and to answer mother's questions.*[2]
- Recommend monitoring number of infant's wet and soiled diapers. *Stools should be yellow in color and infant should have at least six wet diapers a day to determine that infant is receiving sufficient intake.*[6]
- Weigh infant at least every third day initially as indicated and record. *Provides record of appropriate weight gain verifying adequacy of nutritional intake or indicates need for evaluation of insufficient weight gain.*[1] *Note: Most infants lose 5% to 7% of their birth weight in the first few days of life.*[12]
- Educate father/SO about benefits of breastfeeding and how to manage common lactation challenges. *Enlisting support of father/SO is associated with higher ratio of successful breastfeeding at 6 months.*[11]
- Discuss with spouse/SO mother's need for rest, relaxation, and time together with spouse and with other children as appropriate. *Promotes understanding of mother's needs and cooperation with incorporation of new member into family. Spouse and children feel included when they have time alone with mother and are more willing to allow mother time with infant and for herself.*[4]
- Instruct in use of relaxation techniques. *Facilitates release of oxytocin improving milk removal.*[21]
- Promote peer and cultural group counseling for teen mothers. *Provides positive role model that teen can relate to and feel comfortable with discussing concerns and feelings.*[8]
- Discuss importance of adequate nutrition and fluid intake, prenatal vitamins, or other vitamin or mineral supplements, such as vitamin C, as indicated. *During lactation, there is an increased need for energy, and supplementation of protein, minerals, and vitamins is necessary to provide nourishment for the infant and to protect mother's stores, along with extra fluid intake. Alternating different types of fluid, water, juices, decaffeinated tea, and milk can help mother promote sufficient intake. Beer and wine are not recommended for increasing lactation.*[4]
- Address specific problems (e.g., suckling problems, prematurity, anomalies). *Individualized planning can enhance mother's understanding and ability to manage situation.*[1,7]
- Discuss timing of introduction of solid foods and importance of delaying until infant is at least 4 months, preferably 6 months old. *American Academy of Pediatrics and the World Health Organization recommend delaying solids until at least 6 months. If supplementation is necessary, infant can be finger fed, spoon fed, cup fed, or syringe fed.*[10,15]
- Inform mother that the return of menses varies in nursing mothers and usually averages 3 to 36 weeks with ovulation returning in 17 to 28 weeks. *Return of menstruation does not affect breastfeeding, and breastfeeding is not a reliable method of birth control.*[1]

 Diagnostic Studies   Evidence Based Practice   Medications   Pediatric/Geriatric/ Lifespan

- Refer to support groups (e.g., La Leche League, parenting support groups, stress reduction, or other community resources as indicated). *Provides information and visible support for ensuring an effective outcome.*[5]
- Provide bibliotherapy and appropriate Web sites for further information. *Additional resources to assist mother and family to learn and apply new skills.*[1]

DOCUMENTATION FOCUS

Assessment/Reassessment
- Identified assessment factors, both maternal and infant (e.g., is engorgement present, is infant demonstrating adequate weight gain without supplementation).

Planning
- Plan of care, specific interventions, and who is involved in planning.
- Teaching plan.

Implementation/Evaluation
- Mother's/infant's responses to interventions, teaching, and actions performed.
- Changes in infant's weight and output.
- Attainment or progress toward desired outcome(s).
- Modifications to plan of care.

Discharge Planning
- Referrals that have been made and mother's choice of participation.

References

1. Ladewig, P., London, M., Davidson, M. (2009). *Contemporary Maternal-Newborn Nursing Care*. 7th ed. Upper Saddle River, NJ: Prentice Hall.
2. Riodan, J., Auerbach, K. (2010). *Breastfeeding and Human Lactation*. 4th ed. Boston: Jones & Bartlett.
3. Purnell, L. D. (2011). *Guide to Culturally Competent Health Care*. 2nd ed. Philadelphia: F. A. Davis.
4. Lowdermilk, D. L., Cashion, M. C., Perry, S. E. (2011). *Maternity & Women's Health Care*. 10th ed. St. Louis, MO: Mosby.
5. Doenges, M., Moorhouse, M. (1999). *Maternal/Newborn Plans of Care: Guidelines for Individualizing Care*. 3rd ed. Philadelphia: F. A. Davis.
6. Phillips, C. R. (1996). *Family-Centered Maternity and Newborn Care*. 4th ed. St. Louis, MO: Mosby.
7. London, M. L., et al. (2010). *Maternal and Child Nursing Care*. 3rd ed. Upper Saddle River, NJ: Prentice Hall.
8. American Academy of Family Physicians. Breastfeeding (Position paper) with Appendices updates. Retrieved March 2018 from www.aafp.org/about/policies/all/breastfeeding-support .html.
9. Oddy, W. H., et al. (2006). The association of maternal overweight and obesity with breastfeeding duration. *J Pediatr*, 149(2), 185–191.
10. American Academy of Pediatrics. (Revised 2013). Ten steps to support parents' choice to breastfeed their baby. Retrieved March 2018 from https://www.aap.org/en-us/advocacy-and-policy/aap-health-initiatives/Breastfeeding/Documents/tenstepsposter.pdf.
11. Pisacane, A., et al. (2005). A controlled trial of the father's role in breastfeeding promotion. *Pediatrics*, 116(4), e494–e498.
12. Lawrence, R. A., Lawrence, R. M. (2005). *Breastfeeding: A Guide for the Medical Profession*. 6th ed. St. Louis, MO: Mosby.
13. Morbacher, N., Kendall-Tackett, K. (2010). *Breastfeeding Made Simple: Seven Natural Laws for Nursing Mothers*. 2nd ed. Oakland, CA.: New Harbinger.
14. Trenouth, M. J., Campbell, A. N. (1996). Questionnaire evaluation of feeding methods for cleft lip and palate neonates. *Int J Pediatr Dent*, 6(4), 241–244.
15. World Health Organization. (reviewed 2015). Up to what age can a baby stay well nourished by just being breastfed? Retrieved March 2018 from http://www.who.int/features/qa/21/en/.
16. Bramson, L., et al. (2010). Effect of early skin-to-skin mother-infant contact during the first three hours following birth on exclusive breast-feeding during the maternity hospital stay. *J Hum Lact*, 26(2), 130–137.
17. Neifert, M. (2009). *Great Expectations: The Essential Guide to Breastfeeding*. New York: Sterling.
18. Abou-Dakn, M., et al. (2011). Positive effect of HPA lanolin versus expressed breastmilk on painful and damaged nipples during lactation. *Skin Pharmacol Physiol*, 24(11), 27–35.
19. Abou-Dakn, M., Schafer-Graf, U., Wockel, A. (2009). Psychological stress and breast disease during lactation. *Breastfeed Rev*, 17(3), 19–26.
20. Morton, J., et al. (2009). Combining hand techniques with electric pumping increases milk production in mothers of preterm infants. *J Perinatol*, 29(11), 757–764.
21. The Academy of Breastfeeding Medicine Protocol Committee. (2011). Protocol #9: Use of galactogogues in initiating or augmenting maternal milk supply. *Breastfeeding Med*, 6(1), 41–49.

 Acute Care   Collaborative   Community/Home Care   Cultural

interrupted Breastfeeding

Taxonomy II: Nutrition—Class 1 Ingestion (00105) [**Diagnostic Division:** Food/Fluid], Approved 1992; Revised 2013; 2017

DEFINITION: Break in the continuity of providing milk from the breasts, which may compromise breast-feeding success and/or nutritional status of the infant/child.

RELATED FACTORS
Maternal employment
Maternal/infant separation
Need to abruptly wean infant

DEFINING CHARACTERISTICS

Subjective
Nonexclusive breastfeeding
At Risk Population: Hospitalization of child; prematurity
Associated Condition: Contraindications to breastfeeding; infant or maternal illness
Sample Clinical Applications: Prematurity, postpartum depression, conditions requiring hospitalization of infant or mother, occasionally maternal medication or drug use

DESIRED OUTCOMES/EVALUATION CRITERIA

Sample NOC linkages:
Knowledge: Breastfeeding: Extent of understanding conveyed about lactation and nourishment of an infant through breastfeeding
Breastfeeding Maintenance: Continuation of breastfeeding from establishment to weaning for nourishment of an infant/toddler
Parent-Infant Attachment: Parent and infant behaviors that demonstrate an enduring affectionate bond

Client Will (Include Specific Time Frame)
• Identify and demonstrate techniques to sustain lactation until breastfeeding is reinitiated.
• Achieve mutually satisfactory feeding regimen with infant content after feedings and gaining weight appropriately.
• Achieve weaning and cessation of lactation, if desired or necessary.

ACTIONS/INTERVENTIONS

Sample NIC linkages:
Lactation Counseling: Assisting in the establishment and maintenance of successful breastfeeding
Coping Enhancement: Assisting a patient to adapt to perceived stressors, changes, or threats that interfere with meeting life demands and roles
Bottle Feeding: Preparation and administration of fluids to an infant via a bottle

NURSING PRIORITY NO. 1 To identify causative/contributing factors:

• Assess client knowledge and perceptions about breastfeeding and extent of instruction that has been given. *Provides baseline information to develop plan of care for individual situation.*[1,8]
• ∞ Note myths or misunderstandings, especially in some cultures, and in teenage mothers, *who are more likely to have limited knowledge and concerns about body image issues.*[9]

 Diagnostic Studies
 Evidence Based Practice
 Medications
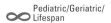 Pediatric/Geriatric/Lifespan

- Encourage discussion of current and previous breastfeeding experience(s). *Useful for determining efforts needed to continue breastfeeding, if desired, while circumstances interrupting process are resolved, if possible.*[2]
- Ascertain cultural expectations or conflicts. *The dominant culture in America has sexualized women's breasts, and mother may be embarrassed by breastfeeding or father/partner may not want mother to breast-feed. Mother may believe her independence will be curtailed by breastfeeding. Studies have shown that in the United States, breastfeeding rates vary not only by race and ethnicity but also by geographic location. For example, the rate of breastfeeding among African American mothers in the Southeast has lagged behind other areas in the country. Other cultures, such as Arab American, may believe that modernization means giving up breastfeeding.*[1,3,19]
- Determine support systems available to mother/family. *Infant's father and maternal grandmother (in addition to caring healthcare providers) are important factors in whether breastfeeding is successful and sustained.*[9]
- Identify factors necessitating interruption or, occasionally, cessation of breastfeeding (e.g., maternal illness, drug use) or desire or need to wean infant. *In general, infants with chronic diseases benefit from breastfeeding, and only a few maternal infections (e.g., HIV, active/untreated tuberculosis for initial 2 weeks of multidrug therapy, active herpes simplex of the breasts, development of chickenpox within 5 days prior to delivery or 2 days after delivery) are hazardous to breastfeeding infants. In addition, use of antiretroviral medications, chemotherapy agents, or maternal substance abuse usually requires weaning of infant. Exposure to radiation therapy requires interruption of breastfeeding for length of time radioactivity is known to be present in breast milk and is therefore dependent on agent used. Note: Mother can "pump and dump" her breastmilk to maintain supply and continue to breastfeed after her condition has resolved (e.g., chicken pox).*[1,8–11,18]
- Determine maternal responsibilities, routines, and scheduled activities. *Caretaking of siblings, employment in or out of the home, and work or school schedules of family members may affect ability to visit hospitalized infant when this is the reason for mother/infant separation.*[6,7]

NURSING PRIORITY NO. 2   To assist mother to maintain breastfeeding, as desired:

- Provide information, as needed, regarding need or decision to interrupt breastfeeding.
- Give emotional support to mother and support her decision regarding cessation or continuation of breastfeeding. *Many women are ambivalent about breastfeeding, and providing information about the pros and cons of both breastfeeding and bottle-feeding, along with support for the mother's/couple's decision, will promote a positive experience.*[1,8]
- ∞ Promote peer counseling for teen mothers. *Provides positive role model teen can relate to and feel comfortable with discussing concerns and feelings.*[9]
- Educate father/significant other (SO) about the benefits of breastfeeding and how to manage common lactation challenges. *Enlisting support of father/SO is associated with higher ratio of successful breastfeeding at 6 months.*[12]
- Discuss and demonstrate use of breastfeeding aids (e.g., infant sling, nursing footstool or pillows, hand expression, manual and/or electric piston-type breast pump). *Enhances comfort and relaxation for breastfeeding. When circumstances dictate that mother and infant are separated for a time, whether due to illness, prematurity, or returning to work or school, the milk supply can be maintained by use of the pump. Storing the milk for future use enables the infant to continue to receive the value of breast milk. Learning the correct technique is important for successful use of the pump.*[1,4,13,15]
- Review techniques for storage and use of expressed breast milk. *Provides safety and optimal nutrition, promoting continuation of the breastfeeding process.*[1]
- Determine if a routine visiting schedule or advance warning can be provided. *When infant remains in the hospital or when working mother continues to nurse, it helps to make preparations so that infant will be hungry and ready to feed when the mother arrives. A sleepy baby can be gently played with to arouse him or her; clothing can be loosened or diaper changed, exposing infant to room air; or if infant is hungry and upset, a calm voice and gentle rocking can calm the infant and prepare him or her to nurse.*[1]

 Acute Care   Collaborative   Community/ Home Care   Cultural

- Provide privacy and calm surroundings when mother breastfeeds in hospital or work setting. *Note: Federal law 2010 requires an employer to provide a place and reasonable break time for an employee to express her breast milk for her baby for 1 year after birth.*[20]
- Problem-solve return-to-work or school issues or periodic infant care requiring bottle or supplemental feeding.[14,15]
- Recommend using expressed breast milk instead of formula or at least partial breastfeeding for as long as mother and child are satisfied. *Prevents temporary interruption in breastfeeding, decreasing the risk of premature weaning.*[13,15]

NURSING PRIORITY NO. 3 To promote successful infant feeding:

- Recommend or provide for infant sucking on a regular basis, especially if gavage feedings are part of the therapeutic regimen. *Reinforces that feeding time is pleasurable and enhances digestion.*[1]
- Explain anticipated changes in feeding needs and frequency. *Growth spurts require increased intake or more feedings by infant.*[13]
- Discuss proper use and choice of supplemental nutrition and alternate feeding methods (e.g., bottle or syringe, finger feeding, cup feeding, or supplemental nursing system feeding). *If infant is not receiving sufficient nourishment, whether by mother's choice to reduce number of feedings (e.g., returning to work) or necessity (e.g., specific maternal illness, medication use), other means for supplementing intake must be taken, and mother needs to be given information regarding method chosen.*[1]
- Review safety precautions when bottle-feeding is necessary/chosen. *Identifying importance of proper flow of formula from nipple, frequency of burping, holding bottle instead of propping, techniques of formula preparation, and sterilization techniques are necessary for successful bottle-feeding.*[1]

NURSING PRIORITY NO. 4 To promote wellness (Teaching/Discharge Considerations):

- Encourage mother to obtain adequate rest, maintain fluid and nutritional intake, continue to take her prenatal vitamins, and schedule breast pumping every 3 hours while awake, as indicated. *Sustains adequate milk production and enhances breastfeeding process when mother and infant are separated for any reason.*[1,8]
- Suggest abstinence or restriction of tobacco, caffeine, alcohol, drugs, and excess sugar, as appropriate, when breastfeeding is reinitiated. *These substances may affect milk production/letdown reflex and can be passed on to the infant.*[1]
- Identify other means of nurturing and strengthening infant attachment, such as skin-to-skin or kangaroo care. *Activities that provide comfort, consolation, and play activities help mother become comfortable with handling the infant, thus enhancing relationship.*[7,15]
- Refer to support groups (e.g., La Leche League, Lact-Aid) or community resources (e.g., public health nurse; lactation specialist; Women, Infants, and Children [WIC] program; and electric pump rental programs). *Additional support may provide assistance, supplies, and education to promote a successful outcome. WIC and other federal programs support breastfeeding through education and enhanced nutritional intake.*[5,15]
- Promote use of bibliotherapy and appropriate Web sites. *Provides additional sources of information.*[5]
- Discuss timing of introduction of solid foods and importance of delaying until infant is at least 4 months, preferably 6 months, old if possible. *American Academy of Pediatrics and the World Health Organization recommend delaying solids until at least 6 months. If supplementation is necessary, infant can be finger fed, spoon fed, cup fed, or syringe fed.*[13,21]

NURSING PRIORITY NO. 5 To assist mother in weaning process, when desired:

- Discuss reducing frequency of daily feedings or breast pumping by once every 2 to 3 days. *Preferred method of weaning, if circumstance permits, to reduce problems associated with engorgement.*[16,17]
- Encourage wearing a snug, well-fitting bra, but refrain from binding breasts *because of increased risk of clogged milk ducts and inflammation.*[15,16]

 Diagnostic Studies   Evidence Based Practice   Medications   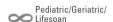 Pediatric/Geriatric/Lifespan

- Recommend expressing some milk from breasts regularly each day over a 1- to 3-week period, if necessary, *to reduce discomfort associated with engorgement until milk production decreases.*[16,17]
- Suggest holding infant differently during bottle-feeding or interactions or having another family member give infant's bottle feeding *to prevent infant rooting for mother's breast and limit stimulation of her nipples.*
- Discuss use of ibuprofen or acetaminophen *for discomfort during weaning process.*[8]
- Suggest use of ice packs to breast tissue (not nipples) for 15 to 20 min at least four times a day *to help reduce swelling during sudden weaning.*[17]

DOCUMENTATION FOCUS

Assessment/Reassessment
- Baseline findings maternal/infant factors, including mother's milk supply, infant nourishment.
- Reason for interruption or cessation of breastfeeding.
- Number of wet and soiled diapers daily, log of intake and output, as appropriate, and periodic weight.

Planning
- Method of feeding chosen.
- Plan of care and who is involved in planning.
- Teaching plan.

Implementation/Evaluation
- Maternal response to interventions, teaching, and actions performed.
- Infant's response to feeding and method.
- Whether infant appears satisfied or still seems to be hungry.
- Attainment or progress toward desired outcome(s).
- Modifications to plan of care.

Discharge Planning
- Referrals, plan for follow-up, and who is responsible.
- Specific referrals made.

References

1. Ladewig, P., London, M., Davidson, M. (2009). *Contemporary Maternal-Newborn Nursing Care.* 7th ed. Upper Saddle River, NJ: Prentice Hall.
2. Riodan, J., Auerbach, K. (2010). *Breastfeeding and Human Lactation.* 4th ed. Boston: Jones & Bartlett.
3. Purnell, L. D. (2011). *Guide to Culturally Competent Health Care.* 2nd ed. Philadelphia: F. A. Davis.
4. Lowdermilk, D. L., Cashion, M. C., Perry, S. (2011). *Maternal and Woman's Health Care.* 10th ed. St. Louis, MO: Mosby.
5. Doenges, M., Moorhouse, M. (1999). *Maternal/Newborn Plans of Care: Guidelines for Individualizing Care.* 3rd ed. Philadelphia: F. A. Davis.
6. Phillips, C. R. (2003). *Family-Centered Maternity and Newborn Care.* Maynard, MA: Jones & Bartlett Learning.
7. Newfield, S. A., et al. (2007). *Cox's Clinical Applications of Nursing Diagnosis: Adult, Child, Women's, Psychiatric, Gerontic and Home Health Considerations.* 5th ed. Philadelphia: F. A. Davis.
8. London, M., et al. (2010). *Maternal and Child Nursing Care.* 3rd ed. Upper Saddle River, NJ: Prentice Hall.
9. American Academy of Family Physicians. Breastfeeding (Position Paper) With Appendices Updates. Retrieved March 2018 from www.aafp.org/about/policies/all/breastfeeding-support.html.
10. Centers for Disease Control and Prevention. (2016). When should a mother avoid breastfeeding?. Retrieved March 2018 from http://www.cdc.gov/breastfeeding/disease/.
11. United States National Library of Medicine. (no date listed). *Toxnet: Drugs and Lactation Database.* (LactMed). Retrieved March 2018 from http://toxnet.nlm.nih.gov/newtoxnet/lactmed.htm.
12. Pisacane, A., et al. (2005). A controlled trial of the father's role in breastfeeding promotion. *Pediatrics,* 116(4), e494–e498.
13. American Academy of Pediatrics. (Updated 2018). Ten steps to support parents' choice to breastfeed their baby. Retrieved March 2018 from https://www.aap.org/en-us/advocacy-and-policy/aap-health-initiatives/Breastfeeding/Documents/tenstepsposter.pdf.
14. U.S. Department of Health and Human Services, Office on Women's Health. (Revised July 2013). Common breastfeeding challenges. Retrieved March 2018 from http://www.womenshealth.gov/breastfeeding/common-challenges/.
15. Smith, A. (edited 2016). Breast infections and plugged ducts. *Breastfeeding Basics.* March 2018 http://www.breastfeedingbasics.com/articles/breast-infections-and-plugged-ducts.

 Acute Care
 Collaborative
 Community/ Home Care
 Cultural

16. Children's Hospitals and Clinics of Minnesota Patient/ Family Education Resources. (reviewed 2018). Breastfeeding: Weaning. Retrieved March 2018 from http://www .childrensmn.org/educationmaterials/childrensmn/article/15846/ breastfeeding-weaning/.

17. Smith, A. (edited 2016). Breastfeeding Basics: Weaning. Retrieved March 2018 from http://www.breastfeeding-basics .com/articles/weaning-your-baby.

18. Hale, T. W. (2010). *Medications and Mothers' Milk: A Manual of Lactational Pharmacology.* 14th ed. Amarillo, TX: Pharmasoft Medical Pub.

19. Wozniki, K. (2010). Breastfeeding rates vary by race, region. Retrieved March 2018 from WebMD Health News. http://www .medicinenet.com/script/main/art.asp?articlekey=114787.

20. U.S. Department of Labor. (revised 2010). Break time for nursing mothers under the FLSA. *Fact Sheet #73.* Retrieved March 2018 from http://www.dol.gov/whd/regs/compliance/whdfs73 .htm.

21. World Health Organization. (2015). Up to what age can a baby stay well nourished by just being breastfed? Retrieved March 2018 from http://www.who.int/features/qa/21/en/index.html.

readiness for enhanced Breastfeeding

Taxonomy II: Nutrition—Class 1 Ingestion (00106) [**Diagnostic Division:** Food/Fluid], Approved 1990; Revised 2010, 2013, 2017

DEFINITION: A pattern of feeding milk from the breasts to an infant or child, which may be strengthened.

DEFINING CHARACTERISTICS

Subjective
Mother expresses desire to enhance ability to exclusively breastfeed
Mother expresses desire to provide breast milk for child's nutritional needs
Sample Clinical Applications: Wellness diagnosis associated with pre-/postnatal client

DESIRED OUTCOMES/EVALUATION CRITERIA

Sample NOC linkages:
Breastfeeding Establishment: Infant: Infant attachment to and sucking from the mother's breast for nourishment during the first 3 weeks of breastfeeding
Breastfeeding Establishment: Maternal: Maternal establishment of proper attachment of an infant to and sucking from the breast for nourishment during the first 3 weeks of breastfeeding
Breastfeeding Maintenance: Continuation of breastfeeding from establishment to weaning for nourishment of an infant/toddler

Client Will (Include Specific Time Frame)
• Verbalize understanding of breastfeeding techniques, good latch, and lactogenesis.
• Demonstrate effective techniques for breastfeeding.
• Demonstrate family involvement and support.
• Attend classes, read appropriate materials, or access resources as necessary.
• Verbalize understanding of the benefits of human milk.

ACTIONS/INTERVENTIONS

Sample NIC linkages:
Lactation Counseling: Assisting in the establishment and maintenance of successful breastfeeding
Teaching: Infant Nutrition (specify months): Instruction on nutrition and feeding practices during the first year of life

NURSING PRIORITY NO. 1 To determine individual learning needs:

- Assess mother's desires/plan for feeding infant. *Provides information for developing plan of care.*[1]
- Assess mother's knowledge and previous experience with breastfeeding. *Accurate knowledge and previous experience can lead to a positive breastfeeding experience.*[1]
- Note cultural and societal influences regarding infant feeding (breastfeeding/bottle-feeding), lactation process, letdown techniques, and maternal food preferences. *In Western cultures, the breast has taken on a sexual connotation, and some mothers may be embarrassed to breastfeed. While breastfeeding may be accepted, in some cultures, certain beliefs may affect specific feeding practices (e.g., in Mexican American, Navajo, Filipino, and Vietnamese cultures, colostrum is not offered to the newborn; breastfeeding begins only after the milk flow is established).*[3]
- ∞ Note myths or misunderstandings, especially in teenage mothers *who are more likely to have limited knowledge and concerns about body image issues.*[6]
- Monitor effectiveness of current breastfeeding efforts. *Determining the actions client is taking provides information about measures that may enhance efforts to be successful in endeavor.*[1]
- Determine support systems available to mother/family. *Presence of adequate support can provide encouragement to mother who may be feeling nervous and unsure about new role.*[1,6]

NURSING PRIORITY NO. 2 To promote effective breastfeeding behaviors:

- Initiate breastfeeding within first hour after birth. *The time of the first feeding is determined by the infant's physiological and behavioral cues. Throughout the first 2 hours after birth, the infant is usually alert and ready to nurse. Early feedings are of great benefit to mother and infant because oxytocin release is stimulated, helping to expel the placenta and prevent excessive maternal blood loss; the infant receives the immunological protection of colostrum; peristalsis is stimulated; lactation is accelerated; and maternal-infant bonding is enhanced.*[2]
- Encourage skin-to-skin contact. Place infant on mother's stomach, skin-to-skin after delivery. *Many full-term infants are alert and capable of latching onto mother's breast without assistance.*[9] *Studies show that early skin-to-skin mother-infant contact is correlated with exclusive breastfeeding while in the hospital.*[10]
- Demonstrate asymmetric latch aiming infant's lower lip as far from base of the nipple as possible, then bringing infant's chin and lower jaw in contact with breast while mouth is wide open and before upper lip touches breast. *This position allows infant to use both tongue and jaw more effectively to obtain milk from the breast.*[9]
- Demonstrate how to support and position infant and use of aids (e.g., infant sling, nursing footstool, or pillows). *The mother should be made as comfortable as possible and given specific instructions for positioning self and baby depending on the type of birth (e.g., cesarean section or vaginal).*[1,5]
- Observe mother's return demonstration/teach back. *Provides practice and the opportunity to correct misunderstandings and add additional information to promote optimal experience for breastfeeding.*[1]
- Keep infant with mother for unrestricted breastfeeding duration and frequency. *Rooming-in offers opportunity for spontaneous encounters for the family to practice handling skills and increase confidence in own ability. It also encourages feeding in response to cues from the baby and increases bonding.*[1]
- Discuss early infant feeding cues (e.g., rooting, lip smacking, sucking fingers or hand) versus the late cue of crying. *Early recognition of infant hunger promotes timely and more rewarding feeding experience for infant and mother.* NOTE: For healthy infants, discourage use of pacifiers and artificial nipples in first month of life *to avoid "nipple confusion" and to establish mother's milk supply.*[6]
- Encourage mother to follow a well-balanced diet containing an extra 500 calories/day, continue her prenatal vitamins, and drink at least 2,000 to 3,000 mL of fluid/day. *There is an increased need for maternal energy, protein, minerals, and vitamins, as well as increased fluid intake, during lactation to restore what the mother loses in secreting milk to provide adequate nutrients for the nourishment of the infant and to protect the mother's own stores.*[4]
- Provide information, as needed, in support of breastfeeding. *Having adequate information about the nutritional, psychological, immunological advantages, contraindications, and disadvantages of breastfeeding helps*

 Acute Care   Collaborative   Community/Home Care   Cultural

the parents to make a decision that is best for the family. Many mothers indicate that if they had had adequate information, they would have chosen to breastfeed.[1]

- ∞ Promote peer counseling for teen mothers. *Provides positive role model teen can relate to and feel comfortable with discussing concerns and feelings.*[6]

NURSING PRIORITY NO. 3 To enhance optimum wellness (Teaching/Discharge Considerations):

- 🏠 Provide for follow-up contact or home visit 48 hours after discharge; repeat visit as necessary. *Provides opportunity to assess adequacy of home situation and breastfeeding efforts as well as support and assistance with problem solving, if needed.*[1]
- Recommend monitoring number of infant's wet diapers (at least six wet diapers in 24 hours suggests adequate hydration) and soiled diapers (breastfed baby's stool will be yellow in color). *Often mothers who are breastfeeding worry about whether infant is getting adequate nutrition because they cannot measure the amount of milk being received, and having this information can allay these fears.*[1]
- Encourage mother and other family members to express feelings and concerns, and active-listen *to determine nature of concerns. Identifying the concerns of the parents promotes problem solving and alleviation of worries and fears. When individuals do not express these concerns, they can become frustrated, which can interfere with successful breastfeeding.*[1]
- 📝 Educate father/significant other (SO) about benefits of breastfeeding and how to manage common lactation challenges. *Enlisting support of father/SO is associated with higher ratio of successful breastfeeding at 6 months.*[8]
- Review techniques for expression and storage of breast milk to help sustain breastfeeding activity. *Having this information enables the mother to successfully manage continuation of breastfeeding while engaging in activities outside the home for specified periods of time.*[1]
- Explain changes in feeding needs and frequency. *Growth spurts require increased intake or more feedings by infant.*[5]
- Review normal nursing behaviors of older breastfeeding infants/toddlers.[5]
- Discuss importance of delaying introduction of solid foods until infant is at least 4 months, preferably 6 months old. *Note:* American Academy of Pediatrics and the World Health Organization recommend delaying solids until at least 6 months.[5,11]
- Recommend avoidance of specific medications or substances (e.g., estrogen-containing contraceptives, bromocriptine, nicotine, alcohol) *known to decrease milk supply. Note: Small amounts of alcohol have not been shown to be detrimental.*[6,7]
- 💊 Emphasize importance of client notifying healthcare providers, dentists, and pharmacists of breastfeeding status.
- Problem-solve return-to-work issues or periodic infant care requiring bottle or supplemental feeding. *Enables mothers who need or desire to return to work (for economic or personal reasons) or who simply want to attend activities without the infant to deal with these issues, thus allowing more freedom while maintaining adequate breastfeeding.*[1]
- Recommend using expressed breast milk instead of formula or at least partial breastfeeding for as long as mother and child are satisfied.[6]
- 💊 Refer to support groups, such as La Leche League, as indicated. Provide mother with phone number of support person or group, prior to leaving hospital. *While the father or SO is the most important support person in Western society, family support systems may be lacking information about other support systems/groups.*[1]
- Refer to ND ineffective Breastfeeding for more specific information, as appropriate.

DOCUMENTATION FOCUS

Assessment/Reassessment
- Identified assessment factors (maternal and infant).
- Number of daily wet and soiled diapers and periodic weight.

 Diagnostic Studies   Evidence Based Practice   Medications ∞ Pediatric/Geriatric/Lifespan

Planning
• Plan of care, specific interventions, and who is involved in the planning.
• Teaching plan.

Implementation/Evaluation
• Mother's response to interventions, teaching plan, and actions performed.
• Effectiveness of infant's efforts to feed.
• Attainment or progress toward desired outcome(s).
• Modifications to plan of care.

Discharge Planning
• Long-term needs, referrals made, and who is responsible for follow-up actions.

References

1. Ladewig, P., London, M., Davidson, M. (2009). *Contemporary Maternal-Newborn Nursing Care*. 7th ed. Upper Saddle River, NJ: Prentice Hall.
2. Riodan, J., Auerbach, K. (2010). *Breastfeeding and Human Lactation*. 4th ed. Boston: Jones & Bartlett.
3. Purnell, L. D. (2011). *Guide to Culturally Competent Health Care*. 2nd ed. Philadelphia: F. A. Davis.
4. Lowdermilk, D., Cashion, M., Perry, S. (2012). *Maternity & Women's Health Care*. 10th ed. St. Louis, MO: Elsevier-Mosby.
5. American Academy of Pediatrics. (Revised 2013). Ten steps to support parents' choice to breastfeed their baby. Retrieved March 2018 from https://www.aap.org/en-us/advocacy-and-policy/aap-health-initiatives/Breastfeeding/Documents/tenstepsposter.pdf.
6. American Academy of Family Physicians. (2011). Breastfeeding (Position Paper) With Appendices Updates. Retrieved March 2018 from https://www.aafp.org/about/policies/all/breastfeeding-support.html.
7. Callen, J., Pinelli, J. (2005). A review of the literature examining the benefits and challenges, incidence and duration, and barriers to breastfeeding in preterm infants. *Adv Neonatal Care*, 5(2), 72–88.
8. Pisacane, A., et al. (2005). A controlled trial of the father's role in breastfeeding promotion. *Pediatrics*, 116(4), e494–e498.
9. Neifert, M. (2009). *Great Expectations: The Essential Guide to Breastfeeding*. New York: Sterling.
10. Bramson, L., et al. (2010). Effect of early skin-to-skin mother-infant contact during the first three hours following birth on exclusive breast-feeding during the maternity hospital stay. *J Hum Lact*, 26(2), 130–137.
11. World Health Organization. Up to what age can a baby stay well nourished by just being breastfed?. Retrieved March 2018 from http://www.who.int/features/qa/21/en/index.html.

---

insufficient Breast Milk Production

Taxonomy II: Nutrition—Class 1 Ingestion (00216) [**Diagnostic Division:** Food/Fluid], Approved 2010; Revised 2017

DEFINITION: Inadequate supply of maternal breast milk to support nutritional state of an infant or child.

RELATED FACTORS
Mother
Insufficient fluid volume
Smoking; alcohol consumption
Malnutrition
Treatment regimen [e.g., medication side effects—contraceptives, diuretics]
Infant
Ineffective latching on to breast, sucking reflex
Insufficient opportunity for suckling at the breast or suckling time at breast
Rejection of breast

 Acute Care   Collaborative   Community/Home Care   Cultural

DEFINING CHARACTERISTICS

Objective
Mother
Absence of milk production with nipple stimulation
Breast milk expressed is less than prescribed volume for infant
Delay in milk production
Infant
Frequently seeks to suckle at breast; prolonged breastfeeding time
Suckling time at breast appears unsatisfactory; frequently crying
Refuses to suckle at breast; unsustained suckling at breast
Voids small amounts of concentrated urine;
Weight gain <500 g in a month
Associated Condition: Pregnancy
Sample Clinical Applications: Conditions resulting in dehydration, such as fluid volume depletion, hemorrhage; malnutrition; premature infant with inability to suck vigorously, or mother not pumping to promote supply; adolescent mother; use/abuse of substances and/or certain medications.

DESIRED OUTCOMES/EVALUATION CRITERIA

Sample NOC linkages:
Knowledge: Breastfeeding: Extent of understanding conveyed about lactation and nourishment of an infant through breastfeeding
Breastfeeding Establishment: Maternal: Maternal establishment of proper attachment of an infant to and sucking from the breast for nourishment during the first 3 weeks of breastfeeding
Breastfeeding Maintenance: Continuation of breastfeeding from establishment to weaning for nourishment of infant/toddler

Client Will [Include Specific Time Frame]
• Develop plan to correct/change contributing factors.
• Engage in techniques to enhance milk production.
• Achieve mutually satisfactory breastfeeding pattern with infant content after feedings and gaining weight appropriately.

ACTIONS/INTERVENTIONS

Sample NIC linkages:
Lactation Counseling: Assisting in the establishment and maintenance of successful breastfeeding

NURSING PRIORITY NO. 1   To identify maternal causative or contributing factors:

• Assess mother's knowledge about breastfeeding and extent of instruction that has been provided. Determine previous breastfeeding experience. *Lack of knowledge, unresolved problems, or stories told by others may cause client to doubt abilities and chances for success.*[8,13]
• 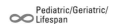 Identify cultural expectations and conflicts about breastfeeding and beliefs or practices regarding lactation, letdown techniques, and maternal food preferences. *Understanding the impact of culture and idiosyncrasies of specific feeding practices is important to determine the effect on infant breastfeeding success.*[8,11,14]
• ∞ Note incorrect myths/misunderstandings, especially in teenage mothers. *Adolescents are more likely to have limited knowledge, difficulty managing time demands of school/work, concerns about body image issues, and feel overwhelmed.*[8,14]

 Diagnostic Studies   Evidence Based Practice   Medications   ∞ Pediatric/Geriatric/Lifespan

- Identify maternal support systems and presence/response of significant others (SOs)/extended family. *Negative attitudes and comments interfere with efforts and may cause client to prematurely abandon attempt to breastfeed.*[14]
- Determine use of supplemental feedings for infant. *Unless medically indicated, routine supplementation increases risk for decrease in mother's milk supply.*[14]
- Perform physical examination, noting appearance of breasts and nipples, marked asymmetry of breasts, obvious inverted or flat nipples, minimal or no breast enlargement during pregnancy. *Inadequate mammary gland tissue, breast surgery that has damaged the nipple, areola enervation results in irremediable primary lactation failure.*[9,13]
- Assess for other causes of primary lactation failure. *Maternal prolactin deficiency/serum prolactin levels, pituitary or thyroid disorders, and anemia may be corrected with medication.*[4,9]
- Review lifestyle for common causes of secondary lactation failure. *Smoking, caffeine/alcohol use, lack of adequate healthy food; birth control pills containing estrogen, becoming pregnant again; medications (e.g., antihistamines, decongestants, diuretics), stress, and fatigue are known to inhibit milk production.*[1,4,9]
- Determine desire/motivation to breastfeed. *Increasing milk supply can be intense, requiring commitment to therapeutic regimen and possible lifestyle changes.*

NURSING PRIORITY NO. 2   To identify infant causative or contributing factors:

- Observe infant at breast to evaluate latching-on skill and presence of suck/swallow difficulties. *Poor latching-on, lack of audible swallowing/gulp are associated with inadequate intake. The infant gets substantial amounts of milk when drinking with an open—pause—close type of suck.*[3] *(Open—pause—close is one suck; the pause described here is not a pause between sucks but rather when swallowing occurs.)*
- Observe signs of inadequate infant intake. *Infant arching and crying at the breast with resistance to latching-on, decreased urinary output/frequency of stools, and inadequate weight gain indicate need for further evaluation and intervention.*[11,13]
- Review feeding schedule—frequency, length of feeding, and taking one or both breasts at each feeding. *Provides information regarding whether sufficient nutrition is being provided.*[10]

NURSING PRIORITY NO. 3   To increase mother's milk supply:

- Instruct on how to differentiate between perceived and actual insufficient milk supply. *Normal breastfeeding frequencies, suckling times, and amounts vary not only between mothers, but also based on infant's needs/moods. Milk production is likely to be a reflection of the infant's appetite rather than the mother's ability to produce milk.*[4,5]
- Provide emotional support to mother. Use one-to-one instruction with each feeding during hospital stay, clinic, or home visit. *Increases likelihood of continuation of breastfeeding efforts and achievement of goals.*[11,14]
- Refer adoptive mothers choosing to breastfeed to a lactation consultant. *Adoptive mothers choosing to breastfeed will require more supportive instruction from a professional consultant to assist with induced lactation techniques.*[14]
- Inform mother how to assess and correct a latch if needed. Demonstrate asymmetric latch, aiming infant's lower lip as far from base of the nipple as possible and then bringing infant's chin and lower jaw in contact with breast while mouth is wide open and before upper lip touches breast. *Correct latching-on is the most effective way to stimulate milk supply.*[2,9]
- Encourage unrestricted frequency and duration of breastfeeding. *Provides stimulation of breast tissue and may increase milk supply naturally.*[9]
- Recommend reducing or stopping supplemental feedings if used. *Gradual tapering off of supplementation can increase frequency/duration of infant's breastfeeding stimulating maternal milk production.*[9,14]
- Demonstrate breast massage technique. *Improves oxytocin release and milk removal to increase milk supply naturally.*[9,14] *Also, gently massaging breast while infant feeds from it can improve the release of higher-calorie hindmilk from the milk glands.*[1,9]

 Acute Care   Collaborative   Community/ Home Care   Cultural

- Use breast pump 8 to 12 times a day. *Expressing with a hospital-grade, double (automatic) pump is ideal for stimulation/reestablishing milk supply.*[1,9]
- Recommend mother adjust the electric pump to her maximum comfortable vacuum. *Enhances milk flow rate and milk yield and minimizes occurrence of tissue damage.*[9]
- Suggest using a breast pump or hand expression after infant finishes breastfeeding. *Continued breast stimulation cues the mother's body that more milk is needed, increasing supply.*[7]
- Encourage use of relaxation techniques during hand or mechanical expression. Facilitates oxytocin release to improve milk removal.[9]
- Monitor increased filling of breasts in response to nursing and/or pumping *to help evaluate effectiveness of interventions.*
- Discuss appropriate/safe use of herbal supplements. *Herbs such as sage, parsley, oregano, peppermint, jasmine, and yarrow may have a negative effect on milk supply if taken in large quantities. A number of herbs have been used for centuries to stimulate milk production, with fenugreek (Trigonella foenum-graecum) being the most commonly recommended herbal galactogogue to facilitate lactation.*[4,9]
- 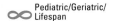 Discuss possible use of prescribed medications (galactogogues) to increase milk production. *Domperidone (Motilium) is approved by the American Academy of Pediatrics for use in breastfeeding mothers and has fewer side effects. Metoclopramide (Reglan) has been shown to increase milk supply anywhere from 72% to 110% depending on how many weeks the mother is postpartum.*[1,6,9]

NURSING PRIORITY NO. 4 To promote optimal success and satisfaction of breastfeeding process for mother and infant:

- Encourage frequent rest periods, sharing household and childcare tasks. *Having assistance can limit fatigue (known to impact milk production) and facilitate relaxation at feeding time.*[12]
- Discuss with spouse/SO mother's requirement for rest, relaxation, and time together with family members. *Enhances understanding of mother's needs, and family members feel included and more willing to support breastfeeding activity/treatment plan.*[11]
- Arrange dietary consult to review nutritional needs and vitamin/mineral supplements, such as vitamin C, as indicated. *During lactation, there is an increased need for energy requiring supplementation of protein, vitamins, and minerals to provide nourishment for the infant.*[11]
- Emphasize importance of adequate fluid intake. *Alternating types of fluids (e.g., water, juice, decaffeinated tea/coffee, milk) enhances intake promoting milk production. Note: Beer and wine are not recommended for increasing lactation.*[11]
- ∞ Encourage peer counseling for teen mothers. *Provides positive role model that teen can relate to and feel comfortable with discussing concerns and feelings.*[14]
- Recommend monitoring number of infant's wet and soiled diapers. *Stools should be yellow in color and infant should have at least six wet diapers a day to determine that infant is receiving sufficient intake.*[12]
- Weigh infant every 3 days, or as directed by primary provider/lactation consultant, and record. *Monitors weight gain verifying adequacy of intake or need for additional interventions.*[11]
- Identify products/programs for cessation of smoking. *Smoking can interfere with the release of oxytocin, which stimulates the letdown reflex, and can negatively affect milk production.*[4,9,11]
- Refer to support groups (e.g., La Leche League International, parenting support groups, stress management class, or other community resources, as indicated). *Provides information and ongoing support increasing likelihood of successful breastfeeding.*[9]

DOCUMENTATION FOCUS

Assessment/Reassessment
- Identified maternal assessment factors—hydration level, medication use, lifestyle choices.
- Cultural factors, support systems.
- Findings of breast examination.

 Diagnostic Studies   Evidence Based Practice   Medications   ∞ Pediatric/Geriatric/Lifespan

- Infant assessment factors—latching-on technique, hydration level/number of wet diapers, weight gain/loss.
- Use of supplemental feedings.

Planning
- Plan of care, specific interventions, and who is involved in planning.
- Individual teaching plan.

Implementation/Evaluation
- Mother's/infant's responses to interventions, teaching, and actions performed.
- Change in infant's weight.
- Attainment or progress toward desired outcomes.
- Modification to plan of care.

Discharge Planning
- Specific referrals made.

References

1. Nagin, M. J. (Updated 2018). Relactation—How to rebuild or increase your milk supply. Retrieved March 2018 from https://www.verywellfamily.com/relactation-increase-milk-supply-431824.
2. Murray, D. (Updated 2018). How to naturally establish or increase a healthy breast milk supply. Retrieved March 2018 from https://www.verywellfamily.com/naturally-increase-your-breast-milk-supply-431842.
3. Iannelli, V. (Updated 2017). Breastfeeding questions and answers. Retrieved March 2018 from https://www.verywellfamily.com/breastfeeding-questions-and-answers-3888935.
4. Murray, D. (Updated 2018). What decreases breast milk supply. Retrieved March 2018 from https://www.verywellfamily.com/things-decrease-breast-milk-supply-431815.
5. Daly, S. E. J., Hartmann, P. E. (1995). Infant demand and milk supply, part 1: Infant demand and milk production in lactating women. *J Hum Lact*, 11(1), 21–26.
6. Kent, J. C., Prime, D. K., Garbin, C. F. (2012). Principles for maintaining or increasing breast milk production. *J Obstet Gynecol Neonatal Nurs*, 41(1), 114–121.
7. Morton, J., et al. (2009). Combining hand techniques with electric pumping increases milk production in mothers of pre-term infants. *J Perinatol*, 29(11), 757–764.
8. Wambach, K. A., Cohen, S. M. (2009). Breast feeding experiences of urban adolescent mothers. *J Pediatr Nurs*, 24(4), 244–254.
9. The Academy of Breastfeeding Medicine Protocol Committee. (2011). Protocol #9: Use of galactogogues in initiating or augmenting maternal milk supply. *Breastfeeding Med*. 6(1), 41–49.
10. Smith, A. (Updated 2016). Increasing Your Milk Supply. Retrieved March 2018 from http://www.breastfeedingbasics.com/article/increasing-your-milk-supply.
11. Ladewig, P., London, M., Davidson, M. (2009). *Contemporary Maternal-Newborn Nursing Care*. 7th ed. Upper Saddle River, NJ: Prentice Hall.
12. Riodan, J., Auerbach, K. (2010). *Breastfeeding and Human Lactation*. 4th ed. Boston: Jones & Bartlett.
13. Lowdermilk, D. L., Cashion, M. C., Perry, S. E. (2011). *Maternity & Women's Health Care*. 10th ed. St. Louis, MO: Mosby.
14. Phillips, C. R. (1996). *Family-Centered Maternity and Newborn Care*. 4th ed. St. Louis, MO: Mosby.

ineffective Breathing Pattern

Taxonomy II: Activity/Rest—Class 4 Cardiovascular/Pulmonary Responses (00032) [**Diagnostic Division:** Respiration], Approved 1980; Revised 1996, 1998, 2010, 2017

DEFINITION: Inspiration and/or expiration that does not provide adequate ventilation.

RELATED FACTORS
Anxiety; [panic attacks]
Body position that inhibits lung expansion; obesity
Fatigue; respiratory muscle fatigue
Hyperventilation
Pain

 Acute Care Collaborative Community/Home Care Cultural

DEFINING CHARACTERISTICS

Subjective
Dyspnea
Orthopnea

Objective
Abnormal breathing pattern
Altered chest excursion; [paradoxical breathing patterns]
Bradypnea; tachypnea
Decrease in inspiratory or expiratory pressure
Decrease in minute ventilation or vital capacity
Use of accessory muscles to breath; use of three-point position
Increase in anterior-posterior chest diameter
Prolonged expiration phases; pursed-lip breathing
Nasal flaring; [grunting]
Associated Condition: Bony or chest wall deformity; hypoventilation syndrome; musculoskeletal, neuro-
logical or neuromuscular impairment; neurological immaturity; spinal cord injury
Sample Clinical Applications: COPD, emphysema, asthma, pneumonia, chest trauma or surgery, SCI,
Guillain-Barré syndrome, traumatic brain injury, cystic fibrosis, drug or alcohol toxicity

DESIRED OUTCOMES/EVALUATION CRITERIA

Sample NOC **linkages:**
Respiratory Status: Ventilation: Movement of air in and out of the lungs
Fatigue Level: Severity of observed or reported prolonged generalized fatigue
Anxiety Level: Severity of manifested apprehension, tension, or uneasiness arising from an unidentifiable
source

Client Will (Include Specific Time Frame)
• Establish a normal, effective respiratory pattern.
• Be free of cyanosis and other signs/symptoms of hypoxia with arterial blood gases (ABGs) within client's
  normal/acceptable range.
• Verbalize awareness of causative factors and initiate needed lifestyle changes.
• Demonstrate appropriate coping behaviors.

ACTIONS/INTERVENTIONS

Sample NIC **linkages:**
Ventilation Assistance: Promotion of an optimal spontaneous breathing pattern that maximizes oxygen
  and carbon dioxide exchange in the lungs
Airway Management: Facilitation of patency of air passages
Respiratory Monitoring: Collection and analysis of patient data to ensure airway patency and adequate
  gas exchange

NURSING PRIORITY NO. 1   To identify etiology/precipitating factors:

• ∞ ⊕ ▨ Identify age and ethnic group of client who may be at increased risk. *Respiratory ailments in general are increased in infants and children with neuromuscular disorders, the frail elderly, and persons living in*

 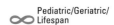

highly polluted environments.[1,2] Smoking (and potential for smoking-related disorders) is prevalent among such groups as Appalachians, African Americans, Chinese men, Latinos, and Arabs. Studies have linked air pollution to heart disease, asthma, and other diseases. Communities of color are especially vulnerable as they tend to live in areas (such as close to freeways or high traffic areas) with high levels of air toxins.[3,4] People most at risk for infectious pneumonias include the very young and frail elderly; those suffering from chronic respiratory or circulatory problems; and those with compromised immune systems from congenital deficiencies, AIDS, cancers, and cancer therapies.[2,5]

- Ascertain if client has history of underlying respiratory disorder or if this is a new condition with potential for breathing problems or exacerbation of preexisting problems (e.g., asthma, other acute upper respiratory infection, lung cancer, neuromuscular disorders, heart disease, sepsis, burns, acute chest or brain trauma). *Important in pointing to cause for current breathing problems.[6]*

- Assess for pregnancy, other abdominal distention, and muscle guarding. *Distended abdomen and muscle tension can impede diaphragmatic excursion and reduce lung expansion.*

- Note current symptoms and how they relate to past history. *Assessing current illness, including history of (1) onset and duration of symptoms; (2) how they are similar to or different from past symptoms; (3) precipitating, relieving, and exacerbating factors; and (4) exposures (e.g., environmental toxins, alcohol or other drugs, source of infection) may help in selecting the correct diagnosis.*

- Note emotional state. *Gasping, crying, anxiety, irritability, struggling, look of fear, report of tingling lips or fingers, withdrawal, and self-focus are responses often associated with respiratory distress. Emotional changes can accompany a condition or precipitate or aggravate ineffective breathing patterns.[5–9]*

- Evaluate client's respiratory status:

   ∞ Note rate and depth of respirations, counting for 1 full minute, if rate is irregular. *Rate may be faster or slower than usual. In infants and younger children, rate increases dramatically relative to anxiety, crying, fever, or disease. Depth may be difficult to evaluate but is usually described as shallow, normal, or deep.[5,7,8]*

   Note client's reports and perceptions of breathing ease. *Client may report a range of symptoms (e.g., air hunger, shortness of breath with speaking, activity, or at rest) and demonstrate a wide range of signs (e.g., tachypnea, gasping, wheezing, coughing).*

   ∞ Observe characteristics of breathing pattern. *May note use of accessory muscles for breathing, sternal retractions (infants and young children), nasal flaring, or pursed-lip breathing. Client may change position in effort to breathe easier. Irregular patterns may be pathological (e.g., prolonged expiration, periods of apnea, obvious agonal breathing) with pronounced alterations in conditions such as severe asthma attack, brainstem damage, or impending respiratory failure.[5–7]*

   Auscultate and percuss chest, describing presence, absence, and character of breath sounds. *Air should be moving freely through air passages (differs from ineffective airway clearance), but ventilatory effort may be insufficient to bring in enough oxygen or to exchange sufficient amounts of carbon dioxide, such as might occur in asthma or congenital heart disease. Abnormal breath sounds are indicative of numerous problems (e.g., obstruction by foreign object, hypoventilation such as might occur with chest or spinal cord injuries, atelectasis, or presence of secretions, improper endotracheal [ET] tube placement, collapsed lung) and must be evaluated and reported for further intervention.[5,8,9]*

   Observe chest size, shape, and symmetry of movement. *Changes in movement of chest wall (such as might occur with chest trauma, chest wall deformities) can impair breathing patterns.*

   ∞ Note color of skin and mucous membranes. *If pallor, duskiness, and/or cyanosis are present, supplemental oxygen and/or other interventions may be required.* (Refer to ND impaired Gas Exchange.)

   Note presence and character of cough. *Cough function may be weak or ineffective in conditions such as extremes in age (e.g., premature infant or elderly); in diseases (e.g., cerebral palsy, muscular dystrophy, SCI, brain injury); after surgery; and/or in mechanical ventilation due to mechanisms affecting muscles of throat, chest, and lungs. Cough that is persistent and constant can interfere with breathing (such as can occur with asthma, acute bronchitis, cystic fibrosis, croup, whooping cough).[1,6–10]* (Refer to ND ineffective Airway Clearance.)

 Acute Care   Collaborative   Community/ Home Care   Cultural

- Assess client's awareness and cognition. *Affects ability to manage own airway and cooperate with interventions such as controlling breathing and managing secretions.*[2,8,9]
- Assist with and monitor results of diagnostic testing (e.g., pulmonary or cardiac function studies, neuromuscular evaluation, sleep studies) *to diagnose presence and severity of lung diseases and degree of respiratory compromise.*
- Review chest radiographs and laboratory data (e.g., ABGs, pulse oximetry at rest and activity *to determine degree of oxygenation, CO_2 retention*) and pulmonary function studies (such as spirometry) *to determine effectiveness of inhalation and exhalation.*[9]

NURSING PRIORITY NO. 2 To provide for relief of causative factors, promoting ease of breathing:[6-11]

- Assist in treatment of underlying conditions, administering medications and therapies as ordered.
- Suction airway to clear secretions as needed. (Refer to ND ineffective Airway Clearance for additional interventions.)
- Maintain emergency equipment in readily accessible location and include age- and size-appropriate airway, ET, and tracheostomy tubes (e.g., infant, child, adolescent, adult).
- Administer oxygen (by cannula, mask, mechanical ventilation) at lowest concentration needed (per ABGs, pulse oximetry) *for underlying pulmonary condition and current respiratory problem.*[11-13] (Refer to ND impaired Gas Exchange for additional interventions.)
- Elevate head of bed or have client sit up in chair; support with pillows *to prevent slumping and promote rest,* or place in position of comfort, as appropriate, *to promote maximal inspiration.*
- Reposition client frequently *to enhance respiratory effort and ventilation of all lung segments, especially if immobility is a factor.*
- Encourage early ambulation using assistive devices, as individually indicated. Involve client in program of exercise training *to prevent onset or reduce severity of respiratory complications and to improve respiratory muscle strength.*[11]
- Direct client in breathing efforts as needed. Encourage slower and deeper respirations and use of the pursed-lip technique, *to assist client in "taking control" of the situation, especially when condition is associated with anxiety and air hunger.*
- Coach client in effective coughing techniques. Place in appropriate position for clearing airways. Splint rib cage and surgical incisions as appropriate. Medicate for pain, as indicated. *Promotes more effective breathing and airway management, especially when client is guarding, as might occur with chest, rib cage, or abdominal injuries or surgeries.* (Refer to NDs acute Pain; chronic Pain for additional interventions.)
- Provide and assist with use of respiratory therapy adjuncts.
- Maintain calm attitude while working with client/significant others (SOs). Provide quiet environment, instruct and reinforce client in the use of relaxation techniques, and administer anti-anxiety medications as indicated *to reduce intensity of anxiety and deal with fear that may be present.* (Refer to NDs Fear; Anxiety for additional interventions.)
- Avoid overfeeding, such as might occur with young infant or client on tube feedings. *Abdominal distention can interfere with breathing as well as increase the risk of aspiration.*
- Ascertain that client possesses and properly operates continuous positive airway pressure machine *when obstructive sleep apnea is causing breathing problems.*
- Maintain emergency equipment in readily accessible location and include age/size-appropriate ET/tracheostomy tubes (e.g., infant, child, adolescent, adult) *when ventilatory support might be needed.*
- Assist with bronchoscopy or chest tube insertion as indicated.

NURSING PRIORITY NO. 3 To promote wellness (Teaching/Discharge Considerations):

- Review with client/SO the type of respiratory condition, treatments, rehabilitation measures, and quality-of-life issues. *Many conditions with impaired breathing are associated with chronic conditions that require lifetime management by client and healthcare providers.*

 Diagnostic Studies   Evidence Based Practice   Medications   Pediatric/Geriatric/Lifespan

- Instruct and reinforce breathing retraining. *Education may include many measures, such as conscious control of breathing rate, effective use of accessory muscles, breathing exercises (diaphragmatic, abdominal breathing, inspiratory resistive, pursed-lip), and assistive devices such as rocking bed.*[6]
- Discuss relationship of smoking to respiratory function. Emphasize importance of smoking cessation and a smoke-free environment.
- Encourage client/SO(s) to develop a plan for smoking cessation. Provide appropriate referrals.
- Encourage self-assessment and symptom management:[6–11]

  Use of equipment to identify respiratory decompensation, such as peak flow meter.

  Appropriate use of oxygen (dosage, route, safety factors).

  Medication regimen, including actions, side effects, and potential interactions of medications, over-the-counter drugs, vitamins, and herbal supplements.

  Home treatments such as metered-dose inhalers, compressor, nebulizer, and chest physiotherapies.

  Dietary patterns and needs; access to foods and nutrients supportive of health and breathing.

  Management of personal environment, including stress reduction, rest and sleep, social events, travel, and recreation issues.

  Avoidance of known irritants, allergens, and sick persons.

  Immunizations against influenza and pneumonia.

  Early intervention when respiratory symptoms occur and what symptoms require reporting to medical providers or seeking emergency care.
- Discuss benefits of exercise for endurance, muscle strengthening, and flexibility training *to improve general health and respiratory muscle function.*
- Refer to physical therapy and pulmonary rehabilitation programs and resources as indicated.[11,12]
- Review energy conservation techniques (e.g., sitting instead of standing to wash dishes, pacing activities, taking short rest periods between activities) *to limit fatigue and improve endurance.*
- Review environmental factors (e.g., exposure to dust, high pollen counts, severe weather, perfumes, animal dander, household chemicals, fumes, secondhand smoke; insufficient home support for safe care) *that may require avoidance/modification of lifestyle or environment to limit impact on client's breathing.*[12–14]
- Reinforce instruction in proper use and safety concerns for home oxygen therapy and/or use of respirator or diaphragmatic stimulator, rocking bed, or apnea monitor, when used. *Protects client's safety, especially when used in the very young or fragile elderly or when a cognitive or neuromuscular impairment is present.*
- Discuss impact of respiratory condition on occupational performance, as well as work environment issues that affect client.
- Provide referrals as indicated by individual situation. *May include a wide variety of services and providers, including support groups, a comprehensive rehabilitation program, occupational nurse, oxygen and durable medical equipment companies for supplies, home health services, occupational and physical therapy, transportation, assisted or alternate living facilities, local and national Lung Association chapters, and Web sites for educational materials.*

DOCUMENTATION FOCUS

Assessment/Reassessment
- Relevant history of problem.
- Respiratory pattern, breath sounds, use of accessory muscles.
- Laboratory values.
- Use of respiratory supports, ventilator settings, etc.

Planning
- Plan of care, specific interventions, and who is involved in the planning.
- Teaching plan.

 Acute Care   Collaborative   Community/ Home Care   Cultural

Implementation/Evaluation
- Response to interventions, teaching, actions performed, and treatment regimen.
- Mastery of skills, level of independence.
- Attainment or progress toward desired outcome(s).
- Modifications to plan of care.

Discharge Planning
- Long-term needs, including appropriate referrals and action taken, available resources.
- Specific referrals provided.

References

1. Bradley, J. S., et al. (2011). The management of community-acquired pneumonia in infants and children older than 3 months of age: Clinical Practice Guidelines by the Pediatric Infectious Diseases Society and the Infectious Diseases Society of America. Retrieved March 2018 from http://www.idsociety.org/uploadedFiles/IDSA/Guidelines-Patient_Care/PDF_Library/2011%20CAP%20in%20Children.pdf.
2. Stanley, M., Blair, K. A., Beare, P. G. (2005). *Gerontological Nursing: Promoting Successful Aging with Older Adults*. 3rd ed. Philadelphia: F. A. Davis.
3. American Lung Association. State of lung disease in diverse communities. (2010). Retrieved October 2015 from http://www.action.lung.org/site/DocServer/state-of-lung-disease-in-diverse-communities-2010.pdf?docID8744.
4. Purnell, L. D. (2011). *A Guide to Culturally Competent Health Care*. 2nd ed. Philadelphia: F. A. Davis.
5. Williams, M. E. (2009). The basic geriatric respiratory examination. Retrieved March 2018 from http://www.medscape.com/viewarticle/712242.
6. Rabe, K. F., et al. (2007). Global strategy for the diagnosis, management, and prevention of chronic obstructive pulmonary disease. *Am J Respir Crit Care Med*, 176, 532–555.
7. Engel, J. (2002). *Mosby's Pocket Guide to Pediatric Assessment*. 4th ed. St. Louis, MO: Mosby.
8. Newfield, S. A., et al. (2007). *Cox's Clinical Applications of Nursing Diagnosis: Adult, Child, Women's, Gerontic, and Home Health Considerations*. 5th ed. Philadelphia: F. A. Davis.
9. Doenges, M. E., Moorhouse, M. F., Murr, A. C. (2016). *Nurse's Pocket Guide: Diagnoses, Prioritized Interventions and Rationales*. 14th ed. Philadelphia: F. A. Davis.
10. Coughlin, L. (2007). Cough: Diagnosis and management of cough: Practice guidelines. *Am Fam Physician*, 75(4), 567–575.
11. Ries, A. L., Bauldoff, G. S., Carlin, B. W. (2007). Pulmonary rehabilitation: Joint ACCP/AACVPR evidence-based clinical practice guidelines. *Chest*, 131(Suppl 5), 4S–42S.
12. Bauldoff, G. S., Diaz, P. T. (2006). Improving outcomes for COPD patients. *Nurs Pract*, 31(8), 26–43.
13. McConville, J. F., Kress, J. P. (2012). Weaning patients from the ventilator. *N Engl J Med*, 367, 2233–2239.
14. Garyi, J. P. (Update 2017). Exercise-induced asthma. Retrieved March 2018 from http://emedicine.medscape.com/article/1938228-overview.

decreased Cardiac Output

Taxonomy II: Activity/Rest—Class 4 Cardiovascular/Pulmonary Responses (00029) [**Diagnostic Division:** Circulation], Approved 1979; Revised 1996, 2000, 2017

DEFINITION: Inadequate blood pumped by the heart to meet the metabolic demands of the body.

RELATED FACTORS
To Be Developed

DEFINING CHARACTERISTICS

Subjective
Altered Heart Rate/Rhythm: Heart palpitations
Altered Preload: Fatigue, weight gain
Altered Afterload: Dyspnea; [feeling breathless]
Altered Contractility: Orthopnea; paroxysmal nocturnal dyspnea [PND]
Behavioral/Emotional: Anxiety

(continues on page 132)

 Diagnostic Studies Evidence Based Practice Medications 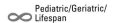 Pediatric/Geriatric/Lifespan

decreased Cardiac Output (continued)

Objective

Altered Heart Rate/Rhythm: Bradycardia; tachycardia; electrocardiogram (ECG) changes [e.g., arrhythmia, conduction abnormality, ischemia]

Altered Preload: Jugular vein distention; edema; weight gain; increase or decrease in central venous pressure (CVP); increase or decrease in pulmonary artery wedge pressure (PAWP); heart murmur

Altered Afterload: Clammy skin; abnormal skin color; prolonged capillary refill; decreased peripheral pulses; alteration in blood pressure; increase or decrease in systemic vascular resistance (SVR); increase or decrease in pulmonary vascular resistance (PVR); oliguria

Altered Contractility: Adventitious breath sounds; coughing; decrease in cardiac index; decrease in ejection fraction; decrease in stroke volume index (SVI) or left ventricular stroke work index (LVSWI); presence of S_3 or S_4 sounds [gallop rhythm]

Behavioral/Emotional: Restlessness

Associated Condition: Alteration in heart rate or rhythm; alteration in preload; alteration in afterload; alteration in stroke volume; alteration in contractility

Sample Clinical Applications: Myocardial infarction (MI), congestive heart failure, valvular heart disease, dysrhythmias, cardiomyopathy, cardiac contusions/trauma, pericarditis, ventricular aneurysm

DESIRED OUTCOMES/EVALUATION CRITERIA

Sample NOC linkages:

Cardiac Pump Effectiveness: Adequacy of blood volume ejected from the left ventricle to support systemic perfusion pressure

Circulation Status: Unobstructed, unidirectional blood flow at an appropriate pressure through large vessels of the systemic and pulmonary circuits

Energy Conservation: Personal actions to manage energy for initiating and sustaining activity

Client Will (Include Specific Time Frame)

- Display hemodynamic stability (e.g., blood pressure, cardiac output, urinary output, peripheral pulses).
- Report or demonstrate decreased episodes of dyspnea, angina, and dysrhythmias.
- Demonstrate an increase in activity tolerance.
- Verbalize knowledge of the disease process, individual risk factors, and treatment plan.
- Participate in activities that reduce the workload of the heart (e.g., stress management or therapeutic medication regimen program, weight reduction, balanced activity/rest plan, proper use of supplemental oxygen, cessation of smoking).
- Identify signs of cardiac decompensation, alter activities, and seek help appropriately.

ACTIONS/INTERVENTIONS

Sample NIC linkages:

Hemodynamic Regulation: Optimization of heart rate, preload, afterload, and contractility

Cardiac Care: Limitation of complications resulting from an imbalance between myocardial oxygen supply and demand for a patient with symptoms of impaired cardiac function

Circulatory Care: Mechanical Assist Devices: Temporary support of the circulation through the use of mechanical devices or pumps

 Acute Care   Collaborative   Community/Home Care   Cultural

NURSING PRIORITY NO. 1   To identify causative/contributing factors:

- Review clients at risk as noted in Related Factors and Defining Characteristics. *In addition to individuals obviously at risk with known cardiac problems, there is a potential for cardiac output problems in persons with trauma; hemorrhage; alcohol and other drug intoxication, withdrawal, chronic use, or overdose; pregnant women with hypertensive states; individuals with chronic renal failure; individuals with brainstem trauma or spinal cord injury at T8 or above.*

- ∞ ⊕ ▧ Note age, gender, and ethnic-related cardiovascular considerations, e.g., *in infants, failure to thrive with poor ability to suck and feed can be an indication of heart problems.[1] Contractile force is naturally decreased in the elderly with reduced ability to raise cardiac output in response to increased demand. Also, arteries are stiffer, veins are more dilated, and heart valves are less competent, often resulting in systemic hypertension and blood pooling.[318] In 2013, the overall prevalence of heart failure (HF) was reported to range from 1% to 12% based on available data from the United States and Europe. In 2017, the American Heart Association estimated the annual incidence of heart failure in persons older than 65 to be 21/1000.[4,19] When in the supine position, pregnant women incur decreased vascular return during the second and third trimesters, potentially compromising cardiac output.[2] Generally, higher-risk populations include African Americans, Hispanics, Native Americans, and recent immigrants from developing nations, Russia, and the former Soviet republics. The higher prevalence of heart failure in African Americans, Hispanics, and Native Americans is directly related to the higher incidence and prevalence of hypertension and diabetes.[5]*

- ▱ Review diagnostic studies, including, but not limited to, chest radiograph, cardiac stress testing, ECG, echocardiogram, cardiac output and ventricular ejection studies, and heart scan or catheterization. *For example, ECG may show previous or evolving MI, left ventricular hypertrophy, and valvular stenosis. Doppler flow echocardiogram showing an ejection fraction (EF) less than 40% is indicative of systolic dysfunction, but many clients with clinical diagnosis of heart failure have a normal EF. Although cardiac output can be high in certain types of heart failure, a client with severe HF will have decreased cardiac output (less than 4 L/m) owing either to an increased hemodynamic burden or to a reduction in oxygen delivery to the myocardium, resulting in impaired contraction. Additional cardiac studies (e.g., radionuclide scans or catheterization) may be indicated to assess left ventricular function, valvular function, and coronary circulation. Chest radiography may show enlarged heart, pulmonary infiltrates.[6–8,12,13]*

- ▱ Review laboratory data, including, but not limited to, complete blood count, electrolytes, arterial blood gases (ABGs), and cardiac biomarkers (e.g., creatine kinase and its subclasses, troponins, myoglobin, and LDH); lactate; brain natriuretic peptide; kidney, thyroid, and liver function studies; and cultures (e.g., blood, wound, secretions), bleeding, and coagulation studies *to identify imbalances, disease processes, and effects of interventions.[6,12]*

NURSING PRIORITY NO. 2   To assess degree of debilitation:

- Assess for signs of poor ventricular function or impending cardiac failure and shock:[2,3,7–12]

  Client reports or demonstrates extreme fatigue, intolerance for activity, sudden or progressive weight gain, swelling of extremities, and progressive shortness of breath.

  Client reports chest pain. *May indicate evolving heart attack; can also accompany congestive heart failure. Chest pain may be atypical in women experiencing an MI and is often atypical in the elderly owing to altered pain perception.*

  Mental status changes. *Confusion, agitation, decreased cognition, and coma may occur due to decreased brain perfusion.*

  Changes in heart rate or rhythm: Tachycardia at rest, bradycardia, atrial fibrillation, or multiple dysrhythmias may be noted. *Heart irritability is common, reflecting conduction defects and/or ischemia.*

  Heart sounds may be distant, with irregular rhythms; murmurs—systolic *(valvular stenosis and shunting)* and diastolic *(aortic or pulmonary insufficiency)* or gallop rhythm (S_3, S_4) noted *when heart failure is present and ventricles are stiff.*

Peripheral pulses may be weak and thready, *reflecting hypotension, vasoconstriction, shunting, and venous congestion.*

∞ Changes in skin color, moisture, temperature, and capillary refill time. *Pallor or cyanosis; cool, moist skin; and slow capillary refill time may be present because of peripheral vasoconstriction and decreased oxygen saturation. Note: Children with chronic heart failure and adults with chronic obstructive pulmonary disease often show clubbing of fingertips.*

Blood pressure changes. *Hypertension may be chronic or blood pressure elevated initially in client with impending cardiogenic, hypovolemic, or septic shock. Later, as cardiac output decreases, profound hypotension can be present, often with narrowed pulse pressure.*

Breath sounds may reveal bilateral crackles and wheezing *associated with congestion. Respiratory distress and failure often occur as shock progresses.*

Edema with neck vein distention is often present, and pitting edema is noted in extremities and dependent portions of body *because of impaired venous return.* Other veins in trunk and extremities can be prominent *owing to venous congestion.*

∞ Urinary output may be decreased or absent, *reflecting poor perfusion of kidneys. Note: Output less than 30 mL/hr (adult) or less than 10 mL/hr (child) indicates inadequate renal perfusion.*

NURSING PRIORITY NO. 3 To minimize/correct causative factors, maximize cardiac output:

Acute/severe phase[7–10,12,15]

- Keep client on bedrest or chairrest in position of comfort. *Decreases oxygen consumption and demand, reducing myocardial workload and risk of decomposition. Note: In congestive state, client may be placed in semi-Fowler's or high Fowler's position to reduce preload and ventricular filling. A supine position may be needed to increase venous return and promote diuresis. May raise legs 20 to 30 degrees in shock situation (Trendelenburg position); however, current studies to support the use of the Trendelenburg position during shock do not reveal any beneficial or sustained changes in systolic blood pressure or cardiac output.*[18]

- Administer supplemental oxygen, as indicated (by cannula, mask, endotracheal or tracheostomy tube with mechanical ventilation), *to improve cardiac function by increasing available oxygen and reducing oxygen consumption. Note: A critically ill client may be on ventilator to support cardiopulmonary function.*[12]

- Monitor vital signs frequently *to evaluate response to treatments and activities.* Perform periodic hemodynamic measurements, as indicated (e.g., arterial, CVP, PAWP, left atrial pressure; cardiac output and cardiac index, oxygen saturation). *These measurements (via central line monitoring) are commonly used in the critically ill to provide continuous, accurate assessment of cardiac function and response to inotropic and vasoactive medications that affect cardiac contractility and systemic circulation (preload and afterload). Note: A multicenter research study evaluating the clinical effectiveness of clinical management guided by a pulmonary artery catheter in adult intensive care patients (N = 1,041) found no clear evidence that management guided by a pulmonary catheter was either beneficial or harmful.*[15,17]

- Monitor cardiac rhythm continuously *to note changes and evaluate effectiveness of medications and devices (e.g., implanted pacemaker/defibrillator).*

- Administer or restrict fluids, as indicated. *Replacement of blood and large amounts of IV fluids may be needed if low output state is due to hypovolemia.* Use infusion pumps for IVs *to monitor IV rates closely to prevent bolus or exacerbation of fluid overload.*

- Assess hourly or periodic urinary output and daily weight, noting 24-hour total fluid balance *to evaluate kidney function and effects of interventions, as well as to allow for timely alterations in therapeutic regimen.*

- Administer medications as indicated (e.g., inotropic drugs *to maintain systemic perfusion and preserve end-organ performance,* antiarrhythmics *to improve cardiac output;* diuretics *to reduce congestion by improving urinary output;* vasopressors and/or dilators as indicated *to manage systemic effects of vasoconstriction and low cardiac output;* pain medications and anti-anxiety agents *to reduce oxygen demand and myocardial workload;* anticoagulants *to improve blood flow and prevent thromboemboli). Note: Randomized clinical trials demonstrate consistent mortality benefit from angiotensin-converting enzyme inhibitors (ACEIs), angiotensin*

 Acute Care   Collaborative   Community/Home Care   Cultural

receptor blockers (ARBs); direct-acting vasodilators, beta blockers, and aldosterone antagonists. Additionally, some data show benefits from two new classes of drugs: ARB/neprilysin inhibitor and sinus node modulator.[7]

- Note reports of anorexia or nausea and limit or withhold oral intake as indicated. *Symptoms may be systemic reaction to low cardiac output, visceral congestion, or reaction to medications or pain.*
- 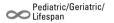 Assist with preparations for and monitor response to support procedures or devices as indicated (e.g., cardioversion, pacemaker, angioplasty and stent placement, coronary artery bypass graft or valve replacement, intra-aortic balloon pump, left ventricular assist device [LVAD]; total artificial heart [TAH], transplantation). *Any number of interventions may be required to correct a condition causing heart failure or to support a failing heart during recovery from myocardial infarction, while awaiting transplantation, or for long-term management of chronic heart failure. Note: The application of LVAD during reperfusion procedures causes reduction of the left ventricular preload, increases regional myocardial blood flow and lactate extraction, and improves general cardiac function.*[6,7]
- Promote rest periods in bed or chair with upper body elevated, as indicated, *to reduce catecholamine-induced stress response and cardiac workload:*[11,15]
  Decrease stimuli, providing quiet environment.
  Schedule activities and assessments *to maximize sleep periods.*
  Assist with or perform self-care activities for client.
  Avoid the use of restraints whenever possible, especially if client is confused.
- Use sedation and analgesics, as indicated, with caution *to achieve desired rest state without compromising hemodynamic responses.*

Postacute/Chronic Phase[6,7,11]

- Provide for adequate rest, positioning client for maximum comfort.
- Encourage changing positions slowly, dangling legs before standing *to reduce risk of orthostatic hypotension.*
- Increase activity levels gradually as permitted by individual condition, noting vital sign response to activity.
- Administer medications, as appropriate, and monitor cardiac responses.
- Encourage relaxation techniques *to reduce anxiety and muscle tension.*
- Refer for nutritional needs assessment and management *to provide for supportive nutrition while meeting diet restrictions (e.g., IV nutrition or total parenteral nutrition, sodium-restricted or other type of diet with frequent small feedings).*
- Monitor intake/output and calculate 24-hour fluid balance. Provide or restrict fluids, as indicated, *to maximize cardiac output and improve tissue perfusion.*[15]

NURSING PRIORITY NO. 4 To enhance safety/prevent complications:[2,14,15]

- Wash hands before and after client contact, maintain aseptic technique during invasive procedures, and provide site care, as indicated, *to prevent hospital-acquired infection.* (Refer to ND risk for Infection for additional interventions.)
- Provide antipyretics and fever control actions as indicated. Adjust ambient environmental temperature *to maintain body temperature in near-normal range.*
- Maintain patency of invasive intravascular monitoring and infusion lines and tape connections *to prevent exsanguination or air embolus.*
- Minimize activities that can elicit Valsalva response (e.g., rectal straining, vomiting, spasmodic coughing with suctioning, prolonged breath-holding during pushing stage of labor) and encourage client to breathe deeply in and out during activities that increase risk of Valsalva effect. *Valsalva response to breath-holding causes increased intrathoracic pressure, reducing cardiac output and blood pressure.*[14]
- Avoid prolonged sitting position for all clients and supine position for sleep or exercise for gravid clients (second and third trimesters) *to maximize vascular return.*[2,15]
- Elevate legs when in sitting position and edematous extremities when at rest. Apply antiembolic hose or sequential compression devices when indicated, being sure they are individually fitted and appropriately applied. *Limits venous stasis, improves venous return, and reduces risk of thrombophlebitis.* (Refer to ND ineffective peripheral Tissue Perfusion for additional interventions.)

 Diagnostic Studies   Evidence Based Practice   Medications   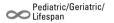 Pediatric/Geriatric/ Lifespan

- Provide skin care, a special bed or mattress (e.g., air, water, gel, foam), and assist with frequent position changes *to prevent the development of pressure ulcers.*
- Provide psychological support *to reduce anxiety and its adverse effects on cardiac function:*
  Maintain calm attitude and limit stressful stimuli.
  Provide and encourage use of relaxation techniques, such as massage therapy, soothing music, or quiet activities.
  Promote visits from family/significant others *to provide positive social interaction.*
  Provide information about testing procedures and client participation.
  Explain limitations imposed by condition and dietary and fluid restrictions.
  Share information about positive signs of improvement.

NURSING PRIORITY NO. 5   To promote wellness (Teaching/Discharge Considerations):[11,16]

- 🏠 Provide information to clients/caregivers on individual condition, therapies, and expected outcomes. Use various forms of teaching according to client needs, desires, and learning style.
- 💊 Direct client and/or caregivers to resources for emergency assistance, financial help, durable medical supplies, and psychosocial support and respite, especially when client has impaired functional capabilities or requires supporting equipment (e.g., pacemaker, LVAD, or 24-hour oxygen).
- 💊 Emphasize importance of regular medical follow-up care *to monitor client's condition and response to treatment and provide the most effective care.*
- Educate client/caregivers about drug regimen, including indications, dose and dosing schedules, potential adverse side effects, or drug/drug interactions. *Client is often on multiple medications, which can be difficult to manage, thus increasing potential that medications can be missed or incorrectly used.*
- Emphasize reporting of adverse and nuisance side effects of medications *so that adjustments can be made in dosing or another class of medication considered.*
- 💊 Discuss significant signs/symptoms that need to be reported to healthcare provider, such as *unrelieved or increased chest pain, dyspnea, fever, swelling of ankles, and sudden unexplained cough; these are all "danger signs" that require immediate evaluation and possible change of usual therapies.*
- Provide instruction for home monitoring of weight, pulse, and blood pressure, as appropriate, *to detect change and allow for timely intervention.*
- 💉 Recommend annual flu shot, and pneumonia vaccination (when needed).
- 💊 Discuss individual's particular risk factors (e.g., smoking, stress, obesity, recent MI) and specific resources for assistance (e.g., written information sheets, direction to helpful Web sites, formalized rehabilitation programs, home interventions) for management of identified factors for:
  Smoking cessation
  Stress management techniques
  Energy conservation techniques
  Nutrition education regarding specific needs (e.g., to improve general health status, reduce or gain weight, lower cholesterol levels, manage sodium)
  Exercise and activity plan
- Refer to NDs Activity Intolerance, decreased Diversional Activity Engagement, ineffective Coping, ineffective Breathing Pattern, compromised family Coping, deficient/excess Fluid Volume, imbalanced Nutrition: less than body requirements, Overweight, acute/chronic Pain, risk for decreased cardiac Tissue Perfusion, ineffective peripheral Tissue Perfusion, Sexual Dysfunction, as indicated.

DOCUMENTATION FOCUS

Assessment/Reassessment
- Baseline and subsequent findings and individual hemodynamic parameters, heart and breath sounds, ECG pattern, presence and strength of peripheral pulses, skin and tissue status, renal output, and mentation.

 Acute Care   Collaborative   Community/ Home Care   Cultural

Planning
- Plan of care and who is involved in planning.
- Teaching plan.

Implementation/Evaluation
- Client's responses to interventions, teaching, and actions performed.
- Status and disposition at discharge.
- Attainment or progress toward desired outcome(s).
- Modifications to plan of care.

Discharge Planning
- Discharge considerations and who will be responsible for carrying out individual actions.
- Long-term needs.
- Specific referrals made.

References

1. Newfield, S. A., et al. (2007). *Cox's Clinical Applications of Nursing Diagnosis: Adult, Child, Women's Psychiatric, Gerontic, and Home Health Considerations*. 5th ed. Philadelphia: F. A. Davis.
2. Ladewig, P., et al. (2001). *Contemporary Maternal-Newborn Nursing Care*. 5th ed. Upper Saddle River, NJ: Prentice Hall.
3. Stanley, M., Beare, P. G. (1999). *Gerontological Nursing: A Health Promotion/Protection Approach*. 2nd ed. Philadelphia: F. A. Davis.
4. Roger, V. L. (2013). Epidemiology of heart failure. *Circ Res*, 113(6), 646–659.
5. Purnell, L. D. (2008). *Guide to Culturally Competent Health Care*. 2nd ed. Philadelphia: F. A. Davis.
6. Dumitru, I., Baker, M. M. (2018). Heart failure. Retrieved March 2018 from http://emedicine.medscape.com/article/163062-workup.
7. 2013 ACCF/AHA guideline for the management of heart failure. (2013). *American College of Cardiology Foundation/American Heart Association Task Force on Practice Guidelines*. Retrieved March 2018 from http://content.onlinejacc.org/article.aspx?articleid=1695825.
8. Chavey, W. E., et al. (2017). Heart failure due to reduced ejection fraction: Medical management. *Am Fam Physician*, 95(1), 13–20.
9. American Heart Association. (2015). Implantable medical devices. Retrieved March 2018 from https://www.heart.org/HEARTORG/Conditions/HeartAttack/PreventionTreatmentofHeartAttack/Implantable-Medical-Devices_UCM_303940_Article.jsp.
10. Cooper, K. L. (2015). Biventricular pacemakers in patients with heart failure. *Crit Care Nurse*, 35(2), 20–24.
11. American Heart Association, the Council on Clinical Cardiology, the Councils on Cardiovascular Nursing, et al. (2007). Core components of cardiac rehabilitation secondary prevention programs: 2007 update. *Circulation*, 115, 2675–2682.
12. Ren, X. (Mike), Lenneman, A. (Updated 2017). Cardiogenic shock. Retrieved March 2018 from http://emedicine.medscape.com/article/152191-overview.
13. Olade, R. B., Safi, A., Badero, A. S. (Updated 2016). Cardiac catheterization of the left heart. Retrieved March 2018 from http://emedicine.medscape.com/article/1819224-overview.
14. Hiner, B. C. (2005). Valsalva maneuver. *Clin Med Res*, 3(2), 55.
15. Kieley, D. G., et al. (2013). Pulmonary hypertension: diagnosis and management. *BMJ*, 346, f2028.
16. Purgason, K. (2006). Broken hearts: Differentiating stress-induced cardiomyopathy from acute myocardial infarction in the patient presenting with acute coronary syndrome. *Dimens Crit Care Nurs*, 25(6), 247–253.
17. Harvey, S. (2005). Assessment of the clinical effectiveness of the pulmonary catheters in the management of patients in intensive care; (PAC-Man): A randomised controlled trial. *Lancet*, 366(9484), 472–477.
18. Halm, M. A. (2012). Trendelenburg position: "Put to bed" or angled toward use in your unit? *Am J Crit Care*, 21(6), 449–452.
19. Benjamin, E. J., et al. (2017). Heart Disease and Stroke Statistics—2017 Update: A Report from the American Heart Association. *Circulation*, 136, 464–468.

 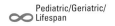

risk for decreased Cardiac Output

Taxonomy II: Activity/Rest—Class 4 Cardiovascular/Pulmonary Responses (00240) [**Diagnostic Division:** Circulation], Approved 2013; Revised 2017

DEFINITION: Susceptible to inadequate blood pumped by the heart to meet the metabolic demands of the body, which may compromise health.

RISK FACTORS
To Be Developed
Associated Condition: Alteration in heart rate or rhythm; alteration in preload; alteration in afterload; alteration in stroke volume; alteration in contractility

DESIRED OUTCOMES/EVALUATION CRITERIA

Sample NOC linkages:
Cardiac Pump Effectiveness: Adequacy of blood volume ejected from the left ventricle to support systemic perfusion pressure
Circulation Status: Unobstructed, unidirectional blood flow at an appropriate pressure through large vessels of the systemic and pulmonary circuits
Energy Conservation: Personal actions to manage energy for initiating and sustaining activity

Client Will (Include Specific Time Frame)
• Display hemodynamic stability (e.g., blood pressure, cardiac output, urinary output, peripheral pulses).
• Verbalize knowledge of the disease process and individual risk factors.
• Participate in activities that reduce risk factors (e.g., stress management or therapeutic medication regimen program, weight reduction, balanced activity/rest plan, proper use of supplemental oxygen, cessation of smoking).

ACTIONS/INTERVENTIONS

Sample NIC linkages:
Cardiac Risk Management: Prevention of an acute episode of impaired cardiac function by minimizing contributing events and risk factors
Hemodynamic Regulation: Optimization of heart rate, preload, afterload, and contractility

NURSING PRIORITY NO. 1   To identify client at risk:

• Identify client at risk: *In addition to an individual obviously at risk because of known cardiac problems, there is a potential for cardiac output issues in others (e.g., person with traumatic injuries and hemorrhage; brainstem trauma; spinal cord injury at T8 or above; alcohol and other drug intoxication, substance withdrawal or overdose; pregnant woman with hypertensive states; individual with chronic renal failure).*
• ∞ 🌐 Note age, gender, and ethnic-related cardiovascular considerations. For example, *in infants, failure to thrive with poor ability to suck and feed can be indications of heart problems;[1] contractile force is naturally decreased in the elderly with reduced ability to increase cardiac output in response to increased demand;[2] when in the supine position, pregnant women incur decreased vascular return during the second and third trimesters, potentially compromising cardiac output;[3] and generally, higher-risk populations include African Americans, Hispanics, Native Americans, and recent immigrants from developing nations, Russia, and the former Soviet republics.[4,5]*

 Acute Care   Collaborative   Community/Home Care   Cultural

- Assess for signs of poor ventricular function or impending cardiac failure:[2,6,7,9,10]

  Note reports of extreme fatigue, intolerance for activity, sudden or progressive weight gain, swelling of extremities, and progressive shortness of breath.

  Evaluate reports of chest pain. *May indicate evolving heart attack; can also accompany congestive heart failure.*

  Observe for mental status changes. *Confusion, agitation, and altered cognition may occur due to decreased brain perfusion.*

  Note changes in heart rate or rhythm: *Heart irritability is common, reflecting conduction defects and/or ischemia.*

  Assess heart sounds. *May become distant, with irregular rhythms; murmurs.*

  Palpate peripheral pulses, *which may become weak and thready.*

  Observe skin, noting color, moisture, temperature, and capillary refill time. *Pallor or cyanosis; cool, moist skin; and slow capillary refill time can occur with peripheral vasoconstriction and decreased oxygen saturation.*

  Evaluate blood pressure changes. *Client may have chronic hypertension. Blood pressure can be elevated initially, followed by hypotension in client with impending cardiogenic, hypovolemic, or septic shock.*

  Auscultate breath sounds. *Bilateral crackles and wheezing can occur associated with congestion.*

  Check for dependent or generalized edema with neck vein distention, *which can occur because of impaired venous return.*

  Observe for changes in urinary output, *which may be decreased or be caused by dehydration, hypovolemia, or poor perfusion of kidneys.*

- Review laboratory data, including, but not limited to, complete blood count, electrolytes, arterial blood gases, cardiac biomarkers (e.g., creatine kinase and its subclasses, troponins, myoglobin, LDH); lactate; brain natriuretic peptide; kidney, thyroid, and liver function studies; cultures (e.g., blood, wound, secretions); bleeding and coagulation studies, *to identify client at risk and promote early intervention, if indicated.*[6,7]

- Refer to ND decreased Cardiac Output for additional assessments and interventions as indicated.

NURSING PRIORITY NO. 2   To minimize risk factors, maximize cardiac output:[6–8,10]

- Provide for adequate rest.
- Increase activity levels gradually as permitted by individual condition, noting vital sign response to activity.
- Administer medications, as appropriate, and monitor cardiac responses.
- Encourage relaxation techniques *to reduce anxiety and muscle tension.*
- Elevate legs when in sitting position and edematous extremities when at rest. Apply antiembolic hose or sequential compression devices when indicated, ensuring they are individually fitted and appropriately applied. *Limits venous stasis, improves venous return, and reduces risk of thrombophlebitis.*
- Avoid prolonged sitting position for all clients and supine position for sleep or exercise for gravid clients (second and third trimesters) *to maximize vascular return.*[2,3]

NURSING PRIORITY NO. 3   To promote wellness (Teaching/Discharge Considerations):[6–8]

- Discuss individual's particular risk factors (e.g., smoking, stress, obesity, recent myocardial infarction) and specific resources for assistance (e.g., written information sheets, direction to helpful Web sites, formalized rehabilitation programs, home interventions) for management of identified risk factors.
- Provide information to clients/caregivers on individual condition, therapies, and expected outcomes.
- Educate client/caregivers about drug regimen, including indications, dose and dosing schedules, potential adverse side effects, or drug/drug interactions.
- Provide instruction for home monitoring of weight, pulse, and blood pressure, as appropriate.
- Discuss significant signs/symptoms that need to be reported to healthcare provider, such as unrelieved or increased chest pain, dyspnea, fever, swelling of ankles, and sudden unexplained cough.

 Diagnostic Studies   Evidence Based Practice   Medications   Pediatric/Geriatric/ Lifespan

- Emphasize importance of regular medical follow-up care *to monitor client's condition and provide early intervention when indicated to prevent complications.*

DOCUMENTATION FOCUS

Assessment/Reassessment
- Baseline and subsequent findings and individual hemodynamic parameters, heart and breath sounds, ECG pattern, presence and strength of peripheral pulses, skin and tissue status, renal output, and mentation.

Planning
- Plan of care and who is involved in planning.
- Teaching plan.

Implementation/Evaluation
- Client's responses to interventions, teaching, and actions performed.
- Status and disposition at discharge.
- Attainment or progress toward desired outcome(s).
- Modifications to plan of care.

Discharge Planning
- Discharge considerations and who will be responsible for carrying out individual actions.
- Long-term needs.
- Specific referrals made.

References

1. Newfield, S. A., et al. (2007). *Cox's Clinical Applications of Nursing Diagnosis: Adult, Child, Women's Psychiatric, Gerontic, and Home Health Considerations.* 5th ed. Philadelphia: F. A. Davis.
2. Stanley, M., Beare, P. G. (1999). *Gerontological Nursing: A Health Promotion/Protection Approach.* 2nd ed. Philadelphia: F. A. Davis.
3. Ladewig, P., et al. (2001). *Contemporary Maternal-Newborn Nursing Care.* 5th ed. Upper Saddle River, NJ: Prentice Hall.
4. Roger, V. L. (2013). Epidemiology of heart failure. *Circ Res.,* 113(6), 646–659.
5. Purnell, L. D. (2008). *Guide to Culturally Competent Health Care.* 2nd ed. Philadelphia: F. A. Davis.
6. Dumitru, I., Baker, M. M. (2018). Heart failure. Retrieved March 2018 from http://emedicine.medscape.com/article/163062-workup.
7. American College of Cardiology Foundation/American Heart Association Task Force on Practice Guidelines. (2013). 2013 ACCF/AHA guideline for the management of heart failure. Retrieved March 2018 from http://content.onlinejacc.org/article.aspx?articleid=1695825.
8. American Heart Association, the Council on Clinical Cardiology, the Councils on Cardiovascular Nursing, et al. Core components of cardiac rehabilitation secondary prevention programs: 2007 update. (2007). *Circulation,* 115, 2675–2682.
9. Ren, X. (Mike), Lenneman, A. (Updated 2017). *Cardiogenic shock.* Retrieved March 2018 from http://emedicine.medscape.com/article/152191-overview.
10. Cheever, K. H. (2005). An overview of pulmonary arterial hypertension: Risks, pathogenesis, clinical manifestations, and management. *J Cardiovasc Nurs,* 20(2), 108–116.

 Acute Care   Collaborative   Community/Home Care   Cultural

ineffective Childbearing Process

Taxonomy II: Sexuality—Class 3 Reproduction (00221) [**Diagnostic Division:** Sexuality], Approved 2010; Revised 2017

DEFINITION: Inability to prepare for and/or maintain a healthy pregnancy, childbirth process, and care of the newborn for ensuring well-being.

RELATED FACTORS

Inadequate maternal nutrition; inconsistent prenatal health visits; insufficient prenatal care
Insufficient knowledge of childbearing process; unrealistic birth plan
Insufficient parental role model or support system
Maternal powerlessness, or low maternal confidence; psychological distress
Domestic violence; substance misuse/[abuse]

DEFINING CHARACTERISTICS

Subjective
During Pregnancy
Inadequate prenatal care and lifestyle [e.g., nutrition, elimination, sleep, exercise, personal hygiene]
Ineffective management of unpleasant symptoms in pregnancy
Unrealistic birth plan
During Labor and Delivery
Inadequate lifestyle for stage of labor
After Birth
Inadequate postpartum lifestyle

Objective
During Pregnancy
Inadequate prenatal care or lifestyle
Insufficient access of support system
Insufficient respect for unborn baby; inadequate preparation of newborn care items or home environment
During Labor and Delivery
Inappropriate response to onset of labor; decrease in proactivity during labor and delivery
Insufficient attachment behavior
Insufficient access of support system
After Birth
Insufficient attachment behavior; inadequate baby care techniques
Inappropriate baby feeding techniques; inappropriate breast care
Unsafe environment for an infant
Insufficient access of support system
Associated Condition: Unplanned or unwanted pregnancy
Sample Clinical Applications: First, second, and third trimester of pregnancy; labor and delivery, postpartum, newborn

DESIRED OUTCOMES/EVALUATION CRITERIA

Sample **NOC** linkages:
Prenatal Health Behavior: Personal actions to promote a healthy pregnancy and a healthy newborn
Maternal Status: Antepartum/Intrapartum/Postpartum [specify]: Extent to which maternal well-being is within normal limits from conception to the onset of labor/from onset of labor to delivery/from delivery of placenta to completion of involution

(continues on page 142)

 Diagnostic Studies   Evidence Based Practice   Medications 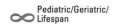 Pediatric/Geriatric/Lifespan

ineffective Childbearing Process (continued)

Knowledge: Infant Care: Extent of understanding conveyed about caring for a baby from birth to first birthday

Client Will (Include Specific Time Frame)
- Demonstrate healthy pregnancy free of preventable complications.
- Engage in activities to prepare for birth process and care of newborn.
- Experience complication-free labor and childbirth.
- Verbalize understanding of care requirements to promote health of self and infant.

ACTIONS/INTERVENTIONS

Sample NIC linkages:

Childbirth Preparation: Providing information and support to facilitate childbirth and to enhance the ability of an individual to develop and perform the parental role

Prenatal Care: Provision of healthcare during the course of pregnancy

Attachment Promotion: Facilitating the development of an effective, enduring relationship between infant and parent

NURSING PRIORITY NO. 1   To determine causative factors and individual needs:

During Pregnancy
- Determine maternal health/nutritional status, usual pregravid weight, and dietary pattern. *Research studies have found a positive correlation between pregravid maternal obesity and increased perinatal morbidity rates (e.g., hypertension and gestational diabetes) associated with preterm births and macrosomia.*[16]
- Note use of alcohol/other drugs, nicotine. *Maternal pregnancy complications and negative effects on the developing fetus are increased with the use of tobacco, alcohol, and illicit drugs. Smoking negatively affects placental circulation; even smoking fewer than 10 cigarettes/day is associated with an increased risk of fetal death, damage in utero, abruptio placenta, placenta previa, and low birth weights.*[4,8,13–15,20] *Note: Prescription medications may also be dangerous to the fetus, requiring a risk/benefit analysis for therapeutic choices and appropriate dosage.*[12]
- Evaluate current knowledge regarding physiological and psychological changes associated with pregnancy. *Provides information to assist in identifying needs and creating individual plan of care.*[2,3]
- Identify involvement/response of child's father to pregnancy. *Helps clarify whether or not father is likely to be supportive or has the potential of posing a threat to the safety and well-being of mother/fetus.*[19]
- Determine family stressors, economic situation/financial needs, and availability/use of resources *to identify necessary referrals. Impact of pregnancy on family with limited resources can create added stress and result in limited prenatal care and preparation for newborn.*[1,2]
- Verify environmental well-being and safety of client/family. *Women experiencing intimate partner violence both prior to and/or during pregnancy are at higher risk for multiple poor maternal and infant health outcomes.*[18,19]
- Determine cultural expectations/beliefs about childbearing, self-care, and so on. Identify who provides support/instruction within the client's culture (e.g., grandmother/other family member, cuerandero/doula, other cultural healer). Work with support person(s) as desired by client, using an interpreter as needed. *Helps ensure quality and continuity of care because support person(s) can reinforce information provided.*[1,2,4]
- Ascertain client's commitments to work, family, and self; roles/responsibilities within family unit; and use of supportive resources. *Helps in setting realistic priorities to assist client in making adjustments, such as*

 Acute Care   Collaborative   Community/Home Care   Cultural

changing work hours, shifting of household chores, curtailing some outside commitments.[12,17] *Note: Initially, even if the pregnancy is planned, the expectant mother may feel ambivalence toward the pregnancy because of personal or professional goals, financial concerns, and/or possible role changes.*[1,2]

- Determine client's/couple's perception of fetus as a separate entity and extent of preparations being made for this infant. *Absence of activities such as choosing a name or nicknaming the baby in utero and home preparations indicate lack of completion of psychological tasks of pregnancy. Note: Cultural or familial beliefs may limit visible preparations out of concern that bad outcome might result.*[2]

During Labor and Delivery

- Ascertain client's understanding and expectations of the labor process and who will participate/provide support.
- Determine presence/appropriateness of birth plan developed by client/couple and any associated cultural expectations/preferences. *Identifies areas to address to ensure that choices made are amenable to the specific care setting, reflect reality of client/fetal status, and accommodate individual wishes. Note: Some cultures or personal values may limit male involvement in the delivery process, necessitating the identification of other support person(s).*[1,6,10]

After Birth

- Determine plan for discharge after delivery and home-care support/needs. *Important to facilitate discharge and ensure client/infant needs will be met.*[3]
- Appraise level of parent's understanding of physiological needs and adaptation to extrauterine life associated with maintenance of body temperature, nutrition, respiratory needs, and bowel and bladder functioning. *Identifies areas of concern/need requiring development of teaching plan and/or demonstration of care activities.*[3,12]
- Assess mother's strengths and needs, noting age, relationship status, and reactions of family members. *Identifies potential risk factors that influence the client's/couple's ability to assume role of parenthood. For example, an adolescent still formulating goals and identity may have difficulty accepting the infant as a person. The single parent who lacks support systems may have difficulty assuming sole responsibility for parenting.*[1,6]
- Ascertain nature of emotional and physical parenting that client/couple received during their childhood. *Parenting role is learned, and individuals use their own parents as role models. Those who experienced a negative upbringing or poor parenting may require additional support to meet the challenges of effective parenting.*

NURSING PRIORITY NO. 2 To promote optimal maternal well-being:

During Pregnancy

- Emphasize importance of maternal well-being including discussion of nutrition, regular moderate exercise, comfort measures, rest, and sexual activity. *Fetal well-being is directly related to maternal health, especially during the first trimester, when developing organ systems are most vulnerable to injury from environmental or hereditary factors:*

  Review nutrition requirements and optimal prenatal weight gain to support maternal-fetal needs. *Dietary focus should be on balanced nutrients and calories to produce appropriate weight gain and to supply vitamins and minerals for healthy fetus. Inadequate prenatal weight gain and/or below normal prepregnancy weight increases the risk of intrauterine growth retardation in the fetus and delivery of a low-birth-weight infant.*[8,12]

  Encourage moderate exercise such as walking, or non-weight-bearing activities (e.g., swimming, bicycling) in accordance with client's physical condition and cultural beliefs. *Nonendurance antepartal exercise tends to shorten labor, increases likelihood of a spontaneous vaginal delivery, and decreases need for oxytocin augmentation.*[4,5] *In some cultures, inactivity may be viewed as a protection for the mother.*[1,6]

  Recommend a consistent sleep and rest schedule (e.g., 1- to 2-hour daytime nap and 8 hours of sleep each night) in a dark, comfortable room. *Provides rest to meet metabolic needs associated with growth of maternal and fetal tissues.*[12]

- Provide necessary referrals (e.g., dietitian, social services, supplemental nutrition assistance programs including the Women, Infants, and Children [WIC] program) as indicated. *May need additional assistance with*

 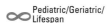

nutritional choices and may have budget or financial constraints. Supplemental federal/state food programs help promote optimal maternal, fetal, and infant nutrition.[12]

- Encourage participation in a smoking-cessation program and alcohol/drug abstinence as appropriate. *Reduces risk of premature birth, stillbirth, low birth weight, congenital defects, drug withdrawal of newborn, and fetal alcohol syndrome.*[14]

- Explain psychological reactions, including ambivalence, introspection, stress reactions, and emotional lability, as being characteristic of pregnancy. *Helps client/couple understand mood swings and may provide opportunity for partner to offer support and affection at these times.*[4] *Note: However, the stressors associated with pregnancy may lead to abuse/exacerbate existing abusive behavior.*[18,19]

- Discuss personal situation and options, providing information about resources available to client. *Partner may be upset about an unplanned pregnancy, financial concern regarding supporting the child, or even jealousy that attention is shifting to the unborn child, creating safety issues for client/family.*[19]

- Identify reportable potential danger signals of pregnancy, such as bleeding, cramping, acute abdominal pain, backache, edema, visual disturbances, headaches, and pelvic pressure. *Helps client distinguish normal from abnormal findings, thus assisting her in seeking timely, appropriate healthcare.*[12] (Refer to ND risk for disturbed Maternal-Fetal Dyad for additional interventions.)

During Labor and Delivery

- Monitor labor progress and maternal and fetal well-being per protocol. Provide continuous intrapartal professional support/doula. *Fear of abandonment can intensify as labor progresses. The client may experience increased anxiety and/or loss of control when left unattended. Doulas can provide client with emotional, physical, and informational support as an adjunct to primary nurse.*[2,8]

- Identify client's support person/coach and ascertain that the individual is providing support the client requires. *Coach may be client's husband/significant other (SO) or doula, and he or she needs to include physical and emotional support for the mother and aid in initiation of bonding with the neonate.*[4]

After Birth

- Promote sleep and rest. *Reduces metabolic rate and allows energy and oxygen to be used for healing process.*[12]

- Ascertain client's perception of labor and delivery, length of labor, and client's fatigue level. *There is a correlation between length of labor and the ability of some clients to assume responsibility for self-care/infant care tasks and activities.*

- Assess client's readiness for learning. Assist client in identifying needs. *The postpartum period provides an opportunity to foster maternal growth, maturation, and competence. However, the client needs time to move from "taking-in" to a "taking-hold" phase, in which her receptiveness and readiness are heightened and she is emotionally and physically ready for learning new information to facilitate mastery of her new role.*[4]

- Provide information about self-care, including perineal care and hygiene; physiological changes, including normal progression of lochial flow; need for sleep and rest; importance of progressive postpartum exercise program; and role changes. *Helps prevent infection, fosters healing and recuperation, and contributes to positive adaptation to physical and emotional changes, enhancing feelings of general well-being.*[12]

- Review nipple and breast care, special dietary needs for lactating mother, factors that facilitate or interfere with successful breastfeeding, use of breast pump and appropriate suppliers, and proper storage of expressed milk. *Prevents nipple cracking and soreness, enhancing comfort, facilitates role of breastfeeding mother, and helps ensure adequate milk supply.*[8]

- Discuss normal psychological changes and needs associated with the postpartal period. *Client's emotional state may be somewhat labile at this time and often is influenced by physical well-being. Anticipating such changes may reduce the stress associated with this transition period that necessitates learning new roles and taking on new responsibilities.*[4,8,12]

- Discuss sexuality needs and plans for contraception. Provide information about available methods, including advantages/disadvantages. *Client/couple may need clarification regarding available contraception methods and the fact that pregnancy could occur even prior to the 4- to 6-week postpartum visit.*[8]

 Acute Care   Collaborative Community/Home Care Cultural

- Reinforce importance of postpartum examination by healthcare provider and interim follow-up as appropriate. *Follow-up visit is necessary to evaluate recovery of reproductive organs, healing of episiotomy/laceration repair, general well-being, and adaptation to life changes.*[12]

NURSING PRIORITY NO. 3 To promote appropriate participation in childbearing process:

During Pregnancy
- Develop nurse-client relationship, maintaining an open attitude toward beliefs of client/couple. *Acceptance is important to developing and maintaining relationship and supporting independence.*[2]
- Explain office visit routine and rationale for ongoing screening and close monitoring (e.g., urine testing, blood pressure monitoring, weight, fetal growth). Emphasize importance of keeping regular appointments. *Reinforces relationship between health assessment and positive outcomes for mother and baby.*[12]
- Suggest father/siblings attend office visits and listen to fetal heart tones as appropriate. *Promotes a sense of involvement and helps make baby a reality for family members.*
- Provide anticipatory guidance regarding health habits/lifestyle and employment concerns:
  Review physical changes to be expected during each trimester. *Questions will continue to arise as new changes occur, regardless of whether changes are anticipated or unexpected, and knowledge of normal variations can be reassuring. Also prepares client/couple for managing common discomforts associated with pregnancy.*[4,12]
  Discuss signs/symptoms requiring evaluation by primary provider during prenatal period (e.g., excessive vomiting, fever, unresolved illness of any kind, decreased fetal movement). *Allows for timely intervention.*[12]
  Identify anticipatory adaptations for SO/family necessitated by pregnancy. *Family members will need to be flexible in adjusting own roles and responsibilities in order to assist client to meet her needs related to the demands of pregnancy, both expected and unplanned, such as prolonged nausea, fatigue, and emotional lability.*[12]
  Provide information about potential teratogens, such as alcohol, nicotine, illicit drugs, the STORCH group of viruses (syphilis, toxoplasmosis, other, rubella, cytomegalovirus, herpes simplex), and HIV. *Helps client make informed decisions/choices about behaviors/environment that can promote healthy offspring. Note: Research supports the attribution of a wide range of negative effects in the neonate from alcohol and recreational drug use and smoking.*[4,8,13–15]
- Provide information about need for additional laboratory studies and diagnostic tests or procedure(s). Review risks and potential side effects. *Aids in making informed decisions and choosing treatment options.*[8,12]
- Discuss signs of labor onset; how to distinguish between false and true labor, when to notify healthcare provider, and when to leave for birth center/hospital as appropriate; and stages of labor and delivery. *Helps ensure timely arrival and enhances coping with labor/delivery process.*[12]
- Determine anticipated infant feeding plan. Discuss physiology and benefits of breastfeeding. *Breastfeeding provides a protective effect against respiratory illnesses, ear infections, gastrointestinal diseases, and allergies, including asthma, eczema, and atopic dermatitis.*[9]
- Encourage attendance at prenatal and childbirth classes. Provide information about father/sibling or grandparent participation in classes and delivery if client desires. *Knowledge gained helps reduce fear of unknown and increases confidence that client/couple can manage the preparation for the birth of their child. Helps family members to realize they are an integral part of the pregnancy and delivery.*[11,12]

During Labor and Delivery
- Support use of positive coping mechanisms. *Enhances feelings of competence and fosters self-esteem.*[12]
- Demonstrate behaviors and techniques (e.g., breathing, focused imagery, music, other distractions; aromatherapy; abdominal effleurage, back or leg rubs, sacral pressure, repositioning, back rest; oral care, linen changes, shower/tub use) that partner can use to assist with pain control and relaxation. *Enhances feeling of well-being. May block pain impulses within the cerebral cortex through conditioned responses and cutaneous stimulation, facilitating progression of normal labor.*[4]

 Diagnostic Studies   Evidence Based Practice   Medications   Pediatric/Geriatric/Lifespan

- Discuss available analgesics, appropriate timing, usual responses and side effects (client and fetal), and duration of analgesia effect in light of current situation. *Allows client to make informed choices about means of pain control and can allay client's fears and anxieties about medication use. Note: If conservative measures are not effective and increasing muscle tension impedes progress of labor, judicious use of medication can enhance relaxation, shorten labor, limit fatigue, and prevent complications.*[4]
- Honor client's decision about the use or nonuse of medication in a nonjudgmental manner. Continue encouragement for efforts and use of relaxation techniques. *Enhances client's sense of control and may prevent or reduce need for medication. Note: Continued support may be needed to help reduce feelings of failure in the client/couple who may have anticipated an unmedicated birth and did not follow through with that plan.*[12]

After Birth

- Monitor and document the client's/couple's interactions with infant. *Presence of bonding acquaintance behaviors (e.g., making eye contact, using high-pitched voice and en face [face-to-face] position as culturally appropriate, calling infant by name, holding infant closely) are indicators of beginning the attachment process.*[2,12]
- Initiate early breast or oral feeding according to facility protocol and client preference. *Initiating feeding for breastfed infants usually occurs in the delivery room; otherwise, 5 to 15 mL of sterile water may be offered in the nursery to assess effectiveness of sucking, swallowing, gag reflexes, and patency of esophagus. If aspirated, sterile water is easily absorbed by pulmonary tissues.*[7,9]
- Provide for unlimited participation of father and siblings. Ascertain whether siblings attended orientation program. *Facilitates family development and ongoing process of acquaintance/attachment and helps family members feel more comfortable caring for newborn.*

NURSING PRIORITY NO. 4   To promote optimal well-being of newborn (Teaching/Discharge Considerations):

- Provide information about newborn interactional capabilities, states of consciousness, and means of stimulating cognitive development. *Helps parents recognize and respond to infant cues during interactional process and fosters optimal interaction, attachment behaviors, and cognitive development in infant. The state of consciousness can be divided into the sleep and the wake states, involving separate predictable behavioral characteristics.*[12]
- Note father's/partner's response to birth and to parenting role. *Client's ability to adapt positively to parenting may be strongly influenced by partner's reaction.*
- Discuss normal variations and characteristics of infant, such as caput succedaneum, cephalohematoma, pseudomenstruation, breast enlargement, physiological jaundice, and milia. *Helps parents recognize normal variations and may reduce anxiety.*[4,12]
- Demonstrate/supervise infant care activities related to feeding and holding; bathing, diapering, and clothing; care of umbilical cord stump; and care of circumcised male infant. *Promotes understanding of principles and techniques of newborn care, fosters parents' skills as caregivers, and enhances self-confidence.*[3,12]
- Note frequency, amount, and length of feeding. Encourage demand feedings instead of scheduled feedings. Note frequency, amount, and appearance of regurgitation. *Hunger and length of time between feedings vary from feeding to feeding, and excessive regurgitation increases replacement needs.*[7,9]
- Evaluate neonate and maternal satisfaction following feedings. *Provides opportunity to answer client questions, offer encouragement for efforts, identify needs, and problem-solve situations.*[7,9]
- Discuss physiological needs and adaptation to extrauterine life, including maintenance of body temperature, nutritional requirements, respiratory needs, and bowel and bladder functioning. *Enhances parents' ability to provide for neonates' well-being.*[3,12]
- Emphasize newborn's need for follow-up laboratory tests, regular evaluations by healthcare provider, and timely immunizations. *Ongoing evaluation is important for monitoring growth and achievement of development milestones. Immunizations are necessary to protect the infant from childhood diseases and associated serious complications.*[12]

 Acute Care   Collaborative   Community/Home Care   Cultural

- Identify manifestations of illness and infection and when to contact healthcare provider. Demonstrate proper technique for taking temperature, administering oral medication, or providing other care activities for infant as required. *Early recognition of illness and prompt use of healthcare facilitate timely treatment and positive outcomes.*[12]
- 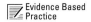Provide oral and written/pictorial information and reliable Web sites about infant care and development, feeding, and safety issues. Offer appropriate resources in client's dominant language reflecting cultural beliefs. *Maximizes learning, providing opportunity to review information as needed to engage in new caretaking role, identify necessary supplies/safety needs, and prepare for feeding method of choice.*[8,12]
- Refer breastfeeding client to lactation consultant/support group (e.g., La Leche League, Lact-Aid) as appropriate. *Provides ongoing support to promote a successful breastfeeding outcome.*[7,9]
- Discuss available community support groups/parenting class as indicated. *Increases parents' knowledge of child rearing and child development and provides a supportive atmosphere while parents incorporate new roles.*

DOCUMENTATION FOCUS

Assessment/Reassessment
- Assessment findings, general health, previous pregnancy experience, any safety concerns.
- Knowledge of pre/postpartum needs and newborn care.
- Cultural beliefs and expectations.
- Specific birth plan and individuals to be involved in delivery.
- Arrangement for postpartum period and preparation for newborn.

Planning
- Plan of care and who is involved in planning.
- Individual teaching plans for pregnancy, labor/delivery, postpartum self-care, and infant care.

Implementation/Evaluation
- Response to interventions, teaching, and actions performed.
- Attainment or progress toward desired outcomes.
- Modifications to plan of care.

Discharge Planning
- Long-term needs and who is responsible for actions to be taken.
- Available resources, specific referrals made.

References

1. Lauderdale, J. (2007). Transcultural perspectives in childbearing. In Andrews, M. M., Boyle, J. S. (eds). *Transcultural Concepts in Nursing Care.* 5th ed. Philadelphia: Wolters Kluwer Health, Lippincott Williams & Wilkins.
2. Purnell, L. D., Paulanka, B. J. (2008). *Transcultural Health Care: Culturally Competent Approach.* 3rd ed. Philadelphia: F. A. Davis.
3. Bastable, S. B. (2005). *Essentials of Patient Education.* Sudbury, MA: Jones and Bartlett.
4. Editorial Staff. (2008). Complications and high-risk conditions of the prenatal period. *Straight A's in Maternal-Neonatal Nursing.* 2nd ed. Philadelphia: Wolters Kluwer, Lippincott Williams & Wilkins.
5. American College of Obstetricians and Gynecologists, Committee on Obstetric Practice. (2002). Exercise during pregnancy and the postpartum period. ACOG Committee Opinion 267. *Obst Gynecol,* 99(1), 171–173.
6. Editorial Staff. (2007). Cultural childbearing practices. *Lippincott Manual of Nursing Practice Pocket Guides: Maternal-Neonatal Nursing.* Philadelphia: Lippincott Williams & Wilkins.
7. Meek, J. Y. (ed). (2002). *The American Academy of Pediatrics New Mothers Guide to Breastfeeding.* New York: Bantam.
8. Holloway, B., Moredich, C., Aduddell, K. (2006). *OB/Peds Women's Health Notes: Nurses' Clinical Pocket Guide.* Philadelphia: F. A. Davis.
9. American Academy of Pediatrics. (2005). Breastfeeding and the use of human milk. *Pediatrics,* 115(2), 496–506.
10. Murry, M., Huelsmann, G. (2009). *Labor and Delivery Nursing: Guide to Evidence-Based Practice.* New York: Springer.
11. Mayo Clinic Staff. (Updated 2017). Childbirth classes: Get ready for labor and delivery. Retrieved March 2018 from http://www.mayoclinic.org/healthy-living/pregnancy-week-by-week/in-depth/pregnancy/art-20044568.

 Diagnostic Studies   Evidence Based Practice   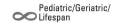 Medications   Pediatric/Geriatric/Lifespan

12. Ricci, S. S., Kyle, T. (2008). *Maternity and Pediatric Nursing.* Philadelphia: Lippincott Williams & Wilkins.
13. Surgeon General. (2005, revised 2007). *Surgeon General's advisory on alcohol use in pregnancy.* Retrieved March 2018 from http://come-over.to/FAS/SurGenAdvisory.html.
14. March of Dimes. (Update 2013, last reviewed 2016). Street drugs and pregnancy. Retrieved March 2018 from http://www.marchofdimes.org/pregnancy/illicit-drug-use-during-pregnancy.aspx#.
15. Acharya, K. S., Groutegut, C. A. (Updated 2017). Psychosocial and environmental pregnancy risks. Retrieved March 2018. from http://emedicine.medscape.com/article/259346-overview.
16. Ehrenberg, H. M. (2009). Maternal obesity, uterine activity, and the risk of spontaneous preterm birth. *Obstet Gynecol*, 113(1), 48–52.
17. March of Dimes. (Updated 2014). Being pregnant at work. Retrieved March 2018 from https://www.marchofdimes.org/pregnancy/being-pregnant-at-work.aspx.
18. Silverman, J. G., et al. (2006). Intimate partner violence victimization prior to and during pregnancy among women residing in 26 U.S. states: Associations with maternal and neonatal health. *Am J Obstet Gynecol*, 195(1), 140–148.
19. March of Dimes. (2008). Abuse during pregnancy. Retrieved March 2018 from http://www.marchofdimes.org/pregnancy/abuse-during-pregnancy.aspx.
20. Shankaran, S., et al. (2007). Impact of maternal substance use during pregnancy on childhood outcome. *Semin Fetal Neonatal Med*, 12(2), 143–150.

readiness for enhanced Childbearing Process

Taxonomy II: Sexuality—Class 3 Reproduction (00208) [**Diagnostic Division:** Sexuality], Approved 2008; Revised 2013

DEFINITION: A pattern of preparing for and maintaining a healthy pregnancy, childbirth process, and care of the newborn for ensuring well-being, which can be strengthened.

DEFINING CHARACTERISTICS
During Pregnancy

Subjective
Expresses desire to enhance prenatal lifestyle [e.g., nutrition, elimination, sleep, exercise, personal hygiene]
Expresses desire to enhance knowledge of childbearing process
Expresses desire to enhance management of unpleasant pregnancy symptoms
Expresses desire to enhance preparation for newborn
During Labor and Delivery

Subjective
Expresses desire to enhance lifestyle appropriate for stage of labor
Expresses desire to enhance proactivity during labor and delivery
After Birth

Subjective
Expresses desire to enhance attachment behavior, baby care/feeding techniques, environmental safety for the baby
Expresses desire to enhance postpartum lifestyle, breast care
Expresses desire to enhance use of support system
Sample Clinical Applications: First, second, and third trimesters of pregnancy; labor and delivery; postpartum; newborn

DESIRED OUTCOMES/EVALUATION CRITERIA

Sample NOC linkages:
Knowledge: Pregnancy: Extent of understanding conveyed about promotion of a healthy pregnancy and prevention of complications

 Acute Care Collaborative Community/Home Care Cultural

Knowledge: Labor & Delivery: Extent of understanding conveyed about labor and vaginal delivery

Knowledge: Infant Care: Extent of understanding conveyed about caring for a baby from birth to first birthday

---

Client Will (Include Specific Time Frame)

• Demonstrate healthy pregnancy free of preventable complications.
• Engage in activities to prepare for birth process and care of newborn.
• Experience complication-free labor and childbirth.
• Display culturally appropriate bonding behaviors.
• Verbalize understanding of care requirements to promote health of self and infant.

ACTIONS/INTERVENTIONS

Sample NIC linkages:

Childbirth Preparation: Providing information and support to facilitate childbirth and to enhance the ability of an individual to develop and perform the parental role

Postpartal Care: Providing care to a woman during the 6-week time period beginning immediately after birth

Parent Education: Infant: Instruction on nurturing and physical care needed during the first year of life

---

NURSING PRIORITY NO. 1   To determine individual needs:

During Pregnancy

• Evaluate current knowledge and cultural beliefs regarding normal physiological and psychological changes of pregnancy, as well as beliefs about activities, self-care, and so on. *Provides information to assist in identifying needs and creating individual plan of care.*[2,3]
• Determine degree of motivation for learning. *Client may have difficulty learning unless the need for it is clear.*[3]
• Identify who provides support/instruction within the client's culture (e.g., grandmother, other family member, curandero or doula, other cultural healer). Work with support person(s) when possible, using interpreter as needed. *Helps ensure quality and continuity of care because support person(s) may be more successful than the healthcare provider in communicating information.*[1,2,4]
• Determine client's commitments to work, family, community, and self; roles and responsibilities within family unit; and use of supportive resources. *Helps in setting realistic priorities to assist client in making adjustments, such as changing work hours, shifting of household chores and responsibilities, prioritizing and curtailing some outside commitments, etc.*[12,17]
• Evaluate the client's/couple's response to pregnancy, individual and family stressors, and cultural implications of pregnancy and childbirth. *The client's/couple's ability to adapt positively depends on support systems, cultural beliefs, resources, and effective coping mechanisms developed in dealing with past stressors. Initially, even if the pregnancy is planned, the expectant mother may feel ambivalent toward the pregnancy because of personal or professional goals, financial concerns, and possible role changes that a child will necessitate.*[1,2]
• Determine client's/couple's perception of fetus as a separate entity and extent of preparations being made for this infant. *Activities such as choosing a name or nicknaming the baby in utero and home preparations indicate completion of psychological tasks of pregnancy. Note: Cultural or familial beliefs may limit visible preparations out of concern that bad outcome may result.*[2]
• Assess economic situation and financial needs. Note use of available resources. *Impact of pregnancy on family with limited resources can create added stress and result in limited prenatal care and preparation for newborn.*
• Determine usual pregravid weight and dietary patterns. *Research studies have found a positive correlation between pregravid maternal obesity and increased perinatal morbidity rates (e.g., hypertension and gestational diabetes) associated with preterm births and macrosomia.*[16]

 Diagnostic Studies   Evidence Based Practice   Medications   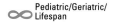 Pediatric/Geriatric/Lifespan

During Labor and Delivery

- Ascertain client's understanding and expectations of the labor process. *The client's/couple's coping skills are most challenged during the active and transition phases as contractions become increasingly intense. Lack of knowledge, misconceptions, or unrealistic expectations can have a negative impact on coping abilities.*
- Review birth plan developed by client/partner. Note cultural expectations/preferences. *Verifies that choices made are amenable to the specific care setting, accommodate individual wishes, and reflect client/fetal status. Note: Some cultures or personal values may limit male involvement in the delivery process, necessitating the identification of other support person(s).*[1,6,10]

After Birth

- Determine plan for discharge after delivery and home care support and needs. *Early planning can facilitate discharge and help ensure that client/infant needs will be met.*[3]
- Ascertain client's perception of labor and delivery, length of labor, and client's fatigue level. *There is a correlation between length of labor and the ability of some clients to assume responsibility for self-care/infant care tasks and activities.*
- Assess mother's strengths and needs, noting age, marital status or relationship, presence and reaction of siblings and other family, available sources of support, and cultural background. *Identifies potential risk factors and sources of support, which influence the client's/couple's ability to assume role of parenthood. For example, the adolescent may still be formulating goals and an identity. She may have difficulty accepting the infant as a person and coping with full-time parenting responsibility. The single parent who lacks support systems may have difficulty assuming sole responsibility for parenting. Cultures in which the extended family members live together may provide more emotional and physical support, facilitating adoption of the new role.*[1,6]
- Appraise level of parents' understanding of infant's physiological needs and adaptation to extrauterine life associated with maintenance of body temperature, nutrition, respiratory needs, and bowel and bladder functioning. *Identifies areas of concern/need, which could require additional information and/or demonstration of care activities.*[3,12]
- Evaluate nature of emotional and physical parenting that client/couple received during their childhood. *Parenting role is learned, and individuals use their own parents as role models. Those who experienced a negative upbringing or poor parenting may require additional support to meet the challenges of effective parenting.*
- Note father's/partner's response to birth and to parenting role. *Client's ability to adapt positively to parenting may be strongly influenced by the father's/partner's reaction.*
- Assess client's readiness and motivation for learning. Assist client/couple in identifying needs. *The postpartal period provides an opportunity to foster maternal growth, maturation, and competence. However, the client needs time to move from a "taking-in" to a "taking-hold" phase, in which her receptiveness and readiness are heightened and she is emotionally and physically ready for learning new information to facilitate mastery of her new role.*[4]

NURSING PRIORITY NO. 2   To promote maximum participation in childbearing process:

During Pregnancy

- Maintain open attitude toward beliefs of client/couple. *Acceptance is important to developing and maintaining relationship and supporting independence.*[2]
- Explain office visit routine and rationale for ongoing screening and close monitoring (e.g., urine testing, blood pressure monitoring, weight, fetal growth). Emphasize importance of keeping regular appointments. *Reinforces relationship between health assessment and positive outcome for mother/baby.*[12]
- Suggest father/siblings attend prenatal office visits and listen to fetal heart tones as appropriate. *Promotes a sense of involvement and helps make baby a reality for family members.*
- Provide information about need for additional laboratory studies and diagnostic tests or procedure(s). Review risks and potential side effects. *Aids in making informed decisions.*[8,12]
- Discuss any medications that may be needed to control or treat medical conditions. *Helpful in choosing treatment options because need must be weighed against possible harmful effects on the fetus.*[12]

 Acute Care   Collaborative   Community/ Home Care   Cultural

- Provide anticipatory guidance, including discussion of nutrition, regular moderate exercise, comfort measures, rest, employment, breast care, sexual activity, and health habits and lifestyle. *Information encourages acceptance of responsibility and promotes self-care:*

Review nutrition requirements and optimal prenatal weight gain to support maternal-fetal needs. *Dietary focus should be on balanced nutrients and calories to produce appropriate weight gain and to supply adequate vitamins and minerals for healthy fetus. Inadequate prenatal weight gain and/or below normal prepregnancy weight increases the risk of intrauterine growth restriction in the fetus and delivery of a low-birth-weight infant.*[8,12]

 Encourage moderate exercise such as walking or non-weight-bearing activities (e.g., swimming, bicycling) in accordance with client's physical condition and cultural beliefs. *Nonendurance, antepartal exercise regimens tend to shorten labor, increase likelihood of a spontaneous vaginal delivery, and decrease need for oxytocin augmentation.*[4,5] *In some cultures, inactivity may be viewed as a protection for mother/child.*[1,6]

Recommend a consistent sleep and rest schedule (e.g., 1- to 2-hour daytime nap and 8 hours of sleep each night) in a dark, cool room. *Provides rest to meet metabolic needs associated with growth of maternal/fetal tissues.*[12]

Identify anticipatory adaptations for significant other (SO)/family necessitated by pregnancy. *Family members will need to be flexible in adjusting own roles and responsibilities in order to assist client to meet her needs related to the demands of pregnancy, both expected and unplanned, such as prolonged nausea, fatigue, and emotional lability.*[12]

Provide or reinforce information about potential teratogens, such as alcohol, nicotine, illicit drugs, the STORCH group of viruses (syphilis, toxoplasmosis, other, rubella, cytomegalovirus, herpes simplex), and HIV. *Helps client make informed decisions and choices about behaviors and environment that can promote healthy offspring. Note: Research supports the fact that alcohol and recreational drug use can lead to a wide range of negative effects in the neonate. Smoking negatively affects placental circulation; even smoking fewer than 10 cigarettes per day is associated with an increased risk of fetal death, damage in utero, abruptio placentae, placenta previa, and low birth weight.*[4,8,13–15]

- Use various methods for learning, including pictures, to discuss fetal development. *Visualization enhances reality of child and strengthens learning process.*[4]
- Discuss signs of labor onset; how to distinguish between false and true labor, when to notify healthcare provider, and when to leave for hospital or birth center; and stages of labor and delivery. *Helps client to recognize onset of labor, to ensure timely arrival, and to cope with labor and delivery process.*[12]
- Review signs/symptoms requiring evaluation by primary provider during prenatal period (e.g., excessive vomiting, fever, unresolved illness of any kind, decreased fetal movement). *Allows for timely intervention.*[12]

During Labor and Delivery

- Identify client's support person/coach and ascertain that the individual is providing support that client requires. *Coach may be client's husband/SO or doula, and support can take the form of physical and emotional support for the mother and aid in initiation of bonding with the neonate.*[4]
- Demonstrate or review behaviors and techniques (e.g., breathing, focused imagery, music, other distraction; aromatherapy; abdominal effleurage, back and leg rubs, sacral pressure, repositioning, back rest; oral and perineal care, linen changes; shower or hot tub use) partner can use to assist with pain control and relaxation. *Enhances feeling of well-being. May block pain impulses within the cerebral cortex through conditioned responses and cutaneous stimulation, facilitating progression of normal labor.*[4]
- Discuss available analgesics, usual responses and side effects (client and fetal), and duration of analgesic effect in light of current situation. *Allows client to make informed choice about means of pain control and can allay client's fears or anxieties about medication use. Note: If conservative measures are not effective and increasing muscle tension impedes progress of labor, judicious use of medication can enhance relaxation, shorten labor, limit fatigue, and prevent complications.*[4]
- Support client's decision about the use or nonuse of medication in a nonjudgmental manner. Continue encouragement for efforts and use of relaxation techniques. *Enhances client sense of control and may prevent or*

 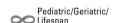

decrease need for medication. Note: Continued support may be needed to help reduce feelings of failure in the client/couple who may have anticipated an unmedicated birth and did not follow through with that plan.[12]

After Birth

- Initiate early breastfeeding or oral feeding according to hospital protocol. *Initial feeding for breastfed infants usually occurs in the delivery room. Otherwise, 5 to 15 mL of sterile water may be offered in the nursery to assess effectiveness of sucking, swallowing, gag reflexes, and patency of esophagus. If aspirated, sterile water is easily absorbed by pulmonary tissues.*[7,9]

- Note frequency and amount and length of feedings. Encourage demand feedings instead of "scheduled" feedings. *Hunger and length of time between feedings vary from feeding to feeding.*[7,9] Note frequency, amount, and appearance of regurgitation. *Excessive regurgitation increases feeding needs.*

- Evaluate neonate/maternal satisfaction following feedings. *Provides opportunity to answer client questions, offer encouragement for efforts, identify needs, and problem-solve solutions.*[7,9]

- Demonstrate and supervise infant care activities related to feeding and holding; bathing, diapering, and clothing; care of circumcised male infant; and care of umbilical cord stump. Provide written and pictorial information for parents to refer to after discharge. *Promotes understanding of principles and techniques of newborn care and fosters parents' skills as caregivers.*[3,12]

- Provide information about newborn interactional capabilities, states of consciousness, and means of stimulating cognitive development. *Helps parents recognize and respond to infant cues during interactional process and fosters optimal interaction, attachment behaviors, and cognitive development in infant. The state of consciousness can be divided into the sleep and the wake states, involving separate and predictable behavioral characteristics.*[12]

- Promote sleep and rest. *Reduces metabolic rate and allows nutrition and oxygen to be used for healing process rather than for energy needs.*[12]

- Provide for unlimited participation for father and siblings. Ascertain whether siblings attended an orientation program. *Facilitates family development and ongoing process of acquaintance and attachment. Helps family members feel comfortable caring for newborn.*

- Monitor and document the client's/couple's interactions with infant. Note presence of bonding (acquaintance) behaviors (e.g., making eye contact, using high-pitched voice and en face [face-to-face] position as culturally appropriate, calling infant by name, holding infant closely).[2,12]

NURSING PRIORITY NO. 3   To enhance optimal well-being:

During Pregnancy

- Emphasize importance of maternal well-being. *Fetal well-being is directly related to maternal well-being, especially during the first trimester, when developing organ systems are most vulnerable to injury from environmental or hereditary factors.*

- Review physical changes to be expected during each trimester. *Questions will continue to arise as new changes occur, regardless of whether changes are expected or unexpected, and knowledge of "what's normal" can be reassuring. Also prepares client/couple for managing common discomforts associated with pregnancy.*[4,12]

- Explain psychological reactions, including ambivalence, introspection, stress reactions, and emotional lability, as being characteristic of pregnancy. *Helps client/couple understand mood swings and may provide opportunities for partner to offer support/affection at these times.*[4]

- Provide necessary referrals (e.g., dietitian, social services, Supplemental Nutrition Assistance Program (SNAP) or the Women, Infants, and Children [WIC] food program) as indicated. *May need additional assistance with nutritional choices and may have budget or financial constraints. Supplemental federally funded food program helps promote optimal maternal, fetal, and infant nutrition.*[12]

- Identify reportable danger signals of pregnancy, such as bleeding, cramping, acute abdominal pain, backache, edema, visual disturbance, headaches, and pelvic pressure. *Helps client to distinguish normal from abnormal findings, thus assisting her in seeking timely, appropriate healthcare.*[12]

 Acute Care   Collaborative   Community/ Home Care   Cultural

- Encourage attendance at prenatal and childbirth classes. Provide information about father/sibling or grandparent participation in classes and delivery as client desires. *Knowledge gained helps reduce fear of unknown and increases confidence that couple can manage the preparation for the birth of their child. Helps family members to realize they are an integral part of the pregnancy and delivery.*[11,12]
- Provide list of appropriate reading materials for client, couple, and siblings regarding adjusting to newborn. *Information helps individual realistically analyze changes in family structure, roles, and behaviors.*[3]

During Labor and Delivery

- Monitor labor progress and maternal and fetal well-being per protocol. Provide continuous intrapartal professional support or a doula. *Fear of abandonment can intensify as labor progresses. The client may experience increased anxiety and/or loss of control when left unattended. Doulas can provide client with emotional, physical, and informational support as an adjunct to primary nurse.*[2,8]
- Reinforce use of positive coping mechanisms. *Enhances feelings of competence and fosters self-esteem.*[12]

After Birth

- Provide information about self-care, including perineal care and hygiene; physiological changes, including normal progression of lochial discharge; need for sleep and rest; importance of progressive postpartal exercise program; and role changes. *Helps prevent infection, fosters healing and recuperation, and contributes to positive adaptation to physical and emotional changes enhancing feelings of general well-being.*[12]
- Review normal psychological changes and needs associated with the postpartal period. *Client's emotional state may be somewhat labile at this time and often is influenced by physical well-being. Anticipating such changes may reduce the stress associated with this transition period that necessitates learning new roles and taking on new responsibilities.*[4,8,12]
- Discuss sexuality needs and plans for contraception. Provide information about available methods, including advantages and disadvantages. *Couple may need clarification regarding available contraceptive methods and the fact that pregnancy could occur even prior to the 4- to 6-week postpartum visit.*[8]
- Reinforce importance of postpartal examination by healthcare provider and interim follow-up as appropriate. *Follow-up visit is necessary to evaluate recovery of reproductive organs, healing of episiotomy or laceration repair, general well-being, and adaptation to life changes.*[12]
- Provide oral and written information about infant care and development, feeding, and safety issues. Offer appropriate references. Elicit cultural beliefs. *Helps prepare for new caretaking role, acquiring necessary items of furniture, clothing, and supplies; helps prepare for breastfeeding and/or bottle feeding.*[8,12]
- Discuss physiology and benefits of breastfeeding, nipple and breast care, special dietary needs, factors that facilitate or interfere with successful breastfeeding, and use of breast pump and appropriate suppliers. *Helps ensure adequate milk supply, prevents nipple cracking and soreness, facilitates comfort, and establishes role of breastfeeding mother.*[8]
- Refer client to support groups (e.g., La Leche League International, Lact-Aid) or a lactation consultant. *Provides ongoing help to promote a successful breastfeeding outcome.*[7,9]
- Identify available community resources as indicated (e.g., WIC program). *WIC and other federal programs support well-being through client education and enhanced nutritional intake for infant.*[12]
- Discuss normal variations and characteristics of infant, such as caput succedaneum, cephalohematoma, pseudomenstruation, breast enlargement, physiological jaundice, and milia. *Helps parents to recognize normal variations and may reduce anxiety.*[4,12]
- Emphasize newborn's need for follow-up evaluation by healthcare provider and timely immunizations. *Ongoing evaluation is important for monitoring growth and development. Immunizations are necessary to protect the infant from childhood diseases with associated serious complications.*[12]
- Identify manifestations of illness and infection and when a healthcare provider should be contacted. Demonstrate proper technique for taking temperature, administering oral medications, or providing other care activities as required. *Early recognition of illness and prompt use of healthcare facilitate treatment and positive outcome.*[12]
- Refer client/couple to community postpartal parent groups. *Increases parents' knowledge of child rearing and child development and provides supportive atmosphere while parents incorporate new roles.*

 Diagnostic Studies   Evidence Based Practice   Medications   Pediatric/Geriatric/Lifespan

DOCUMENTATION FOCUS

Assessment/Reassessment
- Assessment findings, general health, previous pregnancy experience.
- Cultural beliefs and expectations.
- Specific birth plan and individuals to be involved in delivery.
- Arrangements for postpartal recovery period.
- Response to newborn.

Planning
- Plan of care and who is involved in planning.
- Teaching plan.

Implementation/Evaluation
- Response to interventions, teaching, and actions performed.
- Attainment or progress toward desired outcome(s).
- Modifications to plan of care.

Discharge Planning
- Long-term needs and who is responsible for actions to be taken.
- Available resources, specific referrals made.

References

1. Lauderdale, J. (2007). Transcultural perspectives in childbearing. In Andrews, M. M., Boyle, J. S. (eds) *Transcultural Concepts in Nursing Care*. 5th ed. Philadelphia: Wolters Kluwer Health, Lippincott Williams & Wilkins.
2. Purnell, L. D., Paulanka, B. J. (2008). *Transcultural Health Care: Culturally Competent Approach*. 3rd ed. Philadelphia: F. A. Davis.
3. Bastable, S. B. (2005). *Essentials of Patient Education*. Sudbury, MA: Jones and Bartlett.
4. Editorial Staff. (2008). Complications and high-risk conditions of the prenatal period. *Straight A's in Maternal-Neonatal Nursing*. 2nd ed. Philadelphia: Wolters Kluwer, Lippincott Williams & Wilkins.
5. American College of Obstetricians and Gynecologists, Committee on Obstetric Practice. (2002). Exercise during pregnancy and the postpartum period. ACOG Committee Opinion 267. *Obstet Gynecol*, 99(1), 171–173.
6. Editorial Staff. (2007). Cultural childbearing practices. *Lippincott Manual of Nursing Practice Pocket Guides: Maternal-Neonatal Nursing*. Philadelphia: Lippincott Williams & Wilkins.
7. Meek, J. (ed) (2002). *The American Academy of Pediatrics New Mothers Guide to Breastfeeding*. New York: Bantam.
8. Holloway, B., Moredich, C., Aduddell, K. (2006). *OB Peds Women's Health Notes: Nurses Clinical Pocket Guide*. Philadelphia: F. A. Davis.
9. American Academy of Family Physicians. *Breastfeeding, family physicians supporting (Position paper)*. Retrieved March 2018 from http://www.aafp.org/policies/all/breastfeeding-support.html.
10. Murry, M., Huelsmann, G. (2008). *Labor and Delivery Nursing: Guide to Evidence-Based Practice*. New York: Springer.
11. Mayo Clinic Staff. (Update 2017). Childbirth classes: Get ready for labor and delivery. Retrieved March 2018 from http://www.mayoclinic.org/healthy-lifestyle/pregnancy-week-by-week/in-depth/pregnancy/art-20044568.
12. Ricci, S. S., Kyle, T. (2008). *Maternity and Pediatric Nursing*. Philadelphia: Lippincott Williams & Wilkins.
13. Surgeon General. (2005, revised 2007). Surgeon General's advisory on alcohol use in pregnancy. Retrieved March 2018 http://come-over.to/FAS/SurGenAdvisory.html.
14. March of Dimes. (Update 2013, last reviewed 2016). Street drugs and pregnancy. Retrieved March 2018 from http://www.marchofdimes.org/pregnancy/street-drugs-and-pregnancy.aspx.
15. Acharya, K. S., Grotegut, C. A. (Updated 2017). Psychosocial and environmental pregnancy risks. Retrieved March 2018 from http://emedicine.medscape.com/article/259346-overview.
16. Ehrenberg, H. M. (2009). Maternal obesity, uterine activity, and the risk of spontaneous preterm birth. *Obstet Gynecol*, 113(1), 48–52.
17. March of Dimes. (Update 2014). Being pregnant at work. Retrieved March 2018 from https://www.marchofdimes.org/pregnancy/being-pregnant-at-work.aspxp.

 Acute Care
 Collaborative
 Community/ Home Care
 Cultural

risk for ineffective Childbearing Process

Taxonomy II: Sexuality—Class 3 Reproduction (00227) [**Diagnostic Division:** Sexuality], Approved 2010; Revised 2013, 2017

DEFINITION: Susceptible to an inability to prepare for and/or maintain a healthy pregnancy, childbirth process, and care of the newborn for ensuring well-being.

RISK FACTORS

Insufficient knowledge of childbearing process; unrealistic birth plan
Inconsistent prenatal health visits; insufficient prenatal care
Inadequate maternal nutrition
Insufficient parental role model/cognitive readiness for parenting
Substance misuse/[abuse]; domestic violence
Insufficient support system
Low maternal confidence; maternal powerlessness or psychological distress
Associated Condition: Unplanned or unwanted pregnancy
Sample Clinical Applications: First, second, and third trimester of pregnancy; labor and delivery, postpartum, newborn

DESIRED OUTCOMES/EVALUATION CRITERIA

Sample **NOC** linkages:
Prenatal Health Behavior: Personal actions to promote a healthy pregnancy and a healthy newborn
Maternal Status: Antepartum/Intrapartum/Postpartum [specify]: Extent to which maternal well-being is within normal limits from conception to the onset of labor/from onset of labor to delivery/from delivery of placenta to completion of involution
Knowledge: Infant Care: Extent of understanding conveyed about caring for a baby from birth to first birthday

Client Will (Include Specific Time Frame)
• Acknowledge and address individual risk factors.
• Demonstrate healthy pregnancy free of preventable complications.
• Engage in activities to prepare for birth process and care of newborn.
• Experience complication-free labor and childbirth.
• Verbalize understanding of care requirements to promote health of self and infant.

Refer to ND ineffective Childbearing Process *for Interventions and Documentation Focus.*

 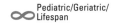

impaired Comfort

Taxonomy II: Comfort—Class 1 Physical Comfort/Class 2 Environmental Comfort/Class 3 Social Comfort (00214)
[**Diagnostic Division:** Pain/Discomfort], Approved 2008; Revised 2010, 2017

DEFINITION: Perceived lack of ease, relief and transcendence in physical, psychospiritual, environmental, cultural, and/or social dimensions.

RELATED FACTORS
Insufficient environmental or situational control
Insufficient privacy
Noxious environmental stimuli
Insufficient resources (e.g., financial, social, knowledge)

DEFINING CHARACTERISTICS

Subjective
Distressing symptoms; feeling of hunger, discomfort; itching; feeling cold, warm
Alteration in sleep pattern, inability to relax
Anxiety, fear; uneasy in situation

Objective
Restlessness; irritability; sighing; moaning; crying
Associated Condition: Illness-related symptoms; treatment regimen
Sample Clinical Applications: Presence of chronic physical or psychological conditions

DESIRED OUTCOMES/EVALUATION CRITERIA

Sample NOC linkages:
Symptom Control: Personal actions to minimize perceived adverse changes in physical and emotional functioning
Comfort Status: Overall physical, psychospiritual, sociocultural, and environmental ease and safety of an individual
Quality of Life: Extent of positive perception of current life circumstances

Client Will (Include Specific Time Frame)
Engage in behaviors or lifestyle changes to increase level of ease.
Verbalize sense of comfort and contentment.
Participate in desirable and realistic health-seeking behaviors.

ACTIONS/INTERVENTIONS

Sample NIC linkages:
Environmental Management: Comfort: Manipulation of the patient's surroundings for promotion of
  optimal comfort
Relaxation Therapy: Use of techniques to encourage and elicit relaxation for the purpose of decreasing
  undesirable signs and symptoms such as pain, muscle tension, or anxiety
Self-Awareness Enhancement: Assisting a patient to explore and understand his/her thoughts, feelings,
  motivations, and behaviors

 Acute Care   Collaborative   Community/Home Care   Cultural

NURSING PRIORITY NO. 1   To assess etiology/precipitating contributory factors:

- Determine the type of discomfort client is experiencing, such as physical pain; feeling of discontent; lack of ease with self, environment, or sociocultural settings; or inability to rise above one's problems or pain (lack of transcendence). Have client rate total comfort using a 0–10 scale, with 10 being as comfortable as possible, or a "general comfort" questionnaire using a Likert-type scale. *A comfort scale is similar to a pain rating scale and can help client identify focus of discomfort (e.g., physical, emotional, social, etc.).*[1,5,10]
- Note cultural or religious beliefs and values that impact perceptions and expectations of comfort.
- Ascertain locus of control. *Presence of external locus of control may hamper efforts to achieve sense of peace or contentment.*
- Discuss concerns with client and active-listen to identify underlying issues (e.g., physical and/or emotional stressors; external factors such as environmental surroundings, social interactions) that could impact client's ability to control own well-being. *Helps to determine client's specific needs and ability to change own situation.*
- Establish context(s) in which lack of comfort is realized: physical—pertaining to bodily sensations; psychospiritual—pertaining to internal awareness of self and meaning in one's life, relationship to a higher order or being; environmental—pertaining to external surroundings, conditions, and influences; sociocultural—pertaining to interpersonal, family, and societal relationships.[1]

Physical
- Determine how client is managing pain and pain components. *Lack of control may be related to other issues or emotions such as fear, loneliness, anxiety, noxious stimuli, and anger.*[1]
- Ascertain what has been tried or is required for comfort or rest (e.g., head of bed up or down, music on or off, white noise, rocking motion, certain person or thing; ability to express and/or manage conflicts).[2]

Psychospiritual
- Determine how psychological and spiritual indicators overlap (e.g., meaningfulness, faith, identity, self-esteem) for client.[1]
- Ascertain if client/significant other (SO) desires support regarding spiritual enrichment, including prayer, meditation, or access to spiritual counselor of choice.[3]

Environmental
- Determine that client's environment respects privacy and provides natural lighting and readily accessible view to outdoors—*an aspect that can be manipulated to enhance comfort.*[1,3]

Sociocultural
- Ascertain meaning of comfort in context of interpersonal, family, and cultural values and societal relationships.[4,10]
- Validate client/SO understanding of client's situation and ongoing methods of managing condition, as appropriate and/or desired by client. *Considers client/family needs in this area and shows appreciation for their desires.*[4]

NURSING PRIORITY NO. 2   To assist client to alleviate discomfort:

- Review knowledge base and note coping skills that have been used previously to change behavior and promote well-being. *Brings these to client's awareness and promotes use in current situation.*[8]
- Acknowledge client's strengths in present situation and build on those strengths in planning for future.

Physical
- Collaborate in treating and managing medical conditions involving oxygenation, elimination, mobility, cognitive abilities, electrolyte balance, thermoregulation, and hydration, *to promote physical stability.*[2,5,6]
- Work with client to prevent pain, nausea, itching, thirst, and other physical discomforts.
- Review medications or treatment regimen *to determine possible changes or options to reduce side effects.*
- Suggest parent be present during procedures *to comfort child.*
- Provide age-appropriate comfort measures (e.g., back rub, change of position, cuddling, use of heat or cold) *to provide nonpharmacological pain management.*

- Discuss interventions and activities to promote ease, such as Therapeutic Touch, massage, healing touch, biofeedback, self-hypnosis, guided imagery, breathing exercises, play therapy, and humor, *to promote relaxation and refocus attention. Note: In recent years, a number of studies have documented emotional and physical health benefits that come from touch. This research is suggesting that touch is truly fundamental to human communication, bonding, and health.*[9,11]
- Assist client to use and modify medication regimen *to make best use of pharmacological pain or symptom management.*
- Assist client/SO(s) to develop plan for activity and exercise within individual ability emphasizing necessity of allowing sufficient time to finish activities.
- Maintain open and flexible visitation with client's desired persons.
- Encourage and plan care to allow individually adequate rest periods *to prevent fatigue.* Schedule activities for periods when client has the most energy *to maximize participation.*
- Discuss routines to promote restful sleep.

Psychospiritual
- Interact with client in therapeutic manner. *The nurse could be the most important comfort intervention for meeting client's needs. For example, assuring client that nausea can be treated successfully with both pharmacological and nonpharmacological methods may be more effective than simply administering antiemetic without reassurance and comforting presence.*[7]
- Encourage verbalization of feelings and make time for listening and interacting.
- Identify ways (e.g., meditation, sharing oneself with others, being out in nature or garden, other spiritual activities) to achieve connectedness or harmony with self, others, nature, and/or a higher power.
- Establish realistic activity goals with client. *Enhances commitment to promoting optimal outcomes.*
- Involve client/SO(s) in schedule planning and decisions about timing and spacing of treatments *to promote relaxation and reduce sense of boredom.*
- Encourage client to do whatever possible (e.g., self-care, sit up in chair, walk). *Enhances self-esteem and independence.*
- Use distraction with music, chatting, texting with family/friends, watching TV or videos, or playing computer games *to limit dwelling on negatives and to transcend unpleasant sensations and situations.*
- Encourage client to make use of beneficial coping behaviors and develop assertiveness skills, prioritizing goals and activities. *Promotes sense of control and improves self-esteem.*
- Offer or identify opportunities for client to participate in experiences that enhance control and independence.

Environmental
- Provide quiet environment and calm activities.
- Provide for periodic changes in the personal surroundings when client is confined. Use the individual's input in creating the changes (e.g., seasonal bulletin boards, color changes, rearranging furniture, pictures).
- Suggest activities, such as bird feeders or baths for bird-watching, a garden in a window box or terrarium, or a fishbowl or aquarium, *to stimulate observation as well as involvement and participation in an activity.*

Sociocultural
- Encourage age-appropriate diversional activities (e.g., TV, radio, computer games, playtime, socialization or outings with others).
- Avoid overstimulation or understimulation (cognitive and sensory).
- Make appropriate referrals to available support groups, hobby clubs, and service organizations.

NURSING PRIORITY NO. 3 To promote wellness (Teaching/Discharge Considerations):

- Provide information about condition, health risk factors, or concerns in desired format (e.g., pictures, TV programs, articles, handouts, audio/visual materials; classes, group discussions, Internet Web sites, other databases) as appropriate. *Use of multiple modalities enhances acquisition and retention of information and gives client choices for accessing and applying information.*

 Acute Care   Collaborative   Community/ Home Care   Cultural

Physical
- Promote overall health measures (e.g., nutrition, adequate fluid intake, appropriate vitamin or iron supplementation).
- Discuss potential complications and possible need for medical follow-up or alternative therapies. *Timely recognition and intervention can promote wellness.*
- Assist client/SO(s) to identify and acquire necessary equipment (e.g., lifts, commode chair, safety grab bars, personal hygiene supplies) to meet individual needs.

Psychospiritual
- Collaborate with others when client expresses interest in lessons, counseling, coaching, and/or mentoring *to meet or enhance emotional and spiritual comfort.*
- Encourage client's contributions toward meeting realistic goals.
- Recommend client take time to be introspective in the search for contentment or transcendence.

Environmental
- Create a compassionate supportive and therapeutic environment incorporating client's cultural, age, and developmental factors.
- Correct environmental hazards that could influence safety and negatively affect comfort.
- Arrange for home visit and evaluation as needed.
- Discuss long-term plan for taking care of environmental needs.

Sociocultural
- Advocate for growth-promoting environment in conflict situations and consider issues from client/family and cultural perspective.
- Identify resources or referrals (e.g., knowledge and skills, financial resources and assistance; personal or psychological support group; social activities).

DOCUMENTATION FOCUS

Assessment/Reassessment
- Individual findings, including client's description of current status or situation, and factors impacting sense of comfort.
- Pertinent cultural or religious beliefs and values.
- Medication use and nonpharmacological measures.

Planning
- Plan of care, specific interventions, and who is involved in planning.
- Teaching plan.

Implementation/Evaluation
- Responses to interventions, teaching, and actions performed.
- Attainment or progress toward desired outcome(s).
- Modifications to plan of care.

Discharge Planning
- Long-term needs and who is responsible for actions to be taken.
- Specific referrals made.

References

1. Kolcaba, K. Y., Fisher, E. M. (1996). A holistic perspective on comfort care as an advance directive. *Crit Care Nurs Q*, 18(4), 66–67.
2. Kolcaba, K., DiMarco, M. A. (2005). Comfort theory and its application to pediatric nursing. *Pediatr Nurs*, 31(3), 187–194.
3. Barclay, L., Lie, D. (2010). New guidelines issued for family support in patient-centered ICU. Retrieved March 2018 from http://www.medscape.org/viewarticle/551738.
4. Malinowski, A., Stamler, L. L. (2002). Comfort: Exploration of the concept in nursing. *J Adv Nurs*, 39(6), 599–606.

 Diagnostic Studies   Evidence Based Practice   Medications 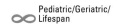 Pediatric/Geriatric/Lifespan

5. Kolcaba, K. (2003). *Comfort Theory and Practice: A Vision for Holistic Health and Research*. New York: Springer.
6. Kaplow, R. (2003). AACN synergy model for patient care: A framework to optimize outcomes. *Crit Care Nurse Suppl*, February, 27–30.
7. Wilson, L., Kolcaba, K. (2004). Practical application of comfort theory in the perianesthesia setting. *J Perianesth Nurs*, 19(3), 164–173.
8. Townsend, M. C. (2005). *Psychiatric Mental Health Nursing Concepts of Care*. 5th ed. Philadelphia: F. A. Davis.
9. Andrade, C., Clifford, P. (2001). *Outcome Based Massage*. 2nd ed. Philadelphia: Lippincott Williams & Wilkins.
10. Kolcaba, K. (2003). *Comfort Theory and Practice*. New York: Springer.
11. Kelter, D. (2010). Hands on research: The science of touch. Retrieved March 2018 from http://emedicine.medscape.com/article/163062-workup.

readiness for enhanced Comfort

Taxonomy II: Comfort—Class 1 Physical Comfort/Class 2 Environmental Comfort/Class 3 Social Comfort (00183) [Diagnostic Division: Pain/Discomfort], Approved 2006; Revised 2013, 2017

DEFINITION: A pattern of ease, relief, and transcendence in physical, psychospiritual, environmental, or social dimensions, which can be strengthened.

DEFINING CHARACTERISTICS

Subjective

Expresses desire to enhance comfort or feeling of contentment

Expresses desire to enhance relaxation

Expresses desire to enhance resolution of complaints

Sample Clinical Applications: Presence of chronic physical or psychological conditions, or any individual seeking improved quality of life

DESIRED OUTCOMES/EVALUATION CRITERIA

Sample NOC linkages:

Comfort Status: Overall physical, psychospiritual, sociocultural, and environmental ease and safety of an individual

Personal Well-Being: Extent of positive perception of one's health status

Quality of Life: Extent of positive perception of current life circumstances

Client Will (Include Specific Time Frame)
• Verbalize sense of comfort or contentment.
• Demonstrate behaviors of optimal level of ease.
• Participate in desirable and realistic health-seeking behaviors.

ACTIONS/INTERVENTIONS

Sample NIC linkages:

Self-Modification Assistance: Reinforcement of self-directed change initiated by the patient to achieve personally important goals

Relaxation Therapy: Use of techniques to encourage and elicit relaxation for the purpose of decreasing undesirable signs and symptoms such as pain, muscle tension, or anxiety

Self-Awareness Enhancement: Assisting a patient to explore and understand his/her thoughts, feelings, motivations, and behaviors

 Acute Care   Collaborative   Community/Home Care   Cultural

NURSING PRIORITY NO. 1 To determine current level of comfort/motivation for growth:

- Determine the type of comfort client is experiencing: (1) relief—as from pain, (2) ease—a state of calm or contentment, or (3) transcendence—a state in which one rises above one's problems or pain.[1]
- Note cultural or religious beliefs and values that impact perceptions of comfort.
- Ascertain motivation and expectations for improvement. *Motivation to improve and high expectations can encourage client to make changes that will improve his or her life. However, presence of external locus of control or unrealistic expectations may hamper efforts.*
- Discuss concerns with client and active-listen to identify underlying issues (e.g., physical or emotional stressors; external factors such as environmental surroundings, social interactions) that could impact client's ability to control own well-being. *Helps to determine client's level of satisfaction with current situation and readiness for change.*
- Establish context(s) in which comfort is realized: (1) physical—pertaining to bodily sensations; (2) psychospiritual—pertaining to internal awareness of self and meaning in one's life; relationship to a higher order or being; (3) environmental—pertaining to external surroundings, conditions, and influences; or (4) sociocultural—pertaining to interpersonal, family, and societal relationships.[1]

Physical
- Verify that client is managing pain and pain components effectively. *Success in this arena usually addresses other issues or emotions (e.g., fear, loneliness, anxiety, noxious stimuli, anger).*[1]
- Ascertain what is used or required for comfort or rest (e.g., head of bed up or down, music on or off, white noise, rocking motion, certain person or thing, ability to express and/or manage conflicts).[2]

Psychospiritual
- Determine how psychological and spiritual indicators overlap (e.g., meaningfulness, faith, identity, self-esteem) for client in enhancing comfort.[1]
- Ascertain that client/significant other (SO) has received desired support regarding spiritual enrichment, including prayer, meditation, or access to spiritual counselor of choice.[3]

Environmental
- Determine that client's environment respects privacy and provides natural lighting and readily accessible view to outdoors—*an aspect that can be manipulated to enhance comfort.*[1,3]

Sociocultural
- Ascertain meaning of comfort in context of interpersonal, family, and cultural values and societal relationships.[4]
- Validate client/SO understanding of client's situation and ongoing methods of managing condition, as appropriate or desired by client. *Considers client/family needs in this area and shows appreciation for their desires.*[4]

NURSING PRIORITY NO. 2 To assist client in developing plan to improve comfort:

- Review knowledge base and note coping skills that have been used previously to change behavior and promote well-being. *Brings these to client's awareness and promotes use in current situation.*[8]
- Acknowledge client's strengths in present situation that can be used to build on in planning for future.

Physical
- Collaborate in treating or managing medical conditions involving oxygenation, elimination, mobility, cognitive abilities, electrolyte balance, thermoregulation, and hydration *to promote physical stability.*[2,5,6]
- Work with client to prevent pain, nausea, itching, thirst, and other physical discomforts.
- ∞ Suggest parent be present during procedures *to comfort child.*
- ∞ Suggest age-appropriate comfort measures (e.g., back rub, change of position, cuddling, use of heat or cold) *to provide nonpharmacological pain management.*
- Participate in interventions and age-appropriate activities, such as Therapeutic Touch, biofeedback, self-hypnosis, guided imagery, breathing exercises, play therapy, and humor, *that promote ease and relaxation and can refocus attention.*

- Assist client to use or modify medication regimen *to make best use of pharmacological pain management.*
- Assist client/SO(s) to develop or modify plan for activity and exercise within individual ability, emphasizing necessity of allowing sufficient time to finish activities.
- Maintain open and flexible visitation with client's desired persons.
- Encourage and plan care to allow individually adequate rest periods *to prevent fatigue.* Encourage client to schedule activities for periods when he/she has the most energy *to maximize effectiveness.*
- Discuss routines to promote restful sleep.

Psychospiritual
- Interact with client in therapeutic manner. *The nurse could be the most important comfort intervention for meeting client's needs. For example, assuring client that nausea can be treated successfully with both pharmacological and nonpharmacological methods may be more effective than simply administering an antiemetic without reassurance and comforting presence.*[7]
- Encourage verbalization of feelings and make time for active-listening and interacting.
- Identify ways (e.g., meditation, sharing oneself with others, being out in nature or garden, other spiritual activities) *to achieve connectedness or harmony with self, others, nature, or a higher power.*
- Establish realistic activity goals with client. *Enhances commitment to promoting optimal outcomes.*
- Involve client/SO(s) in schedule planning and decisions about timing and spacing of treatments *to promote relaxation and desire for involvement in plan.*
- Encourage client to do whatever possible (e.g., self-care, sit up in chair, walk). *Enhances self-esteem and independence.*
- ∞ Use age-appropriate distraction with music, chatting or texting with family/friends, watching TV, and playing video or computer games *to limit dwelling on negatives and to transcend unpleasant sensations and situations.*
- Encourage client to make use of beneficial coping behaviors and assertiveness skills, prioritizing goals and activities. *Promotes sense of control and improves self-esteem.*
- Offer and identify opportunities for client to participate in experiences that enhance control and independence.

Environmental
- Provide quiet environment and calm activities.
- Provide for periodic changes in the personal surroundings when client is confined. Use the individual's input in creating the changes (e.g., seasonal bulletin boards, color changes, rearranging furniture, pictures).
- Suggest activities, such as bird-watching, planting a garden in a window box or terrarium, or populating a fishbowl or aquarium, *to stimulate observation as well as involvement and participation in activity.*

Sociocultural
- ∞ Encourage age-appropriate diversional activities (e.g., TV, radio, playtime, socialization or outings with others).
- Avoid overstimulation or understimulation (cognitive and sensory).
- ⊘ Make appropriate referrals to available support groups, hobby clubs, or service organizations.

NURSING PRIORITY NO. 3   To promote optimum wellness (Teaching/Discharge Considerations):

- ⌂ Provide information about condition, health risk factors, or concerns in desired format (e.g., pictures, TV programs, articles, handouts, audio/visual materials, classes, group discussions, Web sites, other databases), as appropriate. *Use of multiple modalities enhances acquisition and retention of information and gives client choices for accessing and applying information.*

Physical
- Promote overall health measures (e.g., nutrition, adequate fluid intake, appropriate vitamin and iron supplementation).
- ⊘ Discuss potential complications and possible need for medical follow-up or alternative therapies. *Timely recognition and intervention can promote wellness.*

 Acute Care   Collaborative   Community/ Home Care   Cultural

• Assist client/SO(s) to identify and acquire necessary equipment (e.g., lifts, commode chair, safety grab bars, personal hygiene supplies) to meet individual needs.

Psychospiritual

• Collaborate with others when client expresses interest in lessons, counseling, coaching, or mentoring to meet or enhance emotional and spiritual comfort.
• Promote client's contributions toward meeting realistic goals.
• Encourage client to take time to be introspective in the search for contentment or transcendence.

Environmental

• ∞ 🌐 Promote a compassionate, supportive, and therapeutic environment that incorporates client's cultural, age, and developmental factors.
• Review environmental hazards that could influence safety or negatively affect comfort.
• Arrange for home visit and evaluation, as needed.
• Discuss long-term plan for taking care of environmental needs.

Sociocultural

• Advocate for growth-promoting environment in conflict situations and consider issues from client/family and cultural perspective.
• Support client/SO access to resources (e.g., knowledge and skills, financial resources or assistance, personal or psychological support, social systems).

DOCUMENTATION FOCUS

Assessment/Reassessment
• Individual findings, including client's description of current status or situation.
• Motivation and expectations for change.
• Pertinent cultural or religious beliefs and values.
• Medication use and nonpharmacological measures.

Planning
• Plan of care, specific interventions, and who is involved in planning.
• Teaching plan.

Implementation/Evaluation
• Responses to interventions, teaching, and actions performed.
• Attainment or progress toward desired outcome(s).
• Modifications to plan of care.

Discharge Planning
• Long-term needs and who is responsible for actions to be taken.
• Specific referrals made.

References

1. Kolcaba, K. Y., Fisher, E. M. (1996). A holistic perspective on comfort care as an advance directive. *Crit Care Nurs Q*, 18(4), 66–67.
2. Kolcaba, K., DiMarco, M. A. (2005). Comfort theory and its application to pediatric nursing. *Pediatr Nurse*, 31(3), 187–194.
3. Barclay, L., Lie, D. (2007). *New guidelines issued for family support in patient-centered ICU*. Retrieved March 2018 from http://www.medscape.org/viewarticle/551738.
4. Malinowski, A., Stamler, L. L. (2002). Comfort: Exploration of the concept in nursing. *J Adv Nurs*, 39(6), 599–606.
5. Kolcaba, K. (2003). *Comfort Theory and Practice: A Vision for Holistic Health and Research*. New York: Springer.
6. Kaplow, R. (2003). AACN synergy model for patient care: A framework to optimize outcomes. *Crit Care Nurse Suppl (Feb)*, 27–30.
7. Wilson, L., Kolcaba, K. (2004). Practical application of comfort theory in the perianesthesia setting. *J Perianesth Nurs*, 19(3), 164–173.
8. Townsend, M. C. (2005). *Psychiatric Mental Health Nursing Concepts of Care*. 5th ed. Philadelphia: F. A. Davis.

 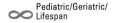

impaired verbal Communication

Taxonomy II: Perception/Cognition—Class 5 Communication (00051) [**Diagnostic Division:** Social Interaction], Approved 1983; Revised 1996, 1998, 2017

DEFINITION: Decreased, delayed, or absent ability to receive, process, transmit, and/or use a system of symbols.

RELATED FACTORS
Alteration in self-concept; low self-esteem
Cultural incongruence
Emotional disturbance; low self-esteem; vulnerability
Insufficient information or stimuli

DEFINING CHARACTERISTICS

Objective
Absence of eye contact; difficulty in selective attending; partial or total visual deficit
Difficulty comprehending or maintaining communication
Difficulty expressing thoughts verbally [e.g., aphasia, dysphasia, apraxia, dyslexia]
Difficulty forming sentences or words [e.g., aphonia, dyslalia, dysarthria]
Difficulty in use of body or facial expressions; inability to use body or facial expressions
Difficulty speaking/verbalizing; stuttering; slurred speech
Inability to speak; inability to speak language of caregiver
Inappropriate verbalization [e.g., incessant, loose association of ideas; flight of ideas]
At Risk Population: Absence of significant other
Associated Condition: Alteration in development; alteration in perception; central nervous system impairment, physiological condition; oropharyngeal defect; physical barrier; treatment regimen
Sample Clinical Applications: Brain injury or stroke, facial trauma, head or neck cancer, radical neck surgery, laryngectomy, cleft lip/palate, dementia, Tourette's syndrome, autism, schizophrenia

DESIRED OUTCOMES/EVALUATION CRITERIA

Sample NOC linkages:
Communication: Reception, interpretation, and expression of spoken, written, and nonverbal messages
Communication: Expressive: Expression of meaningful verbal and/or nonverbal messages
Information Processing: Ability to acquire, organize, and use information

Client Will (Include Specific Time Frame)
• Verbalize or indicate an understanding of the communication difficulty and plans for ways of handling.
• Establish method of communication in which needs can be expressed.
• Participate in therapeutic communication (e.g., using silence, acceptance, restating, reflecting, active-listening, and "I" messages).
• Demonstrate congruent verbal and nonverbal communication.
• Use resources appropriately.

ACTIONS/INTERVENTIONS

Sample NIC linkages:
Communication Enhancement: Speech Deficit: Use of strategies augmenting communication capabilities for a person with impaired speech

 Acute Care   Collaborative   Community/Home Care   Cultural

Communication Enhancement: Hearing Deficit: Use of strategies augmenting communication capabilities for a person with diminished hearing

Active Listening: Attending closely to and attaching significance to a patient's verbal and nonverbal messages

NURSING PRIORITY NO. 1 To assess causative/contributing factors:

- Identify physiological or neurological conditions impacting speech, such as severe shortness of breath, cleft palate, facial trauma, neuromuscular weakness, stroke, brain tumors or infections, dementia, brain trauma, deafness/impaired hearing.
- Review results of diagnostic studies (e.g., speech, language, and hearing evaluations, neurological testing or brain function studies—such as electroencephalogram, computed tomography scan, psychological evaluations) *to assess and delineate underlying conditions affecting verbal communication.*
- Note new onset or diagnosis of deficits that will progress or permanently affect speech.
- Note presence of physical barriers, including tracheostomy/intubation and wired jaws, or problem resulting in failure of voice production or "problem voice" *(pitch, loudness, or quality calls attention to voice rather than what speaker is saying, as might occur with electronic voice box or "talking valves" when tracheostomy in place).*[7,8]
- ∞ Determine age and developmental considerations when performing verbal examination, noting: (1) child too young for language or has developmental delays affecting speech and language skills or comprehension; (2) autism or other mental impairments; and (3) older client doesn't or isn't able to speak, verbalizes with difficulty, or has difficulty hearing or comprehending language or concepts. (The verbal examination should be adapted to the patient's communication skills and should use clear and concrete language, structure, reassurance, and support.)[1-3]
- Obtain history of hearing and speech-related pathophysiology or trauma (e.g., cleft lip/palate, traumatic brain injury, shaken baby syndrome, frequent ear infections affecting hearing, sensorineural changes associated with aging).
- Identify dominant language spoken. *Knowing the client's primary language and fluency in other languages is important to communication. For example, while some individuals may seem to be fluent in conversational English, they may still have limited understanding, especially the language of health professionals, and have difficulty answering questions, describing symptoms, or following directions.*[3,6,16]
- Ascertain whether client is recent immigrant, country of origin, and what cultural, ethnic group client identifies as own *(e.g., recent immigrant may identify with home country and its people, beliefs, and healthcare practices).*[6,16]
- Determine cultural factors affecting communication, such as beliefs concerning touch, eye contact, gestures, and verbal communications. *Certain cultures may prohibit client from speaking directly to healthcare provider; in some cultures, such as Native American, Appalachian, or African American, direct eye contact may be interpreted as disrespectful, impolite, an invasion of privacy, or aggressive. Those from other cultures may shout and gesture when excited.*[5] *Silence and tone of voice have various meanings, and slang words can cause confusion or misunderstandings.*[5]
- Identify environmental barriers, such as recent or chronic exposure to hazardous noise in home, job, recreation, or healthcare setting (e.g., rock music, jackhammer, snowmobile, lawn mower, truck traffic or busy highway, heavy equipment, medical equipment). *Noise not only affects hearing but also increases blood pressure and breathing rate, can have negative cardiovascular effects, disturbs digestion, increases fatigue, causes irritability, and reduces attention to tasks.*[9]
- Investigate client reports of problems such as constantly raising voice to be heard, can't hear someone 2 feet away, conversation in room sounds muffled or dull, too much energy required to listen, or pain or ringing in ears after exposure to noise.[9]

 Diagnostic Studies   Evidence Based Practice   Medications   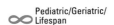 Pediatric/Geriatric/Lifespan

- Determine if client with communication impairment has a speech or language problem or both. *When a speech problem is present, the language code can be correct, but words might be garbled, person may stutter, or there may be problems with voice. Language and speech problems can exist together or by themselves. Language is a code made up of rules (e.g., what words mean, how to make new words, how to combine words, what combinations work in what situations). When a person cannot understand the language code, there is a receptive problem.*[10]
- Determine presence of psychological or emotional barriers, such as history or presence of psychiatric conditions (e.g., bipolar disorder, schizoid or affective behavior); high level of anxiety, frustration, or fear; and presence of angry, hostile behavior. Note effect on speech and communication.[1,4]
- Identify information barriers, such as lack of knowledge or misunderstanding of terms related to client's medical conditions, procedures, treatments, and equipment.[4]
- Assess level of understanding in a sensitive manner. *Individual may be reluctant to say he or she doesn't understand or may be embarrassed to ask for help. Head nodding and smiles do not always mean comprehension.*

NURSING PRIORITY NO. 2   To assist client to establish a means of communication to express needs, wants, ideas, and questions:

- Ascertain that you have client's attention before communicating.
- Establish rapport with client, initiate eye contact, shake hands, address by preferred name, meet family members present, ask simple questions, smile, and engage in brief social conversation if appropriate. *Helps establish a trusting relationship with client/family, demonstrating caring about the client as a person.*[2–4,18]
- Advise other care providers of client's communication deficits (e.g., deafness, aphasia, mechanical ventilation strategies) and needed means of communication (e.g., writing pad, signing, yes/no responses, gestures, picture board) *to minimize client's frustration and promote understanding.*[19]
- Provide and encourage use of glasses, hearing aids, dentures, and electronic speech devices as needed *to maximize sensory perception and improve speech patterns.*[2,4]
- Maintain a calm, unhurried manner and sit at client's eye level if possible. Provide sufficient time for client to respond. *Sitting down conveys that nurse has time and interest in communicating.*
- Pay attention to speaker. Be an active listener.
- ∞ Begin conversation with elderly individual with casual and familiar topics (e.g., weather, happenings with family members) *to convey interest and stimulate conversation and reminiscence.*[2,14]
- Reduce environmental distractions and background noise (e.g., close the door, turn down the radio or television).[14,20,21]
- Refrain from shouting when directing speech to a confused, deaf, or hearing-impaired client. Speak slowly and clearly, pitching voice low *to increase likelihood of being understood.*[2,15,20,21]
- Be honest and let the speaker know when you have difficulty understanding. Repeat part of message that you do understand *so speaker does not have to repeat entire message.*[11]
- Clarify type and special features of aphasia, when present. *Aphasia is a temporary, permanent, or progressive impairment of language affecting production or comprehension of speech and the ability to read or write. Some people with aphasia have problems primarily with expressive language (what is said), while others have problems with receptive language (what is understood). Aphasia can also be global (person understands almost nothing that is said and says little or nothing).*[4,11]
- Note diagnosis of apraxia (impairment in carrying out purposeful movements affecting rhythm and timing of speech), dysarthria (language code can be correct but the right body parts do not move at the right time to produce the right message), or dementia (defect is in decline in mental functions, including memory, attention, intellect, and personality) *to help clarify individual needs, appropriate interventions.*[11,12]
- Determine meaning of words used by the client and congruency of communication and nonverbal messages.
- Evaluate the meaning of words that are used/needed to describe aspects of healthcare (e.g., pain) and ascertain how to communicate important concepts.[5]

 Acute Care   Collaborative   Community/ Home Care   Cultural

- Observe body language, eye movements, and behavioral clues. *For example, client may react with tears, grimacing, stiff posture, turning away, or angry outbursts when pain present.*[13]
- Use confrontation skills, when appropriate, within an established nurse-client relationship *to clarify discrepancies between verbal and nonverbal cues.*[4,15]
- Point to objects or demonstrate desired actions when client has difficulty with language. *Speaker's own body language and gestures can be used to assist client's understanding.*
- Validate meaning of nonverbal communication; do not make assumptions *because they may be wrong.* Be honest; if you do not understand, seek assistance from others.[18]
- Work with confused, brain-injured, mentally disabled, or sensory-deprived client *to correctly interpret his or her environment.* Establish understanding and convey to others meaning of symbolic speech *to reduce frustration.* Teach basic signs such as "eat," "toilet," "more," and "finished" *to communicate basic needs.*[4,15]
- Provide reality orientation by responding with simple, straightforward, honest statements. Associate words with objects using repetition and redundancy *to improve communication patterns.*[2,4,15]
- Assess psychological response to communication impairment and willingness to find alternative means of communication.
- Identify family member who can speak for client and who is the family decision maker regarding healthcare decisions.[5,16]
- Note significant other's (SO's)/parents'/caregiver's speech patterns and interactive manner of communicating with client, including gestures.[20]
- Obtain interpreter with language or signing abilities and preferably with medical knowledge when needed. *Federal law mandates that interpretation services be made available. A trained, professional interpreter who translates precisely and possesses a basic understanding of medical terminology and healthcare ethics is preferred (over a family member) to enhance client and provider interactions.*[6]
- Evaluate ability to read and write, as well as musculoskeletal status, including manual dexterity (e.g., ability to hold a pen and write), and the need or desire for pictures or written communications and instructions as part of treatment plan.
- Plan for and provide alternative methods of communication:[2–4,17,22]
  Provide pad and pencil or a slate board *when client is able to write but cannot speak.*
  Use letter or picture board *when client can't write and picture concepts are understandable to both parties. Note: Studies show that visual aids may improve the accuracy of medication assessment and may be especially beneficial for clients with communication barriers.*[22]
  Establish hand or eye signals *when client can understand language but cannot speak or has physical barrier to writing.*
  Remove isolation mask *when client is deaf and reads lips.*
  Obtain or provide access to typewriter or computer *if communication impairment is long-standing or client is used to this method.*
- Consider form of communication when placing IV. *IV positioned in hand or wrist may limit ability to write or sign.*
- Answer call bell promptly. Anticipate needs and avoid leaving client alone with no way to summon assistance. *Reduces fear, conveys caring to client, and protects nurse from problems associated with failure to provide due care.*[4]
- Refer for appropriate therapies and support services. *Client and family may have multiple needs (e.g., sources for further examinations and rehabilitation services, local community or national support groups and services for disabled, financial assistance with obtaining necessary aids for improving communication).*[4]

NURSING PRIORITY NO. 3 To promote wellness (Teaching/Discharge Considerations):

- Encourage family presence and use of touch. Involve them in plan of care as much as possible. *Enhances participation and commitment to plan, assists in normalizing family role patterns, and provides support and encouragement when learning new patterns of communicating.*[4]

 Diagnostic Studies   Evidence Based Practice   Medications 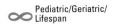 Pediatric/Geriatric/Lifespan

- Review information about condition, prognosis, and treatment with client/SOs, reinforcing that loss of speech does not imply loss of intelligence.
- Teach client and family the needed techniques for communication, whether it be speech or language techniques or alternate modes of communicating. Encourage family to involve client in family activities using enhanced communication techniques. *Reduces stress of difficult situation and promotes earlier return to more normal life patterns.*[4]
- Assess family for possible role changes resulting from client's impairment. Discuss methods of dealing with impairment.
- Use and assist client/SO(s) to learn therapeutic communication skills of acknowledgment, active-listening, and "I" messages. *Improves general communication skills, emphasizes acceptance, and conveys respect.*
- Discuss ways to provide environmental stimuli as appropriate *to maintain contact with reality or reduce environmental stimuli or noise. Unwanted sound affects physical health, increases fatigue, reduces attention to tasks, and makes speech communication more difficult.*[9,14]
- Refer to appropriate resources (e.g., speech or language therapist, support groups [e.g., stroke club], individual/family and/or psychiatric counseling) *to address long-term needs and enhance coping skills.*
- Refer to NDs ineffective Coping, disabled family Coping, Anxiety, Fear for additional interventions.

DOCUMENTATION FOCUS

Assessment/Reassessment
- Assessment findings, pertinent history information (i.e., physical, psychological, or cultural concerns).
- Meaning of nonverbal cues, level of anxiety client exhibits.

Planning
- Plan of care and specific interventions (e.g., type of alternative communication, translator).
- Teaching plan.

Implementation/Evaluation
- Response to interventions, teaching, and actions performed.
- Attainment or progress toward desired outcomes.
- Modifications to plan of care.

Discharge Planning
- Discharge needs, referrals made, additional resources available.

References

1. Szymanski, L., King, B. (1999). Practice parameters for the assessment and treatment of children, adolescents, and adults with mental retardation and comorbid mental disorders. American Academy of Child and Adolescent Psychiatry Working Group on Quality Issues. *J Am Acad Child Adolesc Psychiatry*, 38(12 Suppl), 5S–31S.
2. Stanley, M., Beare, P. G. (1999). *Gerontological Nursing: A Health Promotion Approach*. 2nd ed. Philadelphia: F. A. Davis.
3. Newfield, S. A., et al. (2007). *Cox's Clinical Applications of Nursing Diagnosis: Adult, Child, Women's, Psychiatric, Gerontic, and Home Health Considerations*. 5th ed. Philadelphia: F. A. Davis.
4. Doenges, M. E., Moorhouse, M. F., Murr, A. C. (2010). *Nurse's Pocket Guide: Diagnoses, Interventions, and Rationales*. 12th ed. Philadelphia: F. A. Davis, 193–198.
5. Purnell, L. D. (2009). *Guide to Culturally Competent Health Care*. 2nd ed. Philadelphia: F. A. Davis.

6. Enslein, J., et al. (2002). Evidence-based protocol: Interpreter facilitation for individuals with limited English proficiency. *J Gerontol Nurs*, 28(7), 5–13.
7. American Speech-Language-Hearing Association. *Voice disorders (various pages)*. Index retrieved March 2018 from http://www.asha.org/public/speech/disorders/voice.htm.
8. American Speech-Language-Hearing Association. Speech for patients with tracheostomies or ventilators. Retrieved March 2018 from https://www.asha.org/public/speech/disorders/tracheostomies/.
9. American Speech-Language-Hearing Association. Noise (information sheet). Retrieved March 2018 from http://www.asha.org/uploadedFiles/AIS-Noise.pdf#search=%22Noise%22.
10. American Speech-Language-Hearing Association. What is language? What is speech? Retrieved March 2018 from http://www.asha.org/public/speech/development/language_speech/.

 Acute Care Collaborative Community/ Home Care Cultural

11. National Aphasia Association. (No date). Aphasia Fact Sheet. Retrieved March 2018 from http://www.aphasia.org/Aphasia%20Facts/aphasia_facts.html.

12. National Aphasia Association. (2011). Understanding primary progressive aphasia (PPA). Retrieved March 2018 from http://www.aphasia.org/Aphasia%20Facts/understanding_primary_progressive_aphasia.html.

13. Hahn, J. (1999). Cueing in to patient language. *Reflections*, 25(1), 8–11.

14. Smith, K. (Updated 2011). I can hear you, but I can't understand you. Retrieved March 2018 from http://audioconsult.com/2011/08/i-can-hear-you-…-but-i-can't-understand-you…/.

15. Sendlebach, S., Guthrie, P. F. (2009). Acute confusion/delirium. *J Gerontol Nurs*, 35(11), 11–18.

16. Purnell, L. D. (2009). *Transcultural Health Care: A Culturally Competent Approach.* 3rd ed. Philadelphia: F. A. Davis.

17. Harquez-Rebello, M. C., Tornel-Costa, M. C. (1997). Design of a non-verbal method of communication using cartoons. *Rev Neurol*, 25(148), 2027–2045.

18. No author listed. (2005). Understanding transcultural nursing. *Nursing*, 35(1), 14–23.

19. Kirshner, D. (2016). *Aphasia.* Retrieved March 2018 from http://emedicine.medscape.com/article/1135944-overview.

20. Wallhagen, M. I., Pettengill, E., Whiteside, M. (2006). Sensory impairment in older adults part 1: Hearing loss. *Am J Nurs*, 106(10), 40–49.

21. Sommer, K. D., Sommer, N. W. (2002). When your patient is hearing impaired. *RN*, 65(12), 28–32.

22. Schillinger, D., et al. (2006). Language, literacy, and communication regarding medication in an anticoagulation clinic: A comparison of verbal vs. visual assessment. *J Health Commun*, 11(7), 651–654.

readiness for enhanced Communication

Taxonomy II: Perception/Cognition—Class 5 Communication (00157) **[Diagnostic Division:** Teaching/Learning], Approved 2002; Revised 2013

DEFINITION: A pattern of exchanging information and ideas with others, which can be strengthened.

DEFINING CHARACTERISTICS

Subjective
Expresses desire to enhance communication
Sample Clinical Applications: Brain injury or stroke, head or neck cancer, facial trauma, cleft lip/palate, Tourette's syndrome, autism, foreign-born individual communicating in second language

DESIRED OUTCOMES/EVALUATION CRITERIA

Sample NOC linkages:
Communication: Reception, interpretation, and expression of spoken, written, and nonverbal messages
Communication: Expressive: Expression of meaningful verbal and/or nonverbal messages
Information Processing: Ability to acquire, organize, and use information

Client/SO/Caregiver Will (Include Specific Time Frame)
• Verbalize or indicate an understanding of the communication process.
• Identify ways to improve communication.

ACTIONS/INTERVENTIONS

Sample NIC linkages:
Communication Enhancement: Speech Deficit: Use of strategies augmenting communication capabilities for a person with impaired speech
Communication Enhancement: Hearing Deficit: Use of strategies augmenting communication capabilities for a person with diminished hearing
Active Listening: Attending closely to and attaching significance to a patient's verbal and nonverbal messages

 Diagnostic Studies   Evidence Based Practice   Medications 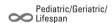 Pediatric/Geriatric/Lifespan

NURSING PRIORITY NO. 1   To assess how client is managing communication and potential difficulties:

- Ascertain circumstances that result in client's desire to improve communication. *Many factors are involved in communication, and identifying specific needs and expectations helps in developing realistic goals and determining likelihood of success.*
- Ascertain motivation and expectations for change. *Motivation to improve and high expectations can encourage client to make changes that will improve his or her life. However, presence of external locus of control or unrealistic expectations may hamper efforts.*
- Evaluate mental status. *Disorientation, acute or chronic confusion, or psychotic conditions may be affecting speech and the communication of thoughts, needs, and desires.*
- Determine client's developmental level of speech and language comprehension. *Provides baseline information for developing plan for improvement.*
- Determine ability to read and write preferred language. *Evaluating grasp of language as well as musculoskeletal status, including manual dexterity (e.g., ability to hold a pen and write), provides information about nature of client's situation. Educational plan can address language skills. Neuromuscular deficits require individual physical or occupational therapeutic program to improve.*
- Determine country of origin, dominant language, whether client is recent immigrant, and what cultural or ethnic group client identifies as own. *Recent immigrant may identify with home country and its people, language, beliefs, and healthcare practices, thus affecting desire to learn language skills and ability to improve interactions in new country.*[1]
- Ascertain if interpreter is needed or desired. *Law mandates that interpretation services be made available. A trained, professional interpreter who translates precisely and possesses a basic understanding of medical terminology and healthcare ethics is preferred over a family member to enhance client and provider interaction and sharing of information.*[1]
- Determine comfort level in expression of feelings and concepts in nonproficient language. *Concern about language skills can impact perception of own ability to communicate effectively.*
- Note any physical challenges to effective communication (e.g., hearing impairment, talking tracheostomy apparatus, wired jaws) or physiological or neurological conditions (e.g., severe shortness of breath, neuromuscular weakness, stroke, brain trauma, deafness, cleft palate, facial trauma). *Client may be dealing with speech or language comprehension or have voice production problems (pitch, loudness, quality) that call attention to voice rather than what speaker is saying. These barriers may need to be addressed to enable client to improve communication skills.*[2,3]
- Clarify meaning of words used by the client to describe important aspects of life and health or well-being (e.g., pain, sorrow, anxiety). *Words can easily be misinterpreted when sender and receiver have different ideas about their meanings. This can affect the way both client and caregivers communicate important concepts. Restating what one has heard can clarify whether an expressed statement has been understood or misinterpreted.*[4]
- Determine presence of emotional lability or frequency of unstable behaviors. *Emotional or psychiatric issues can affect communication and interfere with understanding.*
- Evaluate congruency of verbal and nonverbal messages. *Communication is enhanced when verbal and nonverbal messages are congruent.*[5]
- Determine lack of knowledge or misunderstanding of terms related to client's specific situation. *Indicators of need for additional information; clarification to help client improve ability to communicate.*
- Evaluate need or desire for pictures or written communications and instructions as part of treatment plan. *Alternative methods of communication can help client feel understood and promote feelings of satisfaction with interaction.*

NURSING PRIORITY NO. 2   To improve client's ability to communicate thoughts, needs, and ideas:

- Maintain a calm, unhurried manner. Provide sufficient time for client to respond. *An atmosphere in which client is free to speak without fear of criticism provides the opportunity to explore all the issues involved in making decisions to improve communication skills.*[10]

- Pay attention to speaker. Be an active listener. *The use of active-listening communicates acceptance and respect for the client, establishing trust, and promoting openness and honest expression. It communicates a belief that the client is a capable and competent person.*
- Sit down and maintain eye contact, preferably at the client's level, and spend time with the client. *Conveys message that the nurse has time and interest in communicating.*[10]
- Encourage client to express feelings and clarify meaning of nonverbal clues. *Client may be reluctant to share dissatisfaction with events.*
- Help client identify and learn to avoid use of nontherapeutic communication. *These barriers are recognized as detriments to open communication, and learning to avoid them maximizes the effectiveness of communication between client and others.*
- Obtain interpreter with language or signing abilities as needed. *May be needed to enhance understanding of words and language concepts to ascertain that interpretation of communication is accurate.*[6,10]
- Encourage use of computer/tablet, pad and pencil, slate board, or letter or picture board when interacting or to interface in new situations, as indicated. *When client has physical impairments that interfere with spoken communication, alternative means can provide concepts that are understandable to both parties.*[4,10]
- Obtain or provide access to voice-enabled computer. *Use of these devices may be more helpful when communication challenges are long-standing or when client is used to using them.*[1]
- 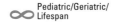 Respect client's cultural communication needs. *Different cultures can dictate beliefs of what is normal or abnormal (i.e., in some cultures, eye-to-eye contact is considered disrespectful, impolite, or an invasion of privacy; silence and tone of voice have various meanings, and slang words can cause confusion).*[4]
- Provide or encourage use of glasses, hearing aids, dentures, or electronic speech devices, as needed. *These devices maximize sensory perception and can improve understanding and enhance speech patterns.*[7]
- Reduce distractions and background noises (e.g., close the door, turn down the radio or television). *A distracting environment can interfere with communication, limiting attention to tasks, and makes speech and communication more difficult. Reducing noise can help both parties hear clearly, improving understanding.*[8]
- Associate words with objects using gestures, repetition and redundancy, point to objects, or demonstrate desired actions. *Speaker's own body language can be used to enhance client's understanding when neurological conditions result in difficulty understanding language.*[9]
- Use confrontation skills carefully, when appropriate, and within an established nurse-client relationship. *Can be used to clarify discrepancies between verbal and nonverbal cues, enabling client to look at areas that may require change.*[10]

NURSING PRIORITY NO. 3 To promote optimum communication:

- Discuss with family/significant other (SO) and other caregivers effective ways in which the client communicates. *Identifying positive aspects of current communication skills enables family members to learn and move forward in desire to enhance ways of interacting.*[10]
- Encourage client and family to familiarize themselves with and use new or developing communication technologies. *Enhances family relationships and promotes self-esteem for all members, as they are able to communicate regardless of problems (e.g., progressive neurological disorder) that could interfere with ability to interact.*[10]
- Reinforce client's/SO's learning and use of therapeutic communication skills of acknowledgment, active-listening, and "I" messages. *Improves general communication skills, emphasizes acceptance, and conveys respect, enabling family relationships to improve.*
- Refer to appropriate resources (e.g., speech therapist, language classes, individual/family or psychiatric counseling). *May need further assistance to overcome challenges as family reaches toward desired goal of enhanced communication.*

 Diagnostic Studies   Evidence Based Practice   Medications   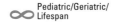 Pediatric/Geriatric/Lifespan

DOCUMENTATION FOCUS

Assessment/Reassessment
• Assessment findings, pertinent history information (i.e., physical, psychological, or cultural concerns).
• Meaning of nonverbal cues, level of anxiety client exhibits.
• Motivation and expectations for change.

Planning
• Plan of care and specific interventions (e.g., type of alternative communication, translator).
• Teaching plan.

Implementation/Evaluation
• Progress toward desired outcome(s).
• Modifications to plan of care.

Discharge Planning
• Discharge needs, referrals made, additional resources available.

References

1. Enslein, J., et al. (2002). Evidence-based protocol: Interpreter facilitation for persons with limited English proficiency. *J Gerontol Nurs*, 28(7), 5–13.
2. American Speech-Language-Hearing Association. Voice disorders (various pages). Index retrieved March 2018 from http://www.asha.org/public/speech/disorders/voice.
3. American Speech-Language-Hearing Association. Speech for patients with tracheostomies or ventilators. Retrieved March 2018 from https://www.asha.org/public/speech/disorders/tracheostomies/.
4. Purnell, L. (2009). *Guide to Culturally Competent Health Care*. 2nd ed. Philadelphia: F. A. Davis.
5. Hahn, J. (1999). Cueing in to client language. *Reflections*, 25(1), 8–11.
6. American Speech-Language-Hearing Association. What is language? What is speech? Retrieved March 2018 from http://www.asha.org/public/speech/development/language_speech.
7. Stanley, M., Beare, P. G. (1999). *Gerontological Nursing: A Health Promotion Approach*. 2nd ed. Philadelphia: F. A. Davis.
8. American Speech-Language-Hearing Association. Noise (information sheet). Retrieved March 2018 from http://www.asha.org/uploadedFiles/AIS-Noise.pdf#search=%22Noise%22.
9. Sendlebach, S., Guthrie, P. F. (2009). Acute confusion/delirium. *J Gerontol Nurs*, 35(11), 11–18.
10. Newfield, S. A., et al. (2007). *Cox's Clinical Applications of Nursing Diagnosis: Adult, Child, Women's, Psychiatric, Gerontic, and Home Health Considerations*. 5th ed. Philadelphia: F. A. Davis.

acute Confusion

Taxonomy II: Perception/Cognition—Class 4 Cognition (00128) [**Diagnostic Division:** Neurosensory], Approved 1994; Revised 2006, 2017

DEFINITION: Reversible disturbances of consciousness, attention, cognition, and perception that develop over a short period of time, and which last less than 3 months

RELATED FACTORS
Alteration in sleep-wake cycle; pain
Dehydration; malnutrition
Impaired mobility; inappropriate use of restraints; sensory deprivation
Urinary retention

DEFINING CHARACTERISTICS

Subjective
Hallucinations [visual or auditory]

 Acute Care Collaborative Community/Home Care Cultural

Objective

Agitation; restlessness

Alteration in cognitive functioning, or level of consciousness

Alteration in psychomotor functioning

Misperception

Inability to initiate goal-directed or purposeful behavior

Inability to follow through with goal-directed or purposeful behavior

Sample Clinical Applications: Brain injury or stroke, respiratory conditions with hypoxia, medication adverse reactions, drug or alcohol intoxication or withdrawal, hyperthermia, infectious processes, malnutrition, eating disorders, fluid and electrolyte imbalances, chemical exposure

DESIRED OUTCOMES/EVALUATION CRITERIA

Sample NOC linkages:

Delirium Level: Severity of disturbance in consciousness and cognition that develops over a short period of time and is reversible

Information Processing: Ability to acquire, organize, and use information

Distorted Thought Self-Control: Self-restraint of disruptions in perception, thought processes, and thought content

Client/Caregiver Will (Include Specific Time Frame)

- Regain and maintain usual reality orientation and level of consciousness.
- Verbalize understanding of causative factors when known.
- Initiate lifestyle or behavior changes to prevent or minimize recurrence of problem.

ACTIONS/INTERVENTIONS

Sample NIC linkages:

Delirium Management: Provision of a safe and therapeutic environment for the patient who is experiencing an acute confusional state

Reality Orientation: Promotion of patient's awareness of personal identity, time, and environment

Delusion Management: Promoting the comfort, safety, and reality orientation of a patient experiencing false, fixed beliefs that have little or no basis in reality

NURSING PRIORITY NO. 1   To assess causative/contributing factors:

- Identify factors present, such as recent surgery or trauma; fluid and electrolyte imbalances; use of large numbers of medications (polypharmacy); intoxication with/withdrawal from a substance (e.g., prescription and over-the-counter [OTC] drugs; alcohol, illicit drugs); history or current seizure activity, episodes of fever, pain, presence of acute infection (especially occult urinary tract infection in elderly client); traumatic events; person with dementia experiencing sudden change in environment, unfamiliar surroundings or people). *Acute confusion is a symptom associated with numerous causes (e.g., hypoxia; metabolic/endocrine/neurological conditions, toxins; electrolyte abnormalities; systemic or central nervous system infections; nutritional deficiencies, acute psychiatric disorders). Note: Delirium due to physical illness is more frequent among the very young and the elderly. Delirium due to drug and alcohol intoxication or withdrawal is more common in persons aged mid-teens to late 30s. Studies show that delirium due to physical illness is more frequent among the very young and those older than 60 years. Delirium due to drug and alcohol intoxication or withdrawal is more common in persons aged mid-teens to late 30s.*[2,11–13]

 Diagnostic Studies   Evidence Based Practice   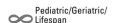 Medications   Pediatric/Geriatric/ Lifespan

- Assess mental status. *Typical symptoms of delirium include anxiety, disorientation, tremors, hallucinations, delusions, and incoherence. Onset is usually sudden, developing over a few hours or days, and resolving over varying periods of time.*[2,11]
- Evaluate vital signs. *Signs of poor tissue perfusion (i.e., hypotension, tachycardia, tachypnea, or fever) may identify underlying cardiovascular or infectious cause for mental status changes. Note: Clients with delirium frequently display elevated blood pressure because of adrenergic overload in the sympathetic nervous system. Heart rate can be either elevated or decreased (particularly in client on certain medications [e.g., beta blockers, calcium channel blockers]).*[11]
- Determine current medications and drug use (especially anti-anxiety agents, barbiturates, certain antipsychotic agents; methyldopa, disulfiram, cocaine, alcohol, amphetamines, hallucinogens, opiates). *Use, misuse, overdose, and withdrawal of many drugs are associated with high risk of confusion and delirium.*[1,11]
- Investigate possibility of alcohol or illicit drug intoxication or withdrawal or prescription or OTC medication toxicity, side effects, or interactions. *Noncompliance with regimen, withdrawal from or overuse of substances, and certain drug combinations increase risk of toxic reactions and adverse reactions or interactions.*[1,2,12]
- Evaluate for exacerbation of psychiatric conditions (e.g., mood disorder, dissociative disorders, dementia). *Identification of the presence of mental illness provides opportunity for correct treatment and medication.*[10,11]
- Assess diet and nutritional status to identify possible deficiencies of essential nutrients and vitamins. *Failure to eat (forgetfulness or lack of food) can lead to deficiencies (e.g., vitamin B_{12}, folate, thiamine, iron) that could affect mental status.*[2,11]
- Evaluate sleep and rest status, noting deprivation or oversleeping. *Discomfort, worry, and lack of sleep and rest can cause or exacerbate confusion.* (Refer to ND Insomnia, disturbed Sleep Pattern as appropriate.)
- Monitor laboratory values (e.g., complete blood count, blood cultures; oxygen saturation and, in some cases, arterial blood gases with carbon monoxide; blood urea nitrogen and creatinine levels; electrolytes; thyroid function studies; liver function studies, ammonia levels; serum glucose; urinalysis for infection and drug analysis; specific drug toxicologies, drug levels [including peak and trough, as appropriate]).[1–7,11]
- Review results of diagnostic studies (e.g., delirium assessment tools, such as the Confusion Assessment Method, delirium index, Mini Mental State Examination, etc.; brain scans or imaging studies, electroencephalogram, lumbar puncture and cerebrospinal fluid studies). *Mental status instruments are helpful because they directly test the client's cognitive performance. However, performance is strongly affected by age, educational level, ethnicity, and language, and they may be difficult for the acutely ill client to perform.*[5,11]

NURSING PRIORITY NO. 2   To determine degree of impairment:

- Talk with client/significant others (SOs) to determine client's physical, functional, cognitive, and behavioral baseline; observed changes; and onset and precipitator of changes *to understand and clarify the current situation.*[1]
- Collaborate with medical and psychiatric providers *to evaluate extent of impairment in orientation, attention span, ability to follow directions, send and receive communication, and appropriateness of response.*[1]
- Note occurrence and timing of agitation, hallucinations, and violent behaviors *(e.g., delirium may occur as early as 1 or 2 days after last drink in an alcoholic; "sundowners syndrome" may occur in intensive care unit, with client oriented during daylight hours but confused during night).*[1,3,15]
- Determine threat to safety of client/others. *Delirium can cause client to become verbally and physically aggressive, resulting in behavior threatening to safety of self and others.*

NURSING PRIORITY NO. 3   To maximize level of function, prevent further deterioration:

- Assist with treatment of underlying problem. *Interventions to establish and maintain normal fluid and electrolyte balance and oxygenation, treat infectious process or pain, detoxify from alcohol and other drugs, and provide psychological interventions can resolve or diminish confusion.*[1–7,9,11,12,14]
- Monitor and adjust medication regimen and note response. Determine which medications can be changed or eliminated when polypharmacy, side effects, or adverse reactions are determined to be associated with current condition.

 Acute Care   Collaborative   Community/Home Care   Cultural

- Implement helpful communication measures:[1–7,9,11,14]

  Use short, simple sentences. Speak slowly and clearly.

  Call client by name and identify yourself at each contact.

  Tell client what you want done, not what to do.

  Orient client to surroundings, staff, and necessary activities as often as needed.

  Acknowledge client's fears and feelings. *Confusion can be very frightening, especially when client knows thinking is not normal.*

  Listen to what client says and try to identify message and emotion or need being communicated.

  Limit choices and decisions until client is able to make them.

  Give simple directions. Allow sufficient time for client to respond, communicate, and make decisions.

  Present reality concisely and briefly and avoid challenging illogical thinking. *Defensive reactions may result.*

  Refer to ND impaired verbal Communication for additional interventions.

- Manage environment, using the following measures:[1–7,9–11,14,15]

  Provide undisturbed rest periods. Eliminate extraneous noise and stimuli. *Preventing overstimulation can help client relax and can result in reduced level of confusion.*

  Provide calm and comfortable environment with good lighting. Encourage client to use vision or hearing aids, when needed, *to reduce disorientation and discomfort from sensory overload or deprivation.*

  Observe client on regular basis, informing client of this schedule.

  Provide adequate supervision (may need one-to-one during severe episode), remove harmful objects from environment, provide siderails and seizure precautions, place call bell and position needed items within reach, clear traffic paths, and ambulate with devices *to meet client's safety needs and reduce risk of falls.*

  Provide clear feedback on appropriate and inappropriate behavior.

  Remove client from situation; provide time-out or seclusion, as indicated, *for protection of client/others.*

  Encourage family/SO(s) to participate in reorientation and provide ongoing normal life input (e.g., current news and family happenings). Provide normal levels of essential sensory and tactile stimulation—include personal items and pictures. *Client may respond positively to well-known person and familiar items.*

- Note behavior that may be indicative of potential for violence and take appropriate actions to prevent injury to client/caregiver. (Refer to ND risk for other-directed Violence.)

- Administer medication cautiously to control restlessness, agitation, and hallucinations. *Depending on the cause of acute delirium, medications could include sedatives, neuroleptics, and antidotes. Sedation with conventional antipsychotic agents (e.g., haloperidol, lorazepam, droperidol) may be used, although many other agents may be tried, including electrolytes, glucose, vitamins, antibiotics, etc. (Note: Sedation should be avoided if it will interfere with, or cloud the results of, serial neurological examinations.)*[2,5–7,11]

- Assist with treatment of alcohol or drug intoxication and/or withdrawal, as indicated.[11,12,14]

- Avoid or limit use of restraints. *May worsen agitation and increase likelihood of untoward complications including injury or death.*[5,12,15]

- Mobilize elderly client (especially after orthopedic injury) as soon as possible. *Older person with low level of activity prior to crisis is at particular risk for acute confusion and may fare better when out of bed.*[4,14,15]

- Establish and maintain elimination patterns. *Disruption of elimination may be a cause for confusion, or changes in elimination may also be a symptom of acute confusion.*[5]

- Consult with psychiatric clinical nurse specialist or psychiatrist for additional interventions related to disruptive behaviors, psychosis, and unresolved symptoms.

- Refer to ND [disturbed Sensory Perception (Specify)] for additional interventions.

NURSING PRIORITY NO. 4   To promote wellness (Teaching/Discharge Considerations):

- Explain reason for confusion, if known. *Acute confusion usually subsides over time as client recovers from underlying cause or adjusts to situation, but it can be frightening to client/SO. Information about cause and treatment to improve condition may be helpful in managing sense of fear and powerlessness.*[13,14]

 Diagnostic Studies   Evidence Based Practice   Medications   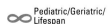 Pediatric/Geriatric/Lifespan

- Educate SO/caregivers to monitor client at home for sudden change in cognition and behavior. *An acute change is a classic presentation of delirium and should be considered a medical emergency. Early intervention can often prevent long-term complications.*[8]
- ∞ Discuss need for ongoing medical review of client's medications to limit possibility of misuse and/or potential for dangerous side effects or interactions. *Medications are frequent precipitants of acute confusion, especially in very young or old.*[2,5,8,9]
- Emphasize importance of keeping vision and hearing aids in good repair and readily available *to improve client's interpretation of environmental stimuli and communication.*
- Provide appropriate referrals. *Additional assistance may be required for client with confusion (e.g., cognitive retraining, substance abuse support groups, medication monitoring program, Meals on Wheels, home health, and adult day care).*[1]

DOCUMENTATION FOCUS

Assessment/Reassessment
- Nature, duration, frequency of problem.
- Current and previous level of function, effect on independence and lifestyle (including safety concerns).

Planning
- Plan of care and who is involved in planning.
- Teaching plan.

Implementation/Evaluation
- Response to interventions and actions performed.
- Attainment or progress toward desired outcomes.
- Modifications to plan of care.

Discharge Planning
- Long-term needs and who is responsible for actions to be taken.
- Available resources and specific referrals.

References

1. Doenges, M. E., Moorhouse, M. F., Murr, A. C. (2010). *Nurse's Pocket Guide: Diagnoses, Prioritized Interventions and Rationales.* 12th ed. Philadelphia: F. A. Davis, 211–215.
2. Alagiakrishnan, K. (Updated 2017). Delerium. Retrieved March 2018 from http://emedicine.medscape.com/article/288890-overview.
3. Stanley, M., Bear, P. G. (1999). *Gerontological Nursing: A Health Promotion/Protection Approach.* 2nd ed. Philadelphia: F. A. Davis, 342–349.
4. Matthiesen, V., et al. (1994). Acute confusion: Nursing intervention in older patients. *Orthop Nurs*, 13(2), 21–27.
5. Sendelbach, S., Guthrie, P. F. (2009). Acute confusion/delirium. *J Gerontol Nurs*, 35(11), 11–18.
6. American Psychiatric Association. (2006). Guideline watch: Practice guideline for the treatment of patients with delirium. *American Psychiatric Association Practice Guidelines for the Treatment of Psychiatric Disorders Compendium.* 2nd ed. Washington, D.C.: American Psychiatric Association.
7. Alexopoulas, G. S. (2007). Treatment of dementia and agitation: A guide for families and caregiver. *J Psychiatr Pract*, 13(3), 12–20.
8. Ackley, B. J., Ladwig, G. B. (2002). *Nursing Diagnosis Handbook: A Guide to Planning Care.* 5th ed. St. Louis, MO: Mosby.
9. Cox, H. C., et al. (2002). *Cox's Clinical Applications of Nursing Diagnosis: Adult, Child, Women's, Psychiatric, Gerontic, and Home Health Considerations.* 4th ed. Philadelphia: F. A. Davis.
10. Doenges, M. E., Townsend, M. C., Moorhouse, M. F. (1999). *Psychiatric Care Plans Guidelines for Individualizing Care.* 3rd ed. Philadelphia: F. A. Davis.
11. Gerstein, P. S. (Updated 2017). Delirium, dementia, and amnesia in emergency medicine. Retrieved March 2018 from http://emedicine.medscape.com/article/793247-overview.
12. Jennings-Ingle, S. (2007). The sobering facts about alcohol withdrawal syndrome. *Nursing Made Incredibly Easy!*, 5(1), 50–60.
13. Spilman, S. K., et al. (2014). Infrequent assessment of pain in elderly trauma patients . *J Trauma Nurs*, 21(5), 229–235.
14. Naylor, M. D., et al. (2005). Cognitively impaired older adults. *Am J Nurs*, 105(2), 52–61.
15. Nall, R. (2016). Sundowner's syndrome: Causes, symptoms, and treatments. Retrieved March 2018 from https://www.medicalnewstoday.com/articles/314685.phpw.

 Acute Care   Collaborative   Community/Home Care   Cultural

chronic Confusion

Taxonomy II: Perception/Cognition—Class 4 Cognition (00129) [**Diagnostic Division:** Neurosensory], Approved 1994; Revised 2017

DEFINITION: Irreversible, progressive, insidious, and long-term alteration of intellect, behavior, and personality, manifested by impairment in cognitive functions (memory, speech, language, decision making, and executive function), and dependency in execution of daily activities.

DEFINING CHARACTERISTICS

Objective
Adequate alertness to surroundings
Alteration in at least one cognitive function other than memory
Alteration in behavior; personality, social functioning
Alteration in short-term or long-term memory
Inability to perform at least one daily activity
Insidious and irreversible onset in cognitive impairment; long-term cognitive impairment; progressive impairment in cognitive functioning
Associated Condition: Cerebral vascular accident; dementia
Sample Clinical Applications: Brain injury or stroke, dementia/Alzheimer's disease, medication adverse reactions, drug or alcohol abuse, malnutrition, eating disorders, chemical exposure

DESIRED OUTCOME/EVALUATION CRITERIA

Sample NOC linkages:
Cognitive Orientation: Ability to identify person, place, and time accurately
Physical Injury Severity: Severity of signs and symptoms of injuries to the body

Client Will (Include Specific Time Frame)
• Maintain usual level of orientation.
• Remain safe and free from harm.

Sample NOC linkages:
Knowledge: Dementia Management: Extent of understanding conveyed about progressive dementia, its course over an extended period of time, and plan for supportive care as the disease progresses
Family/Significant Other (SO) Will (Include Specific Time Frame)
• Verbalize understanding of disease process and prognosis and client's needs.
• Identify and participate in interventions to deal effectively with situation.
• Provide for maximal independence while meeting safety needs of client.

ACTIONS/INTERVENTIONS

Sample NIC linkages:
Dementia Management: Provision of a modified environment for the patient who is experiencing a chronic confusional state
Calming Technique: Reducing anxiety in patient experiencing acute distress
Surveillance: Purposeful and ongoing acquisition, interpretation, and synthesis of patient data for clinical decision making

 Diagnostic Studies   Evidence Based Practice   Medications   Pediatric/Geriatric/Lifespan

NURSING PRIORITY NO. 1   To assess degree of impairment:

- Determine the underlying cause for chronic confusion, as noted in Related Factors. *Helps to sort out possible causes and likelihood for improvement, as well as helping to identify potentially useful interventions and therapies.*[1]
- ✎📝 Review and evaluate responses on diagnostic examinations (e.g., cognitive, functional capacity, behavior, memory impairments, reality orientation, attention span, quality of life). *A combination of tests (e.g., Confusion Assessment Method, Mini-Mental State Examination, Montreal Cognitive Assessment, Alzheimer's Disease Assessment Scale, Brief Dementia Severity Rating Scale, Neuropsychiatric Inventory, Functional Assessment Questionnaire, Clinical Global Impression of Change) is often needed to complete an evaluation of client's overall condition relating to chronic or irreversible condition. Note: Studies show that while a single screening test may identify cognitive decline and functional impairment, many tests serve different clinical and research functions. Therefore, clinical testing will continue to evolve.*[2,3,7]
- Talk with SO(s) regarding baseline behaviors, length of time since onset or progression of problem, their perception of prognosis, and other pertinent information and concerns for client. *The client's SO/primary caregiver is an invaluable and essential source of information, regarding history and current situation, as both cognitive and behavioral symptoms tend to change over time and are often variable from day to day. If history reveals a gradual and insidious decline over months to years, and if memory loss is a prominent part of the confusion, dementia is likely. Conditions that permanently damage brain structure and tissue (e.g., vascular, traumatic, infectious or demyelinating conditions) can lead to dementia in person of any age.*[1-4,8,9]
- Obtain information regarding recent changes or disruptions in client's health or routine. *Decline in physical health or disruption in daily living situation (e.g., hospitalization, change in medications, or moving to new home) can exacerbate agitation or bring on acute confusion.* (Refer to ND acute Confusion.)
- Evaluate client's response to primary care providers as well as receptiveness to interventions. *Awareness of these dynamics is helpful for evaluation of ongoing needs for both client and caregiver as client becomes increasingly dependent on caregivers or resistant to interventions.*
- Determine client and caregiver anxiety level in relation to situation. Note behavior that may be indicative of potential for violence. *The diagnosis of irreversible condition, the organic brain changes, and the day-to-day problems of living with it causes great stress and can potentiate violence.*[4]

NURSING PRIORITY NO. 2   To limit effects of deterioration/maximize level of function:

- 🔄 Assist in treating conditions (e.g., depression, infections, malnutrition, electrolyte imbalances, and adverse medication reactions) *that may contribute to or exacerbate distress, discomfort, and agitation.*[1-6]
- Implement behavioral and environmental management interventions to promote orientation, provide opportunity for client interaction using current cognitive skills, and preserve client's dignity and safety:[6,9,11,12]
  Ascertain interventions previously used or tried and evaluate effectiveness.
  Provide calm environment and minimize relocations; eliminate extraneous noise and stimuli *that may increase client's level of agitation or confusion.*
  Introduce yourself at each contact, if needed. Call client by preferred name.
  Use touch judiciously. Tell client what is being done before touching *to reduce sense of surprise or negative reaction.*
  Be supportive and sensitive to fears, misperceived threats, and frustration with expressing what is wanted.
  Be open and honest when discussing client's disease, abilities, and prognosis.
  Maintain continuity of caregivers and care routines as much as possible.
  Use positive statements, offer guided choices between two options.
  Avoid speaking in loud voice, crowding, restraining, shaming, demanding, or condescending actions toward client.
  Set limits on acting-out behavior *for safety of client/others.*
  Remove from stressors and agitation triggers or danger, move client to quieter place, and offer privacy.

 Acute Care   Collaborative   Community/ Home Care   Cultural

Simplify client's tasks and routines *to accommodate fluctuating abilities and to reduce agitation associated with multiple options or demands.*

Provide for or assist with daily care activities, including bathing, dressing, grooming, toileting, and exercise. *Client may "forget" how to perform activities of daily living.*

Monitor and assist with meeting nutritional needs and feeding and fluid intake and monitor weight. Provide finger food if client has problems with eating utensils or is unable to sit to eat.

Assist with toileting and perineal care, as needed. Provide incontinence supplies.

Allow adequate rest between stimulating events.

Use lighting and visual aids *to reduce confusion.*

Encourage family/SO(s) to provide ongoing orientation/input to include current news and family happenings.

Maintain reality-oriented relationship and environment (e.g., clocks, calendars, personal items, seasonal decorations).

Encourage participation in resocialization groups *to help restore or maintain client's independence and dignity.*

Allow client to reminisce or exist in own reality if not detrimental to well-being.

Avoid challenging illogical thinking *because defensive reactions may result.*

Provide appropriate safety measures. *Client who is confused needs close supervision. Safety measures (such as use of identification bracelet and alarms on unlocked exits, lockup of toxic substances and medication, supervision of outdoor activities and wandering, removal of car or car keys, lowered temperature on hot water tank) can prevent injuries.*[4]

- Avoid use of restraints as much as possible. Investigate use of alternatives (such as bed nets, electronic bed pads, chair alarms, laptop trays), when required. *Although restraints can prevent falls, they can increase client's agitation and distress, resulting in injury or even death.*[7,9,10]

- Administer medications (e.g., antidepressants, anxiolytics, antipsychotics), as ordered, at lowest possible therapeutic dose. Monitor for expected and/or adverse responses, side effects, and interactions. *May be used to manage symptoms of psychosis and aggressive behaviors but need to be used cautiously.*[5,13]

- Implement complementary therapies (e.g., music or dance therapy; animal-assisted therapy; massage, Therapeutic Touch [if touch is tolerated], aromatherapy, bright light treatment) as ordered or desired. Monitor client's response to each modality and modify as indicated. *Use of alternative therapies tailored to the client's preferences, skills, and abilities can be calming and provide relaxation and can be carried out by a wide range of health and social care providers and volunteers.*[11]

- Refer to NDs acute Confusion, impaired Memory, impaired verbal Communication for additional interventions.

NURSING PRIORITY NO. 3 To assist SO(s) to develop coping strategies:

- Determine family dynamics, cultural values, resources, availability, and willingness to participate in meeting client's needs. Evaluate SO's attention to own needs, including health status, grieving process, and respite. *Primary caregiver and other members of family will suffer from the stress that accompanies caregiving and will require ongoing information and support.*

- Discuss caregiver burden when appropriate. Provide educational materials and list of available resources, help lines, Web sites, and so forth, as desired, *to assist SO(s) in dealing and coping with long-term care issues.*[5,7,9] (Refer to NDs caregiver Role Strain, risk for caregiver Role Strain.)

- Involve SO(s) in care and discharge planning. Maintain frequent interactions with SOs *in order to relay information, to change care strategies, try different responses, or implement other problem-solving solutions.*[6]

- Identify appropriate community resources (e.g., Alzheimer's Disease and Related Disorders Association, stroke or other brain injury support groups, senior support groups, specialist day services, home care, respite care; adult placement and short-term residential care; clergy, social services, occupational and physical therapists; assistive technology and telecare; attorney services for advance directives, durable power of attorney) *to provide support for client and SOs and assist with problem solving.*[5,11]

 Diagnostic Studies   Evidence Based Practice   Medications   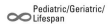 Pediatric/Geriatric/Lifespan

NURSING PRIORITY NO. 4 To promote optimal functioning and safety (Teaching/Discharge Considerations):

- Discuss how client's condition may progress, ongoing age-appropriate treatment needs, and appropriate follow-up. *Intermittent evaluations are needed to determine client's general health, any deterioration in cognitive function, or required adjustment in medication regimen to help the client maintain the highest possible level of functioning.*[6]
- Review medications with SO/caregiver(s), including dosage, route, action, expected and reportable side effects, and potential drug interactions *to prevent or limit complications associated with multiple psychiatric and central nervous system medications.*[5]
- Develop plan of care with family to meet client's and SO's individual needs. *The individual plan is dependent on cultural and belief patterns as well as family resources (personal, emotional, financial).*[6]
- Instruct SO/caregivers to share information about client's condition, functional status, and medications whenever encountering new providers. *Clients often have multiple doctors, each of whom may prescribe medications with potential for adverse effects and overmedication.*
- Provide appropriate referrals (e.g., Meals on Wheels, adult day care, home-care agency, nursing home placement, respite care for family member). *May need additional assistance to maintain the client in the home setting or make arrangements for placement if necessary.*[6]

DOCUMENTATION FOCUS

Assessment/Reassessment
- Individual findings, including current level of function, recent changes, and rate of anticipated changes.
- Client/caregiver response to situation.
- Results of diagnostic testing.

Planning
- Plan of care and who is involved in planning.
- Teaching Plan

Implementation/Evaluation
- Response to interventions and actions performed.
- Attainment or progress toward desired outcomes.
- Modifications to plan of care.

Discharge Planning
- Long-term needs and who is responsible for actions to be taken.
- Available resources, specific referrals made.

References

1. Bostwick, J. M. (2000). The many faces of confusion: Timing and collateral history often holds the key to diagnosis. *Postgrad Med*, 108(6), 60–72.
2. Alzheimer's Disease and Related Disorders Association. (Updated 2015). Tests for Alzheimer's disease and dementia. Retrieved March 2018 from http://www.alz.org/alzheimers_disease_steps_to_diagnosis.asp.
3. Vayda, E. P., Patterson, M. B., Whitehouse, P. J. (2010). The future of dementia: A case of hardening of the categories. *Am J Geriatr Psych*, 18(9), 755–758.
4. Alexopoulas, G. S., et al. (2005). Treatment of dementia and agitation: A guideline for families and caregivers: Expert Consensus Guideline Series. *A Postgraduate Medicine Special Report*, January; 23(1), 18–22.
5. Sommers, M. S., Johnson, S. A., Beery, T. A. (2007). Alzheimer's disease. *Diseases and Disorders: A Nursing Therapeutics Manual*. 3rd ed. Philadelphia: F. A. Davis.
6. Kovach, C. R. (2004). Dementia in older adults. In Stanley, M., Blair, K. A., Gauntlett Beare, P. (eds). *Gerontological Nursing: Promoting Successful Aging With Older Adults*. 3rd ed. Philadelphia: F. A. Davis.
7. Boissonneault, G. (2010). MCI and dementia: Diagnosis and treatment. *JAAPA*, January; 23(1), 18–22.
8. Borbasi, S., et al. (2006). Health professionals' perspective of providing care to people with dementia in the acute setting: Toward better practice. *Geriatr Nurs*, 27(5), 300–308.
9. Kirshner, H. S. (2010). Confusional states and acute memory disorders. Retrieved March 2018 from http://misc.medscape.com/pi/iphone/medscapeapp/html/A1135767-business.html.

 Acute Care   Collaborative   Community/Home Care   Cultural

10. Evans, L. K., Cotter, V. T. (2007). Avoiding restraints in patients with dementia: Understanding, prevention, and management are the keys. *Am J Nurs*, 108(3), 40–49.

11. National Institute for Health and Clinical Excellence. (2006). Dementia: Supporting people with dementia and their carers in health and social care. Retrieved March 2018 from https://www.scie.org.uk/publications/misc/dementia/dementia-guideline.pdf?res=true.

12. Alzheimer's Disease and Related Disorders Association (ADRDA). (2015). Treatments for behavior. Retrieved March 2018 from http://www.alz.org/alzheimers_disease_treatments_for_behavior.asp.

13. Alzheimer's Association. (2015). Treatments for behavior. Retrieved March 2018 from http://www.alz.org/alzheimers_disease_treatments_for_behavior.asp.

risk for acute Confusion

Taxonomy II: Perception/Cognition—Class 4 Cognition (00173) [**Diagnostic Division:** Neurosensory], Approved 2006; Revised 2013, 2017

DEFINITION: Susceptible to reversible disturbances of consciousness, attention, cognition, and perception that develop over a short period of time, which may compromise health.

RISK FACTORS
Alteration in sleep-wake cycle; pain
Dehydration; malnutrition
Impaired mobility; inappropriate use of restraints; sensory deprivation
Urinary retention
At Risk Population: Age ≥60 years; male gender
History of cerebral vascular accident
Associated Condition: Alteration in cognitive functioning; delirium; dementia; impaired metabolic functioning; infection; pharmaceutical agents
Sample Clinical Applications: Brain injury or stroke, respiratory conditions with hypoxia, medication adverse reactions, drug or alcohol intoxication or withdrawal, hyperthermia, infectious processes, malnutrition, eating disorders, fluid and electrolyte imbalances, chemical exposure

DESIRED OUTCOMES/EVALUATION CRITERIA

Sample **NOC** linkages:
Delirium Level: Severity of disturbance in consciousness and cognition that develops over a short period of time and is reversible
Information Processing: Ability to acquire, organize, and use information
Risk Control: Personal actions to prevent, eliminate, or reduce modifiable health threats

Client/Caregiver Will (Include Specific Time Frame)
• Maintain usual level of consciousness and cognition.
• Verbalize understanding of individual risk factor(s).
• Engage in activities or interventions to prevent or reduce risk of confusion.

ACTIONS/INTERVENTIONS

Sample **NIC** linkages:
Reality Orientation: Promotion of patient's awareness of personal identity, time, and environment
Teaching: Disease Process: Assisting the patient to understand information related to a specific disease process
Surveillance: Purposeful and ongoing acquisition, interpretation, and synthesis of patient data for clinical decision making

 Diagnostic Studies   Evidence Based Practice   Medications   Pediatric/Geriatric/Lifespan

NURSING PRIORITY NO. 1 To assess causative/contributing factors:

- ∞ Identify risk factors present, such as recent trauma or fall; use of large numbers of medications (polypharmacy); intoxication with/withdrawal from a substance (e.g., prescription and over-the-counter [OTC] drugs; alcohol, illicit drugs); history or current seizures; episodes of fever, pain, or acute infection; exposure to toxic substances; traumatic events in client's/significant other's (SO's) life; person with dementia experiencing sudden change in environment/unfamiliar surroundings or people; and exacerbation of psychiatric conditions (e.g., mood disorder, dissociative disorders). *Individuals are at risk of developing confusion associated with numerous causes (e.g., hypoxia, abnormal metabolic conditions, ingestion of toxins or medications, electrolyte abnormalities, sepsis/systemic infections, nutritional deficiencies, endocrine disorders, central nervous system infections, other neurological pathology, acute psychiatric disorders). Note: Delirium due to physical illness is more frequent among the very young and the elderly. Delirium due to drug and alcohol intoxication or withdrawal is more common in persons aged mid-teens to late 30s.*[2–5,8]
- Evaluate vital signs for indicators of poor tissue perfusion (i.e., hypotension, tachycardia, tachypnea). *May identify underlying cardiovascular or infectious cause for mental status changes.*
- 📝 Assess mental status. *Typical symptoms of delirium include anxiety, disorientation, tremors, hallucinations, delusions, and incoherence. Onset is usually sudden, developing over a few hours or days, and resolving over varying periods of time.*[2,6,7]
- 💊∞ Determine current medication regimen/drug use—especially anti-anxiety agents, barbiturates, certain antipsychotic agents, methyldopa, disulfiram, cocaine, alcohol, amphetamines, hallucinogens, and opiates, *which are associated with high risk of confusion, disorientation, and delirium;* and OTC medications, such as Benadryl and Tylenol PM, *which can cause an exaggerated response (including "sundowner's syndrome") in elderly individuals.* Note schedule of use (e.g., cimetidine + antacid, digoxin + diuretics). *Combinations can increase risk of adverse reactions/interactions, thus affecting mental status.*[2–5,9]
- Determine client's mobility and functional level. *Conditions or situations that limit client's mobility and independence potentiate prospect of acute confusional state.*
- Ascertain life events (e.g., death of spouse/other family member, absence of known care provider, move from lifelong home, catastrophic natural disaster) *that can affect client's perceptions, attention, and concentration.*[3]
- Assess diet and nutritional status *to identify possible deficiencies of essential nutrients and vitamins that could affect mental status.*[2,5]
- Evaluate sleep and rest status, noting deprivation or oversleeping. (Refer to NDs Insomnia, Sleep Deprivation, as appropriate.)
- 🖊 Monitor laboratory values (e.g., complete blood count, blood cultures; oxygen saturation and, in some cases, arterial blood gases with carbon monoxide; BUN and Cr levels; electrolytes; thyroid function studies; liver function studies, ammonia levels; serum glucose; urinalysis for infection and drug analysis; specific drug toxicologies and drug levels [including peak and trough, as appropriate]) *to identify imbalances that have potential for causing confusion.*[1,2,5,8]

NURSING PRIORITY NO. 2 To maximize level of function, prevent further deterioration, correct existing risk factors:

- 🩺 Assist with treatment of underlying problem (e.g., drug intoxication or substance abuse, infectious processes, hypoxemia, biochemical imbalances, nutritional deficits, pain management) *to reduce potential for confusion.*[1,2,5,8]
- 💊 Monitor and adjust medication regimen and note response. *May identify medications that can be changed or eliminated in client prone to adverse or exaggerated responses to medications (including confusion).*[1,2,5]
- Provide normal levels of essential sensory and tactile stimulation—include personal items and pictures, desired music, activities, and contacts. Encourage family/SO(s) to participate in orientation by providing ongoing input (e.g., current news and family happenings).[1,2]
- Maintain calm environment and eliminate extraneous noise and stimuli *to prevent overstimulation.*

 Acute Care   Collaborative   Community/ Home Care   Cultural

- 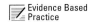 Provide adequate supervision: remove harmful objects from environment, provide siderails and seizure precautions, place call bell and position needed items within reach, clear traffic paths, and ambulate with devices *to meet client's safety needs and reduce risk of falls.*
- Encourage client to use vision or hearing aids and other adaptive equipment when needed *to assist client in interpretation of environment and communication.*
- Avoid or limit use of restraints. *Can cause agitation and increase likelihood of untoward complications.*[4,7]
- Promote early ambulation and recreational activities *to enhance well-being and reduce effects of prolonged bedrest or inactivity.*[1]
- Establish and maintain elimination patterns. *Disruption of elimination may be a cause for confusion or precipitate delerium.*[7]

NURSING PRIORITY NO. 3 To promote wellness (Teaching/Discharge Considerations):

- Explain reason(s) for confusion, if known. *Although acute confusion usually subsides over time as the client recovers from the underlying cause and/or adjusts to a situation, it can initially be frightening to a client/SO. Therefore, information about the cause and appropriate treatment to improve the condition may be helpful in managing a sense of fear and powerlessness.*
- Discuss need for ongoing medical review of client's medications *to limit possibility of misuse or potential for dangerous side effects or interactions.*[1]
- Review ways to maximize sleep (e.g., preferred bedtime rituals; comfortable room temperature, bedding, and pillows; eliminate or reduce extraneous noise or stimuli and interruptions) *to prevent confusional state caused by sleep deprivation.*[1]
- Provide appropriate referrals (e.g., medication monitoring program, nutritionist, substance abuse treatment, support groups, home health and adult day care).[1,2]

DOCUMENTATION FOCUS

Assessment/Reassessment
- Existing conditions and risk factors for individual.
- Current level of function, effect on independence and ability to meet own needs, including food and fluid intake and medication use.

Planning
- Plan of care and who is involved in planning.
- Teaching plan.

Implementation/Evaluation
- Response to interventions and actions performed.
- Attainment or progress toward desired outcomes.
- Modifications to plan of care.

Discharge Planning
- Long-term needs and who is responsible for actions to be taken.
- Available resources and specific referrals.

References

1. Doenges, M. E., Moorhouse, M. F., Murr, A. C. (eds). (2010). Acute confusion. *Nurse's Pocket Guide: Diagnoses, Prioritized Interventions and Rationales.* 12th ed. Philadelphia: F. A. Davis, 211–215.
2. Alagiakrishnan, K. (Updated 2017). Delerium. Retrieved March 2018 from http://emedicine.medscape.com/article/288890-overview.
3. Naylor, M. D., et al. (2005). Cognitively impaired older adults. *Am J Nurs,* 105(2), 52–61.
4. Jennings-Ingle, S. (2007). The sobering facts about alcohol withdrawal syndrome. *Nursing Made Incredibly Easy!,* 5(1), 50–60.
5. American Medical Directors Association (2008, reaffirmed 2014). Delirium and acute problematic behavior in the long-term

 Diagnostic Studies   Evidence Based Practice   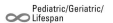 Medications   Pediatric/Geriatric/Lifespan care setting. *Agency for Healthcare Research and Quality Guideline*. Retrieved March 2018 from http://www.guideline.gov/content.aspx?id=12379.

6. Bryson, G. L., Wynand, A. (2006). Evidence-based clinical update: General anesthesia and the risk of delirium and postoperative cognitive dysfunction. *Can J Anaesth*, 53(7), 669–677.

7. Sendelbach, S., Guthrie, P. F. (2009). Acute confusion/delirium. *J Gerontol Nurs*, 35(11), 11–18.

8. Gerstein, P. S. (Updated 2017). Delirium, dementia, and amnesia in emergency medicine. Retrieved March 2018 from http://emedicine.medscape.com/article/793247-overview.

9. Nall, R. (2016). Sundowner's syndrome: Causes, symptoms, and treatments. Retrieved March 2018 from https://www.medicalnewstoday.com/articles/314685.phpw.

Constipation

Taxonomy II: Elimination and Exchange—Class 2 Gastrointestinal Function (00011) [**Diagnostic Division:** Elimination], Approved 1975; Revised 1998, 2017

DEFINITION: Decrease in normal frequency of defecation accompanied by difficult or incomplete passage of stool and/or passage of excessively hard, dry stool.

***Author note: After reviewing current research and all NDs involving constipation, it appears that chronic functional Constipation is actually the more commonly occurring form. To this end the assessment and interventions here reflect only what is presented in the Related Factors and Defining Characteristics. More in-depth assessment and interventions will be found in chronic functional Constipation.

RELATED FACTORS

Abdominal muscle weakness

Average daily physical activity is less than recommended for gender and age

Confusion; depression; emotional disturbance

Eating habit change (e.g., foods, eating times); inadequate dietary habits; insufficient fiber or fluid intake; dehydration

Decrease in gastrointestinal motility

Habitually ignores urge to defecate; irregular defecation habits; inadequate toileting habits

Inadequate dentition or oral hygiene

Obesity

Pharmaceutical agent; laxative abuse

DEFINING CHARACTERISTICS

Subjective

Anorexia

Abdominal pain; pain with defecation

Change in bowel pattern; decrease in frequency or volume of stool; hard, formed stool; liquid stool; inability to defecate

Increase in abdominal pressure; feeling of rectal fullness or pressure; straining with defecation

Indigestion; vomiting; headache; fatigue

Objective

Abdominal tenderness with/without palpable muscle resistance; distended abdomen

Atypical presentations in older adults [e.g., changes in mental status, urinary incontinence, unexplained falls, elevated body temperature]

Borborygmi; hypoactive or hyperactive bowel sounds

Hard, formed stool; presence of soft pastelike stool in rectum; liquid stool; straining with defecation

Bright red blood with stool; liquid stool

Percussed abdominal dullness; palpable abdominal or rectal mass

 Acute Care   Collaborative   Community/Home Care   Cultural

Severe flatus

Associated Condition: Electrolyte imbalance; iron salts

Hemorrhoids; Hirschsprung's disease; postsurgical bowel obstruction; prostate enlargement; tumor

Neurological impairment; pregnancy

Rectal abscess; rectal anal fissure or stricture; rectal ulcer

Rectal prolapse; rectocele

Sample Clinical Applications: Abdominal or pelvic surgeries; hemorrhoids, anal lesions, irritable bowel syndrome, diverticulitis, spinal cord injury (SCI), multiple sclerosis (MS), and other neurological conditions; hypothyroidism, iron deficiency anemia; uremia, kidney dialysis; Alzheimer's disease/other dementias or psychiatric conditions

DESIRED OUTCOMES/EVALUATION CRITERIA

Sample **NOC** linkages:

Bowel Elimination: Formation and evacuation of stool

Nutritional Status: Nutrient Intake: Nutrient intake to meet metabolic needs

Self-Care: Non-Parenteral Medications: Personal actions to administer oral and topical medications to meet therapeutic goals independently with or without assistive device

Client Will (Include Specific Time Frame)

- Establish or regain normal pattern of bowel functioning.
- Verbalize understanding of etiology and appropriate interventions or solutions for individual situation.
- Demonstrate behaviors or lifestyle changes to prevent recurrence of problem.
- Participate in bowel program, as indicated.

ACTIONS/INTERVENTIONS

Sample **NIC** linkages:

Constipation/Impaction Management: Prevention and alleviation of constipation/impaction

Bowel Management: Establishment and maintenance of a regular pattern of bowel elimination

Ostomy Care: Maintenance of elimination through a stoma and care of surrounding tissue

NURSING PRIORITY NO. 1   To identify causative/contributing factors:

- Review medical/surgical history as indicated in Related Factors above *to identify conditions commonly associated with constipation.* (Refer to ND chronic functional Constipation).
- ∞ ▨ Note client's age. *Constipation is more likely to occur in individuals older than 65 years of age, but can occur in any age from infant to elderly. A bottle-fed infant is more prone to constipation than a breastfed infant, especially when formula contains iron. Toddlers are at risk because of developmental factors (e.g., too young, too interested in other things, rigid schedule during potty training), and children and adolescents are at risk because of unwillingness to take breaks from play, poor eating and fluid intake habits, and withholding because of perceived lack of privacy. Many older adults experience constipation as a result of duller nerve sensations, immobility, dehydration, and electrolyte imbalances; incomplete emptying of the bowel; or failing to attend to signals to defecate.*[1–4,7]
- Review daily dietary regimen, noting if diet is deficient in fiber. *Imbalanced nutrition influences the amount and consistency of feces.*
- Assess general oral and dental health. *Dental problems can impact dietary intake (e.g., loss of teeth or other oral conditions can force individuals to eat soft foods or liquids mostly lacking in fiber).*[3]

 Diagnostic Studies   Evidence Based Practice   Medications   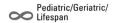 Pediatric/Geriatric/ Lifespan

- Determine fluid intake *to note deficits.*
- Evaluate medication or drug usage *for agents that could slow passage of stool and cause or exacerbate constipation.*
- Note energy and activity level and exercise pattern. *Lack of physical activity or regular exercise is often a factor in constipation.*
- Identify areas of life changes or stressors. *Factors such as pregnancy, travel, traumas, changes in personal relationships, occupational factors, or financial concerns can cause or exacerbate constipation.*[5]
- Determine access to bathroom, privacy, and ability to perform self-care activities.
- Investigate reports of pain with defecation. *Hemorrhoids, rectal fissures or prolapse, skin breakdown, or other abnormal findings may be hindering passage of stool or causing client to hold stool.*[1,4–6]
- Discuss laxative and enema use. Note signs or reports of laxative abuse or overuse of stimulant laxatives. *This is most common among older adults preoccupied with having daily bowel movement.*[4,5,7]
- Auscultate abdomen for presence, location, and characteristics of bowel sounds *reflecting bowel activity.*
- Palpate abdomen for hardness, distension, and masses *indicating possible obstruction or retention of stool.*
- Perform digital rectal examination, as indicated, *to evaluate rectal tone and detect tenderness, blood, or detect fecal impaction.*
- Assist with medical work-up (e.g., x-rays, abdominal imaging, colonoscopy, proctosigmoidoscopy, anorectal function tests; colonic transit studies, stool sample tests) *for identification of possible causative factors.* Refer to ND: chronic functional Constipation for further assessments and interventions regarding dietary issues in constipation.

NURSING PRIORITY NO. 2   To determine usual pattern of elimination:

- Discuss customary elimination habits (e.g., normal urge time [client unable to eliminate unless in own home], passing hard stool after prolonged effort, anal pain, or bleeding). Determine what feature the client finds most distressing. *Helps to identify and clarify client's perception of problem. For example, constipation has been defined as not only infrequent stools, but also straining with bowel movements, hard stools, unproductive urges, and feeling of incomplete evacuation.*[6]
- Note factors that usually stimulate bowel activity and any interferences present. *Client may describe having to sit in a particular position or needing to apply perineal pressure or digital stimulation to start stool. Interferences can include not wanting to use a particular facility or not wanting to interrupt play or an activity.*[6]

NURSING PRIORITY NO. 3   To assess current pattern of elimination:

- Note color, odor, consistency, amount, and frequency of stool following each bowel movement during assessment phase. *Provides a baseline for comparison, promoting recognition of changes. If usual number of weekly bowel movements is decreased to three or less, stool is hard and formed, or client is straining, constipation is likely present.*[2]
- Ascertain duration of current problem and client's degree of concern. *Long-standing condition that client has "lived with" may not cause undue concern, while acute postsurgical constipation can cause great distress. Client's response may/may not be congruent with the severity of condition.*
- Note pharmacological agents client has used (e.g., fiber pills, laxatives, suppositories, enemas) *to determine effectiveness of current regimen and whether laxative use is appropriate and helpful.*

NURSING PRIORITY NO. 4   To facilitate return to usual/acceptable pattern of elimination:

- Promote lifestyle changes.[1–8]
  Limit foods with little or no fiber or diet high in fats (e.g., ice cream, cheese, meats, fast foods, processed foods). Note: Clients with descending or sigmoid colostomy must avoid constipation. Some may find it helpful to create their own dietary bulk laxative by combining unprocessed millers bran, applesauce, and prune juice.

    Acute Care   Collaborative   Community/ Home Care   Cultural

Promote adequate fluid intake, including water, high-fiber fruit and vegetable juices, fruit/vegetable smoothies, and popsicles. Suggest drinking warm, stimulating fluids (e.g., decaffeinated coffee, hot water, tea) *to avoid dehydration; promote moist, soft feces; and facilitate passage of stool.*

Encourage daily activity and exercise within limits of individual ability *to stimulate contractions of the intestines.*

Encourage client to not ignore urge. Provide privacy and routinely scheduled time for defecation (bathroom or commode preferable to bedpan) *to promote psychological readiness and comfort.*

- Provide sitz bath before stools *to relax sphincter* and after stools *for cleansing and soothing effect to rectal area.*[4]
- Review client's current medication regime with physician *to determine if drugs contributing to constipation can be discontinued or changed.*
- Administer stool softeners *(to provide moisture to stool),* mild stimulants *(to cause rhythmic contractions of the bowel),* lubricants *(to enable stool to more easily pass),* saline or hyperosmolar laxatives, or bulk-forming agents *(to draw water into colon)* as ordered or routinely, when appropriate (e.g., for client receiving opiates, decreased level of activity/immobility).[1–3,5–8]
- Apply lubricant/anesthetic ointment to anus, if needed.
- Establish bowel program to include predictable interval timing for colostomy irrigation or toileting, use of particular position for defecation, abdominal massage, colostomy irrigation, biofeedback for pelvic floor dysfunction, and medications as indicated *to provide predictable and effective elimination and reduce evacuation problems when long-term or permanent bowel dysfunction is present.*

NURSING PRIORITY NO. 5 To promote wellness (Teaching/Discharge Considerations):[1,6]

- Discuss client's particular anatomy and physiology of bowel and acceptable variations in elimination.
- Provide information and resources to client/significant other about relationship of diet, fluid, exercise, and healthy elimination.
- Provide social and emotional support *to help client manage actual or potential disabilities associated with long-term bowel management.* Discuss rationale for and encourage continuation of successful interventions.
- Encourage client to maintain elimination diary, if appropriate, *to facilitate monitoring of long-term problem and choice of interventions.*
- Work to implement bowel management program that is easily replicated in home and community settings.
- Identify specific actions to be taken if problem does not resolve *to promote timely intervention, thereby enhancing client's independence.*

DOCUMENTATION FOCUS

Assessment/Reassessment
- Usual and current bowel pattern, duration of the problem, and interventions used.
- Characteristics of stool.
- Individual contributing factors.

Planning
- Plan of care, specific interventions or changes in lifestyle necessary to correct individual situation, and who is involved in planning.
- Teaching plan.

Implementation/Evaluation
- Responses to interventions, teaching, and actions performed.
- Change in bowel pattern, character of stool.
- Attainment or progress toward desired outcomes.
- Modifications to plan of care.

 Diagnostic Studies   Evidence Based Practice   Medications   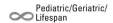 Pediatric/Geriatric/ Lifespan

Discharge Planning
- Individual long-term needs, noting who is responsible for actions to be taken.
- Recommendations for follow-up care.
- Specific referrals made.

References

1. McKay, S. L., Fravel, M., Scanlon, C. (2012). Evidence-based practice: Management of constipation. *J Gerontol Nurs*, 38(7), 9–15.
2. Ferry, R. J. (Updated 2014, last review 2017). Constipation in children (infants). Retrieved March 2018 from http://www.emedicinehealth.com/constipation_in_children/page3_em.htm.
3. Stanley, M., Beare, P. G. (eds). (1999). The aging gastrointestinal system, with nutritional considerations. *Gerontological Nursing: A Health Promotion/Protection Approach*. 7th ed. Philadelphia: F. A. Davis, 180–181.
4. Watson, L. (2010). Childhood constipation. *Community Pract*, 83(7), 40–42.
5. National Digestive Diseases Information Clearinghouse, (Updated 2014 and certain sections in 2017). Constipation. Retrieved March 2018 from http://digestive.niddk.nih.gov/ddiseases/pubs/constipation/.
6. Locke, G. R., Pemberton, J. H., Phillips, S. F. (2000). American Gastroenterological Association: Medical position statement: Guidelines on constipation. *Gastroenterology*, 119(6), 1761–1778.
7. Basson, M. D. (Updated 2018). Constipation in adults. Retrieved March 2018 from http://emedicine.medscape.com/article/184704-overview.
8. CancerConnect.com staff. (Updated 2018). Living with a colostomy. Retrieved March 2018 from http://news.cancerconnect.com/colon-cancertipsliving-with-a-colostomy/.

chronic functional Constipation

Taxonomy II: Elimination and Exchange—Class 2 Gastrointestinal Function (00235) **[Diagnostic Division:** Elimination], Approved 2013; Revised 2017

DEFINITION: Infrequent or difficult evacuation of feces, which has been present for at least 3 of the prior 12 months.

RELATED FACTORS
Decrease in food intake; insufficient food intake; low caloric intake
Food disproportionately high in protein and fat; low-fiber diet
Insufficient fluid intake; dehydration
Habitually ignores urge to defecate
Frail elderly syndrome; immobility; sedentary lifestyle

DEFINING CHARACTERISTICS

Subjective
Pain with defecation
Prolonged straining
[Feeling as though something is blocking stool from passing or stool is still in rectum after bowel movement]

Objective
ADULT: Presence of ≥2 of the following symptoms on Rome III classification system:
Lumpy or hard stools; or straining; or sensation of incomplete evacuation; or sensation of anorectal obstructions; or manual maneuvers to facilitate defecations (digital manipulation, pelvic floor support) in ≥25% of defecations; or ≤3 evacuations per week
CHILD ≥4 years: Presence of ≥2 criteria on Roman III Pediatric classification system for ≥2 months:

 Acute Care   Collaborative   Community/ Home Care   Cultural

≤2 defecations per week; ≥1 episode of fecal incontinence per week; stool retentive posturing; painful or hard bowel movements; presence of large fecal mass in the rectum; large diameter stools that may obstruct the toilet

CHILD ≤4 years: Presence of 2 criteria on Roman III Pediatric classification system for ≥1 month: ≤2 defecations per week; ≥1 episode of fecal incontinence per week; stool retentive posturing; painful or hard bowel movements; presence of large fecal mass in the rectum; large diameter stools that may obstruct the toilet

GENERAL

Distended abdomen; palpable abdominal mass

Fecal impaction

Leakage of stool with digital stimulation

Pain with defecation

Positive fecal occult blood

Prolonged straining

Type 1 or 2 Bristol Stool Chart

Associated Condition: Amyloidosis; anatomic neuropathy; chronic renal insufficiency

Anal fissure or stricture; ischemic, or postinflammatory, or surgical stenosis

Chronic intestinal pseudo-obstruction; colorectal cancer; extra intestinal mass; Hirschsprung's disease; hemorrhoids; inflammatory bowel disease; slow colon transit time

Cerebral vascular accident; diabetes; multiple sclerosis; myotonic dystrophy; paraplegia; Parkinson's disease;

Dermatomyositis; porphyria; scleroderma

Hypercalcemia; hypothyroidism, panhypopituitarism;

Pelvic floor dysfunction; perineal damage; pregnancy; proctitis

Pharmaceutical agent; polypharmacy

Sample Clinical Applications: Abdominal surgeries, hemorrhoids, anal lesions, irritable bowel syndrome, diverticulitis, spinal cord injury (SCI), multiple sclerosis (MS), hypothyroidism, iron deficiency, scleroderma, Alzheimer's disease/dementia

DESIRED OUTCOMES/EVALUATION CRITERIA

Sample NOC linkages:

Bowel Elimination: Formation and evacuation of stool

Gastrointestinal Function: Ability of the gastrointestinal tract to ingest and digest food products, absorb nutrients, and eliminate waste

Client Will (Include Specific Time Frame)

• Establish or regain normal pattern of bowel functioning.

• Document that bowel function has improved, noting an increase in frequency of stools and/or decrease in straining at stool.

• Verbalize understanding of etiology and appropriate interventions or solutions for individual situation.

ACTIONS/INTERVENTIONS

Sample NIC linkages:

Constipation/Impaction Management: Prevention and alleviation of constipation/impaction

Bowel Management: Establishment and maintenance of a regular pattern of bowel elimination

Medication Management: Facilitation of safe and effective use of prescription and over-the-counter drugs

 Diagnostic Studies

 Evidence Based Practice

 Medications

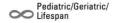 Pediatric/Geriatric/ Lifespan

NURSING PRIORITY NO. 1   To identify causative/contributing factors:

- Review medical/surgical history *to identify conditions commonly associated with functional constipation. Causes may be classified as primary and secondary. Primary causes are related to problems inherent to the intestine; subdivided into normal-transit constipation, slow-transit constipation, and anorectal dysfunction. Secondary causes include (1) gastrointestinal disorders (e.g., intestinal tumors, stenosis; idiopathic megacolon; rectocele, rectal prolapse, anal fissure; irritable bowel syndrome); (2) metabolic and endocrine disorders (e.g., hyper/hypocalcemia, diabetes, hyperparathyroidism, chronic renal insufficiency); (3) neurological conditions (e.g., Parkinson's disease, stroke, dementia syndromes, multiple sclerosis, spinal cord injuries); (4) psychogenic disorders (e.g., anxiety, depression); (5) dehydration; and (6) the use of a variety of medications (e.g., opioids, anti-inflammatories, calcium channel blockers, calcium and iron supplements, anticholinergics, antipsychotics, antihistamines).*[1,2,13] *Note: Functional constipation can also be associated with symptoms arising in the mid- or lower gastrointestinal tract that are not otherwise attributable to anatomic or biochemical defects. There is increasing evidence that a considerable number of individuals with constipation also have a disorder of the process of rectal evacuation.*[4,13]
- ∞ Note client's age, gender, and general health status. *Constipation is more likely to occur in individuals older than 65 years of age, but it may occur in client of any age with chronic or debilitating conditions. Approximately 95% of childhood constipation is functional in nature without any obvious cause. Children with anorectal malformations and Hirschsprung's disease have abnormal peristaltic waves in the colon, which result either in stagnant stool or an overactive colon.*[2,6–8,10] *Note: Prevalence estimates by gender support a female-to-male ratio of 2.2:1.*[13]
- Evaluate current medications or drug usage *for agents that could slow passage of stool and cause or exacerbate constipation (e.g., opioids, anti-inflammatories, calcium channel blockers, calcium and iron supplements, anticholinergics, antidepressants, antipsychotics, antihistamines, anticonvulsants, diuretics, chemotherapy, contrast media, steroids).*[1–3]
- Note interventions client has tried *to relieve current situation (e.g., fiber pills, laxatives, suppositories, enemas)* and document success or lack of effectiveness.
- Assist with medical work-up (e.g., lower GI series x-rays, abdominal imaging [e.g., defecography], colonoscopy, sigmoidoscopy; anorectal function tests [e.g., anal manometry, blood expulsion tests]; colonic transit studies) *for identification of possible causative factors and to show how well food moves through the colon.*[8,9,11]

NURSING PRIORITY NO. 2   To assess current pattern of elimination:[10,11]

- Note color, odor, consistency, amount, and frequency of stool following each bowel movement during assessment phase utilizing elimination diary or calendar. *Provides a baseline for comparison, promoting recognition of changes.*
- Auscultate abdomen for presence, location, and characteristics of bowel sounds *reflecting bowel activity.*
- Palpate abdomen for hardness, distention, and masses, *indicating possible obstruction or retention of stool.*
- Perform digital rectal examination, as indicated, *to evaluate rectal tone and detect tenderness, blood, or fecal impaction.*

NURSING PRIORITY NO. 3   To reduce unacceptable pattern of elimination:

- Collaborate in treatment of underlying medical cause where appropriate (e.g., surgery to repair rectal prolapse, biofeedback to retrain anorectal or pelvic floor dysfunction, medications, and combinations of therapies as indicated) *to improve body and bowel function. Note: Treatment is highly individual. For example, clients with slow-transit constipation tend to benefit from fiber, osmotic laxatives, and stimulant laxatives (e.g., bisacodyl), whereas those with evacuation disorders usually do not need medication other than fiber supplementation following pelvic floor retraining.*[4,12]
- Review client's current medication regimen with physician *to determine if drugs contributing to constipation can be discontinued or changed.*

Acute Care   Collaborative   Community/Home Care   Cultural

- Administer medications, as indicated, such as stool softeners (e.g., docusate sodium [Colase, Surfak]) *to provide moisture to stool,* mild stimulants (e.g., bisacodyl [Dulcolax, Bisco-Lax]) *to cause rhythmic muscle contractions and improve transit time,* osmotic agents (e.g., polyethylene glycol [PEG, Miralax]) *to absorb water in intestine,* and opioid antagonist (e.g., methylanaltrexone [Relistor]) *to treat constipation in client with advanced/ terminal illness necessitating long-term opioid analgesia and/or client who is unresponsive to laxatives.*
- Remove impacted stool digitally, when necessary, after applying lubricant and anesthetic ointment to anus *to soften impaction and decrease rectal pain.*
- Administer enemas (e.g., hyperosmolar agents [e.g., Fleet enema] *to draw water into colon*) or suppositories, as indicated.[4,6]
- Promote lifestyle changes:[1–11]

Instruct in and encourage a personalized dietary program that involves adjustment of dietary fiber and bulk in diet (e.g., fruits, vegetables, whole grains) and fiber supplements (e.g., wheat bran, psyllium) *to improve consistency of stool and increase transit time through colon if slow transit through colon is causing symptoms.*

Promote adequate fluid intake, including water, high-fiber fruit and vegetable juices, fruit/vegetable smoothies, and popsicles. Suggest drinking warm, stimulating fluids (e.g., decaffeinated coffee, hot water, tea) *to avoid dehydration; promote moist, soft feces; and facilitate passage of stool.*

- Instruct in/assist with other means of triggering defecation (e.g., abdominal massage, digital stimulation, placement of rectal stimulant suppositories) *to provide predictable and effective elimination and reduce evacuation problems when long-term or permanent bowel dysfunction is present.*
- Refer for physical therapy or other medical/surgical practitioners for additional interventions as indicated. *Physical therapy may be useful in improving mobility, pelvic floor retraining, and activity levels. Biofeedback treatment with muscle relaxation of anal sphincters and the puborectalis can result in a cure for constipation associated with certain evacuation disorders. Surgical interventions may be used in some instances (e.g., Malone antegrade continence enema procedure, sacral anterior root stimulation) to treat long-term, intractable constipation due to neurogenic bowel.*[5,12]

NURSING PRIORITY NO. 4 To promote wellness (Teaching/Discharge Considerations):[1–11]

- Discuss client's particular anatomy and physiology of bowel and acceptable variations in elimination.
- Provide information and resources to client/significant other about relationship of diet, exercise, fluid, and appropriate use of laxatives, as indicated,
- Provide social and emotional support *to help client manage actual or potential disabilities associated with long-term bowel management.* Discuss rationale for and encourage continuation of successful interventions.
- Encourage client to maintain elimination diary, if appropriate, *to facilitate monitoring of long-term condition and reveal most helpful interventions.*
- Collaborate with medical providers and client/caregiver in designing bowel management program to be easily replicated in home and community settings.
- Identify specific actions to be taken if problem does not resolve (e.g., return to physician for additional testing and interventions) *to promote timely intervention, thereby enhancing client's independence.*

DOCUMENTATION FOCUS

Assessment/Reassessment

- Usual and current bowel pattern, duration of the problem, and interventions used.
- Characteristics of stool.
- Individual contributing factors.

Planning

- Plan of care, specific interventions or changes in lifestyle necessary to correct individual situation, and who is involved in planning.
- Teaching plan.

Diagnostic Studies   Evidence Based Practice   Medications   Pediatric/Geriatric/ Lifespan

Implementation/Evaluation
- Responses to interventions, teaching, and actions performed.
- Change in bowel pattern, character of stool.
- Attainment or progress toward desired outcomes.
- Modifications to plan of care.

Discharge Planning
- Individual long-term needs, noting who is responsible for actions to be taken.
- Recommendations for follow-up care.
- Specific referrals made.

References

1. Longstreth, G. F., et al. (2006). Functional bowel disorders. *Gastroenterology*, 130, 1480–1491.
2. Schmidt, F. M., Santos, V. L. (2014). Prevalence of constipation in the general adult population: An integrative review. *J Wound Ostomy Continence Nurs*, 41(1), 70–76.
3. McKay, S. L., Fravel, M., Scanlon, C. (2012). Evidence-based practice: Management of constipation. *J Gerontol Nurs*, 38(7), 9–15.
4. Mayo Clinic and Mayo Foundation. (1999). Functional gastrointestinal disorders: Novel insights and treatments. Retrieved March 2018 from http://www.medscape.com/viewarticle/717346_1.
5. Surrenti, E., et al. (1995). Audit of constipation in a tertiary referral gastroenterology practice. *Am J Gastroenterol*, 90, 1471–1475.
6. Poggio, J. L., Grossman, J. G., Kucejko, R. J. (Updated 2018). Neurogenic bowel dysfunction. Retrieved March 2018 from http://emedicine.medscape.com/article/321172-overview.
7. Pashankar, D. S. (2005). Management of severe pediatric constipation. *Clin Colon Rectal Surg*, 18(2), 120–127.
8. Levitt, M. A., Wood, R. J. (2017). Severe pediatric constipation. Retrieved March 2018 from https://emedicine.medscape.com/article/937030-overview.
9. Basson, M. D. (Updated 2018). Constipation in adults. Retrieved March 2018 from http://emedicine.medscape.com/article/184704-overview.
10. Ferry, R. J. (2013, last reviewed 2017). Constipation in children. Retrieved March 2018 from http://www.emedicinehealth.com/constipation_in_children/page3_em.htm.
11. Locke, G. R., Pemberton, J. H., Phillips, S. F. (2000). American Gastroenterological Association: Medical position statement: Guidelines on constipation. *Gastroenterology*, 119(6), 1761–1778.
12. Enck, P. (1993). Biofeedback training in disordered defecation. A critical review. *Dig Dis Sci*, 38(11), 1953–1960.
13. Higgins, P. D., Johanson, J. F. (2004). Epidemiology of constipation in North America: A systematic review. *Am J Gastroenterol*, 99(4), 750–759.

risk for chronic functional Constipation

Taxonomy II: Elimination and Exchange—Class 2 Gastrointestinal Function (000236) [**Diagnostic Division:** Elimination], Approved 2013; Revised 2017

DEFINITION: Susceptible to infrequent or difficult evacuation of feces, which has been present nearly 3 of the prior 12 months, which may compromise health.

RISK FACTORS
Decrease in food intake; insufficient food intake; low caloric intake
Depression
Food disproportionately high in protein and fat; low-fiber diet
Insufficient fluid intake; dehydration
Habitually ignores urge to defecate
Frail elderly syndrome; immobility; sedentary lifestyle
Associated Condition: Amyloidosis; anatomic neuropathy; chronic renal insufficiency
Anal fissure or stricture; ischemic, or postinflammatory, or surgical stenosis
Chronic intestinal pseudo-obstruction; colorectal cancer; extra intestinal mass; Hirschsprung's disease; hemorrhoids; inflammatory bowel disease; slow colon transit time

 Acute Care   Collaborative   Community/ Home Care   Cultural

Cerebral vascular accident; diabetes; multiple sclerosis; myotonic dystrophy; paraplegia; Parkinson's disease;

Dermatomyositis; porphyria; scleroderma

Hypercalcemia; hypothyroidism, panhypopituitarism

Pelvic floor dysfunction; perineal damage; pregnancy; proctitis

Pharmaceutical agent; polypharmacy

DESIRED OUTCOMES/EVALUATION CRITERIA

Sample NOC linkages:

Bowel Elimination: Formation and evacuation of stool

Risk Control: Personal actions to understand, prevent, eliminate, or reduce modifiable health threats

Knowledge: Medication: Extent of understanding conveyed about the safe use of medication

Client Will (Include Specific Time Frame)

• Maintain normal pattern of bowel functioning.

• Verbalize understanding of etiology and appropriate interventions or solutions for individual situation.

• Engage in behaviors or lifestyle changes to prevent constipation.

ACTIONS/INTERVENTIONS

Sample NIC linkages:

Constipation/Impaction Management: Prevention and alleviation of constipation/impaction

Bowel Management: Establishment and maintenance of a regular pattern of bowel elimination

Medication Management: Facilitation of safe and effective use of prescription and over-the-counter drugs

NURSING PRIORITY NO. 1 To identify individual risk factors:

• Review medical/surgical history *to identify conditions commonly associated with functional constipation. Note: Causes may be classified as primary and secondary. Primary causes are related to problems inherent to the intestine and are subdivided into normal-transit constipation, slow-transit constipation, and anorectal dysfunction. Secondary causes include gastrointestinal disorders, metabolic and endocrine disorders, neurological conditions, congestive cardiac insufficiency, psychogenic disorders, dehydration, and the use of a variety of medications.*[1,2,5] *Note: Functional constipation can also be associated with symptoms arising in the mid- or lower gastrointestinal tract that are not otherwise attributable to anatomic or biochemical defects. There is increasing evidence that a considerable number of individuals with constipation also have a disorder of the process of rectal evacuation.*[3,5,11]

• ∞ Note client's age, gender, and general health status. *Constipation is more likely to occur in individuals older than 65 years of age, but it may occur in client of any age with chronic or debilitating conditions. Approximately 95% of childhood constipation is functional in nature without any obvious cause.*[3–5]

• Evaluate current medication *for agents that could slow passage of stool and cause or exacerbate constipation (e.g., opioids, anti-inflammatories, calcium channel blockers, calcium and iron supplements, anticholinergics, antidepressants, antipsychotics, antihistamines, anticonvulsants, diuretics, chemotherapy, contrast media, steroids).*[2,6]

• Review daily dietary regimen. *Imbalanced nutrition influences the amount and consistency of feces. Inadequate dietary fiber (vegetable, fruits, whole grains) and highly processed foods (e.g., fast foods, junk foods, packaged snack, or microwavable quick meals) contribute to poor intestinal function.*[1,7–9]

• Determine fluid intake *to note deficits. Most individuals do not drink enough fluids, even when healthy, reducing the speed at which stool moves through the colon. Active fluid loss through sweating, vomiting, diarrhea, or bleeding can greatly increase chances for constipation.*[2,7,9]

 Diagnostic Studies   Evidence Based Practice   Medications   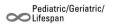 Pediatric/Geriatric/Lifespan

• Note energy and activity level and exercise pattern. *Lack of physical activity or regular exercise is often a factor in constipation.*[2,10]

NURSING PRIORITY NO. 2 To assess current pattern of elimination:

• Discuss usual elimination pattern and use of laxatives *to establish baseline and identify possible areas for intervention or instruction.*
• Note color, odor, consistency, amount, and frequency of stool following each bowel movement during assessment phase. *Provides a baseline for comparison, promoting recognition of changes.*
• Auscultate abdomen for presence, location, and characteristics of bowel sounds *reflecting bowel activity.*
• Palpate abdomen for hardness, distention, and masses, *indicating possible obstruction or retention of stool.*

NURSING PRIORITY NO. 3 To facilitate normal bowel function:

• Promote healthy lifestyle for elimination:[1–10]
  Encourage balanced fiber and bulk (e.g., fruits, vegetables, whole grains) in diet and fiber supplements (e.g., wheat bran, psyllium) *to promote soft consistency of stool and facilitate passage through colon.*
  Promote adequate fluid intake, including water, high-fiber fruit and vegetable juices, fruit/vegetable smoothies, and popsicles. Suggest drinking warm, stimulating fluids (e.g., decaffeinated coffee, hot water, tea) *to avoid dehydration; promote moist, soft feces; and facilitate passage of stool.*
  Encourage daily activity and exercise within limits of individual ability to stimulate contractions of the intestines.
  Encourage client to not ignore urge. Provide privacy and routinely scheduled time for defecation (bathroom or commode preferable to bedpan) *to promote psychological readiness and comfort.*

NURSING PRIORITY NO. 4 Promote wellness (Teaching/Discharge Considerations):[2,8,11]

• Discuss physiology and acceptable variations in elimination. *May help reduce concerns and anxiety about situation.*
• Review individual risk factors or potential problems and specific interventions for prevention of constipation.
• Promote treatment of underlying medical causes where appropriate *to improve organ function, including the bowel.*
• Collaborate with medical providers and client/caregiver in designing bowel management program to be easily replicated in home and community setting.
• Educate client/significant other about safe and risky practices for managing constipation. *Information can assist client to make beneficial choices when need arises.*
• Refer to NDs functional Constipation; Constipation; risk for perceived Constipation for additional interventions as appropriate.

DOCUMENTATION FOCUS

Assessment/Reassessment
• Current bowel pattern, characteristics of stool, medications.
• Individual risk factors.

Planning
• Plan of care and who is involved in planning.
• Teaching plan.

Implementation/Evaluation
• Responses to interventions, teaching, and actions performed.
• Attainment or progress toward desired outcomes.
• Modifications to plan of care.

 Acute Care   Collaborative   Community/ Home Care   Cultural

Discharge Planning
- Individual long-term needs, noting who is responsible for actions to be taken.
- Specific referrals made.

References

1. Longstreth, G. F., et al. (2006). Functional bowel disorders. *Gastroenterology*, 130, 1480–1491.
2. McKay, S. L., Fravel, M., Scanlon, C. (2012). Evidence-based practice: Management of constipation. *J Gerontol Nurs*, 38(7), 9–15.
3. Poggio, J. L., Grossman, J. G., Kucejko, R. J. (Updated 2018). Neurogenic bowel dysfunction. Retrieved March 2018 from http://emedicine.medscape.com/article/321172-overview.
4. Pashankar, D. S. (2005). Management of severe pediatric constipation. *Clin Colon Rectal Surg*, 18(2), 120–127.
5. Higgins, P. D., Johanson, J. F. (2004). Epidemiology of constipation in North America: A systematic review. *Am J Gastroenterol*, 99(4), 750–759.
6. Mayo Clinic and Mayo Foundation. (1999). Functional gastrointestinal disorders: Novel insights and treatments. Retrieved March 2018 from http://www.medscape.com/viewarticle/717346_1.
7. Ferry, R. J. (2013, last reviewed 2017). Constipation in children. Retrieved March 2018 from http://www.emedicinehealth.com/constipation_in_children/page3_em.htm.
8. Locke, G. R., Pemberton, J. H., Phillips, S. F. (2000). American Gastroenterological Association: Medical position statement: Guidelines on constipation. *Gastroenterology*, 119(6), 1761–1778.
9. Watson, L. (2010). Childhood constipation. *Community Pract*, 83(7), 40–42.
10. Marks, J. W. (Updated 2018). Constipation (relief, home remedies, treatment medications). Retrieved March 2018 from https://www.medicinenet.com/constipation/article.htm#constipation_definition_and_facts.
11. Basson, M. D. (Updated 2018). Constipation in adults. Retrieved March 2018 from http://emedicine.medscape.com/article/184704-overview.

perceived Constipation

Taxonomy II: Elimination and Exchange—Class 2 Gastrointestinal Function (00012) [**Diagnostic Division:** Elimination], Approved 1988

DEFINITION: Self-diagnosis of constipation combined with abuse of laxatives, enemas, and/or suppositories to ensure a daily bowel movement.

RELATED FACTORS
Cultural or family health beliefs
Impaired thought process

DEFINING CHARACTERISTICS

Subjective
Expects daily bowel movement
Expects daily bowel movement at same time every day
Laxative, enema, or suppository abuse
Sample Clinical Applications: Irritable bowel, confused states/dementia, hypochondriasis

DESIRED OUTCOMES/EVALUATION CRITERIA

Sample NOC linkages:
Health Beliefs: Personal convictions that influence health behaviors
Bowel Elimination: Formation and evacuation of stool
Knowledge: Health Behavior: Extent of understanding conveyed about the promotion and protection of health

(continues on page 196)

 Diagnostic Studies   Evidence Based Practice   Medications 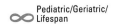 Pediatric/Geriatric/Lifespan

perceived Constipation (continued)

Client Will (Include Specific Time Frame)
- Verbalize understanding of physiology of bowel function.
- Identify acceptable interventions to promote adequate bowel function.
- Decrease reliance on laxatives and/or enemas.
- Establish individually appropriate pattern of elimination.

ACTIONS/INTERVENTIONS

Sample NIC linkages:

Bowel Management: Establishment and maintenance of a regular pattern of bowel elimination

Counseling: Use of an interactive helping process focusing on the needs, problems, or feelings of the patient and significant others (SOs) to enhance or support coping, problem solving, and interpersonal relationships

Medication Management: Facilitation of safe and effective use of prescription and over-the-counter drugs

NURSING PRIORITY NO. 1 To identify factors affecting individual beliefs:

- Determine client's understanding of a "normal" bowel pattern. Compare with client's current bowel functioning. *Helps to identify areas for discussion or intervention. For example, what is considered "normal" varies with the individual, cultural, and familial factors with differences in expectations and dietary habits.[1] In addition, individuals can think they are constipated when, in fact, their bowel movements are regular and soft, possibly revealing a problem with thought processes or perception. Some people believe they are constipated, or irregular if they do not have a bowel movement every day because of ideas instilled from childhood.[2] The elderly client may believe that laxatives or purgatives are necessary for elimination, when in fact the problem may be long-standing habits (e.g., insufficient fluids, lack of exercise and/or fiber in the diet).[3]*
- Discuss client's use of laxatives. *Perceived constipation typically results in self-medicating with various laxatives. Although laxatives may correct the acute problem, chronic use leads to habituation, requiring ever-increasing doses that result in drug dependency and, ultimately, a hypotonic laxative colon.[5]*
- Identify interventions used by client to correct perceived problem *to establish needed changes or interventions or points for discussion and teaching.*

NURSING PRIORITY NO. 2 To promote wellness (Teaching/Discharge Considerations):

- Discuss the following with client/SO/caregiver *to clarify issues regarding actual and perceived bowel functioning and to provide support during behavior modification/bowel retraining:[3,4]*
  Review anatomy and physiology of bowel function and acceptable variations in elimination.
  Identify detrimental effects of habitual laxative or enema use and discuss alternatives.
  Provide information about relationship of diet, hydration, and exercise to improved elimination.
  Encourage client to maintain elimination calendar or diary, if appropriate.
  Provide support by active-listening and discussing client's concerns or fears.
  Provide social and emotional support *to help client manage actual or potential disabilities associated with long-term bowel management.*
  Encourage use of stress-reduction activities and refocusing of attention while client works to establish individually appropriate pattern.
- Offer educational materials and resources for client/SO to peruse at home *to assist him or her in making informed decisions regarding constipation and management options.*

 Acute Care   Collaborative   Community/ Home Care   Cultural

- Refer to medical/psychiatric providers, as indicated. **Client with a fixed perception of constipation where none actually exists may require further assessment and intervention.**
- Refer to ND Constipation for additional interventions, as appropriate.

DOCUMENTATION FOCUS

Assessment/Reassessment
- Assessment findings, client's perceptions of the problem.
- Current bowel pattern, stool characteristics.

Planning
- Plan of care, specific interventions, and who is involved in the planning.
- Teaching plan.

Implementation/Evaluation
- Client's responses to interventions, teaching, and actions performed.
- Changes in bowel pattern, character of stool.
- Attainment or progress toward desired outcome(s).
- Modifications to plan of care.

Discharge Planning
- Referral for follow-up care.

References

1. Pieken, S. R. (2004). Constipation. *Gastrointestinal Health: A Self-Help Nutritional Program to Prevent, Cure, or Alleviate Irritable Bowel Syndrome, Ulcers, Heartburn, Gas, Constipation.* 3rd ed. New York: HarperCollins, 99–104.
2. National Digestive Diseases Information Clearinghouse. (Updated 2014 and certain sections in 2017). Constipation. Retrieved March 2018 from http://digestive.niddk.nih.gov/ddiseases/pubs/constipation/.
3. Stanley, M., Beare, P. G. (eds). (1999). The aging gastrointestinal system with nutritional considerations. *Gerontological Nursing: A Health Promotion/Protection Approach.* 7th ed. Philadelphia: F. A. Davis, 180–181.
4. McKay, S. L., Fravel, M., Scanlon, C. (2012). Evidence-based practice: Management of constipation. *J Gerontol Nurs*, 38(7), 9–15.
5. Basson, M. D. (Updated 2018). Constipation in adults. Retrieved March 2018 from http://emedicine.medscape.com/article/184704-overview.

risk for Constipation

Taxonomy II: Elimination and Exchange—Class 2 Gastrointestinal Function (00015) [Diagnostic Division: Elimination], Submitted 1998; Revised 2013; 2017

DEFINITION: Susceptible to a decrease in normal frequency of defecation accompanied by difficult or incomplete passage of stool, which may compromise health.

RISK FACTORS
Abdominal muscle weakness
Average daily physical activity is less than recommended for gender and age
Confusion; depression; emotional disturbance
Eating habit change (e.g., foods, eating times); inadequate dietary habits; insufficient fiber or fluid intake; dehydration
Decrease in gastrointestinal motility

(continues on page 198)

 Diagnostic Studies   Evidence Based Practice   Medications   Pediatric/Geriatric/Lifespan

risk for Constipation (continued)

Habitually ignores urge to defecate; irregular defecation habits; inadequate toileting habits
Inadequate dentition or oral hygiene
Obesity
Pharmaceutical agent; laxative abuse
Associated Condition: Electrolyte imbalance; iron salts
Hemorrhoids; Hirschsprung's disease; postsurgical bowel obstruction; prostate enlargement; tumor
Neurological impairment; pregnancy
Rectal abscess; rectal anal fissure or stricture; rectal ulcer
Rectal prolapse; rectocele

DESIRED OUTCOMES/EVALUATION CRITERIA

Sample **NOC** linkages:

Bowel Elimination: Formation and evacuation of stool
Risk Control: Personal actions to understand, prevent, eliminate, or reduce modifiable health threats
Knowledge: Medication: Extent of understanding conveyed about the safe use of medication

Client Will (Include Specific Time Frame)
• Maintain effective pattern of bowel functioning.
• Verbalize understanding of risk factors and appropriate interventions or solutions related to individual situation.
• Demonstrate behaviors or lifestyle changes to prevent developing problem.

ACTIONS/INTERVENTIONS

Sample **NIC** linkages:

Constipation/Impaction Management: Prevention and alleviation of constipation/impaction
Bowel Management: Establishment and maintenance of a regular pattern of bowel elimination
Medication Management: Facilitation of safe and effective use of prescription and over-the-counter drugs

NURSING PRIORITY NO. 1 To identify individual risk factors/needs:

• Review medical/surgical history *to identify conditions commonly associated with constipation, including problems with colon or rectum (e.g., obstruction, scar tissue or stricture, diverticulitis, irritable bowel syndrome, tumors, anal fissure), metabolic or endocrine disorders (e.g., diabetes mellitus, hypothyroidism, uremia), limited physical activity (e.g., bedrest, poor mobility, chronic disability), chronic pain problems (especially when client is on pain medications), pregnancy and childbirth, recent abdominal or perianal surgery, and neurological disorders (e.g., stroke, traumatic brain injury, Parkinson's disease, MS, spinal cord abnormalities).*[1–3,8]
• ∞ ⧄ Note client's age. *Constipation is more likely to occur in individuals older than 65 years of age, but it can occur in any age from infant to elderly. A bottle-fed infant is more prone to constipation than a breastfed infant, especially when formula contains iron. Toddlers are at risk because of developmental factors, and children. Adolescents are at risk because of unwillingness to take break from play, poor eating and fluid intake habits, and withholding because of perceived lack of privacy. Many older adults experience constipation as a result of duller nerve sensations, immobility, dehydration, and electrolyte imbalances; incomplete emptying of the bowel; or failing to attend to signals to defecate.*[1–4]
• Discuss usual elimination pattern and use of laxatives *to establish baseline and identify possible areas for intervention or instruction.*[8]

 Acute Care   Collaborative   Community/Home Care   Cultural

- 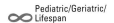Ascertain client's family and cultural beliefs and practices about bowel elimination, such as "must have a bowel movement every day or I need an enema." *These factors reflect familial or cultural thinking about elimination, which affect client's lifetime patterns.*
- Review usual dietary regimen. *Imbalanced nutrition influences the amount and consistency of stool.[2] Inadequate dietary fiber (vegetable, fruits, whole grains) and highly processed foods contribute to poor intestinal function.[1,3,5]*
- Assess general oral and dental health. *Dental problems can impact dietary intake (e.g., loss of teeth can force individuals to eat soft foods that are mostly lacking in fiber).[1,3]*
- Determine fluid intake to note deficits. *Most individuals do not drink enough fluids, even when healthy, reducing the speed at which stool moves through the colon. Active fluid loss through sweating, vomiting, diarrhea, or bleeding can greatly increase chances for constipation.[1–4,6]*
- Evaluate medication or drug usage *for agents that could slow passage of stool and increase risk of constipation (e.g., narcotic pain relievers, antidepressants, anticonvulsants, aluminum-containing antacids, chemotherapy, iron supplements, contrast media, steroids).[1–7]*
- Note energy and activity level and exercise pattern. *Lack of physical activity or regular exercise is often a factor in constipation.[1–5,7]*
- Identify areas of life changes or stressors. *Factors such as pregnancy, travel, traumas, and changes in personal relationships; occupational factors; or financial concerns can cause or exacerbate constipation.[4,7]*
- Determine access to bathroom, privacy, and ability to perform self-care activities.
- Auscultate abdomen for presence, location, and characteristics of bowel sounds *reflecting bowel activity.*

NURSING PRIORITY NO. 2 To facilitate an acceptable pattern of elimination:

- Promote healthy lifestyle for elimination:[1–8]
  Instruct in and encourage balanced fiber and bulk (e.g., fruits, vegetables, whole grains) in diet and fiber supplements (e.g., wheat bran, psyllium) *to improve consistency of stool and facilitate passage through colon.*
  Limit foods with little or no fiber or diet high in fats (e.g., ice cream, cheese, meats, fast food, processed foods).
  Promote adequate fluid intake, including water, high-fiber fruit and vegetable juices, fruit/vegetable smoothies, and popsicles. Suggest drinking warm, stimulating fluids (e.g., decaffeinated coffee, hot water, tea) *to avoid dehydration; promote moist, soft feces; and facilitate passage of stool.*
  Encourage daily activity and exercise within limits of individual ability to stimulate contractions of the intestines.
  Encourage client to not ignore urge. Provide privacy and routinely scheduled time for defecation (bathroom or commode preferable to bedpan) *to promote psychological readiness and comfort.*
- Recommend use of medications (stool softeners, mild stimulants, or bulk-forming agents) as needed and/or routinely when appropriate *to prevent constipation (e.g., client taking pain medications, especially opiates, or who is inactive or immobile).[8]*

NURSING PRIORITY NO. 3 Promote wellness (Teaching/Discharge Considerations):

- Discuss physiology and acceptable variations in elimination. *May help reduce concerns and anxiety about situation.[1,5,7]*
- Review individual risk factors or potential problems and specific interventions for prevention of constipation.[1,5,7]
- Encourage treatment of underlying medical causes where appropriate *to improve organ function, including the bowel.[1,5,7]*
- Educate client/significant other about safe and risky practices for managing constipation. *Information can assist client to make beneficial choices when need arises.[1,5,7]*
- Encourage client to maintain elimination diary, if appropriate, *to help monitor bowel pattern.[1,5,7]*

Diagnostic Studies   Evidence Based Practice   Medications   ∞ Pediatric/Geriatric/Lifespan

- Discuss client's current medication regime with physician *to determine if drugs that may contribute to constipation can be discontinued or changed.*[8]
- Refer to NDs Constipation; chronic functional Constipation; perceived Constipation for additional interventions as appropriate.

DOCUMENTATION FOCUS

Assessment/Reassessment
- Current bowel pattern, characteristics of stool, medications.
- Individual risk factors.

Planning
- Plan of care and who is involved in planning.
- Teaching plan.

Implementation/Evaluation
- Responses to interventions, teaching, and actions performed.
- Attainment or progress toward desired outcomes.
- Modifications to plan of care.

Discharge Planning
- Individual long-term needs, noting who is responsible for actions to be taken.
- Specific referrals made.

References

1. McKay, S. L., Fravel, M., Scanlon, C. (2012). Evidence-based practice: Management of constipation. *J Gerontol Nurs*, 38(7), 9–15.
2. Ferry, R. J. (Updated 2014, last reviewed 2017). Constipation in children (infants). Retrieved March 2018 from http://www .emedicinehealth.com/constipation_in_children/page3_em.htm.
3. Stanley, M. (1999). The aging gastrointestinal system, with nutritional considerations. In Beare, P. G. (ed). *Gerontological Nursing: A Health Promotion/Protection Approach.* 7th ed. Philadelphia: F. A. Davis, 180–181.
4. Watson, L. (2010). Childhood constipation. *Community Pract*, 83(7), 40–42.
5. Locke, G. R., Pemberton, J. H., Phillips, S. F. (2000). American Gastroenterological Association: Medical position statement: Guidelines on constipation. *Gastroenterology*, 119(6), 1761–1766.
6. Marks, J. W. (Updated 2014, last reviewed 2018). Constipation (relief, home remedies, treatment medications). Retrieved March 2018 from http://www.medicinenet.com/constipation/article.htm.
7. Basson, M. D. (Updated 2018). Constipation in adults. Retrieved March 2018 from http://emedicine.medscape.com/article/184704-overview.
8. Wooten, J. M. (2006). OTC laxatives aren't all the same. *RN*, 69(9), 78.

Contamination

Taxonomy II: Safety/Protection—Class 4 Environmental Hazards (00181) **[Diagnostic Division:** Safety**]**, Approved 2006; Revised 2017

DEFINITION: Exposure to environmental contaminants in doses sufficient to cause adverse health effects.

RELATED FACTORS

External
Carpeted flooring; flaking, peeling surface in presence of young children; playing where environmental contaminants are used; inadequate household hygiene practices
Chemical contamination of food or water; ingestion of contaminated material
Unprotected exposure to chemical; or heavy metal, or radioactive material

 Acute Care   Collaborative   Community/Home Care   Cultural

Inadequate municipal services [e.g., trash removal, sewage treatment facilities]

Inadequate or inappropriate use of protective clothing; inadequate personal hygiene practices

Use of environmental contaminants in the home; inadequate breakdown of contaminant; use of noxious material in insufficiently ventilated area or without effective protection

Internal

Concomitant exposure; inadequate nutrition; smoking

DEFINING CHARACTERISTICS

Author Note: Defining characteristics are dependent on the causative agent. Agents cause a variety of individual organ responses as well as systemic responses.

Subjective/Objective

Pesticides: Dermatological, gastrointestinal, neurological, pulmonary, or renal effects of pesticide

Chemicals: [Major chemical agents: petroleum-based agents, anticholinesterases; type I agents act on proximal tracheobronchial portion of the respiratory tract, type II agents act on alveoli, type III agents produce systemic effects]

Dermatological, gastrointestinal, immunological, neurological, pulmonary, or renal effects of chemical exposure

Biologics: [Toxins from living organisms—bacteria, viruses, fungi]

Dermatological, gastrointestinal, neurological, pulmonary, or renal effects of exposure to biologicals

Pollution: [Major locations: air, water, soil; major agents: asbestos, radon, tobacco (smoke), heavy metal, lead, noise, exhaust]

Neurological or pulmonary effects of pollution exposure

Waste: [Categories of waste: trash, raw sewage, industrial waste]

Dermatological, gastrointestinal, hepatic, or pulmonary effects of waste exposure

Radiation: [External exposure through direct contact with radioactive material]

Immunological, genetic, neurological, or oncological effects of radiation exposure

At Risk Population: Children <5 years; female gender; older adults

Exposure to areas with high contaminant level; exposure to atmospheric pollutants, or to bioterrorism, or to disaster, or to radiation; previous exposure to contaminant

Gestational age during exposure

Associated Condition: Pre-existing disease; pregnancy

Sample Clinical Applications: *Escherichia coli* infection, plague, hantavirus, asthma, botulism, cholera, lead or other heavy metal poisoning, chemical burns, asbestosis, carbon monoxide poisoning, radiation sickness

DESIRED OUTCOMES/EVALUATION CRITERIA

Sample NOC linkages:

Symptom Severity: Severity of adverse physical, emotional, and social responses

Knowledge: Personal Safety: Extent of understanding conveyed about prevention of unintentional injuries to self

Risk Control: Environmental Hazards: Personal actions to understand, prevent, eliminate, or reduce the threat of exposure to biological, chemical, physical, biomechanical, or physical hazards in personal environment

(continues on page 202)

 Diagnostic Studies   Evidence Based Practice   Medications   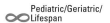 Pediatric/Geriatric/Lifespan

Contamination (continued)

Client Will (Include Specific Time Frame)
• Be free of injury and adverse health effects.
• Verbalize understanding of individual factors that contributed to injury and plans for correcting situation(s) where possible.
• Modify environment, as indicated, to enhance safety.

Sample NOC linkages:
Community Health Status: General state of well-being of a community or population
Community Risk Control: Environmental Hazards: Community actions to monitor, eliminate, or reduce environmental hazards
Community Disaster Response: Community response following a natural or man-made calamitous event

Client/Community Will (Include Specific Time Frame)
• Identify hazards that led to exposure or contamination.
• Correct environmental hazards, as identified.
• Demonstrate necessary actions to promote community safety.

ACTIONS/INTERVENTIONS

In reviewing this ND, it is apparent there is overlap with other diagnoses. We have chosen to present generalized interventions. Although there are commonalities to Contamination situations, we suggest that the reader refer to other primary diagnoses, as indicated, such as ineffective Airway Clearance, ineffective Breathing Pattern, impaired Gas Exchange, impaired Home Maintenance, risk for Infection, risk for Injury, risk for Poisoning, impaired/risk for impaired Skin Integrity, risk for Suffocation, and risk for physical Trauma.

Sample NIC linkages:
Environmental Management: Safety: Monitoring and manipulation of the physical environment to promote safety
Community Health Development: Assisting members of a community to identify a community's health concerns, mobilize resources, and implement solutions
Environmental Risk Protection: Preventing and detecting disease and injury in populations at risk from environmental hazards

NURSING PRIORITY NO. 1 To evaluate degree/source of exposure:

• Ascertain type of contaminant(s) to which client has been exposed (e.g., chemical, biological, air pollutant), the manner of exposure (e.g., inhalation, ingestion, topical), whether exposure was accidental or intentional, and immediate or delayed reactions. *Determines course of action to be taken by all emergency and other care providers. Note: Although exposure history is often difficult to determine, national environmental agencies are working to identify types of chemicals that most humans are exposed to and the effects of those exposures. Since 1999, the Centers for Disease Control and Prevention (CDC) have measured over 300 environmental chemicals in people's blood, urine, breast milk, and meconium.[5] Note: Intentional exposure to hazardous materials requires notification of law enforcement for further investigation and possible prosecution.[1–6]*
• ∞ Note age and gender. *Children (less than 5 years of age) are at greater risk for adverse effects from exposure to contaminants because (1) smaller body size causes them to receive a more concentrated "dose" than adults; (2) they spend more time outside than most adults, increasing exposure to air and soil pollutants; (3) young children spend more time on the floor, increasing exposure to toxins in carpets and low cupboards;*

 Acute Care   Collaborative   Community/ Home Care   Cultural

(4) they consume more water and food per pound than adults, increasing their body weight-to-toxin ratio; and (5) development of fetal, infant, and young children's organ systems can be disrupted. Older adults have a normal decline in function of immune, integumentary, cardiac, renal, hepatic, and pulmonary systems; an increase in adipose tissue mass; and a decline in lean body mass. Females in general have a greater proportion of body fat than men, increasing the chance of accumulating more lipid-soluble toxins.[1-6]

- Ascertain geographical location (e.g., home, work) where exposure occurred. *Individual and/or community intervention may be needed to modify or correct problem.*
- Note socioeconomic status and availability and use of resources. *Living in poverty increases potential for multiple exposures, delayed or lack of access to healthcare, and poor general health, potentially increasing the severity of adverse effects of exposure.*[6]
- Determine factors associated with particular contaminant:

    Pesticides: Determine if client has ingested contaminated foods (e.g., fruits, vegetables, commercially raised meats) or inhaled agent (e.g., aerosol bug sprays, in vicinity of crop spraying).[2,3,9]

    Chemicals: Ascertain if client uses environmental contaminants in the home or at work (e.g., pesticides, chemicals, chlorine household cleaners) and fails to use or inappropriately uses protective clothing.[2,3,9]

     Pollution air/water: Determine if client has been exposed and is sensitive to atmospheric pollutants (e.g., radon, benzene [from gasoline], carbon monoxide, automobile emissions [numerous chemicals], chlorofluorocarbons [refrigerants, solvents], ozone or smog, particles [acids, organic chemicals, particles in smoke], commercial plants [e.g., pulp and paper mills]).[7] *Note: The Environmental Protection Agency (EPA, 2013) identified six pollutants (carbon monoxide, lead, nitrogen oxides, ground-level ozone, particle pollution [often referred to as particulate matter], sulfur oxides) as "criteria" air pollutants because it regulates them by developing human health-based and/or environmentally based criteria for setting permissible levels.*[15]

    Investigate possibility of home-based exposure to air pollution. *Toxins may include carbon monoxide (e.g., poor ventilation, especially in the winter months [poor heating systems, use of charcoal grill indoors, car left running in garage], cigarette or cigar smoke indoors, ozone [spends a lot of time outdoors such as playing children, adults participating in moderate to strenuous work or recreational activities]).*[3,7]

    Investigate possibility of exposure to water pollution in or around the home. *Water pollutants come from many sources (including and not limited to) oil, grease, chemical toxins from paint thinners, cleaning products, pharmaceuticals, personal-care products; pesticides and nutrients from lawns/gardens, heavy metals, viruses, bacteria and nutrients from animal waste; failing septic systems or improper sewage disposal; dirt/groundwater runoff.*[3,7]

    Biologics: Determine if client may have been exposed to biological agents (bacteria, viruses, fungi) or bacterial toxins (e.g., botulinum, ricin). *Exposure occurring as a result of an act of terrorism is relatively rare; however, individuals may be exposed to bacterial agents or toxins through contaminated or poorly prepared foods.*

    Waste: Determine if client lives in area where trash and garbage accumulates or is exposed to raw sewage or industrial wastes that can contaminate soil and water.

    Radiation: Ascertain if client/household member experienced accidental exposure (e.g., occupation in radiography, living near or working in nuclear industries or electrical-generating plants).

- Observe for signs and symptoms of infective agent and sepsis, such as fatigue, malaise, headache, fever, chills, diaphoresis, skin rash, and altered level of consciousness. *Initial symptoms of some diseases may mimic influenza and be misdiagnosed if healthcare providers do not maintain an index of suspicion.*
- Note presence and degree of chemical burns and initial treatment provided.
- Assist with diagnostic studies, as indicated. *Provides information about type and degree of exposure and organ involvement or damage.*
- Identify psychological response (e.g., anger, shock, acute anxiety, confusion, denial) to accidental or mass exposure incident. *Although these are normal responses, they may recycle repeatedly and result in posttrauma syndrome if not dealt with adequately.*
- Alert proper authorities to presence/exposure to contamination, as appropriate. *Depending on agent, there may be reporting requirements to local, state, and national agencies such as the local health department, the Environmental Protection Agency (EPA), and Centers for Disease Control and Prevention (CDC).*

NURSING PRIORITY NO. 2   To assist in treating effects of exposure:

- Implement a coordinated decontamination plan (e.g., removal of clothing, showering with soap and water, other initial decontamination procedures) following consultation with medical toxicologist, hazardous materials team, industrial hygiene, and safety officer *to prevent further harm to client and to protect healthcare providers.*[8,9]
- Ensure availability and proper use of personal protective equipment (PPE) (e.g., high-efficiency particulate air [HEPA] filter masks, special garments, barrier materials, including gloves and face shield) *to protect from exposure to biological, chemical, and radioactive hazards.*[8–10]
- Provide for isolation or group/cohort individuals with same diagnosis or exposure, as resources require. *Limited resources may dictate open wardlike environment; however, the need to control spread of infection still exists. Only plague, smallpox, and viral hemorrhagic fevers require more than standard infection control precautions.*
- Provide therapeutic interventions, as individually appropriate. *Specific needs of the client and the level of care available at a given time and location determine response.*
- Refer pregnant client for individually appropriate diagnostic procedures or screenings. *Helpful in determining effects of teratogenic exposure on fetus allowing for informed choices and preparations. Chemical toxins can include (and are not limited to) lead, arsenic, chlorine, mercury, pesticides.*[16]
- Screen breast milk in lactating client following radiation exposure. *Depending on type and amount of exposure, breastfeeding may need to be briefly interrupted or occasionally terminated.*[12–14]
- Cooperate with and refer to appropriate agencies (e.g., CDC, U.S. Army Medical Research Institute of Infectious Diseases, Federal Emergency Management Agency, Department of Health and Human Services, Office of Emergency Preparedness, EPA) *to prepare for and manage mass casualty incidents.*[9,10]

NURSING PRIORITY NO. 3   To promote wellness (Teaching/Discharge Considerations):

Client/Caregiver
- Identify individual safety needs and injury or illness prevention in home, community, and work setting.
- Install carbon monoxide monitors and other indoor air pollutant detectors in home, as appropriate.
- Review individual nutritional needs, appropriate exercise program, and need for rest. *Essentials for well-being and recovery.*
- Repair, replace, or correct unsafe household items and situations (e.g., storage of solvents in soda bottles, flaking or peeling paint or plaster, filtering unsafe tap water).
- Emphasize importance of supervising infant/child or individuals with cognitive limitations.
- Encourage removal of or proper cleaning of carpeted floors, especially for small children and persons with respiratory conditions. *Carpets hold up to 100 times as much fine particle material as a bare floor and can contain metals and pesticides.*[1]
- Identify commercial cleaning resources, if appropriate, *for safe cleaning of contaminated articles and surfaces.*
- Install dehumidifier in damp areas *to retard growth of molds.*[1]
- Encourage timely cleaning or replacement of air filters on furnace and air-conditioning unit. *Good ventilation cuts down on indoor air pollution from carpets, machines, paints, solvents, cleaning materials, and pesticides.*
- Discuss protective actions for specific "bad air" days. *Measures may include limiting or avoiding outdoor activities, especially in sensitive groups (e.g., children who are active outdoors, adults involved in moderate or strenuous outdoor activities, persons with respiratory diseases).*[6]
- Review effects of secondhand smoke and importance of refraining from smoking in home and car where others are likely to be exposed.
- Recommend periodic inspection of well water and tap water *to identify possible contaminants.*
- Encourage client/caregiver to develop a personal or family disaster plan, to gather needed supplies to provide for self/family during a community emergency, and to learn how specific public health threats might affect client and actions *to reduce the risk to health and safety.*

 Acute Care   Collaborative   Community/ Home Care   Cultural

- Instruct client to always refer to local authorities and health experts for specific up-to-date information for community and to follow their advice.
- Refer to counselor or support groups for ongoing assistance in dealing with traumatic incident and aftereffects of exposure.
- Provide bibliotherapy including written resources and appropriate Web sites *for review and self-paced learning.*
- Refer to a smoking-cessation program, as needed.

Community

- Promote community education programs in different modalities, languages, cultures, and educational levels geared *to increasing awareness of safety measures and resources available to individuals/community.*
- Review pertinent job-related health department and Occupational Safety and Health Administration regulations.
- Refer to local resources that provide information about air quality (e.g., pollen index, "bad air days").
- Encourage community members/groups to engage in problem-solving activities.
- Ascertain that there is a comprehensive disaster plan for the community that includes a chain of command, equipment, communication, training, decontamination area(s), and safety and security plans *to ensure an effective response to any emergency (e.g., flood, toxic spill, infectious disease outbreak, radiation release).*[11]

DOCUMENTATION FOCUS

Assessment/Reassessment

- Details of specific exposure, including location and circumstances.
- Client's/caregiver's understanding of individual risks/safety concerns.

Planning

- Plan of care and who is involved in planning.
- Teaching plan.

Implementation/Evaluation

- Individual responses to interventions, teaching, and actions performed.
- Specific actions and changes that are made.
- Attainment or progress toward desired outcome(s).
- Modifications to plan of care.

Discharge Planning

- Long-term plans for discharge needs, lifestyle and community changes, and who is responsible for actions to be taken.
- Specific referrals made.

References

1. Goldman, L. R. (1998). Linking research and policy to ensure children's environmental health. *Environ Health Perspect*, 106 (13), 957–961.
2. All Family Resources. (1999). Chemical toxins safety. Retrieved March 2018 from http://www.familymanagement .com/childcare/facility/chemical.toxins.safety.html.
3. National Institute of Environmental Health Services. (reviewed 2017). Environmental health topics: Air pollution and water pollution (two articles, see index). Retrieved March 2018 from http://www.familymanagement.com/childcare/facility/chemical .toxins.safety.html.
4. Stabin, M. G., Breitz, H. (2000). Breast milk secretion of radiopharmaceuticals: Mechanisms, findings, and radiation dosimetry. *J Nucl Med*, 41(5), 863–873.
5. Centers for Disease Control and Prevention (CDC). (Updated 2017). Environmental chemicals. Retrieved March 2018 from http://www.cdc.gov/biomonitoring/environmental_chemicals .html.
6. Wilkinson, R., Marmot, M. (2003). *Social Determinants of Health: The Solid Facts.* 2nd ed. Copenhagen, Denmark: World Health Organization.
7. West, L. (2017). The causes and effects of smog. Retrieved March 2018 from https://www.thoughtco.com/ what-is-smog-causes-and-effects-1204194.
8. Gum, R. M., Hoyle, J. D. (2005, updated 2015). CBRNE— Chemical warfare mass casualty management. Retrieved March 2018 from http://emedicine.medscape.com/ article/831375-overview.

 Diagnostic Studies
 Evidence Based Practice
 Medications
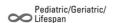 Pediatric/Geriatric/ Lifespan

9. Jagminas, L. (2006, updated 2015). CBRNE—Chemical decontamination (various pages). Retrieved March 2018 from http://emedicine.medscape.com/article/831175-overview.

10. Daller, J. A. (2006, updated 2014, last reviewed 2017). Personal protective equipment. Retrieved March 2018 from http://www.emedicinehealth.com/personal_protective_equipment/article_em.htm.

11. Bauer, J., Steinhauer, R. (2002). A readied response: The emergency plan. *RN*, 65(6), 40.

12. When should a mother avoid breastfeeding? (Updated 2016). *Centers for Disease Control and Prevention*. Retrieved March 2018 from http://www.cdc.gov/breastfeeding/disease/.

13. UAMS College of Pharmacy: Nuclear Pharmacy. (No date). Breastfeeding guidelines following radiopharmaceutical administration. Retrieved March 2018 from https://nuclearpharmacy.uams.edu/nuclear-pharmacy-resources/breastfeeding-guidelines-following-radiopharmaceuticals/.

14. American Academy of Family Physicians. (2014). Breastfeeding (Position paper): Appendix 2: Additional breastfeeding considerations: Section: Toxins and pollutants in infant feeding. Retrieved March 2018 from https://www.aafp.org/about/policies/all/breastfeeding-support.html#.

15. Centers for Disease Control and Prevention (CDC). (2013, updated 2014). EPA criteria pollutants. Retrieved March 2018 from http://www.cdc.gov/air/pollutants.htm.

16. The CPLawyer. (No date). Teratogens. Retrieved March 2018 from https://www.thecplawyer.com/birth-injury/injury-pregnancy/teratogens/.

risk for Contamination

Taxonomy II: Safety/Protection—Class 4 Environmental Hazards (00180) [**Diagnostic Division:** Safety], Approved 2006; Revised 2013; 2017

DEFINITION: Susceptible to exposure to environmental contaminants, which may compromise health.

RISK FACTORS

External

Carpeted flooring; flaking, peeling surface in presence of young children; playing where environmental contaminants are used; inadequate household hygiene practices

Chemical contamination of food or water; ingestion of contaminated material

Unprotected exposure to chemical, or heavy metal, or radioactive material

Inadequate municipal services [e.g., trash removal, sewage treatment facilities]

Inadequate or inappropriate use of protective clothing; inadequate personal hygiene practices

Use of environmental contaminants in the home; inadequate breakdown of contaminant; use of noxious material in insufficiently ventilated area or without effective protection

---

Internal

Concomitant exposure; inadequate nutrition; smoking

At Risk Population: Children <5 years; female gender; older adults

Exposure to areas with high contaminant level; exposure to atmospheric pollutants, or to bioterrorism, or to disaster, or to radiation; previous exposure to contaminant

Gestational age during exposure

Associated Condition: Pre-existing disease; pregnancy

Sample Clinical Applications: *Escherichia coli* infection, plague, hantavirus, asthma, botulism, cholera, lead or other heavy metal poisoning, chemical burns, asbestosis, carbon monoxide poisoning, radiation sickness

DESIRED OUTCOMES/EVALUATION CRITERIA

Sample **NOC** linkages:

Knowledge: Personal Safety: Extent of understanding conveyed about risk reduction and prevention of unintentional injuries to self

Risk Control: Personal actions to understand, prevent, eliminate, or reduce modifiable health threats

 Acute Care Collaborative Community/Home Care Cultural

Client Will (Include Specific Time Frame)
- Verbalize understanding of individual factors that contribute to possibility of injury and take steps to correct situation(s).
- Demonstrate behaviors and lifestyle changes to reduce risk factors and protect self from injury.
- Modify environment as indicated to enhance safety.
- Be free of injury.
- Support community activities for disaster preparedness.

Sample NOC linkages:
Community Health Status: General state of well-being of a community or population
Community Risk Control: Environmental Hazards: Community actions to monitor, eliminate, or reduce environmental hazards
Community Disaster Readiness: Community preparedness to respond to a natural or man-made calamitous event

Community Will (Include Specific Time Frame)
- Identify hazards that could lead to exposure or contamination.
- Correct environmental hazards as identified.
- Demonstrate necessary actions to promote community safety and disaster preparedness.

ACTIONS/INTERVENTIONS

Sample NIC linkages:
Risk Identification: Analysis of potential risk factors, determination of health risks, and prioritization of risk-reduction strategies for an individual or group
Community Health Development: Assisting members of a community to identify a community's health concerns, mobilize resources, and implement solutions
Environmental Risk Protection: Preventing and detecting disease and injury in populations at risk from environmental hazards

NURSING PRIORITY NO. 1 To evaluate degree/source of risk inherent in the home, community, and work site:
- Ascertain type of contaminant(s) and exposure routes posing a potential hazard to client or community (e.g., air, soil, or water pollutants; food source, chemical, biological, radiation) as listed in Risk Factors. *Determines course of action to be taken by client/community/care providers.*
- ∞ ⃠ Note age and gender of client(s) or community base (e.g., community health clinic serving primarily economically disadvantaged children or elderly; school near large industrial plant, family living in smog-prone area). *Young children, frail elderly, and females have been found to be at higher risk for effects of exposure to many toxins.*[1,2] (Refer to ND Contamination.)
- Ascertain client's geographic location at home or work (e.g., lives where crop spraying is routine; works in nuclear plant; contract worker or soldier returning from combat area). *Individual and/or community intervention may be needed to reduce risks of accidental or intentional exposures.*
- Note socioeconomic status and availability and use of resources. *Living in poverty increases the potential for multiple exposures, delayed or lack of access to healthcare, and poor general health.*[3]
- Determine client's/significant other's (SO's) understanding of potential risk and appropriate protective measures.

 Diagnostic Studies   Evidence Based Practice   Medications   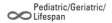 Pediatric/Geriatric/ Lifespan

NURSING PRIORITY NO. 2 To assist client to reduce or correct individual risk factors:

- 🏠 Assist client to develop plan to address individual safety needs and injury or illness prevention in home, community, and work setting.
- Repair, replace, or correct unsafe household items or situations (e.g., flaking or peeling paint or plaster, filtering unsafe tap water).
- Review effects of secondhand smoke and importance of refraining from smoking in home or car *where others are likely to be exposed.*
- 📝 Encourage removal or proper cleaning of carpeted floors, especially for small children and persons with respiratory conditions. *Carpets hold up to 100 times as much fine-particle material as a bare floor and can contain metals and pesticides.*[1]
- Encourage timely cleaning or replacement of air filters on furnace and air-conditioning unit. *Good ventilation cuts down on indoor air pollution from carpets, machines, paints, solvents, cleaning materials, and pesticides.*
- Recommend periodic inspection of well water and tap water *to identify possible contaminants.*
- Encourage client to install carbon monoxide monitors and other air pollutant detectors in home as appropriate.
- Recommend placing dehumidifier in damp areas *to retard growth of molds.*
- Review proper handling of household chemicals:[4,5,9]

    Read chemical labels *to be aware of primary hazards (especially in commonly used household cleaning and gardening products).*

    Follow directions printed on product label (e.g., avoid use of certain chemicals on food preparation surfaces, refrain from spraying garden chemicals on windy days).

    Choose least hazardous products for the job, preferably multiuse products *to reduce number of different chemicals used and stored.* Use products labeled "nontoxic" wherever possible.

    Use form of chemical that most reduces risk of exposure (e.g., cream instead of liquid or aerosol).

    Wear protective clothing, gloves, and safety glasses when using chemicals. Avoid mixing chemicals at all times and use in well-ventilated areas.

    Store chemicals in locked cabinets. Keep chemicals in original labeled containers and do not pour into other containers.

- ∞ Place safety stickers on chemicals *to warn of harmful contents.*
- Review proper food-handling, storage, and cooking techniques.
- ∞ 📝 Stress importance of pregnant or lactating women following fish or wildlife consumption guidelines provided by state, U.S. territorial, or Native American tribes. *Ingestion of noncommercial fish or wildlife can be a significant source of pollutants.*[8]

NURSING PRIORITY NO. 3 To promote wellness (Teaching/Discharge Considerations):

🏠 Home
- Discuss general safety concerns with client/SO/employees *to ensure that people are educated about potential risks, and ways to manage risks.*
- ∞ Stress importance of supervising infant/child or individuals with cognitive limitations *to protect those who are unable to protect themselves.*
- 📞 Post emergency and poison control numbers in a visible location.
- Encourage learning cardiopulmonary resuscitation and first aid for toxic exposures.
- Discuss protective actions for specific "bad air" days (e.g., limiting/avoiding outdoor activities).
- Review pertinent job-related safety regulations. Emphasize necessity of wearing appropriate protective equipment.
- Encourage client/caregiver to develop a personal/family disaster plan, to gather needed supplies to provide for self/family during a community emergency, and to learn how specific public health threats might affect client and actions to promote preparedness and reduce the risk to health and safety.
- Provide information and refer to appropriate resources about potential toxic hazards and protective measures. Provide bibliotherapy including written resources and appropriate Web sites *for client review and self-paced learning.*

 Acute Care   Collaborative   Community/ Home Care   Cultural

- Refer to a smoking-cessation program as needed.

Community
- Promote education programs geared toward increasing awareness of safety measures and resources available to individuals/community.
- Review pertinent job-related health department and Occupational Safety and Health Administration regulations *to safeguard the workplace and the community.*
- Ascertain that there is a comprehensive disaster plan in place for the community that includes a chain of command, equipment, communication, training, decontamination area(s), and safety and security plans *to ensure an effective response to any emergency (e.g., flood, toxic spill, infectious disease outbreak, radiation release).*[6]
- Refer to appropriate agencies (e.g., CDC, U.S. Army Medical Research Institute of Infectious Diseases, Federal Emergency Management Agency, Department of Health and Human Services, Office of Emergency Preparedness, EPA) *to prepare for and manage mass casualty incidents.*[7]

DOCUMENTATION FOCUS

Assessment/Reassessment
- Client's/caregiver's understanding of individual risks and safety concerns.
- Community risks for exposure or contamination.

Planning
- Plan of care and who is involved in planning.
- Teaching plan.

Implementation/Evaluation
- Individual responses to interventions, teaching, and actions performed.
- Specific actions and changes that are made.
- Attainment or progress toward desired outcome(s).
- Modifications to plan of care.

Discharge Planning
- Long-term plans, lifestyle and community changes, and who is responsible for actions to be taken.
- Specific referrals made.

References

1. Goldman, L. R. (1998). Linking research and policy to ensure children's environmental health. *Environ Health Perspect*, 106 (13), 957–961.
2. Centers for Disease Control and Prevention. (Updated 2017). Environmental chemicals. Retrieved March 2018 from http://www.cdc.gov/biomonitoring/environmental_chemicals.html.
3. Wilkinson, R., Marmot, M. (2003). *Social Determinants of Health: The Solid Facts*. 2nd ed. Copenhagen, Denmark: World Health Organization.
4. National Institute of Environmental Health Services. (reviewed 2017). Environmental health topics: Air pollution and water pollution (two articles, see index). Retrieved March 2018 from http://www.familymanagement.com/childcare/facility/chemical.toxins.safety.html.
5. All Family Resources. (1999). Chemical toxins safety. Retrieved March 2018 from www.familymanagement.com/childcare/facility/chemical.toxins.safety.html.
6. Bauer, J., Steinhauer, R. (2002). A readied response: The emergency plan. *RN*, 65(6), 40.
7. Jagminas, L. (2006, updated 2015). CBRNE—Chemical decontamination (various pages). Retrieved March 2018 from http://emedicine.medscape.com/article/831175-overview#showall.
8. American Academy of Family Physicians. Breastfeeding (Position paper): Appendix 2: Additional breastfeeding considerations: Section: Toxins and pollutants in infant feeding. Retrieved March 2018 from https://www.aafp.org/about/policies/all/breastfeeding-support.html#.
9. EPA Science Inventory. (Updated 2004). Risk assessment/risk management for indoor mold. Retrieved March 2018 from https://cfpub.epa.gov/si/si_public_record_report.cfm?dirEntryId=56220.

compromised family Coping

Taxonomy II: Coping/Stress Tolerance—Class 2 Coping Responses (00074) [**Diagnostic Division:** Social Interaction], Submitted 1980; Revised 1996, 2017

DEFINITION: A usually supportive primary person (family member; significant other; or close friend) provides insufficient, ineffective, or compromised support, comfort, assistance, or encouragement that may be needed by the client to manage or master adaptive tasks related to his or her health challenge.

RELATED FACTORS

Coexisting situations affecting the support person; preoccupation by support person with concern outside of family

Exhaustion of support person's capacity; insufficient reciprocal support

Family disorganization

Insufficient information available to support person; misinformation obtained by support person

Insufficient understanding, or misunderstanding of information by support person

Insufficient support given by client to support person

DEFINING CHARACTERISTICS

Subjective

Client complaint or concern about support person's response to health problem

Support person reports inadequate knowledge or understanding that interferes with effective supportive behaviors

Support person reports preoccupation with own reaction to client's need

Objective

Assistive behaviors by support person produce unsatisfactory results

Protective behavior by support person incongruent with client's abilities

Limitation in communication between support person and client

Support person withdraws from client

At Risk Population: Developmental or situational crisis experienced by support person; family role change; prolonged disease that exhausts capacity of support person

Sample Clinical Applications: Chronic conditions (e.g., chronic obstructive pulmonary disease [COPD], AIDS, Alzheimer's disease, pain, renal failure), substance abuse, cancer, depression, hypochondriasis

DESIRED OUTCOMES/EVALUATION CRITERIA

Sample NOC linkages:

Family Coping: Capacity of the family to manage stressors that tax family resources

Family Normalization: Capacity of a family to develop strategies for optimal functioning when a member has a chronic illness or disability

Caregiver-Patient Relationship: Positive interactions and connections between the caregiver and care recipient

Family Will (Include Specific Time Frame)

• Identify resources within themselves to deal with the situation.

• Interact appropriately with the client, providing support and assistance, as indicated.

• Provide opportunity for client to deal with situation in own way.

• Verbalize knowledge and understanding of illness, disability, or condition.

 Acute Care Collaborative Community/ Home Care Cultural

- Express feelings honestly.
- Identify need for and seek outside support.

ACTIONS/INTERVENTIONS

Sample NIC linkages:

Family Involvement Promotion: Facilitating participation of family members in the emotional and physical care of the patient

Family Support: Promotion of family values, interests, and goals

Caregiver Support: Provision of the necessary information, advocacy, and support to facilitate primary patient care by someone other than a healthcare professional

NURSING PRIORITY NO. 1   To assess causative/contributing factors:

- Identify underlying situation(s) that may contribute to the inability of family to provide needed assistance to the client. *Circumstances may have preceded the illness and now have a significant effect (e.g., client was a substance abuser; client had a heart attack during sexual activity, and mate is afraid any activity may cause a repeat).*[1]
- Note cultural factors related to family relationships that may be involved in problems of caring for member who is ill. *Family composition and structure, methods of decision making, and gender issues and expectations will affect how family deals with stress of illness/negative prognosis. Depending on role the ill client has in the family (e.g., mother or father), other members may have difficulty assuming authoritative role and managing the family.*[6]
- Note the length of illness or condition (e.g., cancer, multiple sclerosis) and/or other long-term situations that may exist. *Chronic or unresolved illness, accompanied by changes in role performance or responsibility, often exhausts supportive capacity and coping abilities of significant other (SO)/family.*[1]
- Assess information available to and understood by the family/SO(s). *Access to and understanding of information regarding the specific illness or condition, treatment, and prognosis are essential to family cooperation and care of the client.*[2,3]
- Discuss family perceptions of situation. *Expectations of client and family members may/may not be realistic and may interfere with ability to cope with situation.*[1]
- Identify role of the client in family and how illness has changed the family organization. *Illness affects how client performs usual functions in the family and affects how others in the family take over those responsibilities. These changes may result in dysfunctional behaviors, anger, hostility, and hopelessness.*[1]
- Note factors (beside the client's illness) that are affecting abilities of family members to provide needed support. *Individual members' preoccupation with own needs and concerns can interfere with providing needed care or support during stresses of long-term illness. Additionally, caregivers may incur decreased or lost income or risk losing own health insurance if they alter their work hours to care for client.*[1]

NURSING PRIORITY NO. 2   To assist family to reactivate/develop skills to deal with current situation:

- Listen to client's/SO's comments, remarks, and expression of concern(s). Note nonverbal behaviors and responses and congruency. *Provides information and promotes understanding of client's view of the illness and needs related to current situation.*
- Encourage family members to verbalize feelings openly and clearly. *Promotes understanding of feelings in relationship to current events and helps them to hear what other person is saying, leading to more appropriate interactions.*[5]
- Discuss underlying reasons for client's behavior. *Helps family/SO understand and accept or deal with client behaviors that may be triggered by emotional or physical effects of illness.*[4]

 Diagnostic Studies   Evidence Based Practice   Medications   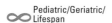 Pediatric/Geriatric/Lifespan

- Assist the family and client to understand "who owns the problem" and who is responsible for resolution. Avoid placing blame or guilt. *When these boundaries are defined, each individual can begin to take care of own self and stop taking care of others in inappropriate ways.*[3,4]
- Encourage client and family to develop problem-solving skills to deal with the situation. *Use of these skills enables each member of the family to identify what he or she sees as the problem to be dealt with and contribute ideas for solutions that are acceptable to him or her, promoting more effective interactions among the family members.*[4]

NURSING PRIORITY NO. 3 To promote wellness (Teaching/Discharge Considerations):

- Provide information for family/SO(s) about specific illness/condition. *Promotes better understanding of need for following therapeutic regimen to provide maximum benefit.*[8]
- Involve client and family in planning care as often as possible. *When family members are knowledgeable and understand needs, commitment to plan is enhanced.*[7,8]
- Promote assistance of family in providing client care, as appropriate. *Identifies ways of demonstrating support while maintaining client's independence (e.g., providing favorite foods, engaging in diversional activities).*[5]
- Refer to appropriate resources for assistance, as indicated (e.g., counseling, psychotherapy, financial, spiritual). *May need additional help, and getting to the appropriate resource provides accurate help for individual situation (e.g., family counseling, financial planning).*[7,8]
- Refer to NDs Anxiety, Death Anxiety, ineffective Coping, readiness for enhanced family Coping, disabled family Coping, Fear, Grieving, as appropriate.

DOCUMENTATION FOCUS

Assessment/Reassessment
- Assessment findings, including current and past coping behaviors, emotional response to situation and stressors.
- Availability and use of support systems.

Planning
- Plan of care, who is involved in planning, and areas of responsibility.
- Teaching plan.

Implementation/Evaluation
- Responses of family members/client to interventions, teaching, and actions performed.
- Attainment or progress toward desired outcome(s).
- Modifications to plan of care.

Discharge Planning
- Long-term plans and who is responsible for actions.
- Specific referrals made.

References

1. Raina, P., et al. (2005). The health and well-being of caregivers of children with cerebral palsy. *Pediatrics*, 115(6), 626–636.
2. Hatzmann, J., et al. (2008). Hidden consequences of success in pediatrics: Parental health-related quality of life. *Pediatrics*, 122(5), 1030–1038.
3. Given, B., Sherwood, P., Given, C. (2008). What knowledge and skills do caregivers need? *Am J Nurs*, 108(9 (Suppl)), S28–S34.
4. Sittner, B. J., Hudson, D. B., DeFrain, J. (2007). Using the concept of family strengths to enhance nursing care. *MCN*, 32(6), 353–357.
5. Yedidia, M., Tiedemann, A. (2008). How do family caregivers describe their needs for professional help? *Am J Nurs*, 108(9 (Suppl)), S35–S37.
6. Dennis, B. P., Small, E. B. (2003). Incorporating cultural diversity in nursing care: An action plan. *ABNF J*, 14(1), 17–26.
7. Feigin, R., Barnetz, Z., Davidson-Arad, B. (2008). Quality of life in family members coping with chronic illness in a relative: An exploratory study. *Fam Syst Health*, 26(3), 267–281.
8. Ammon, S. (2001). Managing patients with heart failure. *Am J Nurs*, 101(12), 34–40.

 Acute Care   Collaborative   Community/Home Care   Cultural

defensive Coping

Taxonomy II: Coping/Stress Tolerance—Class 2 Coping Responses (00071) [**Diagnostic Division:** Ego Integrity], Approved 1988; Revised 2008

DEFINITION: Repeated projection of falsely positive self-evaluation based on a self-protective pattern that defends against underlying perceived threats to positive self-regard.

RELATED FACTORS
Conflict between self-perception and value system; uncertainty
Insufficient confidence in others; insufficient support systems
Insufficient resilience
Unrealistic self-expectations

DEFINING CHARACTERISTICS

Subjective
Denial of problems or weaknesses
Hypersensitive to a discourtesy or criticism
Projection of blame or responsibility
Rationalization of failures

Objective
Alteration in reality testing; reality distortion
Difficulty establishing or maintaining relationships
Grandiosity
Insufficient participation in or follow-through with treatment
Superior attitude toward others; ridicule of others; hostile laughter
Sample Clinical Applications: Eating disorders, substance abuse, chronic illness; bipolar, adjustment, or dissociative disorders

DESIRED OUTCOMES/EVALUATION CRITERIA

Sample NOC linkages:
Acceptance: Health Status: Personal actions to reconcile change in health circumstances
Coping: Personal actions to manage stressors that tax an individual's resources
Social Interaction Skills: Personal behaviors that promote effective relationships

Client Will (Include Specific Time Frame)
• Verbalize understanding of own problems and stressors.
• Identify areas of concern or problems.
• Demonstrate acceptance of responsibility for own actions, successes, and failures.
• Participate in treatment program or therapy.
• Maintain involvement in relationships.

ACTIONS/INTERVENTIONS

Sample NIC linkages:
Self-Awareness Enhancement: Assisting a patient to explore and understand his/her thoughts, feelings, motivations, and behaviors

(continues on page 214)

 Diagnostic Studies Evidence Based Practice Medications Pediatric/Geriatric/Lifespan

defensive Coping (continued)

Coping Enhancement: Facilitation of cognitive and behavioral efforts to manage perceived stressors, changes, or threats that interfere with meeting life demands and roles

Counseling: Use of an interactive helping process focusing on the needs, problems, or feelings of the patient and significant others to enhance or support coping, problem solving, and interpersonal relationships

NURSING PRIORITY NO. 1 To determine degree of impairment:

- Assess ability to comprehend current situation, developmental level of functioning. *Crucial to planning care for this individual. Client will typically have difficulty communicating and responding emotionally in an expected manner in these circumstances.*[1]
- Determine level of anxiety and effectiveness of current coping mechanisms. *Severe anxiety will interfere with ability to cope, and client will need to assess what is working and develop new ways to deal with current situation.*[2]
- ✎ Perform or review results of testing, such as the Taylor Manifest Anxiety Scale and Marlowe-Crowne Social Desirability Scale, as indicated. *Helps to identify coping styles, enabling more accurate therapeutic interventions.*[7]
- Determine coping mechanisms used (e.g., projection, avoidance, rationalization) and purpose of coping strategy (e.g., may mask low self-esteem). *Provides information about how these behaviors affect current situation.*[3]
- Assist client to identify and consider need to address problem differently. *Until client is willing to consider different approaches to dealing with situation, little progress can be expected.*[1]
- Describe all aspects of the problem through the use of therapeutic communication skills such as active-listening. *Provides an opportunity for the client to clarify the situation and begin to look at options for problem solving.*[2]
- Observe interactions with others. *Noting difficulties and ability to establish satisfactory relationships can provide clues to client behaviors that interfere with interactions with others.*[2]
- Note availability of family/friends support for client in current situation. *Significant others may not be supportive when person is denying problems or exhibiting unacceptable behaviors.*[6]
- Note expressions of grandiosity in the face of contrary evidence (e.g., "I'm going to buy a new car" when the individual has no job or available finances). *Evidence of distorted thinking and possibility of mental illness.*[3]
- Assess physical condition. *Defensive coping style has been connected with physical well-being and illnesses, especially chronic health concerns (e.g., congestive heart failure, diabetes, chronic fatigue syndrome).*[5]

NURSING PRIORITY NO. 2 To assist client to deal with current situation:

- Provide explanation of rules of the treatment program and discuss consequences of lack of cooperation. Encourage client participation in setting of consequences and agreement to them. *Promotes understanding and possibility of cooperation on the part of the client, especially when client has been involved in the decisions.*[2]
- Set limits on manipulative behavior; be consistent in enforcing consequences when rules are broken and limits tested. *Providing clear information and following through on identified consequences reduces the ability to manipulate staff or therapist and environment.*[3]
- Develop therapeutic relationship to enable client to test new behaviors in a safe environment. Use positive, nonjudgmental approach and "I" messages. *Promotes sense of self-esteem and enhances sense of control.*
- Encourage control in all situations possible; include client in decisions and planning. *Preserves autonomy, enabling realization of sense of self-worth.*

 Acute Care   Collaborative   Community/Home Care   Cultural

- Acknowledge individual strengths and incorporate awareness of personal assets and strengths in plan. *Promotes use of positive coping behaviors and progress toward effective solutions.*[4]
- Convey attitude of acceptance and respect (unconditional positive regard). *Avoids threatening client's self-concept, preserving existing self-esteem.*[2]
- Encourage identification and expression of feelings. *Provides opportunity for client to learn about and accept self and feelings as normal.*[2]
- Provide or encourage use of healthy outlets for release of hostile feelings (e.g., punching bags, pounding boards). Involve in outdoor recreation program when available. *Promotes acceptable expression of these feelings, which, when unexpressed, can lead to development of undesirable behaviors and make situation worse.*[4]
- Provide opportunities for client to interact with others in a positive manner. *Promotes self-esteem and encourages client to learn how to develop and enhance relationships.*[4]
- Assist client with problem-solving process. Identify and discuss responses to situation, maladaptive coping skills. Suggest alternative responses to situation. *Helps client select more adaptive strategies for coping.*[2]
- Use confrontation judiciously *to help client begin to identify defense mechanisms (e.g., denial, projection) that are hindering development of satisfying relationships.*[2]
- ⊕ Assist with treatments for physical illnesses as appropriate. *Taking care of physical self will enable client to deal with emotional and psychological issues more effectively.*[4]

NURSING PRIORITY NO. 3 To promote wellness (Teaching/Discharge Considerations):

- 🏠 Use cognitive-behavioral therapy. *Helps change negative thinking patterns when rigidly held beliefs are used by client to defend the individual against low self-esteem.*[3]
- Encourage client to learn and use relaxation techniques, guided imagery, and positive affirmation of self. *Enables client to incorporate and practice new behaviors to deal with stressors and view or respond to situation in a more realistic and positive manner.*[4]
- Promote involvement in activities or classes as appropriate. *Client can practice new skills, develop new relationships, and learn new and positive ways of interacting with others.*[1]
- ⊕ Refer to additional resources (e.g., substance rehabilitation, family or marital therapy), as indicated. *Can be useful in making desired changes and developing new coping skills.*[2]
- Refer to ND ineffective Coping for additional interventions.

DOCUMENTATION FOCUS

Assessment/Reassessment
- Assessment findings, client perception of the present situation, presenting behaviors.
- Usual coping methods, degree of impairment.
- Health concerns.

Planning
- Plan of care, specific interventions, and who is involved in development of the plan.
- Teaching plan.

Implementation/Evaluation
- Response to interventions, teaching, and actions performed.
- Attainment or progress toward desired outcome(s).
- Modifications to plan of care.

Discharge Planning
- Referrals and follow-up programming.

 Diagnostic Studies   Evidence Based Practice   Medications   Pediatric/Geriatric/Lifespan

References

1. Soraya, L. (2008). Asperger emotions and adult relationships. Retrieved March 2018 from https://www.psychologytoday.com/blog/aspergers-diary/200809/asperger-emotions-and-adult-relationships.
2. Gordon, B. N. (1981). Child temperament and adult behavior: An exploration of "goodness of fit." *Child Psychiatry Hum Dev*, 11(3), 167–178.
3. Dombeck, M. (Updated 2006). Coping strategies and defense mechanisms: Basic and intermediate defenses. MentalHelp.net. Retrieved March 2018 https://www.mentalhelp.net/articles/coping-strategies-and-defense-mechanisms-basic-and-intermediate-defenses/.
4. Vanderhyder, D. (2008). Stress management for caregivers of Alzheimer's using guided imagery. Retrieved March 2018 from http://caregiverhelp.blogspot.com/2008/06/stress-management-for-caregivers-of.html.
5. Creswell, C., Chalder, T. (2001). Defensive coping styles in chronic fatigue syndrome. *J Psychosom Res*, 51(4), 607–610.
6. Graham, M. (2011). Where to begin: Finding help during chronic illness. Retrieved March 2018 from http://invisibledisabilities.org/coping-with-invisible-disabilities/disability-benefits/finding-help/.
7. Hoyt, D. P., Magoon, T. M. (1954). A validation study of the Taylor Manifest Anxiety Scale. *J Clin Psychol*, 10(4), 357–361.

disabled family Coping

Taxonomy II: Coping/Stress Tolerance—Class 2 Coping Responses (00073) [**Diagnostic Division:** Social Interaction], Submitted 1980; Revised 1996, 2008

DEFINITION: Behavior of primary person (family member, significant other, or close friend) that disables his or her capacities and the client's capacities to effectively address tasks essential to either person's adaptation to the health challenge.

RELATED FACTORS
Ambivalent family relationships
Chronically unexpressed feelings by support person
Differing coping styles between support person and client
Differing coping styles between support persons
Inconsistent management of family's resistance to treatment

DEFINING CHARACTERISTICS

Subjective
[Expresses despair regarding family reactions or lack of involvement]

Objective
Abandonment; depression
Adopts illness symptoms of client; psychosomatic symptoms
Agitation; aggression; hostility; intolerance
Client dependence; family behaviors detrimental to well-being; neglect of relationship of family member
Disregard for client's needs; neglect of basic needs or treatment regimen of client; performing routines without regard for client's needs; prolonged hyperfocus on client; distortion of reality about client's health problems
Impaired ability to structure a meaningful life; impaired individualism
Sample Clinical Applications: Chronic conditions (e.g., chronic obstructive pulmonary disease [COPD], AIDS, Alzheimer's disease, chronic pain, renal failure, brain/spinal cord injury [SCI]), substance abuse, cancer, genetic conditions (e.g., Down syndrome, sickle cell disease, Huntington's disease), depression, hypochondriasis

 Acute Care   Collaborative   Community/ Home Care   Cultural

DESIRED OUTCOMES/EVALUATION CRITERIA

Sample NOC linkages:

Family Normalization: Capacity of a family to develop strategies for optimal functioning when a member has a chronic illness or disability

Family Coping: Capacity of the family to manage stressors that tax family resources

Caregiver Role Endurance: Factors that promote family care provider's capacity to sustain caregiving over an extended period of time

Family Will (Include Specific Time Frame)
- Verbalize more realistic understanding and expectations of the client.
- Visit or contact client regularly.
- Participate positively in care of client, within limits of family's abilities and client's needs.
- Express feelings and expectations openly and honestly as appropriate.
- Access available resources/services to assist with required care.

ACTIONS/INTERVENTIONS

Sample NIC linkages:

Family Therapy: Assisting family members to move their family toward a more productive way of living

Family Support: Promotion of family values, interests, and goals

Family Involvement Promotion: Facilitating participation of family members in the emotional and physical care of the patient

NURSING PRIORITY NO. 1   To assess causative/contributing factors:

- Ascertain pre-illness behaviors and interactions of the family. *Provides comparative baseline for developing plan of care and determining interventions needed.*[4,8]
- Identify current behaviors of the family members (e.g., withdrawal or not visiting, brief visits, ignoring client when visiting; anger and hostility toward client and others; ways of touching between family members; expressions of guilt). *Indicators of extent of problems existing within family. Relationships among family members before and after current illness affect ability to deal with problems of caretaking and lengthy illness.*[1,8]
- Discuss family perceptions of situation. *Expectations of client and family members may not be realistic and may interfere with ability to deal with situation.*[6]
- Note cultural factors related to family relationships that may be involved in problems of caring for member who is ill. *Family composition and structure, methods of decision making, gender issues, and expectations will affect how family perceives situation and deals with stress of illness, negative prognosis.*[7]
- Note other factors that may be stressful for the family (e.g., financial difficulties or lack of community support, as when illness occurs when out of town). *Appropriate referrals can be made to provide information and assistance as needed. If not addressed, these problems can lead to caregiver burnout and compassion fatigue.*[6]
- Determine readiness of family members to be involved with care of the client. *Family members are involved in their lives, jobs, and families and may find it difficult to manage tasks necessary for helping with care of the client.*[5,6]

NURSING PRIORITY NO. 2   To provide assistance to enable family to deal with the current situation:

- Establish rapport with family members who are available. *Promotes therapeutic relationship and support for problem-solving solutions.*[1]

- Acknowledge difficulty of the situation for the family. *Communicates understanding of family's feelings and can reduce blaming and guilt feelings.*[2]
- Active-listen to concerns, note both overconcern and lack of concern. *Identifies accuracy of client's information and measure of concern, which may interfere with ability to resolve situation.*[2]
- Allow free expression of feelings, including frustration, anger, hostility, and hopelessness, while placing limits on acting out or inappropriate behaviors. *Provides opportunity to identify accuracy and validate appropriateness of feelings. Limits or minimizes risk of violent behavior.*[4]
- Give accurate information to SO(s) from the beginning. *Establishes trust and promotes opportunity for clarification and correction of misunderstandings.*[4]
- Act as liaison between family and healthcare providers. *Establishes single contact to provide explanations and clarify treatment plan, enhancing reliability of information.*[4]
-   Provide brief, simple explanations about use and alarms when equipment (such as a ventilator) is required. Identify appropriate professional(s) for continued support and problem solving. *Having information and ready access to appropriate resources can reduce feelings of helplessness and promote sense of control.*[1]
- Provide time for private interaction between client and family/SO(s). *Individuals need to talk about what is happening and process new and frightening information to learn to deal with situation or diagnosis within family relationships.*[3]
- Accompany family when they visit client. *Being available for questions, concerns, and support promotes trusting relationship in which family feels free to learn all they can about situation or diagnosis.*[3]
- Assist SO(s) to initiate therapeutic communication with client. *Learning to use new methods of communication (active-listening and "I" messages) can enhance relationships and promote effective problem solving for the family.*[3]
- Include SO(s) in the plan of care. Provide instruction and demonstrate necessary skills. *Promotes family's ability to provide care and develop a sense of control over difficult situation.*[4,5]
- Refer client to protective services as necessitated by risk of physical harm or neglect. *Removing client from home is sometimes necessary to individual safety. May reduce stress on family to allow opportunity for therapeutic intervention.*[4]

NURSING PRIORITY NO. 3 To promote wellness (Teaching/Discharge Considerations):

- Assist family to identify coping skills being used and how these skills are or are not helping them deal with situation. *When family members know this information, they can begin to enhance those skills that are more effective in promoting healthy family functioning in difficult times.*[4]
- Answer family's questions patiently and honestly. Reinforce information provided by other providers. *Continues trusting relationship with family members and promotes understanding of the situation/prognosis so family members can deal more effectively with what is happening.*[1]
- Reframe negative expressions into positive whenever possible. *A positive frame contributes to supportive interactions and can lead to better outcomes.*[3]
- Respect family needs for withdrawal and intervene judiciously. *Situation may be overwhelming, and time away can be beneficial to continued participation. A brief respite can refresh family members who are serving as caregivers and permit renewed ability to manage situation.*[1]
- Encourage family to deal with the situation in small increments rather than trying to deal with the whole picture. *Reduces likelihood of individual being overwhelmed by possibilities that may face them in potentially disabling or fatal outcomes.*[1]
- Assist the family to identify familiar things that would be helpful to the client (e.g., a family picture on the wall), especially when hospitalized for a long time, such as in hospice or long-term care. *Reinforces and maintains orientation and provides a sense of home and family for client.*[1,5]
- Refer family to appropriate resources as needed (e.g., family therapy, financial counseling, spiritual advisor). *May need additional help to deal with difficult situation or illness.*[6]
- Refer to ND Grieving as appropriate.

 Acute Care   Collaborative   Community/ Home Care   Cultural

DOCUMENTATION FOCUS

Assessment/Reassessment

- Assessment findings, current and past behaviors, family members who are directly involved and support systems available.
- Emotional response(s) to situation or stressors.
- Specific health and therapy challenges.

Planning

- Plan of care, specific interventions, and who is involved in planning.
- Teaching plan.

Implementation/Evaluation

- Responses of individuals to interventions, teaching, and actions performed.
- Attainment or progress toward desired outcome(s).
- Modifications to plan of care.

Discharge Planning

- Ongoing needs, available resources, other follow-up recommendations, and who is responsible for actions.
- Specific referrals made.

References

1. Schulz, R., Sherwood, P. R. (2008). Physical and mental health effects of family caregiving. *Am J Nurs*, 108(9 Suppl), S23–S27.
2. Feigin, R., Barnetz, Z., Davidson-Arad, B. (2008). Quality of life in family members coping with chronic illness in a relative: An exploratory study. *Fam Syst Health*, 26(3), 267–281.
3. Reuman, L. R., Mitamura, C., Tugade, M. M. (2003). Coping and disability. In Wehmeyer, M. L. (ed) *The Oxford Handbook of Positive Psychology and Disability*. Oxford, England: Oxford University Press.
4. Zarit, S., Femia, E. (2008). Behavioral and psychosocial interventions for family caregivers. *Am J Nurs*, 108(9), 47–53.
5. Schumacher, K., Beck, C., Marren, J. (2006). Family caregivers: Caring for older adults, working with their families. *Am J Nurs*, 106(8), 40–49.

6. Sims, D. D. (No date). Mending the family circle: Coping with the death of a loved one. Retrieved March 2018 from http://www.touchstonesongrief.com/touchstones/articles/SURVIVING%20THE%20DEATH%20OF%20A%20LOVED%20ONE.pdf.
7. Gill, C. J. (1995). A brief history: Attitudes and treatment of persons with disabilities. Retrieved March 2018 from http://www.jik.com/ilarts.html#Attitudes.
8. Chawla, B. (2009). Psychosocial difficulties of parents with young children with severe disabilities. *Parenting Journals*. Retrieved March 2018 from http://www.parenting-journals.com/84/prominent-psychosocial-difficulties-that-parents-of-young-children-with-severe-disabilities-may-cope-with-during-their-child%e2%80%99s-early-years/.

---

ineffective Coping

Taxonomy II: Coping/Stress Tolerance—Class 2 Coping Responses (00069) [Diagnostic Division: Ego Integrity], Submitted 1978; Revised 1998

DEFINITION: A pattern of invalid appraisal of stressors with cognitive and or behavioral efforts that fails to manage demands related to well-being, inadequate choices of practiced responses, and/or inability to use available resources.

RELATED FACTORS

High degree of threat; inaccurate threat appraisal
Inability to conserve adaptive energies; inadequate tension release strategies; insufficient sense of control
Inadequate confidence in ability to deal with a situation; inadequate opportunity to prepare for stressor
Inadequate resources; insufficient social support

(continues on page 220)

 Diagnostic Studies   Evidence Based Practice   Medications   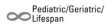 Pediatric/Geriatric/Lifespan

ineffective Coping (continued)

DEFINING CHARACTERISTICS

Subjective
Inability to deal with a situation or ask for help
Alteration in sleep pattern; fatigue; frequent illness
Substance abuse

Objective
Alteration in concentration; inability to attend to information
Change in communication pattern
Destructive behavior toward self or others
Difficulty organizing information
Inability to meet role expectation, basic needs
Insufficient access of social support
Insufficient goal-directed behavior, problem-solution skills, or problem resolution
Ineffective coping strategies
Risk-taking behavior
At Risk Population: Maturational or situational crisis
Sample Clinical Applications: New diagnosis of major illness, chronic conditions, major depression, substance abuse, eating disorders, bipolar disorder, social anxiety disorder, pregnancy, parenting

DESIRED OUTCOMES/EVALUATION CRITERIA

Sample NOC linkages:
Coping: Personal actions to manage stressors that tax an individual's resources
Impulse Self-Control: Self-restraint of compulsive or impulsive behaviors
Decision-Making: Ability to make judgments and choose between two or more alternatives

Client Will (Include Specific Time Frame)
• Assess the current situation accurately.
• Identify ineffective coping behaviors and consequences.
• Verbalize awareness of own coping abilities.
• Verbalize feelings congruent with behavior.
• Meet psychological needs as evidenced by appropriate expression of feelings, identification of options, and use of resources.

ACTIONS/INTERVENTIONS

Sample NIC linkages:
Coping Enhancement: Facilitation of cognitive and behavioral efforts to manage perceived stressors, changes, or threats that interfere with meeting life demands and roles
Decision-Making Support: Providing information and support for a patient who is making a decision regarding healthcare
Impulse Control Training: Assisting the patient to mediate impulsive behavior through application of problem-solving strategies to social and interpersonal situations

 Acute Care Collaborative Community/ Home Care Cultural

NURSING PRIORITY NO. 1   To determine degree of impairment:

- Identify individual stressors (e.g., family, social, work environment, life changes or nursing/healthcare management). *Helps define problem(s), providing a starting point for intervention.*[1]
- Evaluate ability to understand events, provide realistic appraisal of situation. *Necessary information for developing workable plan of care.*[2]
- Identify developmental level of functioning. *Recognizing that people tend to regress to a lower developmental stage during illness or crisis enables more appropriate interventions to be implemented.*[2]
- Assess current functional capacity and note how it is affecting the individual's coping ability. *Promotes identification of strategies that will be helpful in current situation.*
- Determine alcohol intake, drug use, smoking habits, and sleeping and eating patterns. *Substance abuse impairs ability to deal with what is happening in current situation. Identification of impaired sleeping and eating patterns provides clues to extent of anxiety and impaired coping.*[2,3,14]
- Ascertain impact of illness on sexual needs and relationship. *Illnesses, medications, and many treatment regimens can affect sexual functioning, further stressing coping ability.*[2,3]
- Assess level of anxiety and coping on an ongoing basis. *Identifies changes in ability to cope and worsening of ability to understand at an early stage where intervention can be most effective.*[4]
- Note speech and communication patterns. Be aware of negative or catastrophizing thinking. *Identifies existing problems and assesses ability to understand situation and communicate needs.*[7,13]
- Observe and describe behavior in objective terms. Validate observations. *Promotes accuracy and assures correctness of conclusions to arrive at the best possible solutions.*[7]

NURSING PRIORITY NO. 2   To assess coping abilities and skills:

- Ascertain client's understanding of current situation and its impact on life and work. *Client may not understand situation, and being aware of these factors is necessary to planning care and identifying appropriate interventions.*[8]
- Active-listen and identify client's perceptions of what is happening and effectiveness of coping techniques. *Reflecting client's thoughts can provide a forum for understanding perceptions in relation to reality for planning care and determining accuracy of interventions needed.*[2,3]
- Discuss cultural background and whether some beliefs from family may contribute to difficulties coping with situation. *Family of origin can have a positive or negative effect on individual's ability to deal with stressful situations.*[5]
- Evaluate client's decision-making ability. *When ability to make decisions is impaired by illness or treatment regimen, it is important to take this into consideration when planning care to maximize participation and positive outcomes.*[9]
- Determine previous methods of dealing with life problems. *Identifies successful techniques that can be used in current situation. Often client is preoccupied by current concerns and does not think about previous successful skills.*[8]

NURSING PRIORITY NO. 3   To assist client to deal with current situation:

- Call client by name. Ascertain how client prefers to be addressed. *Using client's name enhances sense of self and promotes individuality and self-esteem.*[2]
- Encourage communication with staff/significant others (SOs). *Developing positive interactions between staff, SO(s), and client ensures that everyone has the same understanding.*[8]
- Use reality orientation (e.g., clocks, calendars, bulletin boards) and make frequent references to time and place as indicated. Place needed and familiar objects within sight for visual cues. *Often client can be disoriented by changes in routine and anxiety about illness and treatment regimens, and these measures help the client maintain orientation and a sense of reality.*[9]
- Provide for continuity of care with same personnel taking care of the client as often as possible. *Developing relationships with same caregivers promotes trust and enables client to discuss concerns and fears freely.*[9]

 Diagnostic Studies   Evidence Based Practice   Medications   Pediatric/Geriatric/ Lifespan

- Explain disease process, procedures, or events in a simple, concise manner. Devote time for listening. *May help client to express emotions, grasp situation, and feel more in control.*
- Discuss use of medications as needed. *Short-term use of anti-anxiety medication or antidepressants may be helpful for lifting mood and encouraging individual to develop new coping skills.*[6]
- Provide for a quiet environment and position equipment out of view as much as possible. *Anxiety is increased by noisy surroundings.*
- Schedule activities so periods of rest alternate with nursing care. Increase activity slowly. *Client is weakened by illness and failure to cope with situation. Ensuring rest can promote ability to cope.*[8]
- Assist client in use of diversion, recreation, and relaxation techniques. *Learning new skills can be helpful for reducing stress and will be useful in the future as the client learns to cope more successfully.*
- Emphasize positive body responses to medical conditions, but do not negate the seriousness of the situation (e.g., stable blood pressure during gastric bleed or improved body posture in depressed client). *Acknowledging the reality of the illness while accurately stating the facts can provide hope and encouragement.*[8]
- Encourage client to try new coping behaviors and gradually master situation. *Practicing new ways of dealing with what is happening leads to being more comfortable and can promote a positive outcome as client relaxes and handles illness and treatment regimen more successfully.*[9]
- Confront client when behavior is inappropriate, pointing out difference between words and actions. *Provides external locus of control, enhancing safety while client learns self-control.*[2]
- Assist in dealing with change in concept of body image as appropriate. (Refer to ND disturbed Body Image.) *New view of self may be negative, and client needs to incorporate change in a positive manner to enhance self-image.*[10]

NURSING PRIORITY NO. 4 To provide for meeting psychological needs:

- Treat the client with courtesy and respect. Converse at client's level, providing meaningful conversation while performing care. *Enhances therapeutic relationship.*[2]
- Take advantage of teachable moments. *Individuals learn best and are open to new information when they feel accepted and are in a comfortable environment.*[10]
- Allow client to react in own way without judgment by staff/caregivers. Provide support and diversion as indicated. *Unconditional positive regard and support promote acceptance, enabling client to deal with difficult situation in a positive way.*[8]
- Encourage verbalization of fears and anxieties and expression of feelings of denial, depression, and anger. *Free expression allows for dealing with these feelings, and when the client knows that these are normal reactions, he or she can deal with them better.*[10]
- Help client to learn how to substitute positive thoughts for negative ones (i.e., "I can do this; I am in charge of myself"). *The mind plays a significant role in one's response to stressors, and negative thoughts can actually increase the impact of the stressor.*[13]
- Provide opportunity for expression of sexual concerns. *Important aspect of person that may be difficult to express. Providing an opening for discussion by asking sensitive questions allows client to talk about concerns.*[10]
- Help client to set limits on acting-out behaviors and learn ways to express emotions in an acceptable manner. *Enables client to gain sense of self-esteem, promoting internal locus of control.*[2]

NURSING PRIORITY NO. 5 To promote wellness (Teaching/Discharge Considerations):

- Give updated or additional information needed about events, cause (if known), and potential course of illness as soon as possible. *Knowledge helps reduce anxiety or fear and allows client to deal with reality.*[8]
- Provide and encourage an atmosphere of realistic hope. *Promotes optimistic outlook, energizing client to address situation. Client needs to hear positive things while undergoing difficult circumstances.*[8]
- 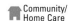 Give information about purposes and side effects of medications and treatments. *Client feels included (promoting sense of control), enabling client to cope with situation in a more positive manner.*[8]

 Acute Care   Collaborative   Community/ Home Care   Cultural

- 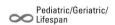 Emphasize importance of follow-up care. *Checkups verify that regimen is being followed accurately and that healing is progressing to promote a satisfactory outcome.*[8]
- Encourage and support client in evaluating lifestyle, occupation, and leisure activities. *Helps client to look at difficult areas that may contribute to anxiety and ability to cope and to make changes gradually without undue or debilitating anxiety.*[8,14]
- Discuss effects of stressors (e.g., family, social, work environment, or nursing/healthcare management) and ways to deal with them. *Addressing these factors will enable client to develop strategies to make changes needed to promote wellness.*[8]
- Provide for gradual implementation and continuation of necessary behavior or lifestyle changes. *Change is difficult, and beginning slowly enhances commitment to plan.*[8]
- Discuss or review anticipated procedures and client concerns, as well as postoperative expectations when surgery is recommended. *Knowledge allays fears and helps client to understand procedures and treatments and expected results. When client has prior information about what to expect during postoperative course, he or she will remain calm, anxiety will be reduced, and client will cope more effectively with situation.*[10,12]
- 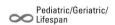 Refer to outside resources and professional therapy as indicated or ordered. *May be necessary to assist with long-term improvement.*[10]
- Determine desire for religious representative or spiritual counselor and facilitate arrangements for visit. *Spiritual needs are an integral part of being human, and determining and meeting individual preferences help client deal with concerns and desires for discussion or assistance in this area.*[11]
- 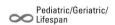 Provide information or consultation as indicated for sexual concerns. Provide privacy when client is not in home. *Individuals are sexual beings, and concerns about role in family/relationship and ability to function are often not readily expressed. Discussion opens opportunity for clarification and understanding and helps to meet need for intimacy.*[10]
- Refer to other NDs as indicated (e.g., Anxiety, impaired verbal Communication, acute/chronic Pain, risk for self/other-directed Violence).

DOCUMENTATION FOCUS

Assessment/Reassessment
- Baseline findings, degree of impairment, and client's perceptions of situation.
- Coping abilities and previous ways of dealing with life problems.

Planning
- Plan of care, specific interventions, and who is involved in planning.
- Teaching plan.

Implementation/Evaluation
- Client's responses to interventions, teaching, and actions performed.
- Medication dose, time, and client's response.
- Attainment or progress toward desired outcome(s).
- Modifications to plan of care.

Discharge Planning
- Long-term needs and actions to be taken.
- Support systems available, specific referrals made, and who is responsible for actions to be taken.

References

1. Sahel, J. A., et al. (2007). Health-related quality of life and utility in patients with age-related macular degeneration. *Arch Ophthalmol*, 125(7), 945–951.
2. McCoy, M. L. (2006). Care of the congestive heart failure patient: The care, cure, and core model. *J Pract Nurs*, 56(1), 5–30.
3. Reuman, L. R., Mitamura, C., Tugade, M. M. (2003). Coping and disability. In Wehmeyer, M. L. (ed). *The Oxford Handbook of Positive Psychology and Disability*. Oxford, England: Oxford University Press.

 Diagnostic Studies Evidence Based Practice Medications 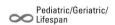 Pediatric/Geriatric/Lifespan

4. Zarit, S., Femia, E. (2008). Behavioral and psychosocial interventions for family caregivers. *Am J Nurs*, 108(9), 47–53.

5. Wilner, A. N. (2008). Patients' cultural and spiritual beliefs influence their diagnosis, treatment and management. *American Psychiatric Association (APA)*. Retrieved March 2018 from http://www.medscape.com/viewarticle/574203_1.

6. Watkins, E. (2003). Combining cognitive therapy with medication in bipolar disorder. *Adv Psychiatr Treat*, 9, 106–110.

7. Rosland, A. M., Heisler, M., Piette, J. D. (2012). The impact of family behaviors and communication patterns on chronic illness outcomes: A systematic review. *J Behav Med*, 35(2), 221–239.

8. Cherif, M., Younis, E. I. (2000). Liver transplantation. *Clin Fam Prac*, 2(1), 117.

9. Liken, M. A. (2001). Caregivers in crisis: Moving a relative with Alzheimer's to assisted living. *Clin Nurs Res*, 10(1), 53–69.

10. Tan, G., Waldman, K., Bostick, R. (2002). Psychosocial issues, sexuality, and cancer. *Sex Disabil*, 20(4), 297–318.

11. Geiter, H. (2002). The spiritual side of nursing. *RN*, 65(5), 43–44.

12. Greene, L. A. (2013). Best and worst ways to cope with stress. Retrieved March 2018 from http://www.health.com/health/gallery/0,,20765943,00.html#stress-busting-solutions.

13. Krull, E. (2016). Replacing your negative thoughts. *PsychCentral*. Retrieved March 2018 from https://psychcentral.com/lib/replacing-your-negative-thoughts/.

14. Franke, J. (1999). Stress, burnout, and addiction. *Tex Med*, 95(3), 43–52.

ineffective community Coping

Taxonomy II: Coping/Stress Tolerance—Class 2 Coping Responses (00077) [**Diagnostic Division:** Social Interaction], Approved 1994; Revised 1998, 2017

DEFINITION: A pattern of community activities for adaptation and problem-solving that is unsatisfactory for meeting the demands or needs of the community.

RELATED FACTORS
Inadequate resources for problem-solving
Insufficient community resources
Nonexistent community systems

DEFINING CHARACTERISTICS

Subjective
Community does not meet expectations of its members
Perceived community vulnerability or powerlessness
Excessive stress

Objective
Deficient community participation
Elevated community illness rate
Excessive community conflict
High incidence of community problems [e.g., homicides, vandalism, robbery, terrorism, abuse, unemployment, poverty, militancy, mental illness]
At Risk Population: History of/exposure to disaster
Sample Clinical Applications: High rate of illness, injury, or violence in community

DESIRED OUTCOMES/EVALUATION CRITERIA

Sample NOC linkages:
Community Competence: Capacity of a community to collectively problem-solve to achieve community goals
Community Health Status: General state of well-being of a community or population

 Acute Care   Collaborative   Community/Home Care   Cultural

Community Disaster Readiness: Community preparedness to respond to a natural or man-made calamitous event

Community Will (Include Specific Time Frame)
- Recognize negative and positive factors affecting community's ability to meet its demands or needs.
- Identify alternatives to inappropriate activities for adaptation and problem-solving.
- Report a measurable increase in necessary or desired activities to improve community functioning.

ACTIONS/INTERVENTIONS

Sample NIC linkages:

Community Health Development: Assisting members of a community to identify a community's health concerns, mobilize resources, and implement solutions
Environmental Management: Community: Monitoring and influencing of the physical, social, cultural, economic, and political conditions that affect the health of groups and communities
Community Disaster Preparedness: Preparing for an effective response to a large-scale disaster

NURSING PRIORITY NO. 1   To identify causative or precipitating factors:

- Evaluate community activities as related to meeting collective needs within the community itself and between the community and the larger society. *Determines what activities are currently available and what needs are not being met, either by the local or county/state entities. Provides information on which to base the steps needed to begin planning for desired changes.*[1]
- Note community reports of community functioning (e.g., immunization status, transportation, water supply, financing), including areas of weakness or conflict. *Community is responsible for identifying needed changes for possible action.*[1]
- Identify effects of Related Factors on community activities. Note immediate needs (e.g., healthcare, food, shelter, funds). *Provides a baseline to determine community needs, and identifying factors that are pertinent to the community allows community to deal with current concerns.*[1,5]
- Plan for the possibility of a disaster when determined by current circumstances. *In relation to threats, terrorist activities, and natural disasters, actions need to be coordinated between the local and the larger community.*[5]
- Determine availability and use of resources. *Helpful to begin planning to correct deficiencies that have been identified. Sometimes even though resources are available, they are not being appropriately or fully used.*[2]
- Identify unmet demands or needs of the community. *Determining deficiencies is a crucial step to developing an accurate plan for correction. Sometimes elected bodies see the problems differently from the general population and conflict can arise; therefore, it is important for communication to resolve the issues that are in question.*[2]

NURSING PRIORITY NO. 2   To assist the community to reactivate/develop skills to deal with needs:

- Determine community strengths. *Promotes understanding of ways in which community is already meeting identified needs, and once identified, they can be built on to develop plan to improve community.*[1]
- Identify and prioritize community goals. *Goals enable the identification of actions to direct the changes that are needed to improve the community. Prioritizing enables actions to be taken in order of importance.*[1]
- Encourage community members/groups to engage in problem-solving activities. *Individuals who are involved in the problem-solving process and make a commitment to the solutions have an investment and are more apt to follow through on their commitments.*[3,5]
- Develop a plan jointly with community to deal with deficits in support. *Working together will enhance efforts and help to meet identified goals.*[3,5]

 Diagnostic Studies   Evidence Based Practice   Medications   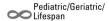 Pediatric/Geriatric/Lifespan

NURSING PRIORITY NO. 3 To promote wellness as related to community health:

- Create plans managing interactions within the community itself and between the community and the larger society. *These activities will meet collective needs.*[1]
- Assist the community to form partnerships within the community and between the community and the larger society. *Promotes long-term development of the community to deal with current and future problems.*[1]
- Provide channels for dissemination of information to the community as a whole (e.g., Web sites, print media; radio and TV reports, community bulletin boards; speakers' bureau; reports to committees, councils, advisory boards on file and accessible to the public). *Having information readily available for everyone provides opportunity for all members of the community to know what is being planned and have input into the planning. Keeping community informed promotes understanding of needs and plans and probability of follow-through to successful outcomes.*[1]
- Make information available in different modalities and geared to differing educational levels and cultural and ethnic populations of the community. *Ensures understanding by all members of the community and promotes cooperation with planning and follow-through.*[1]
- Seek out and evaluate underserved populations, including the homeless. *These members of the community often need to be helped to become productive citizens and be involved in the changes that are occurring.*[3]
- Work with community members to identify lifestyle changes that can be made to meet the goals identified to improve community deficits. *Changing lifestyles can promote a sense of power and encourage members to become involved in improving their community.*[4,5]

DOCUMENTATION FOCUS

Assessment/Reassessment
- Assessment findings, including perception of community members regarding problems.
- Availability and use of resources.

Planning
- Plan of care and who is involved in planning.
- Teaching plan.

Implementation/Evaluation
- Response of community entities to plan, interventions, and actions performed.
- Attainment or progress toward desired outcome(s).
- Modifications to plan of care.

Discharge Planning
- Long-term plans and who is responsible for actions to be taken.

References

1. Lindamer, L. A., et al. (2009). Establishing an implementation network: Lessons learned from community-based participatory research. *Implement Science*. Retrieved March 2018 from http://www.implementationscience.com/content/4/1/17.
2. Hunt, R. (1998). Community-based nursing. *Am J Nurs*, 98(10), 44.
3. Schraeder, C., et al. (1997). Community nursing organizations: A new frontier. *Am J Nurs*, 97(1), 63.
4. Lai, S. C., Cohen, M. N. (1999). Promoting lifestyle changes. *Am J Nurs*, 99(4), 63.
5. Cohn, M. (No date). The importance of community relations. Retrieved March 2018 from http://www.evancarmichael.com/library/martin-cohn/The-Importance-of-Community-Relations.html.

 Acute Care Collaborative Community/ Home Care Cultural

readiness for enhanced Coping

Taxonomy II: Coping/Stress Tolerance—Class 2 Coping Responses (00158) [**Diagnostic Division:** Ego Integrity], Submitted 2002; Revised 2013

DEFINITION: A pattern of valid appraisal of stressors with cognitive and/or behavioral efforts to manage demands related to well-being, which can be strengthened.

DEFINING CHARACTERISTICS

Subjective

Expresses desire to enhance knowledge of stress management strategies and management of stressors
Expresses desire to enhance use of emotion-oriented strategies and problem-oriented strategies
Expresses desire to enhance social support and use of spiritual resources
Awareness of possible environmental change
Sample Clinical Applications: Chronic health conditions (e.g., asthma, diabetes mellitus, arthritis, systemic lupus, multiple sclerosis [MS], AIDS), mental health concerns (e.g., seasonal affective disorder, attention deficit disorder, Down syndrome)

DESIRED OUTCOMES/EVALUATION CRITERIA

Sample NOC linkages:
Coping: Personal actions to manage stressors that tax an individual's resources
Personal Well-Being: Extent of positive perception of one's health status
Quality of Life: Extent of positive perception of current life circumstances

Client Will (Include Specific Time Frame)
• Assess current situation accurately.
• Identify effective coping behaviors currently being used.
• Verbalize feelings congruent with behavior.
• Meet psychological needs as evidenced by appropriate expression of feelings, identification of options, and use of resources.

ACTIONS/INTERVENTIONS

Sample NIC linkages:
Coping Enhancement: Facilitation of cognitive and behavioral efforts to manage perceived stressors, changes, or threats that interfere with meeting life demands and roles
Self-Awareness Enhancement: Assisting a patient to explore and understand his/her thoughts, feelings, motivations, and behaviors
Self-Modification Assistance: Reinforcement of self-directed change initiated by the patient to achieve personally important goals

NURSING PRIORITY NO. 1   To determine needs and desire for improvement:

• Evaluate client's understanding of situation and ability to provide realistic appraisal of situation. *Provides information about client's perception, cognitive ability, and whether the client is aware of the facts of the situation, which reveals essential information for planning care.*[1]
• Determine stressors that may be affecting client. *Accurate identification of situation that client is dealing with provides information for planning interventions to enhance coping abilities.*[1]

 Diagnostic Studies   Evidence Based Practice   Medications   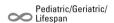 Pediatric/Geriatric/Lifespan

- Ascertain motivation and expectations for change. *Motivation to improve and high expectations can encourage client to make changes that will improve his or her life. However, presence of external locus of control or unrealistic expectations may hamper efforts.*[5]
- Identify social supports available to client. *Available support systems, such as family/friends, can provide client with ability to handle current stressful events, and "talking it out" with an empathic listener will help client move forward to enhance coping skills.*[2]
- Review coping strategies client is aware of and currently using. *The desire to improve one's coping ability is based on an awareness of the status of the stressful situation.*[2]
- Determine use of alcohol or other drugs and smoking habits during times of stress. *Recognition that substituting these actions or old habits for dealing with anxiety increases individual's awareness of opportunity to choose new ways to cope with life stressors.*[6]
- Assess level of anxiety and coping on an ongoing basis. *Provides baseline to develop plan of care to improve coping abilities.*[2]
- Note speech and communication patterns. *Assesses ability to understand and provides information necessary to help client make progress in desire to enhance coping abilities.*[2]
- Evaluate client's decision-making ability. *Understanding client's ability provides a starting point for developing plan and determining what information client needs to develop more effective coping skills.*[1]

NURSING PRIORITY NO. 2   To assist client to develop enhanced coping skills:

- Active-listen and clarify client's perceptions of current status. *Reflecting client's statements and thoughts can provide a forum for understanding perceptions in relation to reality for planning care and determining accuracy of interventions needed.*[4]
- Review previous methods of dealing with life problems. *Enables client to identify successful techniques used in the past, promoting feelings of confidence in own ability.*[2]
- Discuss desire to improve ability to manage stressors of life. *Understanding client's decision to seek new information to enhance life will help client determine what is needed to learn new coping skills.*[2]
- Discuss client's understanding of concept of knowing what can and cannot be changed. *Acceptance of reality that some things cannot be changed allows client to focus energies on dealing with things that can be changed.*[6]
- Help client strengthen problem-solving skills. *Learning the process for problem solving will promote successful resolution of potentially stressful situations that arise.*[4,6]

NURSING PRIORITY NO. 3   To promote optimal well-being (Teaching/Learning Considerations):

- 🏠 Discuss predisposing factors related to individual's response to stress. *Understanding that genetic influences, past experiences, and existing conditions determine whether a person's response is adaptive or maladaptive will give client a base on which to continue to learn what is needed to improve life.*[3]
- Encourage client to develop a stress-management program. *An individualized program of relaxation, meditation, etc., enhances sense of balance in life and strengthens client's ability to manage challenging situations.*[5]
- Recommend involvement in activities of interest, such as exercise/sports, music, and art. *Individuals must decide for themselves what coping strategies are adaptive for them. Most people find enjoyment and relaxation in these kinds of activities.*[6]
- Discuss possibility of doing volunteer work in an area of the client's choosing. *Many individuals report satisfaction in giving of themselves—involvement with caring for others/pets, and client may find sense of fulfillment in service to others.*[1]
- Refer to classes and/or reading material and Web sites, as appropriate. *May be helpful to further learning and pursuing goal of enhanced coping ability.*[1]

 Acute Care   Collaborative   Community/Home Care   Cultural

DOCUMENTATION FOCUS

Assessment/Reassessment
- Baseline information, client's perception of need to enhance abilities.
- Coping abilities and previous ways of dealing with life problems.
- Motivation and expectation for change.

Planning
- Plan of care, specific interventions, and who is involved in planning.
- Teaching plan.

Implementation/Evaluation
- Client's responses to interventions, teaching, and actions performed.
- Attainment or progress toward desired outcome(s).
- Modifications to plan of care.

Discharge Planning
- Long-term needs and actions to be taken.
- Support systems available, specific referrals made, and who is responsible for actions to be taken.

References

1. Cancer Council NSW. (Updated 2016). Your coping toolbox. Retrieved March 2018 from http://www.cancercouncil.com.au/2448/cancer-information/general-information-cancer-information/when-you-are-first-diagnosed/emotions-and-cancer/your-coping-toolbox/.
2. Robinson, L., Smith, M. A., Segal, R. (Updated 2018). Stress management—how to reduce, prevent, and cope with stress. Retrieved March 2018 from http://www.helpguide.org/articles/stress/stress-management.htm.
3. Ryan, R. M., Deci, E. L. (2000). Self-determination theory and the facilitation of intrinsic motivation, social development, and well-being. *Am Psychol*, 55(1), 68–76.
4. Gordon, T. (Updated 2016). Get what you need every time—Method III. Gordon Training International. Retrieved March 2018 from http://www.gordontraining.com/free-parenting-articles/get-what-you-need-every-time-method-iii/.
5. Evans, S., et al. (2009). Using the biopsychosocial model to understand the health benefits of yoga. *J Complement Integr Med*, 6(1), 1–22.
6. Kumarmahi. (No date). Stress Coping Skills. Retrieved March 2018 from https://www.scribd.com/document/16289147/Stress-Coping-Skills-eBook.

readiness for enhanced community Coping

Taxonomy II: Coping/Stress Tolerance—Class 2 Coping Responses (00076) [**Diagnostic Division:** Social Interaction], Approved 1994; Revised 2013

DEFINITION: A pattern of community activities for adaptation and problem-solving for meeting the demands or needs of the community, which can be strengthened.

DEFINING CHARACTERISTICS

Subjective
Expresses desire to enhance problem-solving for identified issue, planning for predictable stressors

Expresses desire to enhance community responsibility for stress management, resources for managing stressors

Expresses desire to enhance communication among community members, between groups and larger community

Expresses desire to enhance availability of community recreation/relaxation programs

(continues on page 230)

 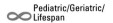

readiness for enhanced community Coping (continued)

DESIRED OUTCOMES/EVALUATION CRITERIA

Sample **NOC** linkages:

Community Competence: Capacity of a community to collectively problem-solve to achieve community goals

Community Health Status: General state of well-being of a community or population

Community Disaster Readiness: Community preparedness to respond to a natural or man-made calamitous event

Community Will (Include Specific Time Frame)

- Identify positive and negative factors affecting management of current and future problems/stressors.
- Have an established plan in place to deal with identified problems and stressors.
- Describe management of challenges in characteristics that indicate effective coping.
- Report a measurable increase in ability to deal with problems and stressors.

ACTIONS/INTERVENTIONS

Sample **NIC** linkages:

Program Development: Planning, implementing, and evaluating a coordinated set of activities designed to enhance wellness, or to prevent, reduce, or eliminate one or more health problems for a group or community

Environmental Management: Community: Monitoring and influencing of the physical, social, cultural, economic, and political conditions that affect the health of groups and communities

Health Policy Monitoring: Surveillance and influence of government and organization regulations, rules, and standards that affect nursing systems and practices to ensure quality care of patients

NURSING PRIORITY NO. 1   To determine existence of and deficits or weaknesses in management of current and future problems/stressors:

- Review community plan for dealing with problems and stressors, untoward events such as natural disaster or terrorist activity. *Provides a baseline for comparisons of preparedness with other communities and developing plan to address concerns.*[4]
- Assess effects of Related Factors on management of problems and stressors. *Identifying social supports available and awareness of the power of the community can enhance the plans needed to improve the community.*[1]
- Identify limitations in current pattern of community activities, such as transportation, water needs, and roads. *Recognition of the factors that can be improved through adaptation and problem solving will make it easier for the community to proceed with planning to make necessary improvements.*[3]
- Evaluate community activities as related to management of problems and stressors within the community itself and between the community and the larger society. *Disasters occurring in a community (or in the country as a whole) affect the local community and need to be recognized and addressed.*[4]

NURSING PRIORITY NO. 2   To assist the community in adaptation and problem-solving for management of current and future needs/stressors:

- Define and discuss current needs and anticipated or projected concerns. *Agreement on scope and parameters of needs is essential for effective planning.*
- Determine community's strengths. *Plan can build on strengths to address areas of weakness.*

 Acute Care
 Collaborative
 Community/ Home Care
 Cultural

- Identify and prioritize goals to facilitate accomplishment. *Helps to bring the community together to meet a common concern or threat, maintain focus, and facilitate accomplishment.*[4]
- Identify and interact with available resources (e.g., persons, groups, financial, governmental, as well as other communities). *Promotes cooperation. Major catastrophes, such as earthquakes, floods, and terrorist activity, affect more than the local community, and communities need to work together to deal with and accomplish reconstruction and future growth.*[5]
- Make a joint plan with the community and the larger community to deal with adaptation and problem-solving. *Promotes management of problems and stressors to enable most effective solution for identified concern.*[2]
- Seek out and involve underserved and at-risk groups within the community, including the homeless. *Supports communication and commitment of community as a whole.*[2]

NURSING PRIORITY NO. 3 To promote optimal well-being of community:

- Assist the community to form partnerships within the community and between the community and the larger society. *Promotes long-term developmental growth of the community.*[4]
- Support development of plans for maintaining these interactions.[5]
- Establish mechanism for self-monitoring of community needs and evaluation of efforts. *Facilitates proactive—rather than reactive—responses by the community.*[5]
- Use multiple formats to disseminate information, such as TV, radio, print media, and billboards, as well as computer bulletin boards, speakers' bureau, and reports to community leaders and groups on file and accessible to the public. *Keeps community informed regarding plans, needs, and outcomes to encourage continued understanding and participation.*[5]

DOCUMENTATION FOCUS

Assessment/Reassessment
- Assessment findings and community's perception of situation.
- Identified areas of concern, community strengths and weaknesses.

Planning
- Plan and who is involved and responsible for each action.
- Teaching plan.

Implementation/Evaluation
- Response of community entities to the actions performed.
- Attainment or progress toward desired outcomes.
- Modifications to plan.

Discharge Planning
- Short- and long-term plans to deal with current, anticipated, and potential problems and who is responsible for follow-through.
- Specific referrals made, coalitions formed.

References

1. Horowitz, C., et al. (2000). Approaches to eliminating socio-cultural disparities in health. *Health Care Financ Rev*, 21(4), 57–74.
2. Schaeder, C., et al. (1997). Community nursing organizations: A new frontier. *Am J Nurs*, 97(1), 63.
3. Lai, S. C., Cohen, M. N. (1999). Promoting lifestyle changes. *Am J Nurs*, 99(4), 63.
4. Gordon, T. Gettwhat you need every time—Method III. Gordon Training International. Retrieved March 2018 from http://www.gordontraining.com/free-parenting-articles/get-what-you-need-every-time-method-iii/.
5. Smith, K. (2002). Public heath nursing. *Encyclopedia of Public Health*. Retrieved March 2018 from http://www.encyclopedia.com/doc/1G2-3404000702.html.

 Diagnostic Studies   Evidence Based Practice   Medications   Pediatric/Geriatric/Lifespan

readiness for enhanced family Coping

Taxonomy II: Coping/Stress Tolerance—Class 2 Coping Responses (00075) [**Diagnostic Division:** Social Interaction], Submitted 1980; Revised 2013

DEFINITION: A pattern of management of adaptive tasks by primary person (family member, significant other, or close friend) involved with the client's health challenge, which can be strengthened.

DEFINING CHARACTERISTICS

Subjective

Expresses desire to acknowledge growth impact of crisis
Expresses desire to choose experiences that optimize wellness
Expresses desire to enhance connection with others who have experienced a similar situation
Expresses desire to enhance health promotion, enrichment of lifestyle
Sample Clinical Applications: Genetic disorders (e.g., Down syndrome, cystic fibrosis, neural tube defects), traumatic injury (e.g., amputation, spinal cord), chronic conditions (e.g., asthma, AIDS, Alzheimer's disease)

DESIRED OUTCOMES/EVALUATION CRITERIA

Sample NOC linkages:

Family Normalization: Capacity of a family to develop strategies for optimal functioning when a member has a chronic illness or disability
Family Coping: Capacity of the family to manage stressors that tax family resources
Family Functioning: Capacity of a family to meet the needs of its members during developmental transitions

Family Will (Include Specific Time Frame)
• Express willingness to look at own role in the family's growth.
• Verbalize desire to undertake tasks leading to change.
• Report feelings of self-confidence and satisfaction with progress being made.

ACTIONS/INTERVENTIONS

Sample NIC linkages:

Normalization Promotion: Assisting parents and other family members of children with chronic illnesses or disabilities in providing normal life experiences for their children and families
Family Support: Promotion of family values, interests, and goals
Family Involvement Promotion: Facilitating participation of family in the emotional and physical care of the patient

NURSING PRIORITY NO. 1   To assess situation and adaptive skills being used by the family members:

• Determine individual situation and stage of growth family is experiencing and demonstrating. *Essential elements needed to identify family needs and develop plan of care for improving communication and interactions. Changes that are occurring may help family adapt, grow, and thrive when faced with these transitional events.*[1,6]

 Acute Care   Collaborative   Community/ Home Care   Cultural

- Ascertain motivation and expectations for change. *Motivation to improve and high expectations can encourage individuals to make changes that will improve their lives; however, presence of external locus of control or unrealistic expectations may hamper efforts.*
- Observe communication patterns of family. Listen to family's expressions of hope, planning, and effect on relationships and life. *Provides clues to difficulties that individuals may have in expressing themselves effectively to others. Beginning to plan for the future with hope promotes changes in relationships that can enhance living for those involved.*[3]
- Note expressions such as "Life has more meaning for me since this has occurred." *Such statements identify change in values that may occur with the diagnosis or stress of a serious or potentially fatal illness.*[1]
- 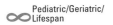Identify cultural or religious health beliefs and expectations. *For example: Navajo parents may define family as nuclear, extended, or clan, and it is important to identify who are the primary child-rearing persons. Beliefs about causes of condition may affect how family interacts with client (e.g., African Americans may believe the condition is punishment for improper behavior and may react with anger and statements of condemnation).*[5]

NURSING PRIORITY NO. 2 To assist family to develop/strengthen potential for growth:

- Provide time to talk with family to discuss their views of the situation. *Provides an opportunity to hear family's understanding and determine how realistic their ideas are for planning how they are going to deal with situation in the most positive manner.*[3]
- Establish a relationship with family/client. *Therapeutic relationships foster growth and enable family to identify skills needed for coping with difficult situation or illness.*[3]
- Provide a role model with whom the family may identify. *Setting a positive example can be a powerful influence in changing behavior, and as family members learn more effective communication skills, consideration for others, warmth, and understanding, family relationships will be enhanced.*[2]
- Discuss importance of open communication and of not having secrets. *Functional communication is clear, direct, open, and honest, with congruence between verbal and nonverbal. Dysfunctional communication is indirect, vague, and controlled, with many double-bind messages. Awareness of this information can enhance relationships among family members.*[3]
- Demonstrate techniques such as active-listening, "I" messages, and problem solving. *Learning these skills can facilitate effective communication and improve interactions within the family.*[2]
- Establish social goals of achieving and maintaining harmony with oneself, family, and community. *Enables client to interact with others in positive ways.*[3]

NURSING PRIORITY NO. 3 To promote optimum family well-being (Teaching/Discharge Considerations):

- 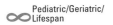Assist family to support the client in meeting own needs within ability or constraints of the illness or situation. *Family members may do too much for client or may not do enough, believing client "wants to be babied." With information and support, they can learn to allow client to take the lead in doing what he or she is able to do.*[3]
- Provide experiences for the family to help them learn ways of assisting and supporting client. *Learning is enhanced when individual participates in hands-on opportunities to try out new activities.*[4]
- 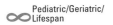Discuss cultural beliefs and practices that may impact family members' interaction with client and dealing with condition. *Preconceived biases may interfere with efforts toward positive growth.*[5]
- 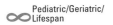Identify other individuals/groups with similar conditions and assist client/family to make contact (groups such as Reach for Recovery, CanSurmount, Al-Anon, and so on). *Provides ongoing support for sharing common experiences, problem-solving, and learning new behaviors.*
- Assist family members to learn new, more effective ways of dealing with feelings and reactions. *Growth process is essential to reach the goal of enhancing the family relationships.*[3]

• Encourage family members to pursue personal interests, hobbies, or leisure activities *to promote individual well-being and strengthen coping abilities.*[6]

DOCUMENTATION FOCUS

Assessment/Reassessment
• Adaptive skills being used, stage of growth.
• Family communication patterns.
• Motivation and expectations for change.

Planning
• Plan of care, specific interventions, and who is involved in planning.
• Teaching plan.

Implementation/Evaluation
• Client's responses to interventions, teaching, and actions performed.
• Attainment or progress toward desired outcome(s).
• Modifications to plan of care.

Discharge Planning
• Identified needs for follow-up care, support systems.
• Specific referral made.

References

1. Garbee, D. D., Gentry, J. A. (2001). Coping with the stress of surgery. *AORN J*, 73(5), 946–951.
2. Gordon, T. Get what you need every time—Method III. Gordon Training International. Retrieved March 2018 from http://www.gordontraining.com/free-parenting-articles/get-what-you-need-every-time-method-iii/.
3. Pychyl, T. A. (2009). Proactive coping: A strategy for self-regulation and enhanced well-being. *Psychol Today*. Retrieved March 2018 from http://www.psychologytoday.com/blog/dont-delay/200903/proactive-coping-strategy-self-regulation-and-enhanced-well-being.
4. Kiser, L. J., et al. (2010). Strengthening family coping resources: The feasibility of a multifamily group intervention for families exposed to trauma. *J Trauma Stress*, 23(6), 802–806.
5. Purnell, L. D. (2011). *Guide to Culturally Competent Health Care*. 2nd ed. Philadelphia: F. A. Davis.
6. Becket, N. (1991). Clinical nurses' characterizations of patient coping problems. *Nurs Diagn*, 2(2), 72–78.

Death Anxiety

Taxonomy II: Coping/Stress Tolerance—Class 2 Coping Responses (00147) [**Diagnostic Division:** Ego Integrity], Approved 1998; Revised 2006, 2017

DEFINITION: Vague uneasy feeling of discomfort or dread generated by perceptions of a real or imagined threat to one's existence.

RELATED FACTORS
Anticipation of: pain, suffering, adverse consequences of anesthesia, impact of death on others
Confronting the reality of terminal disease; fear of the dying process; experiencing dying process; perceived imminence of death
Discussions on the topic of death
Negative thoughts related to death and dying; observations related to death
Uncertainty of prognosis; nonacceptance of own mortality
Uncertainty about: the existence of a higher power, life after death, encountering a higher power

 Acute Care   Collaborative   Community/Home Care   Cultural

DEFINING CHARACTERISTICS

Subjective

Concern about strain on the caregiver; worried about the impact of one's death on significant other

Deep sadness; powerlessness

Fear of: developing a terminal illness, the dying process, pain or suffering related to dying, loss of mental abilities when dying; premature death; prolonged dying process

Negative thoughts related to death and dying

At Risk Population: Discussions on the topic of death; observations related to dying process; experiencing dying process; near-death experience

Associated Condition: Terminal illness

Sample Clinical Applications: Chronic debilitating health conditions, cancer, hospital admission, impending major surgery

DESIRED OUTCOMES/EVALUATION CRITERIA

Sample NOC linkages:

Dignified Life Closure: Personal actions to maintain control when approaching end of life

Hope: Optimism that is personally satisfying and life supporting

Acceptance: Health Status: Personal actions to reconcile significant changes in health circumstances

Client Will (Include Specific Time Frame)

- Identify and express feelings (e.g., sadness, guilt, fear) freely and effectively.
- Look toward or plan for the future one day at a time.
- Formulate a plan dealing with individual concerns and eventualities of dying.

ACTIONS/INTERVENTIONS

Sample NIC linkages:

Dying Care: Promotion of physical comfort and psychological peace in the final phase of life

Spiritual Support: Assisting the patient to feel balance and connection with a greater power

Grief Work Facilitation: Assistance with the resolution of a significant loss

NURSING PRIORITY NO. 1   To assess causative/contributing factors:

- Determine how client sees self in usual lifestyle role functioning and determine perception and meaning of anticipated loss to him/her and significant other(s) (SO(s)). *Provides information that can be compared to changes that are occurring. Understanding these factors are helpful for planning.*[1]
- Ascertain current knowledge of situation. *Identifies misconceptions, lack of information, and other pertinent issues and determines accuracy of knowledge. Healthcare providers may not be anticipating death at this time or in current situation.*[1]
- Determine client's role in family constellation. Observe patterns of communication in family and response of family/SO to client's situation and concerns. *In addition to identifying areas of need or concern, this also reveals strengths useful in addressing the current concerns.*[3]
- Assess impact of client reports of subjective experiences and experience with death (or exposure to death); for example, witnessed violent death, as a child viewed body in casket, etc. *Identifies possible feelings that may be affecting current situation, thus promoting accurate planning.*[2]
- 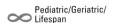 Identify cultural factors or expectations and impact on current situation and feelings. *These factors affect client attitude toward events and impending loss. For instance, in Russia, the head of the family is informed*

first of the impending death, as the head of the family may not want the client to know so he or she will have a peaceful death. Many cultures prefer to keep the client at home instead of in a long-term care facility or hospital. In the United States, hospice is often used to provide palliative care and comfort during the client's final days in any setting.[4]

- ∞ Note age, physical and mental condition, and complexity of therapeutic regimen. *May affect ability to handle current situation. Younger people may handle stress of illness in more positive ways. Older people may be more accepting of possibility of death. Individuals of any age will deal with situation in his/her own way, depending on diagnosis, condition, expectations, and situation.*[8]
- Determine ability to manage own self-care, end-of-life decisions, and other affairs, as well as awareness and use of available resources. *Information will be necessary for determining needs and planning care.*[8]
- Observe behavior indicative of the level of anxiety present (mild to panic). *The level of anxiety affects client's/SO's ability to process information and participate in activities.*[5]
- Note use of drugs (including alcohol), presence of insomnia, excessive sleeping, and avoidance of interactions with others. *Indicators of withdrawal and need for intervention to deal with symptoms or help client deal realistically with diagnosis or illness.*[6]
- Determine sense of futility, feelings of hopelessness, helplessness, and lack of motivation to help self. *Indicators of depression and need for early intervention to help client acknowledge and deal with impending death.*[7,8]
- Listen for expressions of inability to find meaning in life or suicidal ideation. *Signs of depression indicating need for referral to therapist/psychiatrist and possible pharmacological treatment to help client deal with terminal illness or situation.*[7]

NURSING PRIORITY NO. 2 To assist client to deal with situation:

- Provide open and trusting relationship. *Promotes opportunity to explore feelings about impending death.*[2]
- Make time for nonjudgmental discussion of philosophical issues or questions about spiritual impact of illness or situation. *Can help client clarify own position on these issues.*[3]
- Respect client's desire or request not to talk. Provide hope within parameters of the individual situation. *Promotes open environment that encourages client to talk freely about thoughts and feelings. Client may not be ready to talk about situation or concerns about death, or he or she may be denying the reality of what is happening.*[1,8]
- Encourage expressions of feelings (e.g., anger, fear, sadness, etc.). Acknowledge anxiety or fear. Do not deny or reassure client that everything will be all right. Be honest when answering questions and providing information. *Enhances trust and a therapeutic relationship.*[2]
- Use therapeutic communication skills of active-listening. *Technique acknowledges reality of feelings and encourages client to find own solutions.*[2]
- Provide information about normalcy of feelings and individual grief reaction. *Most individuals question their reactions and whether they are normal, and information can provide reassurance.*[3] (Refer to ND Grieving.)
- Identify coping skills currently used and how effective they are. Be aware of defense mechanisms being used by the client. *Provides a starting point to plan care and assists client to acknowledge reality and deal more effectively with what is happening.*[3]
- Review life experiences of loss, noting client strengths and successes. *Provides opportunity to identify and use previously successful skills.*[2]
- Provide a calm, peaceful setting and privacy, as appropriate. *Promotes relaxation and enhances ability to deal with situation.*[8]
- Include family in discussions and decision making, as appropriate. *Involved family members can provide support and ideas for problem-solving.*[7]
- 🌐 Note client's religious or spiritual orientation, involvement in religious or church activities, and presence of conflicts regarding spiritual beliefs. *May benefit by referral to appropriate resource to help client resolve issues, if desired.*[7]
- Assist client to engage in spiritual growth activities, experience prayer or meditation, and practice forgiveness to heal past hurts. Provide information that anger with God is a normal part of the grief process. *May reduce feelings of guilt or conflict, allowing client to move forward toward resolution.*[1]

 Acute Care   Collaborative   Community/Home Care   Cultural

- Refer to therapists, spiritual advisors, or counselors, as appropriate. *Promotes facilitation of grief work.*
- Refer to community agencies and resources. *Assists client/SO in planning for eventualities (legal issues, hospice home care, funeral plans, etc.).*

NURSING PRIORITY NO. 3 To promote independence:

- Support client's efforts to develop realistic steps to put plans into action. *Provides sense of control over situation in which client does not have much control.*[1]
- Direct client's thoughts beyond the present state, encouraging him/her to try to enjoy each day and look to the future, as appropriate. *Being in the moment can help client enjoy this time rather than dwelling on what is ahead.*
- Provide opportunities for client to make simple decisions. *Enhances sense of control.*
- Develop individual plan using client's locus of control. *Incorporating locus of control (internal or external) enhances success of plan by enabling client/family to manage situation more effectively.*[2]
- Treat expressed decisions and desires with respect and convey to others, as appropriate. *Expresses regard for the individual and enhances sense of control in situation that is not controllable.*[8]
- Assist with completion of Advance Directives and cardiopulmonary resuscitation instructions. *Provides opportunity for client to understand options and express desires.*
- Refer to palliative, hospice, or end-of-life care resources, as appropriate. *Provides support and assistance to client and SO/family through potentially complex and difficult process. Choice of type of care is dependent on timing of care (e.g., palliative care interfaces with curative treatment, which hospice does not allow).*[1]

DOCUMENTATION FOCUS

Assessment/Reassessment
- Assessment findings, including client's fears and signs/symptoms being exhibited.
- Responses and actions of family/SOs.
- Availability and use of resources.

Planning
- Plan of care and who is involved in planning.

Implementation/Evaluation
- Client's response to interventions, teaching, and actions performed.
- Attainment or progress toward desired outcome(s).
- Modifications to plan of care.

Discharge Planning
- Identified needs and who is responsible for actions to be taken.
- Specific referrals made.

References

1. Rattan, A. (2012). The question about death and death anxiety. *Scrib.* Access to paid article March 2018 from https://www.scribd.com/document/39578680/Death-Anxiety.
2. Andrews, G., et al. (2002). *The Treatment of Anxiety Disorders: Clinician Guides and Patient Manuals.* 2nd ed. Cambridge, UK: Cambridge University Press.
3. Feifel, H., Branscomb, B. A. (1973). Who's afraid of death? *J Abnorm Psychol,* 81(3), 282–288.
4. Lipson, J. G. (1996). *Culture & Nursing Care: A Pocket Guide.* San Francisco, CA: School of Nursing, UCSF Nursing Press.
5. Kastenbaum, R. (1987). Death-related anxiety. In Michelson, L., Ascher, I. (eds). *Anxiety and Stress Disorders.* New York: Guilford Press.
6. Bruera, E., et al. (1995). The frequency of alcoholism among patients with pain due to terminal cancer. *J Pain Symptom Manage,* 10(8), 599–603.
7. Paice, J. (2002). Managing psychological conditions in palliative care. *Am J Nurs,* 102(11), 36–43.
8. Kouch, M. (2006). Managing symptoms for a "good death." *Nursing,* 36(11), 58–63.

 Diagnostic Studies   Evidence Based Practice   Medications   Pediatric/Geriatric/Lifespan

Decisional Conflict [Specify Level]

Taxonomy II: Life Principles—Class 3 Value/Belief/Action Congruence (00083) [Diagnostic Division: Ego Integrity], Approved 1988; Revised 2006

DEFINITION: Uncertainty about course of action to be taken when choice among competing actions involves risk, loss, or challenge to values and beliefs.

RELATED FACTORS

Conflict with moral obligation
Conflicting information sources; insufficient information
Inexperience with or interference in decision making
Moral principle, rule, or value supports mutually inconsistent actions
Unclear personal values or beliefs; perceived threat to value system

DEFINING CHARACTERISTICS

Subjective

Uncertainty about choices; recognizes undesired consequences of actions being considered
Distress while attempting a decision
Questioning of moral principle, rule, values, or personal beliefs/values while attempting a decision

Objective

Delay in decision making; vacillating among choices
Self-focused
Physical sign of tension or distress
Sample Clinical Applications: Therapeutic options with undesired side effects (e.g., amputation, visible scarring) or conflicting with belief system (e.g., blood transfusion, termination of pregnancy); chronic disease states, dementia, Alzheimer's disease, terminal or end-of-life situations

DESIRED OUTCOMES/EVALUATION CRITERIA

Sample NOC linkages:
Decision-Making: Ability to make judgments; choose between two or more alternatives
Health Beliefs: Personal convictions that influence health behaviors
Psychosocial Adjustment: Life Change: Psychosocial adaptation of an individual to a life change

Client Will (Include Specific Time Frame)
• Verbalize awareness of positive and negative aspect of choices and alternative actions.
• Acknowledge and ventilate feelings of anxiety and distress associated with choice or related to making difficult decision.
• Identify personal values and beliefs concerning issues.
• Make decision(s) and express satisfaction with choices.
• Meet psychological needs as evidenced by appropriate expression of feelings, identification of options, and use of resources.
• Display relaxed manner, calm demeanor, and be free of physical signs of distress.

 Acute Care Collaborative Community/ Home Care Cultural

ACTIONS/INTERVENTIONS

Sample NIC linkages:

Decision-Making Support: Providing information and support for a patient who is making a decision regarding healthcare

Values Clarification: Assisting another to clarify her/his own values in order to facilitate effective decision-making

Coping Enhancement: Facilitation of cognitive and behavioral efforts to manage perceived stressors, changes, or threats that interfere with meeting life demands and roles

NURSING PRIORITY NO. 1   To assess causative/contributing factors:

• ∞Determine usual ability to manage own affairs. Clarify who has legal right to intervene on behalf of child/developmentally delayed adult (e.g., parent, other relative, or court-appointed guardian/advocate). *Family disruption or conflicts can complicate decision-making process. All adults have the right to make their own decisions unless a legal court has ruled the individual is incompetent and a guardian is appointed.*[4]

• Note expressions of indecision, dependence on others, and availability and involvement of support persons (e.g., lack of or conflicting advice). *Care providers need to be sensitive to the physical, cognitive, and emotional effects of illness on decision-making capabilities and whether the individual wants to be involved in making the decision.*[6]

• Ascertain dependency of other(s) on client and/or issues of codependency. *Influence of others may lead client to make decision that is not what is really wanted or in his/her best interest.*[1]

• Active-listen and identify reason for indecisiveness. *Helps client to clarify problem and begin looking for resolution. May talk about uncertainty—and alternative choices that can lead to risky, uncertain outcomes—and the need to make value judgments about losses versus gains.*[2,6]

• ⊕Identify cultural values and beliefs or moral obligations and principles that may be creating conflict for client and complicating decision-making process. *These issues must be addressed before client can be at peace with the decision that is made.*[5]

• Determine effectiveness of current problem-solving techniques. *Provides information about client's ability to make decisions that are needed or desired.*[1]

• Note presence and intensity of physical signs of anxiety (e.g., increased heart rate, muscle tension). *Client may be conflicted about the decision that is required and may need help to deal with anxiety to begin to deal with reality of situation. Different treatment decisions may have more uncertainty and generate more conflict in client.*[2,6]

• Listen for expressions of inability to find meaning in life or reason for living, feelings of futility, or alienation from God or others. (Refer to ND Spiritual Distress, as indicated.) *May need to talk about reasons for feelings of alienation to resolve concerns and may engage in questioning about own values.*[6,10]

• Review information client has to support the decision to be made. *Inaccurate or incomplete information and misinterpretations complicate the process and may result in a poor outcome.*[7,8]

NURSING PRIORITY NO. 2   To assist client to develop/effectively use problem-solving skills:

• Promote safe and hopeful environment, as needed. *Client needs to be protected and supported while he or she regains inner control.*[7]

• Encourage verbalization of conflicts and concerns. *Helps client to clarify these issues so he or she can come to a resolution of the situation.*[7,8]

• Accept verbal expressions of anger or guilt. Set limits on maladaptive behavior. *Verbalization of feelings enables client to sift through feelings and begin to deal with situation. Behavior that is inappropriate is not helpful for dealing with the situation and will lead to feelings of guilt and low self-worth.*[2]

 Diagnostic Studies   Evidence Based Practice   Medications   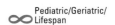 Pediatric/Geriatric/ Lifespan   **239**

- Clarify and prioritize individual goals, noting where the subject of the "conflict" falls on this scale. *Helps to identify importance of problems client is addressing, enabling realistic problem-solving.*[2]
- Identify strengths and use of positive coping skills (e.g., use of relaxation techniques, willingness to express feelings). *Helpful for developing solutions to current situation.*[1]
- Identify positive aspects of this experience and assist client to view it as a learning opportunity. *Reframing the situation can help the client see things in a different light, enabling client to develop new and creative solutions.*[1]
- Correct misperceptions client may have and provide factual information, as needed. *Promotes understanding and enables client to make better decisions for own situation.*[1,6]
- Provide opportunities for client to make simple decisions regarding self-care and other daily activities. Accept choice not to do so. Advance complexity of choices, as tolerated. *Acceptance of what client wants to do, with gentle encouragement to progress, enhances self-esteem and ability to try more. Providing individualized decision support can help the client move to more difficult decisions.*[1,6]
- ∞ Encourage child to make developmentally appropriate decisions concerning own care. *Fosters child's sense of self-worth and enhances ability to learn and exercise coping skills.*[4]
- Discuss time considerations, setting time line for small steps and considering consequences related to not making or postponing specific decisions to facilitate resolution of conflict. *When time is a factor in making a decision, these strategies can promote movement toward solution.*[4]
- Have client list some alternatives to present situation or decisions, using a brainstorming process. Include family in this activity, as indicated (e.g., placement of parent in long-term care facility, use of intervention process with addicted member). *Involving family and looking at different options can promote successful resolution of decision to be made.* Refer to NDs interrupted Family Processes, dysfunctional Family Processes, compromised family Coping, Moral Distress.[7,8]
- Practice use of problem-solving process with current situation and decision. *Promotes identification of different possibilities that may not have been thought of otherwise.*[1]
- Discuss and clarify spiritual concerns, accepting client's values in a nonjudgmental manner. *Client will be willing to consider own situation when accepted as an individual of worth.*[5]

NURSING PRIORITY NO. 3   To promote wellness (Teaching/Discharge Considerations):

- 🏠 Promote opportunities for using conflict-resolution skills, identifying steps as client does each one. *Learning this process can help to solve current dilemma and provide the person with skills he or she can use in the future.*[3]
- Provide positive feedback for efforts and progress noted. *Client needs to hear he or she is doing well, and feedback promotes continuation of efforts.*[2]
- Encourage involvement of family/significant others (SOs), as desired or available. *Provides support for the client and facilitates resolution.*[9]
- Support client for decisions made, especially if consequences are unexpected or difficult to cope with. *Positive feedback promotes feelings of success even when difficult situations occur or outcome is less than desired.*[9]
- Ⓐ Encourage attendance at stress-reduction or assertiveness classes. *Learning these skills can help client achieve a lowered stress level that can promote ability to make decisions.*[4]
- Ⓐ Refer to other resources, as necessary (e.g., clergy, psychiatric clinical nurse specialist or psychiatrist, family or marital therapist, addiction support groups). *May need this additional help to deal with complicated problems and facilitate problem-solving and decision making.*[2]

DOCUMENTATION FOCUS

Assessment/Reassessment
- Assessment findings, behavioral responses, degree of impairment in lifestyle functioning.
- Individuals involved in the conflict.
- Personal values and beliefs.

 Acute Care   Collaborative   Community/ Home Care   Cultural

Planning
- Plan of care, specific interventions, and who is involved in the planning process.
- Teaching plan.

Implementation/Evaluation
- Client's and involved individuals' responses to interventions, teaching, and actions performed.
- Ability to express feelings and identify options.
- Use of resources.
- Attainment or progress toward desired outcome(s).
- Modifications to plan of care.

Discharge Planning
- Long-term needs, actions to be taken, and who is responsible for doing.
- Specific referrals made.

References

1. Tversky, A., Kahneman, D. (No date). The framing of decisions and the psychology of choice. Retrieved March 2018 from http://rangevoting.org/TverskyK81.html.
2. Paul, M. (2009). Relationships: The art of listening. Retrieved March 2018 from http://www.innerbonding.com/show-article/2147/relationships-the-art-of-listening.html.
3. Bolstad, R., Blamlett, M. (No date). Win-Win. Retrieved March 2018 from http://www.nlpca.com/DCweb/winwin.html.
4. Krull, E. (2010). Family conflict power struggles. Psych Central. Retrieved March 2018 from http://blogs.psychcentral.com/family/2010/01/family-conflict-power-struggles/.
5. Purnell, L. D. (2011). *Guide to Culturally Competent Health Care*. 2nd ed. Philadelphia: F. A. Davis.
6. Osborne, H. (2004). Helping patients make difficult decisions. Retrieved March 2018 from http://www.healthliteracy.com/article.asp?PageID=3808.
7. Liken, M. A. (2001). Caregivers in crisis: Moving a relative with Alzheimer's to assisted living. *Clin Nurs Res*, 10(1), 53–69.
8. Liken, M. A. (2001). Experiences of family caregivers of a relative with Alzheimer's disease. *J Psychosoc Nurs*, 39(12), 33–37.
9. Harris, J. C., Halper, J. (2008). *Multiple Sclerosis: Best Practices in Nursing Care*. New York: Bioscience Communications.
10. Zikmund-Fisher, B. J. (2010). Deficits and variations in patients' experience with making 9 common medical decisions: The DECISIONS Survey. *Med Decis Making*, 30(5 Suppl), S85–S95.

---

readiness for enhanced Decision-Making

Taxonomy II: Life Principles—Class 3 Value/Belief/Action Congruence (00184) [Diagnostic Division: Ego Integrity], Submitted 2006; Revised 2013

DEFINITION: A pattern of choosing a course of action for meeting short- and long-term health-related goals, which can be strengthened.

DEFINING CHARACTERISTICS

Subjective

Expresses desire to enhance decision making, risk-benefit analysis of decisions

Expresses desire to enhance congruency of decisions with goal/values, or sociocultural values/goal

Expresses desire to enhance understanding of choices for decision making, meaning of choices

Expresses desire to enhance use of reliable evidence for decisions

Sample Clinical Applications: Any acute or chronic condition, or healthy individual looking to improve well-being

(continues on page 242)

 Diagnostic Studies   Evidence Based Practice   Medications   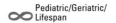 Pediatric/Geriatric/Lifespan

readiness for enhanced Decision-Making (continued)

DESIRED OUTCOMES/EVALUATION CRITERIA

Sample **NOC** linkages:

Decision-Making: Ability to make judgments and choose between two or more alternatives
Health Beliefs: Personal convictions that influence health behaviors
Personal Autonomy: Personal actions of a competent individual to exercise governance in life decisions
Health-Promoting Behavior: Personal actions to sustain or increase wellness

Client Will (Include Specific Time Frame)

- Identify risks and benefit of decisions.
- Express beliefs about the meaning of choices.
- Make decisions that are congruent with personal and sociocultural values and goals.
- Use reliable evidence for decisions.

ACTION/INTERVENTIONS

Sample **NIC** linkages:

Decision-Making Support: Providing information and support for a patient who is making a decision regarding healthcare
Values Clarification: Assisting another to clarify her/his own values in order to facilitate effective decision-making
Teaching: Individual: Planning, implementation, and evaluation of a teaching program designed to address a patient's particular needs

NURSING PRIORITY NO. 1 To assess causative/contributing factors:

- Determine usual ability to manage own affairs. *Provides baseline for understanding client's decision-making process. There may be variations in attitudes toward risk in different areas of the country that will affect this individual's decision-making preferences.*[8]
- Note expressions of decision, dependability, and availability of support persons. *Having support for decision making and having good information regarding pros and cons of choices helps client to feel comfortable with the decisions made.*[8]
- Active-listen and identify reason(s) client would like to improve decision-making abilities and expectations for change. *As client articulates reasons for improvement, they become more clear, and direction is provided.*[2] *Motivation to improve and high expectations can encourage client to make changes that will improve his or her life. However, presence of external locus of control or unrealistic expectations may hamper efforts.*
- Note presence of physical signs of anxiety. *Client may be excited about the quest for improvement, and excitement may be interpreted as anxiety. It is important to clarify meaning of physical signs.*[2]
- Identify cultural values, beliefs, or moral obligations and principles that guide or affect the decision-making process. *Preconceived biases may color decisions and need to be recognized in order to enhance efforts toward growth.*[5]
- Discuss meaning of life, reasons for living, belief in God or higher power, and how these relate to current desire for improvement or growth. *Helps client to clarify beliefs and how they relate to decision-making process.*[6] (Refer to ND readiness for enhanced Spiritual Well-Being.)

NURSING PRIORITY NO. 2 To assist client to improve/effectively use problem-solving skills:

- Promote safe and hopeful environment and help client identify own inner control. *Will help client understand the control he or she has over decisions made.*[1]

 Acute Care
 Collaborative
 Community/ Home Care
 Cultural

- Encourage verbalization of ideas, concerns, and particular decisions that need to be made.[6]
- Correct misperceptions client may have and provide factual information as needed. *Promotes understanding and enables client to make better decisions for own situation.*[1,8]
- Clarify and prioritize individual's goals, noting possible conflicts or "stumbling" blocks that may be encountered. *As client weighs pros and cons of decision making, taking into account negative aspects of situation, decisions will be more realistic and acceptable to client.*[3]
- Discuss dependence on others, involvement of support persons, and possibility for conflicting advice or goals. *While it is appropriate to consider the opinions of others when making choices, one needs to be aware of the potential for conflicting views when seeking advice and make own decisions free of pressure from others.*[8]
- Identify positive aspects of this experience and assist client to view it as a learning opportunity. *As client reframes experience as an opportunity, he or she will be able to use this learning for future situations.*[3]
- Assist client in learning how to find factual information (e.g., use of the library, Internet). *Individual who takes advantage of these resources will benefit from the knowledge gained. Client will need to be cautious in evaluating information to verify accuracy.*[8]
- Discuss the process of performing a risk-benefit analysis to aid in making decisions. *The individual who learns this skill will be able to use it in many areas of life to enhance relationships, both personal and business.*[3]
- Have client list some alternatives to present decisions, using a brainstorming process. Include significant other (SO)/family in this activity if appropriate. *Looking at different options can strengthen the decision-making process.*[7]
- ∞ Encourage children to make age-appropriate decisions. *Learning problem-solving at an early age will enhance sense of self-worth and ability to exercise coping skills.*
- ⊕ Discuss and clarify spiritual beliefs, accepting client's values in a nonjudgmental manner. *Client may be able to decide what is really acceptable or unacceptable in the choice situation related to beliefs or values that have been expressed.*[8]

NURSING PRIORITY NO. 3   To promote optimum well-being (Teaching/Discharge Considerations):

- 🏠 Identify opportunities for using conflict-resolution skills. *Emphasizing each step as it is used will help with learning these skills.*[6]
- Provide positive feedback for efforts, growth in use of skills, and learning efforts. *As individual is moving forward in learning new skills, hearing positive feedback provides reinforcement for individuals to continue efforts.*[3]
- Encourage involvement of family/SOs as desired/appropriate. *Helps all family members to improve conflict-resolution skills. When family works together, relationships are enhanced and family members can live fuller lives.*[4]
- Recommend attending stress-reduction and/or assertiveness classes as desired. *Individual can learn additional skills to enhance decision making, improving ability to make life better.*[2]
- 🔖 Refer to other resources as necessary (e.g., clergy, psychiatrist, clinical psychiatric nurse specialist, family/marital therapist). *May need additional counseling to help with specific concerns.*[4]

DOCUMENTATION FOCUS

Assessment/Reassessment
- Assessment findings, behavioral responses.
- Individuals involved in improving conflict skills.
- Personal values, beliefs, and motivation for change.

Planning
- Plan of care, specific interventions, and who is involved in the planning process.
- Teaching plan.

Implementation/Evaluation
- Client's and involved individual's responses to interventions, teaching, and actions performed.
- Ability to express feelings, identify options, use resources.

 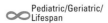

- Attainment or progress toward desired outcomes(s).
- Modifications to plan of care.

Discharge Planning
- Long-term needs, actions to be taken, and who is responsible for doing.
- Specific referrals made.

References

1. Pryor, J., Jannings, W. (2004). Preparing patients to self-manage faecal continence following spinal cord injury. *Int J Ther Rehabil*, 11(2), 79–82.
2. Salem, R. (2003). Empathic listening. Beyond intractability. Retrieved March 2018 from http://www.beyondintractability.org/essay/empathic_listening/.
3. Dunn, S. (Updated 2004). Pros and cons of researching your cancer. *CancerGuide*. Retrieved March 2018 from http://www.cancerguide.org/pros_cons.html.
4. Peterson, R., Green, S. (2009). Families first—keys to successful family functioning: Problem solving. Department of Human Development, Virginia Tech. Retrieved March 2018 from http://www.pubs.ext.vt.edu/350/350-091/350-091.html.
5. Dietrich, C. (2010). Decision making: Factors that influence decision-making, heuristics used, and decision outcomes. Inquiries Journal. Retrieved March 2018 from http://www.inquiriesjournal.com/articles/180/decision-making-factors-that-influence-decision-making-heuristics-used-and-decision-outcomes.
6. Brandt, A. L. (2000). Transition issues for the elderly and their families. Retrieved March 2018 from http://www.ec-online.net/knowledge/articles/brandttransitions.html.
7. Liken, M. A. (2001). Caregivers in crisis: Moving a relative with Alzheimer's to assisted living. *Clin Nurs Res*, 10(1), 53–69.
8. Osborne, H. (2004). Helping patients make difficult decisions. Health Literacy Consulting. Retrieved March 2018 from http://www.healthliteracy.com/article.asp?PageID=3808.

ineffective Denial

Taxonomy II: Coping/Stress Tolerance—Class 2 Coping Responses (00072) [**Diagnostic Division:** Ego Integrity], Approved 1988; Revised 2006

DEFINITION: Conscious or unconscious attempt to disavow the knowledge or meaning of an event to reduce anxiety and/or fear, leading to the detriment of health.

RELATED FACTORS

Anxiety; perceived inadequacy in dealing with strong emotions
Insufficient sense of control; fear of losing autonomy
Excessive stress; ineffective coping strategies
Threat of unpleasant reality
Fear of separation, death
Insufficient emotional support

DEFINING CHARACTERISTICS

Subjective

Minimizes symptoms; displaces source of symptoms
Does not admit impact of disease on life
Displaces fear of impact of the condition
Denies fear of death or invalidism

Objective

Delay in seeking healthcare; refusal of healthcare
Does not perceive relevance of symptoms, danger
Use of dismissive gestures or comments when speaking of distressing event
Inappropriate affect

 Acute Care   Collaborative   Community/Home Care   Cultural

Use of treatment not advised by healthcare professional

Sample Clinical Applications: Chronic illnesses, eating disorders, substance abuse, Alzheimer's disease, terminal conditions, bipolar disorder, body dysmorphic disorder

DESIRED OUTCOMES/EVALUATION CRITERIA

Sample **NOC** linkages:

Acceptance: Health Status: Personal actions to reconcile significant changes in health circumstances

Health Beliefs: Perceived Threat: Personal conviction that a threatening health problem is serious and has potential negative consequences for lifestyle

Psychosocial Adjustment: Life Change: Adaptive psychosocial response of an individual to a significant life circumstance

Client Will (Include Specific Time Frame)

- Acknowledge reality of situation or illness.
- Express realistic concern and feelings about symptoms or illness.
- Seek appropriate assistance for presenting problem.
- Display appropriate affect.

ACTIONS/INTERVENTIONS

Sample **NIC** linkages:

Anxiety Reduction: Minimizing apprehension, dread, foreboding, or uneasiness related to an unidentified source of anticipated danger

Counseling: Use of an interactive helping process focusing on the needs, problems, or feelings of the patient and significant others to enhance or support coping, problem-solving, and interpersonal relationships

Coping Enhancement: Facilitation of cognitive and behavioral effort to manage perceived stressors, changes, or threats that interfere with meeting life demands and roles

NURSING PRIORITY NO. 1   To assess causative/contributing factors:

- Identify situational crisis or problem and client's perception of the situation. *Identification of both reality and client's perception, which may not be the same as the reality, is necessary for planning care accurately.*[1]
- Ascertain cultural values or religious beliefs affecting perception of situation and sense of personal responsibility for crisis. *Client will make choices regarding therapeutic regimen or lifestyle changes incorporating own cultural and social factors. Conflicts may arise when provider and patient disagree on healthcare beliefs and practices. Knowing that lifestyle or choices may have caused or contributed to current situation may limit client's ability to accept outcome or view event realistically.*[5,7]
- Determine stage and degree of denial. *These factors will help identify whether the client is in early stages of denial and may be more amenable to intervention than those who are well entrenched in their beliefs. Treatment needs to begin where the client is and progress from there.*[1,6]
- Compare client's description of symptoms or conditions to reality of clinical picture and impact of illness or problem on lifestyle. *Identifies extent of discrepancy between the two and where treatment needs to start to help client accept reality.*[1]

NURSING PRIORITY NO. 2   To assist client to deal appropriately with situation:

- Develop nurse-client relationship using therapeutic communication skills of active-listening and "I" messages. *Promotes trust in which client can begin to look at reality of situation and deal with it in a positive manner.*[2]

 Diagnostic Studies   Evidence Based Practice   Medications   Pediatric/Geriatric/ Lifespan

- Provide safe, nonthreatening environment. *Allows client to feel comfortable enough to talk freely without fear of judgment and to deal with issues realistically.*[2]
- Encourage expressions of feelings, accepting client's view of the situation without confrontation. Set limits on maladaptive behavior *to promote safety. Helps client to work through and understand feelings. Unacceptable behavior is counterproductive to making progress, as client will view self negatively.*[2]
- Present accurate information as appropriate, without insisting that the client accept what has been presented. *Avoids confrontation, which may further entrench client in denial. Open manner permits client to feel value of self in situation and to begin to accept reality.*[2,7]
- Discuss client's behaviors in relation to illness (e.g., diabetes mellitus, alcoholism, chronic pain conditions, terminal cancer) and point out the results of these behaviors. *Information can help client accept reality and opt to change behaviors.*[3]
- Encourage client to talk with significant others (SO[s]/friends). *May clarify concerns and reduce isolation and withdrawal. Constructive feedback from others facilitates understanding.*[4]
- Involve in group sessions. *Promotes discussion and feedback to enhance learning. Client can hear other views of reality and test own perceptions.*[4]
- Avoid agreeing with inaccurate statements or perceptions. *Prevents perpetuating false reality.*[2]
- Provide positive feedback for constructive moves toward independence. *Promotes repetition of desired behavior.*[4]

NURSING PRIORITY NO. 3   To promote wellness (Teaching/Discharge Considerations):

- Provide written information about illness or situation for client and family. *Provides client/family with reminders and resources they can refer to as they consider options.*[1]
- Involve family members/SO(s) in long-range planning. *Provides support and helps to identify and meet individual needs for the future.*[4]
- Refer to appropriate community resources (e.g., Diabetes Association, MS Society, Alcoholics Anonymous). *May be needed to help client with long-term adjustment.*
- Refer to ND ineffective Coping.

DOCUMENTATION FOCUS

Assessment/Reassessment
- Assessment findings, degree of personal vulnerability and denial.
- Impact of illness or problem on lifestyle.

Planning
- Plan of care and who is involved in the planning.
- Teaching plan.

Implementation/Evaluation
- Client's response to interventions, teaching, and actions performed.
- Use of resources.
- Attainment or progress toward desired outcome(s).
- Modifications to plan of care.

Discharge Planning
- Long-term needs and who is responsible for actions taken.
- Specific referrals made.

 Acute Care   Collaborative   Community/ Home Care   Cultural

References

1. Mayo Clinic Staff (Updated 2017). Denial: When it helps, when it hurts. Retrieved March 2018 from http://www.mayoclinic.org/healthy-lifestyle/adult-health/in-depth/denial/art-20047926.
2. Grinstead, S. F. (2009, updated 2014). Overcoming resistance and denial for effective pain management. Retrieved March 2018 from http://dbhdid.ky.gov/dbh/documents/ksaods/2014/Grinstead1.pdf.
3. Burgess, E. (1994). Denial and terminal illness. *Am J Hosp Palliat Care*, 11(2), 46–48.
4. Robinson, A. W. (1999). Getting to the heart of denial. *Am J Nurs*, 99(5), 38–42.
5. Ngo-Metzger, Q., et al. (2003). Linguistic and cultural barriers to care: Perspectives of Chinese and Vietnamese immigrants. *J Gen Int Med*, 18(1), 44–52.
6. Jacelon, C. S., Henneman, E. A. (2004). Profiles in dignity: Nursing perspectives on nursing and critically ill older patients. *Crit Care Nurse*, 24(4), 30–35.
7. Lawton, G. (2017). Living on the borderline: How I embraced my mixed-race status after years of denial. The Guardian. Retrieved March 2018 from https://www.theguardian.com/lifeandstyle/2017/aug/26/living-on-the-borderline-how-i-embraced-my-mixed-race-status-after-years-of-denial.

---

impaired Dentition

Taxonomy II: Safety/Protection—Class 2 Physical Injury (00048) [**Diagnostic Division:** Food/Fluid], Approved 1998; Revised 2017

DEFINITION: Disruption in tooth development/eruption patterns or structural integrity of individual teeth.

RELATED FACTORS

Barrier to self-care; difficulty accessing dental care
Excessive intake of fluoride or use of abrasive oral cleaning agents
Habitual use of staining substances [e.g., tobacco, coffee, tea, red wine]
Inadequate dietary habits; malnutrition
Pharmaceutical agent
Inadequate oral hygiene
Insufficient knowledge of dental health

DEFINING CHARACTERISTICS

Subjective
Toothache

Objective
Halitosis
Enamel discoloration; erosion of enamel; excessive oral plaque/calculus
Abraded teeth; dental or root caries; tooth fracture; loose tooth; absence of teeth
Premature loss of primary teeth; incomplete tooth eruption for age
Malocclusion; tooth misalignment; facial asymmetry
At Risk Population:
Economically disadvantaged; genetic predisposition
Associated Condition: Bruxism, chronic vomiting; oral temperature sensitivity; pharmaceutical agent
Sample Clinical Applications: Facial trauma or surgery, malnutrition, eating disorders, head or neck cancer, seizure disorder

(continues on page 248)

 Diagnostic Studies   Evidence Based Practice   Medications   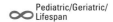 Pediatric/Geriatric/Lifespan

impaired Dentition (continued)

DESIRED OUTCOMES/EVALUATION CRITERIA

Sample NOC linkages:

Oral Health: Condition of the mouth, teeth, gums, and tongue

Self-Care: Oral Hygiene: Personal actions to care for own mouth and teeth independently with or without assistive device

Knowledge: Health Behavior: Extent of understanding conveyed about the promotion and protection of health

Client/SO Will (Include Specific Time Frame)

- Display healthy gums and mucous membranes and teeth that are in good repair.
- Report adequate nutritional and fluid intake.
- Verbalize understanding of appropriate oral hygiene regimen.
- Demonstrate effective dental hygiene skills.
- Follow through on referrals for appropriate dental care.

ACTION/INTERVENTIONS

Sample NIC linkages:

Oral Health Restoration: Promotion of healing for a patient who has an oral mucosa or dental lesion

Teaching: Individual: Planning, implementation, and evaluation of a teaching program designed to address a patient's particular needs

Referral: Arrangement for services by another care provider or agency

NURSING PRIORITY NO. 1   To assess causative/contributing factors:

- Inspect oral cavity. Note presence or absence and intactness of teeth or dentures and appearance of gums. *Provides baseline for planning and interventions in terms of safety, nutritional needs, and aesthetics.*
- Evaluate current status of dental hygiene and oral health *to determine need for instruction or coaching, assistive devices, and/or referral to dental care providers.*
- Note presence of halitosis. *Bad breath may be result of numerous local or systemic conditions, including smoking, periodontal disease, dehydration, malnutrition, ketoacidosis, nasal and sinus infections, and some medications and drugs. Management can include improved mouth care or treatment of underlying conditions.*[11]
- ∞ Document age, developmental and cognitive status, and manual dexterity. Evaluate nutritional and health state, noting presence of conditions such as bulimia or chronic vomiting; musculoskeletal impairments; or problems with mouth (e.g., bleeding disorders, cancer lesions, abscesses, facial trauma). *Factors affecting client's dental health and ability to provide effective oral care.*[1,12]
- Note current situation that will affect dental health (e.g., presence of airway/endotracheal [ET] intubation, facial fractures, jaw surgery, new braces, use of anticoagulants or chemotherapy) that require special mouth care activities.[7,8]
- Document (photograph) facial injuries before treatment *to provide "pictorial baseline" for future comparison and evaluation.*

NURSING PRIORITY NO. 2   To treat/manage dental care needs:

- Ascertain client's usual method of oral care *to provide continuity of care or to build on client's existing knowledge base and current practices in developing plan of care.*
- Assist with or provide oral care, as indicated:[2,8,9,12]
  Offer tap water or saline rinses or diluted alcohol-free mouthwashes.

 Acute Care   Collaborative   Community/Home Care   Cultural

Provide gentle gum massage and tongue brushing with soft toothbrush using fluoride toothpaste *to manage tartar buildup, if appropriate.*

Use foam sticks *to swab gums and oral cavity when brushing is not possible or inadvisable.*

Assist with brushing and flossing when client is unable to do self-care.

Demonstrate and assist with electric or battery-powered mouth care devices (e.g., toothbrush, plaque remover) as indicated.

Assist with or provide denture care when indicated (e.g., remove and clean after meals and at bedtime).

- ∞ Remind client to brush teeth as indicated. *Cues, modeling, or pantomime may be helpful if client is young, elderly, or cognitively or emotionally impaired.*[12]
- ✚ Reposition ET tubes and airway adjuncts routinely, carefully padding and protecting teeth and prosthetics.[7]
- Suction as needed if client is unable to manage secretions.
- Remind client of importance of maintaining good jaw and facial alignment when fractures are present.
- ∞ ▤ Encourage appropriate diet for optimal nutrition, considering client's special needs such as pregnancy, age and developmental concerns, and ability to chew (e.g., liquids or soft foods) and offering low-sugar, low-starch foods and snacks *to minimize tooth decay and improve overall health. Note: Emerging research is revealing important relationships between nutrition, tooth decay, and periodontal disease and chronic health conditions such as heart disease, diabetes, and immune-compromising conditions.*[2,9,13]
- Encourage client to avoid thermal stimuli *when teeth are sensitive* and to use specific toothpastes designed *to reduce sensitivity of teeth.*
- ⚕ Administer antibiotics as needed *to treat oral or gum infections that may be present and to prevent hospital-acquired infection in the critically ill client whose teeth or gums may be colonized by significant bacteria.*[3]
- ⚕ Recommend use of analgesics and topical analgesics as needed *when dental pain is present.*
- ⚕ Administer prophylactic antibiotic therapy prior to some dental procedures *in susceptible individuals* (e.g., presence of prosthetic heart valve, prior infective endocarditis, certain congenital heart defects, cardiac transplant with subsequent valvulopathy) *to reduce risk of infective endocarditis or migration of bacteria to other body organs.*[10]
- ⊕ Direct client to notify dental care provider when bleeding disorder is present or anticoagulant therapy (including aspirin) is being used. *May impact choice of procedure or technique in order to prevent excess bleeding.*
- ⊕ Refer to appropriate care providers (e.g., nutritionist, dental hygienists, dentists, periodontist, oral surgeon).

NURSING PRIORITY NO. 3 To promote wellness (Teaching/Discharge Considerations):

- ⌂ Instruct client/caregiver to inspect oral cavity and in home-care interventions *to provide good oral care and prevent tooth decay and periodontal disease.*[4,5,9]
- ∞ Review or demonstrate proper toothbrushing techniques (e.g., spending several minutes brushing, reaching all tooth surfaces, brushing with bristles at a "45-degree angle" to teeth surfaces) after meals, and daily flossing. Suggest brushing with fluoride-containing toothpaste if client is able to swallow and manage oral secretions. Avoid sharing toothbrushes. Brush child's teeth until he/she can perform alone. *This is the most effective way of reducing oral bacteria and plaque formation and preventing cavities and periodontal disease.*[8]
- Discuss dental and oral health needs, both as client perceives needs and according to professional standards. *Client's perceptions are shaped by self-image, family, and cultural expectations or conditions created by disease or trauma. Current healthcare practices and education are geared toward practices that improve client's appearance and health, including reduced consumption of refined sugars, optimal fluoridation, access to preventative and restorative dental care, prevention of oral cancers, and prevention of craniofacial injuries.*[4,5]
- ∞ Recommend that clients of all ages decrease sugary and high-carbohydrate foods in diet and snacks *to reduce buildup of plaque and risk of cavities caused by acids associated with the breakdown of sugar and starch.*[4]
- ∞ Instruct older client and caregiver(s) concerning their special needs and importance of regular dental care. *Elderly are prone to experience decay around older fillings (also have more fillings in mouth); have receding gums, exposing root surfaces, which decay easily; have reduced production of saliva and use multiple*

 Diagnostic Studies   Evidence Based Practice   Medications   Pediatric/Geriatric/Lifespan

medications that can cause dry mouth with loss of tooth and gum protection; and have loosening of teeth or poorly fitting dentures associated with gum or bone loss. These factors (often compounded by disease conditions and lack of funds) affect nutrient intake, chewing, swallowing, and oral cavity health.[5,12]

- ∞ Advise mother regarding age-appropriate concerns:[1,4–6]

  Instruct mother to refrain from allowing baby to fall asleep with bottle containing formula, milk, or sweetened beverages. Suggest use of water and pacifier during night *to prevent bottle tooth decay.*

  Determine pattern of tooth appearance and tooth loss and compare to norms for primary and secondary teeth.

  Discuss tooth discoloration and needed follow-up. *Brown or black spots on teeth usually indicate decay; gray tooth color may indicate nerve injury; and multiple cavities in adolescent could be caused from repeated vomiting or bulimia.*

  Discuss pit and fissure sealants. *Painted-on tooth surface sealants are becoming widely available to reduce number of cavities and sometimes are available through community dental programs.*

  Determine if school dental health programs are available or recommend regular professional dental examinations as child grows.

  Discuss with children/parents problems associated with oral piercing if individual is contemplating piercing or needs to know what to watch for after piercing. *Common symptoms that occur with piercing of lips, gums, and tongue include pain, swelling, infection, increased flow of saliva, and chipped or cracked teeth requiring diligent oral care or more frequent dental examination to prevent complications.*

  Discuss use of or need for safety devices (e.g., helmets, face mask, mouth guards) *to prevent or limit severity of sports-related facial injuries and tooth damage or loss.*

- ∞ 📝 Discuss with pregnant women special needs and regular dental care. *Pregnant women need additional calcium and phosphorus to maintain good dental health and provide for strong teeth and bones in fetal development. Many women avoid dental care during pregnancy because of concerns for fetal health or for other reasons (including lack of financial resources). However, one research study of 400 women suggests that pregnant women who receive treatment for periodontal disease can reduce their risk of giving birth to a low-birth-weight or preterm baby.*[14]

- 🖐 Review resources that are needed and available for the client to perform adequate dental hygiene care (e.g., toothbrush, paste, clean water, referral to dental care providers, access to financial assistance, personal care assistant).

- 🖐 Encourage cessation of tobacco (especially smokeless) and enrolling in smoking-cessation classes *to reduce risk of oral cancers and other health problems.*

- 🖐 Discuss advisability of dental checkup and care prior to instituting chemotherapy or radiation *to minimize oral, dental, or tissue damage.*

DOCUMENTATION FOCUS

Assessment/Reassessment
- Individual findings, including individual factors influencing dentition problems.
- Baseline photos and description of oral cavity or structures.

Planning
- Plan of care and who is involved in planning.
- Teaching plan.

Implementation/Evaluation
- Responses to interventions, teaching, and actions performed.
- Attainment or progress toward desired outcome(s).
- Modifications to plan of care.

Discharge Planning
- Individual long-term needs, noting who is responsible for actions to be taken.
- Specific referrals made.

 Acute Care   Collaborative   Community/Home Care   Cultural

References

1. Gussy, M. G., et al. (2006). Early childhood caries: Current evidence for aetiology and prevention. *J Paediatr Child Health*, 42, 37–43.
2. Centers for Disease Control and Prevention (CDC). (Updated 2016). Oral health conditions 2011. Retrieved March 2018 from http://198.246.124.29/chronicdisease/resources/publications/aag/pdf/2011/oral-health-aag-pdf-508.pdf.
3. Halyard Health Inc. (2016). Oral care in mechanically ventilated patients: Review of clinical data. Retrieved October 2018 from https://www.halyardhealth.co.uk/media/17600873/hc690-00-uk-oralcompendium.pdf.
4. American Dental Association. (2002). NAS panel reaffirms effectiveness of fluoride. Retrieved March 2018 from https://fluoridealert.org/news/nas-panel-reaffirms-effectiveness-of-fluoride/.
5. A healthy smile for life. (2015). Mount Nittany Health. Retrieved March 2018 from http://www.mountnittany.org/articles/a-healthy-smile-for-life.
6. Engel, J. (2002). *Mosby's Pocket Guide to Pediatric Assessment*. 4th ed. St. Louis, MO: Mosby.
7. Truman, B., et al. (2002). Recommendations on selected interventions to prevent dental caries, oral and pharyngeal cancers, and sports-related craniofacial injuries. *Am J Prev Med*, 23(1 Suppl), 21–54.
8. Stiefel, K. A., et al. (2000). Improving oral hygiene for the seriously ill patient: Implementing research-based practice. *Medsurg Nurs*, 9(1), 40–43.
9. Healthwise Staff. (Updated 2015). Tooth decay: Prevention. Retrieved March 2018 from http://www.webmd.com/oral-health/tc/tooth-decay-topic-overview.
10. Stiles, S., Vega, C. P. (Updated 2008). AHA updates recommendations for antibiotic prophylaxis for dental procedures. Retrieved March 2018 from www.medscape.org/viewarticle/555596.
11. Porter, S. R., Scully, C. (2006). Oral malodour (halitosis). *BMJ*, 333(7569), 632–635.
12. Stein, P. S., Henry, R. G. (2009). Poor oral hygiene in long-term care. *Am J Nurs*, 109(6), 44–50.
13. Palmer, C. A., Burnett, D. J., Dean, B. (2010). It's more than just candy: Important relationships between nutrition and oral health. *Nutr Today*, 45(4), 154–164.
14. Lopez, N. J., Smith, P. C., Guiterrez, J. (2002). Periodontal therapy may reduce the risk of preterm low birth weight in women with periodontal disease: A randomized controlled trial. *J Periodontol*, 73(8), 911–924.

risk for delayed Development

Taxonomy II: Growth/Development—Class 2 Development (00112) [**Diagnostic Division:** Teaching/Learning], Submitted 1998; Revised 2013, 2017

DEFINITION: Susceptible to delay of 25% or more in one or more of the areas of social or self-regulatory behavior, or in cognitive, language, gross, or fine motor skills, which may compromise health.

RISK FACTORS
Inadequate nutrition
Presence of abuse; substance misuse/[abuse]

Individual
At Risk Population:
Behavioral disorder
Economically disadvantaged; maternal functional illiteracy
Exposure to violence or natural disaster
History of adoption; involvement with the foster care system
Inadequate maternal nutrition; insufficient or late-term prenatal care
Maternal age ≤15 years or ≥35 years; maternal substance misuse/[abuse], positive drug screen
Unplanned or unwanted pregnancy
Associated Condition: Brain injury; seizure disorder
Caregiver learning disability or mental health issue
Chronic illness; prenatal infection; recurrent otitis media
Congenital or genetic disorder; endocrine or seizure disorders
Failure to thrive; hearing or vision impairment

(continues on page 252)

 Diagnostic Studies
 Evidence Based Practice
 Medications
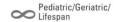 Pediatric/Geriatric/Lifespan

risk for delayed Development (continued)

Treatment regimen

Sample Clinical Applications: Congenital or genetic disorders, prematurity, infection, nutritional problems (malnutrition, anorexia, failure to thrive), toxic exposures (e.g., lead), substance abuse, endocrine disorders, abuse or neglect, developmental delay

DESIRED OUTCOMES/EVALUATION CRITERIA

Sample NOC linkage:

Child Development: [specify age]: Milestones of physical, cognitive, and psychosocial progression by [specify] months or years of age

Client Will (Include Specific Time Frame)

• Perform motor, social, self-regulatory behavior, cognitive, and language skills appropriate for age or within scope of present capabilities.

Sample NOC linkages:

Knowledge: Parenting: Extent of understanding conveyed about provision of a nurturing and constructive environment for a child from 1 year through 17 years of age

Parenting Performance: Parental actions to provide a child a nurturing and constructive physical, emotional, and social environment

Parent/Caregiver Will (Include Specific Time Frame)

• Verbalize understanding of age-appropriate development and expectations.
• Identify individual risk factors for developmental delay or deviation.
• Formulate plan(s) for prevention of developmental deviation.
• Initiate interventions or lifestyle changes promoting appropriate development.

ACTIONS/INTERVENTIONS

Sample NIC linkages:

Developmental Enhancement: Infant, Child [or] Adolescent: Facilitating or teaching parents/caregivers to facilitate the optimal gross motor, fine motor, language, cognitive, social, and emotional growth of child under 1 year of age, preschool and school-age children, or during the transition from childhood to adulthood

Risk Identification: Analysis of potential risk factors, determination of health risks, and prioritization of risk reduction strategies for an individual or group

NURSING PRIORITY NO. 1   To assess for causative/contributing risk factors:

• Identify condition(s) that could contribute to developmental deviations. *This list is extensive and widely variable. Potential for developmental issues might be apparent at birth (e.g., neonatal brain injury, especially that occurring before or at time of birth; prematurity; extremes of maternal age; unwanted or complicated pregnancy; known prenatal substance abuse, etc.). However, risks are not confined to the child's birth events, but also encompass parent/family issues and environment (e.g., family history of developmental disorders; mother with mental illness or retardation; child with acute or chronic severe illness and lengthy hospitalizations; family poverty with inadequate living quarters, nutrition, nurturing, or supervision; family instability or violence; shaken baby syndrome and other maltreatment or child abuse; institutional home or foster system during early life or prior to adoption).*[1,11–13,16,17]

 Acute Care   Collaborative   Community/ Home Care   Cultural

- Participate in screening child's development level by means of observation and history related by concerned parents/other significant others. *Developmental delay occurs when a child fails to achieve one or more developmental milestones within an expected time period; it may be in one or more areas (e.g., cognitive, social and emotional, speech and language, fine motor skills or gross motor skills) and may be the result of one or multiple factors.*[1,13]

- Obtain information from variety of sources. *Parents are often the first ones to think that there is a problem with their baby's development and should be encouraged to have routine well-baby checkups and screening for developmental delays. Teachers, family members, day-care or foster care providers, physicians, and others interacting with a client (older than infant) may have valuable input regarding behaviors that may indicate problems or developmental issues.*[1,2,11–13,16,17]

- Identify cultural beliefs, norms, and values, as they may impact parent/caregiver view of situation. *Culture shapes parenting practices, understanding of health and illness, perceptions related to development, and beliefs about individuals affected by developmental disorders. These cultural implications underscore the importance of having a broad array of tools for assessment and instruction, as well as a good understanding of the child's culture.*[3,12]

- Ascertain nature of required parent/caregiver activities and evaluate caregiver's abilities to perform needed activities.

- Note severity and pervasiveness of situation (e.g., potential for long-term stress leading to abuse or neglect versus situational disruption during period of crisis or transition that may eventually level out). *Situations require different interventions in terms of the intensity and length of time that assistance and support may be critical to the parent/caregiver. A crisis can produce great change within a family, some of which can be detrimental to the individual or family unit.*[4–6]

- Evaluate environment in which long-standing care will be provided. *The physical, emotional, financial, and social needs of a family are impacted and intertwined with the needs of the client. Changes may be needed in the physical structure of the home or family roles, resulting in disruption and stress, placing everyone at risk.*[4,6]

- Refer for and assist with in-depth evaluation, if indicated, using an authoritative text (e.g., Gesell, Mussen-Congor) or assessment tools (e.g., Ages and Stages Questionnaire, Parents Evaluation of Developmental Status, Temperament and Atypical Behavior Scale, Denver II Developmental Screening Test, Bender's Visual Motor Gestalt Test). *Provides guide for comparative measurement as child/individual progresses. Note: Often there is no single diagnostic test for a specific developmental delay. There are tools to evaluate child's skills in certain areas, such as motor development, speech, language, math, etc. However, a diagnosis is often determined over months or years. Also, a child who is delayed in an area at a certain age may "catch up" in later years.*[1,8–12]

NURSING PRIORITY NO. 2 To assist in preventing or limiting developmental delays:

- Note chronological age and review with parents the expectations for "normal development" in infancy and early childhood at clinic visits *to help determine developmental expectations (e.g., when child should roll over, sit up alone, speak first words, attain a certain weight or height) and how the expectations may be altered by child's condition. Ideally, children should be screened for developmental delay at the 9-, 18-, and 24- or 30-month visit, and at 15, 18, and again at 24 months for autism spectrum disorders.*[14,15] *For high-risk individuals, including children affected by biological (e.g., low birth weight) and psychosocial (e.g., foster care, homelessness) risk factors, earlier and more frequent formal developmental screening may be warranted. Note: Pediatrician may screen with a motor quotient (MQ), which is child's age calculated by milestones met divided by chronological age and multiplied by 100. An MQ between 50 and 70 requires further evaluation and intervention.*[1,7,16]

- Describe realistic, age-appropriate patterns of development to parent/caregiver and promote activities and interactions that support developmental tasks where client is at this time. *Important in planning interventions in keeping with the individual's current status and potential. Each child will have own unique strengths and challenges.*[1–3,11,17]

 Diagnostic Studies   Evidence Based Practice   Medications   Pediatric/Geriatric/Lifespan

- Collaborate with related professional resources, as indicated (e.g., physical, occupational, rehabilitation, speech therapists; home health agencies; social services, nutritionist; special education teacher, family therapists; technological and adaptive equipment specialists; vocational counselor). *Multidisciplinary team care increases the likelihood of developing a well-rounded plan of care that meets client/family's specialized and varied needs, minimizing identified risks.*[4,10-12]

NURSING PRIORITY NO. 3   To promote wellness (Teaching/Discharge Considerations):

- Engage in and encourage prevention strategies (e.g., abstinence from drugs, alcohol, and tobacco during pregnancy, referral for treatment programs, referral for violence prevention counseling, anticipatory guidance for potential handicaps [vision, hearing, failure to thrive]). *Promoting wellness starts with preventing complications and acting early to limit severity of anticipated problems. Such strategies can often be initiated by nurses where the potential is first identified, in the community setting.*[1,4]
- Evaluate client's progress on continual basis. Identify target symptoms requiring intervention *to make referrals in a timely manner and/or to make adjustments in plan of care, as indicated.*[2]
- Emphasize importance of follow-up appointments as indicated *to promote ongoing evaluation, support, or management of situation.*[2,12]
- Discuss proactive wellness actions to take (e.g., periodic laboratory studies to monitor nutritional status, getting immunizations on schedule to prevent serious infections) *to avoid preventable complications.*[7]
- Maintain a positive, hopeful attitude. Encourage setting of short-term realistic goals for achieving developmental potential. *Small, incremental steps are often easier to deal with, and successes enhance hopefulness and well-being.*[6]
- Provide information as appropriate, including pertinent reference materials and reliable Web sites. *Bibliotherapy provides opportunity to review data at own pace, enhancing likelihood of retention.*[1,2]
- Encourage attendance at educational programs (e.g., parenting classes, infant stimulation sessions; food buying, cooking, and nutrition; home and family safety, anger management, seminars on life stresses, aging process) *to address specific learning need or desires and interact with others with similar life challenges.*[2,11]
- Refer to available community and national resources if appropriate (e.g., early intervention programs, gifted and talented programs, sheltered workshop, crippled children's services, medical equipment and supplier, caregiver support and respite services). *Can provide assistance to support family and help identify community responsibilities (e.g., services required to be provided to school-age child if developmental disabilities are diagnosed).*[1]

DOCUMENTATION FOCUS

Assessment/Reassessment
- Assessment findings, individual needs, including developmental level.
- Caregiver's understanding of situation and individual role.

Planning
- Plan of care and who is involved in the planning.
- Teaching plan.

Implementation/Evaluation
- Client's response to interventions, teaching, and actions performed.
- Caregiver response to teaching.
- Attainment or progress toward desired outcome(s).
- Modifications to plan of care.

Discharge Planning
- Identified long-term needs and who is responsible for actions to be taken.
- Specific referrals made, sources for assistive devices, educational tools.

 Acute Care   Collaborative   Community/ Home Care   Cultural

References

1. No author. (No date). What is developmental delay and what services are available if I think my child might be delayed?. How Kids Develop Website. Retrieved March 2018 from http://www.howkidsdevelop.com/developDevDelay.html.

2. Volkmar, F., et al. (1999). Practice parameters for the assessment and treatment of children, adolescents, and adults with autism and other pervasive developmental disorders. *J Am Acad Child Adolesc Psychiatry*, 38(12 Suppl), 32s–54s.

3. Valdivia, R. (1999). *The Implications of Culture on Developmental Delay*. Reston, VA: ERIC Clearinghouse on Disabilities and Gifted Education.

4. Doenges, M. E., Moorhouse, M. F., Murr, A. C. (2010). ND: Growth and development, delayed. *Nurse's Pocket Guide: Diagnoses, Interventions, and Rationales*. 12th ed. Philadelphia: F. A. Davis.

5. Engel, J. (2006). *Mosby's Pocket Guide to Pediatric Assessment*. 5th ed. St. Louis, MO: Mosby.

6. Newfield, S. A., et al. (2007). *Cox's Clinical Applications of Nursing Diagnosis: Adult, Child, Women's, Psychiatric, Gerontic, and Home Health Considerations*. 5th ed. Philadelphia: F. A. Davis.

7. Startingpoint.org. (No date). Working with children with special needs. Retrieved March 2018 from http://starting-point.org/SpecialNeeds%20Provider%20brochure.pdf.

8. Schiffman, R. F. (2004). Drug and substance use in adolescents. *MCN Am J Matern Child Nurs*, 29(1), 21–27.

9. Institute for Clinical Systems Improvement. (2005, updated 2013). Healthcare guideline: Preventive services for children and adolescents (Summary of changes). Catalog/Index Retrieved March 2018 from https://www.icsi.org/guidelines__more/catalog_guidelines_and_more/catalog_guidelines/catalog_prevention__screening_guidelines/preventive_services_kids/.

10. Blann, L. E. (2005). Early intervention for children and families with special needs. *MCN Am J Matern Child Nurs*, 30(4), 263–267.

11. Mountstephen, M. (2011). *How to Detect Developmental Delay and What to Do Next: Practical Applications for Home and School*. Philadelphia: Jessica Kinsley.

12. Garzon, D. L., Thrasher, C., Tiernan, K. (2010). Providing optimal care for children with developmental disorders. *Nurse Pract*, 35(10), 30–39.

13. Narad, C., Mason, P. W. (2004). International adoptions: Myths and realities. *Pediatr Nurs*, 30(6), 483–487.

14. American Academy of Pediatrics Council on Children with Disabilities. (2006). Identifying infants and young children with developmental disorders in the medical home: An algorithm for developmental surveillance and screening. *Pediatrics*, 118(1), 405–420.

15. Drotar, D., et al. (2008). Selecting developmental surveillance and screening tools. *Pediatr Rev*, 29(10), e52–e58.

16. Aylward, G. P. (1997). Conceptual issues in developmental screening and assessment. *J Dev Behav Pediatr*, 18(5), 340–349.

17. Harden, B. J. (2004). Safety and stability for foster children: A developmental perspective. *Future Child*, 14(1), 30–47.

Diarrhea

Taxonomy II: Elimination and Exchange—Class 2 Gastrointestinal Function (0013) [**Diagnostic Division:** Elimination], Approved 1975; Nursing Diagnosis Extension and Classification Revision 1998, 2017

DEFINITION: Passage of loose, unformed stools.

RELATED FACTORS
Increase in stress level; anxiety
Laxative or substance abuse

DEFINING CHARACTERISTICS

Subjective
Abdominal pain
Bowel urgency; cramping

Objective
Hyperactive bowel sounds
Loose liquid stools >3 in 24 hours
At Risk Population: Exposure to contaminant or toxin or unsanitary food preparation

(continues on page 256)

 Diagnostic Studies   Evidence Based Practice   Medications   Pediatric/Geriatric/Lifespan

Diarrhea (continued)

Associated Condition: Enteral feedings
Gastrointestinal irritation or inflammation; malabsorption
Parasite
Treatment regimen
Sample Clinical Applications: Inflammatory bowel disease, gastritis, enteral feedings, alcohol abuse, antibiotic use, food allergies or contamination, AIDS, radiation, parasites

DESIRED OUTCOMES/EVALUATION CRITERIA

Sample **NOC** linkages:
Bowel Elimination: Formation and evacuation of stool
Hydration: Adequate water in the intracellular and extracellular compartments of the body
Self-Management: Acute Illness: Personal actions to manage a reversible illness, its treatment, and to prevent complications

Client Will (Include Specific Time Frame)
- Reestablish and maintain normal pattern of bowel functioning.
- Verbalize understanding of causative factors and rationale for treatment regimen.
- Demonstrate appropriate behavior to assist with resolution of causative factors (e.g., proper food preparation or avoidance of irritating foods).

ACTIONS/INTERVENTIONS

Sample **NIC** linkages:
Diarrhea Management: Management and alleviation of diarrhea
Fluid Monitoring: Collection and analysis of patient data to regulate fluid balance
Perineal Care: Maintenance of perineal skin integrity and relief of perineal discomfort

NURSING PRIORITY NO. 1   To assess causative factors/etiology:

- ∞ Note client's age and evaluate client's/caregiver's perception of severity of symptoms. *Acute diarrhea is usually caused by an infection, while chronic diarrhea is usually related to a functional disorder or intestinal disease. Viral diarrhea is most common among young children. Adults tend to average one bout of acute diarrhea each year. Chronic (persistent) diarrhea may be a symptom of a chronic disease and often affects adults more than children. People perceive having diarrhea in many different ways, but generally if client is having loose, watery stools occurring more than three times a day for 3 days or more, the diagnosis of diarrhea can be made. The condition can affect people of all ages, although its effect is more dangerous for infants and frail elderly (due to risk of dehydration).*[1–3]
- Obtain comprehensive history of symptoms *to help in identifying cause and treatment needs:*[1,2,4–6,13,14]
  - Ascertain onset and pattern of diarrhea, noting whether it is acute or chronic. *Acute diarrhea is caused by (1) viral, bacterial, or parasitic infections (e.g., Norwalk virus, rotavirus; salmonella, shigella; giardia, amebiasis, respectively); (2) bacterial food-borne toxins (e.g., Staphylococcus aureus, Escherichia coli); (3) medications (e.g., antibiotics, chemotherapy agents, colchicine, laxatives); and (4) enteral tube feedings. It lasts a few days up to a week. Chronic diarrhea is caused by irritable bowel syndrome, infectious diseases, inflammatory bowel disease, colon cancer and treatments, severe constipation, malabsorption disorders, laxative abuse, and certain endocrine disorders (e.g., hyperthyroidism, Addison's disease). It almost always lasts for more than 3 weeks.*

 Acute Care Collaborative Community/Home Care Cultural

Review history and observe stools for **characteristics** (e.g., soft to watery stools, bloody, greasy), **frequency** (e.g., more than normal number of stools/day), **time of day** (e.g., after meals), **volume**, and **duration**.

Identify any **associated signs/symptoms** (e.g., fever/chills, abdominal cramping, emotional upset, weight loss), **aggravating factors** (e.g., stress, foods), or **mitigating factors** (e.g., changes in diet, use of prescription or over-the-counter [OTC] medications).

Note reports of abdominal or rectal pain. *Pain is often present with inflammatory bowel disease, irritable bowel syndrome, and mesenteric ischemia.*

- Determine recent travel to developing countries or foreign environments, change in drinking water or food intake or consumption of unsafe food, swimming in untreated surface water, or similar illness of family members/others close to client *that may help identify causative environmental factors.*[2,4–6]
- Review medications, noting side effects and possible interactions. *Many drugs (e.g., antibiotics such as cephalosporins, erythromycin, penicillins, quinolones, tetracyclines, digitalis, angiotensin-converting enzyme inhibitors, NSAIDs, hypoglycemia agents, cholesterol-lowering drugs) can cause or exacerbate diarrhea, particularly in the elderly and in those who have had surgery on the intestinal tract.*[1,2,6–8]
- Evaluate diet history, noting food allergies or intolerances, and food and water safety issues, and note general nutritional, fluid, and electrolyte status *that may be causing or exacerbating diarrhea.*
- Auscultate abdomen for presence, location, and characteristics of bowel sounds. *High-pitched, rapidly occurring, and loud or tinkling bowel sounds often accompany diarrhea.*[9]
- Determine if incontinence is present. *May indicate presence of fecal impaction, particularly in the elderly, where impaction may be accompanied by diarrhea.*[3] (Refer to ND bowel Incontinence.)
- Review results of laboratory testing on stool specimens. *Can reveal presence of bacterial or viral infection, parasites, fat, blood, offending drugs, metabolic disorder, malabsorption syndrome, gastroenteritis, colitis, etc.*[1,2,4–6]
- Assist with/prepare for additional evaluation as indicated. *Chronic diarrhea may require more invasive testing, including upper and/or lower gastrointestinal radiographs, ultrasound, endoscopic evaluations, biopsy, etc.*[12]

NURSING PRIORITY NO. 2 To alleviate/limit condition:

- Assist with treatment of underlying conditions (e.g., infections, malabsorption syndrome, cancer) and complications of diarrhea. *Treatments are varied and may be as simple as allowing time for recovery from a self-limiting gastroenteritis or may require complex treatments, including antimicrobials and rehydration, or community health interventions for contaminated food or water sources.*[14]
- Encourage bedrest during an acute episode. *Rest reduces intestinal motility and metabolic rate when infection or hemorrhage is a complication.*[1–6,8,10]
- Restrict solid food intake, if indicated. *May help in short term to allow for bowel rest and reduced intestinal workload, especially if cause of diarrhea is under investigation or vomiting is present. Note: A child's preferred or usual diet may be continued to prevent or limit dehydration, with the possible limitation of fruit, fruit juices, or milk, if these factors are exacerbating the diarrhea.*[5,9,10]
- Limit caffeine and high-fat (e.g., butter, fried foods) or high-protein (e.g., meats) foods known to cause or aggravate diarrhea (e.g., extremely hot or cold foods, chili), milk, and fruits or fruit juices as appropriate.[1–6,8,10]
- Adjust strength and/or rate of enteral tube feedings; change formula as indicated *when diarrhea is associated with tube feedings.*[1–6,8,10]
- Consider change in infant formula. *Diarrhea may be result of or aggravated by intolerance to specific formula.*[9,10]
- Change client's routine medications as appropriate (e.g., stopping magnesium-containing antacid or antibiotic causing diarrhea).[7,8]
- Promote the use of relaxation techniques (e.g., progressive relaxation exercise, visualization techniques) *to decrease stress and anxiety.*[1–6,8,10]
- Administer medications *to treat or limit diarrhea, as indicated, depending on cause. May include use of antidiarrheals, anti-infectives, antispasmodics, etc.*[1–6,8,10,14]

 Diagnostic Studies   Evidence Based Practice   Medications   Pediatric/Geriatric/Lifespan

- Assist client to manage situation:[12]

  Respond to call for assistance promptly.

  Place bedpan in bed with client (if desired) or commode chair near bed *to provide quick access and reduce need to wait for assistance of others.*

  Provide privacy, remove stool promptly, and use room deodorizers *to reduce noxious odors and limit embarrassment.*

  Use incontinence pads, depending on the severity of the problem.

  Provide emotional and psychological support. *Diarrhea can be a source of great embarrassment and can lead to social isolation and feeling of powerlessness. Intimate relationship and sexual activity may be affected and need specific interventions to resolve.*

- Maintain skin integrity:[12]

  Assist as needed with pericare after each bowel movement *to prevent skin excoriation and breakdown.*

  Provide prompt diaper or incontinence pad change and gentle cleansing *because skin breakdown can occur quickly with diarrhea.*

  Apply lotion or skin barrier ointment as needed.

  Provide dry linen as necessary.

  Expose perineum and buttocks to air or use heat lamp with caution if needed *to keep area dry.*

  Refer to ND impaired Skin Integrity.

NURSING PRIORITY NO. 3 To restore/maintain hydration/electrolyte balance:

- Note reports of thirst, less frequent or absent urination, dry mouth and skin, weakness, light-headedness, and headache. *Signs/symptoms of dehydration and need for rehydration.*[1–3,5,6,10]
- ∞ Observe for or question parents about young child crying with no tears, fever, decreased urination or no wet diapers for 6 to 8 hours, listlessness or irritability, sunken eyes, dry mouth and tongue, and suspected or documented weight loss. *Child needs urgent or emergency treatment for dehydration if these signs are present and child is not taking fluids.*[1–3,5,6,10]
- ∞ Note presence of low blood pressure or postural hypotension, tachycardia, poor skin hydration, or turgor. *Presence of these factors indicates severe dehydration and electrolyte imbalance. The frail elderly can progress quickly to this point, especially when vomiting is present or client's normal food and fluid intake is below requirements.*[1–3,5,6,10]
- Monitor total intake and output, including stool output as possible. *Provides estimation of fluid needs.*[1,3,5,6,10]
- ∞ Weigh infant's diapers to determine output.[1–3,5,6,10]
- Offer and encourage water, plus broth or soups that contain sodium, or soft fruits or vegetables that contain potassium *to replace water and electrolytes.*[1–3,5,6,10]
- Recommend oral intake of beverages such as Gatorade, Pedialyte, Infalyte, and Smart Water. *Commercial rehydration solutions containing electrolytes may prevent or correct imbalances.*[1–3,5,6,10]
- Administer IV fluids, electrolytes, and enteral or parenteral feedings, as indicated. *IV fluids may be needed either short term to restore hydration status (e.g., acute gastroenteritis) or long term (severe osmotic diarrhea). Enteral or parenteral nutrition is reserved for clients unable to maintain adequate nutritional status because of long-term diarrhea (e.g., wasting syndrome, malnutrition states).*[1–3,5,6,10]

NURSING PRIORITY NO. 4 To promote return to normal bowel functioning:

- Encourage intake of nonirritating liquids, increasing intake as tolerated and gradually returning to normal diet.[1,2,4–6,10,11,13]
- Recommend products such as natural fiber, plain natural yogurt, and Lactinex *to restore normal bowel flora.*[1,2,4–6,10,11]
- Administer medications as ordered *to treat infectious process, decrease motility, and/or absorb water.*[1,2,4–6,10,11]

 Acute Care   Collaborative   Community/ Home Care   Cultural

NURSING PRIORITY NO. 5   To promote wellness (Teaching/Discharge Considerations):

- Review individual's causative factors and appropriate interventions *to prevent recurrence.*
- Discuss medication regimen, including prescription and OTC drugs, *especially when client has multiple medications with potential for diarrhea as side effect or interaction.*[12]
- ∞ Encourage/refer for vaccines, as indicated. *Vaccines could include those recommended for travelers to susceptible areas of the world (e.g., cholera or typhoid vaccines) and/or could be preventative therapies for infants. For example, currently two oral live-virus vaccines are marketed in the United States for the prevention of rotavirus gastroenteritis, a major cause of severe diarrhea in infants.*[5,13]
- Instruct clients planning to travel outside the United States about traveler's diarrhea and ways to prevent or limit food- and water-borne illness *(e.g., do not drink tap water, use tap water ice cubes, or brush your teeth with tap water; avoid raw fruits and vegetables unless they can be peeled; avoid raw or rare meat or fish; discuss destination with local health department for particular recommendations, such as advisability of use of protective antibiotics).*[12,13]
- Assess home or living environment, if indicated. *Discussion with client/caregivers may be needed regarding (1) sanitation and hygiene (e.g., hand hygiene and laundry practices), (2) safe food storage and preparation (to reduce risk of foodborne infections), and (3) particular risks in select populations (e.g., persons with chronic liver disease should avoid shellfish; persons with impaired immune defenses are at increased risk for diarrhea associated with raw dairy products or unheated deli meats; pregnant women should avoid undercooked meats [infectious diarrhea]).*[12]
- Emphasize importance of hand hygiene *to prevent spread of infectious causes of diarrhea such as Clostridium difficile, S. aureus, etc.*[15]
- Instruct parent/caregiver in signs of dehydration and importance of fluid and electrolyte replacement, as well as simple food and fluids to provide rehydration.

DOCUMENTATION FOCUS

Assessment/Reassessment
- Assessment findings, including characteristics and pattern of elimination.

Planning
- Plan of care and who is involved in planning.
- Teaching plan.

Implementation/Evaluation
- Client's response to treatment, teaching, and actions performed.
- Attainment or progress toward desired outcome(s).
- Modifications to plan of care.

Discharge planning
- Recommendations for follow-up care.

References

1. Hogan, C. M. (1998). The nurse's role in diarrhea management. *Oncol Nurs Forum*, 25(5), 879–885.
2. National Digestive Diseases Information Clearinghouse. (No date). Diarrhea. Retrieved March 2018 from http://www.niddk.nih.gov/health-information/health-topics/digestive-diseases/diarrhea/Pages/facts.aspx.
3. Carnaveli, D. L., Patrick, M. (1993). *Nursing Management for the Elderly*. 3rd ed. Philadelphia: J. B. Lippincott.
4. Acute Gastroenteritis Guideline Team. (2006). Evidence-based clinical guideline for acute gastroenteritis (AGE) in children aged 2 months through 5 years. Cincinnati Children's Hospital Medical Center. Retrieved March 2018 from http://unmfm.pbworks.com/f/Cincinnati_gastroenteritis+guideline+total.pdf.
5. World Gastroenterological Organization. (2012). Acute diarrhea in adults and children. Retrieved March 2018 from http://www.worldgastroenterology.org/guidelines/global-guidelines/acute-diarrhea/acute-diarrhea-english.
6. Guerrant, R. L., et al. (2001). Practice guidelines for the management of infectious diarrhea. *Clin Infect Dis*, 32(3), 331–351.
7. Ratnaike, R. N. (2000). Drug-induced diarrhea in older persons. *Clin Geriatr*, 8(1), 67–76.

 Diagnostic Studies   Evidence Based Practice   Medications   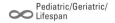 Pediatric/Geriatric/ Lifespan

8. Mayo Clinic Staff. (2013, updated 2016). Antibiotic-associated diarrhea. Retrieved March 2018 from http://www.mayoclinic.org/diseases-conditions/antibiotic-associated-diarrhea/basics/definition/con-20023556.

9. Engel, J. (2006). *Mosby's Pocket Guide to Pediatric Assessment*. 5th ed. St. Louis, MO: Mosby.

10. Larson, C. E. (2000). Evidence-based practice: Safety and efficacy of oral rehydration therapy for the treatment of diarrhea and gastroenteritis in pediatrics. *Pediatr Nurs*, 26(2), 177–179.

11. Peikin, R. (2009). *Diarrhea in Gastrointestinal Health*. 3rd ed. New York: HarperCollins.

12. Doenges, M. E., Moorhouse, M. F., Murr, A. C. (2008). ND Diarrhea, risk for: in Gastrointestinal Disorders-Inflammatory Bowel Disease. *Nursing Care Plans: Guidelines for Individualizing Patient Care*. 8th ed. Philadelphia: F. A. Davis.

13. Guandalini, S., Frye, R. E., Tamer, M. A. (2010, updated 2017). Diarrhea. Retrieved March 2018 from http://emedicine.medscape.com/article/928598-overview.

14. Diskin, A., Guiterrez-Alverez, L. (2006, updated 2017). Emergent treatment of gastroenteritis. Retrieved March 2018 from http://emedicine.medscape.com/article/775277-overview.

15. Martin, L. J. (2006, last reviewed 2017). What Is Clostridium Difficile (C. Diff)? Retrieved March 2018 from https://www.webmd.com/digestive-disorders/clostridium-difficile-colitis#1.

risk for Disuse Syndrome

Taxonomy II: Activity/Rest—Class 2 Activity/Exercise (00040) [**Diagnostic Division:** Activity/Rest], Submitted 1988; Revised 2013, 2017

DEFINITION: Susceptible to deterioration of body systems as the result of prescribed or unavoidable musculoskeletal inactivity, which may compromise health.

AUTHOR NOTE: Complications from immobility can include decreased strength or endurance, activity intolerance, impaired sitting or standing or walking; pressure ulcer, impaired urinary or bowel function; respiratory complications, such as pneumonia; systemic infections; blood clots; orthostatic hypotension; and disorientation, body image disturbance, ineffective coping, and powerlessness.

RISK FACTORS

Pain

Associated Condition: Alteration in level of consciousness

Mechanical or prescribed immobility; paralysis

Sample Clinical Applications: Multiple sclerosis (MS), cerebral palsy, muscular dystrophy, postpolio syndrome, brain injury or stroke, spinal cord injury (SCI), arthritis, osteoporosis, fractures, amputation, dementia

DESIRED OUTCOMES/EVALUATION CRITERIA

Sample **NOC** linkages:

Immobility Consequences: Physiological: Severity of compromise in physiological functioning due to impaired physical mobility

Risk Control: Personal actions to prevent, eliminate, or reduce modifiable health threats

Immobility Consequences: Psycho-Cognitive: Severity of compromise in psycho-cognitive functioning due to impaired physical mobility

Client Will (Include Specific Time Frame)

• Display intact skin and tissues or achieve timely wound healing.

• Maintain or reestablish effective elimination patterns.

• Be free of signs/symptoms of infectious processes.

• Demonstrate absence of pulmonary congestion with breath sounds clear.

• Demonstrate adequate peripheral perfusion with stable vital signs, skin warm and dry, and palpable peripheral pulses.

 Acute Care   Collaborative   Community/Home Care   Cultural

- Maintain usual reality orientation.
- Maintain or regain optimal level of cognitive, neurosensory, and musculoskeletal functioning.
- Express sense of control over the present situation and potential outcome.
- Recognize and incorporate change into self-concept in accurate manner without negative self-esteem.

ACTIONS/INTERVENTIONS

Sample **NIC** linkages:

Surveillance: Purposeful and ongoing acquisition, interpretation, and synthesis of patient data for clinical decision making

Bed Rest Care: Promotion of comfort and safety and prevention of complications for a patient unable to get out of bed

Exercise Promotion: Facilitation of regular physical activity to maintain or advance to a higher level of fitness and health

NURSING PRIORITY NO. 1 To evaluate probability of developing complications:

- Identify underlying conditions/pathology (e.g., cancer, trauma; fractures with casting, immobilization devices; surgery, chronic disease conditions, malnutrition; neurological conditions [e.g., stroke, brain or spinal cord injury, postpolio syndrome, multiple sclerosis]; chronic pain conditions; use of predisposing medications [e.g., steroids]) *that can cause or exacerbate problems associated with inactivity and immobility. Bedrest, immobility, and/or lack of physical activity (for any reason) causes a loss of protein and muscle deterioration. "Disuse syndrome" is a classic pattern of muscular deconditioning and atrophy resulting from inactivity or immobilization. Once muscle is lost, it is difficult to gain it back.*[10]
- Identify potential concerns, including cognition, mobility, and exercise status. *Disuse syndrome can be a complication of and cause for bedridden state. The syndrome can include muscle and bone atrophy, stiffening of joints, brittle bones, reduction of cardiopulmonary function, loss of red blood cells, decreased sex hormones, decreased resistance to infections, increased proportion of body fat in relation to muscle mass, and chemical changes in the brain, which adversely impact client's activities of daily living (ADLs), social life, and quality of life.*[1,2,10]
- 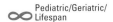 Note client's age. *Age-related physiological changes (e.g., decrease in muscle mass and/or function, increased levels of proinflammatory cytokines, increased production of free radicals or impaired detoxification, malnutrition, low hormone output, reduced neurological drive) accompanied by chronic illness predispose older adults to functional decline related to inactivity and immobility.*[1,3,8–10]
- Determine if client's condition is acute/short term or whether it may be a long-term/permanent condition. *Relatively short-term conditions (e.g., simple fracture treated with cast) may respond quickly to rehabilitative efforts. Long-term conditions (e.g., stroke, aged person with dementia, cancers, demyelinating or degenerative diseases, SCI, psychological problems such as depression or learned helplessness) have a higher risk of complications for the client and caregiver. Note: Studies carried out with intensive-care patients supported that prolonged immobilization leads to disuse atrophy of muscles and other physiological changes that decrease patients' ability to tolerate physical activity. They also found that muscle atrophy begins within hours of immobilization, leading to a 4% to 5% loss of muscle strength for each week of bedrest.*[11,12]
- Assess and document (ongoing) client's functional status, including cognition, vision, and hearing, social support, psychological well-being, and abilities in performance of ADLs *for a comparative baseline, to evaluate response to treatment, and to identify preventative interventions or necessary services.*[8]
- Evaluate client's risk for injury. *Risk is greater in client with cognitive problems, lack of safe or stimulating environment, inadequate mobility aids, and/or sensory-perception problems.*[3]

- Ascertain attitudes of individual/significant other (SO) about condition (e.g., cultural values, stigma). Note misconceptions. *The client may be influenced (positively or negatively) by peer group, cultural, and family role expectations.*
- Evaluate client's/family's understanding and ability to manage care for prolonged period. Ascertain availability and use of support systems. *Caregivers may be influenced by their own physical or emotional limitations, degree of commitment to assisting the client toward optimal independence, or available time.*[3]
- Review psychological assessment of client's emotional status. *Potential problems that may arise from presence of condition need to be identified and dealt with to avoid further debilitation. Common associated psychological changes include depression, anxiety, and avoidance behaviors.*[2,3]

NURSING PRIORITY NO. 2 To identify/provide individually appropriate preventive or corrective interventions:

- Skin:[6,7]

Inspect skin on a frequent basis, noting changes. Monitor skin over bony prominences.

Reposition frequently as individually indicated *to relieve pressure.*

Provide skin care daily and prn, drying well and using gentle massage and lotion *to stimulate circulation.*

Keep skin, clothing, and area clean and dry *to prevent skin irritation and breakdown.*

Initiate use of padding devices (e.g., foam, egg-crate/gel/water/air mattress or cushions) *to reduce pressure on and enhance circulation to compromised tissues.*

Review nutritional status and promote diet with adequate protein, calorie, and vitamin and mineral intake *to aid in healing and promote general good health of skin and tissues.*

Refer to NDs impaired Skin Integrity, impaired Tissue Integrity, and risk for Pressure Ulcer for additional interventions.

- Elimination:[6–8]

Observe elimination pattern, noting changes and potential problems.

Encourage a balanced diet, including fruits and vegetables high in fiber and with adequate fluids *for optimal stool consistency and to facilitate passage through colon.*

Provide or encourage adequate fluid intake, include water and cranberry juice *to reduce risk of urinary infections.*

Maximize mobility at earliest opportunity.

Evaluate need for stool softeners or bulk-forming laxatives.

Implement consistent bowel management or bladder training programs, as indicated.

Monitor urinary output and characteristics *to identify changes associated with infection.*

Refer to NDs Constipation, Diarrhea, bowel Incontinence, impaired Urinary Elimination, and Urinary Retention for additional interventions.

- Respiration:[6,7]

Monitor breath sounds and characteristics of secretions *for early detection of complications (e.g., atelectasis, pneumonia).*

Encourage ambulation and upright position. Reposition, cough, and deep breathe on a regular schedule *to facilitate clearing of secretions and improve lung function.*

Encourage use of incentive spirometry. Suction as indicated *to clear airways.*

Demonstrate techniques and assist with postural drainage when indicated for long-term airway clearance difficulties.

Assist with and instruct family and caregivers in quad coughing techniques or diaphragmatic weight training *to maximize ventilation (in presence of SCI).*

Discourage smoking. Refer for a smoking-cessation program as indicated.

Refer to NDs ineffective Airway Clearance, ineffective Breathing Pattern, impaired Gas Exchange, and impaired spontaneous Ventilation for additional interventions.

Acute Care   Collaborative   Community/Home Care   Cultural

- Vascular (tissue perfusion):[6–8]

Assess cognition and mental status (ongoing). *Changes can reflect state of cardiac health or cerebral oxygenation impairment or be indicative of a mental or emotional state that could adversely affect safety and self-care.*

Determine core and skin temperature. Investigate development of cyanosis and changes in mentation *to identify changes in oxygenation status.*

Evaluate circulation and nerve function of affected body parts on a routine, ongoing basis. *Changes in temperature, color, sensation, and movement can be the effect of immobility, disease, aging, or injury.*

Encourage or provide adequate fluid *to prevent dehydration and impaired circulation.*

Monitor blood pressure before, during, and after activity—sitting, standing, and lying if possible—*to ascertain response to and tolerance of activity.*

Assist with position changes as needed. Raise head gradually. Institute sitting upright on side of bed and arising slowly where appropriate *to reduce incidence of injury that may occur as a result of orthostatic hypotension.*

Maintain proper body position; avoid use of constricting garments and restraints *to prevent vascular congestion.*

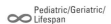 Provide range-of-motion exercise. Refer for and assist with physical therapy exercises *for strengthening, restoration of optimal range of motion, and prevention of circulatory problems related to disuse. Note: Tilt table may be used in physical therapy after neurological insults to improve client's tolerance of upright position and improve functional recovery.*[4,15]

Mobilize quickly and as often as possible, using mobility aids and frequent rest stops to assist client in continuing activity. *Upright position and weight bearing help maintain bone strength, improve circulation, and prevent postural hypotension.*[8,15]

 Institute peripheral vascular support measures (e.g., anti-embolism hose, Ace wraps, sequential compression devices) *to enhance venous return and reduce incidence of deep vein thrombosis. Note: With prolonged bedrest and lack of physical activity, the number of red blood cells declines, which decreases the amount of oxygen being delivered to the tissues. Blood clots and inflammation increase.*[13]

Refer to NDs risk for Activity Intolerance, risk for decreased Cardiac Output, risk for Peripheral Neurovascular Dysfunction, and ineffective peripheral Tissue Perfusion for additional interventions.

- Musculoskeletal (mobility, range of motion, strength, and endurance):[5–8,13]

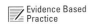 Perform or assist with range-of-motion exercises and involve client in core strengthening and active exercises as soon as possible with physical or occupational therapy *to promote bone health, muscle strengthening, flexibility, optimal conditioning, and functional ability.*

Maximize involvement in self-care *to restore or maintain strength, functional abilities, and early independence in self-care activities.*

Intersperse activity with rest periods. Pace activities as possible *to increase strength and endurance in a gradual manner and reduce failure of planned exercise because of exhaustion or overuse of weak muscles or injured area.*

 Identify need and use of supportive devices (e.g., cane, walker, functional positioning splints) as appropriate *to assist with safe mobility and functional independence.*

Evaluate role of physiological and psychological pain in mobility problem. Implement pain management program as individually indicated.

Avoid or monitor closely the use of restraints and immobilize client as little as possible *to reduce possibility of agitation and injury.*

Refer to NDs risk for Falls; impaired physical Mobility; impaired Sitting, impaired Standing, or impaired Walking; acute Pain; chronic Pain; and chronic Pain Syndrome for additional interventions.

- Sensory Perception:[6–8,13,14]

Orient client as necessary to time, place, person, and situation. Provide cues for orientation (e.g., clock, calendar). *Disturbances of sensory stimulation, interpretation, and thought processes are associated with immobility as well as aging, being ill, disease processes/treatments, and medication effects.*

Avoid or monitor closely the use of restraints and immobilize the client as little as possible *to reduce the possibility of agitation and injury.*

Provide appropriate level of environmental stimulation (e.g., music, TV, radio, personal possessions, visitors). *Needs vary depending on the client, the nature of the current problem, and whether client is at home or in a healthcare facility. Having normal life cues can help with mental stimulation and restoration of health.*

Encourage participation in recreational or diversional activities and a regular exercise program (as tolerated) *to decrease the sensory deprivation associated with immobility and isolation.*

Promote regular sleep hours, use of sleep aids, and usual presleep rituals *to promote normal sleep and rest cycle.*

Refer to NDs chronic Confusion, decreased Diversional Activity Engagement, Insomnia, and [disturbed Sensory Perception] for additional interventions.

- Self-Esteem, Powerlessness, Hopelessness, Social Isolation:[6,7,9]

Determine factors that may contribute to impairment of client's self-esteem and social interactions. *Many factors can be involved, including the client's age, relationship status, and usual health state; presence of disabilities, including pain; financial, environmental, and physical problems; and current situation causing immobility and client's state of mind concerning the importance of the current situation in regard to the rest of client's life and desired lifestyle.*

Ascertain if changes in client's situation are likely to be short term/temporary or long term/permanent. *Can affect both the client and care provider's coping abilities and willingness to engage in activities that prevent or limit effects of immobility.*

Assess living situation (e.g., lives with spouse, parents, alone) and determine factors that may positively or adversely affect client's progress, roles, and/or safety.

Explain or review all care procedures and plans. *Improves knowledge and facilitates decision making. Involves client in own care, enhances sense of control, and promotes independence.*

Encourage questions and verbalization of feelings. *Aids in reducing anxiety and promotes learning about condition and specific needs.*

Acknowledge concerns; provide presence and encouragement.

 Refer for mental, psychological, or spiritual services as indicated *to provide counseling, support, and medications.*

Provide for and assist with mutual goal setting, involving SO(s). *Promotes sense of control and enhances commitment to goals.*

Ascertain that client can communicate needs adequately (e.g., call light, writing tablet, picture or letter board, interpreter).

Refer to NDs impaired Verbal Communication, Powerlessness, ineffective Role Performance, Self-Esteem [specify], impaired Social Interaction, and Social Isolation for additional interventions.

- Body Image:[6,7]

Evaluate for presence or potential for physical, emotional, and behavioral conditions that may contribute to isolation and degeneration. *Disuse syndrome often affects those individuals who are already isolated for one reason or another (e.g., serious illness or injury with disfigurement, frail elderly living alone, individual with severe depression, person with unacceptable behavior or without support system).*

Orient to body changes through discussion and written information *to promote acceptance and understanding of needs.*

Promote interactions with peers and normalization of activities within individual abilities. *Physical activity and social interactions stimulate the production of chemical substances produced by the body that generate increased feelings of well-being, vitality, and alertness.*

Refer to NDs disturbed Body Image, disturbed Personal Identity, situational low Self-Esteem, and Social Isolation for additional interventions.

 Acute Care   Collaborative   Community/ Home Care   Cultural

NURSING PRIORITY NO. 3 To promote wellness (Teaching/Discharge Considerations):

- 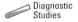 Assist client/caregivers in development of individualized plan of care *to best meet the client's potential, enhance safety, and prevent or limit affects of disuse.*
- Provide information about individual needs and areas of concern (e.g., client's mental status, living environment, nutritional needs). *Information can help client and care providers to understand what long-term goals could be attained, what barriers may need to be overcome, and what constitutes progress or lack of progress requiring further evaluation and intervention.*[6]
- Review therapeutic regimen. *Treatment may be required for underlying condition(s), stress management, medications, therapies, and needed lifestyle changes.*
- Encourage involvement in regular exercise program, including flexibility, resistance and strengthening activities, and active or assistive range of motion *to limit consequences of disuse and maximize level of function.*[2]
- Promote self-care and SO-supported activities *to gain or maintain independence.*
- Recommend suitable balanced nutrition as well as use of supplements if needed *to provide energy for healing and maximal organ function.*
- Refer to appropriate community health providers and resources *to provide necessary assistance (e.g., help with meal preparation, financial help for groceries, dietitian, or nutritionist).*[7]
- Review signs/symptoms requiring medical evaluation/follow-up *to promote timely interventions and limit adverse effects of situation.*[6]
- Identify community support services (e.g., financial, counseling, home maintenance, respite care, transportation).
- Refer to appropriate rehabilitation or home-care and support resources *to help client/care providers learn more about specific condition and acquire needed assistance, adaptive devices, and necessary equipment.*

DOCUMENTATION FOCUS

Assessment/Reassessment

- Assessment findings, noting individual areas of concern, functional level, degree of independence, support systems and available resources.

Planning

- Plan of care and who is involved in planning.
- Teaching plan.

Implementation/Evaluation

- Client's response to interventions, teaching, and actions performed.
- Changes in level of functioning.
- Attainment or progress toward desired outcome(s).
- Modifications to plan of care.

Discharge Planning

- Long-term needs and who is responsible for actions to be taken.
- Specific referrals made, resources for specific equipment needs.

References

1. Eliopoulos, C. (2010). Deconditioning and sarcopenia. *iAdvance Senior Care*. Retrieved March 2018 from https://www.iadvanceseniorcare.com/article/deconditioning-and-sarcopenia.
2. Verbunt, J. A., et al. (2003). Disuse and deconditioning in chronic low back pain: Concepts and hypotheses on contributing mechanisms. *Eur J Pain*, 7, 9–21.
3. Blair, K. A. (1999). Immobility and activity intolerance in older adults. In Stanley, M., Beare, P. G. (eds). *Gerontological Nursing: A Health Promotion/Protection Approach*. 2nd ed. Philadelphia: F. A. Davis.

Diagnostic Studies   Evidence Based Practice   Medications   Pediatric/Geriatric/Lifespan

4. Hannon, R. A. (2014). Activity tolerance and fatigue. In Porth, C. M. (ed). *Porth's Pathophysiology: Concepts of Altered Health States*. 9th ed. Philadelphia: Wolters Klower.

5. Metzlar, D. J., Harr, J. (1996). Positioning your patient properly. *Am J Nurs*, 96(3), 33–37.

6. Doenges, M. E., Moorhouse, M. F., Murr, A. C. (2016). *Nurse's Pocket Guide: Diagnoses, Interventions, and Rationales*. 14th ed. Philadelphia: F. A. Davis.

7. Newfield, S. A., et al. (2007). *Cox's Clinical Applications of Nursing Diagnosis: Adult, Child, Women's, Psychiatric, Gerontic, and Home Health Considerations*. 5th ed. Philadelphia: F. A. Davis.

8. Zisberg, A., et al. (2011). Low mobility during hospitalization and functional decline in older adults. *J Am Geriatr Soc*, 59(2), 266–273.

9. Bortz, W. (2009). Disuse and aging. *J Gerontol A Biol Sci Med Sci*, 108(6), 60–72.

10. Benton, M. J., Whyte, M. D., Dyal, B. W. (2011). Sarcopenic obesity: Strategies for management. *Am J Nurs*, 111(12), 38–44.

11. Needham, M. D. (2008). Mobilizing patients in the intensive care unit: Improving neuromuscular weakness and physical function. *JAMA*, 300(14), 1685–1690.

12. Morris, P. E., Herridge, M. S. (2007). Early intensive care unit mobility: Future directions. *Crit Care Clin*, 23(1), 97–110.

13. Dysautonomia Youth Network of America, Inc. (No date). The importance of physical activity. Retrieved March 2018 from http://www.dynainc.org/living/activity.

14. Parikh, R. (2014). Rethinking hospital restraints. *The Atlantic*. Retrieved March 2018 from https://www.theatlantic.com/health/archive/2014/08/rethinking-hospital-restraints/375647/.

15. Baltz, M. J., Lietz, H. L., Sausser, I. T. (2013). Tolerance of a standing tilt table protocol by patients in an inpatient stroke unit setting: A pilot study. *Crit Care Clin*, 37(1), 9–13.

decreased Diversional Activity Engagement

Taxonomy II: Health Promotion—Class 1 Health Awareness (00097) [**Diagnostic Division:** Activity/Rest], Approved 1980; Revised 2017

DEFINITION: Reduced stimulation interest or participation in recreational or leisure activities.

RELATED FACTORS
Current setting does not allow engagement in activity
Environmental barrier
Impaired mobility; insufficient energy or motivation
Insufficient diversional activity

DEFINING CHARACTERISTICS

Subjective
Boredom; discontent with situation

Objective
Alteration in mood
Current setting does not allow engagement in activities
Physical deconditioning; impaired mobility; frequent naps
At Risk Population: Extremes of age; prolonged hospitalization or institutionalization
Associated Condition: Prescribed immobility; psychological distress; therapeutic isolation
Sample Clinical Applications: Traumatic injuries, chronic pain, prolonged recovery (e.g., postoperative, complicated fractures), cancer therapy, chronic/debilitating conditions (e.g., congestive heart failure [CHF], chronic obstructive pulmonary disease [COPD], renal failure, multiple sclerosis [MS]), awaiting organ transplantation

DESIRED OUTCOMES/EVALUATION CRITERIA

Sample NOC linkages:
Motivation: Inner urge that moves or prompts an individual to positive action(s)

 Acute Care Collaborative Community/Home Care Cultural

Leisure Participation: Use of relaxing, interesting, and enjoyable activities to promote well-being
Social Involvement: Social interactions with persons, groups, or organizations

Client Will (Include Specific Time Frame)
- Recognize own psychological response (e.g., hopelessness and helplessness, anger, depression) and initiate appropriate coping actions.
- Engage in satisfying activities within personal limitations.

ACTIONS/INTERVENTIONS

Sample NIC **linkages:**
Recreation Therapy: Purposeful use of recreational activities to enhance independent function and social skills, as well as reduce or eliminate the effects of illness or disability
Activity Therapy: Prescription of and assistance with specific physical, cognitive, social, and spiritual activities to increase the range, frequency, or duration of an individual's or group's activity
Exercise Promotion: Facilitation of regular physical activity to maintain or advance to a higher level of fitness and health

NURSING PRIORITY NO. 1   To assess precipitating/etiological factors:

- Assess client's physical, cognitive, emotional, and environmental status. *Validates reality of diversional deprivation when it exists or identifies the potential for loss of desired diversional activity in order to plan for prevention or early intervention where possible. Note: Studies show that key problems faced by clients who are hospitalized (or in a long-term facility, or immobilized) for extended periods of time include boredom, stress, and depression. These negative states can impede recovery and lead clients to report symptoms more frequently.*[1,10]
- Observe for restlessness, flat facial expression, withdrawal, hostility, yawning, or statements of boredom as noted above, especially in individual likely to be confined either temporarily or long term. *May be indicative of need for diversional interventions.*
- ∞Note potential impact of current disability or illness on lifestyle (e.g., young child with leukemia, elderly person with fractured hip, individual with severe depression). *Provides comparative baseline for assessments and interventions.*[8]
- ∞Be aware of age and developmental level, gender, cultural factors, and the importance of a given activity in client's life. *Cultural issues include gender roles, communication styles, privacy and personal space; expectations and views regarding time and activities; and control of the immediate environment, family traditions, and social patterns. When illness interferes with individual's ability to engage in usual activities, such as a lifelong dancer with incapacitating osteoporosis (or a woman with strong cultural expectations who is unable to take care of her family), the person may have difficulty engaging in meaningful substitute activities.*[11]
- Determine client's actual ability to participate in available activities, noting attention span, physical limitations and tolerance, level of interest or desire, and safety needs. *Presence of depression or disinterest in life; problems of immobility; protective isolation; and lack of stimulation, developmental delay, or sensory deprivation may interfere with desired activity. However, lack of involvement may not reflect client's actual abilities, but may rather be a matter of misperception about abilities.*[8]

NURSING PRIORITY NO. 2   To motivate and stimulate client involvement in solutions:

- Institute or continue appropriate actions to deal with concomitant conditions such as anxiety, depression, grief, dementia, physical injury, isolation and immobility, malnutrition, acute or chronic pain, etc. *These conditions interfere with the individual's ability to engage in meaningful activities that will stimulate his/her interest.*

 Diagnostic Studies   Evidence Based Practice   Medications   Pediatric/Geriatric/ Lifespan

- Introduce activities at client's current level of functioning, progressing to more complex activities, as tolerated. *Provides opportunity for client to experience successes, reaffirming capabilities and enhancing self-esteem.*[7]
- Establish therapeutic relationship, acknowledging reality of situation and client's feelings. *May be feeling sense of loss when unable to participate in usual activities or to interact socially as desired.*[7]
- Accept hostile expressions while limiting aggressive acting-out behavior. *Permission to express feelings of anger and hopelessness allows for beginning resolution. However, destructive behavior is counterproductive to self-esteem and problem-solving.*[7]
- Involve client and parent/significant other (SO)/caregiver in determining client's needs, desires, and available resources. *Helps ensure that plan is attentive to client's interests and resources, increasing likelihood of client participation.*[2]
- ∞ Encourage parent/caregiver of young child to engage in play with confined child. *Play is essential to young child's development, can help redirect child's attention from pain of condition, and reduce child's boredom and stress.*[3,12]
- Review history of lifelong activities and hobbies client has enjoyed. Discuss reasons client is not doing these activities now and whether client can or would like to resume these activities. *Diversional activities can provide positive and productive avenues into which client can channel thoughts and time.*[4]
- Assist client/caregiver to set realistic goals for diversional activities, communicating hope and patience. *Can help client realize that this situation is not hopeless, that there are choices for improving the current situation, and that the future can hold the promise for improvement.*
- Provide instruction in relaxation techniques (e.g., meditation, sharing experiences, reminiscence, soft music, guided visualization) *to enhance coping skills.*[7]
- Participate in decisions about timing and spacing of visitors and leisure and care activities *to promote relaxation and reduce sense of boredom as well as prevent overstimulation and exhaustion.*[7]
- Encourage client to assist in scheduling required and optional activity choices. *For example, client may want to watch favorite television show at bath time; if bath can be rescheduled later, client's sense of control is enhanced.*[7]
- Encourage mix of desired activities/stimuli (e.g., music, news, educational presentations, movies, computer or Internet access, books or other reading materials, visitors, games, arts and crafts, sensory enrichment [e.g., massage, aromatherapy], grooming and beauty care, cooking, social outings, gardening, discussion groups, as appropriate). *Activities need to be personally meaningful and not physically/emotionally overwhelming for client to derive the most benefit.*[4,9]
- Refrain from making changes in schedule without discussing with client. *It is important for staff to be sensitive and responsible in making and following through on commitments to client.*[7]
- 🏠 Provide change of scenery (indoors and outdoors where possible). Provide for periodic changes in the personal environment when client is confined inside, eliciting the client's input for likes and desires. *Change (e.g., new pictures on the wall, seasonal colors/flowers, altering room furniture, outdoor light and air) can provide positive sensory stimulation, reduce client's boredom, and improve sense of normalcy and control.*[5]
- 🏠 Suggest activities such as bird feeders/baths for bird-watching, a garden in a window box or terrarium, or a fishbowl or aquarium *to stimulate observation as well as involvement and participation in activity (e.g., bird identification, picking out feeders and seeds).*[7]
- 🅐 Involve recreational, occupational, play, music, or movement therapists as appropriate *to help identify enjoyable activities for client and to procure assistive devices or modify activities for individual situation. Assists client to express needs and feelings, share experiences, escape healthcare routines, and participate in self-healing.*[1,6,9]

 Acute Care   Collaborative Community/Home Care   Cultural

NURSING PRIORITY NO. 3 To promote wellness (Teaching/Discharge Considerations):

- Explore options for useful activities using the person's strengths/abilities and interests to engage the client/SO.
- Make appropriate referrals to available resources (e.g., exercise groups, senior activities, hobby clubs, volunteering, companion and service organizations) *to introduce or continue diversional activities in community/home settings.*
- Refer to NDs ineffective Coping, Hopelessness, Powerlessness, and Social Isolation for additional interventions.

DOCUMENTATION FOCUS

Assessment/Reassessment
- Specific assessment findings, including blocks to desired activities.
- Individual choices for activities.

Planning
- Plan of care, specific interventions, and who is involved in planning.

Implementation/Evaluation
- Client's responses to interventions, teaching, and actions performed.
- Attainment or progress toward desired outcome(s).
- Modifications to plan of care.

Discharge Planning
- Long-term needs and who is responsible for actions to be taken.
- Referrals made and available community resources.

References

1. Radziewicz, R. M. (1992). Using diversional activities to enhance coping. *Cancer Nurs*, 15(4), 293–298.
2. Newfield, S. A., et al. (2007). *Cox's Clinical Applications of Nursing Diagnosis: Adult, Child, Women's, Psychiatric, Gerontic, and Home Health Considerations.* 5th ed. Philadelphia: F. A. Davis.
3. Engel, J. (2005). *Mosby's Pocket Guide to Pediatric Assessment.* 6th ed. St. Louis, MO: Mosby.
4. Wheeler, S.L., Houston, K. (2005). The role of diversional activities in the general medical hospital Setting. *Holist Nurs Pract*, 19(2), 87–92.
5. Dossey, B. M. (1998). Holistic modalities & healing moments. *Am J Nurs*, 98(6), 44–47.
6. Coaten, R. (2002). Movement matters: Revealing the hidden humanity within dementia through movement, dance and the imagination. *Dementia*, 1(3), 386–392.
7. Doenges, M. E., Moorhouse, M. F., Murr, A. C. (2014). Psychosocial aspects of care. *Nursing Care Plans: Guidelines for Individualizing Patient Care Across the Life Span.* 9th ed. Philadelphia: F. A. Davis.
8. Heriot, C. S. (1999). Developmental tasks and development in the later years of life. In Stanley, M., Bear, P. G. (eds). *Gerontological Nursing: A Health Promotion/Protection Approach.* 2nd ed. Philadelphia: F. A. Davis.
9. Wheeler, S. L., Houston, K. (2005). The role of diversional activities in the general medical hospital setting. *Holist Nurs Pract*, 19(2), 67–69.
10. Sommers, J., Vodanovich, S. J. (2000). Boredom proneness: Its relationship to psychological and physical-health symptoms. *J Clin Psych*, 56(1), 149–155.
11. Jenko, M., Moffitt, S. (2006). Transcultural nursing principles. *J Hosp Palliat Nurs*, 8(3), 172–180.
12. Gabany, E., Shellenbarger, T. (2010). Caring for families with deployment stress. *Am J Nurs*, 110(11), 36–41.

 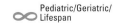

risk for Dry Eye

Taxonomy II: Safety/Protection—Class 5 Physical Injury (00219) **[Diagnostic Division:** Safety], Accepted 2010; Revised 2013, 2017

DEFINITION: Susceptible to eye discomfort or damage to the cornea and conjunctiva due to reduced quantity or quality of tears to moisten the eye, which may compromise health.

RISK FACTORS
Air conditioning; air pollution, excessive wind, low humidity; sunlight exposure
Caffeine intake; vitamin A deficiency
Insufficient knowledge of modifiable factors; prolonged reading; smoking
At Risk Population: Aging; female gender, history of allergy; contact lens wearer
Associated Condition: Autoimmune disease; hormonal change; neurological lesion with sensory or motor reflex loss; ocular surface damage; mechanical ventilation; treatment regimen
Sample Clinical Applications: Any condition where client is unable to protect self from drying of eye tissues, including facial or general trauma or surgery; mechanical ventilation; brain injury, cerebrovascular accident (CVA); neurological conditions such as Parkinson's disease, Bell's palsy; diabetic retinopathy; lupus; rheumatoid arthritis

DESIRED OUTCOMES/EVALUATION CRITERIA

Sample NOC linkages:
Dry Eye Severity: Severity of signs and symptoms of insufficient tears
Risk Control: Visual Impairment: Personal actions to prevent, eliminate, or reduce threats to visual function
Knowledge: Medication: Extent of understanding conveyed about the safe use of medication

Client Will (Include Specific Time Frame)
• Be free of discomfort or damage to eye related to dryness.
• Verbalize understanding of risk factors and ways to prevent dry eye.

ACTIONS/INTERVENTIONS

Sample NIC linkages:
Dry Eye Prevention: Prevention and early detection of dry eye in an individual at risk
Medication Administration: Eye: Preparing and instilling ophthalmic medications

NURSING PRIORITY NO. 1   To identify causative/precipitating factors related to risk:

• Obtain history of eye conditions when assessing client concerns overall. Note reports of dry sensation, burning, itching, pain, foreign body sensation, light sensitivity (photophobia), and blurred or fluctuating vision. *These symptoms can be associated with dry eye syndrome and, if present, require further evaluation and possible treatment.*[1]
• ▧ Note presence of conditions listed in risk factors above *to identify client with possible dry eye syndrome. Dry eye occurs when the quantity and/or quality of tears fails to keep the surface of the eye adequately lubricated. Dry eye is most commonly caused by increased tear evaporation or insufficient aqueous tear production. This can occur because of damage to eye surface (e.g., chemical burn) or be associated with disease conditions, neurological disorders, environmental factors, and electronic devise use. Note: Studies have associated systemic diseases (e.g., rheumatoid arthritis and Sjögren's syndrome, allergies, thyroid disorders) with dry eye,*

 Acute Care   Collaborative   Community/Home Care   Cultural

and some studies have associated dry eye with arterial hypertension and type 2 diabetes, although not all studies are in accord.[1–4,7]

- ∞ ▨ Note client's gender and age. *Note: Studies show a higher incidence of dry eye syndrome in females than males, especially over the age of 50.*[1,2,4]
- Determine client's current situation (e.g., admitted to facility for procedures/surgery, recent neurological event, mechanical ventilation, facial or eye trauma; eye infections, lower eyelid malposition) *that places client at high risk for dry eye associated with low or absent blink reflex and/or decreased tear production.*[5]
- Determine client's history/presence of seasonal or environmental allergies. *which may cause or exacerbate conjunctivitis.*
- Review living and work environment *to identify factors (e.g., exposure to smoke, wind, or chemicals; poor lighting, long periods of computer use or eye-straining work) that can cause or exacerbate dry eyes.*
- 🖊 Assess client's medications, noting use of certain drugs (e.g., antihistamines, beta blockers, antidepressants, and oral contraceptives) *known to decrease tear production.*[1]
- ✥ Refer for diagnostic evaluation and interventions as indicated. *Symptom questionnaire may reveal need for further evaluation.*

NURSING PRIORITY NO. 2 To promote eye health/comfort:

- ✥ Assist in/refer for treatment of underlying cause of dry eyes. *Interventions could range from changing a medication that is causing decreased tear production to surgery to correct an anatomic abnormality of the eyelid that interferes with blinking. Referral may be needed (e.g., to rheumatologist or endocrinologist for treatment of autoimmune condition or diabetes).*[6]
- 🖊 Administer artificial tears, lubricating eyedrops, or ointments as indicated *when client is unable to blink or otherwise protect eyes while in healthcare facility.*[5]

NURSING PRIORITY NO. 3 To promote wellness (Teaching/Discharge Criteria):

- 🏠 Instruct high-risk client in self-management interventions *to prevent or limit symptoms of dry eye:*[6,7]
  Avoid air blowing in eyes *such as might occur with hair dryers, car heaters, air conditioners, or fans directed toward eyes.*
  Wear eyeglasses or safety shield glasses on windy days *to reduce effects of the wind* and goggles while swimming *to protect eyes from chemicals in the water.*
  Take proper care of contact lenses and adhere to prescribed wearing time.
  Add moisture to indoor air, especially in winter.
  Take eye breaks during long reading and computer tasks or when watching TV for long periods of time.
  Blink repeatedly for a few seconds *to help spread tears evenly over eye.*
  Position computer screen below eye level. *This may help slow the evaporation of tears between eye blinks.*
  Cessation of smoking and avoidance of smoking environments. *Smoke can worsen dry eye symptoms.*
  Discuss dietary changes if indicated. *Some physicians and nutritionists recommend a diet high in vitamin A, which is found in liver, carrots, and broccoli, and/or a diet high in omega-3 fatty acids, which are found in fish, walnuts, and vegetable oil, to prevent dry eye associated with vitamin A deficiency.*

DOCUMENTATION FOCUS

Assessment/Reassessment
- Individual risk factors identified.
- Client concerns or difficulty making and following through with plan.

Planning
- Plan of care and who is involved in planning.
- Teaching plan.

 Diagnostic Studies   Evidence Based Practice   Medications 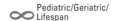 Pediatric/Geriatric/ Lifespan

Implementation/Evaluation
- Response to interventions, teaching, and actions performed.
- Attainment or progress toward outcomes.

Discharge Planning
- Referrals to other resources.
- Long-term need and who is responsible for actions.

References

1. Foster, C. S., et al. (Updated 2017). Dry eye disease (keratoconjunctivitis sicca). Retrieved March 2018 from http://emedicine.medscape.com/article/1210417-overview.
2. Sendecka, M., Baryluk, A., Polz-Dacewicz, M. (2004). Prevalence and risk factors of dry eye syndrome. *Przgl Epidemiol*, 58(1), 227–233.
3. Manaviat, M. R., et al. (2008). Prevalence of dry eye syndrome and diabetic retinopathy in type 2 diabetic patients. *BMC Ophthalmol*, 8, 10.
4. Moss, S. E., Klein, R., Klein, B. E. (2008). Long-term incidence of dry eye in an older population. *Optom Vis Sci*, 85(8), 668–674.
5. Schlessinger, D. A., Ulitsch, E. (2009). The eyes have it. *OR Nurse*, 3(4), 26–32.
6. Mayo Clinic Staff. (2012, update 2015). Dry eyes. Retrieved March 2018 from http://www.mayoclinic.org/diseases-conditions/dry-eyes/basics/definition/con-20024129.
7. Karpeki, P. M. (2015). The evolution of dry eye. Retrieved March 2018 from https://www.reviewofoptometry.com/article/the-evolution-of-dry-eye.

risk for Dry Mouth

Taxonomy II: Safety/Protection—Class 5 Physical Injury (00261) [**Diagnostic Division:** Safety], Approved 2016

DEFINITION: Susceptible to discomfort or damage to the oral mucosa due to reduced quantity and quality of saliva to moisten the mucosa, which may compromise health.

RISK FACTORS
Dehydration
Depression; excessive stress; excitement
Smoking
Associated Condition: Chemotherapy; radiation to the head and neck; oxygen therapy; systemic diseases; pregnancy
Fluid restriction; inability to feed orally
Pharmaceutical agent

DESIRED OUTCOMES/EVALUATION CRITERIA

Sample NOC linkages:
Oral Health: Condition of the mouth, teeth, gums, and tongue
Risk Control: Personal actions to understand, prevent, eliminate, or reduce modifiable health threats

Client/Caregiver Will (Include Specific Time Frame)
- Be free of discomfort or damage to mouth related to dryness.
- Verbalize understanding of risk factors and ways to prevent dry mouth.

Note: Many of the assessments and interventions in this ND are the same or similar to those in ND impaired Oral Mucous Membrane Integrity.

 Acute Care Collaborative Community/Home Care Cultural

ACTIONS/INTERVENTIONS

Sample NIC linkages:

Oral Health Maintenance: Maintenance and promotion of oral hygiene and dental health for the patient at risk for developing oral or dental lesions

NURSING PRIORITY NO. 1   To identify causative/contributing factors:

- 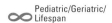 Perform oral screening or comprehensive assessment upon admission to facility using tool (e.g., Oral Health Assessment Tool for Long-Term Care), as indicated. *Use of standardized tool is beneficial in evaluating health of entire mouth including lips, tongue, gums, and other soft tissues.*[4]
- Note presence of diseases/conditions (e.g., Sjögren's syndrome, dementias, diabetes, anemia, cystic fibrosis, rheumatoid arthritis, hypertension, Parkinson's disease, stroke; dehydration [as might occur with fever, vomiting, diarrhea, blood loss, burns]) and treatments (e.g., nerve damage to the head and neck from injury or surgery; damage to the salivary glands as might occur from radiation to the head and neck, or chemotherapy for various cancers). *These factors/conditions are often associated with dry mouth.*[1,2]
- Review client's medications. *Dry mouth is a common side effect of many prescription and nonprescription drugs, including (but not limited to) muscle relaxants, sedatives, antidepressants, psychotropics, anti-anxiety agents; analgesics, antihistamines/decongestants; antileptics, antihypertensives, diuretics; antidiarrheals, antiemetics, bronchodilators.*[3] Note: *In 2013, the Centers for Disease Control and Prevention (CDC) reported that over 400 medications have been implicated in dry mouth.*
- 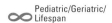 Perform regular oral exams several times/day. Pay attention to client reports of thirst, burning in mouth or tongue; dry throat; problems swallowing or speaking. Observe for dried, flaky, whitish saliva in and around the mouth, thick saliva that sticks to lip, bits of food or other matter on the teeth, tongue, and gums; cracked lips, raw-appearing red tongue, sores in corners of mouth; bad breath. *These signs and symptoms reveal severely dry mouth, reduced saliva, and possible systemic dehydration. Note: If client is receiving radiation therapy for cancer, the symptoms can greatly increase client's discomfort.*[12]
- Determine status of oral hygiene. Observe for chipped, sharp-edged teeth, or malpositioned teeth. Note fit of dentures or other prosthetic appliances when used. *Healthy teeth or well-fitting dentures have a strong effect on oral health and comfort of the oral mucosa, as well as the ability to eat (chewing, swallowing). Note: One recent study reported that people with broken teeth, absent teeth, or loose or ill-fitting dentures were more than 9 times more likely to report at least one oral impact (including dry mouth) than did those with well-fitting dentures.*[11] Conversely, dry mouth can lead to ongoing dental cavities and mouth infections.[11]
- Evaluate lifestyle concerns (e.g., smoking, chewing tobacco, breathing or sleeping with open mouth. *Such factors can cause or exacerbate dry mouth.*
- Determine problems with food and fluid intake (e.g., avoiding eating, reports change in taste, chews painstakingly, swallows numerous times for even small bites; insufficient fluid intake/dehydration; unexplained weight loss). *Malnutrition and dehydration are associated with problems with oral mucous membranes.*[5]

NURSING PRIORITY NO. 2   To correct identified/developing problems:

- Collaborate in treatment of underlying conditions, *which may correct or reduce problem with dry mouth.*
- Adjust medication regimen *to reduce use of drugs with potential for causing or exacerbating painful dry mouth.*
- Provide comfort mouth care (e.g., water; sodium bicarbonate solutions, mucosal coating agents, topical anesthetic gargles). Use petroleum jelly, cocoa butter, or a mild lip balm to keep lips moist. *May improve client comfort by hydration of mucous membrane surfaces.*[5,6,9]
- Avoid mouthwashes containing alcohol *(drying effect)* or hydrogen peroxide *(drying and foul tasting).*[7]

 Diagnostic Studies   Evidence Based Practice   Medications   ∞ Pediatric/Geriatric/Lifespan

- Use lemon/glycerin swabs with caution. *Although some sources mention use of glycerin swabs, the issue appears to be controversial, with some stating that glycerin should not be used as it absorbs water and actually dries the oral cavity and can result in decreased salivary amylase, as well as erosion of tooth enamel.*[5,8]
- Encourage use of chewing gum, hard candy, etc., *to stimulate flow of saliva to neutralize acids and limit bacterial growth.*[2]
- Avoid dry foods, such as crackers, cookies, and toast, or soften them with liquids before eating. Sip liquids with meals to moisten foods and help with swallowing.[8]
- Encourage adequate fluids *to prevent dehydration and oral dryness and limit bacterial overgrowth.*[8]
- Suggest use of vaporizer or room humidifier *to increase humidity if client is mouth breather or ambient humidity is low.*
- Discuss and instruct caregiver(s) in special mouth care required during end-of-life care/hospice *to promote optimal comfort in client who has stopped eating or drinking, who has dry mouth, and may not have sensation of thirst.*[9]

NURSING PRIORITY NO. 3 To promote wellness (Teaching/Discharge Considerations):

- 🏠 ⊛ Recommend regular dental checkups and care and episodic evaluation of oral health prior to certain medical treatments (e.g., chemotherapy, radiation) *to maintain oral health and reduce risks associated with impaired tissues.*
- Review current oral hygiene practices and concerns. Provide informational resources, including reliable Web sites about oral health *to reinforce learning and encourage proper care.*
- Provide nutritional information *to correct deficiencies, reduce mucosal inflammation or gum disease, and prevent dental caries.*
- Emphasize benefit of avoiding alcohol and smoking or chewing tobacco, *which can contribute to mucosal inflammation and gum disease.*
- Discuss need for and demonstrate use of special appliances (e.g., power toothbrushes, dental water jets, flossing instruments, applicators) if indicated. *Enhances independence in self-care.*
- ⊛ Identify community resources (e.g., low-cost dental clinics, smoking-cessation resources, cancer information services or support group, Meals on Wheels, supplemental nutrition program, home-care aide) *to meet individual needs.*

DOCUMENTATION FOCUS

Assessment/Reassessment
- Condition of oral mucous membranes, routine oral care habits and interferences.
- Availability of oral care equipment and products.
- Knowledge of proper oral hygiene and care.
- Availability and use of resources.

Planning
- Plan of care and who is involved in planning.
- Teaching plan.

Implementation/Evaluation
- Responses to interventions, teaching, and actions performed.
- Attainment or progress toward desired outcome(s).
- Modifications to plan of care.

Discharge Planning
- Long-term needs and who is responsible for actions to be taken.
- Specific referrals made, resources for special appliances.

 Acute Care   Collaborative   Community/ Home Care   Cultural

References

1. Friedman, M. (2017). Dental health and dry mouth (various sections). Retrieved May 2018 from https://www.webmd.com/oral-health/guide/dental-health-dry-mouth#1.
2. PDQ® Supportive and Palliative Care Editorial Board. (2014, updated 2016). PDQ oral complications of chemotherapy and head/neck radiation: Various sections. Retrieved May 2018 from https://www.cancer.gov/about-cancer/treatment/side-effects/mouth-throat/oral-complications-hp-pdq#section/_AboutThis_1.
3. Wyatt, A. D. (2016). Oral side effects of medications (various sections). Retrieved May 2018 from https://www.webmd.com/oral-health/guide/oral-side-effects-of-medications#1.
4. University of Iowa College of Nursing, John A. Hartford Foundation Center of Geriatric Nursing Excellence-Academic Institution. (2002, revised 2011). Oral hygiene care for functionally dependent and cognitively impaired older adults. Revised guideline. Retrieved May 2018 from https://www.guidelinecentral.com/summaries/oral-hygiene-care-for-functionally-dependent-and-cognitively-impaired-older-adults/#.
5. Stiefel, K. A., et al. (2000). Improving oral hygiene for the seriously ill patient: Implementing research-based practice. *Medsurg Nurs*, 9(1), 40–46.
6. Farris, C., McEnroe Petitte, D. (2013). Head, neck, and cancer update. *Home Healthc Nurse*, 31(6), 322–328.
7. Winslow, E. H. (1994). Don't use H_2O_2 for oral care. *Am J Nurse*, 94(3), 19.
8. Munro, C., Grap, M. J. (2004). Oral health and care in the intensive care unit: State of science. *Am J Crit Care*, 13(1), 25–33.
9. Schwarz, J. K. (2014). Hospice care for patients who choose to hasten death by voluntarily stopping eating and drinking. *J Hosp Palliat Nurs*, 16(3), 126–131.
10. Porter, J., Nitouva, A., Read, A. (2015). The impact of oral health on the quality of life of nursing home residents. *Health Qual Life Outcomes*, 13, 102–110.
11. Centers for Disease Control and Prevention (CDC). (last updated 2013). Oral health of older Americans. Retrieved May 2018 from https://www.cdc.gov/oralhealth/publications/factsheets/adult_oral_health/adult_older.htm.
12. American Cancer Society (ACS). (2015). Dry mouth. Retrieved May 2018 from https://www.cancer.org/treatment/treatments-and-side-effects/physical-side-effects/mouth-problems/dry-mouth.html.

ineffective adolescent Eating Dynamics

Taxonomy II: Nutrition—Class 1 Ingestion (00269) [**Diagnostic Division:** Food/Fluid] Approved 2016

DEFINITION: Altered eating attitudes and behaviors resulting in over or under eating patterns that compromise nutritional health.

RELATED FACTORS

Altered family dynamics; negative parental influences on eating behaviors
Anxiety; depression; excessive stress
Changes to self-esteem upon entering puberty
Eating disorder; inadequate choice of food
Eating in isolation; excessive family mealtime control; irregular mealtime; stressful mealtimes
Media influence on knowledge of, or eating behaviors of high caloric unhealthy foods
Psychological abuse or neglect

DEFINING CHARACTERISTICS

Subjective

Complains of hunger between meals; poor appetite

Objective

Frequent snacking; frequently eating from fast food restaurants; frequently eating processed food, or poor quality food

(continues on page 276)

 Diagnostic Studies   Evidence Based Practice   Medications   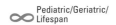 Pediatric/Geriatric/Lifespan

ineffective adolescent Eating Dynamics (continued)

Avoids participation in regular mealtimes; food refusal

Overeating, undereating

Associated Condition: Physical challenge with eating or feeding

Physical or psychological health issues of parents

Sample Clinical Applications: Anorexia, bulimia nervosa, obesity, beriatric surgery, substance abuse, depression, anxiety disorder

DESIRED OUTCOMES/EVALUATION CRITERIA

Sample NOC linkages:

Eating Disorder: Self-Control: Personal actions to eliminate maladaptive behaviors and to adopt and maintain healthy eating patterns and optimum body weight

Nutritional Status: Biochemical Measures: Body fluid components and chemical indices of nutritional status

Client Will (Include Specific Time Frame)

• Make nutritionally adequate choices of food/fluids.

• Assume control over mealtime.

• Identify feelings and underlying dynamics of low self-esteem/changes of puberty.

• Display normalization of laboratory values reflecting appropriate nutrient intake.

Sample NOC linkages:

Knowledge: Eating Disorder Management: Extent of understanding conveyed about an eating disorder, its treatment, and the prevention of disease progression and complications

Parenting Performance: Parental actions to provide a child a nurturing and constructive physical, emotional, and social environment

Parent/Caregiver Will (Include Specific Time Frame)

• Verbalize understanding of under/overinvolved parenting style.

• Identify specific actions that affect eating habits.

• Demonstrate willingness to work together as a family to resolve presenting problems.

Refer to NDs: Nutrition, imbalanced: less than body requirement; Overweight; Obesity as indicated for additional interventions specific to client's situation.

ACTIONS/INTERVENTIONS

Sample NIC linkages:

Nutritional Counseling: Use of an interactive helping process focusing on the need for diet modifications

Family Therapy: Assisting family members to move their family toward a more productive way of living

NURSING PRIORITY NO. 1   To assess causative/contributing factors:

• ✍ Note age and developmental level of client and place in family order. *The adolescent period of development is a period of vulnerability for the development of problems with eating.*[8] *Family order may impact how other members respond to or handle conflict.*

• ✍ Discuss client's perception of the current situation and motivation for change. *Important to understand client's belief and understanding and whether current situation is viewed as a problem.*[6]

 Acute Care   Collaborative   Community/ Home Care   Cultural

- Assess eating habits and nutritional intake. *Helps determine behaviors to be changed and provides basis for planning care.*[1]
- 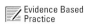 Identify family cultural/religious factors and finances. *Personal beliefs and finances affect choices when developing meal plans.*
- Determine dynamics of family system. *How the family deals with the adolescent is critical to the outcome of the illness. Family-based treatment can be important for the client's recovery.*[2]
- Perform a complete physical exam. *Provides a baseline for comparison as client progresses through treatment.*[3]
- Assess current weight. *to identify deviations from the norm and establish baseline parameters.*[3]
- Evaluate possibility of attention-deficit hyperactivity disorder (ADHD). *Although research has lagged in this area, there are reasons to believe that girls with this disorder may be at increased risk for eating disorders such as body dissatisfaction, showing distress through eating disorders, underweight or overweight.*[5]
- Note issues of self-esteem client may express. *Adolescents often struggle with concerns about their body in relation to others and often believe they are not as worthwhile as their peers.*[6]
- Identify gender of the client. *Although females with eating disorders outnumber males by a significant number, males make up an important aspect of this problem, are more reluctant to seek help, and may need special accommodations, such as an all-male treatment team.*[7]
- Discuss client's/family's eating patterns and attitudes toward food. *Provides information that will be helpful to plan for needed changes and may reveal problems of others needing to be addressed.*[9,10]
- Review lab studies reflecting nutritional status. *Helpful in identifying deficiencies and therapeutic needs.*

NURSING PRIORITY NO. 2   To assist client to develop skills to manage adequate nutritional needs:

- Promote therapeutic nurse/client/family relationship. *A trusting relationship allows the individuals to freely share and be open and honest with self and therapist.*[2]
- Assist client to make achievable goals to maintain healthy eating habits. *Increases likelihood of successful change.*[2]
- Refer to dietician. *Provides information and guidance in determining individual nutritional needs incorporating child's likes and is mindful of dislikes.*
- Discuss frequent use of processed or fast-food sources for meals. *While this may expedite meals for the busy family, they do not provide the nutrition needed for growing children or general health of other family members and are not cost effective.*[10]
- Emphasize need to avoid comparing self with others, encouraging client to look at positive aspects of self. *Adolescents tend to look at friends, TV, models, and others to model themselves after rather than accepting their body as being all right as is.*[10]
- Note perceptions client may express and discuss realities. *Correcting misperceptions helps the adolescent adjust choices of food and activities for more positive results.*[6]
- Address physical/safety issues client presents. *Physical changes in the body that are occurring with client's current eating habits affect how client views self-esteem and contribute to lack of attention to safety issues.*[4]
- Remind family/friends that teasing client about body/eating habits is not to be done. *Teasing can be damaging, regardless of whether client is obese or thin, and is counterproductive.*[2]
- Refer for family therapy as indicated. *May help resolve parent and adolescent issues interfering with relationship and manifesting in unhealthy eating behaviors.*[2]
- Encourage client to become involved in enjoyable physical activities. *Participation in these activities can enhance self-esteem, promote self-reliance and confidence, and lead to improved weight management.*[8]
- Refer to NDs chronic low Self-Esteem for additional interventions.

NURSING PRIORITY NO. 3   To promote wellness (Teaching/Discharge Considerations):

- Involve client in school and social activities. *Continuing scholastic studies will improve sense of accomplishment, and involvement in social groups will provide opportunities to make friends and enjoy activities that may involve eating in accepted manner.*[9]

 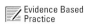

- Talk with adolescent about involvement with social media. *Social media is found to have a negative effect on self-esteem for adolescents, and sharing this information can help the individual change her/his attitude.*[4]
- Identify appropriate online reference sites. *Can provide information and recipes to help with meal planning over time to achieve long-term goals.*
- Identify community support programs and resources as needed. *Useful in sustaining efforts for change.*
- Refer parents to parenting classes, such as effectiveness training, etc., and group therapy. *Will help parents learn how to interact with their growing adolescent as both develop positive relationships.*[11]

DOCUMENTATION FOCUS

Assessment/Reassessment
- Individual findings, including eating habits, attitude toward them, food choices.
- Interactions with others, peers, and family.
- Motivation for change.

Planning
- Plan of care and who is involved in planning.
- Teaching plan.

Implementation/Evaluation
- Responses to interventions, teaching, and changes.
- Attainment or progress toward desired outcomes.
- Modification to plan of care.

Discharge Planning
- Long-term needs and who is responsible for actions.
- Specific referrals made.

References

1. Rikani, A. A., et al. (2013). A critique of the literature on etiology of eating disorder. *Ann Neurosci*, 20(4), 157–161.
2. Robinson, A., Dolhanty, J., Greenberg, L. (2013). Emotion-focused family therapy for eating disorders in children and adolescents. *Clin Psychol Psychother*, 22(1), 75–82.
3. Klein, D., Walsh, B. T. (2004). Eating disorders: Clinical features and pathophysiology. *Physiol Behav*, 81(2), 369–82.
4. Story, M., Neumark-Szainer, D., French, S. (2002). Individual and environmental influences on adolescent eating behaviors. *J Am Diet Assoc*, 102(3 Suppl), S40–S51.
5. Mikami, A. Y., et al. (2008). Eating pathology among adolescent girls with attention-deficit/hyperactivity disorder. *J Abnorm Psychol*, 117(1), 225–235.
6. Chin, S. N. M., Laverty, A. A. Flippidis, F. T. (2018). Trends and correlated of unhealthy dieting behaviors among adolescents in the United States. *BMC Public Health*. Retrieved June 2018, from https://bmcpublichealth.biomedcentral.com/articles/10.1186/s12889-018-5348-2.
7. Crouse, K. (2018). Adam Rippon on quiet starvation in men's figure skating. *New York Times*. Retrieved June 2018, from https://www.nytimes.com/2018/02/13/sports/olympics/figure-skating-adam-rippon.html.
8. Allen, K. L., et al. (2014). Maternal and family factors and child eating pathology: Risk and protective relationships. *J Eat Disord*. Retrieved June 2018, from https://jeatdisord.biomedcentral.com/articles/10.1186/2050-2974-2-11.
9. Reicks, M., et al. (2015). Influence of parenting practices on eating behaviors of early adolescents during independent eating occasions: Implications for obesity prevention. *Nutrients*, 7(10), 8783–8801.
10. Krug, I., et al. (2015). Eating-related environmental factors in underweight eating disorders and obesity: Are there common vulnerabilities during childhood and early adolescence? *Eur Eat Disord Rev*, 21(3), 11.
11. Gerands, S. M., Kremers, C. (2015). The role of food, parenting skills, and the home food environment in children's weight gain and obesity. *Curr Obes Rep*, 4(9), 30–36.

 Acute Care
 Collaborative
 Community/ Home Care
Cultural

ineffective child Eating Dynamics

Taxonomy II: Nutrition—Class 1 Ingestion (00270) [**Diagnostic Division:** Food/Fluid], Approved 2016

DEFINITION: Altered attitudes, behaviors, and influences on child eating patterns resulting in compromised nutritional health

RELATED FACTORS

Eating Habits:
Bribing or forcing child to eat; excessive parental control over child's eating experience; limiting child's eating or rewarding child to eat
Consumption of large volumes of food in a short period of time; inadequate choice of food
Disordered eating habits; eating in isolation; unpredictable eating patterns
Excessive parental control over family meal time; lack of regular mealtimes; stressful mealtimes
Unstructured eating of snacks between meals

Family Process:
Abusive relationship
Anxious, hostile, insecure, or tense parent-child relationship
Disengaged, overinvolved, or underinvolved parenting style

Parental:
Anorexia; inability to support healthy eating patterns
Depression; ineffective coping strategies; substance misuse/[abuse]
Inability to divide eating or feeding responsibility between parent and child
Lack of confidence in child to develop healthy eating patterns or grow appropriately

Environmental:
Media influence on knowledge of, or eating behaviors of, high caloric unhealthy foods

DEFINING CHARACTERISTICS

Subjective
Complains of hunger between meals; poor appetite

Objective
Frequent snacking; frequently eating from fast food restaurants; frequently eating processed food or poor quality food
Avoids participation in regular mealtimes; food refusal
Overeating, undereating
At Risk Population: Economically disadvantaged; homeless
Involved with the foster care system
Life transition
Parental obesity
Associated Condition: Physical challenge with eating or feeding
Physical or psychological health issues of parents
Sample Clinical Applications: Obesity, anorexia, substance abuse

DESIRED OUTCOMES/EVALUATION CRITERIA

Sample NOC linkages:
Eating Disorder Self-Control: Personal actions to eliminate maladaptive behaviors and to adopt and maintain healthy eating patterns and optimum body weight

(continues on page 280)

 Diagnostic Studies   Evidence Based Practice   Medications   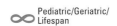 Pediatric/Geriatric/ Lifespan

ineffective child Eating Dynamics (continued)

Child Will (Include Specific Time Frame)
- Ingest appropriate amount of calories/nutrients to meet metabolic needs.
- Achieve/maintain body weight appropriate for height.

Sample NOC linkages:
Knowledge: Eating Disorder Management: Extent of understanding conveyed about an eating disorder, its treatment, and the prevention of disease progression and complications
Parenting Performance: Parental actions to provide a child a nurturing and constructive physical, emotional, and social environment

Parent/Caregiver Will (Include Specific Time Frame)
- Acknowledge that child is having problems with eating.
- Verbalize understanding of under-/overinvolved parenting style.
- Identify specific actions that affect eating habits.
- Demonstrate willingness to work together as a family to resolve presenting problems.

ACTIONS/INTERVENTIONS

Sample NIC linkages:
Parenting Promotion: Providing parenting information, support, and coordination of comprehensive services to high-risk families
Nutritional Counseling: Use of an interactive helping process focusing on the need for diet modifications

NURSING PRIORITY NO. 1   To assess causative/contributing factors:

- Determine individual situation (e.g., bribing or forcing child to eat, excessive parental control over child's eating experience, stressful mealtimes, inappropriate choice of foods). *Provides information to develop plan of care.*[3]
- Assess child's health status, weight, age, stage of growth and development. *Information needed to determine nutritional needs and desired change in weight.*[4]
- Ascertain family functioning and relationships that may affect child's eating disorder. *How family members interact with one another, arguments, or disagreements can affect child's eating behaviors.*[3]
- Note child's eating habits, eating in isolation, unpredictable eating patterns, eating snacks between meals. *These factors can lead to weight gain as child grows.*[5]
- Determine family habits of watching TV and other social media especially while eating. *The influence of media (especially food commercials) on family and child's eating of high calorie unhealthy foods is well documented.*[4]
- Evaluate physical activities of all family members. *Inactivity can contribute to increased risk of obesity. A significant number of children are obese or overweight at an earlier age than in the past.*[1]
- Note environmental factors, including family functioning and parenting style, mother's eating disorder or mental status, relationship between mother and child. *Self-report interviews reveal problem areas for mothers and children to determine needs for intervention.*[3] Note: While primary focus has been directed toward mothers, either or both parents may have issues to be addressed.
- Identify family cultural/religious beliefs and finances. *Personal beliefs and financial resources affect how family views food and impacts meal plans.*

 Acute Care   Collaborative   Community/Home Care   Cultural

NURSING PRIORITY NO. 2 To assist family/child to develop new habits/patterns of family functioning and eating behaviors:

• Develop therapeutic nurse-client relationship. Be attentive, provide encouragement for efforts, use skills of active listening and I messages to maintain open communication. *Promotes trusting situation in which client is able to express self and be honest and open with self and nurse.*
• Discuss eating behaviors with family/child, identifying areas for change. *Realizing how eating patterns affect children can enable parents to be willing to make changes for better nutrition and overall health.*[4]
• Help parents learn new methods of planning and cooking foods. *Learning healthy ways of eating can help parents and children establish nutritionally sound habits of eating.*[4]
• Discuss parental involvement with child's eating behaviors. *Parents may not trust child to make healthy choices for eating, resulting in overinvolvement or anxious behaviors affecting child's eating.*[3]

NURSING PRIORITY NO. 3 To establish nutritionally adequate plan that meets needs of family members:

• Involve parents and child in developing achievable short- and long-term goals. *Increases likelihood of success if all parties agree on the goals.*
• Consult with dietician. *Provides information and guidance in determining individual nutritional needs incorporating child's likes and being mindful of dislikes.*
• Develop a plan, taking into account previously determined problems of family's eating behaviors. *Sitting down as a family at regularly scheduled times in a "media-free zone" that encourages open family communication can reduce stress levels and enhance food intake.*[1]
• Encourage parents to relax and allow child to make own decisions about eating. *Children will eat what they need when given the opportunity to make own choices.*[3]
• Talk about frequent use of processed or "fast food" sources for meals. *While this may expedite meals for the busy family, they do not provide the nutrition needed for growing children as well as general health of other family members, and are not cost effective.*[2]

NURSING PRIORITY NO. 4 To promote wellness (Teaching/Discharge Considerations):

• Emphasize importance of well-balanced nutrition intake within financial concerns. *Individuals may have never learned how to shop for and prepare affordable quality foods.*[1]
• Identify appropriate online reference sites. *Can provide information and recipes to help with meal planning over time to achieve long-term goals.*
• Assist in developing regular exercise and stress reduction programs. *Helps family members learn ways to manage weight and stress levels, improving general well-being.*[6]
• Refer parents to classes in parenting, nutritional food preparation, or therapeutic needs. *Can be helpful when needed to assist family to learn new ways of dealing with issues/problems.*[4]
• Identify community support programs and resources as needed. *Useful in sustaining efforts for change.*

DOCUMENTATION FOCUS

Assessment/Reassessment
• Health status and weight of child and parents.
• Parents' understanding of or perception of problems.

Planning
• Plan of care and who is involved in planning.
• Teaching plan.

Implementation/Evaluation
• Parent/child responses to interventions, teaching, and actions performed.
• Attainment or progress toward desired outcomes.

 Diagnostic Studies   Evidence Based Practice   Medications   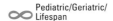 Pediatric/Geriatric/Lifespan

Discharge Planning

• Long-term needs, and who is responsible for actions to be taken.
• Specific referrals made.

References

1. Eneli, I. U., et al. (2015). Rationale and design of the feeding dynamic intervention (FDI) study for self-regulation of energy intake in preschoolers. Contemp Clin Trials. Retrieved June 2018, from https://www.ncbi.nlm.nih.gov/pmc/articles/PMC4400666/.
2. Reicks, M., et al. (2015). Influence of parenting practices on eating behaviors of early adolescents during independent eating occasions: Implications for obesity prevention. *Nutrients*, 7(10), 8783–8801.
3. Allen, K. L., et al. (2014). Maternal and family factors and child eating pathology: Risk and protective relationships. *J Eat Disord*. Retrieved June 2018 from https://jeatdisord.biomedcentral.com/articles/10.1186/2050-2974-2-11.
4. Krug, I., et al. (2015). Eating-related environmental factors in underweight eating disorders and obesity: Are there common vulnerabilities during childhood and early adolescence? *Eur Eat Disord Rev*, 21(3), 11.
5. Gerands, S. M., Kremers, C. (2015). The role of food, parenting skills, and the home food environment in children's weight gain and obesity. *Curr Obes Rep*, 4(9), 30–36.
6. Rikani, A. A., et al. (2013). A critique of the literature on etiology of eating disorder. *Ann Neurosci*, 20(4), 157–161.

ineffective infant Eating Dynamics

Taxonomy II: Nutrition—Class 1 Ingestion (00271) **[Diagnostic Division:** Food/Fluid], Approved 2016

DEFINITION: Altered parental behaviors resulting in over or under eating patterns.

RELATED FACTORS
Abusive relationship

Attachment issues; disengaged parenting style; over-involved or under-involved parenting style

Lack of knowledge of infant's developmental stages or for appropriate methods of feeding infant for each stage of development

Lack of knowledge of parent's responsibility in infant feeding; multiple caregivers

Lack of confidence in child to develop healthy eating habits or to grow appropriately

Media influence on knowledge of, or feeding infant high caloric unhealthy foods

DEFINING CHARACTERISTICS

Objective
Food refusal; poor appetite

Inappropriate transition to solid foods

Overeating or undereating

At Risk Population: Abandonment; involvement with the foster care system

Economically disadvantaged; homeless

History of unsafe eating and feeding experiences

Life transitions

Small for gestational age; prematurity; neonatal intensive care experiences; prolonged hospitalization

Associated Condition: Chromosomal disorders; genetic disorder; neural tube defects; sensory integration problems; congenital heart disease

Cleft lip or palate; physical challenge with eating

Physical or psychological health issues of parents

 Acute Care   Collaborative   Community/Home Care   Cultural

Prolonged enteral feedings

Sample Clinical Applications: Cleft lip/palate, congenital heart disease, premature infant

DESIRED OUTCOMES/EVALUATION CRITERIA

Sample NOC linkages:

Infant Nutritional Status: Amount of nutrients ingested and absorbed to meet metabolic needs and foster growth of an infant

Infant Will (Include Specific Time Frame)
• Ingest appropriate amount of calories/nutrients to meet metabolic needs.
• Achieve/maintain optimum body weight.

Knowledge: Infant Care: Extent of understanding conveyed about caring for a baby from birth to first birthday

Parenting Performance: Infant: Parental actions to provide an infant a safe, nurturing, and positive physical, emotional, spiritual, and social environment from 28 days to first birthday

Parents Will (Include Specific Time Frame)
• Verbalize understanding of infant feeding problems.
• Participate in treatment program as able.
• Attend classes to obtain knowledge about infant needs and developmental issues.
• Verbalize knowledge of appropriate methods of feeding infant at each stage of development.

ACTIONS/INTERVENTIONS

Sample NIC linkages:

Teaching: Infant Nutrition (specify) months: Instruction on nutrition and feeding practices through the 12 months of life

Parenting Promotion: Providing parenting information, support, and coordination of comprehensive services to high-risk families

NURSING PRIORITY NO. 1   To assess causative/contributing factors:

• Identify current situation and specific needs of infant and parents. *Information necessary to define needs and develop plan of care.*
• Assess parents' knowledge of infant feeding needs. *Parents may require basic information or may just need additional information to understand current situation.*[2]
• Note interaction between parent and infant. *Parent may need assistance with handling infant, and caregiver is able to foster appropriate behavior and discourage maladaptive behavior.*[4]
• Obtain baseline weight and weigh on predetermined schedule. *Weight loss can indicate problems with feeding, inability to suck sufficiently and correctly, insufficient quantity of breast milk.*[5]
• Determine sucking dynamics of the breastfed infant, especially preterm infants. *Breastfeeding is the ultimate nutritional goal, and effective sucking is vital to accomplishing adequate intake.*[5]
• Note feeding problems, such as colic, vomiting, slow feeding, or refusal to eat. *Mild to moderately severe issues may be managed by care provider, while more-complicated cases may require referral to specialists.*[1]
• 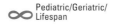 Identify family cultural/religious beliefs and finances. *Personal beliefs and financial resources affect how family views feeding choice (i.e., breast or bottle) and food choices when solids are introduced.*

 Diagnostic Studies   Evidence Based Practice   Medications   ∞ Pediatric/Geriatric/Lifespan

NURSING PRIORITY NO. 2 To promote effective infant eating dynamics:

- Develop positive nurse/family relationship. *Enables family to feel comfortable discussing issues with nurse, being open and honest about concerns and anxieties.*[3]
- Consult with dietician. *Provides information and guidance in determining individual nutritional needs incorporating infant's particular issues.*
- Provide information about normal growth, development, and nutritional needs when no problems are present. *Helps parents understand what to look for as infant progresses.*[1]
- Discuss needs of infant with structural abnormalities, i.e., naso-oropharynx, larynx, and trachea, cleft lip or palate, esophagus, esophageal atresia or stenosis, stricture. *Investigation of individual situation can identify specific needs, difficulty with feeding, child's growth pattern, interaction between parent and child.*[1]
- Provide information about neurodevelopmental disability that has been identified in newborn. *Each situation will need individual assessment regarding how is the problem manifested; the problems with feeding, weight, and development; the emotional climate in the family during feeding or other caregiving.*[1]
- Discuss the basic food rules. *Parents control what, when, and where infant is fed. Infant controls how much they eat in order to learn internal regulation of eating in accordance with physiological signals of hunger and fullness.*[1]
- Give assistance to parents requiring help with management skills. *Setting time limits for meals, ignoring noneating behavior, and using positive reinforcement to motivate infant can promote positive feeding behaviors.*[4]

Refer to ND ineffective infant Feeding Pattern for additional interventions.

NURSING PRIORITY NO. 3 To promote wellness (Teaching/Discharge Considerations):

- Encourage family members to set realistic goals for achieving necessary lifestyle changes. *Depending on the family situation, families will be dealing with problems as infant grows, and having written goals provides reminder of what needs to be done.*[7]
- Discuss methods family can take to make needed changes in family functioning, parenting styles. *Evidence exists to show that associations exist between family characteristics and feeding behavior problems in early childhood.*[3]
- Identify support groups based on individual needs. *Provides opportunity for parents to interact with others addressing similar issues.*
- Refer to community resources (e.g., public health visitor program, home care, day care/respite care, nutrition program/food bank). *Additional support and assistance enhances parents' opportunity for meeting established goals.*
- Refer to parenting classes, individual and family therapy, and/or psychiatric counseling, as indicated. *Additional help will enable family to cope with problems in more positive ways.*[4]
- Suggest participation in group or community activities, e.g., assertiveness classes, volunteer work. *Involvement with others in these activities helps individuals to learn new ways of coping with problems in their own family.*[2]

DOCUMENTATION FOCUS

Assessment/Reassessment
- Individual findings, noting specific family problems and infant issues.
- Underlying dynamics of current situation.
- Family support, availability and use of resources.

Planning
- Plan of care and who is involved in planning.
- Teaching plan.

 Acute Care   Collaborative   Community/ Home Care   Cultural

Implementation/Evaluation

- Response to interventions, teaching, actions performed, and changes that may be indicated.
- Attainment or progress toward desired outcomes.
- Modifications to plan of care.

Discharge Planning

- Long-term needs and goals and who is responsible for actions to be taken.
- Specific referrals made.

References

1. Bernard-Bonnin, A. C. (2006). Feeding problems of infants and toddlers. *Can Fam Physician*, 52(10), 1247–1251.
2. Daily RN (Jalil). (2017). Ineffective infant feeding pattern nursing diagnosis and nursing care plan. Daily RN. Retrieved June 2018 from http://dailyrn.com/ineffective-infant-feeding-pattern-ncp-nd/ml.
3. Yang, H. R. (2017). How to approach feeding difficulties in young children. *Korean J Pediatr*, 60(12), 379–384.
4. Silva, G. A. P., Costa, K. O. A., Giugliani, E. R. J. (2016). Infant feeding: Beyond the nutritional aspects. Retrieved June 2018 from https://www.sciencedirect.com/science/article/pii/S0021755716000474.
5. Geddes, D. T., et al. (2017). Characterisation of sucking dynamics of breastfeeding preterm infants: A cross sectional study. Retrieved June 2018 from https://www.ncbi.nlm.nih.gov/pmc/articles/PMC5693509/.
6. Babbitt, R. L., et al. (1994). Behavioral assessment and treatment of pediatric feeding disorders. *J Dev Behav Pediatr*, 15(4), 278–291.
7. Klein, D., Walsh, B. T. (2004). Eating disorders: Clinical features and pathophysiology. *Physiol Behav*, 81(2), 369–82.

risk for Electrolyte Imbalance

Taxonomy II: Nutrition—Class 5 Hydration (00195) [**Diagnostic Division:** Food/Fluid], Submitted 2008; Revised 2013, 2017

DEFINITION: Susceptible to changes in serum electrolyte levels, which may compromise health.

RISK FACTORS

Diarrhea; vomiting

Excessive or insufficient fluid volume

Associated Condition: Endocrine regulatory dysfunction [e.g., glucose intolerance, increase in IGF-1, androgen, DHEA, and cortisol]; renal dysfunction

Compromised regulatory mechanism [e.g., diabetes insipidus, syndrome of inappropriate secretion of antidiuretic hormone]

Treatment regimen

Sample Clinical Applications: Renal failure, anorexia nervosa, diabetes mellitus, Crohn's disease; gastroenteritis, pancreatitis, traumatic brain injury, cancer, multiple trauma, burns, sickle cell disease

DESIRED OUTCOMES/EVALUATION CRITERIA

Sample NOC linkages:

Electrolyte & Acid/Base Balance: Balance of electrolytes and nonelectrolytes in the intracellular and extracellular compartments of the body

Fluid Balance: Balance of the input and output of fluids in the body

Client Will (Include Specific Time Frame)

- Display laboratory results within normal range for individual.
- Be free of complications resulting from electrolyte imbalance.

(continues on page 286)

 Diagnostic Studies   Evidence Based Practice   Medications   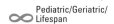 Pediatric/Geriatric/Lifespan

risk for Electrolyte Imbalance (continued)

ACTIONS/INTERVENTIONS

NURSING PRIORITY NO. 1   To assess causative/contributing factors:

- Identify client with current or newly diagnosed condition commonly associated with electrolyte imbalances, such as inability to eat or drink, febrile illness, and active bleeding or other fluid loss, including vomiting, diarrhea, gastrointestinal drainage, and burns. *The nurse taking a history on a new client, in both community health settings and acute care, should be alert to the possibility of electrolyte imbalances either being caused by an underlying condition or actually causing the client's symptoms. Symptoms of electrolyte imbalance depend upon the specific mineral affected but can include fatigue, muscle cramping, weakness, irregular heartbeat, confusion, and blood pressure changes.*[10]
- ∞ Assess specific client risk, noting client age (including premature infants or sick newborn, elderly debilitated client) and chronic disease processes that may lead to electrolyte imbalance, including kidney disease, metabolic or endocrine disorders, chronic alcoholism, cancers or cancer treatments, conditions causing hemolysis such as massive trauma, multiple blood transfusions, and sickle cell disease.[1,18] *Electrolyte excesses are caused by factors that (1) increase electrolyte intake or absorption, (2) shift electrolytes from an electrolyte pool to the extracellular fluid, or (3) decrease electrolyte excretion.*[4] *Electrolyte deficits are caused by factors that (1) decrease electrolyte intake or absorption, (2) shift electrolytes from the extracellular fluid to an electrolyte pool, (3) increase electrolyte excretion, or (4) cause abnormal loss of electrolytes.*[4]
- Review client's medications *for those associated with electrolyte imbalance. Note: There are many such medications, including (but not limited to) diuretics, laxatives, corticosteroids, barbiturates, certain antidepressants (e.g., SSRIs), antihypertensive agents, antiepileptics, some hormones/birth control pills, and some antibiotics and antifungal agents.*

NURSING PRIORITY NO. 2   To identify potential electrolyte deficit:

- Assess mental status, noting client/caregiver report of change—altered attention span, recall of recent events, and other cognitive functions. *Altered mental status is the most common sign of sodium imbalances.*[2,18]
- Monitor heart rate and rhythm by palpation and auscultation. *Weak pulse or thready pulse can be associated with hypokalemia; tachycardia, bradycardia, and other dysrhythmias are associated with various electrolyte imbalances, including potassium, calcium, and magnesium.*[1–3,16]
- Auscultate breath sounds, assess respirations noting rate and depth and ease of respiratory effort, observe color of nailbeds and mucous membranes, and note pulse oximetry or blood gas measurement, as indicated. *Certain electrolyte imbalances, such as hypokalemia, can cause or exacerbate respiratory insufficiency.*[2]

 Acute Care   Collaborative   Community/ Home Care   Cultural

- Review electrocardiogram (ECG). *The ECG reflects electrophysiological, anatomical, metabolic, and hemodynamic alterations and is routinely used for the diagnosis of electrolyte and metabolic disturbances, as well as myocardial ischemia, cardiac dysrhythmias, structural changes of the myocardium, and drug effects.*[1–4]
- Assess gastrointestinal symptoms, noting presence, absence, and character of bowel sounds; presence of acute or chronic diarrhea; and persistent vomiting and high nasogastric tube output. *Any disturbance of gastrointestinal (GI) functioning carries with it the potential for electrolyte imbalances.*[4,5]
- Review client's food intake. Note presence of anorexia/other eating disorders, vomiting, or recent fad or unusual diet, and look for chronic malnutrition. *Can point to potential electrolyte imbalances, either deficiencies or excesses, such as high sodium content.*[5]
- Evaluate motor strength and function. *Neuromuscular function, including steadiness of gait, handgrip strength, reactivity of reflexes, and muscle weakness, can provide clues to electrolyte imbalances, including calcium, magnesium, phosphorus, sodium, and potassium.*[2,4,16]
- Assess fluid intake and output. *Many factors, such as inability to swallow, large diuresis, chronic kidney failure, trauma, or surgery, affect an individual's fluid balance, thereby disrupting electrolyte transport, function, and excretion.*[1–5]
- Review laboratory results for abnormal findings. *Electrolytes include sodium, potassium, calcium, chloride, bicarbonate (carbon dioxide), and magnesium. These chemicals are absolutely essential in many bodily functions, including fluid balance, movement of fluid within and between body compartments, nerve conduction, muscle contraction—including the heart, blood clotting, and pH balance. Excitable cells, such as nerve and muscle, are particularly sensitive to electrolyte imbalances.*[4,6]
- Assess for specific imbalances:

Sodium (Na⁺) *Dominant extracellular cation and cannot freely cross the cell membrane.*[6]

Review laboratory results—normal range in adults is 135 to 145 mEq/L. *Elevated sodium (hypernatremia) can occur if client has an overall deficit of total body water, which occurs via two mechanisms (inadequate fluid intake and water loss),*[7,8] *and can be associated with low potassium, metabolic acidosis, and hypoglycemia.*[2]

Monitor for physical or mental disorders impacting fluid intake. *Impaired thirst sensation and inability to express thirst or obtain needed fluids may lead to hypernatremia.*[7,8]

Note presence of medical conditions that may impact sodium level. *Congestive heart failure, liver and kidney failure, pneumonia, metabolic acidosis, and intestinal conditions resulting in prolonged GI suction are associated with hyponatremia.*[4,6] *Hypernatremia can result from simple conditions such as febrile illness causing fluid loss and/or restricted fluid intake or from complicated conditions such as kidney and endocrine diseases affecting sodium intake or excretion.*[8]

Note presence of cognitive dysfunction such as confusion, restlessness, and abnormal speech *(which may be a cause or effect of sodium imbalance); orthostatic blood pressure changes, tachycardia, or low urine output; or other clinical findings such as generalized weakness, swollen tongue, weight loss, and seizures. Signs suggesting hypernatremia.*[7,8]

Assess for nausea, abdominal cramping, lethargy, and orthostatic blood pressure changes—if fluid volume is also depleted, confusion, decreased level of consciousness, or headache. *Signs and symptoms suggestive of hyponatremia, which can lead to seizures and coma if untreated.*[6]

Review drug regimen. *Drugs such as anabolic steroids, angiotensin, cisplatin, and mannitol may increase sodium level. Drugs such as diuretics, laxatives, theophylline, and triamterene can decrease sodium level.*[4]

Potassium (K⁺) *Most abundant intracellular cation, obtained through diet and excreted via the kidneys.*[9]

Identify at-risk populations. *Extremes of age (premature or elderly); ingestion of unusual diet with high-potassium, low-sodium foods; clients receiving IV potassium boluses or transfusions of whole blood or packed cells; and use of potassium supplements, including over-the-counter (OTC) herbals or salt substitutes, increase possibility of hyperkalemia.*

Review laboratory results—normal range in adults is 3.5 to 5.0 mEq/L.

Obtain ECG as indicated.

 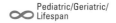

Note presence of medical conditions that may impact potassium level. *Metabolic acidosis, burn or crush injuries, massive hemolysis, diabetes, kidney disease/renal failure, cancer, and sickle cell trait are associated with hyperkalemia.[10] Situations that may lead to hypokalemia are those that decrease potassium intake—excessive fluid resuscitation, fasting, and unbalanced diet or eating disorders/anorexia; shift potassium from the extracellular fluid into cells—alkalosis, some malignancies; or increased potassium loss through diuresis or renal disorders such as acute tubular necrosis, nasogastric suction, and diarrhea.[1,19]*

Evaluate reports of abdominal cramping, fatigue, hyperactive bowel motility, and muscle twitching and cramps followed by muscle weakness. Note presence of depressed reflexes and ascending flaccid paralysis of legs and arms. *Signs/symptoms suggesting hyperkalemia.[2,9]*

Note presence of weakness and fatigue (most common), as well as anorexia, abdominal distention, diminished bowel sounds, palpitations, postural hypotension, muscle cramps and pain (severe hypokalemia), and flaccid paralysis. *May be manifestations of hypokalemia.[1,19]*

Review drug regimen. *Use of potassium-sparing diuretics; other medications, such as NSAIDs, angiotensin-converting enzyme inhibitors, angiotensin-receptor blockers; and heparin and certain antibiotics such as pentamidine may increase potassium level.[6,9,10] Medications such as some pulmonary medications (e.g., albuterol, terbutaline), steroids, certain antimicrobials (e.g., penicillins, aminogylicides), laxatives, and some diuretics may cause hypokalemia.[19]*

Calcium (Ca^{2+}) *Most abundant cation in the body participates in almost all vital processes, working with sodium to regulate depolarization and the generation of action potentials. Disruption of these processes causes cellular irritability and dysfunction.[2,4,10,12,15]*

Laboratory results—normal range for adults is 8.5 to 10.5 mg/dL. *Elevated calcium (hypercalcemia) is associated with excessive urination (polyuria), constipation, lethargy, muscle weakness, anorexia, headache, and coma. Hypocalcemia can lead to cardiac dysrhythmias, hypotension, and heart failure; muscle cramps and facial spasms (positive Chvostek's sign); numbness, tingling sensations, and muscle twitching (positive Trousseau's sign); seizures; or tetany. Low serum albumin levels and vitamin D deficiency may also be associated with hypocalcemia.[4,11]*

Note presence of medical conditions impacting calcium level. *Acidosis, Addison's disease, cancers (e.g., bone, lymphoma, leukemias), hyperparathyroidism, lung disease (e.g., tuberculosis, histoplasmosis), thyrotoxicosis, and polycythemia may lead to an increased calcium level. Chronic diarrhea and intestinal disorders such as Crohn's disease; pancreatitis, alcoholism, renal failure, or renal tubular disease; recent orthopedic surgery or bone healing; history of thyroid surgery or irradiation of upper middle chest and neck; and psychosis may result in hypocalcemia.[2,4,11]*

Review drug regimen. *Drugs such as anabolic steroids, some antacids, lithium, oral contraceptives, vitamins A and D, and amoxapine can increase calcium levels. Drugs such as albuterol, glucocorticoids, and insulin; laxative overuse; and phosphates, trazodone, or long-term anticonvulsant therapy can decrease calcium levels.[4]*

Magnesium (Mg^{2+}) *The second-most abundant intracellular cation after potassium, magnesium controls absorption or function of sodium, potassium, calcium, and phosphorus.[2,4,9,10,13,14]*

Review laboratory results—normal range in adults is 1.5 to 2.0 mEq/L. *Excess magnesium (hypermagnesemia) occurs rarely but affects the central nervous, neuromuscular, and cardiopulmonary systems.*

Note GI and renal function. *Main controlling factors of magnesium are GI absorption and renal excretion.[12] Low levels of potassium (most common), as well as calcium, phosphorus, and magnesium, may be manifest at the same time if GI absorption is impaired.[14] High levels of magnesium, calcium, phosphate, and potassium often occur together in setting of kidney disease.[13,14]*

Note presence of medical condition impacting magnesium level. *Diabetic acidosis, multiple myeloma, renal insufficiency, eclampsia, asthma, certain cardiac dysrhythmias, tumor lysis syndrome, GI hypomotility, adrenal insufficiency, neoplasms with skeletal muscle involvement, extensive soft tissue injury or necrosis, shock, sepsis, severe burns, and cardiac arrest are associated with hypermagnesemia.[4,12,13,15] Conditions resulting in decreased intake (e.g., starvation, alcoholism, parenteral feeding); excess GI losses (e.g., diarrhea, vomiting, nasogastric suction, malabsorption); renal losses (e.g., inherited renal tubular defects among others);*

 Acute Care   Collaborative   Community/ Home Care   Cultural

or miscellaneous other causes, including calcium abnormalities, chronic metabolic acidosis, and diabetic ketoacidosis, can lead to hypomagnesemia.[2,4,12]

Monitor for symptoms of hypermagnesemia. *Presence of nausea, vomiting, weakness, and vasodilation suggest mild to moderate elevation of magnesium level (>3.5–5.0 mEq/L), while the presence of heart blocks, ventilatory failure, and stupor are associated with severe hypermagnesemia (>10.0 mEq/L), which can lead to coma and death.[14]*

Note muscular weakness, tremors, seizures, paresthesia, hypertension, and cardiac abnormalities. *Signs of hypomagnesemia that may lead to potentially fatal complications, including ventricular dysrhythmias, coronary artery vasospasm, and sudden death.[9,13]*

 Review drug regimen. *Drugs such as aspirin and progesterone may increase magnesium level; albuterol, digoxin, diuretics, oral contraceptives, aminoglycosides, proton-pump inhibitors, immunosuppressants, cisplatin, and cyclosporines are some of the medications that may decrease magnesium levels.[4]*

NURSING PRIORITY NO. 3   To prevent imbalances:

- Collaborate in the treatment of underlying conditions *to prevent or limit effects of electrolyte imbalances caused by disease or organ dysfunction.*
- Observe and intervene with elderly hospitalized individuals upon admission and during facility stay. *Elderly are more prone to electrolyte imbalances related to fluid imbalances, the use of multiple medications including diuretics and heart and blood pressure medications, a lack of appetite or interest in eating or drinking, a lack of appropriate dietary and/or medication supervision at home, etc.[2]*
- Provide balanced nutrition to hospitalized client, using best route for feeding and monitoring intake, weight, and bowel function. *Obtaining and utilizing electrolytes and other minerals depend on client receiving them in a readily available route, preferably by oral ingestion, or by GI tube or parenteral route.*
- Measure and report all fluid losses, including emesis, diarrhea, and wound or fistula drainage. *Loss of fluids rich in electrolytes can lead to imbalances.*
- Maintain fluid balance *to prevent dehydration and shifts of electrolytes.*
- Use a pump or controller device when administering IV electrolyte solutions *to provide medication at desired rate and prevent untoward effects of excessive or too rapid delivery.*

NURSING PRIORITY NO. 4   To promote wellness (Teaching/Discharge Considerations):

- Discuss ongoing concerns for clients with chronic health problems, such as kidney disease, diabetes, and cancer; individuals taking multiple medications; and/or clients deciding to take medications or OTC drugs differently than prescribed. *By addressing these issues during each clinic visit, it may be possible to identify client at risk for electrolyte imbalances. Early intervention can help prevent serious complications.*
- Consult with dietitian or nutritionist for specific teaching needs. *Learning how to incorporate foods that increase electrolyte intake or identifying food or condiment alternatives when client is taking in too much of an electrolyte (such as client with renal failure, and not on dialysis, failing to curtail high-potassium foods) increases client's self-sufficiency and likelihood of success.*
- Teach client/caregiver to take or administer drugs as prescribed—especially diuretics, antihypertensives, and cardiac drugs—*to reduce potential of complications associated with medication-induced electrolyte imbalances.*
- Instruct client/caregiver in reportable symptoms. *For example, sudden change in mentation or behavior 2 days after starting a new diuretic could indicate hyponatremia, or an elderly person taking digitalis for atrial fibrillation and a diuretic may be hypokalemic.[2]*
- Provide information regarding calcium supplements, as indicated. *It is popular wisdom to instruct people, women in particular, to take calcium for prevention of osteoporosis. However, calcium absorption cannot take place without vitamins D and K and magnesium. Client taking calcium may need additional information or resources.[16]*
- Review client's medications at each visit *for possible change in dosage or drug choice based on client's response, change in condition, or development of side effects.*

 Diagnostic Studies   Evidence Based Practice   Medications   Pediatric/Geriatric/Lifespan

- Discuss medications with primary care provider *to determine if different pharmaceutical intervention is appropriate. For example, changing to potassium-sparing diuretic or withholding a diuretic in presence of hypokalemia may correct imbalance.*[15]

DOCUMENTATION FOCUS

Assessment/Reassessment
- Identified or potential risk factors for individual.
- Assessment findings, including vital signs, mentation, muscle strength and reflexes, presence of fatigue, respiratory distress.
- Results of laboratory tests and diagnostic studies.

Planning
- Plan of care, specific interventions, and who is involved in the planning.
- Teaching plan.

Implementation/Evaluation
- Client's responses to treatment, teaching, and actions performed.
- Attainment or progress toward desired outcome(s).
- Modifications to plan of care.

Discharge Planning
- Long-term needs, identifying who is responsible for actions to be taken.
- Specific referrals made.

References

1. Lederer, E., et al. (2014; updated 2018). Hypokalemia. Retrieved March 2018 from http://emedicine.medscape.com/article/242008-overview.
2. Workman, M. L. (2006). Interventions for clients with electrolyte imbalances. In Ignatavicius, D. D., Workman, M. L. (eds). *Medical-Surgical Nursing: Critical Thinking for Collaborative Care.* 5th ed. St. Louis, MO: Elsevier Saunders.
3. Wung, S., Kozik, T. (2008). Electrocardiographic evaluation of cardiovascular status. *J Cardiovasc Nurs*, 23(2), 169–174.
4. Leeuwen, A. M., Kranpitz, T. R., Smith, L. (2013). *Davis's Comprehensive Handbook of Diagnostic Tests with Nursing Implications.* 5th ed. Philadelphia, PA: F. A. Davis.
5. Btaiche, I. F., Khalidi, N. (2004). Metabolic complications of parenteral nutrition in adults, part 1. *Am J Health Syst Pharm*, 61(18), 1938–1949.
6. Simon, E. E., Hamrahian, S. M., Teran, F. J. (2014, updated 2018). Hyponatremia. Retrieved March 2018 from http://emedicine.medscape.com/article/242166-overview.
7. Elgart, H. N. (2004). Assessment of fluids and electrolytes. *AACN Clin Issues*, 15(4), 607–621.
8. Lukitsch, I. (2014, updated 2017). Hypernatremia. Retrieved March 2018 from http://emedicine.medscape.com/article/241094-overview.
9. Lederer, E., et al. (2014, updated 2017). Hyperkalemia. Retrieved March 2018 from http://emedicine.medscape.com/article/240903-overview.
10. Muller, A. C., Bell, A. E. (2008). Diagnostic update: Electrolyte update: Potassium, chloride and magnesium. *Crit Care Nurs*, 3(1), 5–7.
11. Felver, L. (2015). Fluid, electrolyte, and acid-base balance. In Potter, P., et al. (eds.), *Essentials for Nursing Practice.* 8th ed. Philadelphia, PA: Mosby Elsevier.
12. Suneja, M., Muster, H. A. (2014; updated 2018). Hypocalcemia. Retrieved March 2018 from http://emedicine.medscape.com/article/241893-overview.
13. Fulop, T., Agarwal, M. (2014; updated 2017). Hypomagnesemia. Retrieved March 2018 from http://emedicine.medscape.com/article/246366-overview.
14. Novello, N. P. (2014; updated 2017). Hypermagnesemia in Emergency Medicine. Retrieved March 2018 from http://emedicine.medscape.com/article/766604-overview.
15. Moe, S. M. (2008). Disorders involving calcium, phosphorus, and magnesium. *Prim Care*, 35(2), 215–237.
16. American Association of Critical Care Nurses (AACN). (2006). The renal system. *AACN Core Curriculum for High Acuity, Progressive, and Critical Care Nursing.* 7th ed. St. Louis, MO: Elsevier.
17. Fitzgerald, M. A. (2008). LAB LOGIC: Hyponatremia associated with SSRI use in a 65-year-old woman. *Nurse Pract*, 33(2), 11–12.
18. Ambalavanan, N. (2014). Fluid, electrolyte, and nutrition management of the newborn. Retrieved March 2018 from http://emedicine.medscape.com/article/976386–overview.
19. Lederer, E., et al. (2014, updated 2017). Hypokalemia. Retrieved March 2018 from http://emedicine.medscape.com/article/242008-overview.

 Acute Care   Collaborative   Community/Home Care   Cultural

impaired urinary Elimination

Taxonomy II: Elimination and Exchange—Class 1 Urinary Function (00016) [**Diagnostic Division:** Elimination], Approved 1973; Revised 2006, 2017

DEFINITION: Dysfunction in urine elimination.

RELATED FACTORS
Multiple causality

DEFINING CHARACTERISTICS

Subjective
Frequent voiding; urinary urgency or hesitancy
Dysuria
Nocturia; [enuresis]

Objective
Urinary incontinence
Urinary retention
Associated Condition: Anatomic obstruction; sensory motor impairment; urinary tract infection
Sample Clinical Applications: Urinary tract infection (UTI), benign prostatic disease (BPH), bladder cancer, interstitial cystitis, spinal cord injury (SCI), multiple sclerosis (MS), pregnancy, childbirth, pelvic trauma, abdominal surgery, dementia, Alzheimer's disease

DESIRED OUTCOMES/EVALUATION CRITERIA

Sample NOC linkages:
Urinary Elimination: Collection and drainage of urine
Urinary Continence: Control of elimination of urine from the bladder
Self-Care: Toileting: Personal actions to toilet self independently with or without assistive device

Client Will (Include Specific Time Frame)
• Verbalize understanding of condition.
• Identify specific causative factors.
• Achieve normal elimination pattern or participate in measures to correct or compensate for defects.
• Demonstrate behaviors or techniques to prevent urinary infection.
• Manage care of urinary catheter or stoma and appliance following urinary diversion.

ACTIONS/INTERVENTIONS

Sample NIC linkages:
Urinary Elimination Management: Maintenance of an optimum urinary elimination pattern
Urinary Catheterization: Insertion of a catheter into the bladder for temporary or permanent drainage of urine
Perineal Care: Maintenance of perineal skin integrity and relief of perineal discomfort

 Diagnostic Studies   Evidence Based Practice   Medications 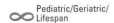 Pediatric/Geriatric/Lifespan

NURSING PRIORITY NO. 1   To assess causative/contributing factors:

- Note presence of physical diagnoses that may be involved, such as UTI or dehydration, surgery (including urinary diversion), neurological conditions (e.g., MS, stroke, Parkinson's disease; paraplegia, tetraplegia), mental or emotional dysfunction (e.g., impaired cognition, delirium, confusion, depression, Alzheimer's disease), prostate disorders, recent or multiple pregnancies, and pelvic trauma.
- Determine pathology of bladder dysfunction relative to identified medical diagnosis. *Identifies direction for further evaluation and treatment options to discover specifics of individual situation. For example, in neurological or demyelinating diseases, such as MS, problem may be failure to store urine, empty bladder, or both.*[1,6]
- ∞ ▨ Note client's age and gender. *Incontinence is twice as common in women as in men and affects at least one in three older women; painful bladder syndrome or interstitial cystitis (PBS/IC) is more common in women.*[3,7]
- Ⓐ Perform physical examination (e.g., cough test *for incontinence,* palpation *for bladder retention and masses,* prostate size, observation for urethral stricture).[8]
- Investigate reports of pain, noting location, duration, and intensity; the presence of bladder spasms; and back or flank pain, *to assist in differentiating between bladder and kidney cause of dysfunction. Note: Bladder pain located suprapubically, vaginally, in the perineum, low back, or medial aspects of the thighs that is relieved by voiding and often recurs with bladder filling suggests presence of PBS/IC.*[7]
- Observe current voiding pattern and time, color, and amount voided, as indicated *to determine type of problem present and to assist in finding likely cause.*
- ▨ Have client complete standardized self-report tool, such as the Pelvic Pain and Urgency/Frequency client symptom survey, as indicated. *Helpful in evaluating the presence and severity of PBS/IC symptoms.*[7,12]
- ▨ Note reports of exacerbations (flare-ups) of symptoms of urgency and frequency, which may/may not be accompanied by pain, pressure, or spasm *to assist in differentiating between bladder and kidney as cause of dysfunction. Note: Clients with PBS/IC void very frequently (has been reported to be up to 60 times/day) with voided volumes usually less than normal.*[7,13,15]
- Determine client's usual daily fluid intake (both amount and beverage choices and use of caffeine). Note condition of skin and mucous membranes and color of urine *to determine level of hydration.*
- ⬭ Review medication regimen to identify drugs that can alter bladder or kidney function (e.g., some antihypertensive agents [e.g., angiotensin-converting enzyme inhibitors (ACE), beta-blockers]; anticholinergics [e.g., antihistamines, antiparkinsonian drugs]; antidepressants, antipsychotics; sedatives, hypnotics, opioids; caffeine; alcohol).[9]
- ⬗ Send urine specimen (midstream clean-voided or catheterized) for culture and sensitivities in presence of signs of UTI—cloudy, foul odor, and/or bloody urine.
- ⬗ Review lab tests *for hyperglycemia, hyperparathyroidism, or other metabolic conditions, as well as changes in renal function, presence of infection/sexually transmitted infection, and cytology revealing cancer.*
- ⬗ Review results of other diagnostic studies (e.g., uroflowmetry; cystometogram; postvoid residual ultrasound (bladder scan), pressure flow, leak point pressure measurement; videourodynamics; electromyography; kidneys, ureters, and bladder imaging) *to identify presence and type of elimination problem.*[10]
- ⬗ Prepare for/review results of bladder cystoscopy and distention test as appropriate *to help identify presence of PBS/IC. Note: Bladder distention test may also be used as initial therapy.*[17]

NURSING PRIORITY NO. 2   To assess degree of interference/disability:

- Ascertain client's previous pattern of elimination and compare with current situation. Note reports of problems (e.g., frequency, urgency, painful urination; leaking or incontinence; changes in size or force of urinary stream; problems emptying bladder completely; nocturia, enuresis) *to assist in identification and treatment of particular dysfunction.*
- Ascertain client's/significant other's (SO's) perception of problem, degree of disability, and impact on self-image (e.g., client may be restricting social, employment, or travel activities; having sexual or relationship difficulties; experiencing depression).

 Acute Care   Collaborative   Community/ Home Care   🌐 Cultural

- Note influence of culture or ethnicity, as well as gender, on client's view of problems of incontinence. *Limited evidence exists to understand and help people cope with the physical and psychosocial consequences of this chronic, socially isolating, and potentially devastating disorder.*[4]
- Have client keep a voiding diary for prescribed number of days to record fluid intake, voiding times, precise urine output, and dietary intake. *Helps determine baseline symptoms, the severity of frequency/urgency, and whether diet is a factor if symptoms worsen.*

NURSING PRIORITY NO. 3 To assist in treating/preventing urinary alteration:

- Encourage fluid intake up to 1,500 to 2,500 mL/day (within cardiac tolerance), including cranberry juice. *Maintains renal function, prevents infection and formation of urinary stones, avoids encrustation around indwelling catheter, or may be used to flush urinary diversion appliance.*
- Regulate liquid intake at prescheduled times *to promote predictable voiding pattern.*
- Discuss possible dietary restrictions (e.g., especially coffee, alcohol, carbonated drinks, citrus, tomatoes, and chocolate) based on individual symptoms.[7]
- Assist with developing toileting routines (e.g., timed voiding, bladder training, prompted voiding, habit retraining) as appropriate. *For adults who are cognitively intact and physically capable of self-toileting, bladder training, timed voiding, and habit retraining may be beneficial.*[3,11] *However, bladder retraining is not recommended for clients with PBS.*[7]
- Encourage client to verbalize fear or concerns (e.g., disruption in sexual activity, inability to work, concern about involvement in social activities). *Open expression allows client to talk about, deal with feelings, and begin to solve the identified problems.*
- Modify medication regimens as appropriate. For example, administer prescribed diuretics in the morning *to lessen nighttime voiding,* and reduce or eliminate use of hypnotics, if possible, *as client may be too sedated to recognize or respond to urge to void.*[3]
- Implement and monitor interventions for specific elimination problem (e.g., pelvic floor exercises or other bladder retraining modalities; medication regimen, antimicrobials [single dose is frequently being used for UTI], sulfonamides, antispasmodics). Evaluate client's response *to modify treatment as needed.*
- Refer to appropriate resources (e.g., medical supply company, ostomy nurse, rehabilitation team) *for assistance, as desired or needed, to promote self-care.*
- Discuss possible surgical procedures and medical regimen as indicated (e.g., client with benign prostatic hypertrophy, bladder or prostatic cancer, PBS/IC). *For example, cystoscopy with bladder hydrodistention for PBS/IC or an electrical stimulator may be implanted to treat chronic urinary urge incontinence, nonobstructive urinary retention, and symptoms of urgency and frequency.*[4,7]
- Refer to specific NDs urinary Incontinence (specify) and [acute/chronic] Urinary Retention for additional interventions/treatment regimens.

NURSING PRIORITY NO. 4 To assist in management of long-term urinary dysfunction:

- Instruct client/SO/caregivers in cues that client needs (e.g., voiding on routine schedule; showing client location of the bathroom; providing adequate room lighting, signs, color coding of door) *assistance in continued continence, especially when in unfamiliar surroundings.*[3,16]
- Keep bladder deflated by use of an indwelling catheter connected to closed drainage. Investigate alternatives when possible. *Measures such as intermittent catheterization, surgical interventions, urinary drugs, voiding maneuvers, and condom catheter may be preferable to the indwelling catheter to provide more effective control and prevent possibility of recurrent infections.*
- Use latex-free catheter and care supplies, if indicated. *Reduces risk of developing sensitivity to latex, which can develop in individuals requiring frequent catheterization or who have long-term indwelling catheters.*
- Check frequently for bladder distention and observe for overflow. *Requires immediate intervention to reduce risk of infection or autonomic hyperreflexia.*

 Diagnostic Studies   Evidence Based Practice   Medications   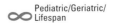 Pediatric/Geriatric/Lifespan

• Recommend a regular bladder or diversion appliance emptying schedule. *Avoids accidents and prevents embarrassment to the individual.*[2]
• Emphasize importance of routine diversion appliance care and assist client to recognize and deal with problems such as alkaline salt encrustation, ill-fitting appliance, malodorous urine, infection, etc. *Provides information and promotes competence in care, increasing self-confidence in dealing with appliance on a regular basis.*[2]

NURSING PRIORITY NO. 5 To promote wellness (Teaching/Discharge Considerations):

• Review expectations and prognosis of underlying condition (e.g., MS, prostate disease). *Provides information to assist client/significant other (SO) to make informed decisions and plan for possible changes.*
• Emphasize importance of keeping perineal area clean and dry. *Reduces risk of infection or skin breakdown.*
• Instruct female clients with UTI to drink large amounts of fluid, void immediately after intercourse, wipe from front to back, promptly treat vaginal infections, and take showers rather than tub baths as appropriate. *These measures can limit risk of or avoid reinfection.*[3]
• Recommend smoking-cessation program as appropriate. *Cigarette smoking can be a source of bladder irritation.*
• Encourage SO(s) who participate in routine care to recognize complications (including latex allergy) necessitating medical follow-up. *Client may be embarrassed to discuss symptoms, and caregivers need to be alert to changes that necessitate evaluation and treatment.*[4]
• Instruct in proper application and care of appliance for urinary diversion. Encourage liberal fluid intake, avoidance of foods and medications that produce strong odor, and use of white vinegar or deodorizer in pouch to promote odor control. *These measures help to ensure patency of device and prevent embarrassing situations for client.*[2]
• Identify sources for supplies and programs or agencies providing financial assistance. *Lack of access to necessities can be a barrier to management of incontinence and having help to obtain needed equipment can assist with daily care.*[4]
• Recommend avoidance of gas-forming foods in presence of ureterosigmoidostomy. *Flatus can cause urinary incontinence.*[1]
• Recommend use of silicone catheter. *Although these catheters are more expensive than rubber catheters, they are more comfortable and generally cause fewer problems with infection when permanent or long-term catheterization is required.*[5,14]
• Demonstrate proper positioning of catheter drainage tubing and bag. *Facilitates drainage and prevents reflux and complications of infection.*
• Refer client/SO(s) to appropriate community resources such as ostomy specialist, support group, sex therapist, psychiatric clinical nurse specialist, etc. *May be necessary to deal with changes in body image and function.*[4]

DOCUMENTATION FOCUS

Assessment/Reassessment
• Individual findings, including previous and current pattern of voiding, nature of problem, effect on desired lifestyle.
• Cultural factors or concerns.

Planning
• Plan of care and who is involved in planning.
• Teaching plan.

Implementation/Evaluation
• Response to interventions, teaching, and actions performed.
• Attainment or progress toward desired outcome(s).
• Modifications to plan of care.

 Acute Care   Collaborative   Community/ Home Care   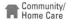 Cultural

Discharge Planning
• Long-term needs and who is responsible for actions to be taken.
• Available resources and specific referrals made.
• Individual equipment needs and sources.

References

1. Newfield, S. A., et al. (2007). *Cox's Clinical Applications of Nursing Diagnosis: Adult, Child, Women's, Psychiatric, Geron- tic, and Home Health Considerations*. 5th ed. Philadelphia: F. A. Davis.
2. Colwell, J. C. (2001). The state of the standard diversion. *J Wound Ostomy Continence Nurs*, 28(1), 6–17.
3. Chang, H. J., Lymn, C., Glass, R. M. (2010). Urinary inconti- nence in older women. *JAMA*, 303(21), 2208.
4. Newman, D. K., Palmer, M. H. (eds.) (2003). The state of the science on urinary incontinence. *Am J Nurs*, 103(Suppl 3), 2–53.
5. SimTech. (2015). The best rubber for medical devices: Silicone vs. latex. Retrieved March 2018 from https://www.simtec- silicone.com/the-best-rubber-for-medical-devices-silicone- vs-latex/.
6. Gray, M. (2005). Overactive bladder: An overview. *J Wound Ostomy Continence Nurs*, 32(3 Suppl), 1–5.
7. Panzera, A. K. (2007). Interstitial cystitis/painful bladder syn- drome. *Urol Nurs*, 27(1), 13–19.
8. Bates, B. (2007). Simple questions can help uncover urinary incontinence. *Urol Nurs*, 37(4), 29.
9. Newman, D. K. (2005). Assessment of the patient with an overactive bladder. *J Wound Ostomy Continence Nurs*, 32(3 Suppl), 5–10.
10. National Kidney and Urologic Diseases Information Clearing- house (Updated 2014). Urodynamic testing. Retrieved March 2018 from http://kidney.niddk.nih.gov/KUDISEASES/pubs/ urodynamic/index.aspx.
11. Milne, J. L., Krissovich, M. (2004). Behavioral therapies at the primary care level: The current state of knowledge. *J Wound Ostomy Continence Nurs*, 31(6), 367–376.
12. Parsons, C. L., Dell, J., Standford, E. J. (2002). Increased prevalence of interstitial cystitis: Previously unrecognized uro- logic and gynecologic cases identified using a new symptom questionnaire and intravesical potassium sensitivity. *Adult Urol*, 60(4), 573–578.
13. Tchetgen, M. B., et al. (2005). Interstitial cystitis. In Vasavada, S. P., et al. (eds). *Female Urology, Urogynecology, and Voiding Dysfunction*. New York: Marcel Dekker.
14. Rull, G. (2016). Catheterising bladders. Retrieved March 2018 from http://www.patient.co.uk/doctor/catheterising- bladders.
15. Interstitial Cystitis Association. (Updated 2015). General IC symptoms. Retrieved March 2018 from https://www.ichelp.org/ about-ic/symptoms-of-ic/general-ic-symptoms/.
16. Registered Nurses Association of Ontario (Updated 2011). Prompting continence using prompted voiding: Guideline Supplement. *Best Practice Guideline*. Retrieved March 2018 from http://rnao.ca/sites/rnao-ca/files/storage/related/7719_ BPG_Continence-Supplement-Only-2011.pdf.
17. National Kidney and Urologic Disease Clearinghouse. (2011). Interstitial cystitis/painful bladder disease. Retrieved March 2018 from file:///C:/Users/Mary's%20PC/Downloads/IC_ PBS_T_508.pdf.

impaired Emancipated Decision-Making

Taxonomy II: Life Principles—Class 3 Values/Belief/Action/Congruence (00242) [**Diagnostic Division:** Ego Integrity], Approved 2013; Revised 2017

DEFINITION: A process of choosing a healthcare decision that does not include personal knowledge and/or consideration of social norms or does not occur in a flexible environment, resulting in decisional dissatisfaction.

RELATED FACTORS
Decrease in understanding of all available healthcare options; insufficient information regarding healthcare options
Inability to adequately verbalize perceptions about healthcare options; insufficient confidence to openly discuss healthcare options
Inadequate time to discuss healthcare options; insufficient privacy to openly discuss healthcare options
Insufficient self-confidence in decision making

(continues on page 296)

 Diagnostic Studies Evidence Based Practice Medications 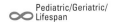 Pediatric/Geriatric/ Lifespan

impaired Emancipated Decision-Making (continued)

DEFINING CHARACTERISTICS

Subjective

Feeling constrained in describing own option

Inability to choose a healthcare option that best fits current lifestyle

Inability to describe how option will fit into current lifestyle

Excessive concern about what others think is the best decision

Excessive fear of what others think about decision

Objective

Delay in enacting chosen healthcare option

Distress when listening to other's opinion

Limited verbalization about healthcare option in other's presence

At Risk Population: Limited decision-making experience; traditional hierarchal family or healthcare systems

Sample Clinical Applications: Any condition/situation requiring healthcare decisions

DESIRED OUTCOMES/EVALUATION CRITERIA

Sample NOC linkages:

Decision-Making: Ability to make judgements and choose between two or more alternatives

Participation in Health Care Decisions: Personal involvement in selecting and evaluating healthcare options to achieve desired outcome

Client Will (Include Specific Time Frame)

- Verbalize concern about healthcare decision making.
- Express understanding of available healthcare options.
- Discuss healthcare options openly and with confidence.
- Participate in decision making freely and openly.

ACTIONS/INTERVENTIONS

Sample NIC linkages:

Decision-Making Support: Providing information and support for a patient who is making a decision regarding healthcare

Health System Guidance: Facilitating a patient's location and use of appropriate health services

NURSING PRIORITY NO. 1 To assess causative/contributing factors (e.g., dementia or delirium):

- Determine usual ability to make decisions and factors that are currently interfering with making a personal choice. *Individual may not have sufficient knowledge or may be influenced by family pressures that may prevent making an independent decision.*[1,3]
- Note expressions of indecision, dependence on others, and availability and involvement of support persons. *Caregivers need to be sensitive to the physical, emotional, and cognitive effects of the situation on decision-making capabilities.*[2]
- Discuss issue of whether individual wants to be involved in decision making. *External influences may pressure person to give up own responsibility for the decision.*[2]

 Acute Care   Collaborative   Community/ Home Care   Cultural

- Identify previous decisions individual has made and environment in which those and current decisions were/are made. *Provides information about client's ability and circumstances surrounding decision making.*[1]
- Active-listen and identify reasons for indecisiveness. *Helps client to clarify problem and begin to look at alternatives for situation.*[1]
- Identify cultural values, beliefs, moral obligations, or ethical concerns that may be creating conflict in current situation. *These issues need to be resolved before client will be comfortable with decision.*[5]
- Review information client has to support the decision to be made. *Provides opportunity to clarify and correct misinformation or inaccurate perceptions that can affect the outcome.*[2]

NURSING PRIORITY NO. 2 To assist client to become empowered and able to make effective decisions:

- Promote safe and hopeful environment as needed, including a therapeutic nurse-client relationship. *Client needs to feel safe and supported to be comfortable in own ability to make satisfactory decisions.*[2]
- Encourage verbalization of conflicts and concerns. *Helps to identify and clarify these issues so individual can reach a satisfying solution.*[1]
- Clarify and prioritize individual goals. *Enables client to look at the importance of the issues of the conflict and reach realistic problem-solving.*[4]
- Identify strengths and use of positive coping skills, relaxation techniques, and willingness to express feelings. *Encourages individual to view themselves as a capable person who can make a desired decision.*[4]
- Discuss time constraints related to the decision to be made. *Healthcare decisions (i.e., breastfeeding) may need to be made quickly depending on the circumstances.*[1]
- Help client to learn the problem-solving process. *Provides a structure for individual to look at alternatives for making a decision in current situation and for other decisions that need to be made in the future.*[6]
- Discuss and clarify spiritual concerns, accepting client's values in a nonjudgmental manner. *Client will be willing to consider own situation when accepted as an individual of worth.*

NURSING PRIORITY NO. 3 To promote independence (Teaching/Discharge Considerations):

- Provide opportunities for practicing problem-solving skills. *Helps client to become more confident and solve current and future situations.*[4]
- Encourage family to become involved as desired/available. *Facilitates understanding of individual's needs and abilities, promoting support and acceptance of ability of family member.*[5]
- Discuss attendance at assertiveness and stress-reduction classes, if able. *Learning these skills helps client to become able to make decisions in a more decisive manner.*[1]
- Refer to other resources as indicated (e.g., public health, support group, clergy, psychiatrist, clinical specialist, psychiatric nurse). *May need additional help to manage difficult decision making.*[4]

DOCUMENTATION FOCUS

Assessment/Reassessment
- Assessment findings, behavioral responses, and degree of impairment in lifestyle functioning.
- Individual involved in the conflict.
- Personal values and beliefs, moral or ethical concerns.

Planning
- Plan of care, specific interventions, and who is involved in the planning process.
- Teaching plan.

Implementation/Evaluation
- Client's and individuals' involved responses to interventions, teaching, and actions performed.
- Ability to express feelings and identify options.

 Diagnostic Studies   Evidence Based Practice   Medications   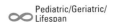 Pediatric/Geriatric/Lifespan

- Use of resources.
- Attainment or progress toward desired outcome(s).
- Modifications to plan of care.

Discharge Planning
- Long-term needs, actions to be taken, and who is responsible for doing.
- Specific referrals made.

References

1. Wittman-Price, R. A. (2006). Exploring the subconcepts of the Wittman-Price Theory of Emancipated Decision-Making in woman's health care. *J Nurs Scholarsh*, 38(4), 377–382.
2. Eggenberger, S. J., Grassley, J., Restrepo, E. (2006). Culturally competent nursing care for families. Listening to the voices of Mexican-American women. *Online J Issues Nurs*, 11(3). Retrieved March 2018 from http://www.nursingworld.org/MainMenuCategories/ANAMarketplace/ANAPeriodicals/OJIN/TableofContents/Volume112006/No3Sept06/ArticlePreviousTopics/CulturallyCompetentNursingCare.html.
3. Karlawish, J. (2008). Measuring decision-making capacity in cognitively impaired individuals. *Neurosignals*, 16(1), 91–98.
4. Paul, M. (2006, updated 2009). Relationships, the art of listening. *Inner Bonding*. Retrieved March 2018 from http://www.innerbonding.com/show-article/2147/relationships-the-art-of-listening.html.
5. Yuvarani, R. (2016). Family influences & decision making. Retrieved March 2018 from http://www.articlesbase.com/marketing-articles/family-influences-decision-making-family-decisionmaking-1014177.html.
6. Liken, M. (2001). Caregivers in crisis: Moving a relative with Alzheimer's to assisted living. *Clin Nurs Res*, 10(1), 53–69.

readiness for enhanced Emancipated Decision-Making

Taxonomy II: Life Principles—Class 3 Values/Belief/Action/Congruence (00243) **[Diagnostic Division:** Ego Integrity], Approved 2013

DEFINITION: A process of choosing a healthcare decision that includes personal knowledge and/or consideration of social norms, which can be strengthened.

DEFINING CHARACTERISTICS

Subjective
Expresses desire to enhance:
Ability to choose healthcare options that best fit current lifestyle; ability to enact chosen healthcare options
Ability to understand all available healthcare options
Ability to verbalize own opinion without constraint; comfort to verbalize healthcare options in the presence of others
Decision making; confidence in decision making
Privacy to discuss healthcare options; confidence to discuss healthcare options openly
Sample Clinical Applications: Any condition/situation requiring healthcare decisions

DESIRED OUTCOMES/EVALUATION CRITERIA

Sample NOC linkages:
Decision-Making: Ability to make judgments and choose between two or more alternatives
Participation in Health Care Decisions: Personal involvement in selecting and evaluating healthcare options to achieve desired outcome

Client Will (Include Specific Time Frame)
- Gather information including opinions of others while making own decision.
- Express comfort with taking adequate time to make decision.

 Acute Care Collaborative Community/ Home Care Cultural

- Make decision that is congruent with lifestyle and personal and sociocultural values and goals.
- Acknowledge comfort with own decision.

ACTIONS/INTERVENTIONS

Sample **NIC** linkages:

Decision-Making Support: Providing information and support for a patient who is making a decision regarding healthcare

Health System Guidance: Facilitating a patient's location and use of appropriate health services

NURSING PRIORITY NO. 1 To determine current decision-making abilities and needs:

- Determine usual ability to manage own affairs and make own decisions. *Provides baseline for understanding client's usual manner of making decisions.*[1]
- Note availability of support person. *Having support can provide individual with positive feedback regarding the validity of the choice.*[3]
- Active-listen and identify reason(s) client is ready to improve decision-making ability. *Provides opportunity for individuals to clarify and understand how decisions are made and how they can help to achieve desired goals.*[1]
- Identify cultural values, beliefs, moral obligations, and ethical principles that guide or affect the decision-making process. *Although individuals believe they are able to look at the issues with an unbiased eye, it has been shown that one's unconscious biases may interfere with making a decision that is desired.*[4]
- Discuss meaning of life and reasons for living and how these relate to desire for improvement. *Cutting-edge research is demonstrating that the mind within the brain affects how these issues impact the individual's decision-making process.*[5]

NURSING PRIORITY NO. 2 To assist client to improve/effectively use problem-solving skills:

- Promote safe and hopeful environment and help client identify own inner control. *Individuals can take into consideration the context and pertinent facts when they feel safe and believe the decision making is in their control and make a rational and well-thought-out decision.*[6]
- Encourage verbalization of ideas, concerns, and particular decisions that need to be made. *Identifying these issues all help client make desired choices.*[6]
- Correct misconceptions and biases client may have. *People often have unconscious biases that can interfere with decision making. Helping to clarify these ideas will make for efficient decisions.*[4]
- Identify positive aspects of this learning opportunity. *Every day individuals make decisions, often without giving thought to what is needed to make a good decision. Decision making can be developed by using rational and lateral thinking.*[6]
- Discuss the process of practicing making decisions. *Decision making is a skill that we use every day at home, work, school, and in every aspect of our lives, so the more one knows about an effective process, the better one's decisions can be.*[6]
- Encourage children to make age-appropriate decisions. *The earlier they learn the problem-solving process, more self-esteem and coping skills will be enhanced.*[7]
- Discuss client's spiritual beliefs and values. *Accepting these in a nonjudgmental manner can help the individual look at what he/she believes in relation to these issues and decision making.*[7]

NURSING PRIORITY NO. 3 To promote optimum independence (Teaching/Discharge Considerations):

- Identify opportunities for using problem-solving skills. *Emphasizing each step as it is used will facilitate the learning process.*[7]

 Diagnostic Studies   Evidence Based Practice   Medications 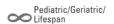 Pediatric/Geriatric/ Lifespan

- Involve family and significant others as desired by client. *Helps all those involved to improve their decision-making skills and enhance relationships, and client can live a fuller life.*[8]
- Recommend client attend assertiveness and/or stress-reduction classes as desired. *Provides opportunity to learn new ways of dealing with problems and enhancing decision-making abilities and life in general.*[8]
- Refer to other resources as necessary (e.g., public health, healthcare providers, clergy, support group, clergy, psychiatrist/clinical specialist psychiatric nurse). *May need additional assistance for specific problems and/or support long-term needs.*[4]

DOCUMENTATION FOCUS

Assessment/Reassessment
- Assessment findings, behavioral responses.
- Motivation for change.
- Personal values, beliefs.

Planning
- Plan of care, specific interventions and actions to be performed.
- Teaching plan.

Implementation/Evaluation
- Response to interventions, teaching, and actions performed.
- Ability to express feelings and confidence in decision-making process.
- Attainment or progress toward desired outcomes.
- Modifications to plan of care.

Discharge Planning
- Long-term needs and who is responsible for actions to be taken.
- Specific referrals made.

References

1. Politi, M. C., et al. (2013). Importance of clarifying patients' desired role in shared decision making to match their level of engagement with their preferences. *BMJ*, (347), f7066.
2. Mazamil, J., Shubeens, A. (2008). An analysis of decision-making power among married and unmarried women. *Stud Home Comm Sci*. Retrieved March 2018 from http://krepublishers.com/02-Journals/S-HCS/HCS-02-0-000-08-Web/HCS-02-1-001-08-Abst-Text/HCS-02-1-043-08-036-Jan-M/HCS-02-1-043-08-036-Jan-M-Tt.pdf.
3. Stepanuk, K. M., et al. (2013). Women's decision-making regarding medication use in pregnancy for anxiety and/or depression. *J Adv Nursing*, 69(11), 2470–2480.
4. Banaji, M. R., Greenwald, A. G. (2013). *Blindspot: Hidden Biases of Good People*. New York: Delacorte Press.
5. Redish, A. D. (2013). *The Mind Within the Brain: How We Make Decisions and How Those Decisions Go Wrong*. New York: Oxford University Press.
6. Welthy, D. (2013). *Decide: Better Ways of Making Better Decisions*. London, UK: Kogan Page.
7. Heath, C., Heath, D. (2013). *Decisive: How to Make Better Choices in Life and Work*. New York: Crown Publishing Group.
8. Miller, W., Rollnick, S. (2008). *Motivational Interviewing in Health Care: Helping Patients Change Behavior*. New York: The Guildford Press.

 Acute Care   Collaborative   Community/Home Care   Cultural

risk for impaired Emancipated Decision-Making

Taxonomy II: Life Principles—Class 3 Values/Belief/Action/Congruence (00244) [Diagnostic Division: Ego Integrity], Approved 2013: Revised 2017

DEFINITION: Susceptible to a process of choosing a healthcare decision that does not include personal knowledge and/or consideration of social norms or does not occur in a flexible environment, resulting in decisional dissatisfaction.

RISK FACTORS

Decrease in understanding of all available healthcare options; insufficient information regarding healthcare options
Inability to adequately verbalize perceptions about healthcare options; insufficient confidence to openly discuss healthcare options
Inadequate time to discuss healthcare options; insufficient privacy to openly discuss healthcare options
Insufficient self-confidence in decision-making
Sample Clinical Applications: Any condition/situation requiring healthcare decisions

DESIRED OUTCOMES/EVALUATION CRITERIA

Sample **NOC** linkages:
Decision-Making: Ability to make judgements and choose between two or more alternatives
Participation in Health Care Decisions: Personal involvement in selecting and evaluating healthcare options to achieve desired outcome

Client Will (Include Specific Time Frame)
• Acknowledge awareness of difficulty in healthcare decision making.
• Seek information for making healthcare decisions.
• Discuss options openly with family/others as appropriate.
• Develop confidence as decisions are made.

ACTIONS/INTERVENTIONS

Sample **NIC** linkages:
Decision-Making Support: Providing information and support for a patient who is making a decision regarding healthcare
Health System Guidance: Facilitating a patient's location and use of appropriate health services

Refer to ND impaired Emancipated Decision Making for Interventions, Documentation, and References.

 Diagnostic Studies   Evidence Based Practice   Medications   Pediatric/Geriatric/ Lifespan

labile Emotional Control

Taxonomy II: Perceptual/Cognition—Class 4 Cognition (00251) **[Diagnostic Division:** Ego Integrity], Approved 2013; Revised 2017

DEFINITION: Uncontrollable outbursts of exaggerated and involuntary emotional expression.

RELATED FACTORS
Alteration in self-esteem
Emotional disturbance; stressors
Fatigue; insufficient muscle strength
Insufficient knowledge of disease or of symptom control
Social distress
Substance misuse/[abuse]

DEFINING CHARACTERISTICS

Subjective
Embarrassment regarding emotional expression
Excessive laughing/crying without feeling happiness
Expression of emotion incongruent with triggering factor

Objective
Absence of eye contact
Difficulty in use of facial expressions
Uncontrollable/involuntary crying, laughing
Withdrawal from social or occupational situations
Associated Condition: Brain injury; functional impairment; mood disorder; musculoskeletal disorder; pharmaceutical agent; physical disability; psychiatric disorder
Sample Clinical Applications: Traumatic brain injury, stroke, multiple sclerosis, psychiatric disorders, substance abuse

DESIRED OUTCOMES/EVALUATION CRITERIA

Sample NOC linkage:
Mood Equilibrium: Appropriate adjustment of prevailing emotional tone in response to circumstances

Client Will (Include Specific Time Frame)
• Acknowledge problem with emotional control.
• Identify feelings that occur with episodes of uncontrollable emotions.
• Follow medication regimen.
• Participate in recommended activities/rehabilitation.

ACTIONS/INTERVENTIONS

Sample NIC linkage:
Mood Management: Providing for safety, stabilization, recovery, and maintenance of a person who is experiencing dysfunctionally depressed or elevated mood

 Acute Care
 Collaborative
 Community/ Home Care
 Cultural

NURSING PRIORITY NO. 1 To assess causative/contributing factors:

- Determine individual factors related to client situation. *Many different physiological/psychological factors may be involved in loss of emotional control for a given person. Identifying these factors will help to develop a plan of care specific to this individual.*[1]
- Assess demographic, clinical, psychiatric, and stroke lesion characteristics. *Identifies individual areas that are affected, possibly related to injury to anterior regions of the cerebral hemispheres.*[2]
- Note when episodes of loss of control occur. *Determines frequency of incidents and factors associated with condition or with first stroke.*[2]
- Identify client's perception of incidents. *Most people are embarrassed by these outbursts, believing they could control them. Individuals with multiple sclerosis are prone to these episodes.*[1]
- Evaluate for depression. *Depression may be a factor for these individuals, but a pseudobulbar affect (PDA) needs to be recognized as different because treatments are different for these conditions.*[1]

NURSING PRIORITY NO. 2 To determine effective control of labile episodes:

- Develop a plan of care to meet the needs of the individual situation. *Provides effective care for specific problems the client is experiencing.*[1]
- Establish a therapeutic nurse/client relationship. *Promotes trust and willingness to share concerns about problems that arise.*
- Note feelings of emotional exhaustion and social isolation. *Client may not recognize that PDA is a medical condition and may tend to remove themselves from situations that trigger the episodes.*[4]
- Assure client that the symptoms are real and need to be treated. *Healthcare providers may not know about this condition, and the client may not recognize that these are symptoms and therefore not report them.*[4]
- Correct misperceptions and provide accurate information. *Promotes understanding and helps client to be proactive in care.*[4]

NURSING PRIORITY NO. 3 To promote wellness (Teaching/Discharge Considerations):

- 🏠 Involve family in treatment plan. *Provides support for the client and promotes understanding of the uncontrollable episodes.*[4]
- 💊 Discuss use of medication. *Tricyclic antidepressants (TCAs) and selective serotonin reuptake inhibitors (SSRIs) are used in clinical practice, but there was no PDA-specific treatment until Nuedexta (a fixed-dose combination of dextromethorphan hydrobromide/quinidine sulfate [DHQ]) was recently approved.*[4,5]
- Encourage involvement in social activities. *Enhances ability to participate with others.*[2]
- ∞ Refer for physical therapy and rehabilitation. *Client may exhibit emotional lability following stroke and can benefit from these activities.*[3]
- ∞ Refer to other resources as necessary, such as group therapy, psychiatric therapy, and assertiveness training. *This additional help will enable client to develop a more positive lifestyle.*[1]

DOCUMENTATION FOCUS

Assessment/Reassessment

- Assessment findings, including triggering or associated factors, impact of condition on life, other pertinent information.

Planning

- Plan of care, specific interventions, and who is involved in planning process.
- Teaching plan.

Implementation/Evaluation

- Response to intervention, teaching, and actions performed.
- Ability to express feelings and control emotions.

 Diagnostic Studies   Evidence Based Practice   Medications 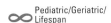 Pediatric/Geriatric/ Lifespan

- Use of resources.
- Attainment or progress toward desired outcomes.
- Modifications to plan of care.

Discharge Planning
- Long-term needs, actions to be taken and who is responsible for doing them.
- Specific referrals made.

References

1. Arnold, C. (Spring 2000, updated 2008). An ocean of emotion: Mood swings, anger, and uncontrollable laughing and crying. InsideMS. Retrieved March 2018 from http://www.nationalms-society.org/NationalMSSociety/media/MSNationalFiles/Brochures/Brochure-MS-and-the-Mind.pdf.
2. Morris, P. L., Robinson, R. G., Raphael, B. (1993). Emotional lability after stroke. *Aust N Z J Psychiatry*, 27(4), 601–605.
3. American Stroke Association. (2014, updated 2016). Pseu-dobulbar affect (PDA). Retrieved March 2018 from http://www.strokeassociation.org/STROKEORG/LifeAfterStroke/RegainingIndependence/EmotionalBehavioralChallenges/Pseudobulbar-Affect-PBA_UCM_467457_Article.jsp.
4. DiSalva, D. (2011). Not all crying is depression: Understanding pseudobulbar affect. *Psychol Today*. Retrieved March 2018 from http://www.psychologytoday.com/blog/neuronarrative/201110/not-all-crying-is-depression-understanding-pseudobulbar-affect.
5. Woodard, T. J., Kim, C., Calderon, F. (2017). Review of the diagnosis and management of pseudobulbar affect. *Mental Health*. Retrieved March 2018 from https://www.uspharmacist.com/article/review-of-the-diagnosis-and-management-of-pseudobulbar-affect.

---

imbalanced Energy Field

Taxonomy II: Activity/Rest—Class 3 Energy Balance (00273) **[Diagnostic Division:** Ego Integrity], Approved 2016

DEFINITION: A disruption in the vital flow of human energy that is normally a continuous whole and is unique, dynamic, creative, and nonlinear

RELATED FACTORS
Anxiety
Discomfort; pain
Excessive stress
Interventions that disrupt the energetic pattern or flow

DEFINING CHARACTERISTICS

Subjective
Expression of the need to regain the experience of the whole

Objective
Arrhythmic, irregular, or dissonant rhythms of the energy field patterns; pulsating to pounding frequency of the energy field patterns; magnetic pull to an area of the energy field
Random or strong or tumultuous or weak energy field patterns; rapid or slow energy field patterns
Blockage or congestion of the energy flow; energy deficit or hyperactivity of the energy flow; pulsations or tingling or unsynchronized rhythms sensed in the energy flow
Temperature differentials of cold or heat in the energy flow
At Risk Population: Crisis states; life transition
Associated Condition: Illness; injury
Sample Clinical Applications: Illness, trauma, cancer, chronic pain, impaired immune system, fatigue, surgical procedures, posttraumatic stress disorder, high-risk pregnancy, labor and delivery, end of life

 Acute Care Collaborative Community/ Home Care Cultural

DESIRED OUTCOMES/EVALUATION CRITERIA

Sample NOC linkages:
Personal Well-Being: Extent of positive perception of one's current health status
Coping: Personal actions to manage stressors that tax an individual's resources
Symptom Control: Personal actions to minimize perceived adverse changes in physical and emotional functioning

Client Will (Include Specific Time Frame)
- Acknowledge feelings of anxiety and distress.
- Verbalize sense of relaxation and well-being.
- Display reduction in severity and/or frequency of symptoms.

ACTIONS/INTERVENTIONS

Sample NIC linkages:
Therapeutic Touch: Attuning to the universal energy field, seeking to act as a healing influence, and using the natural sensitivity of hands passing over the body to gently focus, direct, and modulate the human energy field
Healing Touch: Providing a noninvasive, biofield therapy using touch and compassionate intentionality to influence the energy system of a person, affecting their physical, emotional, mental, and spiritual health and healing
Self-Awareness Enhancement: Assisting a patient to explore and understand his/her thoughts, feelings, motivations, and behaviors
Pain Management: Acute: Alleviation or reduction of pain to a level that is acceptable to the patient in the immediate healing period following tissue damage from an identifiable cause such as trauma, surgery, injury

NURSING PRIORITY NO. 1   To determine causative/contributing factors:

- Review current situation and concerns of client. Encourage client to talk about condition, past history, emotional state, or other relevant information. Note body gestures, tone of voice, and words chosen to express feelings and issues. *Studies demonstrate that biofield, or energy field, therapies (e.g., Healing Touch, Therapeutic Touch [TT]) produce positive outcomes by decreasing levels of anxiety and pain perception and improving sense of well-being and quality of life. Research has also shown significant reduction in PTSD symptoms and depression, as well as reduced cynicism in active duty military, and TT may be beneficial in reducing behavioral symptoms of dementia (e.g., manual manipulation/restlessness, vocalization, pacing).*[8,10–15,20]
- Determine client's motivation and desire for treatment. *Following an explanation of the process and expected results, client may have unrealistic expectations or may understand purpose and believe process will be helpful.*[2,17,18] *Although attitude can affect success of therapy, it is often successful even when the client is skeptical.*[11]
- Note use of medications and other drug use (e.g., alcohol). *May affect client's ability to relax and take full advantage of the therapy process.*[4] *However, it may be helpful in reducing anxiety level in individuals undergoing alcohol withdrawal.*[9]
- Perform or review results of testing, as indicated, such as the State-Trait Anxiety Inventory or the Affect Balance Scale. *Provides measure of the client's anxiety to evaluate need for treatment or intervention.*[3]

NURSING PRIORITY NO. 2   To evaluate energy field:

- Develop therapeutic nurse-client relationship, initially accepting role of healer or guide as client desires. *This relationship is one in which both participants recognize each other as unique and important human beings and in which mutual learning occurs. The role of the nurse and the use of self as a therapeutic tool are recognized.*[4]
- Place client in sitting or supine position with legs and arms uncrossed. Place pillows or other supports to enhance comfort. *Promotes relaxation and feelings of peace, calm, and security, preparing the client to derive the most benefit from the procedure.*[1]
- Center self physically and psychologically. *A quiet mind and focused attention turn to the healing intent.*[6]
- Move hands slowly over the client at level of 2 to 6 inches above skin. *Assesses state of energy field and flow of energy within the system. The feelings that may be noted are tingling, warmth, coolness, comfort, peace, calm, and security.*[5]
- Identify areas of imbalance or obstruction in the field. *Areas of asymmetry; feelings of heat or cold, tingling, congestion or pressure, decreased or disrupted energy flow, pulsation, congestion, heaviness, and decreased flow may be identified.*[7]

NURSING PRIORITY NO. 3   To provide therapeutic intervention:

- Explain the therapy process and answer questions as indicated *to prevent unrealistic expectations. The therapy is the knowledgeable and purposeful patterning of the client environmental energy field to relieve discomfort and anxiety. Providing information that the fundamental focus is on healing and wholeness, not curing signs/symptoms of disease, helps the client to understand the process.*[6,20]
- Discuss findings of evaluation with client. *Including the client in the process by sharing the findings of the nurse combined with sensations the client experienced provides the best opportunity to derive benefit from the procedure.*[2]
- Assist client with exercises to promote "centering." *Deep breathing, guided imagery, and the process of centering increase the potential to self-heal, enhance comfort, and reduce anxiety.*[2]
- Perform the unruffling process, keeping hands 2 to 6 in. from client's body and sweeping them downward and out of the field from head to toe, concentrating on areas of congestion. *Dissipates impediments to free flow of energy within the system and between nurse and client, promoting the reception of healing energy and allowing the client to use own resources for self-healing.*[6]
- Focus on areas of disturbance identified, holding hands over or on skin, or place one hand in back of body with other hand in front. At the same time, concentrate on the intent to help the client heal. *This move allows the client's body to pull or repattern energy as needed and corrects energy imbalances.*[1]
- ∞ Shorten duration of treatment 2 to 3 min as appropriate. *Children, elderly individuals, those with head injuries, and others who are severely debilitated are generally more sensitive to overloading energy fields.*[1,2]
- Make coaching suggestions in a soft voice. *Pleasant images or other visualizations and deep breathing enhance feelings of relaxation and help to relieve anxiety.*[1,2]
- Use hands-on massage or apply pressure to acupressure points as appropriate during the process. *The addition of these methods can enhance the relaxation and benefit client receives from therapy.*[6]
- Note changes in energy sensations as session progresses. Stop when the energy field is symmetrical and there is a change to feelings of peaceful calm. *Signifies energy is balanced, further intervention is not necessary, and client is ready to rest.*[1,2]
- Hold client's feet for a few minutes at end of session. *Assists in "grounding" the body energy, completing the session.*[1]
- Provide client time for a period of peaceful rest following procedure. *Biofield therapy promotes feelings of peace and comfort, relieving anxiety and promoting self-healing.*[1]

NURSING PRIORITY NO. 4   To promote wellness (Teaching/Discharge Considerations):

- Allow period of client dependency, as appropriate. *Period of dependency permits client to strengthen own inner resources at his or her own pace.*[1]

 Acute Care   Collaborative   Community/ Home Care   Cultural

- Encourage ongoing practice of the therapeutic process. *Helping client and family members to learn the skill will promote feelings of control of illness and health. It can be used anytime, anywhere, and with friends and family.*[4,19]
- Instruct in use of stress-reduction activities (e.g., centering/meditation, relaxation exercises, guided imagery). *Continuous use of these activities can promote mind-body-spirit harmony.*[2]
- Discuss importance of integrating techniques into daily activity plan for sustaining or enhancing sense of well-being. *Helps client to understand that making these a way of life will help them in dealing with challenges of illness and promote a healthy lifestyle.*[1]
- Have client practice each step and demonstrate the complete therapeutic process following the session. *Client displays readiness to assume responsibilities for self-healing as he or she learns the process.*[1,2]
- Promote attendance at a support group where members can help each other practice and learn the techniques. *The support of others helps the client to become proficient in new skill.*[2]
- 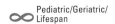 Reinforce that biofield therapies are complementary interventions and stress the importance of seeking timely evaluation and continuing other prescribed treatment modalities as appropriate. *Failure to follow prescribed therapeutic regimen may result in poor outcome and worsening of condition.*
- Refer to other resources as identified (e.g., psychotherapy, clergy, medical treatment of disease processes, hospice). *Encourages the individual to address total well-being and facilitate peaceful death as appropriate.*[6]

DOCUMENTATION FOCUS

Assessment/Reassessment
- Assessment findings, including characteristics and differences in the energy field.
- Client's perception of problem and motivation for treatment.

Planning
- Plan of care and who is involved in planning.
- Teaching plan.

Implementation/Evaluation
- Characteristics of energy work performed.
- Changes in energy field.
- Client's response to interventions (physical, mental, emotional), teaching, and actions performed.
- Attainment or progress toward desired outcomes.
- Modifications to plan of care.

Discharge Planning
- Long-term needs and who is responsible for actions to be taken.
- Specific referrals if made.

References

1. Bach, M. (2016). Therapeutic touch. Taking Charge of Your Health & Wellbeing, University of Minnesota. Retrieved May 2018 from http://takingcharge.csh.umn.edu/explore-healing-practices/therapeutic-touch.
2. Haley, M. A., Coppa, D., Shields, D. (2017). A practice-based theory of healing through Therapeutic Touch: Advancing holistic nursing practice. *J Holistic Nurs*, 35(4), 369–381.
3. Tilton, S. R. (2008). Review of the State-Trait Anxiety Inventory (STAI). *NewsTones*, 48(2), 1–3.
4. Ballen, K. Therapeutic touch healing hospice clients and their families. *Infinity Institute*. Retrieved February 2012 from http://www.infinityinst.com/articles/ttouch_hospice.html.
5. Hayes, J., Cox, C. (1999). The experience of therapeutic touch from a nursing perspective. *Br J Nurs*, 8(18), 1249–1254.
6. Meehan, T. (1998). Therapeutic touch as a nursing intervention. *J Adv Nurs*, 28(1), 117–125.
7. Marnhinweg, G. (1996). Energy field disturbance validation study. *Healing Touch Newsletter*, 6(11).
8. Woods, D. L., Craven, R. F., Whitney, J. (2005). The effect of therapeutic touch on behavioral symptoms of persons with dementia. *Altern Ther Health Med*, 11(1), 66–74.
9. Larden, C. N., Palmer, M. L., Janssen, P. (2004). Efficacy of therapeutic touch in treating pregnant inpatients who have a chemical dependency. *J Holist Nurs*, 22(4), 320–332.
10. Woods, D. L., Dimond, M. (2002). The effect of therapeutic touch on agitated behavior and cortisol in persons with Alzheimer's disease. *Biol Res Nurs*, 4(2), 104–114.

 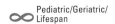

11. Denison, B. (2004). Touch the pain away: New research on therapeutic touch and persons with fibromyalgia syndrome. *Holist Nurs Pract*, 18(3), 142–151.

12. Smith, D. W., et al. (2002). Effects of integrating therapeutic touch into a cognitive behavioral pain treatment program. Report of a pilot clinical trial. *J Holist Nurs*, 20(4), 367–387.

13. Samarel, N., et al. (1998). Effects of dialogue and therapeutic touch on preoperative and postoperative experiences of breast cancer surgery: An exploratory study. *Oncol Nurs Forum*, 25(8), 1369–1376.

14. Giasson, M., Bouchard, L. (1998). Effect of therapeutic touch on the well-being of persons with terminal cancer. *J Holist Nurs*, 16(3), 383–398.

15. Jain, S., et al. (2012). Healing Touch with guided imagery for PTSD in returning active duty military: A randomized controlled trial. *Mil Med*, 177(9), 1015–1021.

16. Healing touch. (2016). *Good Therapy.org*. Retrieved May 2018 from https://www.goodtherapy.org/learn-about-therapy/types/healing-touch.

17. Kurus, M. (2015). Energy healing for your auras, chakras and energy systems. *The Home of Vibrational Health*. Retrieved May 2018 from http://www.mkprojects.com/energy-healing-auras.

18. Wright, D. (2013). Human energy field: What is it and how does it affect your body? *Canadian Positive Psychology Network*. Retrieved May 2018 from http://www.dreampositive.info/human-energy-field-what-is-it-and-how-does-it-affect-your-body/.

19. Chang, P. (2018). Human energy field and DNA–The origin of health. *EnergyFanatics.com*. Retrieved May 2018 from http://energyfanatics.com2017/05/27/human-energy-field-dna.

20. What is healing touch? (2018). *Healing Touch Program*. Retrieved May 2018 from https://www.healingtouchprogram.com/about/what-is-healing-touch.

risk for Falls

Taxonomy II: Safety/Protection—Class 2 Physical Injury (00155) [**Diagnostic Division:** Safety], Submitted 2000; Revised 2013; 2017

DEFINITION: Susceptible to increased susceptibility to falling, which may cause physical harm and compromise health.

RISK FACTORS

Children

Absence of stairway gate or window guard: insufficient automobile restraints

Environment

Use of restraints

Exposure to unsafe weather-related condition

Cluttered environment; use of throw rugs; insufficient anti-slip material in bathroom

Unfamiliar setting; insufficient lighting

Physiological

Alteration in blood glucose level

Decrease in lower extremity strength; difficulty with gait; immobility

Diarrhea; incontinence; urinary urgency

Faintness when extending or turning neck; orthostatic hypotension

Sleeplessness

Other

Alcohol consumption

Insufficient knowledge of modifiable factors

At Risk Population: Age ≥65 years or ≤2 years; male gender when <1 year of age

History of falls; living alone

Associated Condition: Acute illness; anemia; neoplasm; neuropathy; orthostatic hypotension; vascular disease

 Acute Care   Collaborative   Community/Home Care   Cultural

Alteration in cognitive functioning

Arthritis; condition affecting the foot; lower limb prosthesis; use of assistive device

Hearing impairment; impaired balance or vision; proprioceptive deficit

Postoperative recovery period; pharmaceutical agent

Sample Clinical Applications: Amputation, arthritis, osteoporosis, fractures, joint replacement surgery; seizure disorder, cerebrovascular disease, cataracts, dementia, paralysis, hypotension, cardiac dysrhythmias, inner ear infection, alcohol abuse or intoxication; trauma or surgery (general)

DESIRED OUTCOMES/EVALUATION CRITERIA

Sample NOC linkages:

Physical Injury Severity: Severity of signs and symptoms of injuries to the body

Client Will (Include Specific Time Frame)
• Be free of injury.

Knowledge: Fall Prevention: Extent of understanding conveyed about prevention of falls

Fall Prevention Behavior: Personal or family caregiver actions to minimize risk factors that might precipitate falls in the personal environment

Falls Occurrence: Number of times an individual falls

Client/Caregivers Will (Include Specific Time Frame)
• Verbalize understanding of individual risk factors that contribute to possibility of falls.
• Demonstrate behaviors and lifestyle changes to reduce risk factors and protect self from injury.
• Modify environment as indicated to enhance safety.
• Be free of falls.

ACTIONS/INTERVENTIONS

Sample NIC linkages:

Fall Prevention: Instituting special precautions with patient at risk for injury from falling

Environmental Management: Safety: Monitoring and manipulation of the physical environment to promote safety

NURSING PRIORITY NO. 1   To evaluate source/degree of risk:

• Review client's general health status, *noting multiple factors that may affect safety, such as chronic/debilitating conditions, use of more than four prescriptions, recent trauma (especially a fall within the past 3 to 12 months), prolonged bedrest or immobility, unstable balance on standing, and a sedentary lifestyle. Note: Many fall-risk assessment tools have been developed and compared. Best practice interventions in fall reduction have been shown to be (1) the use of a screening tool, (2) visual identification of client at high risk for falls, (3) directed multifactorial interdisciplinary risk factor interventions, and (4) client and care provider education.*[1,9]

• Evaluate client's current disorders/conditions that could enhance risk potential for falls. *Acute, even short-term, situations can affect any client, such as sudden dizziness, positional blood pressure changes, new medication, change in glasses prescription, and recent use of alcohol/other drugs.*[10]

• Assess and document client's fall risk using a fall-risk scale (e.g., Morse Fall Scale [MFS], Functional Ambulation Profile, Tinetti Balance and Gait Assessment, Timed-Up-and-Go [TUG]) upon admission, change in status, transfer, and discharge. *Fall-risk scales are widely used in acute-care and long-term settings and include numbered rating scales for (1) history of falls, (2) secondary diagnosis, (3) use of ambulatory aid,*

 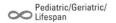

(4) presence of IV, (5) gait and transfer abilities, and (6) mental status. An MFS score greater than 51 indicates the client is at high risk for falls and requires high fall-prevention interventions. A TUG scale greater than 14 seconds combined with three other risk factors (such as support needed for cognition, transportation, and attendance at multiple appointments) places a client at high risk for falls.[1,2,7,8,10]

- ∞ Note client's age/developmental level, gender, decision-making ability, and level of competence. *Infants, young children (e.g., climbing on objects, stairs), young adults (e.g., sports activities), and elderly (e.g., significant vision, cognitive, or mobility impairments; osteoporosis; loss of muscle, fat, and subcutaneous tissue) are at greatest risk because of developmental issues or impaired/lack of ability to self-protect. Note: Tools for adult fall-risk assessment have been found to be unreliable in infants and children. Most falls in this age group occur outside the clinical setting, but assessment of facility environment and developmental issues in hospitalized children must include many factors, such as crib and play area safety, cosleeping issues, lapses of caregiver attention (such as falling asleep while feeding), medical and nursery equipment on which a toddler might climb, etc.[2,9]*

- Assess client's cognitive status (e.g., presence of brain injury, dementia, neurological disorders, visual/hearing/ other sensory impairments). *Affects ability to perceive own limitations or recognize danger. If client is unable to protect self, responsibility falls upon primary care provider(s).*

- Evaluate client's general and hip muscle strength, postural stability, gait and standing balance, gross and fine motor coordination. Review history of past or current physical injuries (e.g., musculoskeletal injuries, orthopedic surgery) *that may be altering coordination, gait, and balance.*

- Review client's ongoing medication regimen, noting number and type of drugs that could impact fall potential. *Studies have confirmed that use of four or more medications (polypharmacy) increases the risk of falls. The probability of using a medication that introduces risk increased that risk from 25% when one medicine was administered to 60% when six or more medicines were being taken.[11]*

- Assess mood, coping abilities, and personality styles. *Individual's temperament, typical behavior, stressors, and level of self-esteem can affect attitude toward safety issues, resulting in carelessness or increased risk-taking without consideration of consequences.[7–9]*

- Determine client's/significant other's (SO's) level of knowledge about and attendance to safety needs. *May reveal lack of knowledge needed to provide for safety, a choice to make a different decision for some reason (e.g., "We can't hire a home assistant"; "I can't watch him every minute"; "It's not manly"), or a lack of resources to attend to safety issues in all settings.[3,9]*

- Evaluate client's use, misuse, or failure to use assistive aids when indicated. *Client may have assistive device but is at high risk for falls while adjusting to altered body state and use of unfamiliar device. Client might refuse to use devices for various reasons (e.g., waiting for help; just doesn't like it for whatever reason).[7–9]*

- Identify hazards in the care setting, home, or other environment. *Determining needs and deficits provides opportunities for environmental redesign and instruction (e.g., concerning clearing of hazards, modification of lighting, equipment placement and space management; intensifying client supervision; obtaining safety equipment; referring for vision evaluation).[7,8,12]*

- ∞ Ascertain caregiver's expectations of client (whether child, cognitively impaired, and/or elderly family member) and compare with actual abilities. *Reality of client's abilities and needs may be different from perception or desires of caregivers.*

- Note socioeconomic status and availability and use of resources in other circumstances. *Can affect current coping abilities and fall risk.*

NURSING PRIORITY NO. 2 To assist client/caregiver to reduce or correct individual risk factors:

- Collaborate in treatment of disease or condition(s) (e.g., acute illness, dementia, incontinence, neurological or musculoskeletal conditions) *to improve client's overall health and thereby reduce potential for falls.*

- Review consequences of previously determined risk factors and client/SO response (e.g., client's current fall and hip fracture caused by failure to make safety provisions for client's impairments).[3]

- Participate in communicating fall risk status when client is in care facility to (1) patient/SO (e.g., verbal reminders of fall-prevention interventions in place to reduce client's risk; visible signage); (2) to staff (e.g.,

 Acute Care   Collaborative   Community/ Home Care   Cultural

consistent use of fall-assessment tool; shift-to-shift report; documentation in client record; (3) within unit/ across units (e.g., hand-off communication to report client's fall risk to receiving unit/facility).*These interventions are found to be part of "best-practice" interventions to reduce fall risk in client while acute care (e.g., hospital, short-stay or rehabilitation unit; extended and long-term care units).*[13]

- 🏠📝 Recommend or implement needed interventions and safety devices *to manage conditions that could contribute to falling and to promote safe environment for individual and others:*[1–9,12]

  Situate bed to enable client to exit toward his or her stronger side whenever possible.

  Place bed in lowest possible position, use raised-edge mattress, pad floor at side of bed, or place mattress on floor as appropriate.

  Use half siderail instead of full siderails or upright pole to assist individual in arising from bed.

  Provide chairs with firm, high seats and lifting mechanisms when indicated.

  Provide appropriate day or night lighting; evaluate vision, encourage use of prescription eyewear.

  Assist with transfers and ambulation; show client/SO ways to move safely.

  Provide and instruct in use of mobility devices and safety devices, like grab bars and call light or personal assistance systems.

  Clear environment of hazards (e.g., obstructing furniture, small items on the floor, electrical cords, throw rugs).

  Lock wheels on movable equipment (e.g., wheelchairs, beds).

  Encourage use of treaded slippers, socks, and shoes, and maintain nonskid floors and floor mats.

  Provide foot and nail care.

- 💊 Provide or encourage use of analgesics before activity if pain is interfering with desired activities. *Balance and movement can be impaired by pain associated with multiple conditions such as trauma or arthritis.*[1,2]

- 💊📝 Follow up with physician to review client's usual medication regimen (e.g., narcotics/opiates, psychotropics, antihypertensives, diuretics), *which can contribute to weakness, confusion, and balance and gait disturbances. May benefit from evaluating drug concentrations of certain medications (e.g., anticonvulsants, tricyclic antidepressants, antiarryhthmics) or may need an adjustment to dose, time of administration, or a change in choice of medication prescribed.*[6–11]

- 💊♾📝 Discuss benefits of supplemental estrogen, calcium, and vitamin D, as indicated. Refer for further evaluation as indicated. *Primary prevention of osteoporosis could be important in reducing falls and risk for fractures.*[12]

- ♾ Refer to physical medicine specialist, physical or occupational therapist, as appropriate. *May require evaluation (e.g., balance, muscle strength) and treatment to improve client's balance, strength, or mobility; to improve or relearn ambulation; and to identify and obtain appropriate assistive devices for mobility, environmental safety, or home modification.*

- 🏠 Perform home visit when appropriate. *Useful in determining client's specific needs and available resources or verifying that home safety issues are addressed, including supervision, access to emergency assistance, and client's ability to manage self-care in the home.*

NURSING PRIORITY NO. 3 To promote safety (Teaching/Discharge Considerations):[1–6]

- 🏠 Educate client/SO/caregivers in fall prevention; address the need for exercise balanced with need for client/ care provider safety. *While fall prevention is necessary, the need to protect the client from harm must be balanced with preserving client's independence. If the client is overly afraid of falling, the lack of activity will result in deconditioning and an even greater risk of falling.*[3]

- Discuss importance of monitoring client/intervening in conditions (e.g., client fatigue; acute illness; depression; objects that block traffic patterns in home; insufficient lighting; unfamiliar surroundings; client attempting tasks that are too difficult for present level of functioning; inability to contact someone when help is needed) *that have been shown to contribute to occurrence of falls.*[7,8]

- Address individual environmental factors associated with falling and create or instruct in a safe physical environment, such as bed height, room lighting, removal of loose carpet or throw rugs, repair of uneven flooring, and installing grab bars in bathrooms.

 Diagnostic Studies
 Evidence Based Practice
 Medications
 Pediatric/Geriatric/ Lifespan

- Refer to community resources as indicated. Provide written material for review and reinforcement of learning. *Client/caregivers may need or desire information (now or later) about financial assistance, home modifications, referrals for counseling, home care, sources for safety equipment, or placement in an extended care facility.*
- Connect client/family with sources of assistance (e.g., neighbors, friends, support groups) *to check on client on regular basis and to assist elderly or handicapped individuals in providing such things as structural maintenance; clearing of snow, gravel, or ice from walks and steps; etc.*
- Promote community awareness about the problems of design of buildings, equipment, transportation, and workplace accidents that contribute to falls.

DOCUMENTATION FOCUS

Assessment/Reassessment
- Individual risk factors noting current physical findings (e.g., bruises, cuts, anemia; use of alcohol, drugs, and prescription medications).
- Client's/caregiver's understanding of individual risks and safety concerns.
- Caregiver's expectations of client's abilities.

Planning
- Plan of care and who is involved in planning.
- Teaching plan.

Implementation/Evaluation
- Individual responses to interventions, teaching, and actions performed.
- Specific actions and changes that are made.
- Attainment or progress toward desired outcomes.
- Modifications to plan of care.

Discharge Planning
- Long-term plans for discharge needs, lifestyle, and home setting and community changes and who is responsible for actions to be taken.
- Specific referrals made.

References

1. National Guideline Clearinghouse. (Updated 2012). Prevention of fall-related injuries in the elderly. Retrieved March 2018 from https://www.guideline.gov/summaries/summary/50433/prevention-of-fallrelated-injuries-in-the-elderly?q=falls.
2. VA National Center for Patient Safety. (Updated 2015). Implementation guide for fall injury reduction. Retrieved March 2018 from https://www.patientsafety.va.gov/docs/fallstoolkit14/falls_implementation_%20guide%20_02_2015.pdf.
3. Henkel, G. (2002). Beyond the MDS. Team approach to falls assessment, prevention & management. *Caring for the Aged*, 3(4), 15–20.
4. Doenges, M. E., Moorhouse, M. F., Geissler-Murr, A. C. (2002). Nursing care plan: Extended care, falls, risk for. *Nursing Care Plans: Guidelines for Individualizing Patient Care.* (CD-ROM). 6th ed. Philadelphia: F. A. Davis.
5. Daus, C. (1999). Maintaining mobility: Assistive equipment helps the geriatric population stay active and independent. *Rehab Manag*, 12(5), 58–61.
6. Horn, L. B. (2000). Reducing the risk of falls in the elderly. *Rehab Manag*, 13(3), 36–38.
7. Bright, L. (2005). Strategies to improve the patient safety outcome indicator: Preventing or reducing falls. *Home Healthc Nurse*, 23(1), 29–36.
8. Poe, S. S., et al. (2005). An evidence-based approach to fall risk assessment, prevention, and management: Lessons learned. *J Nurs Care Qual*, 20(2), 107–116.
9. McWilliams, J. R. (2011). An evidenced-based pediatric fall assessment tool for home health. *Home Healthc Nurse*, 20(29), 98–105.
10. Kemle, K. (2011). Falls in older adults: Averting disaster. Retrieved March 2018 from http://www.clinicaladvisor.com/falls-in-older-adults-averting-a-disaster/article/195485/.
11. Ziere, G., et al. (2006). Polypharmacy and falls in the middle age and elderly population. *Br J Clin Pharmacol*, 61(2), 218–223.
12. Quigley, P. A., Bulat, T., Hart-Hughes, S. (2007). Strategies to reduce risk of fall-related injuries in rehabilitation nursing. *Rehabil Nurs*, 32(3), 120–125.
13. Nailon, R., Conley, D. (2012). Learning Module: Fall risk assessment: Best practices for nursing staff in the acute care setting. Retrieved March 2018 from https://www.unmc.edu/patient-safety/capturefalls/learningmodules/fall-risk-assess-handout.pdf/.

 Acute Care   Collaborative   Community/Home Care   Cultural

dysfunctional Family Processes

Taxonomy II: Role Relationships—Class 2 Family Relationships (00063) **[Diagnostic Division:** Social Interaction], Submitted as dysfunction Family Processes: Alcoholism 1994; Revised: name change 2008, 2013, 2017

DEFINITION: Family functioning which fails to support the well-being of its members.

RELATED FACTORS
Addictive personality; substance misuse/[abuse]
Ineffective coping strategies; insufficient problem-solving skills

DEFINING CHARACTERISTICS

Subjective
Feelings
Abandonment; confuses love and pity; moodiness; failure
Anger, frustration; shame, embarrassment; hurt; unhappiness; guilt
Anxiety, tension, distress; low self-esteem, worthlessness; lingering resentment
Depression; hostility; fear; confusion; dissatisfaction; loss
Emotionally controlled by others; emotional isolation,
Feeling different from others; loss of identity; feeling unloved, misunderstood
Loneliness; powerlessness; insecurity; hopelessness; rejection
Taking responsibility for substance abuser's behavior; vulnerability; mistrust
Roles and Relationships
Family denial; deterioration in family relationships; disturbance in family dynamics; ineffective communication with partner; intimacy dysfunction
Change in role function; disruption in family roles or rituals; inconsistent parenting; perceived insufficient parental support; chronic family problems
Insufficient relationship skills; insufficient cohesiveness
Pattern of rejection; neglect of obligation to family member

Objective
Feelings
Repressed emotions
Roles and Relationships
Closed communication systems
Conflict between partners; diminished ability of family members to relate to each other for mutual growth and maturation; triangulating family relationships
Insufficient family respect for individuality or autonomy of its members
Behavioral
Alteration in concentration; disturbance in academic performance in children; failure to accomplish developmental tasks; difficulty with life-cycle transition
Blaming; inappropriate anger expression; criticizing; verbal abuse of children/partner/parent
Harsh self-judgment; difficulty having fun; self-blaming; social isolation; complicated grieving; seeking of approval or affirmation
Inability to meet the emotional, security, or spiritual needs of its members
Inability to adapt to change; immaturity; stress-related physical illnesses; inability to deal constructively with traumatic experiences
Inappropriate anger expression; blaming; criticizing; verbal abuse of children/partner/parent

(continues on page 314)

dysfunctional Family Processes (continued)

Ineffective communication skills; controlling, contradictory, or paradoxical communication pattern; power struggles

Insufficient problem-solving skills; conflict avoidance; orientation favors tension relief rather than goal attainment; agitation; escalating conflict; chaos

Inability to express or accept a wide range of feelings; difficulty with intimate relationship; decrease in physical contact

Lying; broken promises; unreliable behavior; manipulation; dependency

Rationalization; denial of problems; refusal to get help; inability to accept or receive help appropriately

Substance abuse; enabling substance use pattern; insufficient knowledge about substance abuse; special occasions centered on substance use; nicotine addiction

At Risk Population: Economically disadvantaged

Genetic predisposition to substance misuse/[abuse]; family history of substance misuse/[abuse]; family history of resistance to treatment;

Associated Condition: Biological factors; intimacy dysfunction; surgical procedure

Sample Clinical Applications: Alcohol abuse or withdrawal, prescription or illicit drug abuse, fetal alcohol syndrome

DESIRED OUTCOMES/EVALUATION CRITERIA

Sample **NOC** linkages:

Family Functioning: Capacity of a family to meet the needs of its members during developmental transitions

Family Social Climate: Capacity of a family to provide a supportive milieu as characterized by family member relationships and goals

Substance Addiction Consequences: Severity of change in health status and social functioning due to substance addiction

Family Will (Include Specific Time Frame)
- Verbalize understanding of dynamics of codependence.
- Participate in individual/family treatment programs.
- Identify ineffective coping behaviors and consequences of choices or actions.
- Plan for necessary lifestyle changes.
- Take action to change self-destructive behaviors or alter behaviors that contribute to substance abuse.
- Demonstrate improvement in parenting skills.

ACTIONS/INTERVENTIONS

Sample **NIC** linkages:

Counseling: Use of an interactive helping process focusing on the needs, problems, or feelings of the patient and significant others to enhance or support coping, problem solving, and interpersonal relationships

Substance Use Treatment: Care of patient and family members demonstrating dysfunction as a result of substance abuse or dependence

Family Process Maintenance: Minimization of family process disruption effects

 Acute Care Collaborative Community/ Home Care Cultural

NURSING PRIORITY NO. 1   To assess contributing factors/underlying problem(s):

- Assess current level of functioning of family members. *Information necessary for planning care determines areas for focus and potential for change.*[2]
- Ascertain family's understanding of current situation; note results of previous involvement in treatment. *Family with a member who is addicted to alcohol has often had frequent hospitalizations in the past. Knowing what has brought about the current situation will determine a starting place for this treatment plan.*[2]
- Review family history and explore roles of family members and circumstances involving substance use. *Although one member may be identified as the client, all of the family members are participants in the problem and need to be involved in the solution.*[5]
- Determine history of accidents or violent behaviors within family and current safety issues. *Identifies family at risk and degree of concern or disregard of individual members to determine course of action to prevent further violence.*[2,4]
- Discuss current and past methods of coping. *Family members have developed coping skills to deal with behaviors of client, which may or may not be useful to changing the situation. Skills identified as useful can help to change the present situation. Those identified as not helpful (enabling behaviors) can be targeted for intervention to bring about desired changes and improve family functioning.*[1,2,5]
- Determine extent and understanding of enabling behaviors being evidenced by family members. *Family members may have developed behaviors that support the client continuing the pattern of addiction. Awareness, identification, and knowledge of these behaviors provide opportunity for individuals to begin the process of change.*[2,5]
- Identify sabotage behaviors of family members. *Issues of secondary gain (conscious or unconscious) may impede recovery. Even though family member(s) may verbalize a desire for the individual to be healthy (or substance free), the reality of interactive dynamics is that they may unconsciously not want the individual to recover because this would affect the role(s) of the family member(s) in the relationship.*[2]
- Note presence and extent of behaviors of family, client, and staff that might be "too helpful," such as frequent requests for assistance, excuses for not following through on agreed-on behaviors, and feelings of anger or irritation with others. *Identification of specific behaviors (enabling) can help family members see what they do that complicates acceptance of situation by substance abuser and that need to be changed to facilitate resolution of problem.*[5]

NURSING PRIORITY NO. 2   To assist family to change destructive behaviors:

- Seek mutual agreement on behaviors and responsibilities for nurse and client/family members. *Maximizes understanding of what is expected of each person and minimizes opportunity for manipulation of each individual.*[5]
- Confront and examine denial and sabotage behaviors used by family members. *Identifies specific behaviors that individuals can be aware of and begin to change so they can move beyond blocks to recovery.*[6]
- Discuss use of anger, rationalization, or projection and ways in which these interfere with problem resolution. *Awareness of own feelings can lead to a decision to change; client then has to face the consequences of his or her own actions and may choose to get well.*[6]
- Encourage family to identify and deal with anger. Solve concerns and develop solutions. *Understanding what leads to anger and violence can lead to new behaviors and changes in the family for healthier relationships.*[3]
- Determine family strengths, areas for growth, and individual/family successes. *Family members may not realize they have strengths, and as they identify these areas, they can choose to learn and develop new strategies for a more effective family structure.*[2]
- Remain nonjudgmental in approach to family members and to member who uses alcohol or drugs. *Individual already sees self as unworthy, and judgment on the part of caregivers to family will interfere with ability to be a change agent.*[5]
- Provide information regarding effects of addiction on mood and personality of the involved person. *Family members have been dealing with client's behavior for a time, and information can help them to understand and cope with negative behaviors without being judgmental or reacting angrily.*[2]

 Diagnostic Studies   Evidence Based Practice   Medications   Pediatric/Geriatric/ Lifespan

- Distinguish between destructive aspects of enabling behavior and genuine motivation to aid the user. *Family members often want to help but need to distinguish between behavior that is helpful and that which is not to begin to solve problems of addiction.*[6]
- Identify use of manipulative behaviors and discuss ways to avoid or prevent these situations. *The client often manipulates the people around him or her to maintain the status quo. When family begins to interact in a straightforward, honest manner, manipulation is not possible and healing can begin.*[2]

NURSING PRIORITY NO. 3 To promote wellness (Teaching/Discharge Considerations):

- Provide factual information to client/family about the effects of addictive behaviors on the family and what to expect after discharge from program. *Family may have unrealistic expectations about changes that have occurred in therapy, and having information will help them deal more effectively with the difficulties of continuing the changes as they return to their new life without alcohol or substance.*[5]
- Provide information about enabling behavior and addictive disease characteristics for both the user and nonuser who is codependent. *Education is a prime ingredient in treatment of addiction and can assist family members to deal realistically with these issues.*[6]
- Discuss importance of restructuring life activities, work, and leisure relationships. *Previous lifestyle and relationships supported the substance use, requiring change to prevent relapse.*[7]
- Encourage family to refocus celebrations to exclude substance use. *Because celebrations often include the use of alcohol, this is one area where change can be made that can reduce the risk of relapse.*[7]
- Provide support for family members; encourage participation in group work. *Support is essential to changing client and family behaviors. Participating in group provides an opportunity to practice new skills of communication and behavior.*[5]
- Encourage involvement with/refer to self-help groups, Al-Anon, AlaTeen, Narcotics Anonymous, and family therapy groups. *Regular attendance at a group can provide support; help client see how others are dealing with similar problems; and learn new skills, such as problem solving, for handling family disagreements.*[7]
- Provide bibliotherapy including reliable Web sites, as appropriate. *Reading provides helpful information for making desired changes, especially when client/family members are dedicated to making change and willing to learn new ways of interacting within the family.*[7]
- Refer to NDs compromised/disabled family Coping and interrupted Family Processes as appropriate for additional interventions.

DOCUMENTATION FOCUS

Assessment/Reassessment
- Assessment findings, including history of substance(s) that have been used and family risk factors/safety concerns.
- Family composition and involvement.
- Results of previous treatment involvement.

Planning
- Plan of care and who is involved in planning.
- Teaching plan.

Implementation/Evaluation
- Responses of family members to treatment, teaching, and actions performed.
- Attainment or progress toward desired outcome(s).
- Modifications to plan of care.

Discharge Planning
- Long-term needs and who is responsible for actions to be taken.
- Specific referrals made.

 Acute Care

 Collaborative

 Community/ Home Care

 Cultural

References

1. Messina, J. (No date). *Eliminating manipulation: Tools for handling control issues*. Retrieved March 2018 from http://coping.us/toolsforhandlingcontrol/eliminatemanipulation.html.
2. Friel, J. C., Friel, L. D. (2010). *Adult Children—The Secrets of Dysfunctional Families*. Deerfield Beach, FL: Health Communications, Inc.
3. Pinnacle Recovery. (2017). Types of anger and how it can affect your sobriety. Retrieved March 2018 from https://pinnaclerecoveryut.com/types-of-anger-and-how-it-can-affect-your-sobriety/.
4. Moyer, V. A. (2013). Screening for intimate partner violence and abuse of elderly and vulnerable adults: U.S. Preventive Services Task Force recommendation statement. *Ann of Inter Med*, 158(6), 478–486.
5. Saaticioglu, O., Erim, R., Cakmak, D. (2006). Role of family in alcohol and substance abuse. *Psychiatry Clin Neurosci*, 60(2), 125–132.
6. Nye, C. L., Zucker, R. A., Fitzgerald, H. E. (1999). Early family-based intervention in the path to alcohol problems, rationale and relationship between treatment process characteristics and child and parenting outcomes. *J Stud Alcohol Suppl*, 13, 10–21.
7. Seilhamer, R. A., Jacob, T., Dunn, N. J. (1993). The impact of alcohol consumption on parent-child relationships in families of alcoholics. *J Stud Alcohol*, 54, 189–198.

interrupted Family Processes

Taxonomy II: Role Relationships—Class 2 Family Relationships (00060) [**Diagnostic Division:** Social Interactions], Approved 1982; Revised 1998; 2017

DEFINITION: Break in the continuity of family functioning which fails to support the well-being of its members

RELATED FACTORS
Changes in interaction with community
Power shift among family members; shift in family values

DEFINING CHARACTERISTICS

Subjective
Changes in relationship pattern
Change in availability for affective responsiveness; decrease in mutual support; decrease in available emotional support; change in intimacy
Changes in expression of conflict with, or isolation from, community resources

Objective
Assigned tasks change; ineffective task completion; change in participation for problem solving; changes in participation for decision making
Change in communication pattern; change in family conflict resolution; power alliance changes
Change in stress-reduction behavior; change in somatization
At Risk Population: Changes in interaction with community; power shift among family members; shift in family roles
Associated Condition: Shift in health status of a family member
Sample Clinical Applications: Chronic illness, cancer, surgical procedures, traumatic injury, substance abuse, Alzheimer's disease, pregnancy, adolescent rebellion, conduct disorder

DESIRED OUTCOMES/EVALUATION CRITERIA

Sample NOC linkages:
Family Functioning: Capacity of a family to meet the needs of its members during developmental transitions

(continues on page 318)

 Diagnostic Studies   Evidence Based Practice   Medications   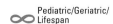 Pediatric/Geriatric/Lifespan

interrupted **Family Processes** (continued)

Family Normalization: Capacity of a family to develop strategies for optimal functioning when a member has a chronic illness or disability

Family Social Climate: Capacity of a family to provide a supportive milieu as characterized by family member relationships and goals

Family Will (Include Specific Time Frame)
- Express feelings freely and appropriately.
- Demonstrate individual involvement in problem-solving processes directed at appropriate solutions for the situation or crisis.
- Direct energies in a purposeful manner to plan for resolution of the crisis.
- Verbalize understanding of illness/trauma, treatment regimen, and prognosis.
- Encourage and allow affected member to handle situation in own way, progressing toward independence.

ACTIONS/INTERVENTIONS

Sample NIC linkages:

Family Process Maintenance: Minimization of family process disruption effects

Family Integrity Promotion: Promotion of family cohesion and unity

Normalization Promotion: Assisting parents and other family members of children with chronic diseases or disabilities in providing normal life experiences for their children and families

---

NURSING PRIORITY NO. 1   To assess individual situation for causative/contributing factors:

- Determine pathophysiology, illness or trauma, and developmental crisis present. *Identifies areas of need for planning care for this family.*[2]
- ∞ Identify family developmental stage (e.g., marriage, birth of a child, children leaving home, death of a spouse). *Developmental stage will affect family functioning; for instance, a couple who are newly married will be dealing with issues of learning how to live with each other, children leaving home may result in problems related to "empty-nest syndrome," or death of a spouse radically changes life for the survivor.*[2,8]
- Note components of family: parent(s), children, male/female, and extended family available. *Affects how individuals deal with current stressors. Relationships among members may be supportive or strained.*[6]
- Observe patterns of communication in this family. Are feelings expressed? Freely? Who talks to whom? Who makes decisions and for whom? Who visits? What is the interaction between family members? *Identifies not only weakness and areas of concern to be addressed, but also strengths that can be used for resolution of problem(s).*[6,9]
- Assess boundaries of family members. Do members share family identity and have little sense of individuality? Do they seem emotionally distant and not connected with one another? *These factors are critical to understanding family dynamics and developing strategies for change. Boundaries need to be clear so individual family members are free to be responsible for themselves.*[6]
- Ascertain role expectations of family members. Who is the ill member (e.g., nurturer, provider)? How does the illness affect the roles of others? *Each person may see the situation in his or her own individual manner; clear identification and sharing of these expectations promote understanding. Family members may expect client to continue to perform usual role or may not allow client to do anything (either action can create problems for the ill member). Realistic planning can provide positive sense of self for the client.*[2,8]
- Determine "family rules" (e.g., adult concerns such as finances, illness, and so on are kept from the children). *Rules may be imposed by adults rather than through a democratic process involving all family members, leading to conflict and angry confrontations. Setting positive family rules with all family members participating can promote a functional family.*[2,3]

 Acute Care   Collaborative   Community/ Home Care   Cultural

- Identify parenting skills and expectations. *Ineffective parenting and unrealistic expectations may contribute to abuse. Understanding normal responses and progression of developmental milestones may help parent cope with changes necessitated by current crisis.*[2,3]
- Note energy direction. Are efforts at resolution/problem solving purposeful or scattered? *Provides clues about interventions that may be appropriate to assist client and family in directing energies in a more effective manner.*[2,9]
- Listen for expressions of despair/helplessness (e.g., "I don't know what to do") to note degree of distress. *Such feelings may contribute to difficulty adjusting to situation (e.g., teenage independence, change in health status of household breadwinner, dependence of aging parent on grown child) and ability to cooperate with plan of care or treatment regimen required.*[4]
- Note cultural and/or religious beliefs and values affecting perceptions and expectations of family members. *These factors affect client/SO reactions and adjustment to situation and may limit choice of interventions and potential for successful resolution. For example, Arab American family relationships often include nuclear and extended family, with families making collective decisions. Men are expected to be responsible for carrying out decisions. Women are usually delegated care for daily needs of the family, while children may have little independence, and birth control may not be allowed for teenagers.*[7]
- Assess support systems available outside of the family. *Having these resources can help the family begin to pull together and deal with current situation and problems they are facing.*[2]

NURSING PRIORITY NO. 2   To assist family to deal with situation/crisis:

- Deal with family members in a warm, caring, and respectful way. *Provides feelings of empathy and promotes individual's sense of worth and competence in ability to handle current situation.*[2]
- Acknowledge difficulties and realities of the situation. *Communicates message of understanding and reinforces that some degree of conflict is to be expected and can be used to promote growth.*[3]
- Encourage expressions of anger. Avoid taking them personally. *Feelings of anger are to be expected when individuals are dealing with a difficult situation. Appropriate expression enables progress toward resolution of the stages of the grieving process when indicated. Not taking their anger personally maintains boundaries between nurse and family.*[2,5]
- Emphasize importance of continuous, open dialogue between family members to facilitate ongoing problem-solving. *Promotes understanding and assists family members to maintain clear communication and resolve problems effectively.*[6,10]
- Provide information, verbal and written, and reinforce as necessary. *Promotes understanding and opportunity to review as needed.*[2]
- Assist family to identify and encourage their use of previously successful coping behaviors. *Most people have developed effective coping skills that, when identified, can be useful in current situation.*[6,10]
- Recommend contact by family members on a regular, frequent basis. *Promotes feelings of warmth and caring and brings family closer to one another, enabling them to manage current difficult situation.*[2]
- Arrange for and encourage family participation in multidisciplinary team conference or group therapy as appropriate. *Participation in family and group therapy for an extended period increases likelihood of success as interactional issues (e.g., marital conflict, "scapegoating" of children) can be addressed and dealt with. Involvement with others can help family members to experience new ways of interacting and gain insight into their behavior, providing opportunity for change.*[2,5]
- Involve family in social support and community activities of their interest and choice. *Involvement with others outside of family constellation provides opportunity to observe how others handle problems and deal with conflict.*[2,8]

NURSING PRIORITY NO. 3   To promote wellness (Teaching/Discharge Considerations):

- Encourage use of stress-management techniques (e.g., appropriate expression of feelings, relaxation exercises). *The relaxation response helps members think more clearly, deal more effectively with conflict, and promote more effective relationships to enhance family interactions.*[4]

- Provide educational materials and information. *Learning about the problems they are facing can assist family members in resolution of current crisis.*[2]
- Refer to classes (e.g., parent effectiveness, specific disease, or disability support groups; self-help groups; clergy, psychological counseling, or family therapy as indicated). *Can assist family to effect positive change and enhance conflict-resolution skills. Presence of substance abuse problems requires all family members to seek support and assistance in dealing with situation to promote a healthy outcome.*[2,3] (Refer to ND dysfunctional Family Processes for additional interventions as appropriate.)
- Assist family to identify situations that may lead to fear or anxiety (e.g., diagnosis of chronic debilitating condition, decline in mental functioning of aging spouse/parent, sexually active teenager). (Refer to NDs Anxiety, Fear.) *Promotes opportunity to provide anticipatory guidance.*[1,5]
- Involve family in mutual goal-setting to plan for the future. *When all members of the family are involved, commitment to goals and continuation of plan are more likely to be maintained.*[3]
- Identify community agencies (e.g., Meals on Wheels, visiting nurse, trauma support group, American Cancer Society, Veterans Administration). *Provides both immediate and long-term support.*[6]

DOCUMENTATION FOCUS

Assessment/Reassessment
- Assessment findings, including family composition, developmental stage of family, and role expectations.
- Family communication patterns.
- Cultural or religious beliefs and values.

Planning
- Plan of care, specific interventions, and who is involved in planning.
- Teaching plan.

Implementation/Evaluation
- Each individual's response to interventions, teaching, and actions performed.
- Attainment or progress toward desired outcome(s).
- Modifications to plan of care.

Discharge Planning
- Long-term needs, noting who is responsible for actions to be taken.
- Specific referrals made.

References

1. LaBier, D. (2013). Why your fears shape so much of your life. *Psychol Today*. Retrieved March 2018 from http://www.psychologytoday.com/blog/the-new-resilience/201303/why-your-fears-shape-so-much-your-life.
2. No author listed. (2009). Stages of family development, education, self improvement, health and medicine. Retrieved March 2018 from http://www.slideshare.net/guest74f230/stages-of-family-development.
3. Aktan, G. B., et al. (1996). Effectiveness of a family skills training program for substance abuse prevention with inner city African-American families. *Subst Use Misuse*, 31(2), 157–175.
4. Reid, M. W. (1977). Counseling the disturbed family. *Aust Fam Physician*, 6(5), 474–479.
5. Rueter, M. A., Koerner, A. F. (2008). The effect of family communication patterns on adopted adolescent adjustment. *J Marriage Fam*, 70(3), 715–727.
6. Gerlach, P. (Updated 2015). Perspective on family role and rule problems. *Break the Cycle*. Retrieved March 2018 from http://sfhelp.org/fam/roles_rules.htm.
7. Fronk, C., Huntington, R., Chadwick, B. A. (1999). Expectations for traditional family roles: Palestinian adolescents in the West Bank and Gaza. *Sex Roles*, 41(9), 705–735.
8. Adjei, N. (2012). Family developmental theory. *Prezi online presentation and transcript*. Retrieved March 2018 from https://prezi.com/yb4qetwov0bw/family-developmental-theory/.
9. Adams, L. (2008). How families resolve conflicts. *The Family Connection Newsletter*, July.
10. DaFoe Whitehead, B., Popenoe, D. (2004). The state of our unions: The social health of marriage in America 2004. *Theology Matters*, 10(2), 1–16.

 Acute Care   Collaborative   Community/Home Care   Cultural

readiness for enhanced Family Processes

Taxonomy II: Role Relationships—Class 2 Family Relationships (00159) [**Diagnostic Division:** Social Interactions], Approved 2002; Revised 2013

DEFINITION: A pattern of family functioning that is sufficient to support the well-being of family members and can be strengthened.

DEFINING CHARACTERISTICS

Subjective

Expresses desire to enhance:

- Balance between autonomy and cohesiveness
- Communication pattern
- Family resilience, growth and safety of family members
- Respect for family members; maintenance of boundaries between family member
- Interdependence with community

Sample Clinical Applications: Chronic health conditions (e.g., asthma, diabetes mellitus, arthritis, systemic lupus, multiple sclerosis [MS], AIDS), mental health concerns (e.g., depression, attention deficit disorder, Down syndrome)

DESIRED OUTCOMES/EVALUATION CRITERIA

Sample NOC linkages:

Family Social Climate: Capacity of a family to provide a supportive milieu as characterized by family member relationships and goals

Family Health Status: Overall health and social competence of a family

Family Resiliency: Capacity of a family to positively adapt and function following significant adversity or crisis

Client Will (Include Specific Time Frame)

- Express feelings freely and appropriately.
- Verbalize understanding of desire for enhanced family dynamics.
- Demonstrate individual involvement in problem solving to improve family communications.
- Acknowledge awareness of and respect for boundaries of family members.

ACTIONS/INTERVENTIONS

Sample NIC linkages:

Family Support: Promotion of family values, interests, and goals

Parent Education: Childrearing Family: Assisting parents to understand and promote the physical, psychological, and social growth and development of their toddler, preschool, or school-age child

Normalization Promotion: Assisting parents and other family members of children with chronic illnesses or disabilities in providing normal life experiences for their children and families

NURSING PRIORITY NO. 1 To determine current status of family:

- Determine family composition, such as parent(s), children, male/female, and extended family involved. *Many family forms exist in society today, such as biological, nuclear, single-parent, step-family, communal, and*

 Diagnostic Studies   Evidence Based Practice   Medications 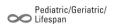 Pediatric/Geriatric/Lifespan *same-sex couple or family. A better way to determine a family may be to determine the attribute of affection, strong emotional ties, a sense of belonging, and durability of membership.*[1,6]

- Identify participating members of family, such as parent(s), children, male/female, and extended family. *Identifies members of family who need to be involved and taken into consideration in developing plan of care to improve family functioning.*[1]
- Note stage of family development. *While the North American middle-class family stages may be described as single, young adult, newly married, family with young children, family with adolescents, grown children, and later life, developmental tasks may vary greatly among cultural groups. This information provides a framework for developing a plan to enhance family processes.*[1]
- Ascertain motivation and expectations for change. *Motivation to improve and high expectations can encourage family to make changes that will improve their life. However, unrealistic expectations may hamper efforts.*[7]
- Observe patterns of communication in the family. Are feelings expressed freely? Who talks to whom? Who makes decisions? For whom? Who visits? When? What is the interaction between family members? *Identifies not only possible weakness or areas of concern to be addressed, but also identifies strengths that can be used for planning improvement in family communication. Effective communication is that in which verbal and nonverbal messages are clear, direct, and congruent.*[1,2]
- Assess boundaries of family members. Do members share family identity and have little sense of individuality? Do they seem emotionally connected with one another? *Individuals need to respect one another, and boundaries need to be clear so family members are free to be responsible for themselves.*[1,3]
- Identify "family rules" that are accepted in the family. *Families interact in certain ways over time and develop patterns of behavior that are accepted as the way "we behave" in this family. "Functional families" rules are constructive and promote the needs of all family members.*[1]
- Note energy direction. *Efforts at problem-solving, resolution of different opinions, and growth may be purposeful or may be scattered and ineffective.*[3]
- Determine cultural and/or religious factors influencing family interactions. *Expectations related to socioeconomic beliefs may be different in various cultures; for instance, traditional views of marriage and family life may be strongly influenced by Roman Catholicism in Italian American and Latino American families. In some cultures, the father is considered the authority figure and the mother is the homemaker. These beliefs may be functional or dysfunctional in any given family and may change with stressors/circumstances (e.g., financial, loss or gain of a family member, personal growth).*[1,3,7]
- Note health of married individuals. *Recent reports have determined that marriage increases life expectancy by as much as 5 years.*[5]

NURSING PRIORITY NO. 2 To assist the family to improve family interactions:

- Establish nurse-family relationship. *Promotes a warm, caring atmosphere in which family members can share thoughts, ideas, and feelings openly and in a nonjudgmental manner.*[3]
- Acknowledge difficulties and realities of individual situation. *Reinforces that some degree of conflict is to be expected in family interactions that can be used to promote growth.*[1,3]
- Emphasize importance of continuous, open dialogue between family members. *Facilitates ongoing expression of open, honest feelings and opinions and effective problem-solving.*[1,4]
- Assist family to identify and encourage use of previously successful coping behaviors. *Promotes recognition of previous successes and confidence in own abilities to learn and improve family interactions.*[2,4]
- Acknowledge differences among family members with open dialogue about how these differences have occurred. *Conveys an acceptance of these differences among individuals and helps to look at how they can be used to strengthen the family process.*[3]
- Identify effective parenting skills already being used and additional ways of handling difficult behaviors that may develop. *Allows the individual family members to realize that some of what has been done already was helpful and helps them to learn new skills to manage family interactions in a more effective manner.*[3]

 Acute Care   Collaborative   Community/ Home Care   Cultural

NURSING PRIORITY NO. 3 To promote optimum well-being (Teaching/Discharge Considerations):

- Involve family members in setting goals and planning for the future. *When individuals are involved in the decision making, they are more committed to carrying through on a plan to enhance family interactions as life goes on.*[2]
- Discuss and encourage use of stress-management techniques. *Relaxation exercises, visualization, and similar skills can be useful for promoting reduction of anxiety and ability to manage stress that occurs in their lives.*[1]
- Encourage participation in learning role-reversal activities. *Helps individuals to gain insight and understanding of other person's feelings and point of view.*[3]
- Provide educational materials and information. *Enhances learning to assist in developing positive relationships among family members.*[4]
- Assist family members to identify situations that may create problems and lead to stress/anxiety. *Thinking ahead can help individuals anticipate helpful actions to handle or prevent conflict and untoward consequences.*[4]
- Refer to classes or community resources as appropriate. *Family effectiveness and self-help groups, psychotherapy, and religious affiliations can provide new information to assist family members to learn and apply to enhancing family interactions.*[4]

DOCUMENTATION FOCUS

Assessment/Reassessment
- Assessment findings, including family composition, developmental stage of family, and role expectations.
- Cultural or religious values and beliefs regarding family and family functioning.
- Family communication patterns.
- Motivation and expectations for change.

Planning
- Plan of care, specific interventions, and who is involved in planning.
- Educational plan.

Implementation/Evaluation
- Each individual's response to interventions, teaching, and actions performed.
- Attainment or progress toward desired outcome(s).
- Modifications to lifestyle and treatment plan.

Discharge Planning
- Long-term needs, noting who is responsible for actions to be taken.
- Specific referrals made.

References

1. No author listed. (2009). Stages of family development. Retrieved March 2018 from http://www.slideshare.net/guest74f230/stages-of-family-development.
2. Gordon, T. (2011). Families need rules. *Parent Programs, Gordon Training International*. Retrieved March 2018 from http://www.gordontraining.com/free-parenting-articles/families-need-rules/.
3. Sophy, C. (2005). Four tips to help you set and enforce family boundaries. Retrieved March 2018 from http://ezinearticles.com/?Four-Tips-To-Help-You-Set-And-Enforce-Family-Boundaries&id=76369.
4. Sittner, B. J., Hudson, D. B., DeFrain, J. (2007). Using the concept of family strengths to enhance nursing care. *Am J Maternal/Child Nurs*, 32(6), 353–357.
5. Kaplan, R. M., Kronick, R. G. (2006). Marital status and longevity in the United States population. *J Epidemiol Community Health*, 60(9), 760–765.
6. Hartley, R., McDonald, P. (1994). The many faces of diversity in Australian families. *Fam Matters*, 37, 6–12.
7. McLeod, D. L., Wright, L. M. (2001). Conversations of spirituality: Spirituality in family systems nursing—Making the case with four clinical vignettes. *J Fam Nurs*, 7(4), 391–415.

 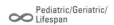

Fatigue

Taxonomy II: Activity/Rest—Class 3 Energy Balance (00093) [Diagnostic Division: Activity/Rest], Approved 1988; Nursing Diagnosis Extension and Classification Revision 1998; Revised 2017

DEFINITION: An overwhelming sustained sense of exhaustion and decreased capacity for physical and mental work at the usual level.

RELATED FACTORS
Anxiety; depression
Environmental barrier
Increase in physical exertion; physical deconditioning; nonstimulating lifestyle
Malnutrition; sleep deprivation; stressors
Demanding occupation

DEFINING CHARACTERISTICS

Subjective
Insufficient energy; impaired ability to maintain usual routines or usual physical activity
Tiredness; nonrestorative sleep pattern
Guilt about difficulty maintaining responsibilities
Alteration in libido
Increase in physical symptoms, rest requirements

Objective
Alteration in concentration
Apathy; lethargy; listlessness; drowsiness
Disinterest in surroundings; introspection
Ineffective role performance
At Risk Population: Demanding occupation
Exposure to negative life events
Associated Condition: Anemia; illness, pregnancy
Sample Clinical Applications: Anemia, hypothyroidism, cancer, multiple sclerosis (MS), Lyme disease, postpolio syndrome, AIDS, chronic renal failure, chronic fatigue syndrome (CFS), depression

DESIRED OUTCOMES/EVALUATION CRITERIA

Sample NOC linkages:
Fatigue: Disruptive Effects: Severity of observed or reported disruptive effects of chronic fatigue on daily functioning
Energy Conservation: Personal actions to manage energy for initiating and sustaining activity
Psychomotor Energy: Personal drive and energy to maintain activities of daily living, nutrition, and personal safety

Client Will (Include Specific Time Frame)
• Report improved sense of energy.
• Identify basis of fatigue and individual areas of control.
• Perform ADLs and participate in desired activities at level of ability.
• Participate in recommended treatment program.

 Acute Care Collaborative Community/Home Care Cultural

ACTIONS/INTERVENTIONS

Sample NIC linkages:
Energy Management: Regulating energy use to treat or prevent fatigue and optimize function
Exercise Promotion: Facilitation of regular physical activity to maintain or advance to a higher level of fitness and health
Nutrition Management: Providing and promoting a balanced intake of nutrients

NURSING PRIORITY NO. 1   To assess causative/contributing factors:

- Identify presence of physical and/or psychological conditions (e.g., pregnancy, infectious processes, blood loss, anemia, autoimmune disorders [e.g., MS, lupus, rheumatoid arthritis], trauma, chronic pain syndromes [e.g., arthritis], cardiopulmonary disorders, cancer or cancer treatments, hepatitis, AIDS, major depressive disorder, anxiety states, substance use or abuse). *Important information can be obtained from knowing if fatigue is a result of an underlying condition or disease process (acute or chronic), whether an exacerbating or remitting condition is in exacerbation, and/or whether fatigue has been present over a long time without any identifiable cause.*
- Note diagnosis or possibility of CFS (also sometimes called chronic fatigue immune dysfunction syndrome [CFIDS], or myalgic encephalomyelitis [ME]). *This condition is difficult to characterize, largely because various studies define it differently. Because no direct tests help in diagnosis, it is one of exclusion. CFS has been defined as a distinct disorder (affecting both children and adults) characterized by chronic (often relapsing but always debilitating) fatigue, lasting for at least 6 months (often for much longer), causing impairments in overall physical and mental functioning, and without an apparent etiology.*[1]
- ∞ Note client's age, gender, and developmental stage. *Some studies show a prevalence of fatigue in females more than in males, and it occurs most commonly in young to middle-aged adults.*[1,9,10]
- Assess general well-being—cardiovascular and respiratory status, musculoskeletal strength, emotional health, and nutritional and fluid status. *Underlying conditions (e.g., anemia, heart failure, depression, malnutrition) may be causing or exacerbating fatigue.*
- Note changes in life (e.g., relationship problems, family illness, injury or death; expanded responsibilities or demands of others, job-related conflicts) that can be causing or exacerbating level of fatigue. *Stress may be the result of dealing with disease or situational crises, dealing with the "unknowns," or trying to meet expectations of others.*[2] *Also, grief and depression can sap energy and cause avoidance of social and/or physical interactions that could stimulate the mind and body. Note: Persons with AIDS and the elderly are especially prone to this fatigue because they experience significant losses, often on a regular or recurring basis.*[3,4]
- Assess sleep pattern—hours and quality of sleep. *Sleep disturbance is both a contributor to and a manifestation of fatigue (e.g., a client with chronic pain or depression may be sleeping long periods but not experience refreshing sleep or may not be able to fall or stay asleep).*
- Determine ability to participate in activities and level of mobility. *While many illness conditions negatively affect client's energy and activity tolerance, if the client is not engaged in light to moderate exercise, he or she may simply adjust to more sedentary activities, which can in turn exacerbate deconditioning and debilitation. However, there are certain conditions (e.g., MS, postpolio syndrome) where the client's ability to do things diminishes as he or she does them (e.g., at the beginning of a walk the client feels okay, but fatigue sets in [out of proportion to the activity] and the client is exhausted as if running a marathon).*[5,6]
- Review medication regimen and use. *Many medications have the potential side effect of causing/exacerbating fatigue (e.g., beta blockers, chemotherapy agents, narcotics, sedatives, muscle relaxants, antiemetics, antidepressants, antileptics, diuretics, cholesterol-lowering drugs, HIV treatment agents, combinations of drugs and/or substances).*

- Assess psychological and personality factors that may affect reports of fatigue level. *Client with severe or chronic fatigue may have issues affecting desire to be active (or work), resulting in over- or underactivity or concerns of secondary gain from exaggerated fatigue reports.*
- Evaluate aspect of "learned helplessness" that may be manifested by giving up. *Can perpetuate a cycle of fatigue, impaired functioning, and increased anxiety and fatigue.*

NURSING PRIORITY NO. 2   To determine degree of fatigue/impact on life:

- Ask client to describe fatigue, noting particular phrases (e.g., drained, exhausted, lousy, weak, lazy, worn out, whole-body tiredness). *Helpful in clarifying client's expressions for symptoms and pattern and timing of fatigue, which varies over time and may also vary in duration, unpleasantness, and intensity from person to person.*[7]
- Have client rate fatigue (using 0 to 10 or a similar scale) and describe its effects on ability to participate in desired activities. *Fatigue may vary in intensity and is often accompanied by irritability, lack of concentration, difficulty making decisions, problems with leisure, and relationship difficulties that can add to stress level and aggravate sleep problems.*[11]
- Assess severity of fatigue using a recognized scale (e.g., Chalder Fatigue Scale, Functional Assessment of Cancer Therapy Fatigue, Multidimensional Assessment of Fatigue, Piper Fatigue Self-Report Scale, Global Fatigue Index), as appropriate. *In initial evaluations, these scales can help determine manifestation, intensity, duration, and emotional meaning of fatigue. The scales can be used in ongoing evaluations to determine current status and estimate response to treatment strategies.*[2,7–9,12]
- Measure blood pressure and heart and respiratory rate before and after activity as indicated. *Physiological response to activity (e.g., changes in blood pressure or heart or respiratory rate) may indicate need for interventions to improve cardiovascular health, pulmonary status, and conditioning.* (Refer to risk for Activity Intolerance for additional interventions.)
- Review availability and current use of assistance with daily activities, support systems, and resources.
- Evaluate need for individual assistance or assistive devices. *Certain conditions causing fatigue (e.g., postpolio syndrome) worsen with overuse of weakened muscles. Client may benefit from support and protection provided by braces, canes, power chairs, etc.*[6,7]

NURSING PRIORITY NO. 3   To assist client to cope with fatigue and manage with individual limitations:

- Accept reality of client's fatigue and avoid underestimating effect on quality of life the client experiences. *Fatigue is subjective and often debilitating (e.g., clients with cancer, AIDS, or MS are prone to more frequent episodes of severe fatigue following minimal energy expenditure and require longer recovery period; postpolio clients often display a cumulative effect if they fail to pace themselves and rest when early signs of fatigue are encountered).*[5,7]
- Active-listen concerns and encourage expression of feelings. *Provides support to help client deal with very frustrating and taxing situation.*
- Treat underlying conditions where possible (e.g., manage pain, depression, or anemia; treat infections; reduce numbers of interacting medications) *to reduce fatigue caused by treatable conditions.*
- Involve client/significant others (SOs)/caregivers(s) in planning care *to incorporate their input, choices, and assistance.*
- Encourage client to do whatever activity possible (e.g., self-care, sit up in chair, walk for 5 minutes), pacing self and increasing activity level gradually. Schedule activities for periods when client has the most energy, *to maximize participation.*
- Structure daily routines and establish realistic activity goals with client, especially when depression is a factor in fatigue. *May enhance client's commitment to efforts and promote sense of self-esteem in accomplishing goals.*
- Instruct client/caregivers in alternate ways of doing familiar activities and methods to conserve energy, such as the following:[2,3,7–9]

 Acute Care   Collaborative   Community/Home Care   Cultural

Sit instead of stand during daily care or other activities.

Adjust the level or height of work surface for ergonomic benefit and to prevent bending over.

Carry several small loads instead of one large load.

Use assistive devices (e.g., wheeled walkers or chairs, power lift recliner chairs, stair-climbers).

Plan steps of activity before beginning so that all needed materials are at hand.

Take frequent short rest breaks and return to activity.

Delegate tasks or duties whenever possible.

Combine and simplify activities.

Ask for and accept assistance.

Say "no" or "later."

- Provide environment conducive to relief of fatigue and avoid temperature and humidity extremes. *Temperature and level of humidity are known to affect exhaustion (especially in clients with MS).*[5]
- Encourage nutritional foods; refer to a dietitian as indicated. *Nutritionally balanced diet with proteins, complex carbohydrates, vitamins, and minerals may boost energy. Frequent, small meals and simple-to-digest foods are beneficial when combating fatigue. Reduced amounts of caffeine and sugar can improve sleep and energy.*[3,7]
- Provide supplemental oxygen as needed. *If fatigue is related to oxygenation/perfusion problems, oxygen may improve energy level and ability to be active.* (Refer to ND Activity Intolerance for additional interventions.)
- Provide diversional activities (e.g., visiting with friends/family, TV/music, doing hobbies or schoolwork). *Participating in pleasurable activities can refocus energy and diminish feelings of unhappiness, sluggishness, and worthlessness, which can accompany fatigue.* (Refer to ND decreased Diversional Activity Engagement for additional interventions.)
- Avoid over/understimulation (cognitive and sensory). *Impaired concentration can limit ability to block competing stimuli and distractions.*
- Assist client/SOs to implement measures to preserve energy over longer periods of time. *Even though the client may continue to experience fatigue, his/her energy level could benefit from such things as (1) planning and organizing work tasks (e.g., delegating, combining activities, simplifying details; spending energy on important/desired tasks); (2) balancing periods of rest and work and resting before fatigue sets in; (3) pacing self and reducing sudden or prolonged strains; (4) limiting work that increases muscle tension and using good body mechanics; and (5) modifying effects of the environment such as temperature extremes and eliminating smoke and harmful fumes.*[2]
- Recommend or implement routines that promote restful sleep, such as the following:

Regular sleep hours at night with beneficial nighttime rituals

Short naps during day hours

A mild, graded exercise program to include strengthening and stretching movements such as yoga or tai chi

Quiet activities in the evening

Meditation and/or visualization

Warm baths

Refer to NDs Insomnia and Sleep Deprivation for additional interventions.
- Instruct in or refer for stress-management skills of visualization, deep breathing, relaxation, and biofeedback *to deal with situation, aid in relaxation, and to reduce boredom, pain, and sense of fatigue.*
- Participate in comprehensive rehabilitation program with physical or occupational therapist and/or an exercise or rehabilitation physiologist. *Collaborative program with short-term achievable goals enhances likelihood of success and may motivate client to adopt a lifestyle for enhancement of health.*[2,7,8]
- Discuss alternative therapies (e.g., massage, acupuncture, osteopathic or chiropractic manipulations), if appropriate. *Complementary therapies may be helpful in reducing muscle tension and pain to promote relaxation and rest.*

 Diagnostic Studies   Evidence Based Practice   Medications   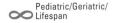 Pediatric/Geriatric/Lifespan

NURSING PRIORITY NO. 4 To promote wellness (Teaching/Discharge Considerations):

- Discuss therapy regimen relating to individual causative factors (e.g., physical and/or psychological illnesses) and help client/SO(s) to understand relationship of fatigue to illness. *Promotes acceptance of situation, allowing client to focus attention on finding ways to live with fatigue.*
- Assist client/SO(s) to develop plan for activity and exercise within individual ability. *Enhances sense of control and commitment to attaining goals.*
- Emphasize necessity of allowing sufficient time to finish activities. *Client is more likely to succeed when he or she does not feel rushed and is allowed to proceed at a measured pace.*
- Instruct client in ways to monitor response to activity and significant signs/symptoms to heed. *Changes in pulse or respiratory rate or development of worsened or unrelenting fatigue is a signal to stop, rest, and then resume activity, possibly modified in some aspect, that will allow the client to proceed.*
- Promote overall health measures (e.g., good nutrition [to include reduced levels of saturated and trans fats, cholesterol, salt and added sugars], adequate fluid intake, appropriate vitamin and iron supplementation).
- Encourage client to develop assertiveness skills and prioritize goals and activities.
- Discuss burnout syndrome when appropriate and actions client can take to change individual situation.
- Assist client to identify appropriate coping behaviors. *Promotes sense of control and improves self-esteem.*
- Identify support groups and resources (e.g., condition-specific groups, reliable Web sites) *to provide information, share experiences, and enhance problem-solving.*
- Refer to community resources for assistance with routine needs (e.g., Meals on Wheels, homemaker or housekeeper services, yard care, transportation options).
- Refer to counseling or psychotherapy as indicated *to deal with stressors and effects of condition.*

DOCUMENTATION FOCUS

Assessment/Reassessment
- Manifestations of fatigue and other assessment findings.
- Degree of impairment and effect on lifestyle.
- Expectations of client/SO relative to individual abilities and specific condition.

Planning
- Plan of care, specific interventions, and who is involved in the planning.
- Teaching plan.

Implementation/Evaluation
- Client's response to interventions, teaching, and actions performed.
- Attainment or progress toward desired outcome(s).
- Modifications to plan of care.

Discharge Planning
- Discharge needs and who is responsible for actions to be taken.
- Specific referrals made.

References

1. Cunha, B. A. (Updated 2017). Chronic fatigue syndrome (CFS). Retrieved March 2018 from http://emedicine.medscape.com/article/235980-overview.
2. Ratini, M. (Reviewed 2017). Cancer-related fatigue. WebMD. Retrieved March 2018 from http://www.webmd.com/cancer/cancer-related-fatigue.
3. Zimmerman, J. (2002). Nutrition for health and healing in HIV. *AIDS Community Research Initiative of America (ACRIA).* Retrieved March 2018 from www.thebody.com/content/art14418.html.
4. Ackley, B. J. (2010). Fatigue. In Ackley, B. J., Ladwig, G. B. (eds). *Nursing Diagnosis Handbook: An Evidence-Based Guide to Planning Care.* 9th ed. St. Louis, MO: Mosby.
5. Lava, N. (Reviewed 2016). Multiple sclerosis fatigue: Causes and treatment. Retrieved March 2018 from http://www.webmd.com/multiple-sclerosis/guide/ms-related-fatigue.
6. National Institute of Neurological Disorders and Stroke. (Updated 2017). Post-polio syndrome fact sheet. Retrieved March 2018 from http://www.ninds.nih.gov/disorders/post_polio/detail_post_polio.htm.

 Acute Care   Collaborative   Community/Home Care   Cultural

7. Keeney, C. E., Head, B. A. (2011). Palliative nursing care of the patient with cancer-related fatigue. *J Hosp Palliat Nurs*, 13(5), 270–278.

8. Veterans Health Administration, Department of Defense. (Last update 2014). Clinical practice guidelines for the management of medically unexplained symptoms: Chronic pain and fatigue. Retrieved March 2018 from https://innovations.ahrq.gov/qualitytools/department-veterans-affairsdepartment-defense-vadod-clinical-practice-guideline-3.

9. Nauert, R. (2016). Chronic fatigue syndrome can hit kids & teens. Retrieved March 2018 from https://psychcentral.com/news/2016/01/26/chronic-fatigue-syndrome-can-hit-kids-teens/98206.html.

10. ter Wolbeek, M., et al. (2006). Severe fatigue in adolescents: A common phenomenon? *Pediatrics*, 117(6), e1078–e1086.

11. Barton-Burke, M. (2006). Cancer-related fatigue and sleep disturbances: Further research on the prevalence of these two symptoms in long-term cancer survivors can inform education, policy, and clinical practice. *Am J Nurs*, 106(3 Suppl), 72–77.

12. Trendall, J. (2005). Concept analysis: Chronic fatigue. *J Adv Nurs*, 32(5), 1126–1131.

Fear [Specify focus]

Taxonomy II: Coping/Stress Tolerance—Class 2 Coping Responses (00148) [**Diagnostic Division:** Ego Integrity], Approved 1980; Revised 1996, 2000, 2017

DEFINITION: Response to perceived threat that is consciously recognized as a danger.

RELATED FACTORS

Language barrier
Learned response [e.g., conditioning, modeling from others]
Response to phobic stimulus
Separation from support system
Unfamiliar setting

DEFINING CHARACTERISTICS

Subjective

Apprehensiveness; excitedness; decrease in self-assurance; increase in tension; nausea
Feelings of alarm, dread, fear, panic, terror
Cognitive: Identifies object of fear; stimulus believed to be a threat
Physiological: Anorexia; fatigue; dry mouth; dyspnea; [palpitations]

Objective

Vomiting; muscle tension; fidgeting; pallor; pupil dilation
Cognitive: Decrease in productivity, learning ability, or problem-solving ability
Behaviors: Increase in alertness; avoidance [or flight] behaviors; attack behaviors; impulsiveness; focus narrowed to the source of fear
Physiological: Diarrhea; increase in perspiration; change in physiological response [e.g., blood pressure, heart rate, respiratory rate, oxygen saturation and end-tidal CO_2]
Associated Condition: Sensory deficit
Sample Clinical Applications: Phobias, hospitalization/diagnostic procedures, diagnosis of chronic or life-threatening condition

DESIRED OUTCOMES/EVALUATION CRITERIA

Sample NOC linkages:
Fear Self-Control: Personal actions to eliminate or reduce disabling feelings of apprehension, tension, or uneasiness from an identifiable source

(continues on page 330)

 Diagnostic Studies
 Evidence Based Practice
 Medications
 Pediatric/Geriatric/Lifespan

Fear [Specify focus] (continued)

Coping: Personal actions to manage stressors that tax an individual's resources

Fear Level: Severity of manifested apprehension, tension, or uneasiness arising from an identifiable source

Client Will (Include Specific Time Frame)

- Acknowledge and discuss fears, recognizing healthy versus unhealthy fears.
- Verbalize accurate knowledge of and sense of safety related to current situation.
- Demonstrate understanding through use of effective coping behaviors (e.g., problem solving) and resources.
- Display lessened fear as evidenced by appropriate range of feelings and relief of signs/symptoms (specific to client).

ACTIONS/INTERVENTIONS

Sample NIC linkages:

Anxiety Reduction: Minimizing apprehension, dread, foreboding, or uneasiness related to an unidentified source or anticipated danger

Coping Enhancement: Facilitation of cognitive and behavioral efforts to manage perceived stressors, changes, or threats that interfere with meeting life demands and roles

NURSING PRIORITY NO. 1 To assess degree of fear and reality of threat perceived by the client:

- Ascertain client's/significant other's (SO's) perception of what is occurring and how this affects life. *Fear is a natural reaction to frightening events, and how client views the event will determine how he or she will react. Fear differs from anxiety in that it is usually unanticipated, is dependent on the termination of the feared object/subject, is often intense, and occurs in self-limiting episodes. Health fears may not be the "fight or flight" type, and may present more like dread and anxiety.*[1,3,9]
- ∞ Determine client's age and developmental level. *Helps in understanding usual or typical fears experienced by individuals (e.g., toddler has entirely different fears than adolescent or older person with dementia being removed from home/usual living situation).*[3,11]
- Note ability to concentrate, level of attention, and degree of incapacitation (e.g., "frozen with fear," inability to engage in necessary activities). *Indicative of extent of anxiety or fear related to what is happening and need for specific interventions to reduce physiological reactions. Presence of severe reaction (panic or phobias) requires more intensive intervention.*[1,4,10]
- Compare verbal and nonverbal responses. *Noting congruencies or incongruencies can help to identify client's misperceptions of situation and what actions may be helpful. Client may be able to verbalize what he/she is afraid of, if asked, providing opportunity to address actual fears.*[1,3]
- Be alert to signs of denial or depression. *Client may deny existence of problem until overwhelmed and unable to deal with situation. Depression may be associated with fear that interferes with productive life and daily activities.*[2]
- Identify sensory deficits that may be present, such as vision or hearing impairment. *Affects reception and interpretation. Inability to correctly sense and perceive stimuli leads to misunderstanding, increasing fear.*[4]
- 📝 Measure vital signs and note physiological responses to situation. *Provides baseline information of extent of response for comparison as needed. Stabilization can indicate effectiveness of interventions by diminished response to identified fear. Note: Fear and acute anxiety can both involve sympathetic arousal (e.g., increased heart rate, respirations, and blood pressure, hyperalertness, antidiuresis, dilation of skeletal blood vessels, constriction of gut blood vessels, and a surge of catecholamine release). These responses can be blunted (e.g., heart rate may not be increased if client is taking certain beta-blocking medications) and should subside as the fear state is reduced.*[6,10]

 Acute Care   Collaborative   Community/ Home Care   Cultural

- Investigate client's reports of subjective experiences (may reflect delusions or hallucinations). *It is important to understand how the client views the situation and identify need for reality orientation and further evaluation.*[4]
- Be alert to and evaluate potential for violence. *Client who is fearful may feel need to protect himself or herself and strike out at closest person. Proactive planning can avert or manage violent behaviors.*[5]
- Assess family dynamics. *Actions and responses of family members may exacerbate or soothe fears of client; conversely, if the client is immersed in illness, whether from crisis or fear, it can take a toll on the family/ involved others.*[1,11] (Refer to NDs Anxiety, readiness for enhanced family Coping, compromised/disabled family Coping, and interrupted Family Processes for additional interventions.)

NURSING PRIORITY NO. 2   To assist client/SOs in dealing with fear/situation:

- Stay with the very fearful client or make arrangements to have someone else be there. *Provides nonthreatening environment in which the presence of a calm, caring person can provide reassurance that individual will be safe. Sense of abandonment can exacerbate fear.*[6]
- Active-listen client concerns. *Conveys message of belief in competence and ability of client. Promotes understanding of issues when client feels listened to so that problem-solving can begin.*[2]
- Acknowledge normalcy of fear, pain, and despair and give "permission" to express feelings appropriately and freely. *Feelings are real, and it is helpful to bring them out in the open so they can be discussed and dealt with.*[6]
- Present objective information when available and allow client to use it freely. Avoid arguing about client's perceptions of the situation. *Limits conflicts when fear response may impair rational thinking.*[6]
- Speak in simple sentences and concrete terms and include written materials as appropriate. *Intense state of fear interferes with reception and interpretation of verbal information; supplementing it with written information facilitates understanding and retention of information.*[4]
- Provide opportunity for questions, answering honestly. *Enhances sense of trust and promotes positive nurse-client relationship in which individual can verbalize fears and begin to problem-solve.*[1]
- ∞ Manage environmental factors, such as loud noises, harsh lighting, changing person's location without knowledge of family/SO, strangers in care area or unfamiliar people, and high traffic flow, *which can cause or exacerbate stress, especially to very young or to older individuals.*
- ∞ Be truthful with client when painful procedures are anticipated; be present and provide physical contact (e.g., hugging, refocusing attention, rocking a child) as appropriate, *to soothe fears and provide assurance.*
- Modify procedures as possible (e.g., substitute oral for intramuscular medications, combine blood draws or use finger-stick method) *to limit degree of stress and avoid overwhelming a fearful individual.*[3]
- Promote client control where possible and help client identify and accept those things over which control is not possible. *Life changes and stressful events are viewed differently by each individual. Providing the client with opportunity to make own decision when possible strengthens internal locus of control. Individual with external locus of control may attribute feelings of anxiety and fear to an external source and may perceive it as beyond his or her control.*[1]
- 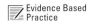 Provide touch, Therapeutic Touch, massage, and other adjunctive therapies as indicated. *Aids in meeting basic human need, decreasing sense of isolation, and assisting client to feel less anxious. Note: Therapeutic touch requires the nurse to have specific knowledge and experience to use the hands to correct energy field disturbances by redirecting human energies to help or heal.*[2,7]
- Encourage contact with a peer who has successfully dealt with a similarly fearful situation. *Provides a role model, which can enhance sense of optimism. Client is more likely to believe others who have had similar experience(s).*[1]

NURSING PRIORITY NO. 3   To assist client in learning to use own responses for problem-solving:

- Acknowledge usefulness of fear for taking care of self. *Provides new idea that can be a motivator to focus on dealing appropriately with situation.*[1]

 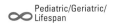

- Explain relationship between disease and symptoms if appropriate. *Providing accurate information promotes understanding of why the symptoms occur, allaying anxiety about them.*[1]
- Identify client's responsibility for the solutions while reinforcing that the nurse will be available for help if desired or needed. *Enhances client's sense of control, self-worth, and confidence in own ability, diminishing fear.*[8]
- Determine internal and external resources for assistance (e.g., awareness and use of effective coping skills in the past; SOs who are available for support). *Provides opportunity to recognize and build on resources client/ SO may have used successfully in the past.*[1]
- Explain actions and procedures within level of client's ability to understand and handle, being aware of how much information client wants *to prevent confusion or overload. Complex and/or anxiety-producing information can be given in manageable amounts over an extended period as opportunities arise and facts are given; individual will accept what he or she is ready for.*[8]
- 💊 Discuss use of anti-anxiety medications and reinforce use as prescribed. *Anti-anxiety agents may be useful for brief periods to assist client to reduce fearful feelings to manageable levels, providing opportunity for initiation of client's own coping skills.*[1]

NURSING PRIORITY NO. 4 To promote wellness (Teaching/Discharge Considerations):

- 🏠 Support planning for dealing with reality. *Assists in identifying areas in which control can be exercised and those in which control is not possible, enabling client to handle fearful situation or feelings.*[1]
- Assist client to learn relaxation, visualization, or guided imagery skills (e.g., imagining a pleasant place, use of music or tapes, deep breathing, meditation, mindfulness). *Promotes release of endorphins and aids in developing internal locus of control, reducing fear and anxious feelings. May enhance coping skills, allowing body to go about its work of healing. Note: Mindfulness is a method of being in the here and now, concentrating on what is happening in the moment.*[7,8]
- 🔵 Encourage regular physical activity. Assist client or refer to physical therapist to develop exercise program within limits of ability. *Provides a healthy outlet for energy generated by feelings and promotes relaxation. Has been shown to raise endorphin levels to enhance sense of well-being.*[2]
- Provide for and deal with sensory deficits in appropriate manner (e.g., speak clearly and distinctly, use touch carefully as indicated by situation). *Hearing or visual impairments and other deficits can contribute to feelings of fear. Recognizing and providing for appropriate contact can enhance communication, promoting understanding.*[4]
- 🔵 Refer to pastoral care, mental healthcare providers, support groups, and community agencies and organizations as indicated. *Provides information, ongoing assistance to meet individual needs, and opportunity for discussing concerns and obtaining further care when indicated.*[2]

DOCUMENTATION FOCUS

Assessment/Reassessment
- Assessment findings, noting individual factors contributing to current situation, and source of fear.
- Manifestations of fear and impact on life and ability to function.

Planning
- Plan of care and who is involved in the planning.
- Teaching plan.

Implementation/Evaluation
- Client's responses to treatment plan, interventions, and actions performed.
- Attainment or progress toward desired outcome(s).
- Modifications to plan of care.

Discharge Planning
- Long-term needs and who is responsible for actions to be taken.
- Specific referrals made.

 Acute Care   Collaborative   Community/ Home Care   Cultural

References

1. Townsend, M. C. (2011). *Psychiatric Mental Health Nursing: Concepts of Care in Evidence-Based Practice*. 7th ed. Philadelphia: F. A. Davis.
2. Doenges, M. E., Moorhouse, M. F., Murr, A. C. (2010). *Nurse's Pocket Guide: Diagnoses, Interventions, and Rationales*. 12th ed. Philadelphia: F. A. Davis.
3. Chang, L. (2005). When health fears are overblown. Retrieved March 2018 from http://www.webmd.com/balance/features/when-health-fears-are-overblown.
4. Newfield, S. A., et al. (2007). *Cox's Clinical Applications of Nursing Diagnosis: Adult, Child, Women's, Psychiatric, Gerontic, and Home Health Considerations*. 5th ed. Philadelphia: F. A. Davis.
5. Lewis, M. I., Dehn, D. S. (1999). Violence against nurses in outpatient mental health settings. *J Psychosoc Nurs*, 37(6), 28.
6. Bay, E. J., Algase, D. L. (1999). Fear and anxiety. A simultaneous concept analysis. *Nurs Diagn*, 10, 103.
7. Olson, M., Sneed, N. (1995). Anxiety and therapeutic touch. *Issues Ment Health Nurs*, 16(2), 97.
8. Kabat-Zinn, J. (1994). *Wherever You Go There You Are, Mindfulness Meditation in Everyday Life*. New York: Hyperion.
9. Kidd, M. (2007). What do patients fear most? Retrieved March 2018 from http://www.medscape.com/view/article/561455.
10. Craig, K. J., Brown, K. J., Baum, A. (2002). Environmental factors in the etiology of anxiety. *In Neuropsychopharmacology: The Fifth Generation of Progress*. Philadelphia: Lippincott, Williams and Wilkins.
11. Hughes, M. (2011). Chronic illness and self-identity. Retrieved March 2018 from https://www.academia.edu/10018819/Chronic_Illness_and_Self-Identity.

ineffective infant Feeding Pattern

Taxonomy II: Nutrition—Class 1 Ingestion (00107) **[Diagnostic Division:** Food/Fluid], Submitted 1992; Revised 2006; 2017

DEFINITION: Impaired ability of an infant to suck or coordinate the suck/swallow response resulting in inadequate oral nutrition for metabolic needs.

RELATED FACTORS
Oral hypersensitivity
Prolonged nil per os (NPO) status

DEFINING CHARACTERISTICS

Subjective
[Caregiver reports infant unable to achieve effective suck.]

Objective
Inability to initiate or sustain an effective suck
Inability to coordinate sucking, swallowing, and breathing
At Risk Population: Prematurity
Associated Condition: Neurological delay or impairment; oral hypersensitivity
Sample Clinical Applications: Prematurity, cleft lip/palate, thrush, hydrocephalus, cerebral palsy, fetal alcohol syndrome, respiratory distress, severe developmental delay

DESIRED OUTCOMES/EVALUATION CRITERIA

Sample NOC linkages:
Swallowing Status: Oral Phase: Preparation, containment, and posterior movement of fluids and/or solids in the mouth
Breastfeeding Establishment: Infant: Infant attachment to and sucking from the mother's breast for nourishment during the first 3 weeks of breastfeeding
Hydration: Adequate water in the intracellular and extracellular compartments of the body

(continues on page 334)

 Diagnostic Studies   Evidence Based Practice   Medications   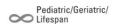 Pediatric/Geriatric/Lifespan

ineffective infant Feeding Pattern (continued)

Infant Will (Include Specific Time Frame)
• Display adequate output as measured by sufficient number of wet diapers daily.
• Demonstrate appropriate weight gain.
• Be free of aspiration.

ACTIONS/INTERVENTIONS

Sample NIC linkages:
Swallowing Therapy: Facilitating swallowing and preventing complications of impaired swallowing
Lactation Counseling: Assisting in the establishment and maintenance of successful breastfeeding
Bottle Feeding: Preparation and administration of fluids to an infant via a bottle

NURSING PRIORITY NO. 1 To identify contributing factors/degree of impaired function:

• Assess infant's suck, swallow, and gag reflexes. *Provides comparative baseline and is useful in determining appropriate feeding method.*
• Note developmental age, structural abnormalities (e.g., cleft lip/palate), mechanical barriers (e.g., endotracheal tube, ventilator). *These factors (infant maturity and structural/mechanical barriers to infant feeding) help to determine plan of care.*[1,2,4,6] *Note: Human milk decreases infections in preterm infants, both during hospitalization and after discharge. Human milk is the feeding of choice.*
• Determine level of consciousness, neurological impairment, seizure activity, and presence of pain. *Provides baseline information and identifies areas of special need.*[1,2]
• Observe parent/infant interactions *to determine level of bonding and comfort that could impact stress level during feeding activity.*
• Note type and scheduling of medications. *May cause sedative effect or otherwise impair feeding activity.*[2]
• Compare birth and current weight and length measurements. *Monitors effectiveness of infant feeding technique.*[1,2,4]
• Assess signs of stress when feeding (e.g., tachypnea, cyanosis, fatigue, lethargy). *Detects areas of increased need for alternate feeding methods and/or rest periods.*[1]
• Note presence of behaviors indicating continued hunger after feeding. *Determines if infant is receiving adequate amount during feeding.*[2,4]

NURSING PRIORITY NO. 2 To promote adequate infant intake:

• Determine appropriate method for feeding (e.g., special nipple or feeding device, gavage or enteral tube feeding) and choice of breast milk or formula to meet infant needs. *Individualizes care and maintains infant health status.*[1]
• Review early infant feeding cues (e.g., rooting, lip smacking, sucking fingers or hand) versus late cue of crying with parents/caregivers. *Early recognition of infant hunger promotes timely and more rewarding feeding experience for infant and mother.*[5]
• Demonstrate techniques or procedures for feeding. Note proper positioning of infant, "latching-on" techniques, rate of delivery of feeding, and frequency of burping. (Refer to ND ineffective Breastfeeding as appropriate.) *Models appropriate feeding methods and increases parental knowledge base and confidence.*[2–4]
• Limit duration of feeding to maximum of 30 minutes based on infant's response (e.g., signs of fatigue) *to balance energy expenditure with nutrient intake.*
• Monitor caregiver's efforts. Provide feedback and assistance as indicated. *Enhances learning and encourages continuation of efforts.*[2,3]

 Acute Care   Collaborative   Community/ Home Care   Cultural

- 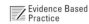 Refer mother to lactation specialist for assistance and support in dealing with unresolved issues (e.g., teaching infant to suck or a decrease in the mother's milk supply). *Provides resource for future needs and problem solving. Begins pattern of resource utilization.*[2–4]
- Emphasize importance of calm/relaxed environment during feeding *to reduce detrimental stimuli and enhance mother/infant's focus on feeding activity.*
- Adjust frequency and amount of feeding according to infant's response. *Prevents infant's frustration associated with under/overfeeding.*
- Advance diet, adding solids or thickening agent as appropriate for age and infant needs. *Provides for infant's nutritional and health needs.*[2,4]
- Alternate feeding techniques (e.g., nipple and gavage) according to infant's ability and level of fatigue. *Individualizes plan of care to enhance successful feeding.*[1]
- Alter medication or feeding schedules as indicated to minimize sedative effects. *Altered states of function and consciousness interfere with feeding and may lead to choking or aspirating.*[1]

NURSING PRIORITY NO. 3   To promote well-being (Teaching/Discharge Considerations):

- Encourage kangaroo care, placing infant skin-to-skin upright, tummy down, on mother's or father's chest. *Skin-to-skin care increases bonding and may promote stable heart rate, temperature, and respiration in infant.*[7]
- Instruct caregiver in techniques to prevent or alleviate aspiration. *Helps parent/caregiver feel more confident and promotes infant safety.*[1,4]
- Discuss anticipated growth and development goals for infant, as well as corresponding caloric needs. *Accommodating infant maturity and development helps to individualize and update plan of care.*[1,2,5]
- Suggest recording infant's weight and nutrient intake periodically. *Monitors effectiveness of infant feeding technique by providing measurable data. Provides positive reinforcement to implementation of plan of care.*[1,2,4]
- 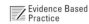 Recommend participation in classes as indicated (e.g., first aid, infant cardiopulmonary resuscitation). *Increases knowledge base for infant safety and caregiver confidence.*[2–4]
- 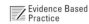 Refer to support groups (e.g., La Leche League, parenting support groups, stress reduction, other community resources as indicated).
- Provide bibliotherapy including appropriate Web sites for further information.

DOCUMENTATION FOCUS

Assessment/Reassessment
- Type and route of feeding, interferences to feeding and reactions.
- Infant's measurements.

Planning
- Plan of care, specific interventions, and who is involved in planning.
- Teaching plan.

Implementation/Evaluation
- Infant's response to interventions (e.g., amount of intake and output, weight gain, response to feeding) and actions performed.
- Caregiver's involvement in infant care, participation in activities, and response to teaching.
- Attainment or progress toward desired outcome(s).
- Modifications to plan of care.

Discharge Planning
- Long-term needs, referrals made, and who is responsible for follow-up actions.

 Diagnostic Studies   Evidence Based Practice   Medications 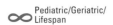 Pediatric/Geriatric/Lifespan

References

1. Creasy, R., et al. (2008). *Maternal-Fetal Medicine: Principles and Practice*. 6th ed. Philadelphia: W. B. Saunders.
2. London, M., et al. (2010). *Maternal & Child Nursing Care*. 3rd ed. Upper Saddle River, NJ: Prentice Hall.
3. Ladewig, P., et al. (2009). *Contemporary Maternal-Newborn Nursing Care*. 7th ed. Upper Saddle River, NJ: Prentice Hall.
4. Lowdermilk, D. (2011). *Maternity and Women's Health Care*. 10th ed. St. Louis, MO: Mosby.
5. American Academy of Family Physicians. (2001, some addendums updated 2014). Breastfeeding (Position paper). Retrieved March 2018 from www.aafp.org/online/en/home/policy/policies/b/breastfeedingpositionpaper.html.
6. Wright, N., Morton, J., Kim, J. (2008). *Best Medicine: Human Milk in the NICU*. Amarillo, TX: Hale.
7. Bergman, J. (2011). The importance of skin-to-skin contact for every newborn. *Breastfeeding Today*, (6), 4–6.

risk for Female Genital Mutilation

Taxonomy II: Safety/Protection—Class 3 Violence (00272) [**Diagnostic Division:** Safety], Approved 2017

DEFINITION: Susceptible to full or partial ablation of the female external genitalia and other lesions of the genitalia, whether for cultural, religious, or any other non-therapeutic reasons, which may compromise health

RISK FACTORS
Lack of family knowledge about impact on physical, reproductive, psychosocial health
At Risk Population: Female gender
Residing in country where practice is accepted; family leaders belong to ethnic group in which practice is accepted
Belonging to family in which any female member has been subjected to practice
Belonging to ethnic group in which practice accepted; favorable attitude of family toward practice
Sample Clinical Applications: Pre/postnatal care, labor and delivery, newborn/well baby care, urinary tract infection (UTI), pelvic inflammatory disease (PID), infertility

DESIRED OUTCOMES/EVALUATION CRITERIA

Sample NOC linkages:
Community Risk Control: Unhealthy Cultural Traditions: Community actions to promote customs, beliefs values, and laws that support member's health and lifestyle modifications within the culture
Health Seeking Behavior: Personal actions to promote wellness, recovery, and rehabilitation
Decision-Making: Ability to make judgements and choose between two or more alternatives

Family/Client Will (Include Specific Time Frame)
• Verbalize understanding of impact of the practice on the health of the child/woman.
• Demonstrate willingness to learn more about the impact of the practice by engaging in conversation with healthcare provider.
• Review information sources about the effect on physical and psychosocial health of the woman.
• Make the decision not to engage in this practice.

Community Will (Include Specific Time Frame)
• Develop resources to eliminate the practice of female genital mutilation.

ACTIONS/INTERVENTIONS

Sample NIC linkages:
Cultural Brokerage: The deliberate use of culturally competent strategies to bridge or mediate between the patient's culture and the biomedical healthcare system
Decision-Making Support: Providing information and support for a patient who is making a decision regarding healthcare

 Acute Care   Collaborative   Community/ Home Care   Cultural

NURSING PRIORITY NO. 1 To assess knowledge and beliefs of family/client and cultural/ethnic group:

- 📝 Note country of origin of family/client. *Although the practice of female genital mutilation (FGM) has declined in some countries, and is banned in a number of others, some type of procedure routinely continues in various regions of Africa and the Middle East.*[3]
- 🌐 Identify cultural/ethnic beliefs of family/client. *FGM has been practiced for over three centuries and may be associated with strong social pressure to continue the practice to conform to tradition, for group identity, marriageability, and right of inheritance.*[2,3]
- Determine how client views the practice. *Often women who grow up in a culture that practices FGM view the procedure as "normal," believing it characterizes womanhood and needs to be done, thereby negatively impacting motivation for change and making it harder to give up custom.*[1]
- Ascertain family/client past experiences with practice including health consequences. *Oftentimes, procedure is performed between first week of life and 8 years of age. Some practices are performed before puberty or at widowhood, and reinfibulation (resuturing after delivery or gynecological procedures of the incised scar tissue resulting from infibulation) may be performed after childbirth. Based on personal experiences, family may have limited understanding of associated risks.*[2]
- 🌐 Determine prevalence of custom in community and use of nonmedical providers to perform procedure.*Community may or may not support the custom, and nonmedically prepared providers may be utilized, increasing the risk of serious complications/death. This provides insight into needs of the community.*

NURSING PRIORITY NO. 2 To assist family/client to make informed decision/modify cultural practices:

- Establish rapport with family/client using their terminology in nonjudgmental manner. *Some women do not view procedure as mutilation, referring to it as "cutting" or "circumcision." Condemning the practice may drive individual(s) away, leading to negative outcome.*[2]
- Provide information about the types of procedures performed in different areas/countries as appropriate. *There are various forms, such as symbolic pricking/piercing or scraping, cutting or removing part or all of the clitoris, or removing the labia minora and majora and suturing the edges closed with only a small hole remaining for urine and menstrual blood to pass (infibulation).*[2,3]
- Discuss complications that can occur, especially with nonmedical practitioners. *Poor surgical skills of most practitioners, absence of anesthesia, and unsterile conditions can result in poor quality of life and even death of the woman. The most common initial complications are bleeding, urine retention, genital tissue swelling, severe pain. Midterm risks include pelvic inflammatory disease (PID), vaginal and urinary tract infections; and long-term problems such as dyspareunia (painful sexual intercourse) and infertility can occur. Adverse obstetric outcomes such as postpartum hemorrhage, stillbirth, and cesarean section are not uncommon. Psychologically, these individuals have higher rates of anxiety disorder and posttraumatic stress response.*[3]
- Provide detailed information in multiple modes, e.g., pamphlets, models, videos, computer programs in individual's primary language. Obtain interpreter as indicated. *Information necessary to make informed decision may be better understood in family/client's primary language.*[1]
- 📝 Include father/husband in educational sessions. *Studies suggest that men who have been educated regarding consequences are less likely to support the practice while those who have not been educated tend to deny reality of physical and obstetrical risks.*[1]
- 🔄 Refer to community services if available for assistance with decision-making. *Support groups and/or counseling can provide individual with accurate information, reliable medical care, psychological support.*
- 📝 Support client once she has made informed decision. If choice is to proceed, encourage a less invasive or symbolic procedure. *In the United States, an individual 18 years of age or older has a legal right to freedom of choice for self, but opting for a less radical procedure can reduce risks and enhance well-being.*[1,3]

 Diagnostic Studies   Evidence Based Practice   Medications   ∞ Pediatric/Geriatric/Lifespan

- ☺ Refer to competent medical providers who perform genital surgery, as indicated. *If client desires some form of procedure, clinicians who are familiar with the medical sequelae and ramifications of female circumcision will be better able to treat these women knowledgeably and with dignity, while helping them to make a decision not to have the procedure done. Note: Some argue FGM is a violation of human rights and against the physician's oath "to do no harm." However, by default, this may drive client to nonmedical providers or to visit country of origin for procedure.*[2,3]

NURSING PRIORITY NO. 3   To reduce the incidence of female genital mutilation:

- ▨ Promote the eradication of this practice. *The World Health Organization has declared FGM illegal and the United Nations calls for its elimination by 2030.*[1]
- Determine additional factors that influence this social change. *Beyond family attitudes, economic benefits to providers, who are often not medically trained but charge substantial fees, cause them to be reluctant to terminate the practice.*[2]
- Encourage religious/community leaders to advocate against practice. *These individuals are generally well respected and influential within their communities.*[1]
- ☺ Develop community-based educational programs addressing concepts of sexuality, marriage practices, legal rights, and federal laws. *Necessary to shift community attitudes supporting practice. Note: In some countries, such as the United States and Canada, the procedure cannot be performed on minors below the age of 18. In a number of other countries, it is totally illegal, with repercussions for the individual performing the procedure, the client, and on occasion anyone aware of and failing to report that the procedure was performed.*[3]
- Educate lawmakers of health and well-being consequences of procedure. *Encourages creation of laws banning practice and allocation of financial resources supporting programs at community level.*
- ☺ Assist in developing emergency care resources and referrals to midwives, gynecologist/obstetrician for pregnant women who have had FGM. *Increases opportunity for a successful delivery of a healthy baby and minimizing injury to the woman. Provides opportunity to discuss reconstructive procedure or at least refraining from reinfibulation.*[3]

DOCUMENTATION FOCUS

Assessment/Reassessment
- Assessment findings, including attitudes/expectations of family/client.
- Religious and cultural/ethnic factors.
- Family/client past experience with practice.
- Community prevalence of custom and providers.
- Available community resources.

Planning
- Plan of care and who is involved in planning.
- Teaching plan.
- Formulation of community action plan.

Implementation/Evaluation
- Client's/family's responses to interventions, teaching, and actions performed.
- Attainment or progress to desire outcomes.
- Client's/family's decision.
- Community's commitment to change.

Discharge Planning
- Long-term plans, and who is responsible for actions to be taken.
- Specific referrals made.

 Acute Care   Collaborative   Community/ Home Care   Cultural

References

1. Odukogbe, A.-T.A., et al. (2017). Female genital mutilation/cutting in Africa. *Transl Androl Urol*, 6(2), 138–148.
2. Horowitz, C. R., Jackson, J. C. (1997). Female circumcision: African women confront American medicine. *J Gen Intern Med*, 12(8), 491–499.
3. Koski, A., Heymann, J. (2017). Thirty-year trends in the prevalence and severity of female genital mutilation: A comparison of 22 countries. *BMJ Glob Health*, 2(4). Retrieved June 2018 from http://gh.bmj.com/content/2/4/e000467.

[deficient hyper/hypotonic Fluid Volume]

DEFINITION: [Decreased intravascular, interstitial, and/or intracellular fluid. This refers to dehydration with changes in sodium.]

[**NOTE:** NANDA has restricted deficient Fluid Volume to address only isotonic dehydration. For client needs related to dehydration associated with alterations in sodium, the authors have provided this second diagnostic label.]

RELATED FACTORS

[Hypertonic dehydration: uncontrolled diabetes mellitus or insipidus, hyperosmolar hyperglycemic syndrome (HHS), increased intake of hypertonic fluids or IV therapy, inability to respond to thirst reflex, inadequate free water supplementation (high-osmolarity enteral feeding formulas), renal insufficiency or failure]

[Hypotonic dehydration: chronic illness, malnutrition, excessive use of hypotonic IV solutions (e.g., D5W), renal insufficiency]

DEFINING CHARACTERISTICS

Subjective

[Reports of fatigue, nervousness, exhaustion]

[Thirst]

Objective

[Increased urine output, dilute urine (initially), or decreased output, oliguria]

[Weight loss]

[Decreased venous filling; hypotension (postural)]

[Increased pulse rate; decreased pulse volume and pressure]

[Decreased skin turgor; dry skin and mucous membranes]

[Increased body temperature]

[Change in mental status (e.g., confusion)]

[Hemoconcentration; altered serum sodium]

Sample Clinical Applications: Diabetes mellitus, diabetic ketoacidosis, renal failure, conditions requiring IV therapy or enteral feeding, heat exhaustion or stroke, presence of draining wounds or fistulas

DESIRED OUTCOMES/EVALUATION CRITERIA

Sample NOC linkages:

Fluid Balance: Balance of the input and output of fluids in the body

Hydration: Adequate water in the intracellular and extracellular compartments of the body

(continues on page 340)

 Diagnostic Studies   Evidence Based Practice   Medications   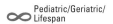 Pediatric/Geriatric/Lifespan

[deficient hyper/hypotonic Fluid Volume] (continued)

Electrolyte and Acid/Base Balance: Balance of electrolytes and nonelectrolytes in the intracellular and extracellular compartments of the body

Client Will (Include Specific Time Frame)

- Maintain fluid volume at a functional level as evidenced by individually adequate urinary output, stable vital signs, moist mucous membranes, and good skin turgor.
- Verbalize understanding of causative factors and purpose of individual therapeutic interventions and medications.
- Demonstrate behaviors to monitor and correct deficit as indicated when condition is chronic.

ACTIONS/INTERVENTIONS

Sample NIC linkages:

Fluid/Electrolyte Management: Regulation and prevention of complications from altered fluid and/or electrolyte levels

Hypovolemia Management: Expansion of intravascular fluid volume in a patient who is volume depleted

Fluid Monitoring: Collection and analysis of patient data to regulate fluid balance

NURSING PRIORITY NO. 1 To assess causative/precipitating factors:

- Note possible medical diagnoses or disease processes *that may lead to fluid deficits: (1) fluid loss (e.g., indwelling tubes, diarrhea, vomiting, fever, excessive sweating, diabetic ketoacidosis; burns, other draining wounds; gastrointestinal obstruction; use of diuretics); (2) limited intake (e.g., extremes of age, limited mobility, client dependent on others for eating and drinking; lack of knowledge related to fluid intake; heat exhaustion or stroke); (3) fluid shifts (e.g., ascites, effusions, burns, sepsis); or (4) environmental factors (e.g., isolation, restraints, very high ambient temperatures, malfunctioning air conditioning).*[5,14,15]
- ∞ Determine effects of age and gender. Obtain weight and measure subcutaneous fat and muscle mass *to ascertain total body water, which is approximately 60% of adult's weight and 75% of infant's weight. Very young and extremely elderly individuals are quickly affected by a fluid volume deficit and are least able to express need. For example, elderly people often have a decreased thirst reflex and/or may not be aware of water needs. Infants/young children and other nonverbal persons cannot describe thirst.*[1,2,15,16] *Worldwide, dehydration (secondary to diarrheal illness) is the leading cause of infant and child mortality.*[3,8]
- Evaluate nutritional status, noting current intake, weight changes, problems with oral intake, and use of supplements/tube feedings. *Factors that can negatively affect fluid intake (e.g., impaired mentation, nausea, wired jaws, immobility, insufficient time for meals, lack of finances restricting availability of food).*
- 🩺 Collaborate with physician to identify or characterize the nature of fluid and electrolyte imbalance(s). *Dehydration is often categorized according to serum sodium concentration. More than one cause may exist at a given time (e.g., increased loss of salt and water caused by diuretics that leads to decreased fluid intake as a result of lethargy and confusion).*[5,9,10]
- Be aware of the difference between signs of **hypovolemia** (e.g., poor skin turgor, dizziness on standing, lethargy, delayed capillary refill, sunken eyeballs, fever, weight loss, little or no urine output) and signs of **dehydration** (e.g., lethargy, weakness, irritability, nausea, vomiting, hyperreflexia, potentially progressing to coma), *which are symptoms of the effect of elevated sodium (hypernatremia) on the central nervous system. Note: Dehydration is not always accompanied by hypovolemia, but it is almost always hypernatremic.*[8,10]
- 💊 Review client's medications, including prescription and over-the-counter drugs, herbals, and nutritional supplements, *to identify medications that can alter fluid and electrolyte balance. These may include diuretics, vasodilators, beta blockers, aldosterone inhibitors, angiotensin-converting enzyme (ACE) inhibitors, and*

 Acute Care   Collaborative   Community/Home Care   Cultural

medications that can cause syndrome of inappropriate secretion of antidiuretic hormone (e.g., phenothiazides, vasopressin, some antineoplastic drugs).[12]

NURSING PRIORITY NO. 2   To evaluate degree of fluid deficit:

* Obtain history of usual pattern of fluid intake and recent alterations. *Intake may be reduced because of current physical or environmental issues (e.g., swallowing problems, vomiting, severe heat wave with inadequate fluid replacement) or a behavior pattern (e.g., elderly person refuses to drink water trying to control incontinence).*
* ✚ Assess vital signs, including temperature (often elevated), pulse (elevated), respirations, and blood pressure (may be low). Measure blood pressure (lying, sitting, standing) *to evaluate orthostatic blood pressure* and monitor invasive hemodynamic parameters as indicated (e.g., central venous pressure) *to determine degree of intravascular deficit and replacement needs.*[7,8]
* Note change in usual mentation, behavior, and functional abilities (e.g., confusion, falling, loss of ability to carry out usual activities, lethargy, dizziness). *These signs indicate either sufficient hypovolemia to impair cerebral perfusion or sufficient dehydration to impair cerebral function.*[9,10]
* ✚ Observe and measure urinary output hourly or for 24 hours as indicated. Note color *(may be dark because of concentration)* and specific gravity *(high number associated with dehydration with usual range being 1.010 to 1.025).*[4]
* Estimate or measure other fluid losses (e.g., gastric, respiratory, and wound losses) *to more accurately determine fluid replacement needs.*
* ✏️📝 Review laboratory data (e.g., hemoglobin/hematocrit; osmolality, electrolytes [sodium, potassium, chloride, bicarbonate]; blood urea nitrogen, creatinine) *to evaluate body's response to fluid loss and to determine replacement needs. Note: The dehydrated client is not always hypovolemic. An abnormal sodium level is a key marker for salt and water imbalance. For example, in* **hypertonic** *dehydration, blood tests may reveal osmolality greater than 300 mOsm/kg and sodium greater than 150 meq/L. The hypernatremia is the* **result** *of dehydration.* **Hypotonic** *dehydration may reveal osmolality less than 250 mOsm/kg and sodium less than 130 meq/L. Hyponatremia is the* **result** *of replacing water without sodium.*[4,11,17]

NURSING PRIORITY NO. 3   To correct/replace fluid losses to reverse pathophysiological mechanisms:

* ⊘ Assist with treatment of underlying conditions causing or contributing to dehydration and electrolyte imbalances (e.g., change antibiotics causing diarrhea; treat fever or infection, malnutrition, or severe depression; discontinue medications contributing to dehydration).
* ⊘📝 Administer fluids and electrolytes as indicated. *Fluid used for replacement depends on the (1) type of dehydration present and (2) degree of deficit determined by age, weight, and type of trauma or condition causing the fluid deficit. Multiple fluid resuscitation formulas (e.g., Parkland, Evans, Brooke, Slater, Monafo burn formulas) exist with variations in both the volumes per weight suggested and the type or types of crystalloid or crystalloid-colloid combinations.*[2,6,9]
* ⊘📝 Establish 24-hr replacement schedule and routes to be used (e.g., IV, PO, tube feeding). *Entire fluid replacement may be done by IV or tube feeding if client is NPO, acutely ill, or severely dehydrated. However, if client is to be rehydrated orally, fluid replacement may be calculated to replace certain amount with meals (e.g., 75% to 80%) with the remainder offered during nonmeal times. Managing oral rehydration in this manner can replace fluids without resorting to IV therapy. These interventions should also be in place to prevent dehydration.*[2,3,5,6,8]
* Spread fluid intake throughout the day *to prevent periods of uncomfortable thirst and to promote client's ability and interest in ingesting fluids.*
* ⊘ Encourage increased intake of water and other fluids based on individual needs (up to 2.5 L/day or amount determined by physician for client's age, weight, and condition).
* Provide a variety of fluids in small frequent offerings, attempting to incorporate client's preferred beverage and temperature (e.g., iced or hot) *to enhance cooperation with regimen.*

 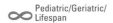

- ∞ Suggest intake of foods with a high water content (e.g., popsicles, gelatin, soup, eggnog, watermelon) and/or electrolyte replacement drinks (e.g., Gatorade, Pedialyte) as appropriate. *Variety may stimulate intake.*
- Limit intake of alcohol and caffeinated beverages that tend to exert a diuretic effect.
- Engage client, family, and all caregivers in fluid management plan. *Everyone is responsible for the prevention or treatment of dehydration and should be involved in the planning and provision of adequate fluid on a daily basis.*
- Provide nutritionally balanced diet and/or enteral feedings (avoiding use of hyperosmolar or excessively high-protein formulas) and provide adequate amount of free water with feedings.
- Maintain accurate intake and output (I&O), calculate 24-hr fluid balance, and weigh regularly (daily, in unstable client) *in order to monitor and document trends. Note: A 1-pound weight loss reflects fluid loss of about 500 mL in an adult.*[7]

NURSING PRIORITY NO. 4   To promote comfort and safety:

- Change position frequently. Bathe infrequently, using mild cleanser or soap, and provide optimal skin care with suitable emollients *to maintain skin integrity and prevent excessive dryness caused by dehydration.*
- Provide frequent oral care and eye protection *to prevent injury from dryness.* Refer to NDs impaired oral Mucous Membrane Integrity, risk for Dry Mouth, and risk for Dry Eye for related interventions.
- Provide for safety measures when client is confused. (Refer to NDs acute Confusion and chronic Confusion for additional interventions.)
- Adjust or discontinue medications (e.g., diuretics, laxatives, steroids, psychotropics, ACE inhibitors) *that may be contributing to dehydration.*[2,5]
- Observe for sudden or marked elevation of blood pressure, restlessness, moist cough, dyspnea, basilar crackles, and frothy sputum. *Too rapid a correction of fluid deficit may compromise the cardiopulmonary system, causing fluid overload and edema, especially if colloids are used in initial fluid resuscitation.*

NURSING PRIORITY NO. 5   To promote wellness (Teaching/Discharge Considerations):

- Discuss factors related to occurrence of deficit as individually appropriate. *Early identification of risk factors can decrease occurrence and severity of complications associated with hypovolemia.*[7]
- Recommend drinking more water when exercising or engaging in physical exertion or during hot weather. Suggest carrying a water bottle when away from home as appropriate.
- Identify and instruct in ways to meet specific fluid and nutritional needs.
- ∞ Offer fluids on a regular basis to infants, young children, and the elderly, *who may not sense/or be able to report thirst.*
- ∞ Instruct client/SO(s) in how to monitor color of urine *(dark urine equates with concentration and dehydration)* and/or how to measure and record I&O *(may include weighing or counting diapers in infant/toddler)* as indicated.
- Review and instruct in medication regimen and administration. Emphasize need for reporting suspected drug interactions/side effects to healthcare provider. *Facilitates timely intervention to prevent or reduce complications.*
- Instruct in signs and symptoms indicating need for emergent or further evaluation and follow-up.

DOCUMENTATION FOCUS

Assessment/Reassessment
- Individual findings, including factors affecting ability to manage (regulate) body fluids and degree of deficit.
- I&O, fluid balance, changes in weight, urine-specific gravity, and vital signs.
- Results of diagnostic studies or laboratory tests.

Planning
- Plan of care and who is involved in the planning.
- Teaching plan.

 Acute Care   Collaborative   Community/Home Care   Cultural

Implementation/Evaluation
* Client's responses to treatment, teaching, and actions performed.
* Attainment or progress toward desired outcome(s).
* Modifications to plan of care.

Discharge Planning
* Long-term needs, noting who is responsible for actions to be taken.
* Specific referrals made.

References

1. Newfield, S. A., et al. (2007). *Cox's Clinical Applications of Nursing Diagnosis: Adult, Child, Women's, Psychiatric, Gerontic, and Home Health Considerations*. 5th ed. Philadelphia: F. A. Davis.
2. Mentes, J. C. (2012). Managing oral hydration. In Boltz, M., Capezuti, E., Fulmer, T. (eds). *Evidence-Based Practice Guideline Hydration Management*. 4th ed. New York: Springer.
3. Huang, L. H., et al. (Updated 2017). Dehydration. Retrieved March 2018 from http://emedicine.medscape.com/article/906999-overview.
4. Van Leeuwen, A. M., Bladh, M. L. (2015). *Davis's Comprehensive Handbook of Laboratory Diagnostic Tests With Nursing Implications*. 6th ed. Philadelphia: F. A. Davis.
5. Robles-Surarez, J., et al. (2012). Hydration status of long term care residents rehospitalized within 30 days of hospital discharge. Retrieved March 2018 from http://www.jnursinghomeresearch.com/406-hydration-status-of-long-term-care-residents-rehospitalized-within-30-days-of-hospital-discharge.html.
6. Oliver, R. I. (2017). Burn resuscitation and early management. Retrieved March 2018 from http://emedicine.medscape.com/article/1277360-overview.
7. Matheny, N. (2010). *Fluid and Electrolyte Balance: Nursing Considerations*. 5th ed. Sudbury, MA: Jones & Bartlett.
8. Mayo Clinic Staff. (Updated 2018). Dehydration. Retrieved March 2018 from http://www.mayoclinic.org/diseases-conditions/dehydration/basics/definition/con-20030056.
9. Astle, S. M. (2005). Restoring electrolyte balance. *RN*, 68(5), 34–39.
10. ASCO Cancer.net. (2016). Dehydration. Retrieved March 2018 from https://www.cancer.net/navigating-cancer-care/side-effects/dehydration.
11. Holley, J. L. (2006). Hypovolemia and dehydration in the oncology patient—A viewpoint of salt and water imbalance. *J Support Oncol*, (4), 455–456.
12. Wotton, K., Crannitch, K., Munt, R. (2008). Prevalence, risk factors and strategies to prevent dehydration in older adults. *Contemp Nurs*, 31(1), 44–56.
13. Mentes, J., Claros, E. (2006). Oral hydration in older adults. *Am J Nurs*, 106(6), 40–49.
14. Mentes, J. (2006). A typology of oral hydration problems exhibited by frail nursing home residents. *J Gerontol Nurs*, 23(1), 13–21.
15. Scholler, D. A. (1989). Changes in total body water with age. *Am J Clin Nutr*, 50(5 Suppl), 1176–1181.
16. Faes, M. C., Spigt, M. G., Rikkert, O. (2007). Dehydration in geriatrics. *Geriatrics and Aging*, 10(9), 590–596.
17. Modric, J. (2013). Dehydration types: Pathophysiology, lab tests and values. Retrieved March 2018 from http://www.ehealthstar.com/dehydration/types-pathophysiology.

deficient [isotonic] Fluid Volume

Taxonomy II: Nutrition—Class 5 Hydration (00027) **[Diagnostic Division:** Food/Fluid], Submitted 1978; Revised 1996; 2017

DEFINITION: Decreased intravascular, interstitial, and/or intracellular fluid. This refers to dehydration, water loss alone without change in sodium.
[NOTE: This diagnosis has been structured to address isotonic dehydration (hypovolemia) when fluids and electrolytes are lost in even amounts and excluding states in which changes in sodium occur. For client needs related to dehydration associated with alterations in sodium, refer to deficient Fluid Volume: hyper/hypotonic.]

RELATED FACTORS
Barrier to accessing fluid; insufficient fluid intake; insufficient knowledge about fluid needs

(continues on page 344)

 Diagnostic Studies　 Evidence Based Practice　 Medications　 Pediatric/Geriatric/Lifespan

deficient [isotonic] Fluid Volume (continued)

DEFINING CHARACTERISTICS

Subjective
Thirst
Weakness

Objective
Alteration in mental status
Alteration in skin or tongue turgor; dry skin and mucous membranes
Decrease in blood pressure; decrease in pulse pressure and pulse volume; decrease in venous filling
Decrease in urine output
Increase in body temperature and heart rate
Increase in hematocrit and urine concentration
Sudden weight loss
At Risk Population: Extremes of age; extremes of weight; factors influencing fluid needs
Associated Condition: Active fluid volume loss: [e.g., hemorrhage; gastric intubation; acute or prolonged diarrhea; wounds; fistulas; ascites; use of hyperosmotic radiopaque contrast agent]
Compromised regulatory mechanism [e.g., fever, thermoregulatory response; renal tubule damage]
Deviations affecting fluid intake or absorption
Excessive fluid loss through normal or abnormal route
Pharmaceutical agent
Sample Clinical Applications: Traumatic injury, hemorrhage, gastroenteritis (with vomiting and diarrhea), malnutrition, uncontrolled diabetes mellitus, severe burns

DESIRED OUTCOMES/EVALUATION CRITERIA

Sample NOC linkages:
Hydration: Adequate water in the intracellular and extracellular compartments of the body
Fluid Balance: Balance of the input and output of fluids in the body
Blood Loss Severity: Severity of signs and symptoms of internal or external bleeding

Client Will (Include Specific Time Frame)
- Maintain fluid volume at a functional level as evidenced by individually adequate urinary output with normal specific gravity, stable vital signs, moist mucous membranes, good skin turgor, prompt capillary refill, and be free of edema.
- Verbalize understanding of causative factors and purpose of individual therapeutic interventions and medications.
- Demonstrate behaviors to monitor and correct deficit, as indicated.

ACTIONS/INTERVENTIONS

Sample NIC linkages:
Fluid/Electrolyte Management: Regulation and prevention of complications from altered fluid and/or electrolyte levels
Hypovolemia Management: Expansion of intracellular fluid volume in a patient who is volume depleted
Shock Prevention: Detecting and treating a patient at risk for impending shock

 Acute Care
 Collaborative
 Community/ Home Care
 Cultural

NURSING PRIORITY NO. 1   To assess causative/precipitating factors:

- Identify relevant diagnoses *that may create a fluid volume depletion (e.g., decreased intravascular plasma volume, such as might occur with rapid blood loss or hemorrhage from trauma; vascular, pregnancy complications, gastrointestinal bleeding disorders); significant fluid (other than blood) loss such as might occur with severe gastroenteritis with vomiting and diarrhea; or extensive burns.*[1,4,12]
- Note presence of other factors (e.g., laryngectomy or tracheostomy tubes, drainage from wounds and fistulas or suction devices; water deprivation or fluid restrictions; decreased level of consciousness; dialysis; hot/humid climate, prolonged exercise; increased metabolic rate secondary to fever; increased caffeine or alcohol) *that may contribute to lack of fluid intake or loss of fluid by various routes.*
- Prepare for and assist with diagnostic evaluations (e.g., imaging studies, x-rays) *to locate source of bleeding or cause for hypovolemia.*
- 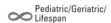 Determine effects of age, gender, weight, subcutaneous fat and muscle mass (influences total body water [TBW], which is approximately 60% of an adult's weight and 75% of an infant's weight).[11] *In general, men have higher TBW than women due to women's higher percentage of body fat and less muscle mass than men, and the elderly's TBW is less than that of a youth. Elderly individuals are often at risk for dehydration because of decreased thirst reflex, impaired renal conservation of water, increased prevalence of chronic conditions, and polypharmacy.*[2,3,8,9] *Infants/young children and other nonverbal persons cannot describe thirst. Worldwide, dehydration (secondary to diarrheal illness) is the leading cause of infant and child mortality.*[4]

NURSING PRIORITY NO. 2   To evaluate degree of fluid deficit:

- 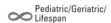 Estimate or measure traumatic or procedural fluid losses. Note possible routes of insensible fluid losses. Determine customary and current weight. *These factors are used to determine degree of volume depletion and method of fluid replacement. In burn injuries, the body surface area method states that dehydration is related to deficit of TBW and assumes that loss of weight is loss of water.*[11]
- Assess vital signs, including temperature (often elevated), pulse and respirations (elevated), and blood pressure (may be low). Measure blood pressure (lying/sitting/standing) if appropriate *to evaluate orthostatic blood pressure* and monitor invasive hemodynamic parameters as indicated (e.g., central venous pressure [CVP]) *to determine degree of intravascular deficit and replacement needs.*[1,6,7]
- Note presence of dry mucous membranes, poor skin turgor, delayed capillary refill, flat neck veins, and reports of thirst or weakness, child crying without tears, sunken eyeballs (or fontanel in infant), fever, weight loss, and little or no urine output. *Assessment signs of dehydration that client/significant other (SO) may notice. In an acute, life-threatening hemorrhage state, cold, pale, moist skin may be noted reflecting body compensatory mechanisms to profound hypovolemia.*[1,6,7]
- Note change in usual mentation, behavior, and functional abilities (e.g., confusion, falling, loss of ability to carry out usual activities, lethargy, dizziness). *These signs indicate sufficient dehydration to cause poor cerebral perfusion or can reflect the effects of electrolyte imbalance. In hypovolemic shock state, mentation changes rapidly and client may present in coma.*
- Observe/measure urinary output (hourly/24-hr totals). Note color *(may be dark greenish brown because of concentration)* and specific gravity *(high number associated with dehydration with usual range being 1.010 to 1.025).*[3,5]
- Review laboratory data (e.g., hemoglobin/hematocrit, prothrombin time, activated partial thromboplastin time; electrolytes [sodium, potassium, chloride, bicarbonate] and glucose; blood urea nitrogen, creatinine) *to evaluate body's response to bleeding/other fluid loss and to determine replacement needs.*[5] *Note: In isotonic dehydration, electrolyte levels may be lower, but concentration ratios remain near normal.*[3]

NURSING PRIORITY NO. 3   To correct/replace losses to reverse pathophysiological mechanisms:

- 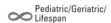 Control blood loss (e.g., gastric lavage with room temperature or cool saline solution, drug administration, prepare for surgical intervention).

 Diagnostic Studies   Evidence Based Practice   Medications   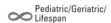 Pediatric/Geriatric/Lifespan

- 🥄 Stop fluid loss (e.g., administer medication to stop vomiting/diarrhea, reduce fever).[1]
- 💊📋 Administer fluids and electrolytes (e.g., blood, isotonic sodium chloride solution, lactated Ringer's solution, albumin, fresh frozen plasma, dextran, hetastarch). *Whether crystalloids (e.g., normal saline) or colloids (e.g., albumin) are best for fluid resuscitation continues to be a matter of discussion. A 2010 large-scale review of studies regarding effects of commonly used resuscitation fluids over the past 50 years supported the conclusion that rapid resuscitation with large-volume crystalloid is deleterious and supported slower, goal-directed resuscitation with low-volume crystalloid.*[1,7,10]
- 🥄 Establish and continually reevaluate 24-hr fluid replacement needs and routes to be used *to prevent peaks and valleys in fluid level and to prevent fluid overload.*[6]
- Control humidity and ambient air temperature as appropriate, especially when major burns are present or in the presence of fever, *to reduce insensible losses.*[12]
- Reduce bedding or clothes and provide a tepid sponge bath.
- 🥄 Assist with hypothermia therapy as indicated *to decrease severe fever and elevated metabolic rate.* (Refer to ND Hyperthermia for additional interventions.)
- Maintain accurate intake and output (I&O) and weigh daily. Measure urine-specific gravity. Monitor blood pressure and invasive hemodynamic parameters as indicated (e.g., CVP) *to evaluate effectiveness of resuscitation measures.*

NURSING PRIORITY NO. 4   To promote comfort and safety:

- Change position frequently. Bathe infrequently, using mild cleanser or soap, and provide optimal skin care with emollients *to maintain skin integrity and prevent excessive dryness caused by dehydration.*
- Provide frequent oral care and eye care *to prevent injury from dryness.*
- Change dressings as needed and use adjunct appliances as indicated for draining wounds *to protect skin and to monitor losses for replacement needs.*
- 🥄 Administer medications (e.g., antiemetics, antidiarrheals *to limit gastric or intestinal losses;* antipyretics *to reduce fever*). (Refer to NDs Diarrhea and Hyperthermia for additional interventions.)
- ➕ Observe for sudden or marked elevation of blood pressure, restlessness, moist cough, dyspnea, basilar crackles, and frothy sputum. *Too rapid a correction of fluid deficit may compromise the cardiopulmonary system, causing fluid overload and edema, especially if colloids are used in initial fluid resuscitation.*

NURSING PRIORITY NO. 5   To promote wellness (Teaching/Discharge Considerations):

- 🏠∞ Discuss factors related to occurrence of fluid deficit as individually appropriate (e.g., reason for hemorrhage, potential for dehydration in children with fever or diarrhea, inadequate fluid replacement when performing strenuous work or exercise, living in hot climate, improper use of diuretics) *to reduce risk of recurrence.*
- ∞ Identify actions (if any) client may take to prevent or correct deficiencies. *Carrying a water bottle when away from home aids in maintaining fluid volume. A client who never takes more than a few sips at a time, even of preferred beverage, may benefit most from being offered frequent small amounts of fluid throughout the day. A client with dementia, on the other hand—one who is able to drink but just forgets—may benefit most from social situations and activities where beverages are served. In cases of mild to moderate dehydration, use of oral solutions (e.g., Gatorade, Rehydralyte), soft drinks, breast milk/formula, or Pedialyte can provide adequate rehydration.*[113]
- Instruct client/SO(s) in how to monitor color of urine (dark urine equates with concentration and dehydration) or how to measure and record I&O (may include weighing or counting diapers in infant/toddler).
- 🥄 Review medications and interactions and side effects, especially medications that can cause or exacerbate fluid loss (e.g., diuretics, laxatives) and those indicated to prevent fluid loss (e.g., antidiarrheals, anticoagulants).[6]

 Acute Care   Collaborative   Community/ Home Care   Cultural

• Discuss signs/symptoms indicating need for emergent or further evaluation and follow-up. *Promotes timely intervention.*

DOCUMENTATION FOCUS

Assessment/Reassessment
• Assessment findings, including degree of deficit and current sources of fluid intake.
• I&O, fluid balance, changes in weight or edema, urine-specific gravity, and vital signs.
• Results of diagnostic studies.

Planning
• Plan of care and who is involved in planning.
• Teaching plan.

Implementation/Evaluation
• Client's responses to interventions, teaching, and actions performed.
• Attainment or progress toward desired outcome(s).
• Modifications to plan of care.

Discharge Planning
• Long-term needs, plan for correction, and who is responsible for actions to be taken.
• Specific referrals made.

References

1. Kolecki, P., Meckhoff, C. R. (Updated 2016). *Hypovolemic shock*. Retrieved March 2018 from http://emedicine.medscape.com/article/760145-overview.
2. Newfield, S. A., et al. (2007). *Cox's Clinical Applications of Nursing Diagnosis: Adult, Child, Women's, Psychiatric, Gerontic, and Home Health Considerations*. 5th ed. Philadelphia: F. A. Davis.
3. Mentes, J. C. (2012). Managing oral hydration. In Boltz, M., Capezuti, E., Fulmer, T. (eds). *Evidence-Based Practice Guideline Hydration Management*. 4th ed. New York: Springer.
4. Huang, L. H., et al. (Updated 2017). *Dehydration*. Retrieved March 2018 from http://emedicine.medscape.com/article/906999-overview.
5. Van Leeuwen, A. M., Bladh, M. L. (2015). *Davis' Comprehensive Handbook of Laboratory & Diagnostic Tests With Nursing Implications*. 6th ed. Philadelphia: F. A. Davis.
6. Mayo Clinic Staff. (Updated 2018). Dehydration. Retrieved March 2018 from http://www.mayoclinic.org/diseases-conditions/dehydration/basics/definition/con-20030056.
7. Diel-Oplinger, L., Kaminski, M. F. (2004). Choosing the right fluid to counter hypovolemic shock. *Nursing*, 34(3), 52–54.
8. Mentes, J., Claros, E. (2006). Oral hydration in older adults. *AJN*, 106(6), 40–49.
9. Collins, M., Claros, E. (2011). Recognizing the face of dehydration. *Nursing*, 41(8), 26–31.
10. Santry, H. P., Alam, H. B. (2014). Fluid resuscitation: Past, present, and the future. *Shock*, 33(3), 229–241.
11. Sterns, R. H. (Updated 2017). General principles of disorders of water balance (hyponatremia and hypernatremia) and sodium balance (hypovolemia and edema). Retrieved March 2018 from paid Web site at http://www.uptodate.com/contents/general-principles-of-disorders-of-water-balance-hyponatremia-and-hypernatremia-and-sodium-balance-hypovolemia-and-edema6.
12. Oliver, R. I. (Updated 2017). Burn resuscitation and early management. Retrieved March 2018 from http://emedicine.medscape.com/article/1277360-overview#aw2aab6b6.
13. Kilgore, C. (2010). Dehydration isn't simple to diagnose or treat. *Caring for the Ages*, 11(2), 6–7.

excess Fluid Volume

Taxonomy II: Nutrition—Class 5 Hydration (00026) [**Diagnostic Division:** Food/Fluid], Approved 1982; Revised 1996, 2013, 2017

DEFINITION: Surplus intake and/or retention of fluid.

RELATED FACTORS
Excessive fluid intake
Excessive sodium intake

DEFINING CHARACTERISTICS

Subjective
Anxiety
Orthopnea; paroxysmal nocturnal dyspnea

Objective
Alteration in respiratory pattern; adventitious breath sounds; dyspnea
Alteration in blood pressure
Alteration in mental status; restlessness
Intake exceeds output; oliguria
Edema; anasarca; weight gain over short period of time
Jugular vein distention; positive hepatojugular reflex; hepatomegaly
Pulmonary congestion; pleural effusion
Presence of S_3 heart sound
Alteration in pulmonary artery pressure (PAP); increase in central venous pressure (CVP)
Decrease in hemoglobin or hematocrit; azotemia; electrolyte imbalance; alteration in urine-specific gravity
Associated Condition: Compromised regulatory mechanism
Sample Clinical Applications: Congestive heart failure, renal failure, cirrhosis of liver, cancer, toxemia of pregnancy, conditions associated with SIADH (e.g., meningitis, encephalitis, Guillain-Barré syndrome), schizophrenia (where polydipsia is a prominent feature)

DESIRED OUTCOMES/EVALUATION CRITERIA

Sample NOC linkages:
Fluid Overload Severity: Severity of signs and symptoms of excess intracellular and extracellular fluids
Fluid Balance: Balance of the input and output of fluids in the body
Electrolyte and Acid/Base Balance: Balance of electrolytes and nonelectrolytes in the intracellular and extracellular compartments of the body

Client Will (Include Specific Time Frame)
• Stabilize fluid volume as evidenced by balanced intake and output (I&O), vital signs within client's normal limits, stable weight, and free of signs of edema.
• Verbalize understanding of individual dietary and fluid restrictions.
• Demonstrate behaviors to monitor fluid status and reduce recurrence of fluid excess.
• List signs that require further evaluation.

  Acute Care   Collaborative   Community/ Home Care   Cultural

---

ACTIONS/INTERVENTIONS

Sample **NIC** linkages:

Hypervolemia Management: Reduction in extracellular or intracellular fluid volume and prevention of complications in a patient who is fluid overloaded

Fluid/Electrolyte Management: Regulation and prevention of complications from altered fluid and/or electrolyte levels

Peritoneal Dialysis [or] Hemodialysis Therapy: Administration and monitoring of dialysis solution into and out of the peritoneal cavity/or management of extracorporeal passage of the patient's blood through a dialyzer

---

NURSING PRIORITY NO. 1   To assess causative/precipitating factors:

• Note presence of medical conditions or situations (e.g., heart failure, chronic kidney disease, renal or adrenal insufficiency, excessive or rapid infusion of IV fluids, cerebral lesions, psychogenic polydipsia, acute stress, anesthesia, surgical procedures, decreased or loss of serum proteins) *that can contribute to excess fluid intake or retention.*[1,2]

• ▨ Determine or estimate amount of fluid intake from all sources: oral, intravenous, enteral, or parenteral feedings, ventilator, etc. *Potential exists for fluid overload due to fluid shifts and changes in electrolyte balance. Note: Severely malnourished client can experience significant fluid shifts and electrolyte imbalances after nutritional support is initiated. This potentially lethal disorder, known as refeeding syndrome, usually is associated with parenteral nutrition, but it also can occur with enteral nutrition, oral intake, or dextrose-containing IV fluids.*[5,11]

• Review nutritional issues (e.g., intake of sodium, potassium, and protein). *Imbalances in these areas are associated with fluid imbalances.*[5]

NURSING PRIORITY NO. 2   To evaluate degree of excess:

• ▨ Compare current weight with admission or previously stated weight. Weigh daily or on a regular schedule, as indicated. *Provides a comparative baseline and evaluates the effectiveness of diuretic therapy when used (i.e., a roughly 1 kilogram [2.2 pounds] change in body weight equates to a 1-liter gain or loss in body fluid volume).*[7,12] *Note: Volume overload can occur over weeks to months in clients with unrecognized renal failure where lean muscle mass is lost and fluid overload occurs with relatively little change in weight.*[4]

• ✚ 🫀 Measure vital signs and invasive hemodynamic parameters (e.g., CVP, PAP/pulmonary capillary wedge pressure) if available for critically ill clients. *Pressures may be high because of excess fluid volume or be low if cardiac failure is occurring.*

• ✚ Note presence of tachycardia and irregular rhythms. Auscultate heart tones for S_3, ventricular gallop. *Signs suggestive of heart failure, which results in decreased cardiac output and tissue hypoxia.*

• Auscultate breath sounds for presence of crackles or congestion. Record occurrence of exertional breathlessness, dyspnea at rest, or paroxysmal nocturnal dyspnea. *Indication of pulmonary congestion and potential of developing pulmonary edema that can interfere with oxygen-carbon dioxide exchange at the capillary level.*[3]

• Note presence and location of edema (e.g., puffy eyelids, swelling ankles and feet if ambulatory or up in chair, sacrum and posterior thighs when recumbent). Determine whether lower extremity edema is new or increasing. *Heart failure and renal failure are associated with dependent edema because of hydrostatic pressures, with dependent edema being a defining characteristic for excess fluid. Generalized edema (e.g., upper extremities and eyelids) is associated with nephrotic syndrome.*[2]

• Assess for presence of neck vein distention/hepatojugular reflux with head of bed elevated 30 to 45 degrees. *Signs of increased intravascular volume.*[5]

• Measure abdominal girth *to evaluate changes that may indicate increasing fluid retention and edema.*[5]

 Diagnostic Studies   Evidence Based Practice   Medications   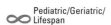 Pediatric/Geriatric/Lifespan

- Evaluate mentation for restlessness, anxiety, confusion, and personality changes. *Signs of decreased cerebral oxygenation (e.g., cerebral edema) or electrolyte imbalance.*[1,8]
- Assess appetite; note presence of nausea/vomiting *to determine the presence of problems associated with an imbalance of electrolytes (e.g., glucose, sodium, potassium, or calcium).* Assess neuromuscular reflexes.[8]
- Observe skin and mucous membranes. *Edematous tissues are prone to ischemia and breakdown or ulceration.*
- Review laboratory data (e.g., blood urea nitrogen/creatinine, hemoglobin/hematocrit, serum albumin, proteins, electrolytes; urine-specific gravity, osmolality, sodium excretion) and chest radiograph. *These tests may be repeated not only to ascertain baseline imbalances, but also to monitor response to therapy.*

NURSING PRIORITY NO. 3 To promote mobilization/elimination of excess fluid:

- Restrict fluid intake as indicated (especially when sodium retention is less than water retention or when fluid retention is related to renal failure).[5]
- Provide for sodium restrictions if needed (as might occur in sodium retention in excess of water retention). *Restricting sodium favors renal excretion of excess fluid and may be more useful than fluid restriction.*[1]
- Set an appropriate rate of fluid intake or infusion throughout 24-hr period. Maintain steady rate of all IV infusions *to prevent exacerbation of excess fluid volume and to prevent peaks and valleys in fluid level.*[5,9]
- Administer medications (e.g., diuretics, cardiotonics, plasma or albumin volume expanders) in order to improve cardiac output and kidney function, thereby *reducing congestion and edema if heart failure is the cause of fluid overload.*
- Evaluate edematous extremities *to enhance venous return and prevent further edema formation.*
- Place in semi-Fowler's position when at bedrest as appropriate. *May promote recumbency-induced diuresis and facilitate respiratory effort when movement of the diaphragm is limited/breathing is impaired because of lung congestion.*
- Prepare for and assist with procedures as indicated (e.g., peritoneal or hemodialysis, ultrafiltration; mechanical ventilation, cardiac resynchronization therapy). *May be done to correct volume overload and electrolyte and acid-base imbalances or to improve cardiac function and support individual during shock state.*[7,10]

NURSING PRIORITY NO. 4 To maintain integrity of skin and tissues:

- Refer to NDs impaired Oral Mucous Membrane Integrity, impaired or risk for impaired Skin/Tissue Integrity, and risk for Pressure Ulcer for related interventions.

NURSING PRIORITY NO. 5 To promote wellness (Teaching/Discharge Considerations):

- Consult dietitian as needed *to develop dietary plan and identify foods to be limited or omitted:*
  Review dietary restrictions and safe substitutes for salt (e.g., lemon juice or spices such as oregano).
  Discuss fluid restrictions and "hidden sources" of fluids (e.g., foods high in water content such as fruits, ice cream, sauces, custard). Use small drinking cup or glass.
  Avoid salty or spicy foods, as they increase thirst or fluid retention. Suck ice chips, hard candy, or slices of lemon *to help allay thirst.*
- Suggest chewing gum and use of lip balm *to reduce discomforts of fluid restrictions.*
- Instruct client/family in ways to keep track of intake. For example, use a marked water bottle or container; refill as needed.[5]
- Measure output, encourage use of voiding record when it is appropriate, or weigh daily and report gain of more than 2 lb/day (or as indicated by individual situation). *If weight is rising daily, fluid is likely being retained.*[5]

 Acute Care   Collaborative   Community/ Home Care   Cultural

- Review drug regimen and side effects of agents used to increase urine output or manage hypertension, kidney disease, or heart failure. *Many drugs have an impact on kidney function and fluid balance, especially in the elderly or those with cardiac and kidney impairments.*
- Emphasize need for mobility, frequent position changes, and early/ongoing ambulation *to prevent stasis and reduce risk of tissue injury.*
- Identify "danger" signs requiring notification of healthcare provider *to ensure timely evaluation and intervention.*[5]

DOCUMENTATION FOCUS

Assessment/Reassessment
- Assessment findings, noting existing conditions contributing to and degree of fluid retention (vital signs; amount, presence, and location of edema; weight changes).
- I&O, fluid balance.
- Results of laboratory tests and diagnostic studies.

Planning
- Plan of care and who is involved in the planning.
- Teaching plan.

Implementation/Evaluation
- Response to interventions, teaching, and actions performed.
- Attainment or progress toward desired outcome(s).
- Modifications to plan of care.

Discharge Planning
- Long-term needs, noting who is responsible for actions to be taken.

References

1. Harrison, T. R., Fauci, A. S. (eds). (1998). *Harrison's Principles of Internal Medicine*. 14th ed. New York: McGraw-Hill.
2. Holcomb, S. (2009). Topics in progressive care: Third-spacing: When body fluid shifts. *Nurs Crit Care*, 4(2), 9–12.
3. Matheny, N. (2010). *Fluid and Electrolyte Balance: Nursing Considerations*. 5th ed. Sudbury, MA: Jones & Bartlett Learning.
4. Veterans Health Administration, Department of Defense. (Updated 2011). VA/DoD clinical practice guideline for management of chronic kidney disease in primary care. Retrieved March 2018 from http://f.i-md.com/medinfo/material/ce3/4eb2 4e6444aeb6583cc40ce3/4eb24e9544aeb6583cc40ce6.pdf.
5. Mentes, J. C., Kang, S. (Updated 2011). Hydration management. Retrieved March 2018 from https://www.guidelinecentral.com/summaries/hydration-management/#section-405.
6. Doenges, M. E., Moorhouse, M. F., Murr, A. C. (2010). Fluid and electrolyte imbalances. *Nursing Care Plans: Guidelines for Individualizing Client Care Across the Life Span*. 8th ed. Philadelphia: F. A. Davis.
7. Riggs, J. M. (2006). Manage heart failure. *Nurs Crit Care*, 1(4), 18–28.
8. Astle, S. M. (2005). Restoring electrolyte balance. *RN*, 68(5), 31–34.
9. Crawford, A., Harris, H. (2011). I.V. fluids: What nurses need to know. *Nursing*, 41(5), 30–38.
10. Streets, A., Vickers, S. M. (2012). Is this patient with heart failure a candidate for ultrafiltration? *Nursing*, 43(6), 30–36.
11. McCray, S., Walker, S., Parrish, C. R. (2005). Much ado about refeeding. *Pract Gastroenterol*, 30(1), 26–44.
12. Davies, H., Leslie, G., Morgan, D. (2015). Effectiveness of daily fluid balance charting in comparison to the measurement of body weight when used in guiding fluid therapy for critically ill adult patients: a systematic review protocol. *JBI Database of Systematic Reviews and Implementation Reports*, 13(3), 111–123.

 Diagnostic Studies   Evidence Based Practice   Medications   Pediatric/Geriatric/Lifespan

risk for deficient Fluid Volume

Taxonomy II: Nutrition—Class 5 Hydration (00028) [**Diagnostic Division:** Food/Fluid], Submitted 1978; Revised 2010, 2013; 2017

DEFINITION: Susceptible to experiencing decreased intravascular, interstitial, and/or intracellular fluid volumes, which may compromise health.

RISK FACTORS
Barrier to accessing fluid
Insufficient fluid intake
Insufficient knowledge about fluid needs
At Risk Population: Extremes of age; extremes of weight; factors influencing fluid needs
Associated Condition: Active fluid volume loss: [e.g., hemorrhage; gastric intubation; acute or prolonged diarrhea; wounds; fistulas; ascites; use of hyperosmotic radiopaque contrast agent]
Compromised regulatory mechanism [e.g., fever, thermoregulatory response; renal tubule damage]
Deviations affecting fluid intake or absorption
Excessive fluid loss through normal or abnormal route
Pharmaceutical agent
Sample Clinical Applications: Conditions with fever, diarrhea, nausea, vomiting; irritable bowel syndrome, draining wounds, dementia, depression, eating disorders

DESIRED OUTCOMES/EVALUATION CRITERIA

Sample NOC linkages:
Fluid Balance: Balance of the input and output of fluids in the body

Client Will (Include Specific Time Frame)
• Maintain fluid volume at a functional level as evidenced by individually adequate urinary output with normal specific gravity, stable vital signs, moist mucous membranes, good skin turgor, and prompt capillary refill.

Sample NOC linkages:
Risk Control: Personal actions to understand, prevent, eliminate, or reduce modifiable health threats
Knowledge: Disease Process: Extent of understanding conveyed about a specific disease process and potential complications

Client/Caregiver Will (Include Specific Time Frame)
• Identify individual risk factors and appropriate interventions.
• Demonstrate behaviors or lifestyle changes to prevent development of fluid volume deficit.

ACTIONS/INTERVENTIONS

Sample NIC linkages:
Fluid Monitoring: Collection and analysis of patient data to regulate fluid balance
Hemodynamic Regulation: Optimization of heart rate, preload, afterload, and contractility
Teaching: Disease Process: Assisting the patient to understand information related to a specific disease process

 Acute Care
 Collaborative
 Community/ Home Care
 Cultural

NURSING PRIORITY NO. 1 To assess causative/contributing factors:

- Note possible conditions/processes *that may lead to fluid deficits (of any type):* (1) fluid loss (e.g., indwelling tubes, diarrhea, vomiting, fever, excessive sweating, diabetic ketoacidosis; burns, other draining wounds; gastrointestinal obstruction; use of diuretics); (2) limited intake (e.g., extremes of age, limited mobility, client dependent on others for eating and drinking; lack of knowledge related to fluid intake; heat exhaustion or stroke); (3) fluid shifts (e.g., ascites, effusions, burns, sepsis); or (4) environmental factors (e.g., isolation, restraints, very high ambient temperatures, malfunctioning air conditioning).[3,6,7]
- ∞ 📝 Determine effects of age, gender, weight, and subcutaneous fat/muscle mass. *These factors affect the ratio of lean body mass to body fat, influencing total body water (TBW). In general, men have higher TBW than women due to women's higher percentage of body fat and less muscle mass than men; the elderly's TBW is known to decline. Elderly individuals are often at risk for dehydration because of reduced water intake (often to less than 1 L/day), decreased thirst reflex, impaired renal conservation of water, increased prevalence of chronic conditions, and polypharmacy.[1,10,11] Infants, children, and developmentally delayed individuals cannot verbalize or self-manage thirst. Worldwide, dehydration (secondary to diarrheal illness) is the leading cause of infant and child mortality.[2,6]*
- ∞ 📝 Assess older client's "hydration habits" *to determine best approach if client has potential for dehydration. Note: A recent study identified four categories of nursing home residents: (1) Can drink (client is functionally capable of consuming fluids, but doesn't for any number of reasons); (2) can't drink (frailty or dysphagia makes this client incapable of consuming fluids safely); (3) won't drink (client may fear incontinence or may have never in life consumed many fluids); and (4) end of life.[7]*
- Evaluate nutritional status, noting current food intake, type of diet (e.g., client is NPO or is on a restricted or pureed diet), and *factors that can negatively affect fluid intake (e.g., impaired mentation, nausea, wired jaws, immobility, insufficient time for meals, lack of finances restricting availability of food).*
- Review client's medications, including prescription, over-the-counter (OTC) drugs, herbals, and nutritional supplements *to identify medications that can alter fluid and electrolyte balance. These may include diuretics, vasodilators, beta blockers, aldosterone inhibitors, angiotensin-converting enzyme blockers, and medications that can cause syndrome of inappropriate secretion of antidiuretic hormone (e.g., phenothiazides, vasopressin, some antineoplastic drugs).[8]*
- Refer to NDs [deficient hyper/hypotonic Fluid Volume] or deficient [isotonic] Fluid Volume for additional interventions.

NURSING PRIORITY NO. 2 To prevent occurrence of deficit:

- Compare current fluid intake to fluid goal. Monitor intake and output balance, if indicated, being aware of changes in intake or output, as well as insensible losses, *to ensure accurate picture of fluid status.[1,3]*
- Assess skin and oral mucous membranes *for signs of dehydration, such as dry skin and mucous membranes, poor skin turgor, delayed capillary refill, and flat neck veins.*
- Monitor vital signs for changes (e.g., orthostatic hypotension, tachycardia, fever) *that may cause or be the effect of dehydration.[3]*
- Weigh client and compare with recent weight history. Perform serial weights to determine trends.
- ✏ Review laboratory data (e.g., hemoglobin/hematocrit, osmolality, electrolytes [e.g., sodium and potassium], blood urea nitrogen/creatinine) as indicated *to evaluate fluid and electrolyte status.[2,3] Note: Faes et al. (2007) state that "three forms of dehydration can be distinguished on the basis of plasma tonicity: hypertonic, isotonic, and hypotonic dehydration. Hypertonic dehydration is easy to diagnose by laboratory tests (e.g., serum sodium levels >150 mmol/L or serum osmolality >300 mOsm/L), but neglects the frequently occurring isotonic and hypotonic dehydration. Isotonic dehydration results from a balanced loss of water and electrolytes (e.g., by vomiting and diarrhea) and hypotonic dehydration results when loss of electrolytes exceeds water loss (e.g., by overuse of diuretics)."[11]*

 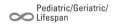

- Offer a variety of fluids and water-rich foods and make them available throughout the day if client is able to take oral fluids. Assist/remind client to drink, as needed. Determine individual fluid needs and establish replacement over 24 hours *to increase client's daily fluid intake.*[9]
- Administer medications as appropriate (e.g., antiemetics, antidiarrheals, antipyretics) *to stop or limit fluid losses. Note: Some practitioners recommend avoidance of antidiarrheal agents (high incidence of side effects including lethargy, respiratory depression, and coma) or OTC antiemetics (due to side effects including drowsiness and this impaired oral rehydration).*[2,3]
- Provide nutritionally balanced diet and/or enteral feedings when indicated (avoiding use of hyperosmolar or excessively high-protein formulas) and provide adequate amount of free water with feedings.[9]
- Provide supplemental IV fluids as indicated.
- Encourage oral intake:[3-6,8]

  Provide water and other fluids to a minimum amount daily (up to 2.5 L/day or amount determined by healthcare provider for client's age, weight, and condition).

  Offer fluids between meals and regularly throughout the day.

  Allow adequate time for eating and drinking at meals.

  Provide fluids in manageable cup, bottle, or with drinking straw.

  Ensure that immobile or restrained client is assisted.

  Encourage a variety of fluids in small frequent offerings, attempting to incorporate client's preferred beverage and temperature (e.g., iced or hot).

  Limit fluids that tend to exert a diuretic effect (e.g., caffeine, alcohol, high-glucose drinks).

  Promote intake of foods with a high water content (e.g., popsicles, gelatin, soup, eggnog, watermelon) or electrolyte replacement drinks (e.g., Smartwater, Gatorade, Pedialyte), as appropriate.

  Encourage client to increase fluids when engaged in physical exertion (such as when working outside or actively participating in sports) during hot weather.
- Review diet orders to remove any nonessential fluid and salt restrictions.

NURSING PRIORITY NO. 3 To promote wellness (Teaching/Discharge Considerations):

- Discuss individual risk factors or potential problems and specific interventions *to reduce risk of heat injury and dehydration (e.g., proper clothing and bedding for infants and elderly and proper clothing for outdoor workers, athletes during hot weather, use of room cooler or fan for comfortable ambient environment; frequent intake of fluid [not just when feeling thirsty]).*[5]
- Review appropriate use of medications and inform client of side effects or interactions of medications *that have potential for causing or exacerbating dehydration.*
- Encourage client/caregiver to maintain diary of fluid intake, number and amount of voidings, and estimate of other fluid losses (e.g., wounds, liquid stools) as necessary *to determine replacement needs.*
- Engage client, family, and all caregivers in fluid management plan. *Enhances cooperation with regimen and achievement of goals.*

DOCUMENTATION FOCUS

Assessment/Reassessment
- Individual findings, including individual risk factors influencing fluid needs or requirements.
- Baseline weight, vital signs.
- Results of laboratory tests.
- Specific client fluid needs and preferences.

Planning
- Plan of care and who is involved in planning.
- Teaching plan.

 Acute Care   Collaborative   Community/Home Care   Cultural

Implementation/Evaluation
• Responses to interventions, teaching, and actions performed.
• Attainment or progress toward desired outcome(s).
• Modifications to plan of care.

Discharge Planning
• Individual long-term needs, noting who is responsible for actions to be taken.
• Specific referrals made.

References

1. Mentes, J. C. (2012). Managing oral hydration. In: Boltz, M., Capezuti, E., Fulmer, T. (eds). *Evidence-Based Practice Guideline Hydration Management*. 4th ed. New York: Springer.
2. Huang, L. H., et al. (Updated 2017). Dehydration. Retrieved March 2018 from http://emedicine.medscape.com/article/906999-overview.
3. Robles-Suarez, J., et al. (2012). Hydration status of long term care residents rehospitalized within 30 days of hospital discharge. Retrieved March 2018 from http://www.jnursinghomeresearch.com/406-hydration-status-of-long-term-care-residents-rehospitalized-within-30-days-of-hospital-discharge.html.
4. Matheny, N. (2010). *Fluid and Electrolyte Balance: Nursing Considerations*. 5th ed. Sudbury, MA: Jones & Bartlett Learning.
5. Gastrolyte Staff. (2010–2018). Dehydration and heat: How hot weather could be dangerous. Retrieved March 2018 from https://gastrolyte.com.au/dehydration/dehydration-and-heat/.
6. Mentes, J., Claros, E. (2006). Oral hydration in older adults. *Am J Nurs*, 106(6), 40–49.
7. Mentes, J. (2006). A typology of oral hydration problems exhibited by frail nursing home residents. *J Gerontol Nurs*, 23(1), 13–21.
8. Wotton, K., Crannitch, K., Munt, R. (2008). Prevalence, risk factors and strategies to prevent dehydration in older adults. *Contemp Nurs*, 31(1), 44–56.
9. Collins, M., Claros, E. (2011). Recognizing the face of dehydration. *Nursing*, 41(8), 26–31.
10. Scholler, D. A. (1989). Changes in total body water with age. *Am J Clin Nutr*, 50(5 Suppl), 1176–1181.
11. Faes, M. C., Spigt, M. G., Rikkert, O. (2007). Dehydration in geriatrics. *Geriatrics and Aging*, 10(9), 590–596.

---

risk for imbalanced Fluid Volume

Taxonomy II: Nutrition—Class 5 Hydration (00025) **[Diagnostic Division:** Food/Fluid], Approved 1998; Revised 2008, 2013, 2017

DEFINITION: Susceptible to a decrease, increase, or rapid shift from one to the other of intravascular, interstitial, and/or intracellular fluid, which may compromise health. This refers to body fluid loss, gain, or both.

RISK FACTORS
To Be Developed
Associated Condition: Apherisis; treatment regimen
Ascites; intestinal obstruction; pancreatitis; sepsis
Burn injury; trauma
Sample Clinical Application: Major surgical procedures, renal dialysis, conditions requiring IV therapy or parenteral or enteral nutrition, heart failure with use of diuretic therapy

DESIRED OUTCOMES/EVALUATION CRITERIA

Sample **NOC** linkages:
Fluid Balance: Water balance in the intracellular and extracellular compartments of the body
Fluid Overload Severity: Severity of excess fluids in the intracellular and extracellular compartments of the body

(continues on page 356)

 Diagnostic Studies   Evidence Based Practice   Medications   Pediatric/Geriatric/Lifespan

risk for imbalanced Fluid Volume (continued)

Risk Control: Personal actions to prevent, eliminate, or reduce modifiable health threats

Client/Caregiver Will (Include Specific Time Frame)
• Demonstrate adequate fluid balance as evidenced by stable vital signs, palpable pulses of good quality, normal skin turgor, moist mucous membranes, individual appropriate urinary output, lack of excessive weight fluctuation (loss or gain), and no edema present.
• Identify individual risk factors and appropriate interventions.
• Demonstrate behaviors or lifestyle changes to prevent development of fluid imbalance.

ACTIONS/INTERVENTIONS

Sample **NIC** linkages:
Fluid Monitoring: Collection and analysis of patient data to regulate fluid balance
Intravenous (IV) Therapy: Administration and monitoring of IV fluids and medication
Hypervolemia Management: Reduction in extracellular and/or intracellular fluid volume and prevention of complications in a patient who is fluid overloaded

NURSING PRIORITY NO. 1   To determine risk/contributing factors:

• Note presence of conditions associated with fluid imbalance (e.g., diabetes insipidus; hyperosmolar nonketotic syndrome; intestinal obstruction; heart, pancreatitis, sepsis, kidney, or liver failure).
• Note current treatment modalities, including (1) major invasive procedures (e.g., surgery, dialysis), (2) use or overuse of certain medications (e.g., heparin, diuretics), (3) use of IV fluids without a delivery device, and (4) plasmapheresis (i.e., aphoresis) therapy. *These modalities can cause/exacerbate fluid imbalances and must be monitored for complications. Note: Therapeutic apheresis refers to extracorporeal therapies used in treatment of a variety of neurological, renal, hematological, and other systemic diseases caused by circulating toxic agents that cannot be cleared by other means. This may be a first-line therapy for conditions (e.g., Guillain-Barre syndrome, myasthenia gravis; therapeutic drug removal) or as a second-line therapy in conjunction with other therapies (e.g., multiple sclerosis unresponsive to steroids).*[7–9]
• Note client's age, current level of hydration, and mentation. *Provides information regarding ability to tolerate fluctuations in fluid level and risk for creating or failing to respond to a problem (e.g., confused client may have inadequate intake, disconnect tubings, or readjust IV flow rate; infant or child may be unable to self-monitor or manage).*[1]

NURSING PRIORITY NO. 2   To prevent fluctuations/imbalances in fluid levels:

• Measure and record intake:
Include all sources (e.g., oral, IV, antibiotic additives, liquids with medications).
• Measure and record output:
Monitor urine output (hourly, or as often as needed). Report urine output less than 30 mL/hr or 0.5 mL/kg/hr *because it may indicate deficient fluid volume or cardiac or kidney failure.*
Observe color of all excretions *to evaluate for bleeding.*
Estimate volume or measure emesis when vomiting.
Measure or estimate amount of liquid stool; weigh diapers or continence pads when indicated.
Inspect dressing(s), weigh dressings, estimate blood loss in surgical sponges, and count dressings or pads saturated per hour. *Note: Small losses can be life-threatening to pediatric clients.*[2]
Measure output from drainage devices (e.g., gastric, wound, chest).

 Acute Care   Collaborative   Community/ Home Care   Cultural

Estimate or calculate insensible fluid losses *to include losses in replacement calculations. Note: Losses from diffusion through skin and via respiratory tract are estimated at about 700 mL/24 hr in adults at ambient temperature,[3] while a diaphoretic episode requiring a full linen change may represent a fluid loss of as much as 1 L.[5]*

Calculate 24-hr fluid balance (noting intake greater than output, or output greater than intake).

- Weigh daily or as indicated, using same scale and clothing, and evaluate changes as they relate to fluid status. *Provides for early detection and prompt intervention as needed.*
- Monitor vital signs:

Evaluate vital signs at rest and with activities. *Blood pressure and heart and respiratory rate often increase initially when either volume deficit or fluid excess is present.[5]*

Evaluate hemodynamic pressures when available. *Central venous pressure and pulmonary artery wedge pressure may be used in critically ill clients to determine fluid balance and fluid volume responsiveness and to guide administration of vasoactive medications. Note: Numerous studies in recent years have weighed the benefits of invasive monitoring for the purpose of evaluating fluid status (and thus cardiac output response to fluid challenge). Research is ongoing into alternate ways and less invasive ways to perform this assessment (including the use of bioreactance, which tracks the phase of the electrical currents traversing the chest).[2,10,11]*

- Maintain IVs on volumetric infusion pumps and rapid infusion devices, as appropriate, *to deliver fluids accurately at desired rates to prevent either under/overinfusion.[5]*
- Assess for peripheral or dependent edema, adventitious breath sounds, and distended neck veins. *Clinical signs of fluid excess. Note: Intravascular volume depletion can be present at the same time as extravascular fluid excess (seen as edema) is present, so hypertension or hypotension could be found.[4,5]*
- Note increased lethargy or reports of dizziness, weakness, and muscle cramping. *Electrolyte imbalances (e.g., sodium, potassium, magnesium, calcium) may be present.[5,6]*
- Review laboratory data (e.g., electrolytes, hemoglobin/hematocrit) and chest radiograph *to determine changes indicative of electrolyte and/or fluid imbalance and fluid needs.[5,6]*
- If fluid volume deficit is possible:

Anticipate fluid replacement needs (e.g., need for blood or plasma transfusion in client with major trauma; planned surgery where blood and fluid loss can be expected; major burn injury; person with heat stroke; vomiting, diarrhea, or inability to take fluids).[5]

Establish and promote oral intake, incorporating beverage preferences when possible. Administer IV fluids (e.g., crystalloids, colloids, blood or blood components) *to support fluid management.[4,5]*

Administer medications (e.g., antidiarrheals, antiemetics, agents to reduce blood loss or promote clotting) as indicated *to reduce fluid loss.[4,5]*

- Refer to NDs [deficient hypertonic/hypotonic Fluid Volume], deficient [isotonic] Fluid Volume, and risk for deficient Fluid Volume for additional interventions.
- If fluid volume excess is possible:

Maintain fluid/sodium restrictions when needed. Offer small amounts of fluid over a 24-hr period.

Administer medications (e.g., diuretics, cardiotonics) *to assist in management of fluid excess or edema.[4,5]*

Assist with or prepare for procedures (e.g., dialysis, apheresis, ultrafiltration, pacemaker, cardiac assist device) *to correct fluid overload situation*[8,9] and monitor for complications associated with fluid imbalances.

Refer to ND excess Fluid Volume for additional interventions.

NURSING PRIORITY NO. 3 To promote wellness (Teaching/Discharge Considerations):

- Engage client, family, and all caregivers in fluid management plan. *Enhances cooperation with regimen and achievement of goals.[5]*
- Discuss individual risk factors or potential problems and specific interventions *to prevent or limit fluid imbalance and complications.*
- Instruct client/significant other in how to measure and record I&O as appropriate.

 Diagnostic Studies   Evidence Based Practice   Medications   Pediatric/Geriatric/Lifespan

- Review and instruct in medications or nutritional regimen (e.g., enteral, parenteral) *to alert to potential complications and ways to manage.*
- Identify signs and symptoms indicating need for prompt evaluation or follow-up by primary healthcare provider *for timely intervention and correction.*[5]

DOCUMENTATION FOCUS

Assessment/Reassessment
- Individual findings, including individual factors influencing fluid needs or requirements.
- Baseline weight, vital signs.
- Specific client preferences for fluids.

Planning
- Plan of care and who is involved in planning.
- Teaching plan.

Implementation/Evaluation
- Responses to interventions, teaching, and actions performed.
- Attainment or progress toward desired outcome(s).
- Modifications to plan of care.

Discharge Planning
- Individual long-term needs, noting who is responsible for actions to be taken.
- Specific referrals made.

References

1. Newfield, S. A., et al. (2007). *Cox's Clinical Applications of Nursing Diagnosis: Adult, Child, Women's, Psychiatric, Gerontic, and Home Health Considerations.* 5th ed. Philadelphia: F. A. Davis.
2. Ackley, B. J., Ladwig, G. B. (2011). *Nursing Diagnosis Handbook: An Evidence-Based Guide to Planning Care.* 9th ed. St. Louis, MO: Mosby Elsevier.
3. Guyton, A. C., Hall, J. E. (2010). *Textbook of Medical Physiology.* 12th ed. Philadelphia: W. B. Saunders.
4. Matheny, N. (2010). *Fluid and Electrolyte Balance: Nursing Considerations.* 5th ed. Philadelphia: J. B. Lippincott.
5. Doenges, M. E., Moorhouse, M. F., Murr, A. C. (2014). Fluid and electrolyte imbalances. *Nursing Care Plans: Guidelines for Individualizing Client Care Across the Life Span.* 9th ed. Philadelphia: F. A. Davis.
6. Astle, S. M. (2005). Restoring electrolyte balance. *RN*, 68(5), 31–34.
7. Stieglitz, E., Huang, J. (2013, updated 2017). Plasmapheresis. Retrieved March 2018 from http://emedicine.medscape.com/article/1895577-overview.
8. Mokrzycki, M. H., Bolagun, R. A. (2011). Therapeutic apheresis: A review of complications and recommendations for prevention and management. *J Clin Apher*, 26(5), 243–248.
9. Mokrzycki, M. H., Bolagun, R. A. (2013). Medications and therapeutic apheresis procedures: Are we doing our best? *J Clin Apher*, 28(1), 73–77.
10. Marik, P. E., Monnet, X., Taboul, J-L. (2011). Hemodynamic parameters to guide fluid therapy. Retrieved March 2018 from http://www.annalsofintensivecare.com/content/1/1/1eDetail.jsp?id=15821.
11. Cheetah Medical. (2013). Clinical application: Tailor fluid management with CHEETAH NICOM to optimize resuscitation. Retrieved March 2018 from http://cheetah-medical.com/fluid.

 Acute Care   Collaborative   Community/ Home Care   Cultural

Frail Elderly Syndrome

Taxonomy II: Health Promotion—Class 2: Health Management (00257) [**Diagnostic Division:** Safety], Approved 2013; Revised 2017

DEFINITION: Dynamic state of unstable equilibrium that affects the older individual experiencing deterioration of one or more domains of health (physical, functional, psychological, or social) and leads to increased susceptibility to adverse health effects, in particular disability.

RELATED FACTORS
Activity intolerance; decrease in energy; decrease in muscle strength; muscle weakness; exhaustion
Anxiety; depression; sadness
Average daily physical activity is less than recommended for gender and age; sedentary lifestyle
Fear of falling; impaired balance; impaired mobility; immobility
Insufficient social support; social isolation
Malnutrition; obesity

DEFINING CHARACTERISTICS
***Author Note: NANDA-I has defined a syndrome as "a clinical judgment concerning a specific cluster of nursing diagnoses [NDs] that occur together and are best addressed together and through similar interventions" (Herdman & Kamitsuru, 2018).[16] Defining Characteristics contain these ND titles.

Subjective
Activity intolerance
Fatigue
Hopelessness

Objective
Bathing, dressing, feeding, or toileting self-care deficit
Decreased cardiac output
Imbalanced nutrition: less than body requirements
Impaired memory
Impaired physical mobility; impaired walking
Social isolation
At Risk Population: Age >70 years; female gender; ethnicity other than Caucasian
Living alone; constricted living space
Economically disadvantaged; low educational level; social vulnerability
History of falls; prolonged hospitalization
Associated Condition: Alteration in cognitive functioning; sensory deficit; psychiatric disorder
Altered clotting process; decrease in serum 25-hydroxyvitamin D concentration; endocrine regulatory dysfunction
Anorexia; sarcopenia; sarcopenic obesity
Chronic illness; suppressed inflammatory response
Unintentional loss of 25% of body weight over 1 year; unintentional loss >10 pounds (>4.5 kg) in 1 year
Walking 15 feet requires >6 seconds (4 meters >5 seconds)
Sample Clinical Applications: Chronic debilitating conditions (e.g., COPD, diabetes, AIDS, Alzheimer's disease, multiple sclerosis [MS]), cancer, terminal illnesses, major depression

(continues on page 360)

 Diagnostic Studies   Evidence Based Practice   Medications 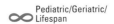 Pediatric/Geriatric/Lifespan

Frail Elderly Syndrome (continued)

DESIRED OUTCOMES/EVALUATION CRITERIA

Sample NOC linkages:

Personal Health Status: Overall physical or psychological, social, and spiritual functioning of an adult 18 years or older

Self-Management: Chronic Disease: Personal actions to manage a chronic disease, its treatment, and to prevent disease progression and complications

Will to Live: Desire, determination, and effort to survive

Client/Caregiver Will (Include Specific Time Frame)

• Acknowledge presence of factors affecting well-being.
• Identify corrective/adaptive measures for individual situation.
• Demonstrate behaviors/lifestyle changes necessary to enhance functional status.

Client Will

Look to the future, expressing a sense of control.

ACTIONS/INTERVENTIONS

Sample NIC linkages:

Self-Care Assistance: Assisting another to perform activities of daily living

Resiliency Promotion: Assisting individuals, families, and communities in development, use, and strengthening of protective factors to be used in coping with environmental and societal stressors

Refer to NDs Activity Intolerance, risk-prone Health Behavior, chronic Confusion, ineffective Coping, impaired Dentition, risk for Falls, Grieving, risk for Loneliness, imbalanced Nutrition: less than body requirements, Relocation Stress Syndrome, Self-Care deficit [specify], chronic low Self-Esteem, risk for Spiritual Distress, and ineffective Health Management, as appropriate, for additional relevant interventions.

NURSING PRIORITY NO. 1 To identify causative/contributing factors:

• Identify presence of "frailty syndrome" (FS). *Demonstrated in elderly person by three or more symptoms together: unintentional weight loss (10 or more pounds within the past year), muscle loss and weakness, a feeling of fatigue, slow walking speed, and low levels of physical activity.[1] Note: The presence of FS is a predictor for hospitalization, disability, decreasing mobility, falls, and even death.[2]*
• Note individual's age and gender. *Fried's (2001) research study of more than 5,000 adults found that chances of frailty rose sharply after the age of 85. Also, women are more likely than men to be frail, possibly because women typically outlive men and "start out with less muscle mass than men and, once they lose it, they may cross the frailty threshold more rapidly than men."[3]*
• Note presence of physical complaints (e.g., fatigue/exhaustion, unintentional weight loss, muscle weakness, slow walking, inability to participate in usual physical activities) and presence of conditions (e.g., heart disease, undetected diabetes mellitus, dementia, stroke, renal failure, long-term period of being bedridden, terminal conditions). *Note: These factors associated with frailty may or may not be recognized by the client, but may be reported or documented by others.*
• Evaluate medication regimen. *Medications that cause electrolyte imbalances (e.g., diuretics) can exacerbate weakness. Drugs that slow reaction time (e.g., sedatives, antidepressants) can interfere with balance and coordination, as can alcohol.[4]*

 Acute Care Collaborative Community/Home Care Cultural

- Determine nutritional status. *Malnutrition (e.g., weight loss, laboratory abnormalities, and identified micro-nutrient deficiencies) and factors contributing to failure to eat (e.g., chronic nausea, loss of appetite, no access to food or cooking, poorly fitting dentures, no one with whom to share meals, depression, financial problems) greatly impact health status and quality of life—especially for the elderly individual.*[2,5–7]
- Assess client's physical and cognitive status *to identify tolerance for activity and/or self-care.*
- Note client's living situation (e.g., lives alone, lives in facility). *Helps identify environmental risk factors such as risk for falls, problem with food shopping or preparation, depression, etc.*
- Evaluate client's level of adaptive behavior and client/caregiver knowledge and skills about health mainte-nance, environment, and safety *in order to instruct, intervene, and refer appropriately.*
- Review with client/significant other (SO) previous and current life situations, including role changes, multiple losses (e.g., death of loved ones, change in living arrangements, finances, independence), social isolation, and grieving *to identify psychological stressors that may be affecting current situation.*
- Ascertain safety of home environment and persons providing care *to identify potential for/presence of neglect-ful or abusive situations and/or need for referrals.*

NURSING PRIORITY NO. 2   To assess degree of impairment:

- Collaborate with multidisciplinary team to determine severity of client's limitations. *Testing may occur over period of time to identify functional and/or nutritional deficits and may include blood work, physi-cal therapy evaluation, and nutritional studies. Note: Studies have associated certain laboratory indicators with frailty, including (but not limited to) anemia, inflammation, and clotting factors.*[6,8]
- Perform nutritional screening and/or refer for comprehensive nutritional assessment. *Studies show that frail person may have weight and muscle loss (sarcopenia) or weight gain/obesity with muscle func-tion impairment and loss of strength (sarcopenic obesity).*[9] *Initial evidence indicates that when obesity and muscle impairment coexist, they act synergistically on the risk of developing multiple health-related outcomes.*[10]

NURSING PRIORITY NO. 3   To assist client to achieve/maintain general well-being:

- Assist with treatment of underlying comorbid medical, functional, cognitive, or psychiatric condi-tions *that could positively influence current situation (e.g., resolution of infection, treating anemia, addressing brain injury, delirium, social isolation, depression).*[11]
- Develop plan of action with client/caregiver *to meet immediate needs for nutrition, safety, and self-care and facilitate implementation of actions.*
- Administer medications as appropriate. *Studies show that optimized management of congestive heart failure and chronic pulmonary disease or improved glycemic control of diabetes results in improved health status, fewer hospitalizations, and reductions in the physical declines associated with the frailty syndrome.*[15]
- Refer to dietitian or nutritionist to assist in planning meals to meet client's specific nutritional needs (e.g., calories, proteins, vitamins, micronutrients), taste, and abilities. *Plans could include offering client's favorite food(s), attending social events (e.g., ice cream social, happy hour), or participating in family-style meals. In addition, interventions may be geared toward treatment of depression, grief, or loss and cultural or environ-mental adaptation measures.*[2,7,12] (Refer to ND imbalanced Nutrition: less than body requirements for addi-tional interventions.)
- Refer to physical and/or occupational therapist as indicated *to improve physical strength, endurance, and stamina. Note: Studies have supported that exercises (e.g., chair aerobics, stretching, resistance training, walking, tai chi) can improve balance and muscle and core strength, promoting physical function and endur-ance and reducing risk of falls.*[2,11]
- Discuss individual concerns about feelings of loss/loneliness and relationship between these feelings and cur-rent decline in well-being. Note desire or willingness to change situation. *Motivation or lack thereof can facili-tate—or impede—achieving desired outcomes.*[12]

 Diagnostic Studies   Evidence Based Practice   Medications   Pediatric/Geriatric/ Lifespan

- Explore mental strengths and successful coping skills the individual has previously used and apply to current situation. Refine or develop new strategies, as appropriate. *Incorporating these into problem-solving builds on past successes.*[13]
- Assist client to develop goals for dealing with life or illness situation. Involve SO in long-range planning. *Promotes commitment to goals and plan, thereby maximizing outcomes.*

NURSING PRIORITY NO. 4   To promote wellness (Teaching/Discharge Considerations):

- Assist client/SO(s) to identify and/or access useful community resources (e.g., support groups, Meals on Wheels, social worker, home care or assistive care, placement services). *Enhances coping, assists with problem solving, and may reduce risks to client and caregiver.*
- Encourage client to talk about positive aspects of life and to keep as physically active as possible *to reduce effects of dispiritedness (e.g., "feeling low," sense of being unimportant, disconnected).*[14]
- Promote socialization within individual limitations *to provide additional stimulation, reduce sense of isolation.*
- Offer opportunities to discuss life goals and support client/SO in setting/attaining new goals for this time in his or her life *to enhance hope for the future.*
- Help client explore reasons for living or begin to deal with end-of-life issues and provide support for grieving. *Enhances hope and sense of control, providing opportunity for client to take charge of own future.*[13,14]
- Assist client/SO/family to understand that frailty commonly occurs near the end of life and cannot always be reversed.[12]
- Discuss appropriateness of and refer to palliative services or hospice care, as indicated.
- Refer to pastoral care, counseling, or psychotherapy *for grief work or other issues as needed.*

DOCUMENTATION FOCUS

Assessment/Reassessment
- Individual findings, including current weight, dietary pattern, food and eating, perceptions of self, motivation for loss, support and feedback from SOs.
- Perception of losses or life changes.
- Ability to perform activities of daily living, participate in care, and meet own needs.
- Motivation for change, support and feedback from SO(s).

Planning
- Plan of care, specific interventions, and who is involved in planning.
- Teaching plan.

Implementation/Evaluation
- Responses to interventions and actions performed, general well-being, weekly weight.
- Attainment or progress toward desired outcome(s).
- Modifications to plan of care.

Discharge Planning
- Long-term needs and who is responsible for actions to be taken.
- Community resources and support groups.
- Specific referrals made.

References

1. Cimons, M. (2013). *Frailty is a medical condition, not an inevitable result of aging (Op-Ed).* Retrieved March 2018 from http://www.livescience.com/41602-frailty-is-medical-condition.html.
2. Cherniak, E. P., et al. (2007). Emerging therapies to treat frailty syndrome in the elderly. *Altern Med Rev*, 12(3), 246–258.
3. Fried, L. P., et al. (2001). Frailty in older adults: Evidence for a phenotype. *J Gerontol A Biol Sci Med Sci*, 56(3), M146–M157.
4. Flinders, D. C. (2007). *Helping elderly patients avoid frailty syndrome.* Retrieved March 2018 from http://www.clinicaladvisor.com/helping-elderly-patients-avoid-frailty-syndrome/article/117361/.

 Acute Care   Collaborative   Community/Home Care   Cultural

5. Rehman, H. U. (2008). Involuntary weight loss in the elderly. *Clin Geriatr Med*, 13, 37–45.

6. Dawodu, S. T., et al. (2003, updated 2015). *Nutritional management in the rehabilitation setting*. Retrieved March 2018 from http://emedicine.medscape.com/article/318180-overview.

7. diMaria-Ghalili, R. A., Amelia, E. (2005). Nutrition in older adults: Interventions and assessment can help curb the growing threat of malnutrition. *Am J Nurs*, 105(3), 40–50.

8. Walston, J., et al. (2002). Frailty and activation of the inflammation and coagulation systems with and without clinical comorbidities: Results from the Cardiovascular Health Study. *Arch Intern Med*, 162(20), 2333–2341.

9. Stenholm, S., et al. (2009). Sarcopenic obesity—definition, etiology and consequences. *Curr Opin Clin Nutr Metab Care*, 11(6), 693–700.

10. Dominguez, L. J., Barbagallo, M. (2007). The cardiometabolic syndrome and sarcopenic obesity in older persons. *J Cardiometab Syndr*, 2(3), 183–189.

11. Ferrucc, L., et al. (2003). The frailty syndrome: A critical issue in geriatric oncology. *Crit Rev Oncol Hematol*, 46(2), 127–137.

12. Robertson, R. G., Montagnini, M. (2004). Geriatric failure to thrive. *Am Family Med*, 70(2), 343–350.

13. Townsend, M. C. (2003). *Psychiatric Mental Health Nursing Concepts of Care*. 4th ed. Philadelphia: F. A. Davis.

14. Butcher, H. K., McGonigal-Kenney, M. (2005). Depression & dispiritedness in later life: A "gray drizzle of horror" isn't inevitable. *Am J Nurs*, 105(12), 52–61.

15. Palace, J. Z., Flood-Sukhdeo, J. (2014). The frailty syndrome. *Today's Geriatric Medicine*, 7(1), 18.

16. Herdman, T. H., Kamitsuru, S. (2018). *NANDA International, Inc. Nursing Diagnosis Definitions and Classification 2018–2020*. 11th ed. New York: Thieme Publishers.

risk for Frail Elderly Syndrome

Taxonomy II: Health Promotion—Class 2 Health Management (00231) **[Diagnostic Division:** Safety], Approved 2013; Revised 2017

DEFINITION: Susceptible to a dynamic state of unstable equilibrium that affects the older individual experiencing deterioration of one or more domain of health (physical, functional, psychological, or social) and leads to increased susceptibility to adverse health effects, in particular disability.

RISK FACTORS

Activity intolerance; decrease in energy; decrease in muscle strength; muscle weakness; exhaustion

Anxiety; depression; sadness

Average daily physical activity is less than recommended for gender and age; sedentary lifestyle

Fear of falling; impaired balance; impaired mobility; immobility

Insufficient social support; social isolation

Malnutrition; obesity

At Risk Population: Age >70 years; female gender; ethnicity other than Caucasian

Living alone; constricted living space;

Economically disadvantaged; low educational level; social vulnerability

History of falls; prolonged hospitalization

Associated Condition: Alteration in cognitive functioning; sensory deficit; psychiatric disorder;

Altered clotting process; decrease in serum 25-hydroxyvitamin D concentration; endocrine regulatory dysfunction

Anorexia; sarcopenia; sarcopenic obesity

Chronic illness; suppressed inflammatory response;

Unintentional loss of 25% of body weight over 1 year; unintentional loss >10 pounds (>4.5 kg) in 1 year;

Walking 15 feet requires >6 seconds (4 meters >5 seconds)

Sample Clinical Applications: Chronic debilitating conditions (e.g., COPD, diabetes, AIDS, Alzheimer's disease, multiple sclerosis [MS]), cancer, terminal illnesses, major depression)

(continues on page 364)

 Diagnostic Studies   Evidence Based Practice   Medications 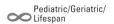 Pediatric/Geriatric/Lifespan

risk for Frail Elderly Syndrome (continued)

DESIRED OUTCOMES/EVALUATION CRITERIA

Sample NOC linkages:

Personal Health Status: Overall physical, psychological, social, and spiritual functioning of an adult 18 years or older

Self-Management: Chronic Disease: Personal actions to manage a chronic disease, its treatment, and prevent disease progression and complications

Client/Caregiver Will (Include Specific Time Frame)
- Identify risk factors that can affect well-being.
- Develop plan to correct/minimize risk factors.
- Engage in behaviors/lifestyle changes necessary to maintain/enhance functional status.

Client Will
- Look to the future, expressing a sense of control.

ACTIONS/INTERVENTIONS

Sample NIC linkages:

Risk Identification: Analysis of potential risk factors, determination of health risks, and prioritization of risk reduction strategies for an individual or group

Health Education: Developing and providing instruction and learning experiences to facilitate voluntary adaptation of behavior conducive to health in individuals, families, groups, or communities

NURSING PRIORITY NO. 1 To identify client at risk:

- Assess client upon admission to care for conditions listed in Risk Factors. *Research shows that frailty in elderly person is demonstrated by three or more symptoms together: unintentional weight loss over a year, along with muscle loss and weakness; a feeling of fatigue/exhaustion, along with slow walking speed; and low levels of physical activity.*[1]
- ∞ Note individual's age and gender. *Fried's (2001) research study of more than 5,000 adults found that chances of frailty rose sharply after the age of 85. Also, women are more likely than men to be frail, possibly because women typically outlive men and "start out with less muscle mass than men and, once they lose it, they may cross the frailty threshold more rapidly than men."*[2]
- Refer to ND: Frail Elderly Syndrome for additional assessment interventions.

NURSING PRIORITY NO. 2 To promote wellness (Teaching/Discharge Considerations):

- Develop plan of action with client/caregiver *to meet immediate needs for safety and self-care.*
- Assist with treatment of underlying comorbid medical, functional, cognitive, or psychiatric conditions *that could positively influence current situation (e.g., resolution of infection, treating anemia, addressing brain injury, delirium, social isolation, depression).*[3]
- Administer medications as appropriate. *Studies show that optimized management of chronic conditions results in improved health status, fewer hospitalizations, and reductions in the physical declines associated with the frailty syndrome.*[4]
- Refer to dietitian or nutritionist to assist in planning meals to meet client's specific nutritional needs (e.g., calories, proteins, vitamins, micronutrients), taste, and abilities. *Plans could include offering client's favorite food(s), attending social events (e.g., ice cream social, happy hour), or participating in family-style meals. In*

 Acute Care   Collaborative   Community/ Home Care   Cultural

addition, interventions may be geared toward treatment of depression, grief or loss, and cultural or environmental adaptation measures.[5–7]

- 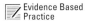 Refer to physical and/or occupational therapist as indicated *to improve physical strength, endurance, and stamina. Note: Studies have supported that exercises (e.g., chair aerobics, stretching, resistance training, walking, tai chi) can improve balance and muscle and core strength, promoting physical function and endurance and reducing risk of falls.*[3,5]
- Encourage client to talk about positive aspects of life and to keep as physically active as possible *to reduce effects of dispiritedness (e.g., "feeling low," sense of being unimportant, disconnected).*
- Promote socialization *to provide additional stimulation and reduce sense of isolation.*
- 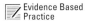 Assist client/significant others to identify and/or access useful community resources (e.g., support groups, Meals on Wheels, social worker, home care or assistive care, placement services). *Enhances coping, assists with problem solving, and may reduce risks to client and caregiver.*
- Refer to ND Frail Elderly Syndrome for additional interventions as indicated.

DOCUMENTATION FOCUS

Assessment/Reassessment
- Identified risk factors.
- Perception of situation and personal significance.

Planning
- Plan of care and who is involved in the planning.
- Teaching plan.

Implementation/Evaluation
- Response to interventions and teaching plan.
- Attainment or progress toward desired outcomes.

Discharge Planning
- Long-term needs and who is responsible for actions to be taken.
- Specific referral made.

References

1. Cimons, M. (2013). Frailty is a medical condition, not an inevitable result of aging (Op-Ed). Retrieved March 2018 from http://www.livescience.com/41602-frailty-is-medical-condition.html.
2. Fried, L. P., et al. (2001). Frailty in older adults: Evidence for a phenotype. *J Gerontol A Biol Sci Med Sci*, 56(3), M146–M157.
3. Ferrucc, L., et al. (2003). The frailty syndrome: A critical issue in geriatric oncology. *Crit Rev Oncol Hematol*, 46(2), 127–137.
4. Palace, J. Z., Flood-Sulchdeo, J. (2014). The frailty syndrome. *Today's Geriatric Medicine*, 7(1), 18.
5. Cherniak, E. P., et al. (2007). Emerging therapies to treat frailty syndrome in the elderly. *Altern Med Rev*, 12(3), 246–258.
6. DiMaria-Ghalili, R. A., Amelia, E. (2005). Nutrition in older adults: Interventions and assessment can help curb the growing threat of malnutrition. *Am J Nurs*, 105(3), 40–50.
7. Robertson, R. G., Montagnini, M. (2004). Geriatric failure to thrive. *Am Family Med*, 70(2), 343–350.

 Diagnostic Studies   Evidence Based Practice   Medications   ∞ Pediatric/Geriatric/Lifespan

impaired Gas Exchange

Taxonomy II: Elimination and Exchange—Class 4 Respiratory Function (00030) [**Diagnostic Division:** Respiration], Submitted 1980; Revised 1996, 1998 by Nursing Diagnosis Extension and Classification; 2017

DEFINITION: Excess or deficit in oxygenation and/or carbon dioxide elimination at the alveoli-capillary membrane.

RELATED FACTORS
To Be Developed

DEFINING CHARACTERISTICS

Subjective
Dyspnea
Visual disturbance
Headache upon awakening
[Sense of impending doom]

Objective
Confusion
Restlessness; irritability
Somnolence
Abnormal arterial blood gases (ABGs) or arterial pH; hypoxia or hypoxemia; hypercapnia; decrease in carbon dioxide (CO_2) level
Cyanosis; abnormal skin color
Abnormal breathing pattern; nasal flaring
Tachycardia; [dysrhythmias]
Diaphoresis
Associated Condition: Alveolar-capillary membrane changes; ventilation-perfusion imbalance
Sample Clinical Applications: Chronic obstructive pulmonary disease (COPD), asthma, pneumonias, tuberculosis, heart failure, sickle cell anemia, acute respiratory distress syndrome (ARDS), high-altitude pulmonary edema, pulmonary emboli (PE); carbon monoxide poisoning

DESIRED OUTCOMES/EVALUATION CRITERIA

Sample NOC linkages:
Respiratory Status: Gas Exchange: Alveolar exchange of carbon dioxide and oxygen to maintain arterial blood gas concentrations
Tissue Perfusion: Pulmonary: Adequacy of blood flow through pulmonary vasculature to perfuse alveoli/capillary unit
Respiratory Status: Ventilation: Movement of air in and out of the lungs

Client Will (Include Specific Time Frame)
• Demonstrate improved ventilation and adequate oxygenation of tissues by ABGs within client's usual parameters and absence of symptoms of respiratory distress (as noted in Defining Characteristics).
• Verbalize understanding of causative factors and appropriate interventions.
• Participate in treatment regimen (e.g., breathing exercises, effective coughing, use of oxygen) within level of ability and situation.

 Acute Care Collaborative Community/ Home Care Cultural

ACTIONS/INTERVENTIONS

Sample NIC linkages:

Respiratory Monitoring: Collection and analysis of patient data to ensure airway patency and adequate gas exchange

Oxygen Therapy: Administration of oxygen and monitoring of its effectiveness

Airway Management: Facilitation of patency of air passages

NURSING PRIORITY NO. 1 To assess causative/contributing factors:

• Note presence of factors and conditions that can cause or be associated in some way with gas exchange problems. *Can be related to multiple factors, including anemias, anesthesia, surgical procedures, high altitude, allergic response, altered level of consciousness, anxiety, fear, aspiration, decreased lung compliance, excessive or thick secretions, immobility, infection, medication and drug toxicity or overdose, neuromuscular impairment of breathing pattern, pain, and smoking.*

• Refer to NDs ineffective Airway Clearance and ineffective Breathing Pattern for additional assessment interventions as appropriate.

NURSING PRIORITY NO. 2 To evaluate degree of compromise:

• ✚ Evaluate respirations:

Observe rate, rhythm, and depth. *Provides insight into the work of breathing and adequacy of alveolar ventilation. For example, increasing both rate and depth of respirations increases alveolar ventilation and occurs normally in response to exercise and stressors.*[1,9]

Note client's reports/perceptions of breathing ease. *Client may report a range of symptoms (e.g., air hunger; shortness of breath with speaking, activity, or at rest).*

Observe for dyspnea on exertion or gasping, changing positions frequently to ease breathing, and tendency to assume three-point position (bending forward while supporting self by placing one hand on each knee) *to maximize respiratory effort.*

Note use of accessory muscles (e.g., scalene muscles, pectoralis minor, sternocleidomastoids, external intercostal muscles) *to assist diaphragm in increasing volume of thoracic cavity, which aids in inspiration.*

∞ Observe infants/young children for nasal flaring and sternal retractions, *indicating increased work of breathing or respiratory distress.*

Note use of abdominal muscles during expiration (normally a passive process) *to reduce thoracic dimensions and overcome airway resistance to expiration.*

• Evaluate lungs:

Auscultate and percuss chest, describing presence or absence of breath sounds; note adventitious breath sounds. *Although air may be heard moving through the lung fields, breath sounds may be faint because of decreased airflow or areas of consolidation. In this nursing diagnosis, ventilatory effort is insufficient to deliver enough oxygen or to get rid of sufficient amounts of carbon dioxide. Abnormal breath sounds are indicative of numerous problems (e.g., hypoventilation such as might occur with atelectasis or presence of secretions, improper endotracheal [ET] tube placement, collapsed lung) and must be evaluated for further intervention.*[2,9]

• Note character and effectiveness of cough mechanism. *Affects ability to clear airways of secretions.*

• Evaluate skin and mucous membrane color, noting areas of pallor or cyanosis, for example, peripheral (nailbeds) versus central (around lips or earlobes) or general duskiness. *Duskiness and central cyanosis are late signs of hypoxemia.*[9]

 Diagnostic Studies   Evidence Based Practice   Medications 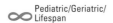 Pediatric/Geriatric/Lifespan

- Evaluate behavior:

  Assess level of consciousness and mentation changes. *Decreased level of consciousness can be an indirect measurement of impaired oxygenation, but it also impairs one's ability to protect the airway, potentially further adversely affecting oxygenation.*

  Note somnolence, restlessness, and reports of headache on arising.

  Assess energy level and activity tolerance, noting reports or evidence of fatigue, weakness, and problems with sleep *that are associated with diminished oxygenation.*

- Monitor vital signs:

  Measure temperature. *A high fever greatly increases metabolic demands and oxygen consumption.*

  Monitor heart rate and rhythm. *Tachycardia and dysrhythmias may be noted as the heart reacts to cardiac ischemia and/or hypoxemia, especially during activity.*

  Monitor blood pressure (BP). *BP can be variable, depending on underlying condition and cardiopulmonary response.*

  Note increased pulmonary artery or right ventricular wedge pressures in the critically ill client with central lines. *Indicative of increased pulmonary vascular resistance.*

- Review pertinent diagnostic data (e.g., ABGs, hemoglobin, red blood cells, electrolytes) and chest radiography. Evaluate oxygen and carbon dioxide at bedside by means of pulse oximetry and end-tidal CO_2 monitoring (capnography). Note results of pulmonary function studies where available *to evaluate lung mechanics, capacities, and function. Blood studies are useful in revealing systemic reasons for problems with oxygenation and/or the results of hypoxemia and acid-base imbalances and to determine response to therapies. Point-of-care tools evaluate ventilation by providing breath-to-breath information. Studies have shown that capnography monitoring improves client outcomes through early recognition of hypoventilation, apnea, and airway obstruction, thus preventing hypoxic episodes. Client in respiratory failure typically shows hypoxemia and metabolic acidosis, and is high risk for developing respiratory acidosis.*[4,6,9,10]

NURSING PRIORITY NO. 3   To correct/improve existing deficiencies:

- Elevate head of bed or position client appropriately. *Elevation or upright position facilitates respiratory function by gravity; however, client in severe distress will seek position of comfort. In ventilated client, prone position may be implemented in some clients to improve pulmonary perfusion and increase oxygen diffusion.*[3]

- Provide airway adjuncts and suction as indicated *to clear or maintain open airway, when client is unable to clear secretions, or to improve gas diffusion when client is showing desaturation of oxygen by oximetry or ABGs.*[3,5]

- Encourage frequent position changes, deep-breathing exercises or directed coughing, use of incentive spirometer, and chest physiotherapy, as indicated. *Promotes optimal chest expansion, mobilization of secretions, and oxygen diffusion.*[3]

- Provide supplemental oxygen (via cannula, mask) using lowest concentration possible *dictated by pulse oximetry, ABGs, and client symptoms/underlying condition.*

- Ensure availability of proper emergency equipment, including ET/tracheostomy set and suction catheters appropriate for age and size of infant/child/adult. Avoid use of face mask in elderly emaciated client.

- Prepare for and assist with intubation and mechanical ventilation. *The decision to intubate and ventilate is made on a clinical diagnosis of respiratory failure, classified as hypoxemic or hypercapnic. Hypoxemic respiratory failure is the most common, associated with acute lung disorders such as pneumothorax, atelectasis, pulmonary edema, pneumonia, ARDS, and smoke inhalation. Hypercapnic respiratory failure can be seen in acute exacerbations of chronic COPD, head trauma, and spinal cord injury.*[4,11]

- Monitor and adjust ventilator settings (e.g., FIO_2, tidal volume, inspiratory and expiratory ratio, sigh, positive end-expiratory pressure) as indicated when mechanical support is being used. *The mode of ventilation (volume or pressure) and ventilator settings are determined by the specific needs of the client, which are determined by clinical evaluation and blood gas parameters.*[11]

- Monitor for carbon dioxide narcosis (e.g., change in level of consciousness, changes in O_2 and CO_2 blood gas levels, flushing, decreased respiratory rate and headaches), *which may occur in clients receiving long-term oxygen therapy.*[6]

 Acute Care   Collaborative   Community/ Home Care   Cultural

- Maintain adequate fluid intake *for mobilization of secretions* but avoid fluid overload *that may increase pulmonary congestion.*
- Provide psychological support, Active-listen questions and concerns. Address client's/significant other's (SO's) fears and anxiety that may be present. Maintain calm attitude while working with client/SOs. *Anxiety is contagious, and associated agitation can increase oxygen consumption and dyspnea.*
- Encourage adequate rest and limit activities to within client tolerance. Promote a calm, restful environment. *Facilitates relaxation and helps limit oxygen needs and consumption.*[3]
- Administer medications as indicated (e.g., inhaled and systemic glucocorticosteroids, antibiotics, bronchodilators, methylxanthines, antitussives/mucolytics, vasodilators). (Medications may be aerosolized or nebulized for enhanced response and limitation of side effects.) *Pharmacological agents are varied and specific to the client but are generally used to prevent and control symptoms, reduce frequency and severity of exacerbations, and improve exercise tolerance.*[11]
- Monitor therapeutic and adverse effects or interactions of drug therapy *to determine efficacy and need for change.*
- Use sedation judiciously *to avoid depressant effects on respiratory functioning.*[12]
- Minimize blood loss from procedures (e.g., blood draws—especially in neonates/infants, hemodialysis) *to limit effects of anemia and related gas diffusion impairment.*
- Assist with procedures as individually indicated (e.g., transfusion, phlebotomy, bronchoscopy) *to improve respiratory function/oxygen-carrying capacity.*
- Keep environment allergen/pollutant free *to reduce irritant effect of dust and chemicals on airways.*

NURSING PRIORITY NO. 4   To promote wellness (Teaching/Discharge Considerations):

- Review risk factors, particularly genetic, environmental, and employment-related conditions (e.g., sickle cell anemia, altitude sickness, exposure to toxins), *to help client/SO prevent complications or manage risk factors.*
- Discuss implications of smoking related to the illness or condition. Encourage client and SO(s) to stop smoking and attend cessation programs as necessary *to reduce health risks and/or prevent further decline in lung function.*[7,12]
- Review oxygen-conserving techniques (e.g., organizing tasks before beginning; sitting instead of standing to perform tasks; eating small meals; performing slower, purposeful movements) *to reduce oxygen demands.*[3]
- Reinforce need for adequate rest, while encouraging activity and exercise (e.g., upper and lower extremity endurance and strength training, and flexibility) *to decrease dyspnea and improve quality of life.*[8]
- Emphasize the importance of good general nutrition *for improving stamina and reducing the work of breathing.*[3,8]
- Refer to dietitian *for nutritional assessment and individual dietary plan as indicated.*[8,12]
- Instruct in the use of relaxation and stress-reduction techniques as appropriate.
- Review job description and work activities *to identify need for job modifications or vocational rehabilitation.*[3]
- Discuss home oxygen therapy use and instruct in safety concerns as indicated *to ensure client's safety, especially when used in the very young and fragile elderly or when cognitive or neuromuscular impairment is present.*[3]
- Identify specific supplier for supplemental oxygen and necessary respiratory devices, as well as other individually appropriate resources, such as home-care agencies, Meals on Wheels, etc., to facilitate independence.[3]

DOCUMENTATION FOCUS

Assessment/Reassessment

- Assessment findings, including respiratory rate, character of breath sounds; frequency, amount, and appearance of secretions; presence of cyanosis; laboratory findings; and mentation level.
- Conditions that may interfere with oxygen delivery or exchange.

 Diagnostic Studies   Evidence Based Practice   Medications   Pediatric/Geriatric/Lifespan

Planning
- Plan of care, specific interventions, and who is involved in the planning.
- Liters of supplemental oxygen, ventilator settings.
- Teaching plan.

Implementation/Evaluation
- Client's responses to treatment, teaching, and actions performed.
- Attainment or progress toward desired outcome(s).
- Modifications to plan of care.

Discharge Planning
- Long-term needs, identifying who is responsible for actions to be taken.
- Community resources for equipment and supplies postdischarge.
- Specific referrals made.

References

1. Seay, S. J., Gay, S. L., Strauss, M. (2002). Tracheostomy emergencies. *Am J Nurs*, 102(3), 59.
2. Newfield, S. A., et al. (2007). *Cox's Clinical Applications of Nursing Diagnosis: Adult, Child, Women's, Psychiatric, Gerontic, and Home Health Considerations*. 5th ed. Philadelphia: F. A. Davis.
3. Doenges, M. E., Moorhouse, M. F., Murr, A. C. (2010). *Nursing Care Plans: Guidelines for Individualizing Client Care Across the Life Span*. 8th ed. Philadelphia: F. A. Davis.
4. Carcillo, J. A., Fields, A. I. (2002). Clinical practice parameters for hemodynamic support of pediatric and neonatal patients in septic shock. *Crit Care Med*, 30(6), 1365–1378.
5. Hess, D. R. (2012). Secretion clearance techniques. In Hess, D. R., et al. (eds). *Respiratory Care: Principles and Practices*. 2nd ed. Sudbury, MA: Jones & Bartlett Learning.
6. Argyle, B. (1996). Blood gas text. *Mad Scientist Software's Blood Gas Tutorial*. Retrieved March 2018 from www.madsci.com/manu/gas_gen.htm.
7. Anderson, N. R. (2006). The role of the home healthcare nurse in smoking cessation: Guidelines for successful intervention. *Home Healthc Nurse*, 24(7), 424–431.
8. McAllister, M. (2005). Promoting physiologic-physical adaptation in chronic obstructive pulmonary disease: Pharmacotherapeutic evidence-based research and guidelines. *Home Healthc Nurse*, 23(8), 523–531.
9. Johnson, K. L., Munro, N. (2004). Diagnostic measures to evaluate oxygenation in critically ill adults: Implications and limitations. *AACN Adv Crit Care*, 15(4), 506–524.
10. Corbo, J., et al. (2005). Concordance between capnography and arterial blood gas measurements of carbon dioxide in acute asthma. *Ann Emerg Med*, 46(4), 323–327.
11. Byrum, D., Crabtree, C. (2009). Mechanical ventilation: Cruise control for the lungs. *Nursing Made Incredibly Easy!*, 7(5), 44–52.
12. Qaseem, A., et al. (2011). Diagnosis and management of stable chronic obstructive pulmonary disease: A clinical practice guideline update. *Ann Intern Med*, 155(3), 179–191.

---

dysfunctional Gastrointestinal Motility

Taxonomy II: Elimination and Exchange—Class 2 Gastrointestinal Function (00196) [**Diagnostic Division:** Elimination], Approved 2008; Revised 2017

DEFINITION: Increased, decreased, ineffective, or lack of peristaltic activity within the gastrointestinal system.

RELATED FACTORS
Anxiety; stressors
Change in water source; unsanitary food preparation
Eating habit change; malnutrition
Sedentary lifestyle; immobility

 Acute Care   Collaborative   Community/Home Care Cultural

DEFINING CHARACTERISTICS

Subjective
Absence of flatus
Abdominal cramping, pain
Diarrhea
Difficulty with defecation
Nausea; regurgitation

Objective
Change in bowel sounds
Acceleration of gastric emptying; diarrhea
Distended abdomen
Increase in gastric residual; bile-colored gastric residual
Hard, formed stool
Vomiting
At Risk Population: Aging
Prematurity
Ingestion of contaminated material
Associated Condition: Decrease in gastrointestinal circulation; gastrointestinal reflux disease
Diabetes mellitus; infection
Enteral feedings; food intolerance
Pharmaceutical agent; treatment regimen
Sample Clinical Applications: Abdominal or intestinal surgery, eating disorders, malnutrition, celiac disease, anemia, anxiety disorders, biliary cancer, cholecystectomy, Crohn's disease, irritable bowel syndrome, gastroesophageal reflux disease (GERD), gastritis, pancreatitis, quadriplegia, peritoneal dialysis, botulism, sepsis, multiple organ dysfunction syndrome, radiation therapy

DESIRED OUTCOMES/EVALUATION CRITERIA

Sample NOC linkages:
Gastrointestinal Function: Ability of the gastrointestinal tract to ingest and digest food products, absorb nutrients, and eliminate waste
Knowledge: Treatment Regimen: Extent of understanding conveyed about a specific treatment regimen

Client Will (Include Specific Time Frame)
• Reestablish and maintain normal pattern of bowel functioning.
• Verbalize understanding of causative factors and rationale for treatment regimen.
• Demonstrate appropriate behaviors to assist with resolution of causative factors.

ACTIONS/INTERVENTIONS

Sample NIC linkages:
Bowel Management: Establishment and maintenance of a regular pattern of bowel elimination
Tube Care: Gastrointestinal: Management of a patient with a gastrointestinal tube
Nutrition Management: Providing and promoting a balanced intake of nutrients

 Diagnostic Studies   Evidence Based Practice   Medications   Pediatric/Geriatric/Lifespan

NURSING PRIORITY NO. 1 To assess causative/contributing factors:

- Note presence of conditions (e.g., congestive heart failure, major trauma, sepsis) affecting systemic circulation and perfusion. *Blood loss or shock can result in hypoperfusion and short- or long-term GI dysfunction.*
- Determine presence of disorders causing localized or diffuse reduction in GI blood flow, such as esophageal varices, GI hemorrhage, pancreatitis, and intraperitoneal hemorrhage, *to identify client at higher risk for ineffective tissue perfusion.*
- Note presence of chronic or long-term disorders, such as GERD, hiatal hernia, inflammatory bowel (e.g., ulcerative colitis, Crohn's disease), malabsorption (e.g., dumping syndrome, celiac disease), and short-bowel syndrome, as may occur after surgical removal of portions of the small intestine. *These conditions are associated with increased, decreased, or ineffective peristaltic activity.*
- ∞ Note client's age and developmental concerns. *Children are prone to infections causing gastroenteritis, manifested by vomiting and diarrhea.[1] Premature or low-birth-weight neonates are at risk for developing necrotizing enterocolitis (NEC). The elderly have concerns associated with decreased motility (e.g., constipation related to slower peristalsis, lack of sufficient fiber and fluid intake, chronic use of laxatives).[18]*
- Note lifestyle issues *that can affect GI function (e.g., people who regularly engage in competitive sports such as long-distance running, cycling; persons with poor sanitary living conditions; people who travel to areas with contaminated food or water; overeating or intake of foods associated with gastric distress or intestinal distention).[4]*
- 💊 Review client's drug regimen. *Medications such as laxatives, antibiotics, anticholesterol agents, opiates, sedatives, and iron preparations may cause or exacerbate intestinal issues. In addition, the likelihood of bleeding increases from use of medications such as NSAIDs, Coumadin, and Plavix.[2,3]*
- Ascertain whether client is experiencing anxiety; acute, extreme, or chronic stress; or other psychogenic factors present in persons with emotional or psychiatric disorders (including anorexia/bulimia, etc.) *that can affect GI function.[4,5]*
- ⬭∞ Review laboratory and other diagnostic studies. *Complete blood count may be done to evaluate for bleeding, inflammation, toxicity, and infection. Metabolic panel may reveal hepatic dysfunction, electrolyte imbalances, or low albumin levels. Computed tomography or other scans and abdominal ultrasound can help identify conditions like kidney or gallstones. X-rays may show bowel dilation or obstruction and stool and gas patterns.[1,9,11,12] Changes in white blood cell count with x-ray evidence of pneumoperitoneum (air in the abdominal cavity) in preterm neonate suggests NEC.[18]*

NURSING PRIORITY NO. 2 To note degree of dysfunction/organ involvement:

- Assess vital signs, noting presence of low blood pressure, elevated heart rate, and fever. *May suggest hypoperfusion or developing sepsis. Fever in presence of bright red blood in stool may indicate ischemic colitis.*
- 📝 Ascertain presence and characteristics of abdominal pain. *Pain is a common symptom of GI disorders and can vary in location, duration, and intensity.[6] Diffuse pain may reflect hypoperfusion of the gastrointestinal tract, which is particularly vulnerable to even small decreases in circulating volume.[7] Mid-epigastric pain immediately following meals and lasting several hours suggests abdominal angina due to atherosclerotic occlusive disease.[19] Tension pain caused by organ distention may develop in presence of bowel obstruction, constipation, or accumulation of pus or fluid. Inflammatory pain is deep and initially poorly localized, caused by irritation of either the visceral or the parietal peritoneum, as in acute appendicitis. Ischemic pain, the most serious type of visceral pain, has sudden onset, is intense, is progressive in severity, and is not relieved by analgesics. (Most common cause is strangulated bowel.)[8]*
- Investigate reports of pain out of proportion to degree of traumatic injury. *May reflect developing abdominal compartment syndrome.[12]*
- Inspect abdomen, noting contour. *Generalized distention may indicate presence of gas or fluid; local bulge could indicate hernia.[7] Distention of the bowel may indicate accumulation of fluids (salivary, gastric, pancreatic, biliary, intestinal) and gases formed from bacteria, swallowed air, or any food or fluid the client has consumed.[9]*

 Acute Care   Collaborative   Community/ Home Care   Cultural

- Auscultate abdomen. *Hypoactive bowel sounds may indicate ileus. Hyperactive bowel sounds may indicate early intestinal obstruction or irritable bowel or GI bleeding. Presence of bruit may indicate blood traveling through narrowed arteries such as aorta.*[9,11]
- Palpate abdomen *to note masses, enlarged organs (e.g., spleen, liver, portions of colon), elicitation of pain with touch, and pulsation of aorta.*[9-11]
- Measure abdominal girth and compare with client's customary waist size/belt length *to monitor development or progression of distention possibly reflecting intra-abdominal bleeding, infection, or edema associated with toxins.*[10,12]
- Note frequency and characteristics of bowel movements. *Bowel movements by themselves are not necessarily diagnostic but need to be considered in total assessment because many different manifestations can occur. For example, diarrhea is the cardinal symptom of gastroenteritis, with severity depending on the causative organism. Both diarrhea and constipation can result from medications. Bloody diarrhea may indicate presence of ulcerative colitis, obstruction, or upper or lower gastrointestinal bleeding.*[1,9,14]
- Note presence of nausea, with or without vomiting, and relationship to food intake or other events, if indicated. *History of nausea and vomiting can provide important information about cause. For example, systemic conditions such as pregnancy, gastroenteritis, cancers, myocardial infarction, hepatitis, systemic infections, drug toxicity are often accompanied by nausea and vomiting. Timing of vomiting may be important, too. For example, vomiting immediately after meals could be indicative of bulimia, or vomiting large amounts several hours after eating can indicate delayed gastric emptying.*[5]
- Evaluate client's current nutritional status, noting ability to ingest and digest food. Inquire about food intolerances. Observe client's reactions to food, such as reluctance or refusal to eat, anorexia, or anxiety—wants to eat but cannot retain food. *Health depends on the intake, digestion, and absorption of nutrients, which both affects and is affected by GI function.*
- Measure intra-abdominal pressure as indicated. *Tissue edema or free fluid collecting in the abdominal cavity leads to intra-abdominal hypertension, which, if untreated, can cause abdominal compartment syndrome with end-stage organ failure.*[12]

NURSING PRIORITY NO. 3 To correct/improve existing dysfunction:

- Collaborate in treatment of underlying conditions *to correct or treat disorders associated with clients' current GI dysfunction.*
- Maintain GI rest when indicated—NPO, fluids only, and gastric or intestinal decompression—*to reduce intestinal bloating and risk of vomiting.*
- Measure GI output periodically and note characteristics of drainage *to manage fluid losses and replacement needs and electrolyte balance.*
- Administer fluids and electrolytes as indicated *to replace losses and to improve GI circulation and function.*
- Encourage early ambulation. *Promotes general circulation and stimulates peristalsis and intestinal function.*
- Collaborate with dietician or nutritionist *to provide diet sufficient in nutrients by best possible route—oral, enteral, or parenteral.*
- Provide small servings of easily digested food and fluids when oral intake is tolerated.
- Encourage rest after meals *to maximize blood flow to digestive system.*
- Manage pain with medications as ordered and nonpharmacological interventions such as positioning, back rub, and heating pad (unless contraindicated) *to enhance muscle relaxation and reduce discomfort.*[7]
- Encourage client to report changes in nature or intensity of pain *as this may indicate worsening of condition, requiring more intensive interventions.*
- Collaborate with physician for medication management. *Oral medications can be absorbed erratically and can change the therapeutic effect or lead to increased side effects of a particular drug.*[15] *Dose modification, discontinuation of certain drugs (e.g., laxatives, opioids, antidepressants, iron supplements), or alternative route of administration may be required over a long period of time to improve client's GI function.*[14,17]

 Diagnostic Studies　　 Evidence Based Practice　　 Medications　　 Pediatric/Geriatric/Lifespan

- Prepare client for procedures and surgery as indicated. *May require a variety of interventions, including endoscopic procedures, appendectomy, bowel resection with/without ostomy, percutaneous transluminal angioplasty, abdominal-aortic bypass graft, mesenteric revascularization, endarterectomy, etc., to treat problem causing or contributing to severe GI dysfunction.*

NURSING PRIORITY NO. 4 To promote wellness (Teaching/Discharge Considerations):

- Provide information regarding cause of GI dysfunction and treatment plans, utilizing best learning methods for client and including written information and bibliography of other resources for postdischarge learning. *May help client/significant other to manage symptoms in a manner more acceptable to them if this is a long-term issue.*
- Discuss normal variations in bowel patterns *to help alleviate unnecessary concern, initiate planned interventions, or seek timely medical care. This may prevent overuse of laxatives or help client understand when food, fluid, or drug modifications are needed.*[14]
- Encourage discussion of feelings regarding prognosis and long-term effects of condition. *Major or unplanned life changes can strain coping abilities, impairing functioning and jeopardizing relationships, and may even result in depression.*
- Discuss value of relaxation and distraction techniques or counseling *if anxiety or other emotional/psychiatric issue is suspected to play a role in GI dysfunction.*[5]
- Identify necessary changes in lifestyle and assist client to incorporate disease management into activities of daily living. *Promotes independence and enhances self-concept regarding ability to deal with change and manage own needs.*
- Review specific dietary changes or restrictions with client. *The client with GI disturbances may need to make various adaptations in food choices and eating habits (e.g., may need to avoid overeating in general, schedule mealtime in relation to activities and bedtime, avoid certain foods [or food element, such as wheat or gluten] and/or alcohol).*
- Suggest healthier variations in preparation of foods, as indicated—broiled instead of fried, spices added to foods instead of salt, addition of higher fiber foods, and use of lactose-free dairy products—*when these factors are affecting GI health.*[11]
- Review use of dietary fiber as a means of managing constipation and incontinence. *Studies have shown that supplementation with dietary fiber from psyllium or gum arabic is associated with a decrease in incontinence and improved stool consistency.*[16]
- Discuss fluid intake appropriate to individual situation. *Water is necessary to general health and GI function. The individual may need encouragement and instruction about how to take in enough fluids or may need fluid restrictions for certain medical conditions.*
- Recommend maintenance of normal weight, or weight loss if client is obese, *to decrease risk associated with GI disorders such as GERD or gallbladder disease.*
- Recommend smoking cessation. *Risk for acquiring or exacerbating certain GI disorders (e.g., Crohn's disease) may be increased with smoking. A recent review of relevant studies revealed various deleterious short- and long-term effects of smoking on the GI circulation and organs.*[13]
- Discuss medication regimen, including reasons for/consequences of failure to take prescribed long-term maintenance therapy (e.g., client with ulcerative colitis may require continuous treatment with 5-aminosalicylates to maintain remission). *Although many reasons are given for failing to take medications as prescribed, including denial of illness, forgetfulness, and costs of prescriptions, nonadherence negatively affects treatment efficacy and client's quality of life.*[17]
- Emphasize importance of avoiding use of NSAIDs (including aspirin), corticosteroids, some over-the-counter drugs, vitamins containing potassium, mineral oil, or alcohol when taking anticoagulants. *These medications can be harmful to GI mucosa and increase risk of bleeding.*[9]
- Refer to NDs Constipation, bowel Incontinence, and Diarrhea for additional interventions, as needed.

Acute Care Collaborative Community/Home Care Cultural

DOCUMENTATION FOCUS

Assessment/Reassessment
- Individual findings, noting nature, extent, and duration of problem; effect on independence and lifestyle.
- Dietary pattern, recent intake, food intolerances.
- Frequency and characteristics of stools.
- Characteristics of abdominal tenderness or pain, precipitators, and what relieves pain.

Planning
- Plan of care and who is involved in planning.
- Teaching plan.

Implementation/Evaluation
- Response to interventions, teaching, and actions performed.
- Attainment or progress toward desired outcome(s).
- Modifications to plan of care.

Discharge Planning
- Long-term needs and who is responsible for actions to be taken.
- Available resources, specific referrals made.

References

1. Sommers, M. S., Johnson, S. A., Beery, T. A. (2007). *Diseases and Disorders: A Nursing Therapeutics Manual*. 3th ed. Philadelphia: F. A. Davis.
2. Neal-Boylan, L. (2007). Health assessment of the very old person at home. *Home Healthc Nurse*, 25(6), 388–398.
3. Tabloski, P. A. (2006). *Gerontological Nursing*. Upper Saddle River, NJ: Pearson Prentice Hall.
4. Pandey, K. R. (2017). Introduction to gastrointestinal physiology (Slide presentation). Retrieved March 2018 from https://www.slideshare.net/dipkari/1-introduction-to-gastrointestinal-physiology.
5. Scorza, K., et al. (2007). Evaluation of nausea and vomiting. *Am Fam Physician*, 76(1), 77–84.
6. Holcomb, S. S. (2008). Acute abdomen: What a pain! *Nursing*, 38(9), 34–40.
7. Sartin, J. S. (2005). Gastrointestinal disorders. In Copstead, L. E. C., Banasik, J. L. (eds). *Pathophysiology*. 3th ed. St. Louis, MO: Elsevier Saunders.
8. Schulman, C. (2002). End points of resuscitation: Choosing the right parameters to monitor. *Dimens Crit Care Nurs*, 21(1), 2–10.
9. Miller, S. K., Alpert, P. T. (2006). Assessment and differential diagnosis of abdominal pain. *Nurs Pract*, 31(7), 39–47.
10. Held-Warmkessel, J., Schiech, L. (2008). Responding to four gastrointestinal complications in cancer patients. *Nursing*, 38(7), 32–38.
11. Hogstel, M. O., Curry, L. C. (2005). *Health Assessment Through the Life Span*. 4th ed. Philadelphia: F. A. Davis.
12. Paula, R. (Updated 2017). Abdominal compartment syndrome. Retrieved March 2018 from http://emedicine.medscape.com/article/829008-overview.
13. Massarratt, S. (2008). Smoking and the gut: Review article. *Arch Iranian Med*, 11(3), 293–305.
14. Hill, R. (2007). Don't let constipation stop you up. *Nursing Made Incredibly Easy!*, 5(5), 40–47.
15. Feigenbaum, K. (2006). Update on gastroparesis. *Gastroenterol Nurs*, 29(3), 239–244.
16. Bliss, D. Z., et al. (2001). Supplementation with dietary fiber improves fecal incontinence. *Nurs Res*, 50(4), 203–213.
17. Turnbough, L., Wilson, L. (2007). Take your medicine: Nonadherence issues in patients with ulcerative colitis. *Gastroenterol Nurs*, 30(3), 212–217.
18. Song, R., Subbarao, G. C., Maheshwari, A. (2012). Hematological abnormalities in neonatal necrotizing enterocolitis. *J Matern Fetal Neonatal Med*, 25(4), 22–25.
19. Aziz, F., Comerota, A. J. (2016). Abdominal angina. Retrieved March 2018 from http://emedicine.medscape.com/article/188618-overview.

 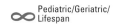

risk for dysfunctional Gastrointestinal Motility

Taxonomy II: Elimination and Exchange—Class 2 Gastrointestinal Function (00197) [**Diagnostic Division:** Elimination], Submitted 2008; Revised 2013, 2017

DEFINITION: Susceptible to increased, decreased, ineffective, or lack of peristaltic activity within the gastrointestinal system, which may compromise health.

RISK FACTORS
Anxiety; stressors
Change in water source; unsanitary food preparation
Eating habit change; malnutrition
Sedentary lifestyle; immobility
At Risk Population: Aging
Prematurity
Ingestion of contaminated material
Associated Condition: Decrease in gastrointestinal circulation; gastrointestinal reflux disease
Diabetes mellitus; infection
Enteral feedings; food intolerance
Pharmaceutical agent; treatment regimen
Sample Clinical Applications: Abdominal or intestinal surgery, eating disorders, malnutrition, celiac disease, anemia, anxiety disorders, biliary cancer, cholecystectomy, Crohn's disease, irritable bowel syndrome, GERD, gastritis, pancreatitis, quadriplegia, peritoneal dialysis, botulism, sepsis, multiple organ dysfunction syndrome, radiation therapy

DESIRED OUTCOMES/EVALUATION CRITERIA

Sample **NOC** linkages:
Gastrointestinal Function: Ability of the gastrointestinal tract to ingest and digest food products, absorb nutrients, and eliminate waste
Knowledge: Treatment Regimen: Extent of understanding conveyed about a specific treatment regimen

Client Will (Include Specific Time Frame)
• Maintain normal pattern of bowel functioning.
• Verbalize understanding of individual risk factors and benefits of managing condition.
• Identify preventive interventions to reduce risk and promote normal bowel pattern.

ACTIONS/INTERVENTIONS

Sample **NIC** linkages:
Bowel Management: Establishment and management of a regular pattern of bowel elimination
Tube Care: Gastrointestinal: Management of a patient with a gastrointestinal tube
Nutrition Management: Providing and promoting a balanced intake of nutrients

NURSING PRIORITY NO. 1   To identify individual risk factors/needs:

• Note presence of conditions affecting systemic circulation and perfusion such as congestive heart failure, major trauma, sepsis, etc. *Blood loss or shock can result in hypoperfusion, and short- or long-term GI dysfunction.*[1]

 Acute Care   Collaborative   Community/Home Care   Cultural

- Determine presence of disorders causing localized or diffuse reduction in GI blood flow (e.g., esophageal varices, intestinal cancer, or obstruction; intestinal surgery; pancreatitis; prior history of bowel obstruction or strangulated hernia; prior abdominal surgery with adhesions) *to identify client at higher risk for changes in peristaltic activity and intestinal dysfunction.*[2,13]
- Note client's age and developmental concerns. *Children are prone to infections causing gastroenteritis manifested by vomiting and diarrhea.*[1] *The elderly have problems associated with decreased motility (e.g., constipation is often a concern related to slower peristalsis, lack of sufficient fiber and fluid intake, chronic use of laxatives).*[3,4] *Premature or low-birth-weight neonates are at risk for developing necrotizing enterocolitis.*[5]
- Assess client's current situation with regard to prior GI history. *Client may have an isolated incident putting him/her at risk (e.g., blunt force trauma to abdomen) or at higher risk for recurrent GI dysfunction associated with history of prior GI problems.*
- Auscultate abdomen *to evaluate peristaltic activity. For example, either hypoactive or hyperactive bowel sounds may indicate developing bowel disorders.*[9,10]
- Palpate abdomen for masses, enlarged organs (e.g., spleen, liver, portions of colon), and elicitation of pain with touch *that could point to changes in organ size or function.*[9–11]
- Note frequency and characteristics of bowel movements. *Bowel movements by themselves are not necessarily diagnostic but need to be considered in total assessment because many different manifestations can occur.*[1,9,12]
- Ascertain presence and characteristics of abdominal pain. *Pain is a common symptom of GI disorders, with location and type aiding in identifying underlying problems.*[8]
- Assess vital signs for changes in blood pressure, heart rate, or body temperature. *May suggest injury or infection of the GI organs or development of a systemic infection/sepsis.*
- Evaluate client's current nutritional status, noting ability to ingest and digest food. *Health depends on the intake, digestion, and absorption of nutrients, which both affects and is affected by GI function.*
- Note lifestyle issues *that can affect GI function (e.g., people who regularly engage in competitive sports such as long-distance running, cycling), persons with poor sanitary living conditions, people who travel to areas with contaminated food or water, overeating or intake of foods associated with gastric distress or intestinal distention, and anorexia or bulimia.*[6]
- Ascertain whether client is experiencing acute, extreme, or chronic anxiety; stress; or other psychogenic factors present in person with emotional or psychiatric disorders (including anorexia and bulimia), *which can affect GI function.*[7]
- Review client's drug regimen. *Medications such as laxatives, antibiotics, anticholesterol agents, opiates, sedatives, and iron preparations may cause or exacerbate intestinal issues. In addition, likelihood of bleeding increases from use of medications such as NSAIDs, Coumadin, and Plavix.*[3,4]
- Review laboratory and other diagnostic studies *to identify if conditions or disorders are present that may affect GI system or GI function.*

NURSING PRIORITY NO. 2 To reduce or correct individual risk factors:

- Discuss normal variations in bowel patterns *so client can initiate planned interventions or seek timely medical care. This may prevent complications, such as overuse of laxatives, or help client understand when regular exercise or food, fluid, or drug modifications are needed to improve or maintain GI health.*
- Collaborate in treatment of underlying conditions *to correct or treat disorders that could impact GI function.*
- Practice and promote hand hygiene and other infection precautions *to prevent transmission of infections that may cause/spread GI illnesses.*
- Maintain GI rest when indicated (e.g., NPO, fluids only, gastric or intestinal decompression after abdominal surgery) *to reduce intestinal bloating and reduce risk of vomiting.*
- Administer fluids and electrolytes as indicated *to replace losses and to maintain GI circulation and function.*

 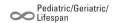

- Administer prescribed prophylactic medications (e.g., antiemetics, proton-pump inhibitors, antihistamines, anticholinergics, antibiotics) *to reduce potential for GI complications such as bleeding, ulceration of stomach mucosa, and viral diarrheas.*
- Collaborate with dietician or nutritionist *to provide diet sufficient in nutrients and provided by best possible route (e.g., oral, enteral, parenteral).*[2,14]
- Emphasize importance of and assist with early ambulation and ongoing exercise following surgery or other procedures. Assist client with mobility issues and refer to physical therapy as indicated *to help reduce GI complications associated with immobility and a sedentary lifestyle.*
- Encourage relaxation and distraction techniques if anxiety is suspected to play a role in GI dysfunction.[7]
- Refer to NDs Constipation, bowel Incontinence, Diarrhea, and dysfunctional Gastrointestinal Motility for additional interventions.

NURSING PRIORITY NO. 3 To promote wellness (Teaching/Discharge Considerations):

- Review measures to maintain bowel health:
  - Use of dietary fiber and/or stool softeners. *Studies have shown that supplementation with dietary fiber from psyllium or gum arabic is associated with a decrease in incontinence and improved stool consistency.*[12,15]
  - Fluid intake appropriate to individual. *Water is necessary to general health and GI function. The individual may need encouragement and instruction about how to take in enough fluids or may need fluid restrictions for certain medical conditions.*
  - Establish or maintain regular bowel evacuation habits, incorporating privacy needs, assistance to bathroom on regular schedule, etc., as indicated.
  - Emphasize benefits of regular exercise in promoting normal GI function.
- Discuss dietary recommendations with client/significant other. *The client with potential for GI disturbances may elect to make adaptations in food choices and eating habits (e.g., to avoid overeating in general, schedule mealtime in relation to activities and bedtime, avoid certain foods and/or alcohol).*
- Instruct in healthier variations in preparation of foods as indicated (e.g., broiled instead of fried, spices added to foods instead of salt, addition of higher fiber foods, lactose-free dairy products) *when these factors may affect GI health.*
- Recommend maintenance of normal weight, or weight loss if client is obese, *to decrease risk associated with GI disorders such as GERD or gallbladder disease.*
- Collaborate with physician in medication management. *Oral medications can be absorbed erratically and can change the therapeutic effect or lead to increased side effects of a particular drug.*[16] *Dose modification, discontinuation of certain drugs (e.g., laxatives, opioids, antidepressants, iron supplements), or alternative route of administration may be required over a long period of time to reduce risk of GI dysfunction.*[12,17]
- Emphasize importance of discussing with physician current and new prescribed medications and/or planned use of certain medications (e.g., NSAIDs [including aspirin], corticosteroids, some over-the-counter drugs, herbals supplements), *which can be harmful to GI mucosa.*
- Recommend smoking cessation. *Risk for acquiring or exacerbating certain GI disorders (e.g., Crohn's disease) may be increased with smoking. Note: A recent review of relevant studies reveals various deleterious short- and long-term effects of smoking on GI circulation and organs.*[19]
- Review food- and water-borne illnesses and contamination and hygiene issues, as indicated, and make needed follow-up referrals. *Many different types of viruses, bacteria, and parasites can cause GI illnesses. This can affect a household, a day-care center, a college dorm, international travelers, or a whole segment of population. Information may be given to individuals, groups, and/or public in general.*
- Refer to appropriate resources (e.g., social services, public health services) for follow-up if client is at risk for ingestion of contaminated water or food sources or would benefit from teaching concerning food preparation and storage.
- Encourage vaccinations. *The Centers for Disease Control and Prevention make recommendations for travelers and/or persons in high-risk areas or situations to receive certain vaccinations. Typhoid vaccine, for*

 Acute Care   Collaborative   Community/ Home Care   Cultural

example, is indicated for travel to areas where a person might be exposed to contaminated food or water. For young children susceptible to severe gastroenteritis, the oral rotavirus vaccine can prevent 85% to 98% of rotavirus gastroenteritis.[18,20]

DOCUMENTATION FOCUS

Assessment/Reassessment
- Individual findings, noting specific risk factors.
- Dietary pattern, recent intake, food intolerances.
- Frequency and characteristics of stools.

Planning
- Plan of care and who is involved in planning.
- Teaching plan.

Implementation/Evaluation
- Response to interventions, teaching, and actions performed.
- Attainment or progress toward desired outcome(s).
- Modifications to plan of care.

Discharge Planning
- Long-term needs and who is responsible for actions to be taken.
- Available resources and specific referrals made.

References

1. Sommers, M. S., Johnson, S. A., Beery, T. A. (2007). *Diseases and Disorders: A Nursing Therapeutics Manual.* 3th ed. Philadelphia: F. A. Davis.
2. Goldberg, S. M. (2008). Identifying intestinal obstruction: Better safe than sorry. *Nurs Crit Care,* 3(5), 18–23.
3. Neal-Boylan, L. (2007). Health assessment of the very old person at home. *Home Healthc Nurs,* 25(6), 388–398.
4. Tabloski, P. A. (ed.) (2006). *Gerontological Nursing.* Upper Saddle River, NJ: Pearson Prentice Hall.
5. Song, R., Subbarao, G. C., Maheshwari, A. (2012). Hematological abnormalities in neonatal necrotizing enterocolitis. *J Matern Fetal Neonatal Med.,* 25(4), 22–25.
6. Pandey, K. R. (2017). Introduction to gastrointestinal physiology (Slide presentation). Retrieved March 2017 from https://www.slideshare.net/dipkari/1-introduction-to-gastrointestinal-physiology.
7. Scorza, K., et al. (2007). Evaluation of nausea and vomiting. *Am Fam Physician,* 76(1), 77–84.
8. Holcomb, S. S. (2008). Acute abdomen: What a pain! *Nursing,* 38(9), 34–40.
9. Miller, S. K., Alpert, P. T. (2006). Assessment and differential diagnosis of abdominal pain. *Nurse Pract,* 31(7), 39–47.
10. Hogstel, M. O., Curry, L. C. (2005). *Health Assessment Through the Life Span.* 4th ed. Philadelphia: F. A. Davis.
11. Held-Warmkessel, J., Schiech, L. (2008). Responding to four gastrointestinal complications in cancer patients. *Nursing,* 38(7), 32–38.
12. Hill, R. (2007). Don't let constipation stop you up. *Nursing Made Incredibly Easy!,* 5(5), 40–47.
13. Paula, R. (Updated 2017). Abdominal compartment syndrome. Retrieved March 2018 from http://emedicine.medscape.com/article/829008-overview.
14. Glare, P. A., et al. (2008). Treatment of nausea and vomiting in terminally ill cancer patients. *Drugs,* 68(18), 2575–2590.
15. Bliss, D. Z., et al. (2001). Supplementation with dietary fiber improves fecal incontinence. *Nurs Res,* 50(4), 203–213.
16. Feigenbaum, K. (2006). Update on gastroparesis. *Gastroenterol Nurs,* 29(3), 239–244.
17. Day, M. W. (2008). Fight back against inflammatory bowel disease. *Nursing,* 38(11), 34–40.
18. Centers for Disease Control and Prevention (CDC). (Updated 2018). Vaccines and immunizations, (Index to various pages). Retrieved March 2018 from https://www.cdc.gov/vaccines/schedules/hcp/.
19. Massarratt, S. (2008). Smoking and the gut: Review article. *Arch Iranian Med,* 11(3), 34–40.
20. Cortese, M. M., Parashar, U. D. (2009). Prevention of rotavirus gastroenteritis among infants and children. Recommendations of the Advisory Committee on Immunization Practices. *Centers for Disease Control and Prevention.* Retrieved March 2018 from http://www.cdc.gov/mmwr/preview/mmwrhtml/rr5802a1.htm.

 Diagnostic Studies   Evidence Based Practice   Medications 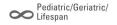 Pediatric/Geriatric/Lifespan

[risk for ineffective Gastrointestinal Perfusion]

Taxonomy II: Activity/Rest Class 4: Cardiovascular/Pulmonary Responses (00202) [**Diagnostic Division:** Circulation], Submitted 2008; Revised 2013

[**DEFINITION:** Susceptible to decrease in gastrointestinal circulation, which may compromise health.]

[RISK FACTORS]

Abdominal aortic aneurysm; abdominal compartment syndrome

Abnormal prothrombin time (PT); abnormal partial thromboplastin time (PTT); coagulopathy (e.g., sickle cell anemia); anemia; disseminated intravascular coagulopathy; hemodynamic instability

Age >60 years; female gender

Cerebral vascular accident; vascular disease; diabetes mellitus

Gastrointestinal (GI) condition (e.g., ulcer, ischemic colitis or pancreatitis); acute gastrointestinal hemorrhage; gastroesophageal varices

Impaired liver function (e.g., cirrhosis, hepatitis)

Myocardial infarction; decrease in left ventricular performance

Renal disease (e.g., polycystic kidney, renal artery stenosis, failure)

Smoking

Trauma; treatment regimen

Sample Clinical Applications: Gastrointestinal (GI) bleed, atherosclerosis, sickle cell anemia, diabetes, pancreatitis, congestive heart failure (CHF), cirrhosis, hemorrhage shock

DESIRED OUTCOMES/EVALUATION CRITERIA

Sample NOC linkages:

Tissue Perfusion: Abdominal Organs: Adequacy of blood flow through the small vessels of the abdominal viscera to maintain organ function

Gastrointestinal Function: Extent to which foods (ingested or tube-fed) are moved from ingestion to evacuation

Client Will (Include Specific Time Frame)

• Demonstrate adequate tissue perfusion as evidenced by active bowel sounds and absence of abdominal pain, nausea, and vomiting.

• Verbalize understanding of condition, therapy regimen, side effects of medication, and when to contact healthcare provider.

• Engage in behaviors or lifestyle changes to improve circulation (e.g., smoking cessation, diabetic glucose control, medication management).

ACTIONS/INTERVENTIONS

Sample NIC linkages:

Surveillance: Purposeful and ongoing acquisition, interpretation, and synthesis of patient data for clinical decision making

Circulatory Care: Arterial Insufficiency: Promotion of arterial circulation

Gastrointestinal Intubation: Insertion of a tube into the GI tract

 Acute Care   Collaborative   Community/Home Care   Cultural

NURSING PRIORITY NO. 1 To assess causative/contributing factors:

- Note presence of conditions affecting systemic circulation/perfusion such as heart failure with left ventricular dysfunction, major trauma with hypotension, surgery with major blood loss, septic shock, and so forth. *Blood loss and hypovolemic or hypotensive shock can result in GI hypoperfusion and bowel ischemia.*[1]
- Determine presence of disorders such as esophageal varices, pancreatitis, abdominal or chest trauma, increase of intra-abdominal pressure or abdominal hypertension, prior history of bowel obstruction or strangulated hernia, or prior abdominal surgery with adhesions *that could cause local or regional reduction in GI blood flow.*[2–5,22]
- Identify client with history of bleeding or coagulation disorders, such as prior GI bleed, sickle cell anemia, or other coagulopathies and cancer, *to identify risk for potential bleeding problems complicating current situation (e.g., client having elective surgical procedure) or exacerbation of comorbidities.*
- Note client's age and gender. *Studies suggest that risk increases with age in both sexes and that risk is higher in men than women when assessing risk for GI bleed and abdominal aortic aneurysm.*[1,6] *Premature or low-birth-weight neonates are at risk for developing necrotizing enterocolitis.*[21]
- Investigate reports of abdominal pain, noting location, intensity, duration, and relationship to activities (e.g., eating, lifting heavy objects), trauma, surgery, or acute or chronic conditions causing displacement of abdominal organs accompanied by abdominal distention (e.g., peritonitis, cirrhosis, ascites, etc.). *Many disorders can result in abdominal pain, some of which can include conditions affecting GI perfusion, such as postprandial abdominal angina due to occlusive mesenteric vascular disease, abdominal compartment syndrome, or other potential perforating disorders such as a duodenal or gastric ulcer or ischemic pancreatitis.*[4,7,8]
- Review routine medication regimen (e.g., NSAIDs, Coumadin, low-dose aspirin such as used for prophylaxis in certain cardiovascular conditions, corticosteroids). *Likelihood of bleeding increases from use of such medications.*[9–11]
- Note history of smoking, *which can potentiate vasoconstriction,* or excessive alcohol use or abuse, *which can cause general inflammation of the stomach mucosa and potentiate risk of GI bleeding or liver involvement and esophageal varices.*
- Auscultate abdomen to evaluate peristaltic activity. *Hypoactive or absent bowel sounds may indicate intraperitoneal injury and bowel perforation and bleeding. Abdominal bruit can indicate abdominal aortic injury or aneurysm.*[5]
- Palpate abdomen for distension, masses, enlarged organs (e.g., spleen, liver, or portions of colon), elicitation of pain with touch, and pulsation of aorta, *which could identify problem in GI organs or circulation system.*[12–14]
- Percuss abdomen for fixed or shifting dullness over regions that normally contain air. *Can indicate accumulated blood or fluid.*[15]
- Measure and monitor progression of abdominal girth as indicated. *Abdominal distention can reflect bowel problems such as ileus or other bowel obstruction. It may also be indicative of organ failure (e.g., heart, liver, kidney) or organ injury or enlargement/displacement with intra-abdominal fluid and gas accumulation. These conditions can cause or exacerbate GI perfusion problems.*[8]
- Note reports of nausea or vomiting along with problems with elimination. *May reflect hypoperfusion of the GI tract, which is particularly vulnerable to even small decreases in circulating volume.*[16]
- Assess client with severe or prolonged vomiting, forceful coughing, lifting and straining activities, or childbirth, *which can result in a tear in the esophageal or stomach wall resulting in hemorrhage.*
- Evaluate stools for color and consistency. Test for occult blood, as indicated. *If bleeding is present, stools may be black or "tarry," currant-colored, or bright red. Consistency can range from normal with occult blood to thick liquid stools.*[1]
- Assess vital signs noting sustained hypotension, *which can result in hypoperfusion of abdominal organs.*
- Test gastric suction contents for blood when tube is used to decompress stomach and/or manage vomiting. *Can help in early identification of bleeding complications.*

 Diagnostic Studies   Evidence Based Practice   Medications   Pediatric/Geriatric/Lifespan

- Review laboratory tests and other diagnostic studies (e.g., complete blood count, bilirubin, liver enzymes, electrolytes, stool guaiac; endoscopy, abdominal ultrasound or computed tomography, aortic angiography, paracentesis) *to identify if conditions or disorders are present that may affect GI perfusion and function.*[8,13]
- Measure intra-abdominal pressure as indicated. *Tissue edema or free fluid collecting in the abdominal cavity leads to intra-abdominal hypertension, which, if untreated, can cause abdominal compartment syndrome with end-stage organ failure.*[23]

NURSING PRIORITY NO. 2   To reduce or correct individual risk factors:

- Collaborate in treatment of underlying conditions *to correct or treat disorders that could affect GI perfusion.*
- Administer fluids and electrolytes as indicated *to replace losses and to maintain GI circulation and function.*
- Administer prescribed prophylactic medications in at-risk clients during illness and hospitalization (e.g., antiemetics, proton-pump inhibitors, antihistamines, anticholinergics, antibiotics) *to reduce potential for stress-related GI complications such as bleeding and ulceration of stomach mucosa.*[17,18]
- Maintain gastric or intestinal decompression; when indicated, measure output periodically and note characteristics of drainage.
- Provide small and easily digested food and fluids when oral intake is tolerated.
- Encourage rest after meals *to maximize blood flow to digestive system.*
- Prepare client for surgery as indicated. *May be a surgical emergency (e.g., gastric resection, bypass graft, mesenteric endarterectomy).*
- Refer to NDs dysfunctional Gastrointestinal Motility, risk for Bleeding, Nausea, and imbalanced Nutrition: less than body requirements for additional interventions.

NURSING PRIORITY NO. 3   To promote wellness (Teaching/Discharge Considerations):

- Discuss individual risk factors (e.g., family history, obesity, age, smoking, hypertension, diabetes, clotting disorders) and potential outcomes of atherosclerosis (e.g., systemic and peripheral vascular disease conditions). *Information necessary for client to make informed choices about remedial risk factors and commit to lifestyle changes as appropriate to prevent onset of complications or manage symptoms when condition is present.*
- Identify necessary changes in lifestyle and assist client to incorporate disease management into activities of daily living. *Promotes independence and enhances self-concept regarding ability to deal with change and manage own needs.*
- Encourage client to quit smoking and join smoking-cessation programs or support groups.
- Establish regular exercise program *to enhance circulation and promote general well-being.*[19]
- Emphasize importance of routine follow-up and laboratory monitoring as indicated. *Important for effective disease management and possible changes in therapeutic regimen.*
- Emphasize importance of discussing with primary care provider current and new prescribed medications and/or planned use of certain medications (e.g., anticoagulants, NSAIDs including aspirin; corticosteroids, some over-the-counter drugs, herbal supplements), *which can be harmful to GI mucosa or cause bleeding.*[20]

DOCUMENTATION FOCUS

Assessment/Reassessment
- Individual findings, noting specific risk factors.
- Vital signs, adequacy of circulation.
- Abdominal assessment, characteristics of emesis/gastric drainage and stools.

Planning
- Plan of care and who is involved in planning.
- Teaching plan.

Implementation/Evaluation
- Response to interventions, teaching, and actions performed.
- Attainment or progress toward desired outcome(s).
- Modifications to plan of care.

Discharge Planning
- Long-term needs and who is responsible for actions to be taken.
- Available resources, specific referrals made.

References

1. Sommers, M. S., Johnson, S. A., Beery, T. A. (2007). *Diseases and Disorders: A Nursing Therapeutics Manual*. 3th ed. Philadelphia: F. A. Davis.
2. Goldberg, S. M. (2008). Identifying intestinal obstruction: Better safe than sorry. *Nurs Crit Care*, 3(5), 18–25.
3. Feigenbaum, K. (2006). Update on gastroparesis. *Gastroenterol Nurs*, 29(3), 239–244.
4. Kelso, L. A. (2008). Cirrhosis: Caring for patients with end-stage liver failure. *Nurse Pract*, 33(7), 24–30.
5. Blank-Reid, C. (2007). Abdominal trauma: Dealing with the damage. *Nursing*, 37(4 Suppl: ED), 4–11.
6. Tan, W. A., Powell, S., Nanjundappa, A. (Updated 2016). Abdominal aortic aneurysm, rupture imaging. Retrieved March 2018 from http://emedicine.medscape.com/article/416397-overview.
7. Aziz, F., Comerota, A. J. (Updated 2016). Abdominal angina. Retrieved March 2018 from http://emedicine.medscape.com/article/188618-overview.
8. Paula, R. (Updated 2017). Compartment syndrome, abdominal. Retrieved March 2018 from http://emedicine.medscape.com/article/829008-overview.
9. Neal-Boylan, L. (2007). Health assessment of the very old person at home. *Home Healthc Nurse*, 25(6), 388–398.
10. Tabloski, P. A. (ed.) (2006). *Gerontological Nursing*. Upper Saddle River, NJ: Pearson Prentice Hall.
11. Estes, K., Thomure, J. (2008). Aspirin for the primary prevention of adverse cardiovascular events. *Crit Care Nurs Q*, 31(4), 324–338.
12. Miller, S. K., Alpert, P. T. (2006). Assessment and differential diagnosis of abdominal pain. *Nurse Pract*, 31(7), 39–47.
13. Hogstel, M. O., Curry, L. C. (2005). *Health Assessment Through the Life Span*. 4th ed. Philadelphia: F. A. Davis.
14. Held-Warmkessel, J., Schiech, L. (2008). Responding to 4 gastrointestinal complications in cancer patients. *Nursing*, 38(7), 32–38.
15. Dietzen, K. K. (2006). Assessment of the Gastrointestinal System. In Ignatavicius, D. D., Workman, M. L. (eds). *Medical-Surgical Nursing: Critical Thinking for Collaborative Care*. 5th ed. St. Louis, MO: Elsevier Saunders.
16. Schulman, J., Schiech, C. (2002). End points of resuscitation: Choosing the right parameters to monitor. *Dimens Crit Care Nurs*, 21(1), 2–10.
17. Singh, H., et al. (2008). Gastrointestinal prophylaxis in critically ill patients. *Crit Care Nurs Q*, 31(4), 291–301.
18. Chey, W. D., Wong, B. C. Y. (2007). American College of Gastroenterology guideline on the management of *Helicobacter pylori* infection. *Am J Gastroenterol*, 102, 1808–1825.
19. Frost, K. L., Topp, R. (2006). A physical activity Rx for the hypertensive patient. *Nurse Pract*, 31(4), 29–37.
20. Turnbough, L., Wilson, L. (2007). Take your medicine: Nonadherence issues in patients with ulcerative colitis. *Gastroenterol Nurs*, 30(3), 212–217.
21. Bin-Nun, A., Bromiker, R., Wilschanski, M. (2005). Oral probiotics prevent necrotizing enterocolitis in very low birth weight neonates. *J Pediatr*, 147(2), 192–196.
22. Cheatham, M. L. (2009). Abdominal compartment syndrome: Pathophysiology and definitions. *Scand J Trauma, Resusc Emer Med*, 17(10).
23. Hunter, J. D., Damani, Z. (2004). Intra-abdominal hypertension and the abdominal compartment syndrome. *Anaesthesia*, 59(9), 899–907.

 Diagnostic Studies   Evidence Based Practice   Medications 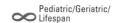 Pediatric/Geriatric/Lifespan

Grieving

Taxonomy II: Coping/Stress Tolerance—Class 2 Coping Responses (00136) [**Diagnostic Division:** Ego Integrity], Approved as anticipatory Grieving 1980; Revised 1996, 2006, 2017

DEFINITION: A normal complex process that includes emotional, physical, spiritual, social, and intellectual responses and behaviors by which individuals, families, and communities incorporate an actual, anticipated, or perceived loss into their daily lives.

RELATED FACTORS
To Be Developed

DEFINING CHARACTERISTICS

Subjective
Anger; pain; distress; suffering; despair; blaming
Alterations in activity level, sleep pattern, dream pattern
Finding meaning in a loss; personal growth
Guilt about feeling relief

Objective
Detachment; disorganization; psychological distress; panic behavior
Maintaining a connection to the deceased
Alterations in immune or neuroendocrine functioning
At Risk Population: Anticipatory loss of significant other or significant object
Death or loss of significant other
Sample Clinical Applications: Cancer, traumatic injuries (e.g., brain or spinal cord), amputation, chronic or debilitating conditions (e.g., renal failure, chronic obstructive pulmonary disease [COPD], multiple sclerosis [MS], amyotrophic lateral sclerosis [ALS]), genetic or birth defects, community disaster

DESIRED OUTCOMES/EVALUATION CRITERIA

Sample NOC linkages:
Grief Resolution: Personal actions to adjust thoughts, feelings, and behaviors to actual or impending loss
Psychosocial Adjustment: Life Change: Adaptive psychosocial response of an individual to significant life circumstance
Caregiver Emotional Health: Emotional well-being of a family care provider while caring for a family member

Client Will (Include Specific Time Frame)
- Identify and express feelings (e.g., sadness, guilt, fear) freely and effectively.
- Acknowledge impact or effect of the grieving process (e.g., physical problems of eating, sleeping) and seek appropriate help.
- Look toward and plan for future 1 day at a time.

Sample NOC linkages:
Community Competence: Capacity of a community to collectively problem-solve to achieve community goals

 Acute Care Collaborative Community/ Home Care Cultural

Community Will (Include Specific Time Frame)
• Recognize needs of citizens, including underserved population.
• Activate or develop plan to address identified needs.

ACTIONS/INTERVENTIONS

Sample NIC linkages:
Grief Work Facilitation: Assistance with the resolution of a significant loss
Grief Work Facilitation: Perinatal Death: Assistance with the resolution of a perinatal loss
Dying Care: Promotion of physical comfort and psychological peace in the final phase of life

NURSING PRIORITY NO. 1   To assess causative/contributing factors:

• Determine circumstances of current situation (e.g., sudden death, prolonged fatal illness, loved one kept alive by extreme medical interventions). *Grief can be anticipatory (mourning the loss of loved one's former self before actual death) or actual. Both types of grief can provoke a wide range of intense and often conflicting feelings. Grief also follows losses other than death (e.g., traumatic loss of a limb, or loss of home by a tornado, loss of known self due to brain injury).*[11]
• Determine significance of loss to community (e.g., school bus accident with loss of life, major storm with damage to community infrastructure, financial failure of major employer).
• Determine client's perception of anticipated or actual loss and meaning to him or her. "What are your concerns?" "What are your fears? Your greatest fear?" "How do you see this affecting you and your lifestyle?" *Identifying the needs to be addressed and acknowledging the client's responses are integral to planning care.*[9] *Some individuals may use anticipatory grieving as a defense against the inevitable loss. While some people may find this helpful when the loss occurs, many people find that intense feelings occur regardless of the period of anticipation.*[2]
• Ascertain response of family/significant others (SOs) to client's situation/concerns. *Family concerns affect client and need to be listened to and appropriate interventions taken. Problems may arise if family completes grieving prematurely and disengages from the dying member, who then feels abandoned at a time when the support is needed.*[2]

NURSING PRIORITY NO. 2   To determine current response:

• Note emotional responses, such as withdrawal, angry behavior, and crying. Provide information about normal stages of grieving. *Awareness allows for appropriate choice of interventions because individuals handle grief in different ways. Knowledge promotes understanding of emotional responses.*[4]
• Observe client's body language and check out meaning with the client. Note congruency of body language with verbalizations. *Body language is open to interpretation and needs to be validated so that misinterpretation does not occur. Client may be saying one thing, but often body language is saying something else; identifying incongruencies can provide opportunity for individual to understand self in relation to grieving process.*[2]
• Note cultural and religious factors and expectations that may impact client's responses to situation. *Beliefs vary with the individual/community and will affect responses to the situation (e.g., Arab Americans may want to pray in silence or private, African Americans may use faith and healers in conjunction with biomedical resources, groups may congregate at site of disaster or at church to grieve together).*[5,8]
• Determine impact on general well-being (e.g., increased frequency of minor illnesses, exacerbation of chronic condition, problems with eating, activity level, sexual desire, role performance [e.g., work, parenting]). *Indicators of severity of feelings client is experiencing and need for specific interventions to resolve these issues.*

 Diagnostic Studies   Evidence Based Practice   Medications   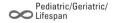 Pediatric/Geriatric/Lifespan

- Note family communication and interaction patterns. *Dysfunctional patterns of communication such as avoidance, preaching, and giving advice, can block effective communication and isolate family members.*[3]
- Discuss with client and family/SOs, and others as appropriate plans that need to be made as well as anticipated adjustments and role changes related to the situation. Encourage and answer questions as needed. *This type of discussion will bring concerns out in the open and help with adaptation to the loss.*[5,11]
- Determine availability and use of community resources and support groups. *Appropriate use of support can help the individual feel less isolated and can promote feelings of inclusion and comfort.*[2]
- Note community plans in place to deal with major loss (e.g., team of crisis counselors stationed at a school to address the loss of classmates, vocational counselors or retraining programs, outreach of services from neighboring communities).

NURSING PRIORITY NO. 3   To assist client/community to deal with situation:

- Provide open environment and trusting relationship. *Promotes a free discussion of feelings and concerns in a safe environment where client can reveal innermost fears and beliefs about anticipated loss.*[2]
- Use therapeutic communication skills of active-listening, silence, and acknowledgment. Respect client desire or request not to talk. *These skills convey belief in ability of client to deal with situation and develop a sense of competence. Client may not be ready to discuss feelings and situation, and respecting client's own time line conveys confidence.*[2]
- ∞ Inform children about the anticipated or actual death or loss in age-appropriate language. *Providing accurate information about loss or change in life situation will help the child begin the mourning process.*[10]
- ∞ Give permission to child to express feelings about situation and ask questions, being careful to provide honest answers within child's understanding. *Adults may be uncomfortable or upset talking about death or loss, and children may be excluded from adult conversation about what is happening.*[10]
- ∞ Provide puppets or play therapy for toddlers/young children. *Young children do not have the ability to express their feelings verbally; use of play may help them express grief and help deal with loss in ways that are appropriate to age.*[2]
- Permit appropriate expressions of anger, fear. Note hostility toward spiritual power or feelings of abandonment. *Anger is a normal part of the grieving process, and talking about these feelings allows individual to think about them and move on, coming to some resolution regarding the anticipated loss.*[2] (Refer to ND Spiritual Distress for additional interventions.)
- Provide information about normalcy of individual grief reaction. *Many people are not familiar with grief and are concerned that what they are experiencing is not normal. Letting them know that grief takes many forms and what they are feeling is all right helps them deal with what is happening.*[6,9]
- Be honest when answering questions, providing information. *Enhances nurse-client relationship, promoting trust and confidence.*[2]
- ∞ Provide assurance to child that cause for situation is not his or her own doing, bearing in mind age and developmental level. *May lessen sense of guilt and affirm there is no need to assign blame to self or any family member.*[2]
- Provide hope within parameters of individual situation. *Assisting client to find the positives will help with management of current situation.* Do not give false reassurance. *Comments such as "Everything will be all right" or "Don't worry" are not helpful and convey lack of understanding to the client.*[2]
- Review past life experiences and previous loss(es), role changes, and coping skills used, noting strengths and successes. *Useful in dealing with current situation and problem-solving existing needs.*[4]
- Discuss control issues, such as what is in the power of the individual to change and what is beyond control. *Recognition of these factors helps client focus energy for maximal benefit and outcome on what can be done.*[4]
- Incorporate family/SO(s) in problem solving. *Encourages family to support and assist client to deal with situation while meeting needs of family members.*[2]
- Determine client's status and role in family (e.g., parent, sibling, child) and address loss of family member role. *Client's illness affects usual activities in the role he or she has in the family and inevitably affects all the other family members as responsibilities are taken over by them.*[2]

 Acute Care   Collaborative   Community/ Home Care   Cultural

- Instruct in use of visualization and relaxation techniques. *These skills can be helpful to reduce anxiety and stress and help client and family members manage grief more effectively.*[7]
- 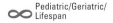 Use sedatives or tranquilizers with caution. *While the use of these medications may be helpful in the short term, dependence on them may retard passage through the grief process.*[2,6]
- Mobilize resources when client is the community. *When anticipated loss affects community as a whole, such as closing of manufacturing plant, impending disaster (e.g., wildfire, hurricane, terrorist concerns), multiple supports will be required to deal with size and complexity of situation. Indeed, when more people are directly or indirectly involved in the anticipated or actual loss, emotions and anxiety tend to be amplified and transmitted, thus complicating the situation.*[1,12]
- Encourage community members/groups to engage in talking about event or loss and verbalizing feelings. Seek out underserved populations to include in process. *Increases likelihood that the needs of the entire community are identified and addressed.*
- Encourage individuals to participate in activities to deal with loss and rebuild community. *Exercising control in a productive manner empowers individuals and promotes rebuilding of life and community.*

NURSING PRIORITY NO. 4   To promote wellness (Teaching/Discharge Considerations):

- Provide information that feelings are okay and are to be expressed appropriately. Set limits regarding destructive behavior. *Talking about feelings can facilitate the grieving process, but destructive behavior can be damaging to self-esteem.*[2]
- Discuss recurring nature of grief reactions. *On birthdays, major holidays, at times of significant personal events, or anniversary of loss, intense grief reactions may occur for a long time after the loss. If these reactions start to disrupt day-to-day functioning, client may need to seek help.*[1] (Refer to NDs such as ineffective community Coping, complicated Grieving.)
- Encourage continuation of usual activities and schedule and involvement in appropriate exercise program, as appropriate and able. *Promotes sense of control and self-worth, enabling client to feel more positive about ability to handle situation.*[2]
- Identify and promote involvement of family and social support systems. *A supportive environment enhances the effectiveness of interventions and promotes a successful grieving process.*[4]
- Discuss and assist with planning for future or funeral, as appropriate. *Involving family members in this discussion ensures that everyone knows what is desired and what is planned, thus avoiding unexpected disagreements.*[4]
- Refer to additional resources, such as pastoral care, counseling or psychotherapy, organized community support groups, as indicated, for both client and family/SO. *Useful for ongoing needs and facilitation of grieving process.*[2,8]
- Identify resources and develop community plan to address anticipated large-scale losses. *Preparation for complex challenges facilitates prompt response as needs occur.*
- Support community efforts to strengthen support and develop plan to foster recovery and growth.

DOCUMENTATION FOCUS

Assessment/reassessment
- Assessment findings, including client's perception of anticipated loss and signs/symptoms that are being exhibited.
- Responses of family/SO(s) or community members, as indicated.
- Availability and use of resources.

Planning
- Plan of care and who is involved in planning.
- Teaching plan.

 Diagnostic Studies   Evidence Based Practice   Medications   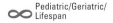 Pediatric/Geriatric/Lifespan

Implementation/Evaluation
- Client's response to interventions, teaching, and actions performed.
- Attainment or progress toward desired outcome(s).
- Modifications to plan of care.

Discharge planning
- Long-term needs and who is responsible for actions to be taken.
- Specific referrals made.

References

1. Lee, J. (2014). Dealing with grief after a disaster—the risk of "complicated grief". Retrieved March 2018 from https://www.choosehelp.com/topics/trauma-therapy/dealing-with-grief-after-a-disaster-2013-the-risk-of-2018complicated-grief2019.html.
2. Townsend, M. C. (2010). *Essentials of Psychiatric Mental Health Nursing: Concepts of Care in Evidence Based Practice*. 5th ed. Philadelphia: F. A. Davis.
3. Kissane, D. W., Bloch, S. (2002). *Family Focused Grief Therapy*. Berkshire, UK: Open University Press.
4. Newfield, S. A., et al. (2007). *Cox's Clinical Applications of Nursing Diagnosis: Adult, Child, Women's, Psychiatric, Gerontic, and Home Health Considerations*. 5th ed. Philadelphia: F. A. Davis.
5. Purnell, L. D., Paulanka, B. J. (2008). *Transcultural Health Care: A Culturally Competent Approach*. 3th ed. Philadelphia: F. A. Davis.
6. No author listed. (Updated 2017). Grief, bereavement, and coping with loss: Treatment. *National Cancer Institute*. Retrieved March 2018 from https://www.cancer.gov/about-cancer/advanced-cancer/caregivers/planning/bereavement-hp-pdq#section/_226.
7. Pearce, J. C. (2004). *The Biology of Transcendence: A Blueprint of the Human Spirit*. Rochester, VT: Park Street Press.
8. Matzo, M., et al. (2002). Teaching cultural consideration at the end of life. End of Life Nursing Education Consortium program recommendations. *J Contin Educ Nurs*, 33(6), 270–278.
9. Neeld, E. H. (2003). *Seven Choices*. 4th ed. Austin, TX: Centerpoint Press.
10. Riely, M. (2003). Facilitating children's grief. *J School Nurs*, 19(4), 212–218.
11. Family Caregiver Alliance: National Center on Caregiving. (No date). Grief and loss. Retrieved March 2018 from http://caregiver.org/grief-and-loss.
12. Eldridge, L. J., Hughes, G. (2014). Anticipatory grief symptoms and purpose: Understanding grief before loss and death. Retrieved March 2018 from https://www.verywell.com/understanding-anticipatory-grief-and-symptoms-2248855.

---

complicated Grieving

Taxonomy II: Coping/Stress Tolerance—Class 2 Coping Responses (00135) [**Diagnostic Division:** Ego Integrity], Approved 1980; Revised 1986, 2004, 2006; 2017

DEFINITION: A disorder that occurs after the death of a significant other, in which the experience of distress accompanying bereavement fails to follow normative expectations and manifests in functional impairment.

RELATED FACTORS
Emotional disturbance
Insufficient social support

DEFINING CHARACTERISTICS

Subjective
Anxiety, anger, disbelief: feeling of emptiness or detachment from others
Feeling dazed or stunned; feeling of shock
Distress about the diseased person; longing or yearning for deceased person
Insufficient sense of well-being; fatigue; mistrust; low levels of intimacy; depression
Nonacceptance of a death; persistent painful memories, distress about the deceased person

 Acute Care   Collaborative   Community/Home Care   Cultural

Objective

Avoidance of grieving

Decrease in functioning in life roles

Excessive stress; separation or traumatic distress

Experiencing symptoms the deceased experienced

Preoccupation with thoughts about a deceased person; rumination; searching for the deceased; self-blame

At Risk Population: Death of a significant other

 [Loss of significant object (e.g., possessions, job, status, home, parts and processes of body)]

Sample Clinical Applications: Death of significant other, traumatic loss, depression, attempted suicide

DESIRED OUTCOMES/EVALUATION CRITERIA

Sample NOC linkages:

Depression Level: Severity of melancholic mood and loss of interest in life events

Grief Resolution: Personal actions to adjust thoughts, feelings, and behaviors to actual or impending loss

Psychosocial Adjustment: Life Change: Adaptive psychosocial response of an individual to significant life circumstance

Client Will (Include Specific Time Frame)

• Acknowledge presence and impact of dysfunctional situation.

• Demonstrate progress in dealing with stages of grief at own pace.

• Participate in work and self-care and activities, as able.

• Verbalize a sense of progress toward resolution of the grief and hope for the future.

ACTIONS/INTERVENTIONS

Sample NIC linkages:

Grief Work Facilitation: Assistance with the resolution of a significant loss

Grief Work Facilitation: Perinatal Death: Assistance with the resolution of a perinatal loss

Coping Enhancement: Facilitation of cognitive and behavioral efforts to manage perceived stressors, changes, or threats that interfere with meeting life demands and roles

NURSING PRIORITY NO. 1   To determine causative/contributing factors:

• Identify loss that is present. Note circumstances of death such as sudden or traumatic (e.g., fatal accident, homicide; large scale natural disaster), related to socially sensitive issue (e.g., AIDS, gun violence in schools, suicide; sexual assault with murder), or associated with unfinished business (e.g., spouse died during time of crisis in marriage, son has not spoken to parent for years). *These situations can sometimes cause individual to become stuck in grief and unable to move forward with life.*[11–13]

• Determine significance of the loss to client (e.g., presence of chronic condition leading to divorce or disruption of family unit and change in lifestyle or financial security). *The more complicated or devastating the loss is to the individual, the more likely she or he will have difficulty reaching resolution.*[15]

• 🌐 Identify cultural or religious beliefs and expectations *that may impact or dictate client's response to loss.*[15]

• Ascertain response of family/significant others (SOs) to situation (e.g., sympathetic or urging client to "just get over it"). Assess needs of SO(s). *Response of family members will affect how client is dealing with situation—functional families are supportive or conflict resolving in nature while dysfunctional families tend to be sullen, hostile, or immediate functioning. This information is important for planning care and choosing resources to enable all members to effectively cope with events.*[6,9]

NURSING PRIORITY NO. 2 To determine degree of impairment/dysfunction:

- Observe for cues of sadness (e.g., sighing, faraway look, unkempt appearance, inattention to conversation, somatic complaints such as exhaustion, headaches). *Indicators of the extent of grief and how individual is dealing with situation.*[12,14]
- Identify stage of grief being expressed: denial, isolation, anger, bargaining, depression, and acceptance. *Helps to establish how client is dealing with grieving and degree of difficulty client is having adjusting to the death or loss.*[10]
- Listen to words and communications indicative of renewed or intense grief (e.g., constantly bringing up death or loss even in casual conversation long after event; outbursts of anger at relatively minor events; expressing desire to die) *indicating person is possibly unable to adjust/move on from feelings of intense grief.*[12] *Note: Complicated grief therapy utilizes the concept of revisiting the loss through storytelling of the death, especially for individuals prone to avoid thinking about the trauma of the loss.*[6]
- Determine level of functioning, ability to care for self, and use of support systems and community resources. *Individual may be incapacitated by depth of loss and be unable to manage day-to-day activities adequately, necessitating intervention and assistance.*[14]
- Be aware of avoidance behaviors (e.g., anger; withdrawal; long periods of sleeping or refusing to interact with family; sudden or radical changes in lifestyle; inability to handle everyday responsibilities at home, work, or school; conflict). *Additional indicators of depth of grieving being experienced and need for more intensive support and monitoring to help client deal effectively with death or loss.*[10–12]
- Determine if client is engaging in reckless or self-destructive behaviors (e.g., substance abuse, heavy drinking, promiscuity, aggression) *to identify safety issues.*[1]
- Identify cultural factors and ways individual(s) has dealt with previous loss(es). *Way of expressing self may reflect cultural background and religious beliefs. Understanding cultural expectations will help put current behavior and responses in context and determine the nature and degree of dysfunction.*[8]
- Perform or refer for psychological testing, as indicated (e.g., Beck's Depression Scale). *Determines degree of depression and possible need for medication.*[2]

NURSING PRIORITY NO. 3 To assist client/others to deal appropriately with loss:

- Encourage verbalization without confrontation about realities. *It is helpful to listen without correcting misperceptions in the beginning, allowing free flow of expression. Provides opportunity for reflection aiding resolution and acceptance.*[2]
- Encourage client to choose topics of conversation and refrain from forcing client to "face the facts." *Talking freely about concerns can help client identify what is important to deal with and how to cope with situation.*[9]
- Active-listen feelings and be available for support or assistance. Speak in a soft, caring voice. *Communicates acceptance and caring, enabling client to seek own answers to current situation.*[2]
- Encourage expression of anger, fear, and anxiety. (Refer to appropriate NDs.) *These feelings are part of the grieving process, and to accomplish the work of grieving, they need to be expressed and accepted.*[9]
- Permit verbalization of anger with acknowledgment of feelings and setting of limits regarding destructive behavior. *Enhances client safety, promotes resolution of grief process by encouraging expression of feelings that are not usually accepted, and supports self-esteem.*[2]
- Acknowledge reality of feelings of guilt or blame, including hostility toward spiritual power. Do not minimize loss; avoid clichés and easy answers. (Refer to ND Spiritual Distress.) *Reinforces that feelings are acceptable and allows client to become aware of own thoughts and begin to deal with feelings.*[1,7]
- Respect the client's needs and wishes for quiet, privacy, talking, or silence. *Individual may not be ready to talk about or share grief and needs to be allowed to make own time line.*[2]
- Give "permission" to be at this point when the client is depressed. *Assures client that feelings are normal and can be a starting point to deal in a positive manner with loss/death that has occurred.*[9]

 Acute Care   Collaborative   Community/Home Care 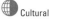 Cultural

- Provide comfort and availability as well as caring for physical needs. *Client needs to know he or she will be supported and helped when not able to care for self.*[2]
- Reinforce use of previously effective coping skills. Instruct in and encourage use of visualization and relaxation techniques. *Identifying and discussing how client has dealt with loss in the past can provide opportunities in the current situation. Use of these techniques helps client to learn to relax and consider options for dealing with loss.*[2]
- ∞ Assist SOs to cope with client's response. Include age-specific interventions. *Family/SO(s) may not understand/be intolerant of client's distress and inadvertently hamper client's progress. Family members, including children, may express their feelings in anger, resulting in punishment for behavior that is deemed unacceptable rather than recognized as the basis in grief.*[10]
- Include family/SO(s) in setting realistic goals for meeting needs of client and family members. *Involving all members enhances the probability that each member will express their needs and hear what the needs of others are, ensuring a more effective outcome.*[2]
- Encourage family members to participate in support group or family-focused therapy as indicated. *Technique of family-focused grief therapy focuses on emotional expression of grief and family functioning to strengthen the family's adaptive capacity and promote cohesiveness.*[3]
- 🥄 Use sedatives or tranquilizers with caution. *While the use of these medications may be of limited benefit in the short term, too much dependence on them may retard passage through the grief process.*[2,4]
- Refer to mental health provider for counseling. *Standard individual psychotherapy identifies and addresses symptoms, relationship problems, and their connections to grief. Research suggests the complicated grief therapy technique may be more effective by supporting the idea of dual processing (i.e., alternating attention between the loss and a focus on restoration and the future).*[6–13]
- Refer to ND Grieving for additional interventions as appropriate.

NURSING PRIORITY NO. 4 To promote wellness (Teaching/Discharge Considerations):

- 🏠 Discuss with client/SO healthy ways of dealing with difficult situations. *Identifying ways individual(s) has dealt with losses in the past will help identify strengths and successes and what might be useful in the current situation.*[2]
- 🌐 Have individual(s) identify familial, religious, and cultural factors that have meaning. *One's family of origin has a major impact on what the individuals learn about these issues and how to deal with losses. Identifying and discussing how they affect the current situation may help bring loss into perspective and facilitate grief resolution.*[5,8]
- Encourage involvement in usual activities, exercise, and socialization within limits of physical ability and psychological state. *Keeping life to a somewhat normal routine can provide individual(s) with some sense of control over events that are not controllable.*
- Suggest client keep a journal of experiences and feelings. *As client writes about what is happening, new insights may occur. Reading over what has been written can help individual see progress that has been made and begin to have hope for the future.*[9]
- Advocate planning for the future as appropriate to individual situation (e.g., staying in own home after death of spouse, returning to sporting activities following traumatic amputation, choice to have another child or to adopt, rebuilding home following a disaster). *Provides a sense of control and purpose and ensures that individual's wishes will be heard and respected.*[10]
- Identify volunteer opportunities (e.g., working with children at risk, raising funds for favorite charity, investigating new employment or relocation opportunities, participating in community reorganization or clean-up). *Exercising control in a productive manner empowers individuals and promotes rebuilding of life and community.*
- Refer to other resources (e.g., pastoral care, family counseling, psychotherapy, organized support groups—widow's group) as indicated. *Provides additional support to resolve situation and continue grief work.*[4]

 Diagnostic Studies   Evidence Based Practice   Medications 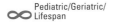 Pediatric/Geriatric/Lifespan

DOCUMENTATION FOCUS

Assessment/Reassessment
- Assessment findings, including meaning of loss to the client, current stage of the grieving process, and responses of family/SOs.
- Cultural or religious beliefs and expectations.
- Availability and use of resources.

Planning
- Plan of care and who is involved in the planning.
- Teaching plan.

Implementation/Evaluation
- Client's response to interventions, teaching, and actions performed.
- Attainment or progress toward desired outcome(s).
- Modifications to plan of care.

Discharge Planning
- Long-term needs and who is responsible for actions to be taken.
- Specific referrals made.

References

1. Lubit, R. H. (Updated 2010). Acute treatment of disaster survivors. Retrieved March 2018 from http://babyhealthcaretips.blogspot.com/2010/01/acute-treatment-of-disaster-survivors.html.
2. Townsend, M. C. (2010). *Essentials of Psychiatric Mental Health Nursing Concepts of Care in Evidence Based Practice*. 5th ed. Philadelphia: F. A. Davis, 585–601.
3. Kissane, D. W., Bloch, S. (2002). *Family Focused Grief Therapy*. Berkshire, UK: Open University Press.
4. Newfield, S. A., et al. (2007). *Cox's Clinical Applications of Nursing Diagnosis: Adult, Child, Women's, Psychiatric, Gerontic, and Home Health Considerations*. 5th ed. Philadelphia: F. A. Davis.
5. Purnell, L. D., Paulanka, B. J. (2008). *Transcultural Health Care: A Culturally Competent Approach*. 3th ed. Philadelphia: F. A. Davis.
6. No author listed. (Updated 2017). Grief, bereavement, and coping with loss: Treatment. *National Cancer Institute*. Retrieved March 2018 from https://www.cancer.gov/about-cancer/advanced-cancer/caregivers/planning/bereavement-hp-pdq#section/_226.
7. Pearce, J. C. (2004). *The Biology of Transcendence: A Blueprint of the Human Spirit*. Rochester, VT: Park Street Press.
8. Matzo, M., et al. (2002). Teaching cultural consideration at the end of life. End of Life Nursing Education Consortium program recommendations. *J Contin Educ Nurs*, 33(6), 270–278.
9. Neeld, E. H. (2003). *Seven Choices*. 4th ed. Austin, TX: Centerpoint Press.
10. Riely, M. (2003). Facilitating children's grief. *J School Nurs*, 19(4), 212–218.
11. Lee, J. (2014). Dealing with grief after a disaster—the risk of "complicated grief". Retrieved March 2018 from https://www.choosehelp.com/topics/trauma-therapy/dealing-with-grief-after-a-disaster-2013-the-risk-of-2018complicated-grief2019.html.
12. No author listed. (2006). Grief becomes complicated, unresolved or stuck. Retrieved March 2018 from https://crumblingwalls.wordpress.com/2006/09/16/grief-becomes-complicated-unresolved-or-stuck/.
13. Kersting, K. (2004). A new approach to complicated grief. *Monitor on Psychology*, 35(10), 51.
14. National Cancer Institute. (Updated 2017). Types of grief reactions. Retrieved March 2018 from https://www.cancer.gov/about-cancer/advanced-cancer/caregivers/planning/bereavement-hp-pdq#section/_164.
15. National Cancer Institute. (Updated 2013). Factors that affect complicated grief. Retrieved March 2018 from https://www.cancer.gov/about-cancer/advanced-cancer/caregivers/planning/bereavement-pdq#section/_31.

 Acute Care   Collaborative   Community/Home Care   Cultural

risk for complicated Grieving

Taxonomy II: Coping/Stress Tolerance—Class 2 Coping Responses (00172) **[Diagnostic Division:** Ego Integrity], Approved 2004; Revised 2006, 2013; 2017

DEFINITION: Susceptible to a disorder that occurs after the death of a significant other, in which the experience of distress accompanying bereavement fails to follow normative expectations and manifests in functional impairment, which may compromise health.

RISK FACTORS
Emotional disturbance
Insufficient social support
At Risk Population: Death of a significant other
[Loss of significant object (e.g., possessions, job, status, home, parts and processes of body)]
Sample Clinical Applications: Death of significant other, traumatic loss, attempted suicide, depression

DESIRED OUTCOMES/EVALUATION CRITERIA

Sample NOC linkages:
Personal Resiliency: Positive adaptation and function of an individual following significant adversity or crisis
Grief Resolution: Personal actions to adjust thoughts, feelings, behaviors to actual or impending loss
Psychosocial Adjustment: Life Change: Adaptive psychosocial response of an individual to significant life circumstance

Client Will (Include Specific Time Frame)
- Acknowledge awareness of individual factors affecting client in this situation.
- Identify emotional responses and behaviors occurring after the death or loss.
- Participate in therapy to learn new ways of dealing with anxiety and feelings of inadequacy.
- Discuss meaning of loss to individual or family.
- Verbalize a sense of beginning to deal with grief process.

ACTIONS/INTERVENTIONS

Sample NIC linkages:
Grief Work Facilitation: Assistance with the resolution of a significant loss
Grief Work Facilitation: Perinatal Death: Assistance with the resolution of a perinatal loss
Coping Enhancement: Facilitation of cognitive and behavioral efforts to manage perceived stressors, changes, or threats that interfere with meeting life demands and roles

NURSING PRIORITY NO. 1   To identify risk/contributing factors:

- Determine loss that has occurred and meaning to client. Note if death was sudden or traumatic (e.g., fatal accident, homicide, large-scale disaster); related to socially sensitive issue (e.g., AIDS, gun violence in schools, suicide, sexual assault with murder); or associated with unfinished business (e.g., spouse died during time of crisis in marriage, son has not spoken to parent for years). *These situations can sometimes cause individual to become stuck in grief and unable to move forward with life.*[1,2]
- ∞ Ascertain circumstances surrounding loss of fetus, infant, or child (e.g., gestational age of fetus, multiple miscarriages, death due to violence or fatal illness). *Repeated losses and/or violent death can increase client's/ significant other's (SO's) sense of futility and compromise resolution of grieving process.*[2,7]

 Diagnostic Studies   Evidence Based Practice   Medications   Pediatric/Geriatric/ Lifespan

- ∞ Meet with both parents following loss of child *to determine how they are dealing with the loss together and individually. Death of a child is often more difficult for parents/family, based on individual values and sense of life unlived.*[2]
- Note stage of grief client is experiencing (e.g., denial, anger, bargaining, depression). *Stages of grief may progress in a predictable manner or stages may be random or revisited.*[3]
- 🏠 Assess client's ability to manage activities of daily living and period of time since loss has occurred. *Feelings of overwhelming sadness, exhaustion, and inertia can occur with active grieving, interfering with life activities; however, when they persist and interfere with normal activities, client may need additional assistance.*[3]
- 🏠 Note availability and use of support systems and community resources.
- Listen to words and communications indicative of renewed or intense grief (e.g., constantly bringing up death or loss even in casual conversation long after event, outbursts of anger at relatively minor events, expressing desire to die), *indicating person is possibly unable to adjust or move on from feelings of intense grief.*[4]
- 🌐 Identify cultural or religious beliefs and expectations that may impact or dictate client's response to loss. *These factors affect current situation and may help bring loss into perspective and promote grief resolution.*[2,5]
- Assess status of relationships or marital difficulties and adjustments to loss. *Responses of family/SOs affect how client deals with situation.*[6]

NURSING PRIORITY NO. 2 To assist client to deal appropriately with loss:

- Discuss meaning of loss to client, Active-listen to responses without judgment. *The more complicated or devastating the loss is to the individual, the more likely she or he will have difficulty reaching resolution.*
- Respect client's desire for quiet, privacy, talking, or silence. *Individual may not be ready to talk about or share grief and needs to be allowed to make own time line.*[3]
- Encourage expression of feelings, including anger, fear, and anxiety. Let client know that all feelings are okay, while setting limits on destructive behavior.[3,6]
- Acknowledge client's sense of relief when death follows a long and debilitating course. *Sadness and loss are still there, but the death may be a release, or client may feel guilty about having a sense of relief.*
- Assist SOs/family to understand and be tolerant of client's feelings and behavior. *Family members may inadvertently hamper client's progress through grief by expressing their feelings in anger for client behavior they deem unacceptable rather than recognizing the basis is grief.*[8]

NURSING PRIORITY NO. 3 To promote wellness (Teaching/Discharge Considerations):

- 🏠 Assist client/SOs to identify successful coping skills they have used in the past. *These can be used in current situation to facilitate dealing with grief.*[3]
- Support client and family in setting goals for meeting needs of members for moving on beyond the grieving process.
- Encourage resuming involvement in usual activities, exercise, and socialization within physical and psychological abilities. *Keeping life to a somewhat normal routine can provide individual with some sense of control over events that are not controllable.*[5]
- Advocate planning for the future as appropriate to individual situation (e.g., staying in own home after death of spouse, returning to sporting activities following traumatic amputation, choice to have another child or to adopt, rebuilding home following a disaster). *Provides a sense of control and purpose and ensures that individual's wishes will be heard and respected.*[8]
- 🄰 Refer to other resources, as needed, such as psychotherapy, family counseling, religious references or pastor, or a grief support group. *Depending upon meaning of the loss, individual may require ongoing support to work through grief.*[5]

 Acute Care   Collaborative   Community/Home Care   Cultural

DOCUMENTATION FOCUS

Assessment/Reassessment
- Assessment findings, including meaning of loss to the client, current stage of the grieving process, psychological status, and responses of family/SOs.
- Cultural or religious beliefs, expectations, and rituals.
- Availability and use of resources.

Planning
- Plan of care and who is involved in the planning.
- Teaching plan.

Implementation/Evaluation
- Client's response to interventions, teaching, and actions performed.
- Attainment or progress toward desired outcome(s).
- Modifications to plan of care.

Discharge Planning
- Long-term needs and who is responsible for actions to be taken.
- Specific referrals made.

References

1. Lee, J. (2014). Dealing with grief after a disaster—the risk of "complicated grief". Retrieved March 2018 from https://www.choosehelp.com/topics/trauma-therapy/dealing-with-grief-after-a-disaster-2013-the-risk-of-2018complicated-grief2019.html.
2. National Cancer Institute. (Updated 2017). Risk factors for complicated grief and other negative bereavement outcomes. Retrieved March 2018 from https://www.cancer.gov/about-cancer/advanced-cancer/caregivers/planning/bereavement-hp-pdq#section/_204.
3. Townsend, M. C. (2010). *Essentials of Psychiatric Mental Health Nursing Concepts of Care in Evidence Based Practice.* 5th ed. Philadelphia: F. A. Davis, 585–601.
4. No author listed. (2006). Grief becomes complicated, unresolved or stuck. Retrieved March 2018 from https://crumblingwalls.wordpress.com/2006/09/16/grief-becomes-complicated-unresolved-or-stuck/.
5. Matzo, M., et al. (2002). Teaching cultural considerations at the end of life. End of Life Nursing Education Consortium program recommendations. *J Contin Educ Nurs,* 33(6), 212–218.
6. Neeld, E. H. (2003). *Seven Choices.* 4th ed. Austin, TX: Centerpoint Press.
7. Kersting, K. (2004). A new approach to complicated grief. *Monitor on Psychology,* 35(10), 51.
8. Riely, M. (2003). Facilitating children's grief. *J School Nurs,* 19(4), 212–218.

risk for disproportionate Growth

Taxonomy II: Growth/Development—Class 1 Growth (00113) [**Diagnostic Division:** Teaching/Learning], Approved 2013

DEFINITION: Susceptible to growth above the 97th percentile or below the 3rd percentile for age, crossing two percentile channels, which may compromise health.

RISK FACTORS

Prenatal
Inadequate maternal nutrition; maternal infection; multiple gestation
Substance abuse; exposure to teratogen
Congenital or genetic disorder

(continues on page 396)

 Diagnostic Studies   Evidence Based Practice   Medications   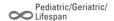 Pediatric/Geriatric/Lifespan

risk for disproportionate Growth (continued)

Individual
Prematurity
Malnutrition; maladaptive feeding behavior by caregiver, or self-feeding; insatiable appetite; anorexia
Infection; chronic illness
Substance abuse (including anabolic steroids)

Environmental
Deprivation, economically disadvantaged
Exposure to violence, natural disasters
Exposure to teratogen; lead poisoning

Caregiver
Presence of abuse (e.g., physical, psychological, sexual)
Mental health issue (e.g., depression, psychosis, personality disorder, substance abuse)
Learning disability; alteration in cognitive functioning
Sample Clinical Applications: Congenital or genetic disorders, prematurity, infection, nutritional problems (malnutrition, anorexia, failure to thrive, excessive intake or obesity), toxic exposures (e.g., lead), abuse or neglect, endocrine disorders, pituitary tumor

DESIRED OUTCOMES/EVALUATION CRITERIA

Sample NOC linkages:
Growth: Normal increase in height and body weight from infancy through adolescence
Weight: Body Mass: Extent to which body weight, muscle, and fat are congruent to height, frame, gender, and age

Client Will (Include Specific Time Frame)
• Receive appropriate nutrition as dictated by individual needs.
• Demonstrate weight and growth stabilizing or progressing toward age-appropriate size.
• Participate in plan of care as appropriate for age and ability.

Sample NOC linkages:
Child Development: [specify age group]: Milestones of physical, cognitive, and psychosocial progression by [specify] months/years of age

Client/Caregiver Will (Include Specific Time Frame)
• Verbalize understanding of potential for growth delay or deviation and plan for prevention.

ACTIONS/INTERVENTIONS

Sample NIC linkages:
Nutritional Monitoring: Collection and analysis of patient data pertaining to nutrient intake
Teaching: Infant [or] Toddler Nutrition [specify age]: Instruction on nutrition and feeding practices during the first, second, or third years of life
Weight Management: Facilitating maintenance of optimal body weight and percent body fat

 Acute Care   Collaborative   Community/Home Care   Cultural

NURSING PRIORITY NO. 1 To assess causative/contributing factors:

- Determine factors or condition(s) existing that could contribute to growth deviation as listed in Risk Factors, including familial history (e.g., pituitary tumors, Marfan's syndrome, genetic anomalies), prematurity with complications, use of certain drugs or substances during pregnancy, maternal diabetes or other chronic illness, poverty or inability to attend to nutritional issues, eating disorders, etc. *Information essential to developing plan of care.*
- Identify nature and effectiveness of parenting and caregiving activities. *Inadequate, inconsistent caregiving; unrealistic or insufficient expectations; lack of stimulation; inadequate limit setting; and lack of responsiveness indicates problems in parent-child relationship.*[4]
- Note severity and pervasiveness of situation (e.g., individual/significant other showing effects of long-term physical or emotional abuse or neglect versus individual experiencing recent-onset situational disruption or inadequate resources during period of crisis or transition).
- Evaluate nutritional status. *Overfeeding or malnutrition (protein and other basic nutrients) on a constant basis prevents individual from reaching healthy growth potential, even if no disorder or disease exists. Malnutrition is the most common cause of growth failure worldwide. In industrialized nations, children continue to have nutritional deficiencies that can impair growth or development.*[12]
- Review results of studies such as skull and hand x-rays; bone scans, such as computed tomography or magnetic resonance imaging; and chest or abdominal imaging *to determine bone age and extent of bone and soft tissue overgrowth and the presence of pituitary or other growth hormone–secreting tumor.* Note laboratory studies (e.g., growth hormone levels, glucose tolerance, thyroid and other endocrine studies, serum transferrin and prealbumin) *to identify pathology.*[8,11,12]
- Determine cultural, familial, and societal values *that may impact situation or parental expectations (e.g., some cultures equate a "plump" baby with a healthy baby; childhood obesity is now a risk for American children and parents are concerned about child's food intake; expectations for "normal growth").*[13]
- Assess cognition, awareness, orientation, and behavior of the client/caregiver. *Actions such as withdrawal or aggression and reactions to environment and stimuli provide information for identifying needs and planning care.*[1]
- Active-listen concerns about body size and ability to perform competitively (e.g., sports, body building) *to ascertain the potential for inappropriate use of anabolic steroids or other drugs.*

NURSING PRIORITY NO. 2 To prevent/limit deviation from growth norms:

- Determine chronological age and note reported losses or alterations in functional level. *Provides comparative baseline.*
- Note familial factors (e.g., parent's body build and stature) *to help determine individual growth expectations (e.g., when child should attain a certain weight and height) and how the expectations may be altered by child's condition.*[12]
- Review expectations for current height and weight percentiles and degree of deviation. Plan for periodic evaluations. *Growth rates are measured in terms of how much a child grows within a specified time. These rates vary dramatically as a child grows (normal growth is a discontinuous process) and must be evaluated periodically over time to ascertain that child has definite growth disturbance. Accelerated or slowed growth rates are rarely normal and warrant further evaluation.*[1]
- Investigate deviations in height, weight, and head size. *Deviations may include weight only (increased or decreased) or height (increased or decreased) and head size (disproportionate to rest of body). These deviations may be seen alone or in combination, all requiring additional testing over time to determine cause and effect on child's growth and development. Some are more urgent than others (e.g., small head size is evaluated further/treated as soon as identified, whereas short stature may require a longer evaluation period to determine if developmental problem exists).*[1]
- Determine if child's growth is above 97th percentile (very tall and large) for age. *Child should be further evaluated for endocrine disorders or pituitary tumor (could result in gigantism). Other disorders may be*

 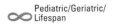

characterized by excessive weight for height (e.g., hypothyroidism, Cushing's syndrome) and abnormal sexual maturation or abnormal body/limb proportions.[2,8]

- Determine if child's growth is below third percentile (very short and small) for age. *Child should have further evaluations for failure to thrive related to intrauterine growth retardation, prematurity or very low birth weight, small parents, poor nutrition, stress or trauma, endocrine disorders (e.g., growth hormone or thyroid deficiency), or medical condition (e.g., intestinal disorders with malabsorption; diseases of heart, kidneys; diabetes mellitus). Treatment of underlying condition may alter or improve child's growth pattern.*[3,9,10]

- Assist with therapies to treat or correct underlying conditions (e.g., Crohn's disease, cardiac problems, or renal disease), endocrine problems (e.g., hyperpituitarism, hypothyroidism, type 1 diabetes mellitus, growth hormone abnormalities), genetic or intrauterine growth retardation, and infant feeding problems and nutritional deficits.

- Include nutritionist and other specialists as indicated (e.g., physical or occupational therapist) in developing plan of care. *Helpful in determining specific dietary needs for growth and weight issues as well as child's personal and cultural preferences, issues with foods (e.g., child who is sensory overresponsive may be bothered by food textures, child with posture problems may need to stand to eat, etc.); child may require assistive devices and appropriate exercise and rehabilitation programs.*[6]

- Note reports of changes in facial features, joint pain, lethargy, sexual dysfunction, or progressive increase in hat, glove, ring, or shoe size in adults, especially after age 40. *Individual should be referred for further evaluation for hyperpituitarism or growth hormone imbalance and acromegaly.*[8]

NURSING PRIORITY NO. 3   To promote wellness (Teaching/Discharge Considerations):

- Provide information regarding growth issues, as appropriate, including pertinent reference materials such as books, audiovisual materials, credible Web sites, etc. *Provides opportunity to review data at own pace, enhancing likelihood of retention, and opportunity to make informed decisions.*

- Discuss with pregnant women and adolescents consequences of substance use or abuse. *Prevention of growth disturbances depends on many factors but includes the cessation of smoking, alcohol, and many drugs that have the potential for causing central nervous system or orthopedic disorders in the fetus.*[5,7]

- Refer for genetic screening as appropriate. *There are many reasons for referral, including (and not limited to) positive family history of a genetic disorder (e.g., fragile X syndrome, muscular dystrophy), pregnant female with exposure to toxins or potential teratogenic agents, women older than 35 years at delivery, previous child born with congenital anomalies, history of intrauterine growth retardation, etc.*

- Address parent/caregiver issues (e.g., parental abuse, learning deficiencies, environment of poverty) *where they could impact client's ability to thrive.*

- Promote client lifestyle that prevents or limits complications (e.g., management of obesity, hypertension, sensory or perceptual impairments), regular medical follow-up, nutritionally balanced meals, socialization for age and development, etc., *to enhance functional independence and quality of life.*

- Recommend involvement in regular monitored exercise and/or sports programs *to enhance muscle tone and strength, and appropriate body building.*

- Review medications being considered (e.g., appetite stimulant, growth hormone, thyroid replacement, antidepressant), noting potential side effects/adverse reactions *to promote adherence to regimen and reduce risk of untoward responses.*

- Identify available community resources as appropriate (e.g., public health programs such as the Women, Infants, and Children program; medical equipment suppliers; nutritionist; substance abuse programs; specialists in endocrine problems/genetics).

- Emphasize importance of periodic reassessment of growth and development (e.g., periodic lab studies to monitor hormone levels, bone maturation, and nutritional status). *Aids in evaluating effectiveness of interventions over time, promotes early identification of need for additional actions, and helps to avoid preventable complications.*

 Acute Care   Collaborative   Community/ Home Care   Cultural

DOCUMENTATION FOCUS

Assessment/Reassessment
- Assessment findings, individual needs, current growth status and trends.
- Caregiver's understanding of situation and individual role.
- Cultural or familial values and expectations.

Planning
- Plan of care and who is involved in the planning.
- Teaching plan.

Implementation/Evaluation
- Client's responses to interventions, teaching, and actions performed.
- Caregiver response to teaching.
- Attainment or progress toward desired outcome(s).
- Modifications to plan of care.

Discharge Planning
- Identified long-term needs and who is responsible for actions to be taken.
- Specific referrals made, sources for assistive devices, educational tools.

References

1. Legler, J. D., Rose, L. C. (1999). Assessment of abnormal growth curves. *Am Fam Physician*, 58(1), 1–9.
2. National Institutes of Health Genetic and Rare Diseases Information Center. (Updated 2010). Gigantism. Retrieved March 2018 from http://rarediseases.info.nih.gov/gard/6506/gigantism/case/28765/case-questions.
3. Child Growth Foundation. (No date). Endocrine gland disorders. Retrieved March 2018 from http://www.childgrowthfoundation.org/Default.aspx?page=ConditionsGHD.
4. Gordon, T. (2000). *Parent Effectiveness Training*. Updated ed. 30th anniversary. New York: Three Rivers Press.
5. Maloni, J. A., et al. (2003). Implementing evidence-based practice: Reducing risk for low birth weight through pregnancy smoking cessation. *J Obstet Gynecol Neonat Nurs*, 32(5), 676–682.
6. Montana Disability & Health Program. (2005). Nutrition for individuals with intellectual or developmental disabilities. Retrieved March 2018 from http://mtdh.ruralinstitute.umt.edu/?page_id=813.
7. Schiffman, R. F. (2004). Drug and substance use in adolescents. *MCN Am J Matern Child Nurs*, 29(1), 21–27.
8. Diaz-Thompson, A., Shim, M., Schwartz, R. A. (Updated 2017). Gigantism and acromegaly. Retrieved March 2018 from http://emedicine.medscape.com/article/925446-overview.
9. Kemp, S., Gungor, N. (Updated 2016). Growth failure. Retrieved March 2018 from http://emedicine.medscape.com/article/920446-overview.
10. Mannheim, J. K. (Updated 2018). Delayed growth. Various pages. Retrieved March 2018 from http://www.nlm.nih.gov/medlineplus/ency/article/003021.htm.
11. Sinha, S. (Updated 2018). Short stature. Retrieved March 2018 from http://emedicine.medscape.com/article/924411-overview.
12. Falkenstern, S. K., Bauer, L. A. (2009). Helping kids grow. *The Nurse Pract*, 34(3), 30–41.
13. Kumanyika, S. K. (2008). Environmental influences on childhood obesity: Ethnic and cultural influences context. *Physiol Behav*, 94(1), 61–70.

risk-prone Health Behavior

Taxonomy II: Health Promotion—Class 2 Health Management (00188) [**Diagnostic Division:** Teaching/Learning], Submitted as impaired Adjustment 1986; Revised 1998; Revised/Renamed 2006, 2008; Revised 2017

DEFINITION: Impaired ability to modify lifestyle and/or actions in a manner that improves the level of wellness.

RELATED FACTORS
Inadequate comprehension; low self-efficacy
Negative perception of health care provider or recommended health care strategy
Social anxiety; insufficient social support; stressors
Smoking; substance misuse/[abuse]

DEFINING CHARACTERISTICS

Subjective
Minimizes health status change
Failure to achieve optimal sense of control

Objective
Failure to take action that prevents health problem
Nonacceptance of health status change
At Risk Population: Family history of alcoholism; economically disadvantaged
Sample Clinical Applications: New diagnosis/life changes for client, Alzheimer's disease, brain injury, personality or psychotic disorders, postpartum depression/psychosis, substance use/abuse

DESIRED OUTCOMES/EVALUATION CRITERIA

Sample NOC linkages:
Acceptance: Health Status: Personal actions to reconcile significant changes in health circumstances
Psychosocial Adjustment: Life Change: Adaptive psychosocial response of an individual to a significant life circumstance
Health Promoting Behavior: Personal actions to sustain or increase wellness

Client Will (Include Specific Time Frame)
• Demonstrate increasing interest or participation in self-care.
• Develop ability to assume responsibility for personal needs when possible.
• Identify stress situations leading to difficulties in adapting to change in health status and specific actions for dealing with them.
• Initiate lifestyle changes that will permit adaptation to present life situations.
• Identify and use appropriate support systems.

ACTIONS/INTERVENTIONS

Sample NIC linkages:
Coping Enhancement: Facilitation of cognitive and behavioral efforts to manage perceived stressors, changes, or threats that interfere with meeting life demands and roles
Counseling: Use of an interactive helping process focusing on the needs, problems, or feelings of the patient and significant others to enhance or support coping, problem solving, and interpersonal relationships
Teaching: Disease Process: Assisting the patient to understand information related to a specific disease process

 Acute Care   Collaborative   Community/ Home Care   Cultural

NURSING PRIORITY NO. 1 To assess degree of impaired function:

- Perform a physical and/or psychosocial assessment. *Determines the extent of the limitation(s) of the present condition.*[1]
- Listen to the client's perception of inability or reluctance to adapt to situations that are occurring at present. *Perceptions are reality to the client and need to be identified so they may be addressed and dealt with.*[3]
- Survey (with the client) past and present significant support systems (family, church, groups, organizations). *Identifies helpful resources that may be needed in current situation or change in health status.*[2]
- Explore the expressions of emotions signifying impaired adjustment by client/significant others (SOs). *Overwhelming anxiety, fear, anger, worry, passive or active denial can be experienced by the client who is having difficulty adjusting to a change in health or a feared diagnosis.*[4]
-   Note child's interaction with parent/caregiver. *Interactions can be indicative of problems when family is dealing with major health issues and change in family functioning. Development of coping behaviors is limited at this age, and primary caregivers provide support for the child and serve as role models.*[5]
- Determine whether child displays problems with school performance, withdraws from family/peers, or demonstrates aggressive behavior toward others/self. *Indicators of poor coping and need for specific interventions to help child deal with own health issues or what is happening in the family.*[6]

NURSING PRIORITY NO. 2 To identify the causative/contributing factors relating to the impaired adjustment:

- Listen to client's perception of factors leading to the present dilemma, noting onset, duration, presence or absence of physical complaints, and social withdrawal. *Change often creates a feeling of disequilibrium, and the individual may respond with irrational or unfounded fears. Client may benefit from feedback that corrects misperceptions about how life will be with the change in health status.*[7]
- Note substance use or abuse (e.g., smoking, alcohol, prescription medications, street drugs) *that may be used as a coping mechanism, exacerbate health problem, or impair client's comprehension of situation.*
- Identify possible cultural beliefs or values influencing client's response to change. *Different cultures deal with change of health issues, such as cancer, chronic obstructive pulmonary disease, and diabetes mellitus, in different ways (i.e., some cultures may believe they should be quiet and stoic when sick; some may seem passive or expect the family to care for the client; others may be assertive and direct their care more frequently).*[12]
- Assess affective climate within family system and how it determines family members' response to adjustment to a major health challenge. *Families who are high-strung and nervous may interfere with client's dealing with illness in a rational manner, while those who are more sedate and phlegmatic may be more helpful to the client in accepting the current circumstances.*[2]
- Determine lack of or inability to use available resources. *The high degree of anxiety that usually accompanies a major lifestyle change often interferes with ability to deal with problems created by the change or loss. Helping client learn to use these resources enables him or her to take control of own illness.*[8]
- Discuss normalcy of anger as life is being changed and encourage channeling anger to healthy activities. *The increased energy of anger can be used to accomplish other tasks and enhance feelings of self-esteem.*[2]
- Review available documentation and resources to determine actual life experiences (e.g., medical records, statements of SOs, consultants' notes). *In situations of great stress (physical or emotional), the client may not accurately assess occurrences leading to the present situation.*[9]

NURSING PRIORITY NO. 3 To assist client in coping/dealing with impairment:

- Organize a team conference (including client and ancillary services). *Individuals who are involved and knowledgeable can focus on contributing factors that are affecting client's adjustment to the current situation and can plan for management as indicated.*[10]
- Explain disease process or causative factors and prognosis as appropriate, promote questioning, and provide written and other resource materials. *Enhances understanding, clarifies information, and provides opportunity to review information at individual's leisure.*

 Diagnostic Studies   Evidence Based Practice   Medications   Pediatric/Geriatric/ Lifespan

- ∞ Share information with adolescent's peers with client's permission and involvement when illness or injury affects body image or function. *Peers are primary support for this age group, and sharing information promotes understanding and compassion.*[5]
- Provide an open environment encouraging communication. *Supports expression of feelings concerning impaired function so they can be dealt with realistically.*[2]
- Use therapeutic communication skills (e.g., Active-listening, acknowledgment, silence, "I" statements). *Promotes open relationship in which client can explore possibilities and solutions for changing lifestyle situation.*[13]
- Acknowledge client's efforts to adjust: "You have done your best." *May reduce feelings of blame or guilt and defensive responses.*[11]
- Discuss and evaluate resources that have been useful to the client in adapting to changes in other life situations. *Vocational rehabilitation, employment experiences, and psychosocial support services may be useful in current situation.*[11]
- Develop a plan of action with client to meet immediate needs (e.g., physical safety and hygiene, emotional support of professionals and SOs) and assist in implementation of the plan. *Provides a starting point to deal with current situation for moving ahead with plan for adjusting to change in life circumstances and for evaluation of progress toward goals.*
- Reinforce structure in daily life. Include exercise as part of routine. *Routines help the client focus. Exercise improves sense of wellness and enhances immune response.*
- Review with client coping skills used in previous life situations and role changes. *Identifies the strengths that may be used to facilitate adaptation to change or loss that has occurred.*[8]
- Refine or develop new coping strategies as appropriate. *Strengthens skills for dealing with change in health or lifestyle.*
- Identify with and problem-solve the client frustrations in daily care. *Focusing on the smaller factors of concern gives the individual the ability to perceive the impaired function from a less threatening perspective (one-step-at-a-time concept). Also promotes sense of control over situation.*
- Involve SO(s) in long-range planning for emotional, psychological, physical, and social needs. *Change that is occurring when illness is long term or permanent indicates that lifestyle changes will need to be dealt with on an ongoing basis, which may be difficult for client and family to adjust to.*[12]
- Refer for individual/family counseling as indicated. *May need additional assistance to cope with current situation.*

NURSING PRIORITY NO. 4   To promote wellness (Teaching/Discharge Considerations):

- Identify strengths the client perceives in present life situation. Keep focus on the present. *Unknowns of the future may be too overwhelming when diagnosis or injury means permanent changes in lifestyle and long-term management.*
- Assist SOs to learn methods of managing present needs. (Refer to NDs specific to client's deficits.) *Promotes internal locus of control and helps develop plan for long-term needs reflecting changes required by illness or changes in health status.*[2]
- Pace and time learning sessions to meet client's needs, providing for feedback during and after learning experiences (e.g., self-catheterization, range-of-motion exercises, wound care, therapeutic communication). *Promotes skill and enhances retention, thereby improving confidence.*[1]
- Refer to other resources in the long-range plan of care. *Long-term assistance may include such elements as home care, transportation alternatives, occupational therapy, or vocational rehabilitation that may be useful for making indicated changes in life and assisting with adjustment to new situation as needed.*[2]
- Assist client/SO(s) to see appropriate alternatives and potential changes in locus of control. *Often major change in health status results in loss of sense of control, and client needs to begin to look at possibilities for managing illness and what abilities can make life go on in a positive manner.*

 Acute Care   Collaborative   Community/ Home Care   Cultural

DOCUMENTATION FOCUS

Assessment/Reassessment
- Reasons for and degree of impairment.
- Client's/SO's perception of the situation.
- Effect of behavior on health status or condition.

Planning
- Plan for adjustments and interventions for achieving the plan and who is involved.
- Teaching plan.

Implementation/Evaluation
- Client responses to the interventions, teaching, and actions performed.
- Attainment or progress toward desired outcome(s).
- Modifications to plan of care.

Discharge Planning
- Resources that are available for the client and SO(s) and referrals that are made.

References

1. Klopf, J., Kofler-Westergren, B., Mitterauer, B. (2007). Towards an action-oriented criteria in risk assessment. *Int J Forensic Ment Health*, 6(1), 47–56.
2. Tucker, J. S., et al. (2006). Affective and behavioral responses to health-related social control. *Health Psychol*, 25(6), 715–722.
3. Locher, J. L., et al. (2002). Effects of age and causal attribution to aging on health-related behaviors associated with urinary incontinence in older women. *Gerontologist*, 42(4), 515–521.
4. Koton, S., et al. (2004). Triggering risk factors for ischemic stroke: A case-crossover study. *Neurology*, 63(11), 2006–2010.
5. Pinhas-Hamiel, O., et al. (1996). Increased incidence of non-insulin-dependent diabetes mellitus among adolescents. *J Pediatr*, 128(8), 608–615.
6. Deckelbaum, R. J., Williams, C. L. (2001). Childhood obesity: The health issue. *Obesity Res*, 9(5), S239–S243.
7. Badger, J. M. (2001). Burns: The psychological aspect. *Am J Nurs*, 101(11), 38–41.
8. Bartol, T. (2002). Putting a patient with diabetes in the driver's seat. *Nursing*, 32(2), 53–55.
9. Konigova, R. (1992). The psychological problems of burned patients. The Rudy Hermans Lecture 1991. *Burns*, 18(3), 189–199.
10. Grady, K. L. (2006). Management of heart failure in older adults. *J Cardiovasc Nurs*, 21(5 Suppl), S10–S14.
11. Burke, V., et al. (2008). Changes in cognitive measures associated with a lifestyle program for treated hypertensives: A randomized controlled trial (ADAPT). *Health Educ Res*, 23(2), 202–217.
12. Chang, M., Kelly, A. E. (2007). Patient education: Addressing cultural diversity and health literacy issues. *Urol Nurs*, 27(5).
13. Pilgrim, G. (2010). Therapeutic communication techniques. Retrieved March 2018 from http://www.buzzle.com/articles/therapeutic-communication-techniques.html.

deficient community Health

Taxonomy II: Health Promotion—Class 2 Health Management (00215) [**Diagnostic Division:** Teaching/Learning], Approved 2010

DEFINITION: Presence of one or more health problems or factors that deter wellness or increase the risk of health problems experienced by an aggregate.

RELATED FACTORS
Insufficient access to healthcare providers; insufficient resources [e.g., financial, social, knowledge]
Insufficient community experts
Inadequate program budget, outcome data, or evaluation plan
Inadequate social support or consumer satisfaction with program
Program incompletely addresses health program

(continues on page 404)

 Diagnostic Studies   Evidence Based Practice   Medications   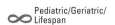 Pediatric/Geriatric/Lifespan

deficient community Health (continued)

DEFINING CHARACTERISTICS

Subjective

[Community members/agencies verbalize overburdening of resources to meet therapeutic needs of all members]

[Community members/agencies verbalize inability to meet therapeutic needs of all members]

Objective

Health problem experienced by aggregates or populations

Program unavailable to prevent, reduce, or eliminate health problem(s) of an aggregate or population

Program unavailable to enhance wellness of an aggregate or population

Risk of hospitalization experienced by aggregates or populations

Risk of physiological or psychological states experienced by aggregates or populations

Sample Clinical Applications: HIV/AIDS, substance abuse, sexually transmitted infections, teen pregnancy, prematurity, acute lead poisoning, influenza, severe acute respiratory syndrome (SARS)

DESIRED OUTCOMES/EVALUATION CRITERIA

Sample NOC linkages:

Community Competence: Capacity of a community to collectively problem-solve to achieve community goals

Community Health Status: General state of well-being of a community or population

Community Risk Control: Communicable Disease: Community actions to eliminate or reduce the spread of infectious agents that threaten public health

Community Will (Include Specific Time Frame)

• Identify both strengths and limitations affecting community programs for meeting health-related goals.

• Participate in problem-solving of factors interfering with regulating and integrating community programs.

• Develop plans to address identified community health needs.

ACTIONS/INTERVENTIONS

Sample NIC linkages:

Community Health Development: Assisting members of a community to identify a community's health concerns, mobilize resources, and implement solutions

Program Development: Planning, implementing, and evaluating a coordinated set of activities designed to enhance wellness, or to prevent, reduce, or eliminate one or more health problems for a group or community

Health Policy Monitoring: Surveillance and influence of government and organization regulations, rules, and standards that affect nursing systems and practices to ensure quality care of patients

NURSING PRIORITY NO. 1 To identify causative/precipitating factors:

• Determine healthcare providers' understanding, terminology, and practice policies relating to community (populations and aggregate). *Population-based practice considers the broad determinants of health, such as income/ social status, housing, employment/working conditions, social support networks, education, neighborhood*

 Acute Care Collaborative Community/ Home Care Cultural

safety/violence issues, physical environment, personal health practices and coping skills, cultural customs/ values, and community capacity to support family and economic growth.[6]

- Investigate health problems, unexpected outbreaks or acceleration of illness, and health hazards in the community. *Identifying specific problems allows for population-based interventions emphasizing primary prevention, promoting health, and preventing problems before they occur.*[2,6,7]
- Evaluate strengths and limitations of community healthcare resources for wellness, illness, or sequelae of illness. *Knowledge of currently available resources and ease of access provide a starting point to determine needs of the community and plan for future needs.*
- Note reports from members of the community regarding ineffective or inadequate community functioning. *Provides feedback from people who live in the community and avail themselves of resources, thus presenting a realistic picture of problem areas.*
- Determine areas of conflict among members of community. *Cultural or religious beliefs, values, social mores, and lack of a shared vision may limit dialogue or creative problem-solving if not addressed.*[5,7]
- Ascertain effect of related factors on community. *Issues of safety, poor air quality, lack of education or information, and lack of sufficient healthcare facilities affect citizens and how they view their community—whether it is a healthy, positive environment in which to live or lacks adequate healthcare or safety resources.*[1]
- Determine knowledge and understanding of treatment regimen. *Citizens need to know and understand what is being proposed to correct the identified deficiencies before they are willing to be involved and actively support goals of the treatment regimen.*
- Note use of resources available to community for developing and funding programs. *May require creative program planning to utilize/maximize resources to meet multiple needs.*

NURSING PRIORITY NO. 2   To assist community to develop strategies to improve community functioning and management:

- Foster cooperative spirit of community without negating individuality of members/groups. *As individuals feel valued and respected, they are more willing to work together with others to develop a plan for identifying and improving healthcare for the community.*
- Involve community in determining healthcare goals and prioritizing them to facilitate planning process. *The goal is healthy people in a healthy community, and as community members become involved and see that by prioritizing the identified goals, progress can be seen as individuals become healthier and needed services become readily available.*[2]
- Link people to needed services and ensure the provision of healthcare to extent possible. Plan together with community health and social agencies to problem-solve solutions identified and anticipated problems and needs. *Interventions may be directed at an entire population within a community, the systems that affect the health of those populations, and/or the individuals and families within at-risk populations. Working together promotes a sense of involvement and control, helping people implement more effective problem-solving.*[2,3]
- Identify specific populations at risk or underserved (e.g., chronically ill or disabled persons; elder adults; mentally ill persons; substance abusers; veterans; economically disadvantaged families; rural, migrant, immigrant, and homeless persons; racial and ethnic minorities) to actively involve them in the planning and evaluation processes. *These groups are often marginalized and frequently lack knowledge of available services, may be suspicious or lack interest in available programs, or lack resources to access services. Being part of the solution enhances sense of being heard, empowering these groups and promoting continued participation in the process.*[3,4,7,8]
- Network with others involved in educating healthcare providers and healthcare consumers regarding community needs. Create a teaching plan and form a speakers' bureau. Provide accurate information and demonstrate desired action. Present information in a culturally appropriate manner. *Disseminating information to community members regarding value of treatment or preventive programs helps people know and understand the importance of these actions and be willing to support the programs.*[1,3,7]

 Diagnostic Studies   Evidence Based Practice   Medications   Pediatric/Geriatric/ Lifespan

NURSING PRIORITY NO. 3 To promote wellness (Teaching/Discharge Considerations):

• Assist community to develop a plan for continued assessment of community needs and functioning (e.g., access to adequate healthcare; education regarding disease prevention, public health threats, and immunization; local warning system and evacuation plan in event of disaster; emergency contact numbers; planning for community members with special needs [elderly, handicapped, low-income persons]; violence prevention, personal or property protection; water, sanitation, toxic substance management; mobilization of local, state, and national resources). *Promotes proactive approach in planning for the future and continuation of efforts to improve healthy behaviors and necessary services. Note: Networks may be internal to the agency (e.g., with epidemiologists; public health nurses and educators; in-house laboratories; plumbing, electrical, and building inspectors) community-wide (e.g., with nongovernmental organizations, industry, academia, labs), or within the government's public health/environmental protection system (Environmental Protection Agency, the Centers for Disease Control and Protection, other federal agencies; state offices such as State Engineer and Attorney General; local agencies).*[1,4,7]

• Encourage community to form partnerships within the community and between the community and the larger society. *Aids in long-term planning for anticipated and projected needs and concerns to ensure the quality and accessibility of health services.*[1]

DOCUMENTATION FOCUS

Assessment/Reassessment
• Assessment findings, including members' perceptions of community problems, healthcare resources.
• Community use of available resources.

Planning
• Plan and who is involved in planning process.
• Teaching plan.

Implementation/Evaluation
• Community's response to plan, interventions, and actions performed.
• Attainment or progress toward desired outcome(s).
• Modifications to plan.

Discharge Planning
• Long-term goals and who is responsible for actions to be taken.
• Specific referrals made.

References

1. American Public Health Association. (2012, update 2017). Environmental health competency project: Draft recommendations for non-technical competencies at the local level. Retrieved March 2018 from https://www.cdc.gov/nceh/ehs/Corecomp/CoreCompetencies.htm.
2. Health.gov. (2018). 2018 physical activity guidelines advisory committee submits Scientific Report. Retrieved March 2018 from https://health.gov/news/blog-bayw/2018/03/2018-physical-activity-guidelines-advisory-committee-submits-scientific-report/.
3. Healthy People 2010 Toolkit: A Field Guide to Health Planning. (2002). Washington, DC: Public Health Foundation.
4. Centers for Disease Control and Prevention (CDC). (last review 2016). Strategic Priority #1: Improve health security at home and around the world. Retrieved March 2018 from http://www.cdc.gov/about/organization/mission.htm.
5. Bokinskie, J. C., Evanson, T. A. (2009). The stranger among us: Ministering health to migrants. *J Christian Nurs*, 26(4), 202–209.
6. Keller, L. O., Schaffer, M. A., Lia-Hoagberg, M. A. (2002). Assessment, program planning, and evaluation in population-based public health practice. *J Public Health Manage & Pract*, 8(5), 30–43.
7. de Chesnay, M., Anderson, B. A. (2012). Chapter 1: Vulnerable populations: Vulnerable people. *Caring for the Vulnerable: Perspectives in Nursing Theory, Practice, and Research*. 3rd ed. Burlington, MA: Jones & Bartlett Learning.
8. Phillips, C. D., McLeroy, K. R. (2004). Health in rural America: Remembering the importance of place. *Am J Public Health*, 94(10), 1661–1663.

 Acute Care Collaborative Community/Home Care Cultural

readiness for enhanced Health Literacy

Taxonomy II: Health Promotion—Class 1 Health Awareness (00262) [**Diagnostic Division:** Teaching/Learning], Approved 2016

DEFINITION: A pattern of using and developing a set of skills and competencies (literacy, knowledge, motivation, culture, and language) to find, comprehend, evaluate, and use health information and concepts to make daily health decisions to promote and maintain health, decrease health risks, and improve overall quality of life, which can be strengthened.

DEFINING CHARACTERISTICS

Subjective
Expresses desire to obtain sufficient information to navigate the healthcare system
Expresses desire to enhance:
• Ability to read, write, speak, and interpret numbers for everyday health needs
• Awareness of civic and/or government processes that impact public health, and social support for health
• Health communication with healthcare providers
• Knowledge of current determinants of health on social and physical environments
• Personal healthcare decision-making;
• Understanding of healthcare information, customs, and beliefs to make healthcare decisions
Sample Clinical Applications:

DESIRED OUTCOMES/EVALUATION CRITERIA

Sample NOC linkages:
Health Literacy Behavior: Personal actions to obtain, understand, and evaluate information related to health, illness, and available services to make care decisions

Client Will (Include Specific Time Frame)
• Identify personal health needs/goals.
• Identify quality informational resources to enhance knowledge and support decision-making.
• Verbalize understanding of health information received/accessed.
• Make informed healthcare decisions relevant to needs.
• Engage in preventive health practices.

ACTIONS/INTERVENTIONS

Sample NIC linkages:
Health Literacy Enhancement: Assisting individuals with limited ability to obtain, process, and understand information related to health and illness

NURSING PRIORITY NO. 1 To determine level of health literacy and motivation for change:

• Determine client's health status and client's perception of how healthy he/she is at this time. *Client may perceive self as healthy when actually the client has some serious symptoms he/she is not aware of or is minimizing.*
• Ascertain current ability and knowledge about own healthcare and healthcare system. *Ability to verbalize health needs, report symptoms, know where to get healthcare and follow guidance from the caregiver is vital in accomplishing health goals. Belief in the ability to accomplish desired action is predictive of performance.*[3]

 Diagnostic Studies   Evidence Based Practice   Medications   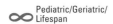 Pediatric/Geriatric/Lifespan

- Determine cultural beliefs that may influence client's view of the healthcare system and the client's own care. *These beliefs can have strong influence on client's desire to change.*[4]
- Active-listen client's concerns and issues that may be affecting client's desire to make changes. *Factors such as health insurance and access to care, family problems, and economic situation may motivate client as well as interfere with plan for change.*
- Determine sources client currently uses to access information and how client actually uses the information. *Sources used vary widely depending on multiple factors such as client's age, language proficiency, accessibility of technology. Individuals may be very adept at getting information but may not know how to use it in the context of their own health, to understand insurance papers, or to pay their bills.*[4]
- Determine the ability of the individual to understand the medical information and instructions the client is given/accessing. *Many adults are challenged by what is termed "low health literacy," a significant number reading at a fifth grade level, economically disadvantaged, elderly, and having a low English proficiency or are non-native speakers of English.*[3,4]
- Note social factors such as inadequate access to healthcare, educational disparities, and socioeconomic status that can influence client's behavior regarding healthcare. *Access and participation in health resources and education programs are not spread evenly across underserved populations, affecting choice of interventions.*[1]

NURSING PRIORITY NO. 2   To assist client to develop plan for change:

- Provide guidance that fits with client's cultural, dietary, and/or religious values. During interactions with client, be sensitive to body language, mode of dress, gender "rules" (e.g., female shaking hands with male, direct eye contact), and when asking sensitive questions to clarify understanding or dispelling preconceived ideas. *These strategies help put client at ease, enhance trust, and can improve nurse-client relationship.*[4]
- Assist client to develop a plan addressing individual needs/weaknesses. *Identifying specific areas for improvement aids in choice of interventions.*
- Discuss with the client/family what areas of the client's life he/she has control over, such as choosing foods, cooking, safe place to exercise. *Making these decisions promotes sense of self-esteem, helping to improve health practices.*
- Focus energies on promoting informed lifestyle choices, preventive health programs, risk factor modification as appropriate. *Patient self-management relies on these factors to improve health, especially in management of chronic diseases.*[1]
- Educate client/family in the use of web portals and public access resource sites as needed. *Persons with limited health literacy are less likely to use these resources, which may be due to ethnic/cultural or racial differences or level of comfort in sharing private health information.*[2]
- Acknowledge efforts the client is making to maintain consistent positive outcomes of interventions. *These actions improve self-care efforts, patient satisfaction, coping skills, and perceptions of social support.*[1]

NURSING PRIORITY NO. 3   To promote optimum health literacy:

- Reduce the use of health industry jargon, provide health materials in several languages and provide interpreters when needed. *These changes will help client to understand the information the client is given.*[4]
- Deliver health information in a clear, engaging, and personally relevant manner. Have client repeat back what you have told him/her. *Can help client to understand, feel empowered, and respected. Provides an opportunity to clarify and correct misunderstandings.*[4]
- Improve print communication by using plain and clear language, organizing ideas clearly, and using logical layout and design. *Facilitates reading and comprehension of potentially complicated consumer health information.*[4]
- Promote client/family involvement in consumer education and health literacy. *Low literacy and numeracy (basic math skills) means that health communication is poorly understood. Individuals who are actively involved in seeking, understanding, and acting on health information learn how to navigate the system for maximum well-being.*[1]

 Acute Care   Collaborative   Community/ Home Care   Cultural

- Provide information about other community resources that can enhance learning and improve health literacy. *Programs such as smoking cessation, nutrition/weight loss, healthy exercise provide opportunities for skill training, problem-solving.*[1]
- Encourage client to do breast self-examination/mammogram, testicular and prostate exams, regular dental examination, keep immunizations current. *These actions contribute to maintaining wellness and encourage health literacy.*[1]
- Assist client to prepare for healthcare encounters—write list of questions, list of all medications taken (prescription, over-the-counter, vitamins/herbals), and obtaining results of diagnostic testing. *Role-playing and collecting necessary information can improve client confidence and facilitate meaningful interaction with provider.*[4]
- Suggest SO/family member accompany client to healthcare appointments as appropriate. *Helpful for writing down/remembering information presented.*[4]

DOCUMENTATION FOCUS

Assessment/Reassessment
- Personal health status.
- Goals and motivation for change.
- Pertinent social factors, cultural beliefs, religious values impacting health and use of healthcare system.
- Primary language, literacy/reading level.
- Availability and use of resources/health services.

Planning
- Plan of care and who is involved in planning.
- Individual learning needs.

Implementation/Evaluation
- Response to interventions, teaching and actions performed.
- Attainment or progress toward desired outcomes.
- Modifications to plan.

Discharge Planning
- Short- and long-term needs and who is responsible for actions.
- Available resources, specific referrals made.

References

1. Adams, R. J. (2010). Improving health outcomes with better patient understanding and education. *Risk Manag Healthc Policy*. June 2018 from. https://www.ncbi.nlm.nih.gov/pmc/articles/PMC3270921/. 3, 61–72.
2. Coughlin, S. S., et al. (2018). Health literacy and patient web portals. *Int J Medical Informatics*. June 2018 from https://www.sciencedirect.com/science/article/pii/S1386505618300790. 113, 43–48.
3. Pisano, S. (2008). The Health Literacy & Plain Language Resource Guide. *Health Literacy Innovations*. June 2018 from https://www.amerihealthcaritas.com/pdf/health-literacy-guide.pdf.
4. What Is Health Literacy? Fact Sheets 1-5. (2013). *Center for Health Care Strategies. Inc*. June 2018 from https://www.chcs.org/media/CHCS_Health_Literacy_Fact_Sheets_2013.pdf.

 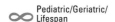

ineffective Health Maintenance

Taxonomy II: Health Promotion—Class 2 Health Management (00099) [**Diagnostic Division:** Safety], Approved 1982; Revised 2017

DEFINITION: Inability to identify, manage, and/or seek out help to maintain health.
[Author note: This diagnosis contains components of other NDs. We recommend subsuming health maintenance interventions under the "basic" nursing diagnosis when a single causative factor is identified (e.g., deficient Knowledge [specify], ineffective Health Management, chronic Confusion, impaired Verbal Communication, ineffective Coping, compromised family Coping, risk for delayed Development).]

RELATED FACTORS
Complicated grieving; spiritual distress
Impaired decision-making
Ineffective communication skills or coping strategies
Insufficient resources

DEFINING CHARACTERISTICS

Objective
Absence of adaptive behaviors to environmental changes
Absence of interest in improving health behaviors; pattern of lack of health-seeking behavior
Inability to take responsibility for meeting basic health practices; insufficient knowledge about basic health practices
Insufficient social support
At Risk Population: Developmental delay
Associated Condition: Alteration in cognitive functioning, perceptual disorders; decrease in fine or gross motor skills
Sample Clinical Applications: Chronic conditions (e.g., multiple sclerosis [MS], rheumatoid arthritis, chronic pain), brain injury or stroke, spinal cord injury or paralysis, laryngectomy, dementia, Alzheimer's disease, developmental delay

DESIRED OUTCOMES/EVALUATION CRITERIA

Sample NOC linkages:
Health Promoting Behavior: Personal actions to sustain or increase wellness
Knowledge: Health Behavior: Extent of understanding conveyed about the promotion and protection of health
Participation in Health Care Decisions: Personal involvement in selecting and evaluating healthcare options to achieve desired outcome

Client Will (Include Specific Time Frame)
• Identify necessary health maintenance activities.
• Verbalize understanding of factors contributing to current situation.
• Assume responsibility for own healthcare needs within level of ability.
• Adopt lifestyle changes supporting individual healthcare goals.

Sample NOC linkages:
Risk Detection: Personal actions to identify personal health threats
Social Support: Reliable assistance from others

 Acute Care
 Collaborative
 Community/ Home Care
Cultural

SO/Caregiver Will (Include Specific Time Frame)
- Verbalize ability to cope adequately with existing situation and provide support and monitoring as indicated.

ACTIONS/INTERVENTIONS

Sample **NIC** linkages:

Health System Guidance: Facilitating a patient's location and use of appropriate health services
Support System Enhancement: Facilitation of support to patient by family, friends, and community
Health Education: Developing and providing instruction and learning experiences to facilitate voluntary adaptation of behavior conducive to health in individuals, families, groups, or communities

NURSING PRIORITY NO. 1   To assess causative/contributing factors:

- Recognize differing perceptions regarding health issues between healthcare providers and clients. Explore ways to partner. *Awareness that healthcare provider's goals may not be the same as a client's goals can provide opportunities to explore and communicate. Left undone, the door is open for frustration on both sides, affecting client care experience and/or perceived outcome of care. Note: For example, one study found that healthcare staff rated client's self-responsibility as the most important variable (out of 17) while the patients rated it 11th.*[13,14]
- Identify health practices and beliefs in client's personal and family history, including health values, religious or cultural beliefs, and expectations regarding healthcare. *Clients and healthcare providers do not always view a health risk in the same way. The client may not view current situation as a problem or may be unaware of routine health maintenance practices and needs. Note: In one study researchers found that information designed to meet unique characteristics of the individual through culturally relevant tailoring increased the adherent rate of interventions significantly.*[11,12]
- Note client's age (e.g., very young or elderly age); cognitive, emotional, physical, and developmental status; and level of dependence and independence. *Client's status may range from complete dependence (dysfunctional) to partial or relative independence and determines type of interventions/support needed.*
- Note whether impairment is related to an acute or sudden onset situation or a progressive illness or long-term health problem. *Determines type and intensity and length of time support may be required.*[4]
- Ascertain client's ability and desire to learn. Determine barriers to learning (e.g., can't read, speaks or understands different language, is overcome with stress or grief). *The client may not be physically, emotionally, or mentally capable at present because of current situation or may need information in small, manageable increments.*[1]
- Assess communication skills and ability or need for interpreter. Identify support person requiring or willing to accept information. *Ability to understand is essential to identification of needs and planning care. May need to provide the information to another individual if client is unable to comprehend.*[9]
- Evaluate medication regimen and also for substance use/abuse (e.g., alcohol/other drugs) as indicated. *Can affect client's understanding of information or desire and ability to accept responsibility for self.*[6]
- Note client's desire and level of ability to meet health maintenance needs as well as self-care activities of daily living. *Care may begin with helping client make a decision to improve situation, as well as identifying factors that are currently interfering with meeting needs.*[3]
- Note setting where client lives (e.g., long-term/other residential care facility, rural versus urban setting; homebound, or homeless). *Socioeconomic status and geographic location contribute to an individual's ability to achieve or maintain good health.*[10]
- Ascertain recent changes in lifestyle. *For instance, a man whose spouse dies and who has no skills for taking care of his own/family's health needs may need assistance to learn how to manage new situation, or a newly unemployed individual without healthcare benefits may require referral to public assistance agencies.*[8]

 Diagnostic Studies   Evidence Based Practice   Medications   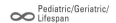 Pediatric/Geriatric/Lifespan

- Determine level of adaptive behavior, knowledge, and skills about health maintenance, environment, and safety. *Will determine beginning point for planning and intervening to help client learn necessary skills to maintain health in a positive manner.*[7]
- Evaluate home environment, as indicated, *to note individual adaptation needs (e.g., supplemental humidity, air purifier, change in heating system).*[1]
- Note client's use of professional services and resources (i.e., appropriate or inappropriate, nonexistent).[9]

NURSING PRIORITY NO. 2 To assist client/caregiver(s) to maintain and manage desired health practices:

- Discuss with client/significant others (SOs) beliefs about health and reasons for not following prescribed plan of care. *Determines client's view about current situation and potential for change. Provides opportunity for discussion about alternate plan of care that client may find more suitable or may help identify a compromise that could improve client's participation in a particular course of treatment.*
- Identify realistic health goals and develop plan with client/SO(s) for self-care. *Allows for incorporating existing disabilities with client's/SO's desires, adapting and organizing care as necessary.*[1]
- Involve comprehensive specialty health teams when available or indicated (e.g., pulmonary, psychiatric, enterostomal, IV therapy, nutritional support, substance abuse counselors).
- Provide time to active-listen concerns of client/SO(s). *Provides opportunity to clarify expectations and misconceptions.*
- Provide anticipatory guidance *to maintain and manage effective health practices during periods of wellness and to identify ways client can adapt when progressive illness or long-term health problems occur.*[9,11]
- Encourage socialization, "buddy system," and personal involvement *to enhance support system, provide pleasant stimuli, and limit permanent regression.*[2]
- Provide for communication and coordination between healthcare facility teams and community healthcare providers *to promote continuation of care and maximize outcomes.*[2]
- Monitor adherence to prescribed medical regimen *to problem-solve difficulties in adherence and alter the plan of care as needed.*[1]

NURSING PRIORITY NO. 3 To promote wellness (Teaching/Discharge Considerations):

- Provide information about individual healthcare needs, using client's preferred learning style (e.g., pictures, words, video, Internet). *Can help client to understand own situation and enhance cooperation with the plan of care.*[8]
- ∞ Limit amount of information presented at one time, especially when dealing with elderly or cognitively impaired client. Present new material through self-paced instruction when possible. *Allows client time to process and store new information.*[8]
- Help client/SO(s) prioritize healthcare goals. Provide a written copy to those involved in planning process *for future reference/revision as appropriate. Promotes planning to enable the client to maintain a healthy and productive lifestyle.*[10]
- Assist client/SO(s) to develop stress-management skills. *Knowing ways to manage stress helps individual to develop and maintain a healthy lifestyle.*[3]
- Identify ways to make adaptations in certain circumstances *to meet client's changing needs and abilities and environmental concerns.*[5]
- Identify signs and symptoms requiring further screening, evaluation, and follow-up. Essential to identify developing problems that could interfere with maintaining well-being.[10,11]
- Make referral as needed for community support services (e.g., homemaker or home attendant, Meals on Wheels, skilled nursing care, community or free clinic, Well-Baby Clinic, senior citizen healthcare activities). *Client may need additional assistance to maintain self-sufficiency.*[9]
- Refer to social services as indicated. *May need assistance with financial, housing, or legal concerns (e.g., conservatorship).*[2]

 Acute Care   Collaborative   Community/ Home Care   Cultural

- Refer to support groups as appropriate (e.g., senior citizen groups, Alcoholics or Narcotics Anonymous, Red Cross, Salvation Army). *Provides information and help for specific needs or at times of crisis.*[9]
- Assist with referral for hospice service for client with terminal illness, where indicated. *Will help client and family deal with end-of-life issues in a positive manner.*[3,4]

DOCUMENTATION FOCUS

Assessment/Reassessment
- Assessment findings, including individual abilities, family involvement, and support factors.
- Cultural or religious beliefs, healthcare values, and expectations.
- Availability and use of resources.

Planning
- Plan of care and who is involved in planning.
- Teaching plan.

Implementation/Evaluation
- Responses of client/SO(s) to plan, interventions, teaching, and actions performed.
- Attainment or progress toward desired outcome(s).
- Modifications to plan of care.

Discharge Planning
- Long-term needs and who is responsible for actions to be taken.
- Specific referrals made.

References

1. Bohny, B. (1997). A time for self-care: Role of the home healthcare nurse. *Home Healthc Nurs*, 15(4), 281–286.
2. Callaghan, P., Morrissey, G. (1993). Social support and health: A review. *J Adv Nurs*, 18(2), 203–210.
3. Dossey, B. M., Dossey, L. (1998). Body-mind-spirit: Attending to holistic care. *Am J Nurs*, 98(8), 35–38.
4. Gregory, C. M. (1997). Caring for caregivers: Proactive planning eases burden on caregivers. *AWHONN Lifelines*, 1(2), 51–53.
5. Lai, S. C., Cohen, M. N. (1999). Promoting lifestyle changes. *Am J Nurs*, 99(4), 63–67.
6. Larsen, L. S. (1998). Effectiveness of counseling intervention to assist family caregivers of chronically ill relatives. *J Psychosoc Nurs*, 36(8), 26–32.
7. MacNeill, D., Weis, T. (1998). Case study: Coordinating care. *Contin Care*, 17(4), 78.
8. McCrory Pocinki, K. (1991). Writing for an older audience: Ways to maximize understanding and acceptance. *J Nutr Elder*, 11(1–2), 69–77.
9. Stuifbergen, A. (1997). Health promotion: An essential component of rehabilitation for persons with chronic disabling conditions. *Adv Nurs Sci*, 19(4), 138–147.
10. U.S. Department of Health and Human Services: Public Health Foundation. (2010). *Healthy People 2020*. Retrieved March 2018 from https://www.healthypeople.gov/sites/default/files/HP2020_brochure_with_LHI_508_FNL.pdf.
11. Palo Alto Medical Foundation. (No date 1). Health maintenance guidelines (various pages). Retrieved March 2018 from http://www.pamf.org/preventive/healtheval.html.
12. Kreuter, M. W., et al. (2005). Cultural tailoring for mammography and fruit and vegetable intake among low-income African-American women in urban public health centers. *Prev Med*, 4(1), 53–61.
13. Quill, T., et al. (2006). What is most important for you to achieve? An analysis of patient responses when receiving palliative care consultation. *J Palliat Med*, 9(2), 382–388.
14. Antoniazzi, M., Celinski, M., Alcock, J. (2002). Self-responsibility and coping with pain: Disparate attitudes toward psychosocial issues in recovery from work place injury. *Disabil Rehabil*, 24(18), 948–953.

Diagnostic Studies   Evidence Based Practice   Medications   Pediatric/Geriatric/Lifespan

ineffective family Health Management

Taxonomy II: Health Promotion—Class 2 Health Management (00080) [Diagnostic Division: Teaching/Learning],
Submitted 1992; Revised 2013, 2017

DEFINITION: A pattern of regulating and integrating into family processes a program for the treatment of illness and its sequelae that is unsatisfactory for meeting specific health goals.

RELATED FACTORS

Difficulty managing complexity of treatment regimen or healthcare systems
Decisional conflict; family conflicts

DEFINING CHARACTERISTICS

Subjective
Difficulty with prescribed regimen

Objective
Inappropriate family activities for meeting health goal
Acceleration of illness symptoms of a family member
Failure to take action to reduce risk factors; decrease in attention to illness
At Risk Population: Economically disadvantaged
Sample Clinical Applications: Chronic conditions (e.g., chronic obstructive pulmonary disease [COPD], multiple sclerosis [MS], arthritis, chronic pain, substance abuse, end-stage liver or renal failure) or new diagnoses necessitating lifestyle changes

DESIRED OUTCOMES/EVALUATION CRITERIA

Sample **NOC** linkages:
Family Health Status: Overall health and social competence of family unit
Family Normalization: Capacity of a family to develop strategies for optimal functioning when a member has a chronic illness or disability
Family Participation in Professional Care: Capacity of a family to be involved in decision-making, care delivery, and evaluation of care provided by healthcare personnel

Family Will (Include Specific Time Frame)
• Identify individual factors affecting regulation/integration of treatment program.
• Participate in problem-solving of identified concerns.
• Engage in mutual goal-setting for care/treatment plan.
• Verbalize acceptance of need or desire to change actions to achieve agreed-on outcomes or health goals.
• Demonstrate behaviors/changes in lifestyle necessary to maintain therapeutic regimen.

ACTIONS/INTERVENTIONS

Sample **NIC** linkages:
Family Involvement Promotion: Facilitating participation of family members in the emotional and physical care of the patient
Family Mobilization: Utilization of family strengths to influence patient's health in a positive direction
Health System Guidance: Facilitating a patient's location and use of appropriate health services

 Acute Care
 Collaborative
 Community/ Home Care
 Cultural

NURSING PRIORITY NO. 1   To identify causative/precipitating factors:

- Ascertain family's perception of efforts to date. *Perceptions are more important than facts, and by getting family's point of view, realistic goals can be set and family can look to the future.*[2]
- Evaluate family functioning and activities, including frequency and effectiveness of family communication, promotion of autonomy, adaptations to meet changing needs, health of home environment and lifestyle, problem-solving abilities, and ties to the community. *Understanding the family and the context in which it lives allows for more personalized support of the family and choosing coping strategies in partnership with the family to meet individualized goals.*[7]
- Note family health goals and agreement of individual members. *Presence of conflict interferes with problem-solving and needs to be addressed before family can move forward to meet goals.*[2]
- Determine understanding and value of the treatment regimen to the family. *Individual members may misunderstand either the cause of the illness or the prescribed regimen and may disagree with what is happening, thereby promoting dissension within the family group and causing distress for the client.*[1]
- Identify cultural values and religious beliefs affecting view of situation and willingness to make necessary changes. *May influence choice of interventions.*
- Identify availability and use of resources. *Knowing who is available to help and support the family will help in planning care to maximize positive outcomes.*[2]

NURSING PRIORITY NO. 2   To assist family to develop strategies to improve management of therapeutic regimen:

- Provide family-centered education addressing management of condition/chronic illness, treatment plan, and self-care needs. *Accurate information helps family make informed decisions, see the connection between illness and treatment, facilitate treatment adherence, and improve client outcomes.*[3,8]
- Encourage incorporation of care strategies into family's lifestyle. *Assisting family to manage needs on a daily basis can instill confidence, decrease anxiety, and provide a degree of predictability to daily life.*[8]
- Assist family members to recognize inappropriate family activities. Help the members identify both togetherness and individual needs and behavior. *Effective interactions can be enhanced and perpetuated when these factors are identified and used to improve family behaviors.*[2]
- Make a plan jointly with family members to deal with complexity of healthcare regimen or system and other related factors. *Enhances commitment to plan, optimizing outcomes when family and caregivers work together to plan therapeutic regimen.*[2,5] *Engaging all family members as able empowers family to build new competencies and shared confidence in own abilities, enabling more effective coping.*[6]
- Identify community resources as needed using the three strategies of education, problem-solving, and resource linking to address specific deficits. *Providing information and helping family members learn effective problem-solving techniques and how to access needed resources can help them deal successfully with the chronically ill family member.*[4]

NURSING PRIORITY NO. 3   To promote wellness as related to future health and well-being of family members (Teaching/Discharge Considerations):

- Help family identify criteria to promote ongoing self-evaluation of situation and effectiveness and family progress. *Involvement promotes sense of control and provides the opportunity to be proactive in meeting needs.*[2]
- Assist family to plan for potential problems or complications. *Helping families anticipate likely challenges allows them to plan more effective coping strategies.*[6]
- Make referrals to and/or jointly plan with other health, social, and community resources. *Problems often are multifaceted, requiring involvement of numerous providers or agencies to plan appropriate regimen to meet family/individual needs.*[3]
- Encourage involvement in disease/condition support groups. *Family resiliency is gained/supported through contact with other families dealing with similar challenges and from learning from one another.*[6]

 Diagnostic Studies   Evidence Based Practice   Medications   Pediatric/Geriatric/Lifespan

• Provide contact person or case manager for one-on-one assistance as needed. *Having a single contact to coordinate care, provide support, and assist with problem-solving maintains continuity and prevents misunderstandings and errors in managing the family's regimen.*[1]
• Refer to NDs caregiver Role Strain and ineffective Health Management, as indicated.

DOCUMENTATION FOCUS

Assessment/Reassessment
• Individual findings, including nature of problem and degree of impairment, family values, health goals, and level of participation and commitment of family members.
• Cultural values, religious beliefs.
• Availability and use of resources.

Planning
• Plan of care and who is involved in planning.
• Teaching plan.

Implementation/Evaluation
• Response to interventions, teaching, and actions performed.
• Attainment or progress toward desired outcome(s).
• Modifications of plan of care.

Discharge Planning
• Long-term needs, plan for meeting and who is responsible for actions.
• Specific referrals made.

References

1. Newfield, S. A., et al. (2007). *Cox's Clinical Applications of Nursing Diagnosis: Adult, Child, Women's, Psychiatric, Gerontic, and Home Health Considerations.* 5th ed. Philadelphia: F. A. Davis.
2. Healthy People 2010 Toolkit: A Field Guide to Health Planning. (2002). Washington, DC: Public Health Foundation.
3. Bombardier, C. H., Wadwhani, R., LaRotonda, C. (2005). Health promotion in people with multiple sclerosis. *Phys Med Rehab Clin North Am*, (16), 557–570.
4. Larsen, L. S. (1998). Effectiveness of counseling intervention to assist family caregivers of chronically ill relatives. *J Psychosoc Nurs*, 36(8), 26–32.
5. Gance-Cleveland, B. (2005). Motivational interviewing as a strategy to increase families' adherence to treatment regimens. *J Spec Pediatr Nurs*, 10(3), 151–155.
6. Walsh, F. (2003). Family resilience: A framework for clinical practice. *Fam Process*, 42(1), 10–11.
7. Jokinen, P. (2004). The family life-path theory: A tool for nurses working in partnership with families. *J Child Health Care*, 8(2), 124–133.
8. Kumar, C., Edelman, M., Ficorelli, C. (2005). Children with asthma. *MCN*, 30(5), 305–311.

 Acute Care   Collaborative   Community/ Home Care   Cultural

ineffective Health Management

Taxonomy II: Health Promotion—Class 2 Health Management (00078) [**Diagnostic Division:** Teaching/Learning], Submitted 1994; Revised 2008; 2017

DEFINITION: Pattern of regulating and integrating into daily living a therapeutic regimen for the treatment of illness and its sequelae that is unsatisfactory for meeting specific health goals.

RELATED FACTORS

Difficulty managing complex treatment regimen or healthcare systems
Decisional conflicts
Excessive demands; family conflict; insufficient social support
Family pattern of healthcare
Inadequate number of cues to action
Insufficient knowledge of therapeutic regimen
Perceived barrier, benefit, susceptibility or seriousness of condition
Powerlessness
Insufficient social support

DEFINING CHARACTERISTICS

Subjective
Difficulty with prescribed regimen

Objective
Failure to include treatment regimen in daily living, or take action to reduce risk factors
Ineffective choices in daily living for meeting health goal
[Unexpected acceleration of illness symptoms; development of avoidable complications]
At Risk Population: Economically disadvantaged
Sample Clinical Applications: Chronic conditions (e.g., cancer, chronic obstructive pulmonary disease [COPD], multiple sclerosis [MS], arthritis, chronic pain, end-stage heart, liver, or renal failure) or new diagnoses necessitating lifestyle changes

DESIRED OUTCOMES/EVALUATION CRITERIA

Sample NOC linkages:
Health Promoting Behavior: Personal actions to sustain or increase wellness
Health Beliefs: Personal convictions that influence health behaviors
Adherence Behavior: Self-initiated actions to promote optimal wellness, recovery, and rehabilitation

Client Will (Include Specific Time Frame)
• Verbalize acceptance of need or desire to change actions to achieve agreed-on health goals.
• Verbalize understanding of factors and blocks involved in individual situation.
• Participate in problem solving of factors interfering with integration of therapeutic regimen.
• Demonstrate behaviors or changes in lifestyle necessary to maintain therapeutic regimen.
• Identify and use available resources.

(continues on page 418)

 Diagnostic Studies   Evidence Based Practice   Medications   Pediatric/Geriatric/Lifespan

ineffective Health Management (continued)

ACTIONS/INTERVENTIONS

Sample NIC linkages:

Self-Modification Assistance: Reinforcement of self-directed change initiated by the patient to achieve personally important goals

Health System Guidance: Facilitating a patient's location and use of appropriate health services

Patient Contracting: Negotiating an agreement with an individual that reinforces a specific behavior change

---

NURSING PRIORITY NO. 1 To identify causative/contributing factors:

- Determine whether client has acute or chronic illness; note any comorbidities and complexity of care needs. *These factors affect how client views and manages self-care. Client may be overwhelmed, in denial, depressed, or have complications exacerbating care needs. For example, diabetes is considered a biopsychosocial illness, meaning there are not only biological factors, including cause of illness and the toll it takes on the body, but also psychological, social, and economic components for the client dealing with a chronic progressive disease over a long time, usually with comorbidities.[10] Furthermore, people tend to become passive and dependent in long-term, debilitating illnesses and may find it difficulty to expend energy to follow through with therapeutic regimen.[13]*
- Ascertain client's knowledge/understanding of condition and treatment needs. *Provides a baseline so planning care can begin where the client is in relation to condition or illness and current regimen.[1]*
- Determine client's/family's health goals and patterns of healthcare. *Provides information about current behaviors and misperceptions that may be potential areas of conflict, values, or financial considerations.[1]*
- Identify health practices and beliefs in client's personal and family history, including health values, religious or cultural beliefs, and expectations regarding healthcare. *The client may not view current situation as a problem or be unaware of health management needs. For instance, those from a Hispanic culture may believe the future is in God's hands; or women may delay Pap smears and mammograms because of modesty.[14] In addition, expectations of others may dictate client's adaptation to situation and willingness to modify life. Note: In one study, researchers found that information designed to meet unique characteristics of the individual through culturally relevant tailoring significantly increased adherence rate with interventions.[1,8,9]*
- Identify client locus of control. *Those with an internal locus of control (e.g., expressions of responsibility for self and ability to control outcomes, such as "I didn't quit smoking") are more likely to take charge of situation, whereas individuals with an external locus of control (e.g., expressions of lack of control over self and environment, such as "Nothing ever works out" or "What bad luck to get lung cancer") may perceive difficulties as beyond his/her control and will look to others or external source to solve his/her problems and take care of them.[7]*
- Identify individual perceptions and expectations of treatment regimen. Active-listen client's concerns and comments. *May reveal client's thinking about regimen, misinformation, unrealistic expectations, or other factors that may be interfering with client's willingness to follow therapeutic regimen.[1,10,15]*
- Determine issues of secondary gain for the client/significant others (SOs). *Marital/family concern or attention, school or work issues, or financial considerations may cause client to subconsciously desire to remain ill or disabled, or SO to support the status quo. This can interfere with complying with prescribed treatment plans, prolong recovery time, and create frustrating medical-legal issues.[11]*
- Review complexity of treatment regimen (e.g., number of expected tasks, such as taking medication several times/day, visiting multiple healthcare providers with treatment or follow-up appointments; abundant, often conflicting information sources). Evaluate how difficult tasks might be for client (e.g., must stop smoking or must follow strict dialysis diet even when feeling well, must manage limitations while remaining active in life roles). *These factors are often involved in lack of participation in treatment plan.[12]*

 Acute Care   Collaborative   Community/ Home Care   Cultural

- Determine who (e.g., client, SO, other) manages the medication regimen and whether individual knows what the medications are and why they are prescribed and any factors that interfere with taking medications or lead to lack of adherence (e.g., depression, active alcohol or other drug use, low literacy, lack of support, lack of belief in treatment efficacy). *Forgetfulness is the most common reason given for not complying with the treatment plan.*[17]
- Note availability and use of support systems, resources for assistance and caregiving or respite care services. *Client may not have, be aware of, or know how to access available resources.*[6]

NURSING PRIORITY NO. 2 To assist client/SO(s) to develop strategies to improve management of therapeutic regimen:

- Use therapeutic communication skills to assist client to problem-solve solution(s). *Active-listening promotes accurate identification of the problem, ensuring that problem-solving is directed to the correct solution.*[7]
- Explore client involvement in or lack of mutual goal-setting. *Understanding client's willingness to be involved (or not) provides insight into the reasons for actions and suggests appropriate interventions.*[7]
- Have client identify consequences of current behaviors/ineffective management of condition. *May help client visualize the "cost" of lack of commitment to therapeutic regimen.*
- Use client's locus of control to develop individual plan to adapt regimen. *For client with internal control, encourage client to take control of own care, and for those with external control, begin with small tasks and add as tolerated.*[7]
- Establish graduated goals or modified regimen as necessary. *Specifying steps to take requires discussion and the use of critical-thinking skills to determine how to best reach the agreed-on goals.*[4] *For example, client with COPD who smokes a pack of cigarettes a day may be willing to reduce that amount but not give up smoking altogether. This choice may improve quality of life, and success with this goal may encourage progression to more advanced goals.*
- Contract with the client for participation in care, as appropriate. *By making a contract, client commits self to therapeutic regimen and is more likely to follow through because of commitment.*[6]
- Accept client's evaluation of own strengths and limitations while working together to improve abilities. State belief in client's ability to cope and/or adapt to situation. *Individuals may minimize own strengths or exaggerate limitations when faced with the difficulties of a chronic illness. By helping in concrete ways, client can begin to accept reality of strengths. Stating your belief in positive terms lets client hear someone else's evaluation and begin to accept that he/she can manage the situation.*[3]
- Acknowledge individual efforts and capabilities. *Positive reinforcement encourages continuation of desired behaviors and facilitates movement toward attainment of desired outcomes.*[5,7]
- Provide information and help client to know where and how to find it on own. Reinforce previous instructions and rationale, using a variety of learning modalities, including role-playing, demonstration, written materials, etc. *Incorporating multiple modalities promotes retention of information. Developing client's skill at finding own information encourages self-sufficiency and sense of self-worth.*[2]

NURSING PRIORITY NO. 3 To promote optimal health (Teaching/Discharge Considerations):

- 🏠 Emphasize importance of client knowledge and understanding of the need for treatment or medication as well as consequences of actions and choices. *Reinforces client's role in success of therapeutic regimen, encouraging continuation of competent behaviors.*[1]
- Promote client/caregiver/SO participation in planning and evaluating process. *Enhances commitment to plan and promotes competent self-management, optimizing outcomes.*[1]
- Assist client to develop strategies for monitoring symptoms and response to therapeutic regimen. *Promotes early recognition of changes, allowing proactive response.*[5]
- Mobilize support systems, including family/SO(s), social services, financial assistance, etc. *Success of therapeutic regimen is enhanced by using support systems effectively, avoiding or reducing stress and worry of dealing with unresolved problems.*[2]
- Provide for continuity of care in and out of the hospital or care setting, including long-range plans. *Supports trust and facilitates progress toward goals as client illness is dealt with over time.*[13,16]

 Diagnostic Studies   Evidence Based Practice   Medications   Pediatric/Geriatric/Lifespan

- Refer to counseling or therapy (group and individual) as indicated. *Client may need additional help to deal with stress and anxiety of chronic condition or illness.*[1]
- Identify home- and community-based nursing services. *These agencies can provide services for assessment, follow-up care, and education in client's home to promote more effective management of therapeutic regimen.*[1]

DOCUMENTATION FOCUS

Assessment/Reassessment

- Assessment findings, including underlying dynamics of individual situation, client's perception of problem or needs, locus of control.
- Cultural values or religious beliefs.
- Family involvement and needs.
- Individual strengths and limitations.
- Availability and use of resources.

Planning

- Plan of care and who is involved in planning.
- Teaching plan.

Implementation/Evaluation

- Response to interventions, teaching, and actions performed.
- Attainment or progress toward desired outcome(s).
- Modifications to plan of care.

Discharge Planning

- Long-term needs and who is responsible for actions to be taken.
- Available resources, specific referrals made.

References

1. Newfield, S. A., et al. (2007). *Cox's Clinical Applications of Nursing Diagnosis: Adult, Child, Women's, Psychiatric, Geron-tic, and Home Health Considerations*. 5th ed. Philadelphia: F. A. Davis.
2. U.S. Department of Health and Human Services: Public Health Foundation. (2010). Healthy People 2020 (various pages). Retrieved March 2018 from https://www.healthypeople.gov/sites/default/files/HP2020_brochure_with_LHI_508_FNL.pdf.
3. Stuifbergen, A. (1997). Health promotion: An essential compo-nent of rehabilitation for persons with chronic disabling condi-tions. *Adv Nurs Sci*, 19(4), 147–148.
4. Larsen, L. S. (1998). Effectiveness of counseling intervention to assist family caregivers of chronically ill relatives. *J Psycho-soc Nurs*, 36(8), 26–32.
5. Lai, S. C., Cohen, M. N. (1999). Promoting lifestyle changes. *Am J Nurs*, 99(4), 63–67.
6. Miller, J. F. (1999). *Coping with Chronic Illness: Overcoming Powerlessness*. 3rd ed. Philadelphia: F. A. Davis.
7. Townsend, M. C. (2011). *Psychiatric Mental Health Nurs-ing Concepts of Care in Evidence-Based Practice*. 7th ed. Philadelphia: F. A. Davis.
8. Purnell, L. D. (2009). *Guide to Culturally Competent Health Care*. 2nd ed. Philadelphia: F. A. Davis.
9. Krueter, M. W., et al. (2005). Cultural tailoring for mammogra-phy and fruit and vegetable intake among low-income African-American women in urban public health centers. *Prev Med*, 41(1), 53–61.
10. Zinzer, K. A., Mulhern, J. L., Kareem, A. A. (2011). The implementation of the Chronic Care Model with respect to dealing with the biopsychosocial aspects of the chronic disease of diabetes. *Adv Skin Wound Care*, 24(10), 475–484.
11. Dersh, J., et al. (2004). The management of secondary gain and loss in medicolegal settings: Strengths and weaknesses. *J Occup Rehabil*, 14(4), 267–279.
12. Corser, W., Dontje, K. (2011). Self-management perspectives of heavily comorbid primary care adults. *Prof Case Manag*, 16(1), 6–15.
13. Smith, J. S. (2006). The psychology of burns. *J Trauma Nurs*, 13(3), 105–106.
14. Kotelnikov, V. Personal beliefs, values and basic assumptions and attitudes—Understanding what drives you and others. *E-Coach*. Retrieved May 2018 from http://www.1000ventures.com/business_guide/crosscuttings/character_beliefs-values.html.
15. Sherry, D. C., et al. (2003). Noncompliance in heart trans-plantation: A role for advanced practice nurses. Medscape Nurses. Retrieved May 2018 from http://www.medscape.com/viewarticle/459038.
16. Laws, M. B., et al. (2012). Lecture or listen: When patients waver on meds. Retrieved May 2018 from https://news.brown.edu/articles/2012/02/aids.
17. Hassan, N. B., et al. (2006). Identification of psychosocial fac-tors in noncompliance in hypertensive patients. *J Hum Hyper-tens*, 20(1), 23–29.

 Acute Care Collaborative Community/ Home Care Cultural

readiness for enhanced Health Management

Taxonomy II: Health Promotion—Class 2 Health Management (00162) [**Diagnostic Division:** Teaching/Learning], Approved 2002; Revised 2010, 2013

DEFINITION: A pattern of regulating and integrating into daily living a therapeutic regimen for treatment of illness and its sequelae, which can be strengthened.

DEFINING CHARACTERISTICS

Subjective

Expresses desire to enhance:
- Management of illness, symptoms, or risk factors
- Management of prescribed regimens
- Immunization/vaccination status
- Choices of daily living for meeting goals

Sample Clinical Applications: Diabetes mellitus, congestive heart failure (CHF), chronic obstructive pulmonary disease (COPD), asthma, multiple sclerosis (MS), systemic lupus, HIV positive, AIDS, premature newborn

DESIRED OUTCOMES/EVALUATION CRITERIA

Sample NOC linkages:

Adherence Behavior: Self-initiated actions to promote optimal wellness, recovery, and rehabilitation

Knowledge: Treatment Regimen: Extent of understanding conveyed about a specific treatment regimen

Participation in Health-Care Decisions: Personal involvement in selecting and evaluating health care options to achieve desired outcomes

Client Will (Include Specific Time Frame)
- Assume responsibility for managing treatment regimen.
- Demonstrate proactive management by anticipating and planning for eventualities of condition or potential complications.
- Identify and use additional resources, as appropriate.
- Remain free of preventable complications and progression of illness and sequelae.

ACTIONS/INTERVENTIONS

Sample NIC linkages:

Health System Guidance: Facilitating a patient's location and use of appropriate health services

Health Education: Developing and providing instruction and learning experiences to facilitate voluntary adaptation of behavior conducive to health in individuals, families, groups, or communities

Anticipatory Guidance: Preparation of patient for an anticipated developmental or situational crisis

NURSING PRIORITY NO. 1   To determine motivation for continued growth:

- Ascertain client's beliefs about health and his/her ability to maintain health. *Belief in ability to accomplish desired action is predictive of performance.*
- Verify client's level of knowledge and understanding of therapeutic regimen. Note specific health goals and what measures client has been using to achieve his/her goals. *Provides opportunity to ensure accuracy and completeness of information for future learning.*[1]

 Diagnostic Studies   Evidence Based Practice   Medications   Pediatric/Geriatric/Lifespan

- Determine source(s) individuals use when seeking health information and what is done with this information (e.g., incorporated into self-management, used as basis for seeking healthcare). *The manner in which people access and use healthcare information varies widely, with variables including age, race/culture, location, literacy, and computer use. Although the Internet is utilized by many individuals to learn about their health and healthcare needs, studies show that the most common and trusted sources of information are still healthcare professionals. Many people supplement information received from healthcare professionals with information from TV, radio, newspapers, magazines, and family/friends/coworkers.*[9,10]
- Determine individual's perceptions of adaptation to treatment, anticipated changes, or possible threats to well-being. *How client sees the situation is important to discussing what is happening in regard to the treatment regimen and planning for the future.*[1]
- Identify individual's expectations of long-term treatment needs and anticipated changes. *Knowing expectations identifies understanding and acceptance of what is realistic for own situation.*[3]
- Determine influence of cultural beliefs on client/caregiver(s) participation in regimen. *These factors influence the way people view health issues and management. For instance, people of Mexican heritage may believe that good health means being free of pain or that their future health is in God's hands; therefore, they may have difficulty adhering to a long-term healthcare regimen.*[7]

NURSING PRIORITY NO. 2 To assist client/SO(s) to develop plan to meet individual needs:

- Active-listen concerns to identify underlying issues (e.g., physical or emotional stressors, external factors such as environmental pollutants or other hazards) *that could impact client's ability to control own health.*
- Identify steps necessary to reach desired health goal(s). *Understanding the process enhances commitment and the likelihood of achieving the goals.*[4]
- Discuss resources presently used by client *to note whether changes can be arranged (e.g., increased hours of home-care assistance, access to case manager to support complex or long-term program). Helps with planning for improved therapeutic regimen.*[3]
- Accept client's evaluation of own strengths/limitations while working together to improve abilities. *Promotes sense of self-esteem and confidence to continue efforts to manage therapeutic regimen, such as diabetes and MS, more effectively.*[6]
- Incorporate client's cultural values or religious beliefs that support attainment of health goals. Problem-solve conflicts *to facilitate growth.*
- Provide information and bibliotherapy. Help client/significant others (SOs) identify and evaluate resources they can access on their own. *Promotes sense of confidence in own ability to learn about illness or condition. When referencing the Internet and nontraditional or unproven resources, the individual must exercise some restraint and determine the reliability of the source and information provided before acting on it.*[5]
- Acknowledge individual's efforts, capabilities, and skills to acquire or maintain interpersonal, self-care, and coping skills. *Provides positive reinforcement, encouraging continued progress toward desired goals to enhance therapeutic regimen.*[3,5,8]

NURSING PRIORITY NO. 3 To promote optimum health management (Teaching/Discharge Considerations):

- Promote client/caregiver choices and involvement in planning for and implementing added tasks or responsibilities. *Being involved in planning and knowing that he/she can make own choices promotes commitment to program and enhances probability that client will follow through with change.*[1,8]
- Assist in implementing strategies for monitoring progress and responses to therapeutic regimen. *Promotes proactive problem-solving, enabling client/caregiver to identify problems as they arise and deal appropriately with them so regimen is maintained.*[1,8]
- Identify additional community resources and support groups. *Provides additional opportunities for role modeling, skill training, anticipatory problem-solving, etc.*[2,6]

 Acute Care   Collaborative   Community/ Home Care   Cultural

DOCUMENTATION FOCUS

Assessment/Reassessment
- Findings, including dynamics of individual situation.
- Individual strengths and additional needs.
- Cultural values or religious beliefs.

Planning
- Plan of care and who is involved in planning.
- Teaching plan.

Implementation/Evaluation
- Response to interventions, teaching, and actions performed.
- Attainment or progress toward desired outcome(s).
- Modifications to plan of care.

Discharge Planning
- Short- and long-term needs and who is responsible for actions.
- Available resources, specific referrals made.

References

1. Newfield, S. A., et al. (2007). *Clinical Applications of Nursing Diagnosis: Adult, Child, Women's, Psychiatric, Gerontic, and Home Health Considerations.* 5th ed. Philadelphia: F. A. Davis.
2. U.S. Department of Health and Human Services: Public Health Foundation. (2010). Healthy People 2020. Retrieved March 2018 from https://www.healthypeople.gov/sites/default/files/HP2020_brochure_with_LHI_508_FNL.pdf.
3. Bombardier, C. H., Wadwhani, R., LaRotondan, C. (2005). Health promotion in people with multiple sclerosis. *Phys Med Rehabil Clin North Am,* (16), 557–570.
4. Larsen, L. S. (1998). Effectiveness of counseling intervention to assist family caregivers of chronically ill relatives. *J Psychosoc Nurs,* 36(8), 26–32.
5. Lai, S. C., Cohen, M. N. (1999). Promoting lifestyle changes. *Am J Nurs,* 99(4), 63–67.
6. Miller, J. F. (1999). *Coping with Chronic Illness: Overcoming Powerlessness.* 3rd ed. Philadelphia: F. A. Davis.
7. Purnell, L. D. (2009). *Guide to Culturally Competent Health Care.* 2nd ed. Philadelphia: F. A. Davis.
8. Agency for Healthcare Research and Quality. (2013, last review 2014). Self-management support. Retrieved March 2018 from https://www.ahrq.gov/professionals/prevention-chronic-care/improve/self-mgmt/self/index.html.
9. Dart, J., Gallois, C., Yellowlees, P. (2008). Community health information sources: A survey in three disparate communities. *Aust Health Rev,* 32(1), 186–196.
10. Cutilli, C. C. (2010). Patient Education Center: Seeking health information: What sources do your patients use? *Orthop Nurs,* 29(3), 214–219.

impaired Home Maintenance

Taxonomy II: Activity/Rest—Class 5 Self-Care (00098) [**Diagnostic Division:** Safety], Approved 1980; Revised 2017

DEFINITION: Inability to independently maintain a safe growth-promoting immediate environment.

RELATED FACTORS
Inadequate role model; insufficient support system
Insufficient family organization or planning
Insufficient knowledge of home maintenance, neighborhood resources

(continues on page 424)

 Diagnostic Studies   Evidence Based Practice   Medications   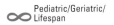 Pediatric/Geriatric/Lifespan

impaired Home Maintenance (continued)

DEFINING CHARACTERISTICS

Subjective
Difficulty maintaining a comfortable [safe] environment; impaired ability to maintain home
Request for assistance with home maintenance
Excessive family responsibilities

Objective
Unsanitary environment
Pattern of disease or infection caused by unhygienic conditions
Insufficient equipment for maintaining home; insufficient cooking equipment, clothing, or linen
At Risk Population: Financial crisis
Associated Condition: Alteration in cognitive functioning
Sample Clinical Applications: Chronic conditions (e.g., AIDS, multiple sclerosis [MS], rheumatoid arthritis), depression, dementia, developmental delay

DESIRED OUTCOMES/EVALUATION CRITERIA

Sample NOC linkages:
Self-Care: Instrumental Activities of Daily Living [IADLs]: Personal actions to perform activities needed to function in the home or community independently with or without assistive device
Family Functioning: Capacity of a family to meet the needs of its members during developmental transitions
Safe Home Environment: Physical arrangements to minimize environmental factors that might cause physical injury in the home

Client/Caregiver Will (Include Specific Time Frame)
• Identify individual factors related to difficulty in maintaining a safe environment.
• Verbalize plan to eliminate health and safety hazards.
• Adopt behaviors reflecting lifestyle changes to create and sustain a healthy and growth-promoting environment.
• Demonstrate appropriate, effective use of resources.

ACTIONS/INTERVENTIONS

Sample NIC linkages:
Home Maintenance Assistance: Helping the patient/family to maintain the home as a clean, safe, and pleasant place to live
Environmental Management: Safety: Monitoring and manipulation of the physical environment to promote safety
Support System Enhancement: Facilitation of support to patient by family, friends, and community

NURSING PRIORITY NO. 1   To assess causative/contributing factors:

• Identify presence of or potential for conditions such as diabetes, fractures, spinal cord injury, amputation, MS, arthritis, stroke, Parkinson's disease, dementia, and mental illness, *which can compromise client's/significant other's (SO's) functional abilities in taking care of home.*[3]

 Acute Care   Collaborative   Community/ Home Care   Cultural

- Note personal or environmental factors (e.g., family member with multiple care tasks, addition of family member(s) [e.g., new baby, ill parent moving in]; substance abuse; poverty/inadequate financial resources; absence of family/support systems; lifestyle of self-neglect; client comfortable with home environment or has no desire for change) *that can contribute to neglect of home cleanliness or repair.*[2,5]
- Determine problems in the household and degree of discomfort or unsafe conditions noted by client/SO. *Some safety problems may be immediately obvious (e.g., lack of heat, water; need for laundry, garbage disposal, etc.), while other problems may be more subtle and difficult to manage (e.g., lack of sufficient finances for home repairs, lack of knowledge about food storage, indoor air and fire safety, rodent control). Client/SO may need assistance or teaching regarding safety of his/her environment, especially if it is negatively impacting the client's health.*[2,6]
- Assess client's/SO's level of cognitive, emotional, and physical functioning *to ascertain client's needs and caregiver's capabilities when developing plan of care for preventive, supportive, and therapeutic care.*[1,2]
- Identify lack of interest or knowledge or misinformation *to determine need for health education/home safety program or other intervention.*
- Identify support systems available to client/SO(s) *to determine needs and initiate referrals (e.g., companionship, daily care, respite care, homemaking, running errands, meal preparation or meal-service program, financial assistance).*[1]
- Determine financial resources to meet needs of individual situation. *May need referral to social services for funds, necessary equipment, home repairs, transportation, etc.*[2]

NURSING PRIORITY NO. 2 To help client/SO(s) to create/maintain a safe, growth-promoting environment:

- Coordinate planning with multidisciplinary team and client/SO as appropriate. *Coordination and cooperation of team improves motivation and maximizes outcomes.*
- Assist client/SO(s) to develop plan for restoring/maintaining a clean, healthful environment. *Activities such as sharing of household tasks or repairs between family members, contract services, exterminators, and trash removal can promote ongoing maintenance.*
- Educate and assist client/family to address lifestyle adjustments that may be required, such as personal/home hygiene practices, elimination of substance abuse or unsafe smoking habits, proper food storage, stress management, etc. *Individuals may not be aware of impact of these factors on their health or welfare; they may be overwhelmed and in need of specific assistance for varying periods of time.*
- Discuss home environment or perform home visit as indicated *to determine client's ability to care for self, to identify potential health and safety hazards, and to determine adaptations that may be needed (e.g., wheelchair-accessible doors and hallways, safety bars in bathroom, safe place for child play, clean water available, working cook stove or microwave, screens on windows).*[2]
- Assist client/SO(s) to identify and acquire necessary equipment and services (e.g., chair or stair lifts; commode chair; safety grab bar; structural adaptations; service animals; aids for hearing, seeing, mobility; trash removal; cleaning supplies) *to meet individual needs.*[3]
- Identify resources available for appropriate assistance (e.g., visiting nurse, budget counseling, homemaker, Meals on Wheels, physical or occupational therapy, social services).[2]
- Discuss options for financial assistance with housing needs. *Client may be able to stay in home with minimal assistance or may need significant assistance over a wide range of possibilities, including removal from the home.*[2]

NURSING PRIORITY NO. 3 To promote wellness (Teaching/Discharge Considerations):

- Evaluate client at each community contact or before facility discharge *to determine if home maintenance needs are ongoing in order to initiate appropriate referrals.*[3]
- Discuss environmental hazards *that may negatively affect health or ability to perform desired activities.*

 Diagnostic Studies   Evidence Based Practice   Medications   Pediatric/Geriatric/Lifespan

- Discuss long-term plan *for taking care of environmental needs (e.g., assistive personnel, specialized controls for electrical equipment, trash removal, and pest control services).*[4]
- Provide information necessary for the individual situation. *Helps client/family decide what can be done to improve situation.*[3]
- Identify ways to access/use community resources and support systems (e.g., extended family, neighbors, church group, seniors program).
- Refer to NDs caregiver Role Strain, compromised family Coping, ineffective Coping, risk for Injury, deficient Knowledge [specify], and Self-Care deficit [specify] for additional interventions as appropriate.

DOCUMENTATION FOCUS

Assessment/Reassessment
- Assessment findings include individual (cognitive, emotional, and physical functioning) and environmental factors, specific safety concerns.
- Availability and use of support systems.

Planning
- Plan of care and who is involved in planning; support systems and community resources identified.
- Teaching plan.

Implementation/Evaluation
- Client's/SO's responses to interventions, teaching, and actions performed.
- Attainment or progress toward desired outcome(s).
- Modifications to plan of care.

Discharge Planning
- Long-term needs and who is responsible for actions to be taken.
- Specific referrals made, equipment needs/resources.

References

1. Townsend, M. C. (2011). *Psychiatric Mental Health Nursing Concepts of Care in Evidence-Based Practice*. 7th ed. Philadelphia: F. A. Davis.
2. Newfield, S. A., et al. (2007). *Cox's Clinical Applications of Nursing Diagnosis: Adult, Child, Women's, Mental Health, Gerontic, and Home Health Considerations*. 5th ed. Philadelphia: F. A. Davis.
3. Bombardier, C. H., Wadhwani, R., LaRontonda, C. (2005). Health promotion in people with multiple sclerosis. *Phys Med Rehab Clin North Am*, (16), 557–570.
4. Schmelling, S. (2005). Home, adapted home. *Rehab Manag*, 18(6), 12–19.
5. Gibbons, S., Lauder, W., Ludwick, R. (2006). Self-neglect: A proposed new NANDA diagnosis. *Int J Nurs Terminol Classif*, 17(1), 10–18.
6. Centers for Disease Control and Prevention (CDC). (2007). Healthy homes; Health issues related to community design (fact sheets). Retrieved March 2018 from http://www.cdc.gov/healthyplaces/factsheets/health_issues_related_to_community_design_factsheet_final.pdf.

 Acute Care   Collaborative   Community/Home Care   Cultural

Hopelessness

Taxonomy II: Self-Perception—Class 1 Self-Concept (00124) [**Diagnostic Division:** Ego Integrity], Submitted 1986; Revised 2017

DEFINITION: Subjective state in which an individual sees limited or no alternatives or personal choices available and is unable to mobilize energy on own behalf.

RELATED FACTORS

Prolonged activity restriction; social isolation
Deteriorating physiological condition
Chronic stress
Loss of belief in spiritual power or transcendent values

DEFINING CHARACTERISTICS

Subjective
Despondent verbal cues [Believes things will not change]

Objective
Passivity; decrease in verbalization
Decrease in affect, appetite, or response to stimuli
Decrease in initiative; inadequate involvement in care
Alteration in sleep pattern
Turning away from speaker; shrugging in response to speaker; poor eye contact
At Risk Population: History of abandonment
Associated Condition: Deterioration in physiological condition
Sample Clinical Applications: Chronic conditions, terminal diagnoses, infertility

DESIRED OUTCOMES/EVALUATION CRITERIA

Sample NOC linkages:
Depression Self-Control: Personal actions to minimize melancholy and maintain interest in life events
Hope: Optimism that is personally satisfying and life supporting
Quality of Life: Extent of positive perception of current life circumstances

Client Will (Include Specific Time Frame)
• Recognize and verbalize feelings.
• Identify and use coping mechanisms to counteract feelings of hopelessness.
• Involve self in and control (within limits of the individual situation) own self-care and activities of daily living.
• Set progressive short-term goals that develop, foster, and sustain behavioral changes and positive outlook.
• Participate in diversional activities of own choice.

ACTIONS/INTERVENTIONS

Sample NIC linkages:
Hope Inspiration: Enhancing the belief in one's capacity to initiate and sustain actions
Emotional Support: Provision of reassurance, acceptance, and encouragement during times of stress
Mood Management: Providing for safety, stabilization, recovery, and maintenance of a patient who is experiencing dysfunctionally depressed or elevated mood

 Diagnostic Studies   Evidence Based Practice   Medications   Pediatric/Geriatric/Lifespan

NURSING PRIORITY NO. 1 To identify causative/contributing factors:

* Review familial/social history and physiological history contributing to current problems. *History of poor coping abilities, disorder of familial relating patterns, emotional problems, language or cultural barriers (leading to feelings of isolation), recent or long-term illness of client or family member, and multiple social and/or physiological traumas to individual or family members can all affect client's feelings of hopelessness.*[2,5]
* Identify current familial, social, and physical factors contributing to sense of hopelessness. *Issues such as a newly diagnosed chronic/terminal disease, lack of support system, recent job loss, loss of spiritual or religious faith, and recent multiple traumas can result in an individual giving up. Identification of the issues involved in each person's situation is necessary to appropriately plan for care.*[2]
* Determine client's locus of control (internal or external) and associated cultural factors influencing self-view. Note expressions of responsibility for self versus expressions of lack of control over self and environment. *Individuals view life change and stressful events differently. Those with internal locus of control tend to be more optimistic about their ability to deal with adversity even in the face of current difficulties. Individual with external locus of control may attribute feelings of hopelessness to an external source, perceiving it as beyond his or her control, and will look to others to solve problems and take care of them.*[2,5]
* Identify coping behaviors and defense mechanisms displayed previously and in current situation as well as client's perception of effectiveness then and now. *It is important to identify client's strengths and encourage their use as client begins to deal with what is currently happening.*[2]
* Have client describe events that lead to feeling inadequate or having no control. *Identifies sources of frustration and defines problem areas so action can be taken to learn how to deal with them in more positive ways.*[6]
* Discuss problem and duration of alcohol or drug abuse as indicated. *Behavior may be an effort to provide psychological numbing in an attempt to lessen pain of situation or may have preceded and contributed to sense of hopelessness. Client may feel hopeless about stopping behavior and believe that it is impossible.*[2]
* Determine presence of suicidal ideation, availability of plan, and means to follow through with plan. (Refer to ND risk for Suicide.) *Hopelessness is identified as a central underlying factor in the predisposition to suicide, and the client sees no other way out of a hopeless situation.*[7]
* Perform physical examination and review results of lab tests and diagnostic studies. *Current situation may be the result of a decline in physical well-being or progression of a chronic condition, or physical symptoms may be associated with effects of depression (e.g., loss of appetite, lack of sleep).*[7]

NURSING PRIORITY NO. 2 To assess level of hopelessness:

* Note behaviors indicative of hopelessness as listed in Defining Characteristics. *Identifies problem areas to be addressed in developing an effective plan of care and suggests possible resources needed.*[6]
* Evaluate and discuss use of defense mechanisms (useful or not). *Identifying behaviors such as increased sleeping, dependence on medications, illness behaviors, eating disorders, denial, forgetfulness, daydreaming, ineffectual organizational efforts, exploiting own goal-setting, and regression can provide accurate information for client to begin changing behavior or inaccurate beliefs.*[6]
* Evaluate degree of hopelessness using psychological testing such as Beck's Depression Scale. Note client's feelings about life not being worth living and other signs of hopelessness and worthlessness. *Identifying the degree of hopelessness and possible suicidal thoughts is crucial to instituting appropriate treatment to protect client.*[10]

NURSING PRIORITY NO. 3 To assist client to identify feelings and to begin to cope with problems as perceived by the client:

* Establish a therapeutic and facilitative relationship showing positive regard for the client. Answer questions truthfully. *Enhances trust so that client may feel safe to disclose feelings, talk openly about concerns, and feel understood and listened to.*[2,3,10]
* Encourage client to verbalize and explore feelings and perceptions of what is happening. *Talking about feelings of anger, helplessness, powerlessness, confusion, despondency, isolation, and grief (which can lead to a sense*

 Acute Care   Collaborative   Community/ Home Care   Cultural

of hopelessness and the belief that nothing can be done) provides opportunity for reflection and enables client to begin to understand self and that there are actions that can be helpful.[3]

- ∞ Provide opportunity for children to "play out" feelings (e.g., puppets or art for preschooler, peer discussions for adolescents). *Provides insight into perceptions and can give direction for developing coping strategies.*[2]
- ∞ Engage teens and parents in discussions and arrange to do activities with them. *Parents can make a difference in their children's lives by being with them, discussing sensitive topics, and going different places with them.*[3,4]
- Express hope to client and encourage significant others and other health-team members to do so as well. Avoid expressions of false hope. *Client may not identify positives in own situation and may find it difficult to accept them from others, but will hear them. False reassurances will undermine sense of security.*[2]
- Help client recognize areas in which he or she has control versus those that are not within his or her control. *Often the individual who is feeling hopeless is focusing on issues that cannot be changed. When the client begins to focus energy in those areas where he or she has control, a sense of hope can be nurtured.*[6]
- Use client's locus of control to develop individual plan of care. *Tailoring care to the individual's ability will maximize effectiveness. For instance, client with internal control can take control of own destiny, and those with external control may need to begin with small tasks and add as tolerated, moving toward learning to take more control of personal choices.*[13]
- Encourage client to identify short-term goals. Promote activities to achieve goals and facilitate contingency planning. *Dealing with situation in manageable steps enhances chances for success, promotes sense of control, and encourages belief that there is hope for resolution of situation/moving forward.*[6]
- Discuss current options with client and list actions that can be taken. Correct misconceptions expressed by the client. *Encourages use of own actions, validates reality, and promotes sense of control of the situation.*[2]
- Endeavor to prevent situations that might lead to feelings of isolation or lack of control in client's perception. *Client will interpret these occurrences as further proof that there is no hope.*[6]
- 🏠 Promote client control in establishing time, place, and frequency of treatment/therapy sessions. Involve family members in the appointments as appropriate. *Allows individual to assume control over own situation, engendering positive feelings of ability to manage what is happening. Involvement of family members provides source of support and encouragement for client.*[2]
- Encourage risk-taking in situations in which the client can succeed. *Succeeding in new ventures can improve self-esteem and hope for more successful actions.*[2]
- Help client begin to develop new coping mechanisms. *New skills need to be learned and used effectively to counteract hopelessness.*[3]
- Encourage structured and controlled increase in physical activity as tolerated. *Promotes the release of endorphins, enhancing sense of well-being.*[2]
- Demonstrate and encourage use of relaxation exercises, guided imagery. *Anxious feelings create tension, and learning to relax can help client begin to look at possibilities of feeling more hopeful.*[9]
- 💊 Discuss safe use of prescribed antidepressants. *May require short-term use to elevate mood while client pursues other therapeutic measures to regain sense of hope.*[2]

NURSING PRIORITY NO. 4 To promote wellness (Teaching/Discharge Considerations):

- 🏠 Provide positive feedback for actions taken to deal with and overcome feelings of hopelessness. *Encourages changes in thinking patterns and continuation of desired behaviors.*[10,12]
- Assist client/family to become aware of factors or situations leading to feelings of hopelessness. *Helps individuals to identify precipitating events and provides opportunities to avoid or modify situation, promoting sense of control over life.*[8]
- Discuss initial signs of hopelessness. *Helps client to identify behaviors such as procrastination, increased need for sleep, decreased physical activity, or withdrawal from social or familial activities and how they have affected thinking and ability to deal with current situation. Awareness provides the opportunity to begin to change.*[9]
- Facilitate client's incorporation of personal loss. *Often prior losses in individual's life result in feelings of hopelessness and lack of control in current events. Hopelessness means a loss of hope rather than just an*

 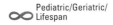

absence of hope. Enhancing grief work and promoting resolution of feelings help client to begin to feel hope again and look forward to life.[9]

- Encourage client/family to develop support systems in the immediate community. *Having support nearby provides individuals with assistance and advocacy for moving forward, enabling them to look toward future with hope.*[4,6]
- Help client to become aware of, nurture, and expand spiritual self. (Refer to ND Spiritual Distress.) *Spiritual needs are an integral part of being human. Acknowledging and learning about spiritual aspect of self can help client look toward the future with hope for improved sense of well-being.*[11]
- Encourage and facilitate interaction with religious representative or spiritual counselor as indicated. *Client's sense of hopelessness may include the loss of spiritual connectedness, or client may view spiritual being as responsible for current situation.*[1]
- Introduce the client into a support group before the individual therapy is terminated for continuation of therapeutic process. *Provides for a smooth transition so client feels accepted and comfortable in the presence of others.*[6]
- Emphasize need for continued monitoring of medication regimen by healthcare provider. *Necessary to evaluate effectiveness and prevent or minimize possible side effects. Antidepressant agents are not to be discontinued abruptly without consulting healthcare provider.*[2]
- Refer to other resources for assistance as indicated (e.g., clinical nurse specialist, psychiatrist, social services, Alcoholics or Narcotics Anonymous, Al-Anon, or Alateen). *May need additional help to develop hope for the future, sustain efforts for change.*[2]

DOCUMENTATION FOCUS

Assessment/Reassessment
- Assessment findings, including what has been lost in hopelessness, degree of impairment, locus of control, use of coping skills.
- Cultural or religious beliefs and expectations.
- Spiritual concerns.
- Availability and use of resources or support systems.

Planning
- Plan of care and who is involved in planning.
- Teaching plan.

Implementation/Evaluation
- Responses to interventions, teaching, and actions performed.
- Attainment or progress toward desired outcome(s).
- Modifications to plan of care.

Discharge Planning
- Identified long-term needs, client's goals for change, and who is responsible for actions to be taken.
- Specific referrals made.

References

1. Geiter, H. (2002). The spiritual side of nursing. *RN*, 65(5), 43–44.
2. Reznikoff, P. T. M. (1982). Perceived peer and family relationships, hopelessness and locus of control as factors in adolescent suicide attempts. *Suicide Life Threat Behav*, 12(3), 141–150.
3. Gordon, T. (No date). Families need rules. *Gordon Training International*. Retrieved March 2018 from http://www.gordon-training.com/free-parenting-articles/families-need-rules/.
4. Clark, C. M. (Last modified 2005). Relations between social support and physical health. *Rochester Institute of Technology*.

Retrieved March 2018 from http://www.personalityresearch.org/papers/clark.html.
5. McLeod, D., Wright, L. M. (2001). Conversations of spirituality: Spirituality in family systems nursing—Making the case with four clinical vignettes. *J Fam Nurs*, 7(4), 391–415.
6. Kwon, P. (2002). Hope, defense mechanisms, and adjustment: Implications for false hope and defensive hopelessness. *J Pers*, 70(2), 207–231.
7. Ghosh, T. B., Victor, B. S. (1994). Suicide. In Hales, R. R., et al. (eds). *The American Psychiatric Press Textbook of Psychiatry*. 2nd ed. Washington, DC: American Psychiatric Press.

 Acute Care   Collaborative   Community/Home Care   Cultural

8. Drew, B. (1990). Differentiation of hopelessness, helplessness, and powerlessness using Erik Erikson's "Roots of Virtue." *Arch Psychiatr Nurs*, 4, 332–337.

9. Patterson, B. (2009, no update). A Buddhist approach to grief counseling. Navigating Life's Changes. Retrieved March 2018 from http://bethspatterson.com/a-buddhist-approach-to-grief-counseling/.

10. Beck, A. T., Brown, G., Berchick, R. J. (1990). Relationship between hopelessness and ultimate suicide: A replication with psychiatric out-patients. *Am J Psychiatry*, 147, 190–195.

11. Sharma, Y. R. S. (2007). Scientific research studies on spiritual science and philosophy. *SelfGrowth.com*. Retrieved March 2018 from http://www.articlesfactory.com/articles/metaphysical/scientific-research-studies-on-spiritual-science-and-philosophy.html.

12. Seligman, M. (No date). Positive health. *Authentic Happiness, University of Pennsylvania*. Retrieved March 2018 from https://www.authentichappiness.sas.upenn.edu/learn/positivehealth.

13. Kunert, P. K. (2002). Stress and adaptation. In Porth, C. M. (ed). *Pathophysiology: Concepts of Altered Health States*. Philadelphia: J. B. Lippincott.

readiness for enhanced Hope

Taxonomy II: Self–Perception Class 1 Self—Concept (00185) [**Diagnostic Division:** Ego Integrity], Approved 2006; Revised 2017

DEFINITION: A pattern of expectations and desires for mobilizing energy on one's own behalf, which can be strengthened.

DEFINING CHARACTERISTICS

Subjective

Expresses desire to enhance: hope; belief in possibilities; congruency of expectation with goal; ability to set achievable goals; problem solving to meet goals

Expresses desire to enhance: sense of meaning in life; connectedness with others; spirituality

Sample Clinical Applications: Any acute or chronic condition, or healthy individual looking to improve well-being

DESIRED OUTCOMES/EVALUATION CRITERIA

Sample NOC linkages:

Hope: Optimism that is personally satisfying and life supporting

Quality of Life: Extent of positive perception of current life circumstances

Personal Well-Being: Extent of positive perception of one's health status

Client Will (Include Specific Time Frame)

• Identify and verbalize feelings related to expectations and desires.

• Verbalize belief in possibilities for the future.

• Discuss current situation and desire to enhance hope.

• Set short-term goals that will lead to behavioral changes to meet desire for enhanced hope.

ACTIONS/INTERVENTIONS

Sample NIC linkages:

Hope Inspiration: Enhancing the belief in one's capacity to initiate and sustain actions

Self-Awareness Enhancement: Assisting a patient to explore and understand his/her thoughts, feelings, motivations, and behaviors

Spiritual Growth Facilitation: Facilitation of growth in patient's capacity to identify, connect with, and call upon the source of meaning, purpose, comfort, strength, and hope in their lives

 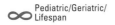

NURSING PRIORITY NO. 1   To determine needs and desire for improvement:

- Review familial and social history to identify past situations (e.g., illness, emotional conflicts, alcoholism) that have led to decision to improve life. *When trials of life have been resolved, individuals may look toward making life better.*[1]
- Determine current physical condition of client/significant other (SO). *Treatment regimen and indicators of healing can influence ability and promote positive feelings of hope.*[2]
- Ascertain client's perception of current state and expectations or goals for the future (e.g., general well-being, prosperity, independence). *Perception is more important than reality in individual's mind and may help client pursue realistic goals for self.*[3]
- Identify spiritual beliefs/cultural values that guide or influence client's spirituality and view of self. *Influences sense of hope and connectedness.*[4]
- Determine meaning of life or reasons for living, belief in God or higher power. *Helps client to clarify beliefs and how they relate to desire for improvement in life.*
- Ascertain motivation and expectations for change. Note congruency of expectations with desires for change. *Motivation to improve and high expectations can encourage client to make changes that will improve his or her life. However, presence of unrealistic expectations may hamper efforts.*[3,4]
- Note degree of involvement in activities and relationships with others. *Interactions with others can promote a sense of connectedness and enjoyment of relationships.*[3]

NURSING PRIORITY NO. 2   To assist client to achieve goals and strengthen sense of hope:

- Establish a therapeutic relationship, showing positive regard and hopefulness for the client. *Enhances feelings of worth and comfort, inspiring client to continue pursuit of goals.*[3]
- Help client recognize areas that are in his or her control versus those that are not. *To be most effective, client needs to expend energy in those areas where he or she has control and let the others go.*[2]
- Assist client to develop manageable short-term goals. *Success at short-term goals can lead to attainment of long-term goals too.*[2]
- Identify activities to achieve goals and facilitate contingency planning. *Promotes dealing with situation in manageable steps, enhancing chances for success and sense of control.*[5]
- Explore interrelatedness of relationship between unresolved emotions, anxieties, fears, and guilt. *Provides opportunity to address issues that may be limiting individual's ability to improve life situation.*[5]
- Assist client to acknowledge current coping behaviors and defense mechanisms that may hamper moving toward goals. *Allows client to focus on coping mechanisms that are more successful in problem-solving.*[3]
- Encourage client to concentrate on progress not perfection. *If client can accept that perfection is difficult or not always the desirable outcome, he/she may be able to view accomplishments with pride.*[3]
- Involve client in care and explain all procedures, answering questions truthfully. *Enhances trust and relationship, promoting hope for a positive outcome.*[2]
- Express hope to client and encourage SO(s) and other health team members to do so. *Enhances client's sense of hope and belief in possibilities of a positive outcome.*[1]
- Identify ways to strengthen sense of interconnectedness or harmony with others *to support sense of belonging and connection that promotes feelings of wholeness and hopefulness.*[1]

NURSING PRIORITY NO. 3   To promote optimum wellness:

- Demonstrate and encourage use of relaxation techniques, guided imagery, and meditation activities. *Learning to relax can decrease tension, resulting in refreshment of body and mind and enabling individual to perform and think more successfully.*[3]
- Provide positive feedback for efforts taken to improve situation, growth in use of skills, and learning efforts. *Acknowledges client's efforts as individual is moving forward in learning new skills and reinforces gains.*[3]
- Explore ways that beliefs give meaning and value to daily living. *As client's understanding of these issues improves, hope for the future is strengthened.*[1]

 Acute Care   Collaborative   Community/ Home Care   Cultural

- Encourage life review by client. *Acknowledges own successes, identifies opportunity for change, and clarifies meaning in life.*[5]
- Identify ways for spiritual expression, strengthening spirituality. *There are many options for enhancing spirituality through connectedness with self and others (e.g., volunteering, mentoring, involvement in religious activities).*[5] (Refer to ND readiness for enhanced Spiritual Well-Being.)
- Encourage client to join groups with similar or new interests. *Expanding knowledge and making friendships with new people will widen horizons for the individual.*
- Refer to community resources and support groups and spiritual advisor as indicated.

DOCUMENTATION FOCUS

Assessment/Reassessment
- Assessment findings, including client's perceptions of current situation, relationships, sense of desire for enhancing life.
- Cultural or spiritual values and beliefs.
- Motivation and expectations for improvement.

Planning
- Plan of care and who is involved in planning.
- Teaching plan.

Implementation/Evaluation
- Responses to interventions, teaching, and actions performed.
- Attainment or progress toward desired outcome(s).
- Modifications to plan of care.

Discharge Planning
- Identified long-term needs, individual goals for change, and who is responsible for actions to be taken.
- Specific referrals made.

References

1. Laudet, A. B., Morgen, K., White, W. L. (2006). The role of social supports, spirituality, religiousness, life meaning and affiliation with 12-step fellowships in quality of life satisfaction among individuals in recovery from alcohol and drug problems. *Alcohol Treat Q*, 24(1–2), 33–73.
2. Davison, S. N., Simpson, C. (2006). Hope and advance care planning in patients with end stage renal disease: Qualitative interview study. *BMJ*, 333, 886–889.
3. Saltz, L. B. (2008). Progress in cancer care—The hype, hope and the gap between perception and reality. *J Clin Oncol*, 26(31), 520–521.
4. Blagen, M., Yang, J. (2008). Courage and hope as factors for client change: Important cultural implications and spiritual considerations. *American Counseling Association: Vistas Online*. Retrieved March 2018 from https://www.counseling.org/Resources/Library/VISTAS/2008-V-Online-MSWord-files/Blagen.pdf.
5. Rousseau, P. (2000). Hope in the terminally ill. *West J Med*, 173(2), 117–118.

 Diagnostic Studies   Evidence Based Practice Medications Pediatric/Geriatric/Lifespan

risk for compromised Human Dignity

Taxonomy II: Self-Perception—Class 1 Self-Concept (00174) [**Diagnostic Division:** Ego Integrity], Submitted 2006; Revised 2013

DEFINITION: Susceptible for perceived loss of respect and honor, which may compromise health.

RISK FACTORS
Loss of control over body function; exposure of the body
Humiliation; invasion of privacy
Disclosure of confidential information; stigmatization
Dehumanizing treatment; intrusion by clinician
Insufficient comprehension of health information
Limited decision-making experience
Cultural incongruence
Sample Clinical Applications: Chronic conditions (e.g., multiple sclerosis [MS], stroke, quadriplegia, amyotrophic lateral sclerosis [ALS])

DESIRED OUTCOMES/EVALUATION CRITERIA

Sample **NOC** linkages:
Client Satisfaction: Protection of Rights: Extent of positive perception of protection of a client's legal and moral rights provided by nursing staff
Client Satisfaction: Cultural Needs Fulfillment: Extent of positive perception of integration of cultural beliefs, values, and social structures into nursing care

Client Will (Include Specific Time Frame)
• Verbalize awareness of specific problem.
• Identify positive ways to deal with situation.
• Demonstrate problem-solving skills.
• Express desire to increase participation in decision-making process.
• Express sense of dignity in situation.

ACTIONS/INTERVENTIONS

Sample **NIC** linkages:
Cultural Brokerage: The deliberate use of culturally competent strategies to bridge or mediate between the patient's culture and the biomedical healthcare system
Patient Rights Protection: Protection of healthcare rights of a patient, especially a minor, incapacitated, or incompetent patient unable to make decisions
Emotional Support: Provision of reassurance, acceptance, and encouragement during times of stress

NURSING PRIORITY NO. 1   To determine individual situation as perceived by client:

• Determine client's perception and specific factors that could lead to sense of loss of dignity. *Human dignity is a totality of the individual's uniqueness—mind, body, and spirit—and all components must be considered.*[4]
• Note names, labels, or items used by staff, friends/family that stigmatize the client. *Human dignity is threatened by insensitive as well as inadequate healthcare and lack of client participation in care decisions.*[4]
• Identify cultural beliefs or values and degree of importance to client. *Individuals cling to their basic beliefs and values, especially during times of stress, which may result in conflict with current circumstances.*[7]

 Acute Care   Collaborative   Community/ Home Care   Cultural

- Identify client's/significant other's (SO's) healthcare goals and expectations. *Clarifies client's (or SO's/ family's) vision, provides framework for planning care, and identifies possible conflicts.*[2]
- Note availability of support systems. *Client who feels loved and valued will be able to manage difficult circumstances better when the support of family and friends surrounds individual.*[2]
- Ascertain response of family/SOs to client's situation. *It is important that family supports and values client to enable him or her to manage situation. If they are not supportive or conflicts arise, client may need to separate self from family members who are negative.*[3]

NURSING PRIORITY NO. 2   To assist client to deal with situation in positive ways:

- Ask client by what name he or she would like to be addressed. *Name is important to a person's identity and recognizes his or her individuality. Many older people prefer to be addressed in a formal manner (e.g., Mr. or Mrs.).*[2,7]
- Active-listen feelings, encouraging client to verbalize concerns. Be available for support and assistance. *Can help client to discover underlying reasons for feelings and seek solutions to problems.*[5]
- Respect the client's needs and wishes for quiet, privacy, talking, or silence. *Conveys respect and concern for client's dignity.*[3]
- Provide for privacy when discussing sensitive or personal issues. *Demonstrates respect for client and promotes sense of safe environment for free exchange of thoughts and feelings.*[3]
- Use understandable terms when talking to client/family about the medical condition, procedures, and treatments (component of informed consent). *Many people do not understand medical terms and may be hesitant to ask what is meant.*[6]
- ∞ Encourage family/SO(s) to treat client with respect and understanding, especially when the client is older and may be irritable and difficult to deal with. *Everyone should be treated with respect and dignity, regardless of individual abilities or frailty.*[4]
- Include client and family in decision making, especially regarding end-of-life issues. *Helps the individual feel respected or valued and involved in the care process.*[2]
- Involve facility or local ethics committee as appropriate *to facilitate mediation or resolution of conflicts between client/family and staff or client and family members.*[5]
- Protect client's privacy when providing personal care and during procedures. *Prevents embarrassment over unnecessary exposure and conveys a message of caring and preserves client dignity.*

NURSING PRIORITY NO. 3   To promote wellness (Teaching/Discharge Considerations):

- 🏠 Discuss client's rights as an individual. *While hospitals and other care settings have a Client's Bill of Rights, a broader view of human dignity is stated in the U.S. Constitution.*[1,6]
- Assist with planning for the future, taking into account client's desires and rights. *As the client plans for the future, the needs of the self as a human who has dignity are considered and incorporated to preserve that dignity.*[4]
- 🌐 Incorporate familial, religious, and cultural factors that have meaning for client in planning process. *When these issues are addressed and incorporated in plan of care, they add to the feelings of inclusion for the client.*[4,7]
- 🔵 Refer to other resources (e.g., pastoral care, counseling, organized support groups, classes), as appropriate. *May need additional assistance to deal with illness/situation.*

DOCUMENTATION FOCUS

Assessment/Reassessment
- Assessment findings, including individual risk factors, client's perceptions, and concerns about involvement in care.
- Individual cultural or religious beliefs and values, healthcare goals.
- Responses and involvement of family/SOs.

 Diagnostic Studies   Evidence Based Practice   Medications   Pediatric/Geriatric/ Lifespan

Planning
- Plan of care and who is involved in planning.
- Teaching plan.

Implementation/Evaluation
- Client's response to interventions, teaching, and actions performed.
- Attainment or progress toward desired outcome(s).
- Modifications to plan of care.

Discharge Planning
- Long-term needs and who is responsible for actions to be taken.
- Specific referrals made.

References

1. Bush, G. W. (2002). Champion aspirations for human dignity. Retrieved March 2018 from https://georgewbush-whitehouse.archives.gov/nsc/nss/2006/sectionII.html.
2. Schulman, A. (2009). Bioethics and the question of human dignity. *University of Notre Dame Press*. Retrieved March 2018 from https://www3.nd.edu/~undpress/excerpts/P01307-ex.pdf.
3. Cheshire, W. P. (2007). Grey matters when eloquence is inarticulate. *The Center for Bioethics & Human Dignity. Trinity International University*. Retrieved March 2018 from https://cbhd.org/content/grey-matters-when-eloquence-inarticulate.
4. Moran, G. (No date). Dignity, uniqueness, rights (white paper). Retrieved March 2018 from http://www.nyu.edu/classes/gmoran/EXC-RIGH.pdf.
5. Phatak, O. (2010). Therapeutic communication techniques. Retrieved March 2018 from http://www.buzzle.com/articles/therapeutic-communication-techniques.html.
6. No author listed. (No date). Patient's Bill of Rights. Retrieved March 2018 from http://www.healthsourceglobal.com/docs/patient%20bill%20of%20rights_merged.pdf.
7. Chang, M., Kelley, A. (2007). Patient education: Addressing cultural diversity and health literacy issues. *Urol Nurs*, 27(5), 411–417.

---

neonatal Hyperbilirubinemia

Taxonomy II: Nutrition—Class 4 Metabolism (00230) **[Diagnostic Division:** Safety**],** Approved 2008; Revised 2010, 2017

DEFINITION: The accumulation of unconjugated bilirubin in the circulation (less than 15 ml/dl) that occurs after 24 hours of life.

RELATED FACTORS
Deficient feeding pattern
Infant with inadequate nutrition
Delay in meconium passage

DEFINING CHARACTERISTICS

Objective
Yellow-orange skin color; yellow sclera, mucous membranes
Bruised skin
Abnormal blood profile [e.g., hemolysis; total serum bilirubin in high-risk range on age in hour-specific nomogram]
At Risk Population: ABO incompatibility; blood type incompatibility between mother and infant; Rhesus (Rh) incompatibility
Age ≤7 days; premature infant, or infant with low birthweight; infant who is breastfed
American Indian or East Asian ethnicity
Significant bruising during birth
Maternal diabetes mellitus; populations living at high altitudes

 Acute Care   Collaborative   Community/Home Care Cultural

Associated Condition: Prenatal infection; bacterial or viral infection; sepsis
Infant with liver malfunction, enzyme deficiency; internal bleeding
Sample Clinical Applications: Newborn, premature infant

DESIRED OUTCOMES/EVALUATION CRITERIA

Sample NOC linkages:
Newborn Adaptation: Adaptive response to the extrauterine environment by a physiologically mature newborn during the first 28 days

Infant Will (Include Specific Time Frame):
• Display decreasing bilirubin levels with resolution of jaundice.
• Be free of central nervous system (CNS) involvement or complications associated with therapeutic regimen.

Sample NOC linkages:
Knowledge: Treatment Procedure: Extent of understanding conveyed about a procedure required as part of a treatment regimen

Parent/Caregiver Will (Include Specific Time Frame):
• Verbalize understanding of cause, treatment, and possible outcomes of hyperbilirubinemia.
• Demonstrate appropriate care of infant.

ACTIONS/INTERVENTIONS

Sample NIC linkages:
Infant Care: Newborn: Provision of care to the infant during the transition from birth to extrauterine life and subsequent period of stabilization
Phototherapy: Neonate: Use of light therapy to reduce bilirubin levels in newborn infants
Lactation Counseling: Assisting in the establishment and maintenance of successful breastfeeding

NURSING PRIORITY NO. 1   To assess causative/contributing factors:

• Determine infant and maternal blood group and blood type. *ABO incompatibility is more often seen in newborns who have type A blood because of the higher frequency of type A compared to type B in most populations. Incidence figures are difficult to compare because authors of different studies do not use the same definitions for significant neonatal hyperbilirubinemia or jaundice. For example, Woodgate and Jadine (2015) report an estimated 50% of term and 80% of preterm infants develop jaundice, typically 2 to 4 days after birth. However, Munniti (2011) reports that ABO incompatibility generally presents as neonatal jaundice due to a Coombs' positive hemolytic anemia and occurs in 0.5% to 1% of newborns.*[1,2,9]
• Note gender, race, and place of birth. *Risk of developing jaundice is higher in males, infants of East Asian or American Indian descent, and those living at high altitudes. Incidence is lower for African American infants.*[2]
• Review intrapartal record for specific risk factors, such as low birth weight (LBW) or intrauterine growth retardation, prematurity, abnormal metabolic processes, vascular injuries, abnormal circulation, sepsis, or polycythemia. *The risk of significant neonatal jaundice is increased in LBW or premature infants, presence of congenital infection, or maternal diabetes.*[2] *Studies suggest neonates at 36 to 37 weeks' gestation are four to five times more likely to develop hyperbilirubinemia than those born at 40 weeks.*[3] *Also, certain clinical conditions may cause a reversal of the blood-brain barrier, allowing bound bilirubin to separate either at the level of the cell membrane or within the cell itself, increasing the risk of CNS involvement.*

 Diagnostic Studies   Evidence Based Practice   Medications   Pediatric/Geriatric/Lifespan

- 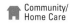Note use of instruments or vacuum extractor for delivery. Assess infant for presence of birth trauma, cephalohematoma, and excessive ecchymosis or petechiae. *Resorption of blood trapped in fetal scalp tissue and excessive hemolysis may increase the amount of bilirubin being released and cause jaundice.[7]*
- 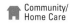Review infant's condition at birth, noting need for resuscitation or evidence of excessive ecchymosis or petechiae, cold stress, asphyxia, or acidosis. *Asphyxia and acidosis reduce affinity of bilirubin to albumin increasing the amount of unbound circulating (indirect) bilirubin, which may cross the blood-brain barrier, causing CNS toxicity.[2]*
- Evaluate maternal and prenatal nutritional levels; note possible neonatal hypoproteinemia, especially in the preterm infant. *One gram of albumin carries 16 mg of unconjugated bilirubin; therefore, lack of sufficient albumin (hypoproteinemia) in the newborn increases risk of jaundice.*
- Assess infant for signs of hypoglycemia such as jitteriness, irritability, and lethargy. Obtain heelstick glucose levels as indicated. *Hypoglycemia necessitates use of fat stores for energy-releasing fatty acids, which compete with bilirubin for binding sites on albumin.*
- Determine successful initiation and adequacy of breastfeeding. *Poor caloric intake and dehydration associated with ineffective breastfeeding increase risk of developing hyperbilirubinemia.[1]*
- Evaluate infant for pallor, edema, or hepatosplenomegaly. *These signs may be associated with hydrops fetalis, Rh incompatibility, and in utero hemolysis of fetal RBCs.*
- 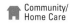Evaluate for jaundice in natural light, noting sclera and oral mucosa, yellowing of skin immediately after blanching, and specific body parts involved. Assess oral mucosa, posterior portion of hard palate, and conjunctival sacs in dark-skinned newborns. *Detects evidence/degree of jaundice generally first noted on face and progressing to trunk and then extremities.[1,6] Clinical appearance of jaundice is evident at bilirubin levels greater than 5 mg/dL in the full-term infant. Estimated degree of jaundice is as follows: face, 4 to 8 mg/dL; trunk, 10 to 12 mg/dL; groin, 8 to 16 mg/dL; arms/legs, 11 to 18 mg/dL; and hands/feet, 15 to 20 mg/dL. Note: Yellow underlying pigment may be normal in dark-skinned infants.[1,6,7]*
- 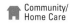Note infant's age at onset of jaundice. *Aids in differentiating type of jaundice (i.e., physiological, breast milk induced, or pathological). Physiological jaundice usually appears between the second and third days of life, as excess RBCs needed to maintain adequate oxygenation for the fetus are no longer required in the newborn and are hemolyzed, thereby releasing bilirubin.[2,6] Breast milk jaundice usually appears between the fourth and the seventh days of life, affecting approximately 14% of breastfed infants.[6] Pathological jaundice occurs within the first 24 hours of life or when the total serum bilirubin level rises by more than 5 mg/dL per day.[2,7]*

NURSING PRIORITY NO. 2   To evaluate degree of compromise:

- 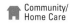Review laboratory studies, including total serum bilirubin and albumin levels, hemoglobin/hematocrit, and reticulocyte count, *to monitor severity of problem and need for, or effectiveness, of therapy.[2] Note: Excessive unconjugated bilirubin has an affinity for extravascular tissue, including the basal ganglia of brain tissue.[7]*
- 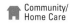Calculate plasma bilirubin-albumin–binding capacity. *Aids in determining risk of kernicterus and treatment needs.[1] When total bilirubin value divided by total serum protein level is less than 3.7, the danger of kernicterus is very low. However, the risk of injury is dependent on factors such as degree of prematurity, presence of hypoxia or acidosis, and drug regimen (e.g., sulfonamides, chloramphenicol).[7]*
- Assess infant for progression of signs and behavioral changes associated with bilirubin toxicity. *Early-stage toxicity involves neurodepression (lethargy, poor feeding, high-pitched cry, diminished or absent reflexes), late-stage hypotonia, and neuro-hyperreflexia (twitching, convulsions, opisthotonos, fever). Behavior changes associated with kernicterus usually occur between the 3rd and 10th days of life and rarely occur prior to 36 hours of life.*
- Evaluate appearance of skin and urine, noting brownish-black color. *An uncommon side effect of phototherapy, particularly in presence of cholestatic jaundice, involves exaggerated pigment changes (bronze baby syndrome), which may occur if conjugated bilirubin levels rise. The changes in skin color may last for 2 to 4 months but are not associated with harmful sequelae.*

 Acute Care   Collaborative   Community/ Home Care   Cultural

NURSING PRIORITY NO. 3 To correct hyperbilirubinemia and prevent associated complications:

- Keep infant warm and dry; monitor skin and core temperature frequently. *Prevents cold stress and the release of fatty acids that compete for binding sites on albumin, thus increasing the level of freely circulating bilirubin.*
- Initiate early oral feedings within 4 to 6 hours following birth, especially if infant is to be breastfed. *Establishes proper intestinal flora necessary for reduction of bilirubin to urobilinogen and decreases reabsorption of bilirubin from bowel by promoting passage of meconium stool.*[7]
- Encourage frequent breastfeeding—8 to 12 times per day. Assist mother with pumping of breasts as needed to maintain milk production. *Interruption of breastfeeding is rarely necessary unless serum levels reach 20 mg/ dL; however, breastfeeding support may increase frequency and efficacy of intake.*[2,5–7]
- Administer small amounts of breast milk substitute (L-aspartic acid or enzymatically hydrolyzed casein) for 24 to 48 hours if indicated. *Use of feeding additives is under investigation with mixed results for inhibition of beta-glucuronidase leading to increased fecal excretion of bilirubin.*[4,5]
- Apply transcutaneous jaundice meter, as indicated. *Provides noninvasive screening of jaundice, quantifying skin color in relation to total serum bilirubin.*
- Initiate phototherapy per protocol, using fluorescent bulbs placed above the infant or a fiberoptic pad or blanket (except for newborn with Rh disease). *Primary therapy for neonates with unconjugated hyperbilirubinemia. Three separate processes work to convert bilirubin isomers to water-soluble isomers and the formation of lumirubin. The photoisomers are then excreted in urine, stool, and bile.*[2]
- Apply eye patches ensuring correct fit during periods of phototherapy *to prevent retinal injury.* Remove eye covering during feedings or other care activities as appropriate *to provide visual stimulation and interaction with caregivers/parents.*[8]
- Avoid application of lotion or oils to skin of infant receiving phototherapy *to prevent dermal irritation or injury.*[8]
- Reposition infant every 2 hours *to ensure all areas of skin are exposed to bili light when fiberoptic pad or blanket is not used.*[8]
- Cover male groin with small pad *to protect from heat-related injury to testes.*[8]
- Monitor infant's weight loss, urine output and specific gravity, and fecal water loss from loose stools associated with phototherapy *to determine adequacy of fluid intake.*[2] *Note: Infant may sleep for longer periods in conjunction with phototherapy, increasing risk of dehydration if frequent feeding schedule is not maintained.*
- Administer intravenous immunoglobulin (IVIG) to neonates with Rh or ABO isoimmunization. *Rate of hemolysis in Rh disease or other cases of immune hemolytic jaundice usually exceeds the rate of bilirubin reduction related to phototherapy. IVIG inhibits antibodies that cause red cell destruction, helping to limit the rise in bilirubin levels.*[2–5]
- Administer enzyme induction agent (phenobarbital) as appropriate. *May be used on occasion to stimulate hepatic enzymes to enhance clearance of bilirubin.*[2]
- Assist with preparation and administration of exchange transfusion. *Exchange transfusions are occasionally required in cases of severe hemolytic anemia unresponsive to other treatment options or in the presence of acute bilirubin encephalopathy, as evidenced by hypertonia, arching, retrocollis, opisthotonos, fever, and high-pitched cry.*[1,2] *Procedure removes serum bilirubin and provides bilirubin-free albumin, increasing binding sites for bilirubin, and it treats anemia by providing RBCs that are not susceptible to maternal antibodies.*
- Document events during transfusion, carefully recording amount of blood withdrawn and injected (usually 7–20 mL at a time). *Helps prevent errors in fluid replacement. Amount of blood exchanged is approximately 170 mL/kg of body weight. A double-volume exchange ensures that between 75% and 90% of circulating RBCs are replaced.*

NURSING PRIORITY NO. 4 To promote wellness (Teaching/Discharge Considerations):

- Provide information about types of jaundice and pathophysiological factors and future implications of hyperbilirubinemia. *Promotes understanding, corrects misconceptions, and may reduce fear and feelings of guilt.*

- Review means of assessing infant status (feedings, intake/output, stools, temperature, serial weights if scale available) and for monitoring increasing bilirubin levels (e.g., observing blanching of skin over bony prominence or behavior changes), especially if infant is to be discharged early. *Enables parents to monitor infant's progress and to recognize signs of increasing bilirubin levels. Note: Persistence of jaundice beyond 2 weeks in formula-fed infant or 3 weeks in breastfed infant requires further evaluation.*[7]
- Provide parents with 24-hour emergency telephone number and name of contact person, stressing importance of reporting increased jaundice or changes in behavior. *Promotes independence and provides for timely evaluation and intervention.* Refer to lactation specialist *to enhance or reestablish breastfeeding process.*[6]
- Arrange appropriate referral for home phototherapy program if necessary. *Lack of available support systems may necessitate use of visiting nurse to monitor home phototherapy program.*
- Provide written explanation of home phototherapy, safety precautions, and potential problems. *Home phototherapy is recommended only for full-term infants after the first 48 hours of life whose serum bilirubin levels are between 14 and 18 mg/dL, with no increase in direct-reacting bilirubin concentration.*
- Make appropriate arrangements for follow-up testing of serum bilirubin at same laboratory facility. *Treatment is discontinued once serum bilirubin concentrations fall below 14 mg/dL. Untreated or chronic hyperbilirubinemia can lead to permanent damage, such as high-pitch hearing loss, cerebral palsy, or mental retardation.*[7]
- Discuss possible long-term effects of hyperbilirubinemia and the need for continued assessment and early intervention. *Neurological damage associated with kernicterus includes cerebral palsy, mental retardation, sensory difficulties, delayed speech, learning difficulties, and death.*

DOCUMENTATION FOCUS

Assessment/Reassessment
- Assessment findings, risk or related factors.
- Adequacy of intake—hydration level, character and number of stools.
- Laboratory results—bilirubin trends.

Planning
- Plan of care, specific interventions, and who is involved in the planning.
- Teaching plan and resources provided.

Implementation/Evaluation
- Client's responses to treatment and actions performed.
- Parents' understanding of teaching.
- Attainment or progress toward desired outcome(s).
- Modifications to plan of care.

Discharge Planning
- Long-term needs, identifying who is responsible for actions to be taken.
- Community resources for equipment and supplies postdischarge.
- Specific referrals made.

References

1. Munniti, M. T. (2011). Management of pregnancy with ABO incompatibility. *The Foundation for Excellence in Women's Health*. Retrieved March 2018 from https://exxcellence.org/pearls-of-exxcellence/list-of-pearls/management-of-pregnancy-with-abo-incompatibility/.
2. Hansen, T. W. R. (Updated 2017). Neonatal jaundice. Retrieved March 2018 from http://emedicine.medscape.com/article/974786-overview.
3. Sarici, S. U., et al. (2004). Incidence, course, and prediction of hyperbilirubinemia in near-term and term newborns. *Pediatrics*, 113(4), 775–780.
4. Gourley, G. R., et al. (2005). A controlled, randomized, double-blind trial of prophylaxis against jaundice among breastfed newborns. *Pediatrics*, 116(2), 385–391.
5. Canadian Paediatric Society Position Statement. (2007). Guidelines for detection, management and prevention of

 Acute Care   Collaborative   Community/Home Care   Cultural

hyperbilirubinemia in term and late preterm newborn infants (35 or more weeks' gestation). *Paediatr Child Health*, 12(Suppl B), 1B–12B.

6. Deshpande, P. G., Waggle, S. (Updated 2018). Breast milk jaundice. Retrieved March 2018 from http://emedicine.medscape.com/article/973629-overview.

7. Porter, M. L., Dennis, B. L. (2002). Hyperbilirubinemia in the term newborn. *Am Fam Physician*, 65(4), 599–606.

8. Springhouse (eds.). (2008). Phototherapy. *Lippincott's Nursing Procedures*. 5th ed. Philadelphia: Lippincott Williams & Wilkins.

9. Woodgate, P., Jardine, L. A. (2015). Neonatal jaundice: phototherapy. *BMJ Clin Evid*. Retrieved March 2018 from https://reference.medscape.com/medline/abstract/25998618.

---

risk for neonatal Hyperbilrubinemia

Taxonomy II: Nutrition—Class 4 Metabolism (00230) **[Diagnostic Division:** Safety], Approved 2010; Revised 2013, 2017

DEFINITION: Susceptible to the accumulation of unconjugated bilirubin in the circulation (less than 15 ml/dl) that occurs after 24 hours of life, which may compromise health.

RISK FACTORS
Deficient feeding pattern
Infant with inadequate nutrition
Delay in meconium passage
At Risk Population: ABO incompatibility; blood type incompatibility between mother and infant; Rhesus (Rh) incompatibility
Age ≤7 days; premature infant or infant with low birthweight; infant who is breastfed
American Indian or East Asian ethnicity
Significant bruising during birth
Maternal diabetes mellitus; populations living at high altitudes
Associated Condition: Prenatal infection; bacterial, or viral infection; sepsis
Infant with liver malfunction, enzyme deficiency; internal bleeding
Sample Clinical Applications: Newborn, premature infant

DESIRED OUTCOMES/EVALUATION CRITERIA

Sample NOC linkages:
Newborn Adaptation: Adaptive response to the extrauterine environment by a physiologically mature newborn during the first 28 days

Infant Will (Include Specific Time Frame)
• Be free of signs of hyperbilirubinemia with normal bilirubin level
• Establish effective feeding pattern

Sample NOC linkages:
Risk Control: Personal actions to understand, prevent, eliminate, or reduce modifiable health threats

Parent/Caregiver Will (Include Specific Time Frame)
• Verbalize understanding of cause, treatment, and possible outcomes of hyperbilirubinemia.
• Demonstrate appropriate care of infant.

(continues on page 442)

 Diagnostic Studies   Evidence Based Practice   Medications   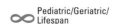 Pediatric/Geriatric/Lifespan

risk for neonatal Hyperbilirubinemia (continued)

ACTIONS/INTERVENTIONS

Sample NIC linkages:

Infant Care: Newborn: Provision of care to the infant during the transition from birth to extrauterine life and subsequent period of stabilization

Lactation Counseling: Assisting in the establishment and maintenance of successful breastfeeding

Bottle Feeding: Preparation and administration of fluids to an infant via a bottle

NURSING PRIORITY NO. 1   To determine individual risk factors:

- Determine infant and maternal blood group and blood type. *ABO incompatibility is more often seen in newborns who have type A blood because of the higher frequency of type A compared to type B in most populations. Incidence figures are difficult to compare because authors of different studies do not use the same definitions for significant neonatal hyperbilirubinemia or jaundice.*[1,7]

- Note gender, race, and place of birth. *Risk of developing jaundice is higher in males, infants of East Asian or American Indian descent, and those living at high altitudes. Incidence is lower for African American infants.*[2]

- Review intrapartal record for specific risk factors, such as low birth weight (LBW) or intrauterine growth retardation, prematurity, abnormal metabolic processes, vascular injuries, abnormal circulation, sepsis, or polycythemia. *The risk of significant neonatal jaundice is increased in LBW or premature infants, presence of congenital infection, or maternal diabetes.*[2] *Studies suggest neonates at 36 to 37 weeks' gestation are four to five times more likely to develop hyperbilirubinemia than those born at 40 weeks.*[3] *Also, certain clinical conditions may cause a reversal of the blood-brain barrier, allowing bound bilirubin to separate either at the level of the cell membrane or within the cell itself, increasing the risk of central nervous system (CNS) involvement.*

- Note use of instruments or vacuum extractor for delivery. Assess infant for presence of birth trauma, cephalohematoma, and excessive ecchymosis or petechiae. *Resorption of blood trapped in fetal scalp tissue and excessive hemolysis may increase the amount of bilirubin being released and cause jaundice.*[4]

- Review infant's condition at birth, noting need for resuscitation or evidence of excessive ecchymosis or petechiae, cold stress, asphyxia, or acidosis. *Asphyxia and acidosis reduce affinity of bilirubin to albumin increasing the amount of unbound circulating (indirect) bilirubin, which may cross the blood-brain barrier, causing CNS toxicity.*[2]

- Evaluate maternal and prenatal nutritional levels; note possible neonatal hypoproteinemia, especially in preterm infant. *One gram of albumin carries 16 mg of unconjugated bilirubin; therefore, lack of sufficient albumin (hypoproteinemia) in the newborn increases risk of jaundice.*

- Assess infant for signs of hypoglycemia such as jitteriness, irritability, and lethargy. Obtain heelstick glucose levels as indicated. *Hypoglycemia necessitates use of fat stores for energy-releasing fatty acids, which compete with bilirubin for binding sites on albumin.*

- Determine successful initiation and adequacy of breastfeeding. *Poor caloric intake and dehydration associated with ineffective breastfeeding increase risk of developing hyperbilirubinemia.*[1]

- Examine infant for pallor, edema, or hepatosplenomegaly. *These signs may be associated with hydrops fetalis, Rh incompatibility, and in utero hemolysis of fetal RBCs.*

- Evaluate for jaundice in natural light, noting sclera and oral mucosa, yellowing of skin immediately after blanching, and specific body parts involved. Assess oral mucosa, posterior portion of hard palate, and conjunctival sacs in dark-skinned newborns. *Detects evidence/degree of jaundice generally first noted on face and progressing to trunk and then extremities.*[1,6] *Clinical appearance of jaundice is evident at bilirubin levels greater than 5 mg/dL in full-term infant. Estimated degree of jaundice is as follows: face, 4 to 8 mg/dL; trunk, 10 to 12 mg/dL;*

 Acute Care   Collaborative   Community/ Home Care   Cultural

groin, 8 to 16 mg/dL; arms/legs, 11 to 18 mg/dL; and hands/feet, 15 to 20 mg/dL. Note: Yellow underlying pig-ment may be normal in dark-skinned infants.[1,4,6]

NURSING PRIORITY NO. 2   To prevent onset of hyperbilirubinemia:

- Review laboratory studies, including total serum bilirubin and albumin levels, hemoglobin/hematocrit, and reticulocyte count, as indicated.
- Keep infant warm and dry; monitor skin and core temperature frequently. *Prevents cold stress and the release of fatty acids that compete for binding sites on albumin, thus increasing the level of freely circulating bilirubin.*
- Initiate early oral feedings within 4 to 6 hours following birth, especially if infant is to be breastfed. *Estab-lishes proper intestinal flora necessary for reduction of bilirubin to urobilinogen and decreases reabsorption of bilirubin from bowel by promoting passage of meconium stool.*[4]
- Encourage frequent breastfeeding—8 to 12 times per day. Assist mother with pumping of breasts as needed to maintain milk production for hospitalized preterm infant. *Breastfeeding support may increase frequency and efficacy of intake.*[2,4,5]
- Administer intravenous immunoglobulin (IVIG) to neonates with Rh or ABO isoimmunization. *Rate of hemolysis in Rh disease or other cases of immune hemolytic jaundice usually exceeds the rate of bilirubin reduction related to phototherapy. IVIG inhibits antibodies that cause red cell destruction, helping to limit the rise in bilirubin levels.*[2,5]

NURSING PRIORITY NO. 3   To promote wellness (Teaching/Discharge Considerations):

- Review means of assessing infant status (feedings, intake/output, stools, temperature, serial weights if scale available) and for monitoring increasing bilirubin levels (e.g., observing blanching of skin over bony promi-nence or behavior changes), especially if infant is to be discharged early. *Enables parents to monitor infant for early signs of increasing bilirubin levels.*[4]
- Provide parents with 24-hour emergency telephone number and name of contact person, stressing importance of reporting signs of jaundice or changes in infant's behavior. *Promotes independence and provides for timely evaluation and intervention.*
- Refer to lactation specialist as indicated *to assist with establishing/enhancing breastfeeding process.*
- Review proper formula preparation/storage and demonstrate feeding techniques *to meet nutritional and fluid needs.*
- Make arrangements for follow-up testing of serum bilirubin at same laboratory facility.

DOCUMENTATION FOCUS

Assessment/Reassessment
- Assessment findings, risk or related factors.
- Adequacy of intake—hydration level, character and number of stools.
- Laboratory results—bilirubin level.

Planning
- Plan of care, specific interventions, and who is involved in the planning.
- Teaching plan and resources provided.

Implementation/Evaluation
- Parents understanding of teaching.
- Attainment or progress toward desired outcome(s).
- Modifications to plan of care.

Discharge Planning
- Home care needs and who is responsible for actions to be taken.
- Any referrals made.

 Diagnostic Studies   Evidence Based Practice   Medications   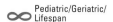 Pediatric/Geriatric/Lifespan

References

1. Munniti, M. T. (2011). Management of pregnancy with ABO incompatibility. *The Foundation for Excellence in Women's Health*. Retrieved March 2018 from https://exxcellence.org/pearls-of-exxcellence/list-of-pearls/management-of-pregnancy-with-abo-incompatibility/.

2. Hansen, T. W. R. (Updated 2017). Neonatal jaundice. Retrieved March 2018 from http://emedicine.medscape.com/article/974786-overview.

3. Sarici, S. U., et al. (2004). Incidence, course, and prediction of hyperbilirubinemia in near-term and term newborns. *Pediatrics*, 113(4), 775–780.

4. Porter, M. L., Dennis, B. L. (2002). Hyperbilirubinemia in the term newborn. *Am Fam Physician*, 65(4), 599–606.

5. Canadian Paediatric Society. (2007). Position Statement: Guidelines for detection, management and prevention of hyperbilirubinemia in term and late preterm newborn infants (35 or more weeks' gestation). *Paediatr Child Health*, 12(Suppl B), 1B–12B.

6. Deshpande, P. G., Waggle, S. (Updated 2018). Breast milk jaundice. Retrieved March 2018 from http://emedicine.medscape.com/article/973629-overview.

7. Woodgate, P., Jardine, L. A. (2015). Neonatal jaundice: phototherapy. *BMJ Clin Evid*. Retrieved March 2018 from https://reference.medscape.com/medline/abstract/25998618.

Hyperthermia

Taxonomy II: Safety/Protection—Class 6 Thermoregulation (00007) [**Diagnostic Division:** Safety], Submitted 1986; Revised 2013; 2017

DEFINITION: Core body temperature elevated above the normal diurnal range due to failure of thermoregulation.

RELATED FACTORS

Dehydration; increase in metabolic rate
Inappropriate clothing
Vigorous activity

DEFINING CHARACTERISTICS

Objective
Abnormal posturing; seizure
Flushed skin; skin warm to touch; vasodilation
Hypotension; tachycardia; tachypnea; apnea
Irritability; lethargy; stupor; coma
Infant does not maintain suck
At Risk Population: Exposure to high environmental temperature
Decrease in sweat response
Illness, sepsis; trauma; ischemia
Pharmaceutical agent
Sample Clinical Applications: Infectious diseases, head trauma, hyperthyroidism, heat exhaustion or heatstroke, surgical procedure, anesthesia

DESIRED OUTCOMES/EVALUATION CRITERIA

Sample NOC linkages:
Thermoregulation: Balance among heat production, heat gain, and heat loss
Thermoregulation: Newborn: Balance among heat production, heat gain, and heat loss during the first 28 days of life
Risk Control: Personal actions to understand, prevent, eliminate, or reduce modifiable health threats

 Acute Care
 Collaborative
 Community/Home Care
 Cultural

Client Will (Include Specific Time Frame)
- Maintain core temperature within normal range.
- Be free of complications such as irreversible brain or neurological damage and acute renal failure.
- Identify underlying cause or contributing factors and importance of treatment as well as signs/symptoms requiring further evaluation or intervention.
- Demonstrate behaviors to monitor and promote normothermia.
- Be free of seizure activity.

ACTIONS/INTERVENTIONS

Sample NIC linkages:

Temperature Regulation: Attaining and/or maintaining body temperature within a normal range
Fever Treatment: Management of symptoms and related conditions associated with an increase in body temperature mediated by endogenous pyrogens
Malignant Hyperthermia Precautions: Prevention or reduction of hypermetabolic response to pharmacological agents used during surgery

NURSING PRIORITY NO. 1 To assess causative/contributing factors:

- Identify underlying cause. *These factors can include **excessive heat production** such as occurs with strenuous exercise, fever, shivering, tremors, convulsions, hyperthyroid state, and infection or sepsis and malignant hyperpyrexia, heatstroke, and sympathomimetic drugs; **impaired heat dissipation** such as occurs with heatstroke, dermatological diseases, burns, and inability to perspire such as occurs with spinal cord injury and certain medications (e.g., diuretics, sedatives, certain heart and blood pressure medications); and **loss of thermoregulation** such as may occur in infections, brain lesions, and drug overdose.*[1,8,9]
- ∞ Note chronological and developmental age of client. *Infants, young children, and elderly persons are most susceptible to damaging hyperthermia. Environmental factors and relatively minor infections can produce a much higher temperature in infants and young children than in older children and adults. Infants, children, or impaired individuals are not able to protect themselves and cannot recognize and/or act on symptoms of hyperthermia. Elderly persons have age-related risk factors (e.g., poor circulation, inefficient sweat glands, skin changes caused by normal aging, chronic diseases).*[1-4,9]

NURSING PRIORITY NO. 2 To evaluate effects/degree of hyperthermia:

- ➕∞ Monitor core temperature by appropriate route (e.g., tympanic, rectal). Note presence of temperature elevation (>98.6°F [37°C]) or fever (100.4°F [38°C]). *Rectal and tympanic temperatures most closely approximate core temperature; however, shell temperatures (oral, axillary, touch) are often measured at home and are predictive of fever. Rectal temperature measurement may be the most accurate but is not always expedient (e.g., client declines, is agitated, has rectal lesions or surgery). Abdominal temperature monitoring may be done in the premature neonate.*[1-4]
- Assess whether body temperature reflects heatstroke. *Defined as body temperature higher than 105°F (40.5°C) that is associated with neurological dysfunction and is potentially life threatening.*[9,11]
- Assess neurological response, noting level of consciousness and orientation, reaction to stimuli, reaction of pupils, and presence of posturing or seizures. *High fever accompanied by changes in mentation (from confusion to delirium) may indicate septic state or heatstroke.*[1-3,5]
- Monitor blood pressure and invasive hemodynamic parameters if available (e.g., cardiac output, arterial pressures). *Hyperdynamic state (high central venous pressure, low systemic vascular resistance, tachycardia, elevated blood pressure, which may later fall) can occur, especially in person with preexisting cardiovascular*

 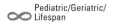

disease if heat-related illness (e.g., heatstroke or malignant hyperthermia reaction to anesthesia) has rendered the client critically ill.[1-3,5]

- Monitor heart rate and rhythm. *Tachycardia, dysrhythmias, and electrocardiogram changes are common due to electrolyte and acid-base imbalance, dehydration, specific action of catecholamines, and direct effects of hyperthermia on blood and cardiac tissue.*[1-3,5]
- *Monitor respirations. Hyperventilation may initially be present, but ventilatory effort may eventually be impaired by seizures and hypermetabolic state (shock and acidosis).*
- Auscultate breath sounds *to note presence and progression of adventitious sounds such as crackles (rales), especially when heart failure or pneumonia is present.*[1-3,5]
- Monitor and record all sources of fluid loss such as urine *(oliguria or renal failure may occur due to hypotension, dehydration, shock, and tissue necrosis),* vomiting and diarrhea, wounds or fistulas, and insensible losses *(potentiates fluid and electrolyte losses).*[1-3,5]
- Note presence or absence of sweating. *The body attempts to increase heat loss by evaporation, conduction, and diffusion. Evaporation is decreased by environmental factors of high humidity and high ambient temperature as well as body factors producing loss of ability to sweat or sweat gland dysfunction (e.g., spinal cord transection, cystic fibrosis, dehydration, vasoconstriction).*[8,9]
- Monitor laboratory studies such as arterial blood gases, electrolytes and cardiac and liver enzymes *(may reveal tissue degeneration)*; glucose *(hypoglycemia)*; blood urea nitrogen/creatinine *(acute renal failure)*; and urinalysis *(myoglobinuria, proteinuria, and hemoglobinuria can occur as products of tissue necrosis).*[1,11]

NURSING PRIORITY NO. 3   To assist with measures to reduce body temperature/restore normal body/organ function:[1-3,5,8,9,11]

- Administer antipyretics, orally or rectally (e.g., acetaminophen, ibuprofen), as ordered.
  Avoid use of aspirin products in children *(may cause Reye's syndrome or liver failure)*[13] or in individuals with a clotting disorder or receiving anticoagulant therapy.
- Promote cooling by means of:
  Limiting clothing and dress in lightweight, loose-fitting clothes. *Encourages heat loss by radiation and conduction.*
  Cooling the environment with air-conditioning or fans. *Promotes heat loss by convection.*
  Provide cool or tepid sponge baths, spray bottle, or immersion if temperature is greater than 104°F (40°C) *(heat loss by evaporation and conduction)* or local ice packs, especially in groin and axillae *(areas of high blood flow). Note: Immersion in very cold/ice water is good for exertional heatstroke (such as with athletes or military recruits in training) but use with caution in treatment of classic heatstroke (such as in elderly client or client with alcoholism), which has been associated with a high mortality rate.*[12] *In pediatric clients, alcohol sponge baths are contraindicated because they increase peripheral vascular constriction and central nervous system depression; cold water sponges or immersion can increase shivering, producing heat.*[13]
  Keep clothing and linens dry *to reduce shivering.*
  Monitor use of hypothermia blanket and wrap extremities with bath towels *to minimize shivering.* Turn off hypothermia blanket when core temperature is within 1° to 3° of desired temperature *to allow for downward drift.*
  Administer medications (e.g., dantrolene, chlorpromazine, diazepam) as ordered, *to manage hyperthermia and control shivering and seizures.*
  Assist with internal cooling methods in presence of malignant hyperthermia *to promote rapid core cooling.*
- Provide hydration:
  Offer or force plenty of fluids by appropriate route even if client is not thirsty *to replace fluids lost through perspiration and respiration.*
  Avoid alcohol and caffeinated beverages *(increases fluid loss by diuresis).*
  Administer replacement IV fluids and electrolytes *to support circulating volume and tissue perfusion and treat acid-base imbalance.*

 Acute Care   Collaborative   Community/Home Care   Cultural

- Promote client safety (e.g., maintain patent airway, padded siderails, quiet environment, mouth care for dry mucous membranes, skin protection from cold when hypothermia blanket is used, observation of equipment safety measures).
- Maintain bedrest *to reduce metabolic demands and oxygen consumption.*
- Provide supplemental oxygen *to offset increased oxygen demands and consumption.*
- Administer medications as indicated to treat underlying cause, such as antibiotics *(for infection)*, dantrolene *(for malignant hyperthermia)*, and beta blockers *(for thyroid storm).*
- Provide high-calorie diet and enteral or parenteral nutrition *to meet increased metabolic demands.*

NURSING PRIORITY NO. 4   To promote wellness (Teaching/Discharge Considerations):

- Instruct parents in how to measure child's temperature, at what body temperature to give antipyretic medications, and what symptoms to report to physician. *Low-grade fever enhances immune system functioning in presence of infection and is not harmful as long as individual is not dehydrated or susceptible to febrile seizures.*[3] *Fever may be treated at home to relieve the general discomfort and lethargy associated with fever. Fever is reportable, however, especially in infants or very young children with or without other symptoms and in older children or adults, if it is unresponsive to antipyretics and fluids because it often accompanies a treatable infection (viral or bacterial).*[13]
- Review with client/significant other specific cause of hyperthermia. *Helps to identify those factors that client can control (if any), such as correction of underlying disease process (e.g., thyroid suppression medication), ways to protect oneself from excessive exposure to environmental heat (e.g., proper clothing, restriction of activity, scheduling outings during cooler part of day), and understanding of family traits (e.g., malignant hyperthermia reaction to anesthesia is often familial).*[7,9]
- Discuss importance of adequate fluid intake at all times and ways to improve hydration status when ill or when under stress (e.g., exercise, hot environment).
- Instruct families/caregivers (of young children, persons who are outdoors in very hot climate, elderly living alone) in dangers of heat exhaustion and heatstroke and ways to manage hot environments. Caution parents to avoid leaving young children in unattended car, emphasizing the extreme hazard to the child in a very short period of time depending on outdoor temperature and humidity, whether the car is parked in direct sunlight, and air and surface temperatures in the car. *Heat injuries can be immediately life threatening. Being aware of environmental hazards and hydration levels can save one's life.*[6,10]
- Recommend avoidance of hot tubs/saunas as appropriate (e.g., client with cardiac conditions compromised by decreased cardiac output associated with peripheral vasodilation, pregnancy that may affect fetal development or increase maternal cardiac workload).
- Review signs/symptoms of hyperthermia (e.g., flushed skin, increased body temperature, increased respiratory and heart rate; fainting, loss of consciousness, seizures). *Indicates need for prompt intervention.*
- Identify community resources, especially for elderly clients, to address specific needs *(e.g., provision of fans for individual use, location of cooling rooms—usually in a community center—during heat waves, daily telephone contact to assess wellness).*

DOCUMENTATION FOCUS

Assessment/Reassessment
- Temperature and other assessment findings, including vital signs and state of mentation.

Planning
- Plan of care, specific interventions, and who is involved in the planning.
- Teaching plan.

Implementation/Evaluation
- Responses to interventions, teaching, and actions performed.
- Attainment or progress toward desired outcome(s).
- Modifications to plan of care.

 Diagnostic Studies   Evidence Based Practice   Medications   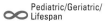 Pediatric/Geriatric/Lifespan

Discharge Planning
• Specific referrals made and those responsible for actions to be taken.

References

1. Stoppler, M. C. (Updated 2015). Heatstroke. Retrieved March 2018 from http://www.medicinenet.com/heat_stroke/article.htm.
2. Sur, D. K., Bukont, E. L. (2007). Evaluating fever of unidentifiable source in young children. *Am Fam Physician*, 75(12), 1805–1811.
3. Engel, J. (2006). *Mosby's Pocket Guide to Pediatric Assessment*. 5th ed. St. Louis, MO: Mosby.
4. Kare, J., Shneiderman, A. (2001). Hyperthermia and hypothermia in the older population, 23(3), 39–52.
5. Doenges, M. E., Moorhouse, M. F., Murr, A. C. (2014). Sepsis/Septicemia. *Nursing Care Plans: Guidelines for Individualizing Patient Care Across the Life Span*. 9th ed. Philadelphia: F. A. Davis.
6. Occupational Safety and Health Administration (OSHA). (2014, updated 2017). Protecting workers from heat stress. Retrieved March 2018 from https://www.osha.gov/Publications/osha3154.pdf.
7. Malignant Hyperthermia Association of the United States. (Updated 2013). Guideline statement for malignant hyperthermia in the perioperative environment. Retrieved March 2018 from http://www.ast.org/uploadedFiles/Main_Site/Content/About_Us/Guideline_Malignant_Hyperthermia.pdf.
8. Cunha, J. P. (2015, last review 2017). Heat cramps. Retrieved March 2018 from http://www.emedicinehealth.com/heat_cramps/article_em.htm.
9. Hyperthermia: Too hot for your health. (2015). *National Institute on Aging*. Retrieved March 2018 from https://www.nia.nih.gov/health/publication/hyperthermia.
10. Grundstein, A., Dowd, J., Meentemeyer, V. (2001). Quantifying the heat related hazard for children in motor vehicles. *American Meteorological Society*, 91(9), 1183.
11. Schraga, E. D., Kates, L. W. (2011, updated 2017). Cooling techniques for hyperthermia. Retrieved March 2018 from http://emedicine.medscape.com/article/149546-overview.
12. Casa, D. J., et al. (2007). Cold water immersion: The gold standard for exertional heatstroke treatment. *Exerc Sport Sci Rev*, 35(3), 141–149.
13. Ferry, R. (2015, last review 2018). Fever in children. Retrieved March 2018 from http://www.emedicinehealth.com/fever_in_children/article_em.htm.

Hypothermia

Taxonomy II: Safety/Protection—Class 6 Thermoregulation (00006) [**Diagnostic Division:** Safety], Submitted 1986; Revised 1988, 2013, 2017

DEFINITION: Core body temperature below the normal diurnal range due to failure of thermoregulation.

RELATED FACTORS
Alcohol consumption; malnutrition
Decrease in metabolic rate; inactivity
Economically disadvantaged
Excessive conductive, convective, evaporative, or radiative heat transfer
Low environmental temperature
Insufficient caregiver knowledge of hypothermia prevention; insufficient clothing

Neonates
Early bathing of newborn; delay in breastfeeding
Increase in oxygen demand

DEFINING CHARACTERISTICS

Objective
Acrocyanosis, cyanotic nailbeds; peripheral vasoconstriction; hypoxia
Bradycardia; tachycardia
Decrease in blood glucose level; hypoglycemia
Decrease in ventilation

 Acute Care Collaborative Community/Home Care Cultural

Increase in metabolic rate; increase in oxygen consumption

Peripheral vasoconstriction; shivering; piloerection

Skin cool to touch; slow capillary refill

Neonates

Infant with insufficient energy to maintain sucking; or with insufficient weight gain (<30 g/d)

Irritability

Jaundice, pallor

Respiratory distress; metabolic acidosis

At Risk Population: Economically disadvantaged

Extremes of age

Extremes of weight; increased body surface-to-weight ratio; insufficient supply of subcutaneous fat

High-risk or unplanned out-of-hospital birth

Associated Condition: Damage to hypothalamus; increase in pulmonary vascular resistance (PVR); ineffective vascular control; inefficient nonshivering thermogenesis

Immature stratum corneum

Radiation therapy; trauma

Sample Clinical Applications: Dementia, malnutrition, anorexia nervosa, brain trauma, stroke, endocrine disorders, some surgical procedures (e.g., craniotomy), alcohol intoxication, abuse or neglect, prematurity, near drowning

DESIRED OUTCOMES/EVALUATION CRITERIA

Sample **NOC** linkages:

Thermoregulation: Balance among heat production, heat gain, and heat loss

Thermoregulation: Newborn: Balance among heat production, heat gain, and heat loss during the first 28 days of life

Client Will (Include Specific Time Frame)

• Display core temperature within normal range.

• Be free of complications such as cardiac failure, respiratory infection or failure, and thromboembolic phenomena.

Sample **NOC** linkages:

Personal Safety Behavior: Personal actions to prevent unintentional physical injury to self

Client/Caregiver Will (Include Specific Time Frame)

• Maintain safe environment.

• Identify underlying cause or contributing factors that are within caregiver control.

• Verbalize understanding of specific interventions to prevent hypothermia.

• Demonstrate behaviors to monitor and promote normothermia.

ACTIONS/INTERVENTIONS

Sample **NIC** linkages:

Hypothermia Treatment: Heat loss prevention, rewarming, and surveillance of a patient whose core body temperature is abnormally low as a result of noninduced circumstances

Temperature Regulation: Attaining or maintaining body temperature within a normal range

 Diagnostic Studies   Evidence Based Practice   Medications   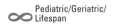 Pediatric/Geriatric/Lifespan

NURSING PRIORITY NO. 1   To assess causative/contributing factors:

• Note underlying cause, for example, (1) ***decreased heat production*** *such as occurs with hypopituitary, hypo-adrenal, and hypothyroid conditions, and hypoglycemia and neuromuscular inefficiencies seen in extremes of age;* (2) ***increased heat loss*** *(e.g., exposure to cold weather, winter outdoor activities; cold water drenching or immersion; improper clothing, shelter, or food for conditions; vasodilation from medications, drugs, or poisons; skin-surface problems such as burns or psoriasis; fluid losses, dehydration; surgery, open wounds, exposed skin or viscera; multiple rapid infusions of cold solutions or transfusions of banked blood; overtreatment of hyperthermia);* and (3) ***impaired thermoregulation.*** *The hypothalamus is sensitive to blood temperature changes of as little as 0.5°C and also reacts to nerve impulses received from nerve endings in the skin. Hypothalamus failure might occur with central nervous system (CNS) trauma or tumor; intracranial bleeding or stroke; toxicological and metabolic disorders; and Parkinson's disease and multiple sclerosis.*[1,2]

• ∞ Note contributing factors: **age of client** (e.g., premature neonate, child, elderly person), **concurrent or coexisting medical problems** (e.g., brainstem injury, CNS trauma; near drowning, sepsis, hypothyroidism), **other factors** (e.g., alcohol or other drug use or abuse, homelessness), **nutrition status** (e.g., thin, tall person loses heat easier than short stature, overweight person), and **living condition and relationship status** (e.g., aged or cognitive impaired client living alone).[1,2,6]

NURSING PRIORITY NO. 2   To prevent further decrease in body temperature:

• 🏠 **Mild-to-moderate hypothermia:1–6**
• Remove wet clothing and bedding.
• Add layers of clothing and wrap in warm blankets.
• Increase physical activity if possible.
• Provide warm liquids after shivering stops if client is alert and can swallow.
• Provide warm nutrient-dense food (carbohydrates, proteins, fats) and fluids (hot, sweet liquids are easily digestible and absorbable).
• Avoid alcohol, caffeine, and tobacco *to prevent vasodilation, diuresis, or vasoconstriction, respectively.*
• Place in warm ambient temperature environment and protect from drafts; provide external heat sources.
• ∞ 📝 Provide barriers to heat loss, as well as active rewarming for newborns, especially preterm and/or low-birth-weight infants, monitoring temperature closely. *Measures might include use of protective hats, open radiant warmer or Isolette, and/or heating blanket. Note: Wariki and Mori's study (2010) found that plastic wraps or bags were effective in reducing heat losses in infants less than 28 weeks' gestation. Stockinet caps were not effective in reducing heat losses. Skin-to-skin care was shown to be effective in reducing the risk of hypothermia when compared to conventional incubator care for infants. The transwarmer mattress reduced the incidence of hypothermia on admission to NICU in very low-birth-weight infants.*[7]
• 🏠 **Severe hypothermia:1–6**
• Remove client from causative or contributing factors.
• Dry the skin, cover with blankets or vapor barrier, and provide shelter with warm ambient temperature; use radiant lights.
• Warm the person's trunk first, not hands and feet. *Warming extremities first can cause shock.*
• Avoid immersing in warm water or applying hot objects or excessive pressure directly to skin (e.g., uninsulated hot water bottles, blood pressure cuffs, etc.).
• Keep individual lying down. Avoid jarring *(can trigger an abnormal heart rhythm).*

NURSING PRIORITY NO. 3   To evaluate effects of hypothermia:

• ➕ Measure core temperature with low register thermometer (measuring below 34.4°C [94°F]).
• Assess respiratory effort *(rate and tidal volume are reduced when metabolic rate decreases and respiratory acidosis occurs).*
• Auscultate lungs, noting adventitious sounds. *Pulmonary edema, respiratory infection, and pulmonary embolus are potential complications of hypothermia.*

 Acute Care   Collaborative   Community/Home Care   Cultural

- Monitor heart rate and rhythm. *Cold stress reduces pacemaker function, and bradycardia (unresponsive to atropine), atrial fibrillation, atrioventricular blocks, and ventricular tachycardia can occur. Ventricular fibrillation occurs most frequently when core temperature is 27.7°C (82°F) or below.*[1,2,4]
- Monitor blood pressure, noting hypotension. *Can occur due to vasoconstriction, and shunting of fluids as a result of cold injury effect on capillary permeability.*
- Measure urine output. *Oliguria or renal failure can occur due to a low flow state and/or following hypothermic osmotic diuresis.*
- Note CNS effects (e.g., mood changes, sluggish thinking, amnesia, complete obtundation) and peripheral CNS effects (e.g., paralysis—30.9°C [87.7°F]; dilated pupils—below 30°C [86°F]; flat electroencephalogram—20°C [68°F]).[1,2,4]
- Monitor laboratory studies such as arterial blood gases *(respiratory and metabolic acidosis)*, electrolytes *(hyperkalemia initially, followed by hypokalemia after hypothermia-induced diuresis)*, complete blood count *(increased hematocrit, decreased white blood cell count)*, cardiac enzymes *(myocardial infarct may occur owing to electrolyte imbalance, cold stress catecholamine release, hypoxia, or acidosis)*, coagulation profile *(late hypothermia associated with increased prothrombin time and partial prothrombin time)*, and glucose *(hyperglycemia occurs initially, followed by hypoglycemia)*, as well as pharmacological profile *(for toxicology [alcohol/other drugs]; possible cumulative drug effects).*[2]

NURSING PRIORITY NO. 4 To restore normal body temperature/organ function:

- Assist with surface warming. Cover head, neck, and thorax, leaving extremities uncovered as appropriate *to maintain peripheral vasoconstriction.* Note: Do not institute surface rewarming prior to core rewarming in severe hypothermia *(causes afterdrop of temperature by shunting cold blood back to heart, in addition to rewarming shock as a result of surface vasodilation).*[1–4]
- Assist with core rewarming measures, such as warmed IV solutions and warm-solution lavage of body cavities (gastric, peritoneal, bladder) or cardiopulmonary bypass if indicated to normalize core temperature. Rewarm no faster than 1°F to 2°F per hour *to avoid sudden vasodilation, increased metabolic demands on heart, and hypotension (rewarming shock).*[2]
- Protect skin and tissues by repositioning, applying lotion or lubricants, and avoiding direct contact with heating appliance or blanket. *Impaired circulation can result in severe tissue damage.*
- Keep client quiet; handle gently *to reduce potential for fibrillation in cold heart.*[2]
- Provide cardiopulmonary resuscitation as necessary, with compressions initially at one-half the normal heart rate. *Severe hypothermia causes slowed conduction, and cold heart may be unresponsive to medications, pacing, and defibrillation.*[2,4,5]
- Maintain patent airway. Assist with intubation if indicated. Provide heated, humidified oxygen when used.
- Turn off warming blanket when temperature is within 1°F to 3°F of desired temperature *to accommodate drift and avoid hyperthermia situation.*
- Administer IV fluids with caution *to prevent overload as the vascular bed expands.*[2] *Cold heart is slow to compensate for increased volume.*
- Avoid vigorous pharmacological therapy. *As rewarming occurs, organ function returns, correcting endocrine abnormalities, and tissues become more receptive to the effects of drugs previously administered, creating risk for overdose.*
- Perform range-of-motion exercises, provide support hose or sequential compression device, reposition, encourage coughing and deep-breathing exercises, and avoid restrictive clothing or restraints *to reduce effects of circulatory stasis.*
- Provide well-balanced, high-calorie diet or feedings *to replenish glycogen stores and nutritional balance.*

NURSING PRIORITY NO. 5 To promote wellness (Teaching/Discharge Considerations):

- Review specific risk factors or causes of hypothermia. Note that hypothermia can be accidental or intentional *(e.g., when induced-hypothermia therapy is used after cardiac arrest or brain injury),* requiring interventions to protect client from adverse affects.[5]

 Diagnostic Studies   Evidence Based Practice   Medications   Pediatric/Geriatric/ Lifespan

- Identify factors that client can control (if any), such as protection from environment and adequate heat in home, layering of clothing and blankets, minimizing heat loss from head with hat or scarf, appropriate cold weather clothing, avoidance of alcohol or other drugs if anticipating exposure to cold, potential risks for future hypersensitivity to cold, etc.
- Discuss signs/symptoms of early hypothermia (e.g., changes in mentation, somnolence, impaired coordination, slurred speech) *to facilitate recognition of problem and timely intervention. Information may be especially important if client works or plays outdoors (e.g., camping, skiing, hiking).*[1,2]
- Identify assistive community resources, as indicated (e.g., social services, emergency shelters, clothing suppliers, food bank, public service company, financial resources). *Individual/significant other may be in need of numerous resources if hypothermia was associated with inadequate housing, homelessness, or malnutrition.*

DOCUMENTATION FOCUS

Assessment/Reassessment
- Findings, noting degree of system involvement.
- Graph temperature.

Planning
- Plan of care and who is involved in planning.
- Teaching plan.

Implementation/Evaluation
- Responses to interventions, teaching, and actions performed.
- Attainment or progress toward desired outcome(s).
- Modifications to plan of care.

Discharge Planning
- Long-term needs, identifying who is responsible for each action.
- Specific referrals made.

References

1. Curtis, R. (Updated 2015). Outdoor Action guide to hypothermia and cold weather injuries. *Princeton University Outdoor Action*. Retrieved March 2018 from https://www.princeton.edu/~oa/safety/hypocold.shtml.
2. Li, J., et al. (2014, updated 2017). Hypothermia. Retrieved March 2018 from http://emedicine.medscape.com/article/770542-overview.
3. Doenges, M. E., Moorhouse, M. F., Murr, A. C. (2014). Surgical intervention: Risk for imbalanced body temperature. *Nursing Care Plans: Guidelines for Individualizing Client Care Across the Life Span*. 9th ed. Philadelphia: F. A. Davis, 772.
4. State of Alaska. (2005, updated 2014). Cold Injury Guidelines. Retrieved March 2018 from http://dhss.alaska.gov/dph/Emergency/Documents/ems/documents/Alaska%20DHSS%20EMS%20Cold%20Injuries%20Guidelines%20June%202014.pdf.
5. Calver, P., et al. (2005). The big chill: Improving the odds after cardiac arrest. Retrieved March 2018 from http://www.modernmedicine.com/modern-medicine/content/big-chill-improving-odds-after-cardiac-arrest?page=full.
6. Soreide, E., Smith, C. E. (2004). Hypothermia in trauma victims—Friend or foe? *Indian J Crit Care Med (IJCCM)*, 8(2), 116–119.
7. Wariki, W. M. V., Mori, R. (last update 2010). Interventions to prevent hypothermia at birth in preterm and/or low birthweight infants. *The World Health Organization (WHO)*. Retrieved March 2018 from https://extranet.who.int/rhl/topics/newborn-health/care-newborn-infant/interventions-prevent-hypothermia-birth-preterm-and/or-low-birth-weight-infants.

 Acute Care   Collaborative   Community/Home Care   Cultural

risk for Hypothermia

Taxonomy II: Safety/Protection—Class 6 Thermoregulation (00253) [**Diagnostic Division:** Safety], Approved 2013; Revised 2017

DEFINITION: Susceptible to a failure of thermoregulation that may result in a core body temperature below the normal diurnal range, which may compromise health.

RISK FACTORS

Alcohol consumption; malnutrition
Decrease in metabolic rate; inactivity
Economically disadvantaged
Excessive conductive, convective, evaporative, or radiative heat transfer
Low environmental temperature
Insufficient caregiver knowledge of hypothermia prevention; insufficient clothing
Neonates
Early bathing of newborn; delay in breastfeeding
Increase in oxygen demand
At Risk Population: Economically disadvantaged
Extremes of age
Extremes of weight; increased body surface-to-weight ratio; insufficient supply of subcutaneous fat
High-risk or unplanned out-of-hospital birth
Associated Condition: Damage to hypothalamus; increase in pulmonary vascular resistance (PVR); ineffective vascular control; inefficient nonshivering thermogenesis
Immature stratum corneum
Radiation therapy; trauma; radiation therapy
Sample Clinical Applications: Dementia, malnutrition, anorexia nervosa, brain trauma, stroke, endocrine disorders, some surgical procedures (e.g., craniotomy), alcohol intoxication, abuse or neglect, prematurity, near-drowning

DESIRED OUTCOMES/EVALUATION CRITERIA

Sample NOC linkages:
Thermoregulation: Balance among heat production, heat gain, and heat loss
Thermoregulation: Newborn: Balance among heat production, heat gain, and heat loss during the first 28 days of life

Client Will (Include Specific Time Frame)
• Display core temperature within normal range.
• Be free of complications such as cardiac failure, respiratory infection or failure, and thromboembolic phenomena.

Sample NOC linkages:
Risk Control: Hypothermia: Personal actions to understand, prevent, eliminate, or reduce the threat of low body temperature

Client/Caregiver Will (Include Specific Time Frame)
• Maintain safe environment.
• Identify underlying cause or contributing factors that can be controlled.

(continues on page 454)

 Diagnostic Studies   Evidence Based Practice   Medications   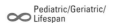 Pediatric/Geriatric/Lifespan

risk for Hypothermia (continued)

- Verbalize understanding of specific interventions to prevent hypothermia.
- Demonstrate behaviors to monitor and promote normothermia.

ACTIONS/INTERVENTIONS

Sample NIC linkages:

Temperature Regulation: Attaining or maintaining body temperature within a normal range

Risk Identification: Analysis of potential risk factors, determination of health risks, and prioritization of risk reduction strategies for an individual or group

NURSING PRIORITY NO. 1 To assess risk factors:

- Note presence of risk factors as related to current situation, for example (1) *decreased heat production, such as occurs with hypopituitary, hypoadrenal, and hypothyroid conditions, and hypoglycemia and neuromuscular inefficiencies seen in extremes of age;* (2) *increased heat loss (e.g., exposure to cold weather, winter outdoor activities; cold water drenching or immersion; improper clothing, shelter, or food for weather conditions; problems such as could occur with burns; fluid losses, dehydration; surgery, open wounds, exposed skin or viscera);* and (3) *impaired thermoregulation as might occur with central nervous system trauma or tumor, intracranial bleeding or stroke, toxicological and metabolic disorders, and Parkinson's disease and multiple sclerosis.*[1,2]
- ∞ Note age of client (e.g., premature neonate, child, elderly person) and other associated conditions, such as nutrition status (e.g., thin, tall person loses heat easier than short stature, overweight person) and living condition and relationship status (e.g., aged or cognitively impaired client living alone or homeless alcoholic).[1-3]
- Measure core temperature with low-register thermometer (measuring below 94°F [34.4°C]) *to identify client approaching hypothermia range as listed in Risk Factors.*
- Monitor for change in vital signs and mental status.

NURSING PRIORITY NO. 2 To prevent hypothermia (Teaching/Discharge Considerations):

- 🏠 Review specific risk factors or causes of hypothermia *to assist client/caregivers in identifying safety concerns.*
- Identify factors that client can control (if any), such as protection from environment and adequate heat in home, layering clothing and blankets, minimizing heat loss from head with hat or scarf, appropriate cold weather clothing, avoidance of alcohol or other drugs if anticipating exposure to cold, potential risks for future hypersensitivity to cold, etc.
- Discuss signs/symptoms of early hypothermia (e.g., changes in mentation, somnolence, impaired coordination, slurred speech) *to facilitate recognition of problem and timely intervention. Information may be especially important if client works or plays outdoors (e.g., camping, skiing, hiking).*[1,2]
- 🔄 Identify assistive community resources, as indicated (e.g., social services, emergency shelters, clothing suppliers, food bank, public service company, financial resources). *Individual/significant other may be in need of numerous resources if risk for hypothermia is associated with inadequate housing, homelessness, or malnutrition.*

DOCUMENTATION FOCUS

Assessment/Reassessment
- Individual risks identified.
- Available resources.

 Acute Care   Collaborative   Community/ Home Care   Cultural

Planning
• Plan of care and who is involved in planning.
• Teaching plan.

Implementation/Evaluation
• Responses to interventions, teaching, and actions performed.
• Attainment or progress toward desired outcome(s).
• Modifications to plan of care.

Discharge Planning
• Long-term needs, identifying who is responsible for each action.
• Specific referrals made.

References

1. Curtis, R. (Updated 2015). Outdoor Action guide to hypothermia and cold weather injuries. *Princeton University Outdoor Action*. Retrieved March 2018 from https://www.princeton.edu/~oa/safety/hypocold.shtml.

2. Li, J., et al. (2014, updated 2017). Hypothermia. Retrieved March 2018 from http://emedicine.medscape.com/article/770542-overview.

3. Soreide, E., Smith, C. E. (2004). Hypothermia in trauma victims—Friend or foe? *Indian J Crit Care Med*, 8, 116–119.

---

risk for perioperative Hypothermia

Taxonomy II: Safety/Protection—Class 6 Thermoregulation (00254) [**Diagnostic Division:** Safety], Approved 2013; Revised 2017

DEFINITION: Susceptible to an inadvertent drop in core body temperature below 36°C (96.8°F) occurring 1 hour before to 24 hours after surgery, which may compromise health.

RISK FACTORS
Excessive conductive, convective, or radiative heat transfer
Low environmental temperature
At Risk Population: American Society of Anesthesiologists (ASA) Physical Status classification score >1
Low body weight
Low preoperative temperature (<36°C [96.8°F])
Associated Condition: Cardiovascular complications; diabetic neuropathy
Combined regional and general anesthesia; surgical procedure
Sample Clinical Applications: Surgical procedures where therapeutic hypothermia is not planned

DESIRED OUTCOMES/EVALUATION CRITERIA

Sample **NOC** linkages:
Thermoregulation: Balance among heat production, heat gain, and heat loss

Client Will (Include Specific Time Frame)
• Display core temperature within normal range.
• Be free of complications such as cardiac failure, respiratory infection or failure, thromboembolic phenomena, and delayed healing.

(continues on page 456)

 Diagnostic Studies   Evidence Based Practice   Medications   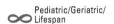 Pediatric/Geriatric/Lifespan

risk for perioperative Hypothermia (continued)

Sample NOC linkages:

Risk Control: Hypothermia: Personal actions to understand, prevent, eliminate, or reduce the threat of low body temperature

Care Provider Will (Include Specific Time Frame)
• Identify client condition/situations that may lead to problems with temperature regulation.
• Engage in protective actions to control body temperature.

ACTIONS/INTERVENTIONS

Sample NIC linkages:

Temperature Regulation: Perioperative: Attaining and maintaining desired body temperature throughout the surgical event

---

NURSING PRIORITY NO. 1 To identify risk factors affecting current situation:

• Ascertain type of surgical procedure client is having. *Helps in identifying elements of risk. For example, some procedures carry higher risk of hypothermia (e.g., laparoscopic abdominal procedure with carbon dioxide insufflation; large volume liposuction; extensive surgical procedure of any sort with prolonged exposure of body surfaces and long period of anesthesia).*[1–3]

• Assess client conditions/comorbidities (e.g., diabetes, impaired skin and tissue integrity, respiratory, cardiac, vascular, neurological disorders) *that may place client at higher risk for perioperative complications, including hypothermia.*[4]

• ∞ Note client's body type and age. *Very thin, malnourished, or dehydrated individuals, as well as those who are very young or elderly, are more susceptible to perioperative hypothermia. The body's ability to regulate temperature may lessen with age.*[5,6]

• Note client's medication regimen. *Medications including some vasodilators, antipsychotics, and sedatives can impair the body's ability to regulate its temperature.*[6]

NURSING PRIORITY NO. 2 To maintain appropriate body temperature/prevent hypothermia complications:

• Measure client's temperature preoperatively and confirm that continuous monitoring of temperature is occurring during procedure. Report preoperative temperature below ideal range to surgical team/anesthesiologist.

• Implement preventive warming techniques in the operating room. *Evidence supports commencement of active warming preoperatively and monitoring it throughout the intraoperative period. Single strategies such as forced-air warming are more effective than passive warming (e.g., blankets from a warmer); however, combined strategies, including preoperative commencement, use of warmed fluids plus forced-air warming, and other active strategies, were more effective in vulnerable groups.*[13]

Consider administering warmed IV fluids. *A large-scale study published in 2015 reported that use of warmed intravenous fluids (kept at temperatures between 37°C [98.6°F] and 41°C [105.8°F]) kept the core temperature of study participants about half a degree warmer than that of participants given room temperature intravenous fluids at 30, 60, 90, and 120 minutes and at the end of surgery. Warmed intravenous fluids also further reduced the risk of shivering compared with room temperature intravenous fluids.*[7]

Use heated blankets from warming cabinet. *Note: While easy to use and effective, blankets on top of client can limit access to surgical site. Also, adding too many layers of warmed cotton blankets is ineffective in raising the patient's body temperature. The first blanket can reduce heat loss by 33%, but adding another blanket only adds another 18% reduction in heat loss. Adding three or more blankets adds no further warming.*[8]

 Acute Care   Collaborative   Community/Home Care   Cultural

Use conductive warming devices. *One type of warming pad is an electrical resistive/conductive device that warms underneath the client's body. The anesthesiologist can select one of five preset temperatures. Because the client is warming from underneath, blankets need not be placed on top, allowing for greater surgical access.*[9]

 Provide forced-air warming blanket. *Warm air is pumped through a hose into a disposable blanket that covers the client. Heat transfer results from the movement of warm air across the surface of the patient's skin, which allows forced-air blankets to transfer more heat at a lower temperature. Note: Recent studies show some evidence that forced air warming increases body temperature by 0.5° to 1° compared with extra insulation (mostly reflective blankets in these studies).*[7,13–15]

 Use warm water garment or mattress. *Research has shown that circulating water garments and energy transfer pads warm about 50% better than forced air because they warm both over and under the body. Note: Care must be exercised when the mattress is used, as the heat of the fluid mattress combined with body weight and static position increases the risk of pressure ulcers or necrosis.*[10,11]

 Increase operating room temperature, as indicated. *It is currently thought that optimal operating room temperatures for the client should be no less than 20°C (68°F) to reduce risk of hypothermia complications while still providing comfortable environment for scrubbed personnel under surgical lights. Recovery room temperatures of 20°C to 24°C (68°F to 75°F) may be ideal for rewarming client.*[12]

DOCUMENTATION FOCUS

Assessment/Reassessment
- Findings, noting degree of system involvement.
- Graph temperature.

Planning
- Plan of care.

Implementation/Evaluation
- Responses to interventions and actions performed.
- Attainment of desired outcome(s).
- Modifications to plan of care.

References

1. Shermak, M. A., Mahaffey, G. (2010). Preventing liposuction complications. *OR Nurse 2105*, 4(1), 14–19.
2. Conner, R. (ed) (2008). Recommended practices for endoscopic minimally invasive surgery. *Perioperative Standards and Recommended Practices*. Denver: AORN, Inc.
3. Paulikas, C. A. (2008). Prevention of unplanned perioperative hypothermia. *AORN J*, 88(3), 358–364.
4. Fletcher, H. C. (2014). Preventing skin injury in the OR. *OR Nurse 2015*, 8(3), 28–34.
5. Lynch, S., Dixon, J., Leary, D. (2010). Reducing the risk of unplanned perioperative hypothermia. *AORN J*, 92(5), 553–562.
6. Madrid, E., et al. (2016). Body warming of people undergoing surgery to avoid complications and increase comfort after surgery. Retrieved March 2018 from http://www.cochrane.org/CD009016/ANAESTH_body-warming-people-undergoing-surgery-avoid-complications-and-increase-comfort-after-surgery.
7. Campbell, G., et al. (2015). Warming of intravenous and irrigation fluids for preventing inadvertent perioperative hypothermia. Cochrane Libr. Retrieved March 2018 from http://cochranelibrary-wiley.com/doi/10.1002/14651858.CD009891.pub2/abstract.
8. Weirich, T. L. (2008). Hypothermia warming protocols: Why are they not widely used in the OR? *AORN J*, 87(2), 333–344.
9. Mathias, J. M. (2006). Taking steps to keep OR patients warm. *OR Manager*, 22(12), 14–16.
10. Sessler, D., Todd, M. (2000). Perioperative heat balance. *Anesthesiology*, 92(2), 578–596.
11. Zangrillo, A., et al. (2006). Temperature management during off-pump coronary artery bypass graft surgery: A randomized clinical trial on the efficacy of a circulating water system versus a forced-air system. *J Cardiothorac Vasc Anesth*, 20(6), 788–792.
12. Good, K. K., et al. (2006). Postoperative hypothermia—the chilling consequences. *AORN J*, 83(5), 1054–1066.
13. Moola, S., Lockwood, C. (2011). Effectiveness of strategies for the management and/or prevention of hypothermia within the adult perioperative environment. *Int J Evid Based Healthc*, 9(4), 337–345.
14. Stevens, M. H. (2011). Forced-air warming: An effective tool in fighting SSI. *Infection Control Today*. Retrieved March 2018 from http://www.infectioncontroltoday.com/articles/2011/03/forced-air-warming-an-effective-tool-in-fighting-ssi.aspx.
15. Chapman, S. (2015). Keeping people warm during surgery: What's the evidence? *Evidently Cochrane*. Retrieved March 2018 from http://www.evidentlycochrane.net/keeping-people-warm-during-surgery-whats-the-evidence/.

 Diagnostic Studies   Evidence Based Practice   Medications   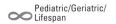 Pediatric/Geriatric/Lifespan

risk for complicated Immigration Transition

Taxonomy II: Coping/Stress Tolerance—Class 1 Posttrauma Responses (00260) [**Diagnostic Division:** Social Interaction], Approved 2016

DEFINITION: Susceptible to experiencing negative feeling (loneliness, fear, anxiety) in response to unsatisfactory consequences and cultural barriers to one's immigration transition, which may compromise health.

RISK FACTORS
Available work below educational preparation
Cultural barriers or insufficient social support in host country; insufficient knowledge about process to access resources in host country
Unsanitary or overcrowded housing; multiple nonrelated persons within household
Language barriers in host country
Overt discrimination; abusive landlord
Parent-child conflicts related to enculturation in host country
At Risk Population: Forced migration; unfulfilled expectations of immigration; illegal status in host country
Hazardous work conditions with inadequate training; labor exploitation
Precarious economic situation
Separation from family and friends in home country

DESIRED OUTCOMES/EVALUATION CRITERIA

Sample NOC linkages:
Relocation Adaptation: Adaptive and behavioral response of a cognitively intact individual to a required change in living environment
Quality of Life: Extent of positive perception of current life circumstances
Hope: Optimism that is personally satisfying and life supporting

Client Will (Include Specific Time Frame)
• Verbalize understanding of current situation.
• Develop plan to address identified issues.
• Engage in activities to overcome issues impacting transition to new life.
• Express optimism about outcome of transition.

ACTIONS/INTERVENTIONS

Sample NIC linkages:
Relocation Stress Reduction: Assisting the individual to prepare for and cope with movement from one environment to another
Coping Enhancement: Facilitation of cognitive and behavioral efforts to manage perceived stressors, changes, or threats that interfere with meeting life demands and roles
Hope Inspiration: Enhancing the belief in one's capacity to initiate and sustain actions

NURSING PRIORITY NO. 1   To determine underlying dynamics of individual situation:

• Ascertain circumstances of migration, nature of the involuntary move and acculturation since arrival. *These individuals/families face multiple consequences and barriers that are specific to their situation and require unique solutions.*[1]

 Acute Care Collaborative Community/ Home Care Cultural

- ∞ 📝 Note age of immigrants. *A growing number of older people are immigrating and face economic disadvantages. Midlife women who immigrate show more depressive symptoms than nonimmigrants.[2,3] Young children are more likely to have health rated as "poor" or "fair," and their health tends to decline more rapidly as they age versus native born children.[4]*
- Determine primary language and ability to speak, read, and understand the language of the host country. *Acculturation is slowed when dominant language of the host country is not understood by client/family members.[1]*
- Note level of stress being experienced (e.g., anxiety, difficulty sleeping, changes in eating habits, depression, hopelessness). *Difficulties encountered with relocation can impair coping and general well-being.*
- Identify current coping strategies and past skills used. *Bringing to mind previous situations where the individual functioned successfully can help client to use these skills in the current situation and provides opportunity to learn new skills.[1]*
- Determine financial situation and access to and use of available resources. *Provides insight for client/family needs and possible options to lessen stressors and facilitate integration in the new environment.[1]*

NURSING PRIORITY NO. 2 To promote integration of immigrants into new environment:

- Obtain services of an interpreter, bilingual written materials/videos as indicated. *May be needed for clients to adequately understand plan of care and what is needed to improve their situation.[1]*
- Allow sufficient time for discussions, information exchanges, and teaching. *Lack of/weak language skills may impede communications. If client feels rushed he/she may falsely indicate understanding.*
- Identify resources for English as second language (ESL) classes, if needed/desired. *Learning dominate language of the host country can facilitate self-actualization by improving opportunities for employment, continuing education, and meeting needs of family members.*
- Designate a primary or 'family nurse,' as appropriate, who can coordinate the team aiding the family. *Additional services can empower the family to develop a well-functioning daily life and adaptation to their new environment.[1]*
- Make home visits as appropriate, noting family communication pattern/interactions, conflicts, safety concerns. *Provides opportunity to observe client/family in more relaxed surrounding, identify issues to be addressed, answer questions, and impart needed information.[1]*
- Discuss changes from previous life to new circumstances and expectations for the future. *Acculturation is a complex social and psychological process implying cultural learning and behavioral adaptation to a nonnative country.[1]*
- 🌐 Identify cultural differences/value conflicts and similarities. *Transition is complicated when long-held beliefs/values and traditional family roles are in conflict with those of host country. Recognizing and addressing conflicts while accepting that differences will exist allows client to build on similarities facilitating adaptation.*
- Provide useful resources as desired for immigrants to learn new lifestyle, i.e., food, dress, language, and manner of interacting. *Can assist in efforts to "blend in" and relate to others.[1]*
- Encourage participation in community activities, sporting events, neighborhood gatherings, governmental affairs as interested. *Provides opportunity to socialize and learn various aspects of new society, facilitating adjustment to new life.[1]*
- ∞ Assist immigrants, especially seniors, to navigate the problems of income, public benefits, and other means of managing living in a new country. *While these problems affect most immigrants, seniors are a growing proportion of immigrants with all the resultant problems of managing how to survive on lower incomes.[3]*
- 🌐 Identify cultural/religious resources, ethnic organizations, support groups. *Provides mentors in new culture that may be able to introduce immigrants to local business, engage in religious practices, and visit other facilities where immigrants can find support and guidance as they progress toward acculturation.*

 Diagnostic Studies   Evidence Based Practice   Medications   Pediatric/Geriatric/Lifespan

NURSING PRIORITY NO. 3   To assist immigrants to enhance quality of life in new situation:

• Encourage client/family to identify positives in life to build on. *Assists client/family to find hope for the future.*
• Identify community resources/programs such as emergency housing, utilities, transportation, nutrition assistance program (food stamps)/ pantries, clothing/home goods assistance. *Helps to provide basic necessities to enable client/family to begin to settle into their new home.*[1]
• Refer to vocational counselor/resources as indicated. *Helpful for evaluating marketable skills, developing resume, preparing for interview, obtaining additional education as appropriate to gain employment and provide for family.*
• Provide assistance with health/behavioral issues that may occur, identifying healthcare and counseling resources available to client/family. *The changes incurred with the transition from the old to the new country markedly increase stressors, impacting role performance of family members and family cohesiveness, negatively affecting both physical and psychological well-being of client/family.*[2]

DOCUMENTATION FOCUS

Assessment/Reassessment
• Individual findings regarding immigrant's circumstances.
• Immigrant's perception of what has happened, specific stressors.
• Language(s) spoken, fluency with language of host country.
• Perceived cultural barriers.
• Safety concerns.

Planning
• Plan of care and who is involved in planning.
• Teaching plan.

Implementation/Evaluation
• Response to interventions, teaching, actions performed.
• Attainment or progress toward desired outcomes.
• Modifications to plan of care.

Discharge Planning
• Long-term needs and goals, and who is responsible for actions to be taken.
• Specific referrals made.

References

1. Samarasinghe, K. L. (2011). A conceptual model facilitating the transition of involuntary migrant families. *ISRN Nursing.* Retrieved June 2018 from https://www.hindawi.com/journals/isrn/2011/82420.
2. Im, E. O., et al. (2015). Immigration transition and depressive symptoms: Four major ethnic groups of midlife women in the United States. *Health Care Women Int*, 36(4), 439–456.
3. O'Neil, K., Tienda, M. (2014). Age at immigration and the incomes of older immigrants, 1994–2010. *J Gerontol B Psychol Sci Soc Sci*, 70(2), 291–302.
4. Reardon-Anderson, J., Capps, R., Fix, M. E. (2002). The health and well-being of children in immigrant families. *The Urban Institute: Washington, D.C.* Retrieved June 2018 from http://webarchive.urban.org/publications/310584.html.

 Acute Care   Collaborative   Community/Home Care   Cultural

ineffective Impulse Control

Taxonomy II: Perception/Cognition—Class 4 Cognition (00222) [**Diagnostic Division:** Ego Integrity], Approved 2010; Revised 2017

DEFINITION: A pattern of performing rapid, unplanned reactions to internal or external stimuli without regard for the negative consequences of these reactions to the impulsive individual or to others.

RELATED FACTORS

Hopelessness; mood disorder
Smoking; substance use/[abuse]

DEFINING CHARACTERISTICS

Subjective

Inability to save money or regulate finances
Asking personal questions despite discomfort of others

Objective

Acting without thinking
Sensation seeking; sexual promiscuity
Inappropriate sharing of personal details; overly familiar with strangers
Irritability; temper outbursts
Gambling addiction
Violent behavior
Associated Condition: Alteration in development or cognitive functioning
Organic brain disorder; personality disorder
Sample Clinical Applications: Eating disorders, addictions—substance/sexual, bipolar disorders, dementia, attention deficit hyperactivity disorder (ADHD), oppositional defiant disorder, traumatic brain injury, Down syndrome, Asperger's syndrome

DESIRED OUTCOMES/EVALUATION CRITERIA

Sample NOC linkages:
Impulse Self-Control: Self-restraint of compulsive or impulsive behaviors
Mood Equilibrium: Appropriate adjustment of prevailing emotional tone in response to circumstances
Self-Management: Autism Spectrum Disorder Management: Personal actions to manage autism, use positive behavior practices, its treatment, and to prevent complications

Client Will (Include Specific Time Frame)
- Acknowledge problem with impulse control.
- Identify feelings that precede desire to engage in impulsive actions.
- Verbalize desire to learn new ways of controlling impulsive behavior.
- Participate in anger management therapy.

ACTIONS/INTERVENTIONS

Sample NIC linkages:
Impulse Control Training: Assisting the patient to mediate impulsive behavior through application of problem-solving strategies to social and interpersonal situations
Anger Control Assistance: Facilitation of the expression of anger in an adaptive, nonviolent manner

 Diagnostic Studies   Evidence Based Practice   Medications   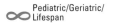 Pediatric/Geriatric/Lifespan

NURSING PRIORITY NO. 1   To assess causative/contributing factors:

• Investigate causes/individual factors that may be involved in client's situation. *Impulse disorders are a group of mental health disorders generally believed to be the result of biological, social, and psychological factors. It is theorized that unbalanced neurotransmitters in the brain may be a cause, as well as the hormone imbalances implicated in violent and aggressive behavior.*[1–4,7,9]

• Evaluate for underlying neurological conditions. *Presence of traumatic brain injury, strokes, brain tumors, etc., may result in poor impulse control, affecting therapeutic choices.*[11]

• Explore individual's inability to control actions. *Healthy people are aware of an impulse and are able to make a decision about whether to follow the urge. The key differentiation between healthy impulsiveness and an impulse disorder is the negative consequences that follow.*[1,7,9]

• Note negative consequences incurred by client's impulsive actions, such as repeat detentions or suspensions from school, loss of employment, financial ruin, arrests/convictions, and civil litigation. *Regardless of the form of the impulsive disorder—predisposition to rapid unplanned reactions (e.g., ADHD, bipolar, substance use, explosive behavior) or impaired ability to resist impulses (e.g., compulsive buying, kleptomania, pathological gambling, pyromania)—individuals with poor control engage in the activity even if they know that there will be negative consequences.*[1–3,7,9,10]

• Ascertain degree of anxiety client experiences when having an impulse to act on the desire. *Not acting on the impulse creates intense anxiety or arousal in the individual. Engaging in the behavior produces release of the anxiety and possibly pleasure or gratification. This may be followed by remorse, regret, or conversely, satisfaction.*[1–3,7]

• Identify behaviors indicative of ADHD for further evaluation. *This diagnosis needs to be made by a physician based on reports of behaviors of inattention, hyperactivity, and impulsivity by multiple sources (e.g., parent, teachers, employer) in more than one setting and lasting at least 6 months.*[4]

• Evaluate for co-occurring psychiatric conditions. *The presence of comorbidities has treatment implications and, if left untreated, will complicate and/or limit successful outcomes for impulse control therapy.*[4,7,9]

NURSING PRIORITY NO. 2   To assist client to develop strategies to manage impulsive behaviors:

• Collaborate with treatment of condition, as indicated. *Individuals with impulsive control disorders do not necessarily present for treatment. Those with kleptomania, fire starters, and compulsive gamblers usually come to the attention of court authorities and may be referred for mental health services.*[1–5,7,9]

• Encourage client to make the decision to change and set personally achievable goals. *Making this decision can enable the client to enter therapy and be willing to stay with the program.*[2,4,7]

• Encourage client to identify negative consequences of behavior by expressing own feelings and anxieties regarding the adverse impact on his/her life. *Helps individual begin to understand problems of impulsive behavior.*[7]

• Help client take responsibility and control in situation. *Recognizing own control over impulsive behavior can help client begin to manage problems.*[3,4,7]

• ∞ Develop a treatment plan for child with ADHD in conjunction with the parents, teachers, and physician. *Medications and behavioral therapy can be helpful, along with monitoring the child and setting goals that are realistic and achievable.*[4]

• ∞ Organize a routine schedule for the child with Autism spectrum disorder. *Deficits in cognitive functioning make it difficult for the child to see the big picture, process information, see the consequences of an action, and understand the concept of time.*[5,6]

• ∞ Plan for problem with "melt downs," tantrums, or rage in children with Autism spectrum disorder. *These children do not recognize feelings, and parents and caregivers need to maintain a calm manner, remove child in a nonpunitive fashion, move closer, redirect, etc. These actions are calming; however, the child may begin acting out and need to go to a safe room where he or she can regain control.*[5,6]

• Discuss issue of hypersexuality. *It can be difficult to determine whether this term applies to an individual because people have differing definitions for what is too much sexual behavior.*[8]

 Acute Care   Collaborative   Community/ Home Care   Cultural

- Determine use of medications. *No specific medications have been approved by the FDA for use with impulse control disorders, but some medications such as selective serotonin reuptake inhibitor (SSRI) antidepressants are being used successfully.*[1,4,7]

NURSING PRIORITY NO. 3 To promote wellness (Teaching/Discharge Considerations):

- Involve in cognitive/behavioral therapy. *Having client identify behavioral patterns that result in negative consequences or harmful effects for self or others allows the individual to recognize and avoid these situations and use techniques that facilitate self-restraint.*[3–5,7]
- Discuss the use of exposure therapy. *This helps the client build up a tolerance for the trigger situation while using self-control.*[3,7]
- Encourage client to become involved in group or community activities. *Provides opportunity to learn new social skills and feel better about self.*[7]

DOCUMENTATION FOCUS

Assessment/Reassessment
- Individual findings, including type of situation involved in client's loss of control.
- Negative consequences incurred due to behavior.
- Client awareness of consequences of actions.

Planning
- Plan of care, specific interventions, and who is involved in planning.
- Individual teaching plan.

Implementation/Evaluation
- Responses to interventions, teaching, and actions performed.
- Attainment or progress toward desired outcome(s).
- Any modifications to plan of care.

Discharge Planning
- Long-term needs and who is responsible for actions to be taken.
- Specific referrals made.

References

1. Bose, D. (2009). Impulse control disorders. Retrieved March 2018 from http://www.buzzle.com/articles/impulse-control-disorder.html.
2. No author listed. (No date). Impulse control disorders. *Disorders.org*. Retrieved March 2018 from http://www.disorders.org/impulse-control-disorders/.
3. Aboujaoude, E., Koran, L. M. (eds.) (2010). *Impulse Control Disorders*. New York, NY: Cambridge University Press.
4. National Institute of Mental Health (NIMH). (Revised 2016). Attention deficit hyperactivity disorder (ADHD). Retrieved March 2018 from http://www.nimh.nih.gov/health/topics/attention-deficit-hyperactivity-disorder-adhd/index.shtml.
5. No author. (2018). Asperger/autism spectrum diagnosis in adults. *The Asperger/Autism Network (AANE)*. Retrieved March 2018 from http://www.aane.org/resources/adults/aspergerautism-spectrum-diagnosis-adults/.
6. Hutten, M. (No date). Aspergers children who worry excessively: Tips for parents. *My Aspergers Child*. Retrieved March 2018 from http://www.myaspergerschild.com/2012/06/aspergers-children-who-worry.html.
7. No author. (No date). Impulse control disorders (various pages). *PsychSolve*. Retrieved March 2018 from https://www.newharbinger.com/psychsolve/impulse-control-disorders.
8. Kaplan, M., Krueger, R. (2010). Diagnosis, assessment, and treatment of hypersexuality. *J Sex Res*, 47(2), 181–198.
9. Grant, J. E., Levine, L., Kim, D. (2005). Impulse control disorders in adult psychiatric inpatients. *Am J Psychiatry*, 162(11), 2184–2188.
10. Grant, J. E., et al. (2010). Introduction to behavioral addictions. *Am J Drug Alcohol Abuse*, 36(5), 233–241.
11. Yudofsky, S. C., Silver, J. M. (1985). Psychiatric aspects of brain injury: Trauma, stroke and tumor. In Hales, R. E., Frances, A. J. (eds). *Psychiatric Update—American Psychiatric Association Annual Review*, Vol. IV, Washington, DC: American Psychiatric Press.

 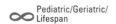

bowel Incontinence

Taxonomy II: Elimination and Exchange—Class 2 Gastrointestinal Function (00014) [**Diagnostic Division:** Elimination], Approved 1975; Revised 1998, 2017

DEFINITION: Involuntary passage of stool.

RELATED FACTORS
Incomplete emptying of the bowel
Inadequate dietary habits
Difficulty with toileting self-care
Environmental factor [e.g., inaccessible bathroom]
Generalized decline in muscle tone; immobility;
Laxative abuse

DEFINING CHARACTERISTICS

Subjective
Inability to expel formed stool despite recognition of rectal fullness
Bowel urgency; inability to delay defecation
Inability to recognize rectal fullness

Objective
Constant passage of soft stool
Fecal staining
Does not recognize or inattentive to urge to defecate
Associated Condition: Abnormal increase in abdominal or intestinal pressure; colorectal lesion; dysfunctional rectal sphincter; impaired reservoir capacity
Alternation in cognitive functioning; upper or lower motor nerve damage
Chronic diarrhea; impaction
Pharmaceutical agent
Sample Clinical Applications: Hemorrhoids, rectal prolapse, anal/gynecological surgery, childbirth injuries/uterine prolapse, spinal cord injury (SCI), stroke, multiple sclerosis (MS), ulcerative colitis, dementia

DESIRED OUTCOMES/EVALUATION CRITERIA

Sample NOC linkages:
Bowel Continence: Control of passage of stool from the bowel
Bowel Elimination: Formation and evacuation of stool
Neurological Status: Ability of the peripheral and central nervous system to receive, process, and respond to internal and external stimuli

Client Will (Include Specific Time Frame)
• Verbalize understanding of causative or controlling factors.
• Identify individually appropriate interventions.
• Participate in therapeutic regimen to control incontinence.
• Establish and maintain as regular a pattern of bowel functioning as possible.

 Acute Care Collaborative Community/ Home Care Cultural

ACTIONS/INTERVENTIONS

Sample **NIC** linkages:
Bowel Incontinence Care: Promotion of bowel continence and maintenance of perineal skin integrity
Bowel Incontinence Care: Encopresis: Promotion of bowel continence in children
Bowel Training: Assisting the patient to train the bowel to evacuate at specific intervals

NURSING PRIORITY NO. 1 To assess causative/contributing factors:

- Determine type of bowel incontinence present, as possible: *(1) loss of anal sphincter control (such as might occur with sphincter trauma), (2) stool seepage (as may occur with fistula and prolapse), or (3) poor bowel control (as might occur with inflammatory bowel disease, following intestinal surgery; chronic constipation with weakening musculature; laxative abuse, parasitic infection, toxins).*[8]
- Determine historical aspects of incontinence with preceding/precipitating events. *Common factors are (1) structural changes in the sphincter muscle (e.g., hemorrhoids, rectal prolapse; prostate, anal, or gynecological surgery; vaginal delivery with inadequate repair of obstetric sphincter disruption); (2) injuries to sensory nerves (e.g., SCI, multiple sclerosis); major trauma; stroke, tumor, or radiation therapy; (3) strong-urge or severe prolonged diarrhea (e.g., ulcerative colitis, Crohn's disease, infectious diarrhea); (4) dementia (e.g., acute or chronic cognitive impairment, not necessarily related to sphincter control); (5) result of toxins (e.g., salmonella); (6) aging, particularly in menopausal women; and (7) effects of improper diet or type and rate of enteral feedings.*[1-8]
- Note client's age and gender. *Bowel incontinence is more common in children, women of childbirth age, and elderly adults (difficulty responding to urge in a timely manner, problems walking or undoing zippers, decrease of maximum squeeze pressure); it is more common in boys than girls, but more common in elderly women than elderly men.*[1,2,7]
- Review medication regimen, including over-the-counter drugs. *Laxative abuse and drugs with a side effect of diarrhea (e.g., antibiotics) or constipation (e.g., sedatives, hypnotics, opioids, muscle relaxants) may impact bowel control.*
- Review diagnostic studies. *Pelvic and/or anal ultrasound may be used to identify structural abnormalities; endoscopy may be used to visualize lower gastrointestinal tract; manometry may be used to measure pressure and strength of anal muscles; and nerve studies may be used to check for nerve damage. Blood tests and stool cultures may be done to identify presence of bacteria and toxins.*[1-3,5,6]

NURSING PRIORITY NO. 2 To determine current pattern of elimination:

- Ascertain timing and characteristic aspects of incontinent occurrence, noting preceding or precipitating events. *Helps to identify patterns or worsening trends. Interventions are different for a sudden acute accident than for chronic long-term incontinence problems. Note: Client may have passive incontinence and be unaware that stool is being passed (related to poorly functioning sphincter muscle) or urge incontinence in which the individual is aware but unable to prevent passage of stool (sphincter muscle normal). Problem may have been present for a long time, either because of client/caregiver sense of embarrassment or failure to realize that effective treatment may be available.*[2,5]
- Determine stool characteristics, including **consistency** (may be liquid, hard formed, or hard at first and then soft), **amount** (may be a small amount of liquid or entire solid bowel movement), and **frequency**. *Provides information that can help differentiate type of incontinence present and provides comparative baseline for response to interventions.*
- Note where bowel accidents occur and what client is experiencing at the time. *Changes in usual routines or surrounding environment, general health condition, and the addition of emotional stressors can cause or exacerbate incontinence behaviors.*[5]

 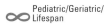

NURSING PRIORITY NO. 3　To promote control/management of incontinence:

- Assist in treatment of underlying conditions. *While incontinence is a symptom and not a disease, appropriate treatment can often correct the problem or at least improve the client's quality of life.*[2]
- 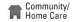 Administer medications, as indicated, such as stool softeners or bulk formers and laxatives (*may be used when the cause is constipation*) or antidiarrheals, including cholinergics (*may be used to decrease intestinal secretions and bowel motility if diarrhea is cause for incontinence*).[1,2]
- 🏠 Establish a toileting program as early as possible *to maximize success of program and preserve comfort and self-esteem.*[1–5,7]

　Take client to the bathroom or place on commode or bedpan at specified intervals, taking into consideration individual needs and incontinence patterns.

　Use the same type of facility for toileting as much as possible.

　Make sure bathroom is safe for impaired person (good lighting, support rails, good height for getting onto and up from stool).

　Provide time and privacy for elimination.

　Demonstrate techniques and assist client/caregiver to practice contracting abdominal muscles, leaning forward on commode *to increase intra-abdominal pressure during defecation,* and left to right abdominal massage *to stimulate peristalsis.*

- Encourage and instruct client/caregiver in providing diet high in natural bulk and fiber, with fruits, vegetables, grains, and reduced fatty foods. Identify and eliminate problem foods *to avoid diarrhea, constipation, or gas formation.*[2]
- Adjust enteral feedings and/or change formula, as indicated, *to reduce diarrhea effect.*[7]
- Encourage adequate fluid intake (at least 2,000 mL/d) within client's need and tolerance, including fruit juices *to help manage constipation.* Encourage warm fluids after meals *to promote intestinal motility.* Avoid caffeine and alcohol *to reduce diarrhea.*[7]
- Recommend walking and a regular exercise program, pelvic floor exercises, and biofeedback, as individually indicated, *to improve abdominal and pelvic muscles and strengthen rectal sphincter tone.*[2,7]
- Encourage or provide perineal care with frequent gentle cleansing and use of emollients after incontinent stools *to reduce excoriation of skin.*[6]
- Provide incontinence aids or pads until control is obtained. Change pads frequently *to reduce incidence of skin rashes or breakdown.*[6]
- Refer to ND Diarrhea *if incontinence is due to uncontrolled diarrhea* and ND Constipation *if incontinence is due to impaction.*

NURSING PRIORITY NO. 4　To promote wellness (Teaching/Discharge Considerations):

- 🏠 Review and encourage continuation of successful interventions as individually identified.
- 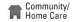 Instruct in use of suppositories or laxatives or stool softeners, when indicated, *to stimulate timed defecation.*
- Identify foods (e.g., daily bran muffins or prunes) *that promote soft stool consistency and bowel regularity.* Recommend avoidance of problem foods dependent on individual reactions.
- Refer client/caregivers to outside resources when condition is long term or chronic *to obtain care assistance and emotional support and respite.*
- Encourage scheduling of social activities within time frame of bowel program, as indicated (e.g., avoid a 4-hr excursion with no access to appropriate facilities if bowel program requires toileting every 3 hr), *to maximize social functioning and success of bowel program.*

DOCUMENTATION FOCUS

Assessment/Reassessment

- Current and previous pattern of elimination, physical findings, character of stool, actions tried.

 Acute Care　 Collaborative　🏠 Community/Home Care　🌐 Cultural

Planning
- Plan of care and who is involved in planning.
- Teaching plan.

Implementation/Evaluation
- Client's/caregiver's responses to interventions, teaching, and actions performed.
- Changes in pattern of elimination, characteristics of stool.
- Attainment or progress toward desired outcome(s).
- Modifications to plan of care.

Discharge Planning
- Identified long-term needs, noting who is responsible for each action.
- Specific bowel program at time of discharge.

References

1. Ferzandi, T. R., Demtchouk, V. (2015, updated 2016). Fecal incontinence (various pages). Retrieved March 2018 from http://emedicine.medscape.com/article/268674-overview#a0102.
2. Cleveland Clinic. (Updated 2016). Fecal (bowel) incontinence. Retrieved March 2018 from http://www.clevelandclinic.org/health/health-info/docs/4700/4787.asp.
3. Bowel incontinence. *Patient & Public Information*. (1996, updated 2008). Arlington Heights, IL: American Society of Colon and Rectal Surgeons.
4. Doenges, M. E., Moorhouse, M. F., Murr, A. C. (2010). Spinal cord injury (acute rehabilitative phase). *Nursing Care Plans: Guidelines for Individualizing Client Care Across the Life Span*. 8th ed. Philadelphia: F. A. Davis.
5. Monickan, D. (1989). *Special Care Problems: Bowel Incontinence*. 5th ed. Philadelphia: Department of Veterans Affairs, Veterans Health Services and Research Administration, Office of Geriatrics and Extended Care.
6. Langemo, D., et al. (2011). Incontinence and incontinence-associated dermatitis. *Adv Skin Wound Care*, 24(3), 126–140.
7. Lal, S. K. (2010, update 2016). Bowel incontinence. Retrieved March 2018 from http://www.nlm.nih.gov/medlineplus/ency/article/003135.htm.
8. Bharucha, A. E., et al. (2015). Epidemiology, pathophysiology, and classification of fecal incontinence: State of the science summary for the National Institute of Diabetes and Digestive and Kidney Diseases (NIDDK) workshop. *Am J Gastroenterology*, 110(1), 27–36.

functional urinary Incontinence

Taxonomy II: Elimination and Exchange—Class 1 Urinary Function (00020) **[Diagnostic Division:** Elimination], Approved 1986; Revised 1998; 2017

DEFINITION: Inability of usually continent person to reach the toilet in time to avoid unintentional loss of urine.

RELATED FACTORS
Alteration in environmental factor
Weakened supporting pelvic structure

DEFINING CHARACTERISTICS

Subjective
Sensation of need to void

Objective
Voiding prior to reaching toilet; time required to reach toilet is too long after sensation of urge
Completely empties bladder
Early morning urinary incontinence

(continues on page 468)

 Diagnostic Studies   Evidence Based Practice   Medications   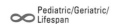 Pediatric/Geriatric/Lifespan

functional urinary Incontinence (continued)

Associated Condition: Alteration in cognitive functioning; impaired vision; neuromuscular impairment; psychological disorder

Sample Clinical Applications: Diabetes mellitus, congestive heart failure (CHF) (diuretic use), arthritis, bladder prolapse or cystocele, stroke; dementia; depression

DESIRED OUTCOMES/EVALUATION CRITERIA

Sample NOC linkages:

Urinary Elimination: Collection and discharge of urine

Urinary Continence: Control of elimination of urine from the bladder

Self-Care: Toileting: Personal actions to toilet self independently with or without assistive device

Client/Caregiver Will (Include Specific Time Frame)
- Verbalize understanding of condition and identify interventions to prevent incontinence.
- Alter environment to accommodate individual needs.
- Report voiding in individually appropriate amounts.
- Void at acceptable times and places.

ACTIONS/INTERVENTIONS

Sample NIC linkages:

Prompted Voiding: Promotion of urinary continence through the use of timed verbal toileting reminders and positive social feedback for successful toileting

Urinary Habit Training: Establishing an individual toileting schedule to preempt involuntary bladder emptying for persons with limited cognitive or physical ability

Self-Care Assistance: Toileting: Assisting another with elimination

NURSING PRIORITY NO. 1   To assess causative/contributing factors:

- ∞ Identify or differentiate client with functional incontinence (e.g., bladder and urethra are functioning normally, but client either cannot get to toilet or fails to recognize need to urinate in time to get to the toilet) from other types of incontinence. *Many causes are transient and reversible but can often occur in elderly hospitalized client. Note: A mnemonic to help remember the functional contributors to incontinence is as follows: DIAPPERS: D–delirium; I–infection (urinary); A–atrophic urethritis or vaginitis; P–pharmacological agents; P–psychiatric illness; E–excess urine output (due to excess fluid intake, alcoholic or caffeinated beverages, diuretics, peripheral edema, congestive heart failure, metabolic disorders such as hyperglycemia or hypercalcemia); R–reduced mobility; S–stool impaction.*[5]
- Determine if client is voluntarily postponing urination. *Often the demands of the work setting (such as restrictions on bathroom breaks, working alone [e.g., pharmacist, nurse, teacher], or demands of the job [heavy workload and unable to find time for a bathroom break]) make it difficult for individuals to go to the bathroom when the need arises, resulting in frequent urinary tract infections and incontinence.*[1,5]
- Evaluate cognition. *Delirium or acute confusion or psychosis can affect mental status—orientation to place, recognition of urge to void, or its significance.*[1,5]
- Note presence and type of functional impairments (e.g., poor eyesight, mobility difficulties, dexterity problems, self-care deficits) *that can hinder ability to get to bathroom.*[4]
- Identify environmental conditions that interfere with timely access to bathroom or successful toileting process. *Unfamiliar surroundings, poor lighting, improperly fitted chair walker, low toilet seat, absence of safety bars, and travel distance to toilet may affect self-care ability.*

 Acute Care   Collaborative   Community/Home Care   Cultural

- Review medical history for conditions known to increase urine output or alter bladder tone. *For example, diabetes mellitus, prolapsed bladder, and multiple sclerosis can affect frequency of urination and ability to hold urine until individual can reach the bathroom.*[1]
- Note use of medications or agents that can increase urine formation. *Diuretics, alcohol, and caffeine are several substances that can increase amount and frequency of voiding.*
- Test urine for presence of glucose. *Hyperglycemia can cause polyuria and overdistention of the bladder, resulting in problem with continence.*

NURSING PRIORITY NO. 2 To assess degree of interference/disability:

- Determine the frequency and timing of continent and incontinent voids. Note time of day or night when incontinence occurs, as well as timing issues (e.g., difference between the time it takes to get to bathroom and remove clothing and involuntary loss of urine). *Information will be used to plan program to manage incontinence.*[2]
- Initiate voiding diary. Note time of day or night when incontinence occurs as well as timing issues (e.g., difference between the time it takes to get to bathroom and remove clothing and involuntary loss of urine).
- Measure or estimate amount of urine voided or lost with incontinent episodes *to help determine options for managing problem.*
- Ascertain effect on lifestyle (including socialization and sexuality) and self-esteem. *There is a general belief that incontinence is an inevitable result of aging and that nothing can be done about it. However, individuals with incontinence problems are often embarrassed, withdraw from social activities and relationships, and hesitate to discuss the problem—even with their healthcare provider.*[1]

NURSING PRIORITY NO. 3 To assist in treating/preventing incontinence:

- Remind client to void when needed and schedule voiding times (e.g., cognitive decline, client who ambulates slowly because of physical limitations) *to reduce incontinence episodes and promote comfort.*[4,6]
- Administer prescribed diuretics in the morning. *The effect of these medications diminishes by bedtime, thus resulting in fewer nighttime voidings.*
- Reduce or eliminate use of hypnotics, if possible. *Client may be too sedated to recognize or respond to urge to void.*[3,5]
- Provide means of summoning assistance and respond immediately to summons. *Ready placement of a call light when hospitalized or a bell in the home setting enables client to obtain toileting help, as needed. Quick response to summons can promote continence.*[3]
- ∞ Use night lights to mark bathroom location. *Elderly person may become confused upon arising and be unable to locate bathroom in the dark. Lighting will facilitate access, reducing the possibility of accidents.*[3]
- Provide cues such as adequate room lighting, signs, and color coding of door. *Assists disoriented client to find the bathroom.*
- Remove throw rugs and excess furniture in travel path to bathroom. *Reduces risk of falls and facilitates access to bathroom.*
- Adapt clothes for quick removal. *Velcro fasteners, full skirts, crotchless panties or no panties, and suspenders or elastic waists instead of belts on pants facilitate toileting once urge to void is noted.*[3]
- Provide raised toilet seat or easily accessible bedside commode, urinal, or bedpan as indicated. *Facilitates toileting when individual has difficulty with movement.*[1]
- Schedule voiding on regular time schedule (e.g., every 2–3 hr). Encourage client to resist ignoring urge to urinate or have a bowel movement. *Emptying bladder on a regular schedule or when feeling urge reduces risk for incontinence. Since urge to void may be difficult to differentiate from urge to defecate, advise client to respond to urge.*[1,6]
- Assist client to assume normal anatomic position *for ease of complete bladder emptying.*[3]
- Restrict fluid intake 2 to 3 hr before bedtime. *May reduce need to waken to void during the night.*[1,6]

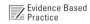

Diagnostic Studies   Evidence Based Practice   Medications   Pediatric/Geriatric/Lifespan

- Include physical or occupational therapist in determining ways to alter environment, appropriate assistive devices. *Useful in meeting individual needs of client.*
- Refer to urologist or continence specialist as indicated for interventions such as pelvic floor strengthening exercises, biofeedback techniques, vaginal weight training. *May be useful/needed to meet individual needs of client.*

NURSING PRIORITY NO. 4   To promote wellness (Teaching/Discharge Considerations):

- Discuss with client/significant other need for prompted and scheduled voidings *to manage continence when client is unable to respond immediately to urge to void.*[1]
- Suggest limiting intake of coffee, tea, and alcohol. *Diuretic effect of these substances impacts voiding pattern and can contribute to incontinence.*[1]
- Maintain positive regard when incontinence occurs. *Reduces embarrassment associated with incontinence, need for assistance, and use of bedpan.*
- Promote participation in developing long-term plan of care. *Encourages involvement in follow-through of plan, thus increasing possibility of success and confidence in own ability to manage program.*
- Refer to NDs reflex/stress/urge urinary Incontinence for additional interventions, as appropriate.

DOCUMENTATION FOCUS

Assessment/Reassessment
- Current elimination pattern, assessment findings, and effect on lifestyle and self-esteem.

Planning
- Plan of care and who is involved in planning.
- Teaching plan.

Implementation/Evaluation
- Response to interventions, teaching, and actions performed.
- Attainment or progress toward desired outcome(s).
- Modifications to plan of care.

Discharge Planning
- Long-term needs and who is responsible for actions to be taken.
- Specific referrals made.

References

1. Newman, D. K., Palmer, M. H. (eds). (2003). The state of the science on urinary incontinence. *Am J Nurs*, 3(Suppl), 2–53.
2. Wyman, J. F. (2003). Treatment of urinary incontinence in men and older women: The evidence shows the efficacy of a variety of techniques. *Am J Nurs*, 103(suppl), 26–35.
3. Newfield, S. A., et al. (2007). *Cox's Clinical Applications of Nursing Diagnosis: Adult, Child, Women's, Psychiatric, Gerontic, and Home Health Considerations.* 5th ed. Philadelphia, PA: F. A. Davis.
4. Pringle-Specht, J. K. (2005). Nine myths of incontinence in older adults. *Am J Nurs*, 105(6), 58–68.
5. Vasavada, S. P., Carmel, M. E., Rackley, R. (Updated 2017). Urinary incontinence. Retrieved March 2018 from http://emedicine.medscape.com/article/452289-overview.
6. Lazarou, G. (No date). Bladder control problems. Retrieved March 2018 from http://www.emedicinehealth.com/bladder_control_problems/article_em.htm.

 Acute Care   Collaborative   Community/Home Care Cultural

overflow urinary Incontinence

Taxonomy II: Elimination and Exchange—Class 1 Urinary Function (00176) [**Diagnostic Division:** Elimination], Approved 2006; Revised 2017

DEFINITION: Involuntary loss of urine associated with overdistention of the bladder.

RELATED FACTORS
Fecal impaction

DEFINING CHARACTERISTICS

Subjective
Involuntary leakage of small volume of urine
Nocturia

Objective
Bladder distention
High post-void residual volume
Associated Condition: Bladder outlet or urethral obstruction; detrusor external sphincter dyssynergia; detrusor hypocontractility
Severe pelvic organ prolapse
Treatment
Sample Clinical Applications: Uterine or bladder prolapse, benign prostatic hypertrophy, diabetes mellitus, multiple sclerosis (MS), spinal cord injury (SCI), Parkinson's disease; pelvic urinary stones

DESIRED OUTCOMES/EVALUATION CRITERIA

Sample NOC linkages:
Urinary Continence: Control of elimination of urine from the bladder
Urinary Elimination: Collection and discharge of urine
Knowledge: Disease Process: Extent of understanding conveyed about a specific disease process and potential complications

Client Will (Include Specific Time Frame)
• Verbalize understanding of causative factors and appropriate interventions for individual situation.
• Demonstrate techniques or behaviors to alleviate or prevent overflow incontinence.
• Void in sufficient amounts with no palpable bladder distention, experience no postvoid residuals greater than 50 mL, and have no dribbling or overflow.

ACTIONS/INTERVENTIONS

Sample NIC linkages:
Urinary Incontinence Care: Assistance in promoting continence and maintaining perineal skin integrity
Urinary Catheterization: Intermittent: Regular periodic use of a catheter to empty the bladder

NURSING PRIORITY NO. 1   To assess causative/contributing factors:

• Review client's history for (1) bladder outlet obstruction (e.g., prostatic hypertrophy, urethral stricture, urinary stones or tumors), (2) nonfunctioning detrusor muscle (i.e., sensory or motor paralytic bladder due to

 Diagnostic Studies   Evidence Based Practice   Medications   Pediatric/Geriatric/Lifespan

underlying neurological disease), or (3) atonic bladder that has lost its muscular tone (i.e., chronic overdistention) *to identify potential for or presence of conditions associated with overflow incontinence.*[5,6]

- ∞ Note client's age and gender. *Urinary incontinence due to overflow bladder is more common in older men because of the prevalence of obstructive prostate gland enlargement. However, age and sex are not factors in other conditions affecting overflow bladder incontinence, such as nerve damage from diseases such as diabetes, alcoholism, Parkinson's disease, MS, or spina bifida.*[1,5,6]
- Review medication regimen *for drugs that can cause or exacerbate retention and overflow incontinence (e.g., anticholinergics, calcium channel blockers, psychotropics, anesthesia, opiates, sedatives, alpha and beta blockers, antihistamines, neuroleptics).*[2,4,5]

NURSING PRIORITY NO. 2 To determine degree of interference/disability:

- Note client reports of symptoms common to overflow incontinence:[3,5,6]
  Feeling no need to urinate, while simultaneously losing urine; frequent leaking or dribbling.
  Feeling the urge to urinate but not being able to.
  Feeling as though the bladder is never completely empty.
  Passing a dribbling stream of urine, even after spending a long time at the toilet.
  Frequently getting up at night to urinate.
- Prepare for or assist with urodynamic testing (e.g., uroflowmetry *to assess urine speed and volume*; cystometrogram *to measure bladder pressure and volume*; bladder scan *to measure retention or postvoid residual, leak point pressure*).[1,5]

NURSING PRIORITY NO. 3 To assist in treating/preventing overflow incontinence:

- Collaborate in treatment of underlying conditions (e.g., medications or surgery for prostatic hypertrophy or severe pelvic prolapse; use of medications, to relax urinary sphincter; altering dose or discontinuing medications contributing to retention). *If the underlying cause of the overflow problem can be treated or eliminated, client may be able to return to normal voiding pattern.*
- Collaborate with physician regarding client's medications (e.g., anticholinergics, antidepressants, antipsychotics, sedatives, narcotics, alpha-adrenergic blockers) *that could be discontinued or altered to reduce/limit their effects on cognition and/or innervation and function of the bladder.*[9]
- Administer medications, as indicated. *Anticholinergics (e.g., oxybutinin [Ditropan]) or β₃ blockers (e.g., mirabegron [Myrbetriq]) are often used to reduce bladder spasms that are impeding urine outflow. For some men with an enlarged prostate, treatment with an alpha-adrenergic blocker (e.g., finasteride [Proscar], tamulosin [Flomax]) can help relax the muscle at the base of the urethra and allow urine to pass from the bladder.*[5,9]
- Administer stool softeners, laxatives, enema/other treatments as indicated. *Chronic constipation is a factor in weakening muscles that control urination. Fecal impaction can be a cause of urinary retention and overflow incontinence, especially in elderly clients.*[6]
- Demonstrate and encourage use of gentle massage over bladder (Credé's maneuver). *May facilitate bladder emptying when cause is detrusor weakness.*
- Implement intermittent or continuous catheterization. *Bladder catheterization may be a temporary measure or a permanent solution for overflow incontinence. Short-term use may be required while acute conditions are treated (e.g., infection, surgery for enlarged prostate); long-term use is required for permanent conditions (e.g., SCI or other neuromuscular conditions resulting in permanent bladder dysfunction). Note: Sterile intermittent catheterization is preferred when possible in overflow incontinence to promote the return to normal bladder emptying and to reduce risk of infection and other complications associated with long-term indwelling catheter.*[5,7,8,10]
- Refer to NDs urge urinary Incontinence, stress urinary Incontinence, and [acute/chronic] Urinary Retention for additional interventions.

 Acute Care   Collaborative   Community/ Home Care   Cultural

NURSING PRIORITY NO. 4 To promote wellness (Teaching/Discharge Considerations):

- 🏠 Identify and continue client's successful self-management of incontinence, where possible. *Continuation of successful strategies (e.g., allowing plenty of time for voiding, double voiding, self-catherization) can reduce risk of recurrence/failure of continence.*
- Establish regular schedule for bladder emptying whether voiding or using catheter.
- Emphasize need for adequate fluid intake, including use of acidifying fruit juices or ingestion of vitamin C *to discourage bacterial growth and stone formation.*
- 🔵 Instruct client/significant others in clean intermittent self-catheterization techniques *to prevent reflux or increased renal pressures and to enhance independence.*
- 🔵 Review signs/symptoms of complications requiring prompt medical evaluation *to promote timely intervention and prevent complications.*

DOCUMENTATION FOCUS

Assessment/Reassessment
- Current elimination pattern, assessment findings, and effect on lifestyle and sleep.

Planning
- Plan of care and who is involved in planning.
- Teaching plan.

Implementation/Evaluation
- Response to interventions, teaching, and actions performed.
- Attainment or progress toward desired outcome(s).
- Modifications to plan of care.

Discharge Planning
- Long-term needs and who is responsible for actions to be taken.
- Specific referrals made.

References

1. Merkelj, I. (2001). Urinary incontinence in the elderly. *South Med J*, 94(10), 952–957.
2. National Association for Continence (NAFC). (2017). Continence management (various pages). Retrieved March 2018 from http://www.nafc.org/management.
3. Gray, M. (2005). Overactive bladder: An overview. *J Wound Ostomy Continence Nurs*, 32(3 Suppl), 1–5.
4. Goode, P. S., Burgio, K. L. (2001). Managing incontinence in the geriatric patient. In Kursh, E. D., et al. (ed). *Office Urology: The Clinician's Guide*. Totawa, NJ: Humana Press.
5. DerSarkissian, C. (Updated 2016). Overflow incontinence. Retrieved March 2018 from http://www.webmd.com/urinary-incontinence-oab/overflow-incontinence.
6. Lazarou, G. (No date). Bladder control problems. Retrieved March 2018 from http://www.emedicinehealth.com/bladder_control_problems/article_em.htm.
7. Terpenning, M. S., Allada, R., Kauffman, C. A. (1989). Intermittent urethral catheterization in the elderly (Evidence Level IV: Nonexperimental study). *J Am Geriatr Soc*, 37(5), 411–416.
8. Dowling-Castronovo, A., Bradway, C. (2012). Urinary incontinence (UI) in older adults admitted to acute care. In Capezuti, E., et al. (eds). *Evidence-Based Geriatric Nursing Protocols for Best Practice*. 4th ed. New York, NY: Springer.
9. Allbaugh, J., Bernier, F. (reviewers) (Updated 2018). Urinary incontinence (sections on overflow incontinence and medications). Simon Foundation for Continence. Retrieved March 2018 from https://simonfoundation.org/category/causes-of-incontinence/.
10. Vasavada, S. P., Carmel, M. E., Rackley, R. R. (Updated 2017). Urinary incontinence treatment & management. Retrieved March 2018 from https://emedicine.medscape.com/article/452289-treatment#d11.

 Diagnostic Studies   📊 Evidence Based Practice   💊 Medications   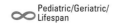 Pediatric/Geriatric/Lifespan

reflex urinary Incontinence

Taxonomy II: Elimination and Exchange—Class 1 Urinary Function (00018) [Diagnostic Division: Elimination], Submitted 1986; Revised 1998, 2017

DEFINITION: Involuntary loss of urine at somewhat predictable intervals when a specific bladder volume is reached.

RELATED FACTORS

To Be Developed

DEFINING CHARACTERISTICS

Subjective

Absence of urge to void, or of voiding sensation

Sensation of urgency to void without voluntary inhibition of bladder contraction

Sensations associated with bladder fullness

Objective

Predictable pattern of voiding

Inability to voluntarily inhibit or initiate voiding

Incomplete emptying of bladder with lesion above pontine micturition center

Associated Condition: Neurological impairment above levels of sacral or pontine micturition centers

Sample Clinical Applications: Spinal cord injury (SCI), multiple sclerosis (MS), bladder or pelvic cancer, Parkinson's disease, dementia

DESIRED OUTCOMES/EVALUATION CRITERIA

Sample NOC linkages:

Urinary Continence: Control of the elimination of urine from the bladder

Neurological Status: Autonomic: Ability of the autonomic nervous system to coordinate visceral and hemostatic function

Urinary Elimination: Collection and discharge of urine

Client Will (Include Specific Time Frame)

• Verbalize understanding of condition or contributing factors.

• Establish bladder regimen appropriate for individual situation.

• Demonstrate behaviors or techniques to manage condition and prevent complications.

• Void at acceptable times and places.

ACTIONS/INTERVENTIONS

Sample NIC linkages:

Urinary Incontinence Care: Assistance in promoting continence and maintaining perineal skin integrity

Urinary Catheterization: Intermittent: Regular periodic use of a catheter to empty the bladder

NURSING PRIORITY NO. 1 To assess degree of interference/disability:

• Identify pathology of problem (e.g., pelvic cancer, central nervous system disorder, SCI, stroke, Parkinson's disease, diabetes with bladder neuropathy, brain tumor) *that results in either hypotonic or spastic neurogenic*

 Acute Care
 Collaborative
 Community/ Home Care
 Cultural

bladder, thereby affecting bladder storage, emptying, and control. Note: The causes of reflex incontinence are often mixed (e.g., most people with reflex incontinence experience symptoms of urinary frequency, urgency, and nocturia). In this situation, the bladder empties urine as it fills.[3–5,7–9]

- Ascertain whether client experiences any sense of bladder fullness or awareness of incontinence. *Individuals with reflex incontinence have little, if any, awareness of need to void. Loss of sensation of bladder filling can result in overfilling, inadequate emptying (retention), and/or constant dribbling.*[5,8,9] (Refer to NDs [acute/chronic] Urinary Retention and overflow urinary Incontinence for additional interventions.)
- Review voiding diary, if available, or record frequency and time of urination. Compare timing of voidings, particularly in relation to certain factors (e.g., liquid intake and medications). *Aids in targeting interventions to meet individual situation.*[1]
- Measure amount of each voiding during assessment phase. *Incontinence often occurs once a specific bladder volume is reached and may indicate need for insertion of a permanent or intermittent catheter.*[2,8]
- Determine postvoid residual volume (via handheld bladder scan) in client with incomplete emptying or on scheduled catheterization *to evaluate for urinary retention when attempting toilet training, to establish schedule for intermittent catheterization, and to avoid unnecessary catheterization.*[6] *Note: Often the bladder is not completely emptied because there is no voluntary control of the bladder.*[8]
- Refer to urologist or appropriate specialist for testing. *Urinalysis, ultrasound, radiographs, and urine flowmetry are standard to measure urine flow. A urodynamic evaluation measuring bladder capacity, pressure, and rate of urinary flow may also be indicated.*

NURSING PRIORITY NO. 2 To assist in managing incontinence:

- Evaluate client's ability to manipulate or use urinary collection device or catheter. *Type and degree of neurological impairment (i.e., SCI, MS, dementia) may interfere with client's ability to be self-sufficient.*[7]
- Collaborate in treatment of underlying cause or management of incontinence. *Of all the types of urinary incontinence, reflex incontinence is probably the most difficult to treat; however, this condition may be treated with medications, neuromodulation (electrical stimulation of specific nerves to influence the nerve circuit that controls urination), bladder surgery, or indwelling bladder catheters. Note: In recent years, intradetrusor injections of onabotulinumtoxinA (Botox) have transformed the management of neurogenic detrusor overactivity, and neuromodulation (controlled stimulation of the peripheral or central nervous system with electricity) offers promise for managing both storage and voiding dysfunction.*[8–10]
- Involve client/significant other/caregiver in creating plan of care *to develop mutually agreed-upon goals and ensure individual needs are met, enhancing commitment to plan.*[1–8]
- Encourage minimum of 1,500 to 2,000 mL of fluid intake daily. *Reduces risk of bladder and kidney infection/stone formation.*
- Remind or assist client to go to toilet before the expected time of incontinence *in an attempt to stimulate the reflexes for voiding.*[1]
- Set alarm to awaken during night, if necessary, to maintain catheterization schedule or use external catheter or collection device, as appropriate. *Developing a regular time to empty the bladder may prevent urinary retention or overflow incontinence during the night.*
- Implement continuous or intermittent catheterization schedule, if condition indicates, *to prevent bladder overdistention and detrusor muscle damage. Note: Experience has shown that intermittent catheterization is preferable to indwelling catheters in young persons (both male and female) with SCI. It is also a valuable alternative for individuals with chronic urinary retention due to an obstructed, weak, or nonfunctioning bladder.*[1,4,7]

NURSING PRIORITY NO. 3 To promote wellness (Teaching/Discharge Considerations):

- 🏠 Encourage continuation of regularly timed bladder program. *May be able to establish a schedule that takes advantage of whatever ability remains, even though the neurological impairment is affecting bladder sensation.*

 Diagnostic Studies Evidence Based Practice 💊 Medications ∞ Pediatric/Geriatric/Lifespan

- Suggest use of incontinence pads/pants during day and with social contact, if appropriate. *Depending on client's activity level, amount of urine loss, manual dexterity, and cognitive ability, these devices provide security and comfort and protect the skin and clothing from urine leakage, reduce odor, and are generally unnoticeable under clothing.*[7,8]
- Emphasize importance of perineal care following voiding and frequent changing of incontinence pads, if used. *Maintains cleanliness and prevents skin irritation or breakdown and odor.*[7,8]
- Encourage limited intake of coffee, tea, and alcohol, as well as avoidance of citrus foods, artificial sweeteners, tomatoes, and spicy foods. *Diuretic effect of these beverages may affect predictability of voiding pattern, and the acidic, spicy, or highly sweet substances can irritate the bladder.*[11]
- Instruct in proper care of catheter and cleaning techniques when used. *Reduces risk of infection.*[7,8]
- Review signs/symptoms of urinary complications and need for medical follow-up. *Provides immediate attention preventing exacerbation of problem or extension of infection into kidneys.*

DOCUMENTATION FOCUS

Assessment/Reassessment
- Findings including degree of disability and effect on lifestyle.
- Availability of resources or support person.

Planning
- Plan of care and who is involved in planning.
- Teaching plan.

Implementation/Evaluation
- Responses to treatment plan, interventions, and actions performed.
- Attainment or progress toward desired outcome(s).
- Modifications to plan of care.

Discharge Planning
- Long-term needs and who is responsible for actions to be taken.
- Available resources, equipment needs and sources.

References

1. Newman, D. K., Palmer, M. H. (eds). The state of the science on urinary incontinence. *Am J Nurs*, (2003). 103(Suppl), 20.
2. Newfield, S. A., et al. (2007). *Cox's Clinical Applications of Nursing Diagnosis: Adult, Child, Women's, Psychiatric, Gerontic, and Home Health Considerations.* 5th ed. Philadelphia: F. A. Davis.
3. Beers, M. H., Berkow, R. (eds). (1999). *The Merck Manual of Diagnosis and Therapy.* 17th ed. Whitehouse Station, NJ: Merck Research Laboratories.
4. Gray, M. (2005). Assessment and management of urinary incontinence. *Nurse Pract*, 30(7), 32–43.
5. Vasavada, S. P., Carmel, M. E., Rackley, R. (Updated 2017). Urinary incontinence. Retrieved March 2018 from http://emedicine.medscape.com/article/452289-overview.
6. Verathon. (2018). BladderScan BVI 9400 product information page. Retrieved March 2018 from https://verathon.com/bladderscan-bvi-9400/.
7. No author listed. (Updated 2015). Living with spinal cord injury-bladder care. Retrieved March 2018 from http://www.webmd.com/brain/tc/living-with-a-spinal-cord-injury-bladder-care.
8. Stoppler, M. C. (2017). Urinary incontinence. Retrieved March 2018 from http://www.emedicinehealth.com/incontinence/article_em.htm.
9. Paniker, J. N., Fowler, C. J., Kessler, T. M. (2015). Lower urinary tract dysfunction in the neurological patient: Clinical assessment and management. *Lancet Neurol*, 14(7), 720–732.
10. Healthline. (2017). What is reflex incontinence? Retrieved March 2018 from https://www.healthline.com/health/overactive-bladder/reflex-incontinence.
11. Pathak, N. (2017). Diet, drugs, and urinary incontinence symptoms. Retrieved March 2018 from https://www.webmd.com/urinary-incontinence-oab/urinary-incontinence-diet-medications-chart#1.

 Acute Care Collaborative Community/ Home Care Cultural

risk for urge urinary Incontinence

Taxonomy II: Elimination and Exchange—Class 1 Urinary Function (00022) [**Diagnostic Division:** Elimination], Approved 1998; Revised 2008, 2013, 2017

DEFINITION: Susceptible to involuntary passage of urine occurring soon after a strong sensation or urgency to void, which may compromise health.

RISK FACTORS

Alcohol consumption; caffeine intake
Fecal impaction; involuntary sphincter relaxation
Ineffective toileting habits
Associated Condition: Atrophic urethritis or vaginitis
Bladder infection; decrease in bladder capacity
Impaired bladder contractility; detrusor hyperactivity with impaired bladder contractility
Treatment regimen
Sample Clinical Applications: Abdominal trauma/surgery, pelvic inflammatory disease (PID); pregnancy; childbirth; pelvic surgery; obesity; enlarged prostate, prostate surgery; recurrent urinary tract infections (UTIs), diabetes, stroke, multiple sclerosis, Parkinson's disease, spinal cord injury

DESIRED OUTCOMES/EVALUATION CRITERIA

Sample NOC linkages:
Urinary Continence: Control of elimination of urine from the bladder
Risk Control: Personal actions to understand, prevent, eliminate, or reduce modifiable health threats

Client Will (Include Specific Time Frame)
• Identify individual risk factors and appropriate interventions.
• Demonstrate behaviors or lifestyle changes to prevent development of problem.

ACTIONS/INTERVENTIONS

Sample NIC linkages:
Urinary Bladder Training: Improving bladder function for those with urge incontinence by increasing the bladder's ability to hold urine and the patient's ability to suppress urination
Urinary Habit Training: Establishing an individualized toileting schedule to preempt involuntary bladder emptying for persons with limited cognitive or physical ability
Self-Care Assistance: Toileting: Assisting another with elimination

NURSING PRIORITY NO. 1   To assess potential for developing incontinence:

• Note presence of diagnoses often associated with urgent voiding (e.g., UTI; pregnancy; pelvic or gynecological surgery; prostatitis, or prostate surgery; obesity; bladder tumors or stones; nerve damage from conditions such as diabetes, stroke, Parkinson's, MS; certain cancers, including the bladder and prostate; recent or lengthy use of indwelling urinary catheter). *Such conditions can affect bladder capacity; pelvic, bladder, or urethral musculature tone; and/or innervation.*[1–3,10]
• Ask client about urgency (more than just normal desire to void). *Urgency (also called overactive bladder [OAB]) is a sudden, compelling need to void that is difficult to defer, can occur frequently (e.g., eight or more times in 24 hr), and may be accompanied by leaking or urge incontinence.*[11–14]
• Note factors that may affect ability to respond to urge to void in a timely manner. *Impaired mobility, use of sedation, or cognitive impairments may result in client failing to recognize need to void or moving too slowly to make it to the bathroom, with subsequent loss of urine.*[2,10]

 Diagnostic Studies   Evidence Based Practice   Medications   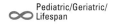 Pediatric/Geriatric/Lifespan

- Determine use or presence of bladder irritants. *A significant intake of alcohol, caffeine, acidic or spicy food, and fluids can result in increased output or urge symptoms and contribute to the possibility of incontinence.*[5]
- Review client's medications for affect on bladder function, such as beta blockers and cholinergic drugs *(can increase detrusor tone)*; neuroleptics, antidepressants, sedatives, and opiates *(can cause detrusor relaxation)*; muscle relaxants and psychoactive drugs *(can cause sphincter relaxation)*; and diuretics *(can increase urine production).*[7]
- Measure amount of urine voided, especially noting amounts less than 100 mL or greater than 550 mL, *to determine bladder capacity and effectiveness of bladder contractions to facilitate emptying.*[6]
- Prepare for and assist with appropriate testing (e.g., urinalysis, noninvasive bladder scanning, urine culture, urine and serum glucose, voiding cystometrogram). *Accurate assessment and diagnosis can determine voiding pattern and identify pathology that may lead to the development of incontinence.*[2,4,8]

NURSING PRIORITY NO. 2   To prevent occurrence of problem:

- Assist in treatment of underlying conditions that may contribute to urge incontinence. *Urgency symptoms may resolve with treatment of medical problem (e.g., UTI; recovery from pelvic surgery, childbirth, or pelvic trauma; use of estrogen-based oral or topical products for atrophic vaginitis; etc.).*
- Record intake along with frequency and degree of urgency of voiding. *May reveal developing incontinence problem when need to void is more frequent and urgent relative to normal fluid intake.*
- Ascertain client's awareness and concerns about developing problem and whether lifestyle is affected (e.g., daily activities, socialization, sexual patterns). *Provides information regarding the degree of concern client is experiencing and need for preventive measures to be instituted.*
- Regulate liquid intake at prescheduled times (with and between meals). *Promotes a predictable voiding pattern to establish a bladder-training program to prevent incontinence.*[4]
- Establish schedule for voiding (habit training) based on client's usual voiding pattern. *Can successfully reduce risk for incontinence.*
- Manage bowel elimination *to prevent continence problems associated with constipation or fecal impaction.*
- Provide assistance or devices, as indicated, for clients who are mobility impaired. *Providing means of summoning assistance and placing bedside commode, urinal, or bedpan within client's reach can promote sense of control in self-managing voiding.*[5]
- Encourage regular pelvic floor strengthening exercises (Kegel exercises or use of vaginal cones). *Can improve pelvic musculature tone and strength, preventing or halting incontinence. Note: Studies reveal a positive effect on urge incontinence using a combination of behavioral interventions (including pelvic muscle exercises) and medications in older women.*[4,6,9]

NURSING PRIORITY NO. 3   To promote wellness (Teaching/Discharge Considerations):

- Provide information to client/significant other about potential for urge incontinence (also called OAB) and lifestyle measures to prevent development of incontinence, as individually indicated.
- Recommend limiting intake of coffee, tea, and alcohol. *These substances have an irritating effect on the bladder and may contribute to incontinence.*[10]
- Suggest wearing loose-fitting or especially adapted clothing. *Facilitates response to voiding urge, especially in elderly or infirm individuals, enabling them to reach the toilet without loss of urine.*[6]
- Emphasize importance of perineal care after each voiding. *Reduces risk of ascending infection and incontinence-related dermatitis.*[5]
- Identify signs/symptoms indicating urinary complications and need for medical follow-up care. *Helps client be aware and seek intervention in a timely manner to prevent more serious problems from developing.*

DOCUMENTATION FOCUS

Assessment/Reassessment

- Individual findings, including specific risk factors and pattern of voiding.

 Acute Care   Collaborative   Community/ Home Care   Cultural

Planning
- Plan of care, specific interventions, and who is involved in planning.
- Teaching plan.

Implementation/Evaluation
- Response to interventions, teaching, and actions performed.
- Attainment or progress toward desired outcome(s).
- Modifications to plan of care.

Discharge Planning
- Discharge needs and who is responsible for actions to be taken.
- Specific referrals made.

References

1. Vasavada, S. P., Carmel, M. E., Rackley, R. (Updated 2017). *Urinary incontinence*. Retrieved March 2018 from http://emedicine.medscape.com/article/452289-overview.
2. Booth, C. (2002). Introduction to urinary incontinence. *Hosp Pharmacist*, 9(3), 65–68.
3. Sampsell, C. M., et al. (ed). (2000). Continence for women: Evaluation of AWHONN's third research utilization project. *J Obstet Gynecol Neonatal Nurs*, 29, 9–17.
4. Newman, D. K., Palmer, M. H. (eds). The state of the science on urinary incontinence. *Am J Nurs*, (2003). 3(Suppl), 2–53.
5. Newfield, S. A., et al. (2007). ND: Urinary Incontinence. *Cox's Clinical Applications of Nursing Diagnosis: Adult, Child, Women's, Psychiatric, Gerontic, and Home Health Considerations*. 5th ed. Philadelphia: F. A. Davis.
6. Wyman, J. F. (2003). Treatment of urinary incontinence in men and older women: The evidence shows the efficacy of a variety of techniques. *Am J Nurs*, 103(Suppl), 26–35.
7. Cleveland Clinic Staff. (2014). Are your medications causing or increasing incontinence? Retrieved March 2018 from https://health.clevelandclinic.org/are-your-medications-causing-or-increasing-incontinence/.
8. Verathon. (2018). BladderScan BVI 9400 product information page. Retrieved March 2018 from https://verathon.com/bladderscan-bvi-9400/.
9. Burgio, K. L., Locher, J. L., Goode, P. S. (2000). Combined behavioral and drug therapy for urge incontinence in older women. *Obstet Gynecol Surv*, 55(8), 485–486.
10. Stoppler, M. C. (Reviewed 2017). Urinary incontinence. Retrieved March 2018 from http://www.emedicinehealth.com/incontinence/article_em.htm.
11. Gray, M. (2005). Assessment and management of urinary incontinence. *Nurse Pract*, 30(7), 32–43.
12. Gray, M. (2005). Overactive bladder: An overview. *J Wound Ostomy Continence Nurs*, 32(3 Suppl), 1–5.
13. Newman, D. K. (2005). Assessment of the patient with an overactive bladder. *J Wound Ostomy Continence Nurs*, 32(3 Suppl), 5–10.
14. Bergman, S. (Updated 2016). Urge Incontinence (various pages). Retrieved March 2018 from http://www.webmd.com/urinary-incontinence-oab/america-asks-11/urge?page=1.

stress urinary Incontinence

Taxonomy II: Elimination and Exchange—Class 1 Urinary Function (00017) [**Diagnostic Division:** Elimination], Approved 1986; Revised 2006; 2017

DEFINITION: Sudden leakage of urine with activities that increase intra-abdominal pressure.

RELATED FACTORS
Weak pelvic floor muscles

DEFINING CHARACTERISTICS

Subjective
Involuntary leakage of small volume of urine [e.g., with sneezing, laughing, coughing, on exertion]

(continues on page 480)

 Diagnostic Studies   Evidence Based Practice   Medications 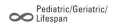 Pediatric/Geriatric/Lifespan

stress urinary Incontinence (continued)

Objective

Involuntary leakage of small volume of urine in the absence of detrusor contraction or an overdistended bladder

Associated Condition: Degenerative changes in pelvic floor muscles

Increase in intra-abdominal muscles

Intrinsic urethral sphincter deficiency

DESIRED OUTCOMES/EVALUATION CRITERIA

Sample NOC linkages:

Urinary Continence: Control of elimination of urine from the bladder

Symptom Control: Personal actions to minimize perceived adverse changes in physical and emotional functioning

Client Will (Include Specific Time Frame)

- Verbalize understanding of condition and interventions for bladder conditioning.
- Demonstrate behaviors or techniques to strengthen pelvic floor musculature.
- Remain continent even with increased intra-abdominal pressure.

ACTIONS/INTERVENTIONS

Sample NIC linkages:

Pelvic Muscle Exercise: Strengthening and training the levator ani and urogenital muscles through voluntary, repetitive contraction to decrease stress, urge, or mixed types of urinary incontinence

Urinary Incontinence Care: Assistance in promoting continence and maintaining perineal skin integrity

Urinary Habit Training: Establishing an individualized toileting schedule to preempt involuntary bladder emptying for persons with limited cognitive or physical ability

NURSING PRIORITY NO. 1   To assess causative/contributing factors:

- Identify physiological causes of increased intra-abdominal pressure (e.g., obesity, gravid uterus; repeated heavy lifting [occupational risk]), contributing history (e.g., multiple births, bladder or pelvic trauma/fractures), surgery (e.g., radical prostatectomy, bladder or other pelvic surgeries that may damage sphincter muscles), and participation in high-impact athletic or military field activities (particularly women). *Identification of specifics of individual situation provides for developing an accurate plan of care.*[2,6,7]
- Assess for urine loss (usually in small amounts) with coughing, sneezing, or sports activities; relaxed pelvic musculature and support, noting inability to start and stop stream while voiding; and bulging of perineum when bearing down. *Severity of symptoms may indicate need for more specialized evaluation.*
- ∞ Note client's sex and age. *Note: The majority of clients with stress urinary incontinence are women, although men who undergo surgical prostatectomy may also experience it. Although pregnancy and childbirth are known to cause stress incontinence in younger women, it is also common in older women, possibly related to loss of estrogen and weakened muscles in the pelvic organs.*[11]
- Review client's medications (e.g., alpha-blockers, angiotensin-converting enzyme inhibitors, loop diuretics) *for those that may cause or exacerbate stress incontinence. Note: The urge incontinence effect with these agents is usually transient.*[1,7]
- Assess for mixed incontinence (consisting of two or more kinds of incontinence), noting whether bladder irritability, reduced bladder capacity, or voluntary overdistention is present. *The most common*

 Acute Care   Collaborative   Community/Home Care   Cultural

combinations are urge with stress incontinence and urge or stress with functional incontinence. These impact treatment choices.[1,11] (Refer to NDs urge and reflex urinary Incontinence; [acute/chronic] Urinary Retention.)

NURSING PRIORITY NO. 2 To assess degree of interference/disability:

- Observe voiding patterns, time and amount voided, and note the stimulus provoking incontinence. Review voiding diary if available. *Provides information that can help determine type of incontinence and type of treatment indicated.*
- 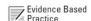 Prepare for and assist with testing or refer to urology specialist as indicated. *Diagnosing urinary incontinence often requires comprehensive evaluation (e.g., measuring bladder filling and capacity, leak-point pressure, rate of urinary flow, pelvic ultrasound, cystogram/other scans) to differentiate stress incontinence from other types.*[1–12]
- Determine effect on lifestyle (including daily activities, participation in sports or exercise and recreation, socialization, sexuality) and self-esteem. *Untreated incontinence can have emotional and physical consequences. Client may limit or abstain from sports or recreational activities. Urinary tract infections, skin rashes, and sores can occur. Self-esteem is affected, and the client may suffer from depression and withdraw from social functions.*[6]
- Ascertain methods of self-management. *Client may already be limiting liquid intake, voiding before any activity, or using undergarment protection.*
- Perform bladder scan to determine postvoid residuals as indicated. *Presence of volumes greater than 200 mL (or 150 mL in elder clients) suggests incomplete emptying of bladder, requiring further evaluation.*[8]

NURSING PRIORITY NO. 3 To assist in treating/preventing incontinence:

- Implement nonsurgical treatment techniques:
  Keep a voiding diary, as indicated. *The use of a frequency/volume chart is helpful in bladder training. A review of urine output in relation to fluid intake record can reveal need to modify fluid intake in client who is resistant to fluid management efforts. The contribution of dietary items that may precipitate incontinence may become obvious after reviewing the voiding log.*[12]
  Practice timed voidings (e.g., 3-hr intervals during the day) *to keep bladder relatively empty.*
  Extend time between voidings to 3- to 4-hr intervals. *May improve bladder capacity and retention time.*[12]
  Limit use of coffee, tea, and alcohol. *Diuretic effect of these substances may lead to bladder distention, increasing likelihood of incontinence.*[4]
  Encourage weight loss as indicated *to reduce pressure on intra-abdominal and pelvic organs.*[1]
  Void before physical exertion such as exercise or sports activities *to reduce potential for incontinence.*[9]
  Encourage regular pelvic floor strengthening exercises (Kegel exercises). *These exercises involve tightening the muscles of the pelvic floor and need to be done numerous times throughout the day.*[2]
  Avoid or limit heavy lifting and high-impact aerobics or sports *to decrease incontinence associated with elevated intra-abdominal pressures.*[4]
  Incorporate "bent-knee sit-ups" into exercise program. *Increasing abdominal muscle tone can help relieve stress incontinence.*[3]
- Assist with medical treatment of underlying urological condition, as indicated. *Stress incontinence may be treated with surgical intervention (e.g., bladder neck suspension, pubovaginal sling to reposition bladder and strengthen pelvic musculature; prostate surgery) and nonsurgical therapies (e.g., behavioral modification, pelvic muscle exercises, medications, use of pessary, vaginal cones; electrical stimulation; biofeedback).*[7,9,11]
- Administer medications, as indicated, such as tolterodine (Detrol), oxybutynin (Ditropan), fesoterodine (Toviaz), darifenacin (Enablex), solifenacin (VESIcare), trospium (Sanctura). *May improve bladder tone and capacity and increase effectiveness of bladder sphincter and proximal urethra contractions.*[1,5,11]

 Diagnostic Studies   Evidence Based Practice   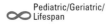 Medications   ∞ Pediatric/Geriatric/Lifespan

NURSING PRIORITY NO. 4 To promote wellness (Teaching/Discharge Considerations):

- Suggest use of incontinence pads or undergarments as needed. *Considering client's activity level, amount of urine loss, physical size, manual dexterity, and cognitive ability to determine specific product choices best suited to individual situation and needs may be necessary when leakage continues to occur in spite of other measures.*

- Emphasize importance of perineal care following voiding and frequent changing of incontinence pads. Recommend application of oil-based emollient. *Prevents infection and protects skin from irritation.*

- Discuss participation in incontinence management for activities such as heavy lifting and strenuous sports activities that increase intra-abdominal pressure. *Substituting swimming or other low-impact exercises may help reduce frequency of incontinence and maintain active life.*

- Recommend or refer for behavioral training, as indicated. *An important part of pelvic floor biofeedback therapy is consistent practice of the pelvic floor muscle exercises at home. With biofeedback, an individual can learn to stop using the incorrect muscles and start using the correct ones.*[10,11]

DOCUMENTATION FOCUS

Assessment/Reassessment
- Findings including pattern of incontinence and physical factors present.
- Effect on lifestyle and self-esteem.
- Client understanding of condition.

Planning
- Plan of care and who is involved in the planning.
- Teaching plan.

Implementation/Evaluation
- Responses to interventions, teaching, actions performed, and changes that are identified.
- Attainment or progress toward desired outcome(s).
- Modifications to plan of care.

Discharge Planning
- Long-term needs, referrals, and who is responsible for specific actions.
- Specific referrals made.

References

1. Shenot, P. J. (Updated 2016). Urinary incontinence in adults. *The Merck Manual for Health Care Professionals.* Retrieved March 2018 from http://www.merckmanuals.com/professional/genitourinary_disorders/voiding_disorders/urinary_incontinence.html.

2. Wyman, J. F. (2003). Treatment of urinary incontinence in men and older women: The evidence shows the efficacy of a variety of techniques. *Am J Nurs,* 103(Suppl), 26–35.

3. Newfield, S. A., et al. (2007). ND: Urinary Incontinence, stress. *Cox's Clinical Applications of Nursing Diagnosis: Adult, Child, Women's, Psychiatric, Gerontic, and Home Health Considerations.* 5th ed. Philadelphia: F. A. Davis.

4. Newman, D. K., Palmer, M. H. (eds). (2003). The state of the science on urinary incontinence. *Am J Nurs,* 3(Suppl), 2–53.

5. Booth, C. (2002). Introduction to urinary incontinence. *Hosp Pharmacist,* 9(3), 65–68.

6. Carls, C. (2007). The prevalence of stress urinary incontinence in high school and college-age female athletes in the Midwest: Implications for education and prevention. *Urol Nurs,* 27(1), 21–24.

7. Vasavada, S. P., Carmel, M. E., Rackley, R. (Updated 2017). Urinary incontinence. Retrieved March 2018 from http://emedicine.medscape.com/article/452289-overview.

8. Verathon. (2018). BladderScan 9400 product information page. Retrieved March 2018 from https://verathon.com/bladderscan-bvi-9400/.

9. Bray, B., Van Sell, S. L., Miller-Anderson, M. (2007). Stress incontinence: It's no laughing matter. *RN,* 70(4), 25–29.

10. National Association for Continence. (2017). Continence management (various pages). Retrieved March 2018 from http://www.nafc.org/urinary-incontinence.

11. Palmer, M. H., Willis-Gray, M. G. (2017). Overactive bladder in women. *Am J Nurs,* 117(4), 34–41.

12. Rovner, E. S., Wein, A. J. (2004). Treatment options for stress urinary incontinence. *Rev Urol,* 6(3 Suppl), S29–S47.

 Acute Care   Collaborative   Community/Home Care   Cultural

urge urinary Incontinence

Taxonomy II: Elimination and Exchange—Class 1 Urinary Function (00019) [**Diagnostic Division:** Elimination], Approved1986; Revised 2006; 2017

DEFINITION: Involuntary passage of urine occurring soon after a strong sense of urgency to void.

RELATED FACTORS
Alcohol consumption; caffeine intake
Fecal impaction; involuntary sphincter relaxation
Ineffective toileting habits

DEFINING CHARACTERISTICS

Subjective
Urinary urgency; involuntary loss of urine with bladder contractions or spasms
Inability to reach toilet in time to avoid urine loss
Associated Condition: Atrophic urethritis or vaginitis
Bladder infection; decrease in bladder capacity
Impaired bladder contractility; detrusor hyperactivity with impaired bladder contractility
Treatment regimen
Sample Clinical Applications: Abdominal trauma/surgery, pelvic inflammatory disease (PID); pregnancy; childbirth; pelvic surgery; obesity; enlarged prostate, prostate surgery; recurrent urinary tract infections (UTIs), diabetes, stroke, multiple sclerosis, Parkinson's disease, spinal cord injury

DESIRED OUTCOMES/EVALUATION CRITERIA

Sample NOC linkages:
Urinary Continence: Control of elimination of urine from the bladder
Cognition: Ability to execute complex mental processes
Self-Care: Toileting: Personal actions to toilet self independently with or without assistive device

Client Will (Include Specific Time Frame)
• Verbalize understanding of condition.
• Demonstrate behaviors or techniques to control or correct situation.
• Report increase in interval between urge and involuntary loss of urine.
• Void every 3 to 4 hr in individually appropriate amounts.

ACTIONS/INTERVENTIONS

Sample NIC linkages:
Urinary Bladder Training: Improving bladder function for those with urge incontinence by increasing the bladder's ability to hold urine and the patient's ability to suppress urination
Urinary Habit Training: Establishing an individualized toileting schedule to preempt involuntary bladder emptying for persons with limited cognitive or physical ability
Urinary Incontinence Care: Assistance in promoting continence and maintaining perineal skin integrity

 Diagnostic Studies   Evidence Based Practice   Medications 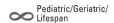 Pediatric/Geriatric/ Lifespan

NURSING PRIORITY NO. 1   To assess causative/contributing factors:

- Note presence of conditions often associated with urgent voiding (e.g., UTI; pregnancy; pelvic or gynecological surgery; prostatitis or prostate surgery; obesity; bladder tumors or stones; nerve damage from conditions such as diabetes, stroke, Parkinson's, MS; certain cancers, including the bladder and prostate; recent or lengthy use of indwelling urinary catheter) *affecting bladder capacity, pelvic musculature tone, or innervation.*[7,8,13]
- Ask client about urgency (more than just normal desire to void). *Urgency (also called overactive bladder [OAB]) is a sudden, compelling need to void that is difficult to defer, can occur frequently (e.g., eight or more times in 24 hr), and may be accompanied by leaking or urge incontinence.*[6–8,13]
- Note factors that may affect ability to respond to urge to void in timely manner. *Impaired mobility, use of sedation, or cognitive impairments may result in client failing to recognize need to void or moving too slowly to make it to the bathroom, with subsequent loss of urine.*
- Determine use or presence of bladder irritants. *A significant intake of alcohol, caffeine, acidic or spicy food, and fluids can result in increased output or urge symptoms and can contribute to the possibility of incontinence.*[5]
- Review client's medications for affect on bladder function, such as beta blockers and cholinergic drugs *(can increase detrusor tone)*; neuroleptics, antidepressants, sedatives, and opiates *(can cause detrusor relaxation)*; muscle relaxants and psychoactive drugs *(can cause sphincter relaxation)*; and diuretics *(can increase urine production).*[15]
- Assess for cloudy, odorous urine associated with acute, painful urgency symptoms. *Incontinence often reflects presence of infection.*[1]
- Test urine for glucose. *Presence of glucose in urine causes polyuria, resulting in overdistention of the bladder and inability to hold urine until reaching the bathroom.*[2]
- Assist with appropriate diagnostic testing (e.g., pre/postvoid bladder scanning; pelvic examination *for strictures, impaired perineal sensation or musculature*; urinalysis, uroflowmetry voiding pressures; cystoscopy, cystometrogram) *to determine anatomic and functional status of bladder and urethra.*[2,3,8]
- Assess for concomitant stress or functional incontinence. *Older women often have a mix of stress and urge incontinence, whereas individuals with dementia or disabling neurological disorders tend to have urge and functional incontinence.* (Refer to NDs stress/functional urinary Incontinence for additional interventions.)

NURSING PRIORITY NO. 2   To assess degree of interference/disability:

- Measure amount of urine voided, especially noting amounts less than 100 mL or greater than 550 mL. *Bladder capacity may be impaired, or bladder contractions facilitating emptying may be ineffective.* (Refer to ND [acute/chronic] Urinary Retention.)
- Record frequency of voiding during a typical day and typical night. *Maintaining a voiding diary identifies degree of difficulty being experienced by client.*[2,4]
- Note length of warning time between initial urge and loss of urine. *Overactivity or irritability shortens the length of time between urge and urine loss and helps clarify the type of incontinence.*
- Ascertain if client experiences triggers (e.g., sound of running water, putting hands in water, seeing a restroom sign, "key-in-the lock" syndrome).[8]
- Ascertain effect on lifestyle including daily activities, sleep, socialization, sexuality, and self-esteem. *There is a considerable impact on the quality of life of individuals with an incontinence problem, affecting socialization and view of themselves as sexual beings and sense of self-esteem.*[2]

NURSING PRIORITY NO. 3   To assist in treating/preventing incontinence:

- Implement continence management interventions:
  Establish voiding schedule (habit and bladder training) based on client's usual voiding pattern. *Bladder retraining program is often successful in the control of urge incontinence. Note: One review of multiple studies revealed a strongly positive effect on continence using a combination of behavioral interventions*

 Acute Care   Collaborative   Community/ Home Care   Cultural

(including pelvic muscle exercises) and medications in older women. However, it appears that clients have difficulty sustaining the effort of behavioral modification, and thus the positive effect is lost.[1,4,9,14]

Recommend consciously delaying voiding by using distraction (e.g., slow, deep breathing), self-statements (e.g., "I can wait"), and contracting pelvic muscles when exposed to triggers. *Behavioral techniques for urge suppression.*[2,9]

 Combine pelvic floor strengthening exercise with biofeedback, as appropriate. *Enhances effectiveness of training and success at controlling incontinence.*[4,9]

Instruct client to tighten pelvic floor muscles before arising from bed. *Helps prevent loss of urine as abdominal pressure changes.*[4,13]

Set alarm to awaken during night, if indicated. *May be useful in maintaining continence during training schedule.*[4]

Manage fluid intake (e.g., increase fluid intake to 1,500 to 2,000 mL/d or as indicated) *to prevent dehydration and promote good urine flow*[4] *(e.g., reduce fluid intake if indicated). Note: Too much water can also increase bladder irritation, so amount of intake needs to be determined by individual response.*[12]

Regulate liquid intake at prescheduled times, and limit fluids 2 to 3 hr prior to bedtime. *Promotes a predictable voiding pattern and can help limit nocturia.*

Modify diet, as indicated (e.g., reduce acidic/citrus juices, chocolate and caffeine-containing drinks, carbonated beverages, spicy foods, artificial sweeteners), *to reduce bladder irritants.*[12]

Suggest limiting intake of coffee, tea, and alcohol *to reduce diuretic effect, urge symptoms, and nighttime incontinence.*[12]

Manage bowel elimination *to prevent continence problems associated with constipation or fecal impaction.*

- Offer assistance to cognitively impaired client (e.g., prompt client or take to bathroom on regularly timed schedule) *to reduce frequency of incontinence episodes and promote comfort.*

- Provide assistance or devices, as indicated, for clients who are mobility impaired. *Providing means of summoning assistance and placing bedside commode, urinal, or bedpan within reach helps to avoid unintended loss of urine and promotes sense of control over situation.*[4]

- Collaborate in treating underlying cause. *Urgency symptoms may resolve with treatment of medical problem (e.g., infection; recovery from surgery, childbirth, or pelvic trauma) or may be resistant to resolution (e.g., incontinence associated with neurogenic bladder).*

- Refer to specialist or treatment program, as indicated, for additional or specialized interventions (e.g., biofeedback, use of vaginal cones, electronic stimulation therapy). *Significant reduction in incontinence episodes is reported with use of combined therapies (e.g., electronic stimulation therapy plus pelvic muscle exercises).*[12–14]

- 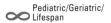 Administer medications (e.g., antibiotics, antimuscarinics [oxybutynin (Ditropan), tolterodine (Detrol), solifenacin (VESIcare)]) *to reduce incidence of UTIs and reduce voiding frequency and urgency by blocking overactive detrusor contractions.*[6,10,13]

- Discuss possible surgical interventions. *Urinary incontinence surgery includes a variety of procedures, from minimally invasive injections of bulking agents to major surgical interventions to change position of or enlarge the bladder, add support to weakened pelvic muscles, replace the urinary sphincter, or implant a sacral nerve stimulator that acts as a bladder pacemaker.*[2,11,13]

NURSING PRIORITY NO. 4 To promote wellness (Teaching/Discharge Considerations):

- Provide information to client/significant others (SOs) about potential for urge incontinence (also called overactive bladder [OAB]) and lifestyle measures to prevent or limit incontinence.

- Encourage comfort measures (e.g., use of incontinence pads or adult briefs, wearing loose-fitting or especially adapted clothing) *to prepare for or manage urge incontinence symptoms over the long term as well as to enhance sense of security and confidence in abilities to be socially active.*[5]

- Emphasize importance of perineal care after each voiding. *Prevents skin irritation and reduces potential for bladder infection and incontinence-related dermatitis.*[5]

 Diagnostic Studies   Evidence Based Practice   Medications Pediatric/Geriatric/ Lifespan

• Identify signs/symptoms indicating urinary complications and need for medical follow-up care. *Helps client be aware of and seek intervention in a timely manner to prevent more serious problems from developing.*[4]

DOCUMENTATION FOCUS

Assessment/Reassessment
• Individual findings, including pattern of incontinence, effect on lifestyle and self-esteem.

Planning
• Plan of care, specific interventions, and who is involved in planning.
• Teaching plan.

Implementation/Evaluation
• Response to interventions, teaching, and actions performed.
• Attainment or progress toward desired outcome(s).
• Modifications to plan of care.

Discharge Planning
• Discharge needs and who is responsible for actions to be taken.
• Specific referrals made.

References

1. Wyman, J. F. (2003). Treatment of urinary incontinence in men and older women: The evidence shows the efficacy of a variety of techniques. *Am J Nurs*, 103(Suppl), 26–35.
2. Booth, C. (2002). Introduction to urinary incontinence. *Hosp Pharmacist*, 9(3), 65–68.
3. Beers, M. H., Berkow, R. (eds). (1999). *The Merck Manual of Diagnosis and Therapy*. 17th ed. Whitehouse Station, NJ: Merck Research Laboratories.
4. Newman, D. K., Palmer, M. H. (eds). (2003). The state of the science on urinary incontinence. *Am J Nurs*, 103(3 Suppl), 2–53.
5. Newfield, S. A., et al. (2007). ND: Urinary incontinence. *Cox's Clinical Applications of Nursing Diagnosis: Adult, Child, Women's, Psychiatric, Geronatic, and Home Health Considerations*. 5th ed. Philadelphia: F. A. Davis.
6. Gray, M. (2005). Assessment and management of urinary incontinence. *Nurse Pract*, 30(7), 32–43.
7. Gray, M. (2005). Overactive bladder: An overview. *J Wound Ostomy Continence Nurs*, 32(3 Suppl), 1–5.
8. Newman, D. K. (2005). Assessment of the patient with an overactive bladder. *J Wound Ostomy Continence Nurs*, 32(3 Suppl), 5–10.
9. Wyman, J. F. (2005). Behavioral interventions for the patient with overactive bladder. *J Wound Ostomy Continence Nurs*, 32(3 Suppl), 11–15.
10. Mauk, K. L. (2005). Pharmacology update: Medications for bladder management. *ARN Network*, 21(3), 3–10.
11. NHS. (Reviewed 2016). Urinary incontinence: Surgery and procedures. Retrieved March 2018 from https://www.nhs.uk/conditions/urinary-incontinence/surgery/#surgery-and-procedures-for-stress-incontinence.
12. Stoppler, M. C. (Last reviewed 2017). Urinary incontinence. Retrieved March 2018 from http://www.emedicinehealth.com/incontinence/article_em.htm.
13. Bergman, S. (Updated 2016). Urge Incontinence (various pages). Retrieved March 2018 from http://www.webmd.com/urinary-incontinence-oab/america-asks-11/urge?page=1.
14. Burgio, K. L., Locher, J. L., Goode, P. S. (2000). Combined behavioral and drug therapy for urge incontinence in older women. *Obstet Gynecol Surv*, 55(8), 485–486.
15. Cleveland Clinic Staff. (2014). Are your medications causing or increasing incontinence? Retrieved March 2018 from https://health.clevelandclinic.org/are-your-medications-causing-or-increasing-incontinence/.

 Acute Care Collaborative Community/ Home Care Cultural

risk for Infection

Taxonomy II: Safety/Protection—Class 1 Infection (00004) [**Diagnostic Division:** Safety], Submitted 1986; Revised 1986, 2013, 2017

DEFINITION: Susceptible to invasion and multiplication of pathogenic organisms, which may compromise health.

RISK FACTORS

Alteration in skin integrity; stasis of body fluid
Inadequate vaccination
Insufficient knowledge to avoid exposure to pathogens
Malnutrition; obesity
Smoking
At Risk Population: Exposure to disease outbreak
Associated Condition: Alteration in pH of secretions; decrease in ciliary action; decrease in hemoglobin; leukopenia
Chronic illness; immunosuppression; suppressed inflammatory response
Invasive procedure
Sample Clinical Applications: Immune suppressed conditions (e.g., HIV positive, AIDS, cancer), chronic obstructive pulmonary disease (COPD), long-term use of steroids (e.g., asthma, rheumatoid arthritis, systemic lupus erythematosus [SLE]), diabetes mellitus, malnutrition, surgical or invasive procedures, substance abuse, burns, pregnancy/preterm labor

DESIRED OUTCOMES/EVALUATION CRITERIA

Sample **NOC** linkages:
Knowledge: Infection Management: Extent of understanding conveyed about infection, its treatment, and the prevention of disease progression and complications
Risk Control: Personal actions to understand, prevent, eliminate, or reduce modifiable health threats
Infection Severity: Severity of signs and symptoms of infection

Client Will (Include Specific Time Frame)
• Verbalize understanding of individual causative or risk factor(s).
• Identify interventions to prevent or reduce risk of infection.
• Demonstrate techniques and lifestyle changes to promote safe environment.
• Achieve timely wound healing, be free of purulent drainage or erythema, and be afebrile.

ACTIONS/INTERVENTIONS

Sample **NIC** linkages:
Infection Protection: Prevention and early detection of infection in a patient at risk
Infection Control: Minimizing the acquisition and transmission of infectious agents
Surveillance: Purposeful and ongoing acquisition, interpretation, and synthesis of patient data for clinical decision making

NURSING PRIORITY NO. 1   To determine risk/contributing factors:

- Assess for presence of host-specific factors that affect immunity:[1,7–9]

  Extremes of age: *Newborns and the elderly are more susceptible to disease and infection than the general population. Studies reported by the Centers for Disease Control and Prevention (CDC) in 2015 showed that between 1 and 3 million infections occur annually in nursing homes and assisted living facilities.*[1,18]

  Presence of underlying disease: *Client may have disease that directly impacts immune system (e.g., cancer, AIDS, autoimmune disorder) or may be weakened by prolonged disease conditions (e.g., diabetes, kidney disease, heart failure) or treatments.*

  Certain treatment settings/modalities: *Client in acute/critical-care setting and/or on mechanical ventilation may have a prolonged exposure to risk factors for infection, including problems with breathing and circulation, GI motility disorders, and use of analgesics and sedatives, causing a higher rate of acquired infections. Note: The National and State Healthcare-Associated Infections Progress Report (2015) to the CDC reported progress in prevention of some healthcare-associated infections. For example, catheter-associated urinary tract infection (CAUTI) (decreased by 43% between 2014 and 2015. However, in that same time frame, central line–associated bloodstream infections (CLABSI) increased over 21%.*[17,20]

  Lifestyle: *Personal habits or living situations, such as persons sharing close quarters and/or equipment (e.g., college dorm, group home, long-term care facility, day care, correctional facility); persons/groups with inadequate vaccination protection; and IV drug use, shared needles, and unprotected sex can increase susceptibility to infections.*

  Nutritional status: *Malnutrition weakens the immune system; elevated serum glucose levels (e.g., administration of total parenteral nutrition or poorly controlled diabetes mellitus) provide growth media for pathogens.*

  Trauma: *Loss of skin or mucous membrane integrity or invasive surgical or diagnostic procedures; premature rupture of amniotic membranes; urinary catheterizations; and parenteral injection, sharps, and needlesticks are common paths of pathogen entry.*

  Certain medications: *Steroids and chemotherapeutic agents directly affect the immune system. Long-term or improper antibiotic treatment can disrupt body's normal flora and result in increased susceptibility to antibiotic-resistant organisms.*

  Presence or absence of immunity: *Natural immunity may be acquired as a result of development of antibodies to a specific agent following infection, preventing recurrence of specific disease (e.g., chicken pox). Active immunization (via vaccination; e.g., measles, polio) and passive immunization (e.g., antitoxin or immunoglobulin administration) can prevent certain communicable diseases.*

  Environmental exposure: *May be accidental or intentional. Exposure can occur in different ways, such as use of specific microorganisms (in laboratories, biotechnological industries, acts of bioterrorism). Accidental exposure can result from exposure to contaminants arising from commonplace processes (e.g., waste water recycling) or through animal contact (e.g., agriculture, animal food processing) and through contact with humans (e.g., healthcare, education, mass transit, close contact living, etc.).*[21]

- Observe skin/tissues surrounding injuries (e.g., knife cuts, toe injuries, insect or animal bites); also inspect insertion sites of invasive lines, sutures, surgical incisions, and wounds. *Redness, warmth, swelling, pain, and red streaks are signs of developing localized infection that may have systemic implications if treatment is delayed.*[4,5,9,12]

- Assess and document skin conditions around insertions of orthopedic pins, wires, and tongs. *Direct connection to bone increases the risk of infections in bone sites that can lead to osteomyelitis, bone loss, and long-term delays of healing.*[4,5,9,12]

- Review laboratory values (e.g., white blood cell count and differential, blood, urine, sputum, or wound cultures) *to identify presence of pathogens and treatment options.*

- Refer to NDs risk for Aspiration, risk for Contamination, risk for urinary tract Injury, risk for impaired Oral Mucous Membranes, and risk for impaired Skin or Tissue Integrity for related assessments and interventions.

 Acute Care   Collaborative   Community/Home Care   Cultural

NURSING PRIORITY NO. 2 To reduce/correct existing risk factors:

Healthcare environment

- Practice and emphasize constant and proper hand-washing techniques (using antibacterial soap and running water) before and after all care contacts and after contact with items likely to be contaminated. Wear gloves where appropriate to minimize contamination of hands and discard after each client. Wash hands after glove removal. Instruct client/significant others (SOs)/visitors to wash hands, as indicated. *This is a first-line defense against healthcare-associated infections (HAIs).*[1,10]
- Provide a clean, well-ventilated environment (may require turning off central air-conditioning and opening window for good ventilation, room with negative air pressure, etc.).
- Post visual alerts in healthcare settings instructing clients/SOs to inform healthcare providers if they have symptoms of respiratory infections or influenza-like symptoms. *Can limit or prevent transmission to and from client and may reveal additional cases.*[1,3,6,7,10]
- Monitor client's visitors/caregivers for respiratory illnesses. Offer masks and tissues to client/visitors who are coughing or sneezing *to limit exposures and reduce cross-contamination.*[1]
- Encourage parents of sick children to keep them away from childcare settings and school until afebrile for 24 hr.
- Provide for isolation as indicated (e.g., contact, droplet, and airborne precautions). Educate staff in infection-control procedures. *Reduces risk of cross-contamination.*[1,13]
- Emphasize proper use of personal protective equipment by staff/visitors as dictated by agency policy *for particular exposure risk (e.g., airborne, droplet, splash risk), including mask or respiratory filter of appropriate particulate regulator, gowns, aprons, head covers, face shields, and protective eyewear.*[1,3,8]
- Include information in preoperative teaching about ways *to reduce potential for postoperative infection (e.g., respiratory measures to prevent pneumonia, wound or dressing care, avoidance of others with infection).*[4,14]
- Encourage early ambulation, deep breathing, coughing, position changes, and early removal of endotracheal and/or nasal or oral feeding tubes *for mobilization of respiratory secretions and prevention of aspiration and respiratory infections.*[10,11]
- Monitor and assist with use of adjuncts (e.g., respiratory aids such as incentive spirometry) *to prevent pneumonia.*[10,11]
- Maintain adequate hydration and electrolyte balance *to prevent imbalances that would predispose to infection.*
- Provide or encourage balanced diet, emphasizing proteins to feed the immune system. *Immune function is affected by protein intake; the balance between omega-6 and omega-3 fatty acid intake; and adequate amounts of vitamins A, C, and E and the minerals zinc and iron. A deficiency of these nutrients puts the client at an increased risk of infection.*
- Handle and properly package tissue and fluid specimens.[1,2]
- Administer prophylactic antibiotics and immunizations as indicated.
- Assist with medical procedures (e.g., wound or joint aspiration, incision and drainage of abscess, bronchoscopy) as indicated.
- Administer and monitor medication regimen (e.g., antimicrobials, drip infusion into osteomyelitis, subeschar clysis, topical antibiotics) and note client's response *to determine effectiveness of therapy and presence of side effects.*

Medical devices

- Maintain sterile technique for invasive procedures (e.g., IV, urinary catheter, tracheostomy care, pulmonary suctioning).[1,2]
- Use disposable equipment whenever possible. Disinfect or sterilize reusable equipment and surfaces according to manufacturer recommendations.[1-3]
- Dispose of needles and sharps in approved containers *to reduce risk of needlestick or sharps injury.*[1,3]
- Choose proper vascular access device based on anticipated treatment duration and solution or medication to be infused and best available aseptic insertion techniques; cleanse incisions and insertion sites daily/per facility protocol with appropriate solution *to reduce potential for catheter-related bloodstream infections.*[12]

   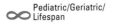

- Maintain appropriate hang times for parenteral solutions (IVs, additives, nutritional solutions) *to reduce opportunity for contamination and bacterial growth.*
- 🅐 📋 Assist with monitoring client on ventilator for signs of bacterial infections and wean from mechanical ventilator as soon as possible *to reduce risk of ventilator-associated pneumonia.*[13]
- Fill bubbling humidifiers or nebulizers with sterile water—not distilled or tap water. Use heat and moisture exchangers instead of a heated humidifier with mechanical ventilator.[11,13]

Skin/Tissues

- Change surgical or other wound dressings as needed or indicated, using proper technique for changing and disposing of contaminated materials.[1,3,4,14,19]
- 📋 Cleanse incisions and insertion sites as indicated with appropriate antimicrobial topical or solution *to prevent growth of bacteria.*[4,19]
- Separate touching surfaces of excoriated skin (e.g., in herpes zoster, burns, weeping dermatitis) and apply appropriate skin barriers. Use gloves when caring for open lesions *to minimize autoinoculation or transmission of viral diseases.*[4]
- 📋 Perform or instruct in daily mouth care. Include use of antiseptic mouthwash for individuals in acute or long-term care settings *at high risk for healthcare-associated infections, especially in client on a ventilator.*[13,22]
- Provide regular urinary catheter and perineal care when client requires assistance with these actions. *Reduces risk of ascending urinary tract infection.*
- Cover perineal and pelvic region dressings or casts with plastic when using bedpan *to prevent contamination when wound is in perineal or pelvic region.*
- 📋 Discuss routine or preoperative antiseptic body shower or scrubs when indicated (e.g., orthopedic, plastic surgery) *to reduce bacterial colonization.*[10,19]

Community

- Recommend individuals/staff isolate self at home when ill *to prevent spread of infection to others, including coworkers.*[1,6]
- Alert infection control officer/proper authorities to presence of specific infectious agents and number of cases as required. *Provides for case finding and helps curtail outbreak.*[6,16]
- Group/cohort individuals with same diagnosis or exposure as resources require. *Limited resources (as may occur with an outbreak or epidemic) may dictate a wardlike environment, but need for regular precautions to control spread of infection still exists.*[6]
- 🅐 Encourage contacting healthcare provider for prophylactic therapy as indicated following exposure to individuals with infectious disease (e.g., tuberculosis, hepatitis, influenza).

NURSING PRIORITY NO. 3   To promote wellness (Teaching/Discharge Considerations):

- 🏠 Review individual nutritional needs, appropriate exercise program, and need for rest *to enhance immune system function and healing.*[5,6]
- Instruct client/SO(s) in techniques to protect the integrity of skin, care for lesions, temperature measurement, and prevention of spread of infection in the home setting. *Provides basic knowledge for self-help and self-protection.*[2,5]
- 💊 Emphasize necessity of taking medications such as antivirals or antibiotics as directed (e.g., dosage and length of therapy). *Premature discontinuation of treatment when client begins to feel well may result in return of infection and potentiate drug-resistant strains.*[15]
- 💊 Discuss importance of not taking antibiotics prescribed for another person or using "leftover" drugs unless specifically instructed by healthcare provider. *Inappropriate use can lead to development of drug-resistant strains or secondary infections.*[5]
- 🅐 Discuss the role of smoking and secondhand smoke in respiratory infections and in postoperative healing. Refer to smoking cessation programs as indicated.[19]
- Promote safer-sex practices and reporting sexual contacts of infected individuals *to prevent the spread of HIV or other sexually transmitted infections.*[1,5,15]

 Acute Care   Collaborative   Community/Home Care   Cultural

- Encourage high-risk persons, including healthcare workers, to have influenza and pneumonia vaccinations *to reduce individual risk as well as help prevent spread of flu and viral pneumonias to others.*[1,6,16]
- Promote childhood immunization program. Encourage adults to update immunizations as appropriate.[7]
- Discuss precautions with client engaged in international travel and refer for immunizations *to reduce incidence and transmission of global infections.*[8]
- Review use of prophylactic antibiotics if appropriate *(e.g., before dental work for clients with history of rheumatic fever, heart valve replacements).*[5]
- Identify resources available to the individual (e.g., substance abuse or rehabilitation, needle-exchange program as appropriate; available or free condoms).
- Provide information and involve in appropriate community and national education programs *to increase awareness of and prevention of communicable diseases.*[1,5,6]
- Refer to NDs ineffective Health Maintenance and impaired Home Maintenance for additional interventions as appropriate.

DOCUMENTATION FOCUS

Assessment/Reassessment
- Individual risk factors that are present, including recent and current antibiotic therapy.
- Wound and/or insertion sites, character of drainage or body secretions.
- Signs/symptoms of infectious process.

Planning
- Plan of care, specific interventions, and who is involved in planning.
- Teaching plan.

Implementation/Evaluation
- Responses to interventions, teaching, and actions performed.
- Attainment or progress toward desired outcome(s).
- Modifications to plan of care.

Discharge Planning
- Discharge needs and who is responsible for actions to be taken.
- Specific referrals made.

References

1. Swan, J., McDonald, M. (2012, updated 2018). Infection control. Retrieved March 2018 from https://wildirismedical education.com/courses/infection-control-training.
2. Friedman, M. M. (2002). Improving infection control in home care: From ritual to science-based practice. *Home Healthc Nurse*, 18(2), 99–106.
3. World Health Organization. (No date). Hospital hygiene and infection control. Retrieved March 2018 from www.who.int/ water_sanitation_health/medicalwaste/148to158.pdf.
4. Thompson, J. (2000). A practical guide to wound care. *RN*, 63(1), 48–52.
5. Androwich, I., Burkhart, L., Gettrust, K. V. (1996). *Community and Home Health Nursing.* Albany, NY: Delmar.
6. Doenges, M. E., Moorhouse, M. F., Murr, A. C. (2010). Care plan: Disaster considerations; and ND infection, risk for, in numerous care plans. *Nursing Care Plans: Guidelines for Individualizing Client Care Across the Life Span.* 8th ed. Philadelphia: F. A. Davis.
7. Goldrick, B. A., Goetz, A. M. (2006). 'Tis the season for influenza. *Nurse Pract*, 31(12), 24–33.
8. Hunter, A., Denman-Vitale, S., Garzon, L. (2007). Global infections: Recognition, management, and prevention. *Nurse Pract*, 32(2), 34–41.
9. Romero, D. V., Treston, J., O'Sullivan, A. L. (2006). Hand-to-hand combat: Preventing MRSA infection. *Adv Wound Care*, 19(6), 328–333.
10. Houghton, D. (2006). HAI prevention: The power is in your hands. *Nurs Manage*, 37(5 Suppl), 1–7.
11. Lorente, L., et al. (2006). Ventilator-associated pneumonia using a heated humidifier or a heat and moisture exchanger: A randomized controlled trial. *Crit Care*, 10(4), R116.
12. Rosenthal, K. (2006). Guarding against vascular site infection. *Nurs Manage*, 37(4), 54–66.
13. Klompas, M., et al. (2015). The preventability of ventilator-associated events. The CDC prevention epicenters wake up and breathe collaborative. *Am J Respir Crit Care Med*, 191(3), 292–301.

 Diagnostic Studies   Evidence Based Practice   Medications   Pediatric/Geriatric/Lifespan

14. Odom-Forren, J. (2006). Preventing surgical site infections. *Nursing*, 36(6), 59–63.
15. Kirton, C. (2005). The HIV/AIDS epidemic: A case of good news/bad news. *Nursing Made Incredibly Easy!*, 3(2), 28–40.
16. Lashley, F. R. (2006). Emerging infectious diseases at the beginning of the 21st century. *Online J Issues Nurs*, 11(1). Retrieved March 2018 from http://www.medscape.com/viewarticle/528306.
17. Nseir, S., et al. (2010). Intensive care unit–acquired infection as a side effect of sedation. *Crit Care*, 14(2), R30.
18. Centers for Disease Control and Prevention: National Healthcare Safety Network. (Updated 2015, last reviewed 2017). Tracking infections in long-term care facilities. Retrieved March 2018 from https://www.cdc.gov/longtermcare/index.html.
19. Alexander, J. W., Solomkin, J. S., Edwards, M. J. (2011). Updated recommendations for control of surgical site infections. *Ann Surg*, 253(6), 1082–1093.
20. Centers for Disease Control and Prevention (CDC). (2013, updated 2018). National 2015 standardized infection ratios (SIRs) calculated using historical baselines). *CDC's Healthcare-associated infections*. Retrieved March 2018 from https://www.cdc.gov/hai/surveillance/data-reports/2015-SIR-report.html.
21. Haagmus, J. A., Tariq, D. J., Heederik, D. J. (2012). Infectious disease risks associated with occupational exposure: A systematic review of the literature. *Occup Environ Med*, 69(2), 140–146.
22. Booker, S., et al. (2013). Mouth care to reduce ventilator-associated pneumonia. *Am J Nurs*, 113(10), 24–30.

risk for Injury

Taxonomy II: Safety/Protection—Class 2 Physical Injury (00035) [**Diagnostic Division:** Safety], Approved 1978, Revised 2013; 2017

DEFINITION: Susceptible to physical damage due to environmental conditions interacting with the individual's adaptive and defensive resources, which may compromise health.

RISK FACTORS

Compromised nutritional source; malnutrition
Exposure to pathogen or toxic chemical; nosocomial agent
Immunization level within community
Insufficient knowledge of modifiable factors
Physical barrier
Unsafe mode of transport
At Risk Population: Extremes of age
Impaired primary defense mechanisms
Associated Condition: Abnormal blood profile; tissue hypoxia
Alteration in cognitive or psychomotor functioning
Alteration in sensation; effector or sensory integration dysfunction
Autoimmune or immune dysfunction; biochemical dysfunction
Sample Clinical Applications: Burns, seizure disorder, dementia, AIDS, influenza, cataracts, glaucoma, Parkinson's disease, substance abuse, malnutrition, developmental delay, para/quadraplegia, neuropathy.
[Note: In reviewing this ND, it is apparent there is much overlap with other diagnoses. We have chosen to present generalized interventions. Although there are commonalities to injury situations, we suggest that the reader refer to other primary diagnoses as indicated, such as risk for Bleeding; risk for acute Confusion; chronic Confusion; risk for Contamination; risk for Falls; ineffective Health Maintenance; impaired Home Maintenance; risk for Infection; impaired physical Mobility; impaired/risk for impaired Parenting; ineffective Protection; risk for Poisoning; impaired/risk for impaired Skin/Tissue Integrity; Rape-Trauma Syndrome; risk for Pressure Ulcer; ineffective Tissue Perfusion [specify]; risk for Trauma; risk for self and other-directed Violence; Wandering for additional interventions.]

 Acute Care   Collaborative   Community/Home Care   Cultural

DESIRED OUTCOMES/EVALUATION CRITERIA

Sample NOC linkage:
Physical Injury Severity: Severity of signs and symptoms of injuries to the body

Client Will (Include Specific Time Frame)
• Be free of injury.

Sample NOC linkages:
Personal Safety Behavior: Personal actions to prevent unintentional physical injury to self
Risk Control [specify]: Personal actions to understand, prevent, eliminate, or reduce modifiable health threats [e.g., alcohol/drug use, altered visual function, sun exposure]

Client/Caregivers Will (Include Specific Time Frame)
• Verbalize understanding of individual factors that contribute to possibility of injury.
• Demonstrate behaviors, lifestyle changes to reduce risk factors and protect self from injury.
• Modify environment as indicated to enhance safety.

ACTIONS/INTERVENTIONS

Sample NIC linkages:
Surveillance: Purposeful and ongoing acquisition, interpretation, and synthesis of patient data for clinical decision making
Risk Identification: Analysis of potential risk factors, determination of health risks, and prioritization of risk reduction strategies for an individual or group
Environmental Management: Safety: Monitoring and manipulation of the physical environment to promote safety

NURSING PRIORITY NO. 1 To evaluate degree/source of risk inherent in the individual situation:

• Identify client at risk (e.g., acute illness, surgery, trauma; chronic illness conditions with weakness, immunosuppression, abnormal blood profiles, or prolonged immobility; acute or chronic confusion, dementia, head injury; use of multiple medications; use of alcohol or other drugs; mental illness, emotional liability; cultural, familial, and socioeconomic factors adversely affecting lifestyle and home; exposure to environmental chemicals or other hazards).
• ⊞📝 Perform thorough assessments regarding safety issues when planning for client care and discharge. *Failure to accurately assess and intervene or refer regarding these issues can place the client at needless risk and creates negligence issues for the healthcare practitioner. Note: Research has identified 34 safe practices that evidence shows can work to reduce or prevent adverse events and medical errors regarding client safety, including (and not limited to) adequate numbers of nursing personnel; ensuring that written documentation of the client's preference for life-sustaining treatments is prominently displayed in chart; evaluating each person upon admission, and regularly thereafter, for the risk of developing pressure ulcers; employing clinically appropriate strategies to prevent malnutrition; vaccinating healthcare workers against influenza to protect both them and clients; and standardizing methods for labeling, packaging, and storing medications.*[14]
• ∞📝 Note age, developmental stage, and gender. *Children, young adults, elderly persons, and men are at greater risk for injury, which may reflect client's ability or desire to protect self and influences choice of interventions or teaching.*[15,16]

 Diagnostic Studies
 Evidence Based Practice
 Medications
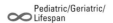 Pediatric/Geriatric/Lifespan

- Evaluate developmental level, decision-making ability, level of cognition, competence, and independence. *Determines client's/significant other's (SO's) ability to attend to safety issues.*
- Assess mood, coping abilities, and personality styles (i.e., temperament, aggression, impulsive behavior, level of self-esteem). *May result in carelessness or increased risk-taking without consideration of consequences.*[1,2]
- Evaluate individual's emotional and behavioral response to violence in surroundings (e.g., neighborhood, television, peer group). *May affect client's view of and regard for own or others' safety.*[1,2,15]
- ∞ Assess muscle strength and gross and fine motor coordination *to identify risk for falls. Note: The frequency of falls increases with age and frailty level. Risk factors for falls lie in four categories: (1) biological, (2) behavioral, (3) environmental, and (4) socioeconomic. In each of these areas, some risk factors can be modified to decrease fall risk. Protective factors for falls in older age are related to behavioral change and environmental modification.*[17]
- Observe client for signs of injury and ascertain age of injury (e.g., old or new bruises, history of fractures, frequent absences from school or work). Determine potential for abusive behavior by intimate partner/family members/peers. *Client or care providers may require further evaluation or investigation for abuse; prevention strategies may be indicated.*[5,7]
- Ascertain knowledge of safety needs and injury prevention and motivation to prevent injury in home, community, and work settings. *Information may reveal areas of misinformation, lack of knowledge, and need for teaching.*[6]
- Note socioeconomic status and availability and use of resources.

NURSING PRIORITY NO. 2   To assist client/caregiver to reduce or correct individual risk factors:

- Provide healthcare within a culture of safety (e.g., adherence to nursing standards of care and facility safe-care policies) *to prevent errors resulting in client injury, to promote client safety, and to model safety behaviors for client/SO. Note: A culture of safety encompasses the following elements: shared beliefs and values about the healthcare delivery system; recruitment and training with patient safety in mind; organizational commitment to detecting and analyzing patient injuries and near misses; open communication regarding patient injury results, both within and outside the organization; and the establishment of a just culture.*[14]

    Practice hand hygiene at all times and device safety when client has IV lines and catheters *to prevent healthcare-associated infections and potential for bloodborne pathogens.*

    Administer medications and infusions using the "6 rights" system (right client, right medication, right route, right dose, right time, right documentation).[8]

    Inform and educate client/SO regarding all treatments and medications.

    Adhere to measures to prevent blood clots, especially in client with abnormal blood profile, surgical procedures, or immobility.

    Monitor environment for potentially unsafe conditions or hazards, modify as needed.

    ∞ Prevent falls:[6,9]

    Orient or reorient client to environment, as needed.

    Place confused elderly client or young child near nurses' station *to provide for frequent observation.*

    Instruct client/SO to request assistance, as needed; make sure call light is within reach and client knows how to operate.

    Utilize bed/chair alarms *that alert when client is trying to get up alone.*

    Maintain bed or chair in lowest position with wheels locked. Provide covered cribs for enclosed bed or wall bed on floor, where indicated.

    Provide seat raisers for chairs and use stand-assist, repositioning, or lifting devices as indicated *to prevent injury to both client and care providers.*

    Ensure that all floors are clear of tripping hazards and that pathway to bathroom is unobstructed and properly lighted.

    Place assistive devices (e.g., walker, cane, glasses, hearing aid) within reach and ascertain that client is using them appropriately.

    Safety-lock exit and stairwell doors *when client can wander away.*

 Acute Care   Collaborative   Community/ Home Care   Cultural

- Avoid use of restraints as much as possible when client is confused. *Restraints can increase client's agitation and risk of entrapment and death.*
- Provide client/SO information regarding client's specific disease or condition and consequences of continuing unhealthy behaviors (e.g., increase in oral cancer among teenagers using smokeless tobacco; fetal alcohol syndrome or neonatal addiction in prenatal women using tobacco, alcohol, or other drugs) *to enhance decision making and clarify expectations and individual needs.*
- Review consequences of previously determined risk factors that client is reluctant to modify. *Many consequences could occur, such as oral cancer in teenager using smokeless tobacco; occurrence of spontaneous abortion, fetal alcohol syndrome, or neonatal addiction in prenatal woman using drugs; fall related to failure to use assistive equipment; toddler getting into medicine cabinet; binge drinking while skiing; health and legal implications of illicit drug use; and working too many hours for safe operation of machinery or vehicles.*
- Determine if risk-prone behavior is occurring or likely to occur *to initiate appropriate wellness counseling and referrals.*
- Review client's history of immunization and understanding of the importance of immunization to self/family. Refer to ND readiness for enhanced Health Management *to determine changes or adaptations that may be desired/required.*
- Review client's level of physical activity in his or her lifestyle *to determine changes or adaptations that may be required by current situation.*
- Refer to physical or occupational therapist as appropriate *to identify high-risk tasks; conduct site visits; select, create, and modify equipment or assistive devices; and provide education about body mechanics and musculoskeletal injuries in addition to providing therapies as indicated.*[6]
- Perform home assessment and recommend actions (or take steps) to correct unsafe conditions, such as:[1–4,8,9,13,14]

  locking up medications and poisonous substances;

  using window grates or locks and safety gates at top and bottom of stairs *to prevent young children from falling;*

  installing handrails on stairs/steps, ramps, and bathtub safety products (e.g., grab bars/handles, nonskid mats or stickers);

  using electrical outlet covers or lockouts;

  locking exterior doors *to prevent confused individual from wandering off while SO is engaged in other household activities;*

  removing matches, smoking materials, and knobs from the stove *so young children or confused individuals do not turn on burner and leave it unattended;*

  properly placing lights, alarms (e.g., fire, carbon monoxide, and intruder), and fire extinguishers;

  discussing safe use of oxygen; and

  obtaining medical alert device or home monitoring service.

- Review specific employment concerns or worksite issues and needs (e.g., ergonomic chairs and workstations, properly fitting safety equipment and footwear, regular use of safety glasses or goggles and ear protectors, safe storage of hazardous substances, number of hours worked per shift/week).
- Demonstrate and encourage use of techniques to reduce or manage stress and vent emotions such as anger and hostility. *Identifying and dealing with emotions appropriately enables individual to maintain control of behavior and avoid possibility of violent outbursts.*[2,5,7]
- Discuss importance of self-monitoring of factors that can contribute to occurrence of injury (e.g., fatigue, anger, irritability). *Client/SO may be able to modify risk through monitoring of actions or postponement of certain actions, especially during times when client is likely to be highly stressed.*
- Encourage participation in self-help programs, such as assertiveness training, anger management, and positive self-image *to enhance self-esteem.*
- Review expectations caregivers have of children, cognitively impaired, and/or elderly family members. Discuss concerns about discipline practices.[13]
- Discuss need for and sources of supervision (e.g., before- and after-school programs, elderly day care).

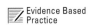 Diagnostic Studies   Evidence Based Practice   Medications   Pediatric/Geriatric/Lifespan

NURSING PRIORITY NO. 3 To promote wellness (Teaching/Discharge Considerations):

- Identify individual needs and resources for safety education (e.g., home hazard information, fall prevention, water safety [including burns or drowning hazards], firearm safety, cardiopulmonary resuscitation/first aid).[3,10,11]
- Emphasize importance of correct use of baby gates, cabinet door locks, child safety seats, car seat belts, bicycle or other helmets, regular use of sports safety equipment, etc.
- Provide instruction or refer to classes for back safety and proper use of injury-prevention devices. Recommend use of ergonomic bed and chair as appropriate.
- Provide telephone numbers and other contact numbers as individually indicated (e.g., doctor, 911, poison control, police, elder advocate).
- Provide bibliotherapy including written resource lists and reliable Web sites *for later review and self-paced learning.*
- Refer to professional resources as indicated (e.g., counseling or psychotherapy, budget counseling, substance recovery, anger management, parenting classes).
- Refer to or assist with community education programs *to increase awareness of safety measures and resources available to the individual. Note: Many evidence-based programs are being implemented nationally to promote safe environments for children, adolescents, and adults. These may include (and are not limited to) education about bullying and Internet safety issues, suicide prevention, use of helmets when riding bicycles or skateboarding, drowning prevention, gun safety, substance abuse, and intimate partner violence and anger management.*[2–5,7,9,11,12]
- Promote community awareness about the problems of the design of buildings, equipment, transportation, and workplace practices that contribute to accidents.[4]
- Identify community resources, neighbors, or friends to assist elderly or handicapped individuals in providing such things as structural maintenance, removal of snow and ice from walks and steps, etc.
- Identify emergency escape plans and routes for home and community *to be prepared in the event of natural or human-caused disaster (e.g., fire, hurricane, earthquake, toxic chemical release).*[4]

DOCUMENTATION FOCUS

Assessment/Reassessment
- Individual risk factors, noting current physical findings (e.g., bruises, cuts).
- Client's/caregiver's understanding of individual risks and safety concerns.
- Availability and use of resources.

Planning
- Plan of care and who is involved in planning.
- Teaching plan.

Implementation/Evaluation
- Individual responses to interventions, teaching, and actions performed.
- Specific actions and changes that are made.
- Attainment or progress toward desired outcome(s).
- Modifications to plan of care.

Discharge Planning
- Long-term plans for discharge needs, lifestyle and community changes, and who is responsible for actions to be taken.
- Specific referrals made.

 Acute Care   Collaborative   Community/Home Care   Cultural

References

1. Gorman-Smith, D., Henry, D. B., Tolan, P. H. (2004). Exposure to community violence and violence perpetration: The protective effects of family functioning. *J Clin Child Psychol*, 33(3), 439–449.

2. Centers for Disease Control and Prevention. (2012, updated 2015). Understanding youth violence. Injury Center: Violence Prevention. Retrieved March 2018 from http://www.cdc.gov/ViolencePrevention/pdf/YV-FactSheet-a.pdf.

3. Emergency Nurses Association. (2012, revised 2013). Firearm safety and injury prevention: Position statement. Retrieved March 2018 from https://www.ena.org/docs/default-source/resource-library/practice-resources/position-statements/firearminjuryprevention.pdf?sfvrsn=95bf0ad8_10.

4. Doenges, M. E., Moorhouse, M. F., Murr, A. C. (2010). Care plan: Disaster considerations; and ND infection, risk for, in numerous care plans. *Nursing Care Plans: Guidelines for Individualizing Client Care Across the Life Span*. 8th ed. Philadelphia: F. A. Davis.

5. Centers for Disease Control and Prevention. (2010, updated 2017). Intimate partner violence. National Center for Injury Prevention and Control. Retrieved March 2018 from http://www.cdc.gov/violenceprevention/pdf/nisvs_report2010-a.pdf.

6. Nelson, A., et al. (2003). Safe patient handling & movement. *Am J Nurs*, 103(3), 32–43.

7. Centers for Disease Control and Prevention. (2016). Stop SV: A technical package to prevent sexual violence. National Center for Injury Prevention and Control. Retrieved March 2018 from https://www.cdc.gov/violenceprevention/pdf/SV-Prevention-Technical-Package.pdf.

8. Gozdan, M. J. (2009). Using technology to reduce medication errors. *Nursing*, 39(6), 57–58.

9. Mayo Clinic Staff. (Updated 2017). Intracranial hematoma (various pages). Retrieved March 2018 from https://www.mayoclinic.org/diseases-conditions/intracranial-hematoma/symptoms-causes/syc-20356145.

10. Lassman, J. (2002). Water safety. *J Emerg Nurs*, 28(3), 241–243.

11. Dolman, M. (2014). Drowning risks in natural water settings. Retrieved March 2018 from https://www.lawyer.com/a/drowning-accidents-in-natural-water-settings.html.

12. Centers for Disease Control and Prevention. (Updated 2017). Preventing suicide. Retrieved March 2018 from http://www.cdc.gov/features/preventingsuicide/.

13. Safety for older consumers' home safety checklist. Consumer Product Safety Commission (CPSC) document no. 701. Retrieved February 2015 from http://www.cpsc.gov/PageFiles/122038/701.pdf.

14. National Quality Forum (NQF). (2010). Safe Practices for Better Health Care—2010 Update. Retrieved March 2018 from www.willjoelfriedman.com/printAndSound/tbSafePractices_20091023_website.pdf.

15. Schwebel, D. C., Barton, B. K. (2005). Contributions of multiple risk factors to child injury. *J Pediatr Psychol*, 30(7), 553–561.

16. Ristolainen, L., et al. (2009). Gender differences in sport injury risk and types of injuries: A retrospective twelve-month study on cross-country skiers, long distance runners and soccer players. *J Sports Sci Med*, 8, 443–451.

17. World Health Organization. (2007). WHO global report on falls prevention in older age. Section 2.5. Retrieved March 2018 from http://www.who.int/ageing/publications/Falls_prevention7March.pdf.

---

risk for corneal Injury

Taxonomy II: Safety/Protection—Class 5 Physical Injury (00245) **[Diagnostic Division:** Safety**],** Submitted: 2013; Revised 2017

DEFINITION: Susceptible to infection or inflammatory lesion in the corneal tissue that can affect superficial or deep layers, which may compromise health.

RISK FACTORS

Exposure of the eyeball

Insufficient knowledge of modifiable factors

At Risk Population: Prolonged hospitalization

Associated Condition: Blinking <5 times per minute; periorbital edema

Glasgow Coma Scale <6

Oxygen therapy; tracheostomy; intubation; mechanical ventilation

Pharmaceutical agent

Sample Clinical Applications: Any condition where client is unable to protect self from drying of eye tissues, including facial or general trauma or surgery; mechanical ventilation; brain injury, CVA; neurological conditions such as Parkinson's disease, Bell's palsy; diabetic retinopathy; lupus; rheumatoid arthritis

(continues on page 498)

 Diagnostic Studies Evidence Based Practice Medications 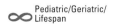 Pediatric/Geriatric/Lifespan

risk for corneal Injury (continued)

DESIRED OUTCOMES/EVALUATION CRITERIA

Sample NOC linkage:
Risk Control: Personal actions to understand, prevent, eliminate, or reduce modifiable health threats

Client/Caregiver Will (Include Specific Time Frame)
• Identify/monitor personal risk factors.
• Engage in risk control strategies.

Sample NOC linkage:
Dry Eye Severity: Severity of signs and symptoms of insufficient tears

Client Will (Include Specific Time Frame)
Be free of discomfort or damage to corneal tissues.

ACTIONS/INTERVENTIONS

Sample NIC linkages:
Risk Identification: Analysis of potential risk factors, determination of health risks, and prioritization of risk reduction strategies for an individual or group
Eye Care: Prevention or minimization of threats to eye or visual integrity

NURSING PRIORITY NO. 1 To identify causative/precipitating factors related to risk:

• Obtain history of eye conditions when assessing client concerns overall. Listen for reports of eye pain, foreign body sensation, light sensitivity (photophobia), and blurred vision. *These symptoms can be associated with corneal injury and, if present, require further evaluation and possible treatment.*[1]
• Note presence of conditions (e.g., recent neurological event, facial trauma or burns; use of contact lenses, failure to use safety glasses in high-risk employment situation) or treatment environments (e.g., intubated client on mechanical ventilation; use of therapeutic hypothermia; sedated, anesthetized, or obtunded client with absent blink reflex) *to identify client at high risk for corneal injury. Note: It has been reported that 60% of sedated/paralyzed patients on mechanical ventilation in intensive care units have incomplete closure of the eyelids (lagophthalmos), predisposing them to corneal dryness and inflammation.*[2,3]
• Obtain history of events from client/others when trauma (e.g., facial blunt force trauma, car crash with airbag deployment, accidental or intentional gun shot wounds; accidents with fireworks or hot metal) has occurred. *Eye injury (including corneal abrasions and lacerations) may not be immediately discovered but should be suspected.*[4]
• Evaluate current drug regimen, noting pharmaceutical agents (e.g., topical drugs, preservatives in eye drops; beta blockers, antihistamines, phenothiazides; diuretics, steroids, sedatives, neuromuscular blocking agents, antiparkinsonian agents, topical anesthetics) *that can contribute to dry eye, thereby increasing risk of corneal inflammation or injury in high-risk clients.*[5]

NURSING PRIORITY NO. 2 To promote eye health/comfort:

• Refer for diagnostic evaluation and interventions as indicated. *A standard eye exam and visual acuity testing may be performed, and other diagnostic studies (e.g., radiography, computed tomography, magnetic resonance imaging) may be indicated to locate foreign bodies or associated orbital, cranial, or facial trauma.*[4]

 Acute Care   Collaborative   Community/ Home Care   Cultural

- Assist in/refer for treatment of underlying conditions that might be affecting corneal health.
- Perform routine assessment of eyes and preventive interventions in critically ill client:[2,7,8]
Evaluate client's ability to maintain eyelid closure on daily basis and as needed.
Perform actions to maintain eyelid closure in client that cannot do it for self (e.g., taping).
Perform eye care (e.g., cleaning with saline-soaked gauze, administration of eye-specific lubricant, where indicated).
Observe for developing complications.
Ascertain that client undergoing anesthesia has proper eye protection (e.g., lubricant, eyelids taped, goggles), especially when placed in prone position. *The cornea is easily abraded because of reduced lacrimation during anesthesia, if face masks are improperly applied, or if surgical drapes are manipulated while the eyes remain open. In some positions, such as prone, a significant amount of pressure can be applied to the eyes.*

NURSING PRIORITY NO. 3   To promote wellness (Teaching/Discharge Criteria):

- Instruct high-risk client/caregivers in self-management interventions *to prevent corneal inflammation symptoms:*[1,5,6,9]
Avoid rubbing eyes with fingers or harsh cloths.
Protect eyes from blowing air or oxygen; discuss benefit of redirecting air flow.
Wear protective eyewear in situations or sports where objects may fly into eyes or face.
Wear protective eyewear that gives 180-degree protection while using a grinding wheel or hammering on metal.
Wear sunglasses that block ultraviolet radiation when in bright sunlight or under sunlamps.
Follow prescribed wear time for contact lenses.
Add moisture to indoor air, especially in winter, to *reduce corneal irritation associated with dryness.*
Blink repeatedly for a few seconds when using computer for any length of time *to prevent dryness and help spread tears evenly over eye.*
- Instruct in use of eye drops or ointments as indicated *to prevent inflammation/infection or to protect corneal surface.*
- Refer to appropriate healthcare provider concerning glasses, contact lenses, or other safety eyewear and offer information about suppliers.

DOCUMENTATION FOCUS

Assessment/Reassessment
- Individual risk factors identified.
- Client concerns or difficulty making and following through with plan.

Planning
- Plan of care and who is involved in planning.
- Teaching plan.

Implementation/Evaluation
- Response to interventions, teaching, and actions performed.
- Attainment or progress toward outcomes.

Discharge Planning
- Referrals to other resources.
- Long-term need and who is responsible for actions.

 Diagnostic Studies   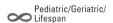 Evidence Based Practice   Medications   Pediatric/Geriatric/ Lifespan

References

1. Verma, A., Khan, F. H. (2014, updated 2017). Corneal abrasion. Retrieved March 2018 from http://emedicine.medscape.com/article/1195402-overview.
2. Johnson, K., Rolls, K. (2014). Eye care for critically ill adults. *IC Manual: Best Practice Guidelines for Intensive Care*. Chatswood, NSW, Australia: Agency for Clinical Innovation.
3. Schlessinger, D. A., Ulitsch, E. (2009). The eyes have it. *OR Nurse*, 3(4), 26–32.
4. Adesina, A., Silverberg, M. A. (2013, updated 2016). Corneal laceration. Retrieved March 2018 from http://emedicine.medscape.com/article/798005-overview.
5. Foster, C. S., et al. (Updated 2017). Dry eye disease (keratoconjunctivitis sicca) (various pages). Retrieved March 2018 from http://emedicine.medscape.com/article/1210417-overview#showall.
6. Mayo Clinic Staff. (2014, updated 2015). Dry eye. Retrieved March 2018 from https://www.mayoclinic.org/diseases-conditions/dry-eyes/symptoms-causes/syc-20371863.
7. Cucchiara, R. F., Faust, J. P. (1994). Patient positioning. In Miller, R. D. (ed.). *Anesthesia*. New York: Churchill Livingstone, 1057–1073.
8. Roth, S., et al. (1996). Eye injuries after nonocular surgery. A study of 60,965 anesthetics from 1988 to 1992. *Anesthesiology*, 85(5), 1020–1027.
9. Dahl, A. A. (2014, updated 2017). Corneal abrasion. Retrieved March 2018 from http://www.emedicinehealth.com/corneal_abrasion/article_em.htm.

risk for urinary tract Injury

Taxonomy II: Safety/Protection—Class 2 Physical Injury (00250) **[Diagnostic Division:** Safety], Approved 2013; Revised 2017

DEFINITION: Susceptible to damage of the urinary tract structures from use of catheters, which may compromise health.

RISK FACTORS

Confusion

Deficient patient or caregiver knowledge regarding care of urinary catheter

Obesity

At Risk Population: Extremes of age

Associated Condition: Anatomical variation in the pelvic organs; detrusor sphincter dyssynergia

Long-term use of urinary catheter; multiple catheterizations

Impaired cognition; medullary injury; condition preventing ability to secure catheter [e.g., burn, trauma, amputation]

Use of large-caliber urinary catheter; retention balloon inflated to ≥30 mL

DESIRED OUTCOMES/EVALUATION CRITERIA

Sample NOC linkages:

Physical Injury Severity: Severity of signs and symptoms of injuries to the body

Client Will (Include Specific Time Frame)
• Be free of injury.

Sample NOC linkages:

Personal Safety Behavior: Personal actions to prevent unintentional physical injury to self
Knowledge: Treatment Procedure: Extent of understanding conveyed about a procedure required as part of a treatment regimen

 Acute Care Collaborative Community/Home Care Cultural

Client/Caregivers Will (Include Specific Time Frame)
- Verbalize understanding of individual factors that contribute to possibility of injury.
- Demonstrate behaviors and lifestyle changes to reduce risk factors and protect from injury.

ACTIONS/INTERVENTIONS

Sample **NIC** linkages:

Urinary Catheterization: Insertion of a catheter into the bladder for temporary or permanent drainage of urine

Urinary Catheterization: Intermittent: Regular periodic use of a catheter to empty the bladder

NURSING PRIORITY NO. 1   To assess causative/contributing factors:

- Identify conditions potentially affecting client need for/response to catheterization (e.g., acute illness, presence of infection, surgery, trauma including skin and tissue problems; chronic illness, including neurological conditions with paralysis or weakness; prolonged immobility; acute or chronic confusion, dementia, sedation, or use of multiple medications affecting mental acuity). *These conditions could require indwelling catheter for varying lengths of time with attendant potential for complications. Risk factors include longer duration of catheterization, bacterial colonization of the drainage bag, errors in catheter care, catheterization late in the hospital course, and immunocompromised or debilitated states. Note: About 80% of hospital-acquired urinary tract infections (UTIs) are related to urethral catheterization.*[1]
- Determine type of catheterization client is likely to require. *Client might require one-time or intermittent, long-term single catheterization for any number of reasons (e.g., relief of acute urinary retention, management of voiding issues associated with multiple sclerosis or spinal cord injury). These procedures may be done by either the client or a caregiver. Indwelling urinary catheters are generally used when longer-term urinary management issues are expected. Use of indwelling catheter should be limited to (1) urinary retention, (2) close monitoring of urine output in critically ill patients, (3) fluid challenge in patients with acute renal insufficiency, (4) open wound in sacral or perineal area in client with urinary incontinence, and (5) comfort care in terminally ill client.*[2,3]
- Note client's age, developmental level, decision-making ability, level of cognition, competence, and independence. *Determines client's/significant other's (SO's) ability to attend to safety issues and influences choice of interventions or teaching about catheterization.*
- Check for allergies to latex and select appropriate catheter (e.g., coated). *Latex allergic reactions are implicated in the development of urethritis and urethral stricture or anaphylaxis. Materials that are commonly used for the long term (such as silver alloy or hydrogel coated) may be used to overcome irritation and microscopic lacerations or stricture development associated with latex.*[4,5]

NURSING PRIORITY NO. 2   To reduce potential for complications:

- Avoid catheterization when possible. Refer to NDs pertaining to impaired urinary Elimination and Incontinence for related interventions. *Studies have shown that urinary catheters often are placed unnecessarily, remain in use without physician awareness, and are not removed promptly when no longer needed.*[2,6,7]
- Perform catheterization using best practices:
  Use strict aseptic technique when inserting indwelling catheter (clean technique may be implemented for long-term intermittent catheterization). *Note: The Centers for Disease Control and Prevention's 2009 recommendations stated, "In the acute care hospital setting, insert urinary catheters using aseptic technique and sterile equipment," but "In the non-acute care setting, clean (i.e., non-sterile) technique for intermittent*

Diagnostic Studies   Evidence Based Practice   Medications   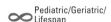Pediatric/Geriatric/Lifespan *catheterization is an acceptable and more practical alternative to sterile technique for patients requiring chronic intermittent catheterization."*[8]

∞ ✍ Select the smallest bore catheter possible that will allow for adequate drainage, using size guidelines. *Appropriate selection of catheter size will help reduce the likelihood of bladder spasm. Adult sizes are typically 14 Fr or 16 Fr. Guidelines are available for each pediatric age group from neonate (5–6 Fr) to adolescent (10, 12, 14 Fr). Note: Large-size catheters (18 Fr or larger) can increase erosion of the bladder neck and urethral mucosa, cause the formation of strictures, and impede adequate drainage of periurethral gland secretions.*[3,9–11]

Ascertain good urine is established before inflating balloon. *Ensures that catheter has been correctly inserted into the bladder. Note: If the balloon is opened before catheter is completely inserted into the bladder, bleeding, damage, and even rupture of the urethra can occur.*[13]

Inflate balloon, using correct amount of sterile liquid (usually 10 cc, but check actual balloon size). *Balloon size is relevant to levels of bladder irritation. Although balloons are thin walled to reduce irritation to the bladder, it is still important to use the smallest size possible, usually with a 5- to 10-mL capacity. The use of 30-mL balloons is not recommended.*[12,13]

✍ Secure catheter to thigh or abdomen, as indicated. Inspect the skin underneath the securement device with each reapplication to monitor for irritation or dermatitis. *Catheter/tubing can be held in place with adhesive tapes, safety pins, sutures, or nonadhesive devices. Latex-free nonadhesive products secure with a soft hook-and-loop closure strap. There are many reasons for this intervention, including (1) reducing bladder irritability/spasms, (2) preventing metal erosion or inflammation, (3) managing discomfort related to catheter movement and traction, (4) preventing inadvertent migration of balloon from bladder into urethra or accidental removal of catheter, (5) avoiding obstruction of urine flow secondary to catheter kinking, and (6) preventing retention of urine and risk for catheter-associated UTIs. [Note: Studies continue to report that catheter securement practices are inadequate in spite of guidelines. One small study published in 2016 reported that the overall prevalence of catheter securement was only 18%, although 87% of those were secured correctly. Securement policies and products were in place and available.]*[14–19]

✍ Position the collection bag level *to facilitate gravity drainage of the bladder and to prevent reflux of urine into the bladder. Note: A Belly Bag® abdominal drainage bag may be chosen over affixing tubing to leg in some instances (e.g., extremity trauma such as burns or amputation). The bag fastens around the waist by means of a woven belt with a quick release buckle. An anti-reflux valve behind the catheter port prevents reflux urine flow.*[13,18]

✍ Perform ongoing evaluation of catheter function and monitor color and characteristics of urine *to assess for developing complications. A properly maintained closed drainage system and unobstructed urine flow are essential for prevention of urinary tract infection.*[5]

• Ascertain if client is experiencing discomfort or pain (e.g., bladder spasms). *Bladder spasms are caused by the irritation of the bladder, bladder neck, or urethral mucosa. Spasms are a distressing complication but are usually self-limiting when procedure is followed (e.g., proper size and insertion of catheter, appropriate size and inflation of balloon). Note: Contractions may intensify when large indwelling urinary catheters with large-capacity balloons are inserted.*[10,19,20]

NURSING PRIORITY NO. 3   To promote wellness (Teaching/Discharge Instructions):

• 🏠 Review individual needs regarding catheter self-management with client/SO[21] *to reduce risk of complications:*

Always wash hands before and after handling catheter.

Make sure that urine is flowing out of the catheter into collection bag.

Keep urine collection bag below level of bladder.

Make sure that catheter tubing does not get twisted or kinked.

Check for inflammation or signs of infection (e.g., pus or irritated, swollen, red, or tender skin) in the area around the catheter.

Clean the area around the catheter twice a day using soap and water. Dry with clean towel afterward.

 Acute Care   Collaborative   Community/ Home Care   Cultural

Do not apply powder or lotion to the skin around the catheter.

Do not tug or pull on the catheter.

Follow physician instructions regarding catheter cleaning and/or replacement (if long-term indwelling), frequency of catheterization (if intermittent).

• Instruct client/caregiver in techniques to protect the integrity of skin. Refer to NDs risk for impaired Skin/Tissue Integrity and risk for Pressure Ulcer for related interventions.

• 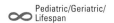 Instruct client/caregiver in reportable problems, such as leaking, sediment in urine, absence of urine, presence of pain, etc. *In a review of 37 studies regarding catheter problems, between 90% and 100% of patients who undergo long-term catheterization developed bacteriuria. About 80% of nosocomial (healthcare-associated) UTIs were related to urethral catheterization; only 5% to 10% are related to genitourinary manipulation. Minor complications were also common. For example, the frequency of urine leakage occurred in approximately 52% in short-term catheterization.*[22,23]

• Identify resources available to the individual (e.g., urinary catheters, samples and supplies, and various types of assistance and support).

DOCUMENTATION FOCUS

Assessment/Reassessment

• Individual risk factors, noting current physical findings.
• Client's/caregiver's understanding of individual risks and safety concerns.

Planning

• Plan of care and who is involved in planning.
• Teaching plan.

Implementation/Evaluation

• Individual responses to interventions, teaching, and actions performed.
• Specific actions and changes that are made.
• Attainment or progress toward desired outcome(s).
• Modifications to plan of care.

Discharge Planning

• Long-term plans for discharge needs, lifestyle and community changes, and who is responsible for actions to be taken.
• Specific referrals made.

References

1. Brusch, J. L. (2013, updated 2017). Catheter-related urinary tract infection (UTI). Medscape. Retrieved March 2018 from http://emedicine.medscape.com/article/2040035-overview#showall.
2. Jain, P., Parada, A., Smith, L. G. (1995). Overuse of the indwelling urinary tract catheter in hospitalized medical patients. *Arch Intern Med*, 155(13), 1425–1429.
3. Hart, S. (2008). Urinary catheterization. *Nurs Stand*, 22(27), 44–48.
4. Crippa, M., et al. (2006). Prevention of latex allergy among health care workers and in the general population: Latex protein content in devices commonly used in hospitals and general practice. *Int Arch Occup Environ Health*, 79(7), 550–557.
5. Schumm, K., Lam, T. B. (2008). Types of urethral catheters for management of short-term voiding problems in hospitalised adults. *Cochrane Database Syst Rev*, April 16(2), CD004013.
6. Saint, S., et al. (2000). Are physicians aware of which of their patients have indwelling urinary catheters? *Am J Med*, 109(6), 476–480.
7. Fakih, M. G., et al.(2008). Effect of nurse-led multidisciplinary rounds on reducing the unnecessary use of urinary catheterization in hospitalized patients. *Infect Control Hosp*, 29(9), 815–819.
8. Centers for Disease Control and Prevention (CDC). (2009). Guideline for prevention of catheter-associated urinary tract infections, 2009. Retrieved March 2018 from https://www.cdc.gov/infectioncontrol/pdf/guidelines/cauti-guidelines.pdf.
9. Carlson, D., Mowery, B. D. (1997). Standards to prevent complications of urinary catheterization in children: Should and should-knots. *J Soc Pediatr Nurs*, 2(1), 37–41.
10. Winson, L. (1997). Catheterization: A need for improved patient management. *Br J Nurs*, 6(21), 1229–1252.

 Diagnostic Studies   Evidence Based Practice   Medications   ∞ Pediatric/Geriatric/Lifespan

11. Astra Tech Staff. (No date). A parent's guide to intermittent catheterization. Torrence, CA.: Astra Tach.

12. Westbrook, I. P. (2000). Catheter design and selection. In Downey, P. (ed). *Introduction to Urological Nursing*. Hoboken, NJ: John Wiley & Sons.

13. Thangavelu-Veluswamy, A., Thangavelu, D. (Last review 2017). Foley catheter. Retrieved March 2018 from https://www.emedicinehealth.com/foley_catheter/article_em.htm#when_to_seek_medical_care_for_foley_catheter_complications.

14. Macaulay, M. (1994). Urinary drainage systems. In Laker, C. (ed). *Urological Nursing*. London, UK: Scutari Press.

15. Appah, Y., Hunter, K. F., Moore, K. N. (2016). Securement of the indwelling urinary catheter: A prevalence study. *J Wound Ostomy Continence Nurs*, 43(2), 173–177.

16. Gray, M. L. (2008). Securing the indwelling catheter. *Am J Nurs*, 108(12), 44–50.

17. Siegel, T. J. (2008). The ins and outs of urinary catheters. Evidence-based management. *Advance Nurs Pract*, 16(8), 57–60.

18. Care Pathways. (No date). Belly Bag® urinary drainage bag. Retrieved March 2018 from http://www.carepathways.com/estore-cat-Incon.cfm?Title=Belly+Bag+Urinary+Drainage+Bag.

19. Kelly, T. W., Griffiths, G. L. (1983). Balloon problems with foley catheters. *Lancet*, 2(8362), 1310.

20. Sulzbach, L. M. (2002). Ask the Experts (questions regarding catheter management). *Crit Care Nurse*, 22(3), (84), 87.

21. Healthwise Staff. (2014). Care for an indwelling urinary catheter: Fact sheet for public education. Retrieved March 2018 from http://www.webmd.com/a-to-z-guides/care-for-an-indwelling-urinary-catheter-topic-overview.

22. Brusch, J. L. (Updated 2017). Catheter-related urinary tract infection (UTI). Retrieved March 2018 from https://emedicine.medscape.com/article/2040035-overview.

23. Hollingsworth, J. M., et al. (2013). Determining the noninfectious complications of indwelling urethral catheters: A systematic review and meta-analysis. *Ann Intern Med*, 159(6), 401–410.

Insomnia

Taxonomy II: Activity/Rest—Class 1 Sleep/Rest (00095) [**Diagnostic Division:** Activity/Rest], Approved 2006: Revised 2017

DEFINITION: A disruption in amount and quality of sleep that impairs functioning.

RELATED FACTORS

Alcohol consumption

Anxiety; depression; fear; grieving

Average daily physical activity is less than recommended for gender and age; frequent naps; inadequate sleep hygiene

Environmental barrier [e.g., ambient noise, daylight/darkness exposure, ambient temperature/humidity, unfamiliar setting]

Physical discomfort; stressors

DEFINING CHARACTERISTICS

Subjective

Alteration in sleep pattern; nonrestorative sleep pattern, difficulty initiating sleep or maintaining sleep state; early awakening

Compromised health status; decrease in quality of life; increase in accidents

Dissatisfaction with sleep; sleep-disturbance producing next-day consequences

Objective

Alteration in concentration

Alteration in mood/affect

Increase in absenteeism

Associated Condition: Hormonal change; pharmaceutical agent

Sample Clinical Applications: Chronic pain, substance use or abuse, hyperthyroidism, pulmonary diseases (e.g., COPD, asthma), sleep apnea, restless leg syndrome, depression, Alzheimer's disease, senile dementia, anxiety disorders, bipolar disorders, pregnancy—prenatal or postnatal period

 Acute Care Collaborative Community/ Home Care Cultural

DESIRED OUTCOMES/EVALUATION CRITERIA

Sample NOC linkages:
Fatigue Level: Severity of observed or reported prolonged generalized fatigue
Sleep: Natural periodic suspension of consciousness during which the body is restored
Rest: Quality and pattern of diminished activity for mental and physical rejuvenation

Client Will (Include Specific Time Frame)
- Verbalize understanding of sleep impairment.
- Identify individually appropriate interventions to promote sleep.
- Adjust lifestyle to accommodate chronobiological rhythms.
- Report improvement in sleep or rest pattern.
- Report increased sense of well-being and feeling rested.

ACTIONS/INTERVENTIONS

Sample NIC linkages:
Sleep Enhancement: Facilitation of regular sleep/wake cycles
Relaxation Therapy: Use of techniques to encourage and elicit relaxation for the purpose of decreasing undesirable signs and symptoms such as pain, muscle tension, or anxiety
Environmental Management: Manipulation of the patient's surroundings for therapeutic benefit, sensory appeal, and psychological well-being

NURSING PRIORITY NO. 1   To identify causative/contributing factors:

- Identify presence of factors that can contribute to insomnia (e.g., chronic pain, arthritis, dyspnea; movement disorders; dementia; obesity; pregnancy, menopause; psychiatric disorders); metabolic diseases (e.g., hyperthyroidism and diabetes); prescribed and over-the-counter (OTC) drugs; alcohol, stimulant, or other recreational drug use; circadian rhythm disorders (e.g., shift work, jet lag); environmental factors (e.g., noise, no control over thermostat, uncomfortable bed); major life stressors (e.g., grief, loss, finances).[1–5,9,10]
- ∞ ▨ Note client age. *Increased sleep latency (time required to fall asleep), decreased sleep efficiency, and increased awakenings are common in the elderly. Two primary sleep disorders that increase with age are sleep apnea and periodic limb movements in sleep.*[2,9]
- ∞ Observe parent-infant interactions and provision of emotional support. Note mother's sleep-wake pattern. *Lack of knowledge of infant cues or problem relationships may create tension interfering with sleep. Structured sleep routines based on adult schedules may not meet child's needs.*[6]
- Ascertain presence and frequency of enuresis, incontinence, or need for frequent nighttime voidings, thus interrupting sleep.[2,9]
- ✎ Assist with or review psychological assessment, noting individual and personality characteristics *if anxiety disorders or depression could be affecting sleep.*[2,8,9,13]
- Determine recent traumatic events in client's life (e.g., a death in family, loss of job). *Physical and emotional trauma often affects client's sleep patterns and quality for a short period of time. This disruption can become long term and require more intensive assessment and intervention.*[2,3]
- 🥄 Review client's medication regimen, including prescription (e.g., beta blockers [e.g., metoprolol, propranolol], sedative antidepressants [e.g., amitriptyline], sedative neuroleptics [e.g., chlorpramazine, clozapine]; other antidepressants [e.g., floxetine]; steroids, antihypertensives, bronchodilators, weight-loss drugs, thyroid preparations, sedatives), OTC products (e.g., decongestants), and herbal remedies. *Use or timing may be interfering with falling asleep or staying asleep requiring adjustments such as change in dose or time medication is taken or choice of drug prescribed.*[7,9,10]

 Diagnostic Studies   Evidence Based Practice   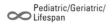 Medications   ∞ Pediatric/Geriatric/Lifespan

- Note caffeine and alcohol intake. *May interfere with falling asleep or duration and quality of sleep.*
- Assist with diagnostic testing (e.g., polysomnography, daytime multiple sleep latency testing, actigraphy, full-night sleep studies) *to determine cause and type of sleep disturbance. Note: Insomnia is a clinical diagnosis. Diagnostic studies are indicated principally for clarification of comorbid disorders.*[14]

NURSING PRIORITY NO. 2   To determine sleep pattern and dysfunction(s):

- Review sleep diary (where available); observe or obtain feedback from client/significant others (SOs) regarding client's sleep problems, usual bedtime, rituals or routines, number of hours of sleep, time of arising, and environmental needs *to determine usual sleep pattern and provide comparative baseline.*
- Listen to subjective reports of sleep quality (e.g., client never feels rested or feels excessively sleepy during day). *Provides opportunity to address misconceptions or unrealistic expectations and plan for interventions.*
- Determine type of insomnia (e.g., transient, short term, chronic). *Transient episodes are occasional restless nights caused by such factors as jet lag, first night in a new bed, and so forth. Short-term insomnia lasts a few weeks and arises from temporary stressful experience, such as pressures at work, loss of job, and death in family, and usually resolves over time as client adapts to stressor. Chronic insomnia lasts for more than 6 months and can be caused by many physical and psychological factors as well as use/misuse of medications and drugs.*[9,13]
- Investigate whether client snores and in what position(s) this occurs. Also determine if obese individual experiences loud periodic snoring, along with unusual nighttime activities (e.g., sitting upright, sleepwalking), and morning headaches, sleepiness, and/or depression. *Sleep studies may need to be done to rule out obstructive sleep disorder.*[2,4,14]
- Note alteration of habitual sleep time, such as change of work pattern or rotating shifts or change in normal bedtime (hospitalization). *Helps identify circumstances that are known to interrupt sleep patterns resulting in mental and physical fatigue, affecting concentration, interest, energy, and appetite.*[5]
- Observe physical signs of fatigue (e.g., restlessness, hand tremors, thick speech, drowsiness).
- Assist with diagnostic testing (e.g., electroencephalogram, electrooculogram, electromyogram; psychological assessment/testing, chronological chart). *Polysomnography tests (the three electrical tests noted above) are performed in a sleep laboratory to measure several parameters of sleep, including brain wave activity, eye movement, and leg muscle tone. These tests may be performed after initial clinical evaluation or symptom management fails to discover or resolve a particular sleep disturbance or point to appropriate interventions and treatments.*[1,2,4]

NURSING PRIORITY NO. 3   To assist client to establish optimal sleep/rest patterns:

- Collaborate in treatment of underlying medical and psychiatric problem (e.g., obstructive sleep apnea, pain, gastroesophageal reflux disease, lower urinary tract infection/prostatic hypertropy; depression, bipolar disorder; complicated grief).
- Assist client with implementing measures to manage sleep problems when in facility care:[9,11,14]
   Arrange care to provide for uninterrupted periods of rest. *Allows for longer periods of sleep, especially during night.*
   Provide quiet environment and comfort measures (e.g., back rub, washing hands and face, cleaning and straightening sheets). *Promotes relaxation and readiness for sleep.*
   Administer pain medications (if required) 1 hr before sleep *to relieve discomfort and take maximum advantage of analgesic and sedative effect.*
   Discuss and implement effective age-appropriate bedtime rituals (e.g., going to bed at same time each night, drinking warm milk, rocking, story reading, cuddling, favorite blanket or toy) *to enhance client's relaxation, reinforce that bed is a place to sleep, and promote sense of security for child or confused elder.*[6,9]
- Limit fluid intake in evening if nocturia is a problem *to reduce need for nighttime elimination.* Suggest avowing chocolate and caffeinated or alcoholic beverages, especially prior to bedtime. *Substances known to impair falling asleep or staying asleep. Alcohol may help individual fall asleep, but ensuing sleep is fragmented.*[6]

 Acute Care   Collaborative   Community/ Home Care   Cultural

- Explore other sleep aids (e.g., warm bath or milk, light protein snack before bedtime, soothing music, favorite TV show). *Nonpharmaceutical aids may enhance falling asleep free of concern of medication side effects such as morning hangover or drug dependence.*
- 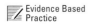 Develop behavioral program for insomnia, such as:[1–5,9,10,14,15]

  establishing regular sleeping and waking-up time, and maintaining a routine at bedtime and arising;

  thinking relaxing thoughts when in bed;

  avoiding napping in the daytime;

  exercising daily, but not immediately before bedtime;

  avoiding heavy meals at bedtime;

  using bed only for sleeping or sex;

  wearing comfortable, loose-fitting clothing to bed;

  refraining from reading or watching TV in bed;

  getting out of bed if not asleep in 15 to 30 min and participating in relaxing activity until sleepy;

  getting up at the same time each day—even on weekends and days off;

  getting adequate exposure to bright light during day; and

  individually tailoring a stress-reduction program, music therapy, and/or relaxation routine.
- Recommend and assist with implementing program to "reset" sleep clock (chronotherapy when client has delayed sleep-onset insomnia). *These sleep-wake problems are common among shift workers and airplane travelers. Shift workers can benefit by adhering to a set routine and ensuring that noises and interruptions are kept to a minimum. Those who travel across time zones can benefit by adjusting their sleep time to match the time zone of their arrival and avoiding caffeine and alcohol.[5]*
- Use barbiturates or other sleeping medications sparingly. *Research indicates long-term use of these medications, especially in the absence of cognitive behavioral therapy (CBT), fails to show long-term benefit and can actually induce sleep disturbances.[16]*
- Encourage routine use of continuous positive airway pressure therapy when indicated *to obtain optimal benefit of treatment for sleep apnea.*
- Monitor effects of therapeutic use of amphetamines or stimulants (such as may be used for attention deficit disorder or narcolepsy). *Use of these medications can induce or potentiate sleep disturbances.[7]*
- Administer and monitor effects of prescribed medications to promote sleep (e.g., *benzodiazepines* such as zolpidem [Ambien], zaleplon [Sonata], eszopiclone [Lunesta]), *antidepressants* (e.g., trazodone [Desyrel], nefazodone [Serzone]), and *melatonin agonists* (e.g., ramelteon [Rozerem]). *Many medications may be tried to manage insomnia. While most are effective in the short term, many lose effectiveness over time. The client may have adverse side effects or develop tolerance and misuse the drug. Many drug regimens are most effective when combined with CBT, in which the client can be weaned off medications at some point.[9,14]*
- Refer to sleep specialist as indicated or desired. *Follow-up evaluation and intervention may be needed when insomnia is having a serious impact on client's quality of life, productivity, and safety (e.g., on the job, at home, on the road). Note: Studies show that the most effective treatment for primary insomnia is CBT. Techniques are used to ameliorate factors that perpetuate or exacerbate chronic insomnia, such as poor sleep habits, hyperarousal, irregular sleep schedules, inadequate sleep hygiene, and misconceptions about sleep and the consequences of insomnia.[2,12,16]*

NURSING PRIORITY NO. 4 To promote wellness (Teaching/Discharge Considerations):

- Assure client that occasional sleeplessness should not threaten health. *Knowledge that occasional insomnia is universal and usually not harmful may promote relaxation and relief from worry, which can perpetuate the problem.[4]*
- Assist client to develop individual program of relaxation. Demonstrate techniques (e.g., biofeedback, self-hypnosis, visualization, progressive muscle relaxation). *Methods that reduce sympathetic response and decrease stress can help induce sleep, particularly in persons suffering from chronic and long-term sleep disturbances.[3]*
- Encourage participation in regular exercise program during day *to aid in stress control and release of energy. Note: Exercise at bedtime may stimulate rather than relax client and actually interfere with sleep.[2]*

 Diagnostic Studies   Evidence Based Practice   Medications   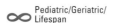 Pediatric/Geriatric/Lifespan

- Investigate use of environmental sleep aids (e.g., sleep mask, darkening shades or curtains, earplugs, monotonous sounds [white noise]) *to block out ambient light and noise.*
- Assist individuals with insomnia associated with shift work to develop individual schedule *to take advantage of peak performance times as identified in chronobiological chart.*
- Recommend midmorning nap if one is required. *Napping, especially in the afternoon, can disrupt normal sleep patterns.*
- Assist client to deal with grieving process if grief is causing or exacerbating insomnia. (Refer to ND Grieving.)

DOCUMENTATION FOCUS

Assessment/Reassessment
- Assessment findings, including specifics of sleep pattern (current and past) and effects on lifestyle and level of functioning.
- Medications, interventions, and previous therapies tried.
- Results of testing.

Planning
- Plan of care and who is involved in planning.
- Teaching plan.

Implementation/Evaluation
- Client's response to interventions, teaching, and actions performed.
- Attainment or progress toward desired outcome(s).
- Modifications to plan of care.

Discharge Planning
- Long-term needs and who is responsible for actions to be taken.
- Specific referrals made.

References

1. Insomnia (various pages). (2018). *National Sleep Foundation*. Retrieved March 2018 from https://sleepfoundation.org/insomnia/content/what-causes-insomnia.
2. Krishnan, P., Hawranik, P. (2008). Diagnosis and management of geriatric insomnia: A guide for nurse practitioners. *Nurse Pract*, 20(12), 590–599.
3. Newfield, S. A., et al. (2007). *Cox's Clinical Applications of Nursing Diagnosis: Adult, Child, Women's, Psychiatric, Gerontic, and Home Health Considerations*. 5th ed. Philadelphia: F. A. Davis.
4. Brain basics: Understanding sleep. (Updated 2017). *National Institute of Neurological Disorders and Stroke*. Retrieved March 2018 from www.ninds.nih.gov/disorders/brain_basics/understanding_sleep.htm.
5. Nazario, B. (2011). Sleep and the night shift: Could you have work sleep disorder? Retrieved March 2018 from http://www.webmd.com/sleep-disorders/excessive-sleepiness-10/night-shift-sleep.
6. London, M., et al. (2010). *Maternal and Child Nursing Care*. 3rd ed. Upper Saddle River, NJ: Prentice Hall.
7. Vallerand, A. H., Sanoski, C. A., with Deglin, J. H. (2016). *Davis's Drug Guide for Nurses*. 15th ed. Philadelphia: F. A. Davis.
8. Townsend, M. C. (2011). *Psychiatric Mental Health Nursing: Concepts of Care in Evidence-Based Practice*. 7th ed. Philadelphia: F. A. Davis.
9. Xlong, G. L., Gentilli, A. (Updated 2017). Geriatric sleep disorder. Retrieved March 2018 from http://emedicine.medscape.com/article/292498-overview.
10. Hertz, G., Cataletto, M. E. (Updated 2018). Sleep dysfunction in women. Retrieved March 2018 from http://emedicine.medscape.com/article/1189087-overview.
11. Turkowski, B. B. (2006). Managing insomnia. *Orthop Nurs*, 25(5), 339–345.
12. Nadolski, M. (2005). Getting a good night's sleep: Diagnosing and treating insomnia. *Plast Surg Nurs*, 25(4), 167–173.
13. Spielman, A. J., Caruso, L. S., Glovinsky, P. B. (1987). A behavioral perspective on insomnia treatment. *Psychiatr Clin North Am*, 10(4), 541–543.
14. Chawla, J., et al. (2015, updated 2017). Insomnia. Retrieved March 2018 from http://emedicine.medscape.com/article/1187829-overview.
15. Schutte-Rodin, S., et al. (2008). Clinical guideline for the evaluation and management of chronic insomnia in adults. *J Clin Sleep Med*, 15(4), 487–504.
16. Morin, C. M., et al. (2009). Cognitive behavioral therapy, singly and combined with medication, for persistent insomnia. *JAMA*, 301(19), 2005–2015.

 Acute Care   Collaborative   Community/Home Care   Cultural

deficient Knowledge

Taxonomy II: Perception/Cognition—Class 4 Cognition (00126) [**Diagnostic Division:** Teaching/Learning], Approved 1980; Revised 2017

DEFINITION: Absence of cognitive information related to specific topic or its acquisition.

RELATED FACTORS
Insufficient information; insufficient knowledge of resources
Insufficient interest in learning
Misinformation presented by others

DEFINING CHARACTERISTICS

Subjective
Insufficient knowledge

Objective
Inaccurate follow-through of instruction or performance on a test
Inappropriate behavior
[Development of preventable complication]
Associated Condition: Alteration in cognitive functioning or memory
Sample Clinical Applications: Any newly diagnosed disease or traumatic injury, progression of or deterioration in a chronic condition

DESIRED OUTCOMES/EVALUATION CRITERIA

Sample NOC linkages:
Knowledge: [specify—78 choices]: Extent of understanding conveyed about a specific disease process, its treatment, the promotion and protection of health, maintaining optimal health, etc.
Information Processing: Ability to acquire, organize, and use information
Client Satisfaction: Teaching: Extent of positive perception of instruction provided by nursing staff to improve knowledge, understanding, and participation in care

Client Will (Include Specific Time Frame)
- Participate in learning process.
- Identify interferences to learning and specific action(s) to deal with them.
- Exhibit increased interest and assume responsibility for own learning by beginning to look for information and ask questions.
- Verbalize understanding of condition or disease process and treatment.
- Identify relationship of signs/symptoms to the disease process and correlate symptoms with causative factors.
- Perform necessary procedures correctly and explain reasons for the actions.
- Initiate necessary lifestyle changes and participate in treatment regimen.

ACTIONS/INTERVENTIONS

Sample NIC linkages:
Teaching: Individual: Planning, implementation, and evaluation of a teaching program designed to address a patient's particular needs
Learning Facilitation: Promoting the ability to process and comprehend information
Learning Readiness Enhancement: Improving the ability and willingness to receive information

 Diagnostic Studies   Evidence Based Practice   Medications   Pediatric/Geriatric/Lifespan

NURSING PRIORITY NO. 1 To assess readiness to learn and individual learning needs:

- Ascertain level of knowledge, including anticipatory needs. *Learning needs can include many things (e.g., disease cause and process, factors contributing to symptoms, procedures for symptom control, needed alterations in lifestyle, ways to prevent complications). Client may or may not ask for information or may express inaccurate perceptions of health status and needed behaviors to manage self-care.*[1]
- Engage in active listening. *Conveys expectation of confidence in client's ability to determine learning needs and best ways of meeting them.*[5]
- Determine client's ability and readiness and barriers to learning. *Client may not be physically, emotionally, or mentally capable at this time and may need time to work through and express emotions before learning.*[1]
- Be alert to signs of avoidance. *May need to allow client to suffer the consequences of lack of knowledge before client is ready to accept information.*[1]
- Identify significant others (SOs)/family members requiring information. Providing appropriate information to others can provide reinforcement for learning, as everyone will understand what is to be expected.[4]

NURSING PRIORITY NO. 2 To determine other factors pertinent to the learning process:

- ∞ 🌐 Note personal factors (e.g., age, developmental level, gender, social and cultural influences, religion, life experiences, level of education, emotional stability) *that affect ability and desire to learn and assimilate new information, take control of situation, and accept responsibility for change.*[2,11]
- Determine blocks to learning, including (1) language barriers (e.g., can't read or write, speaks or understands a different language than that spoken by teacher); (2) physical factors (e.g., cognitive impairment, sensory deficits [e.g., aphasia, dyslexia, hearing or vision impairment]); (3) physical constraints (e.g., acute illness, activity intolerance, impaired thought processes); (4) complexity of material to be learned (e.g., caring for colostomy, giving own insulin injections); (5) forced change in lifestyle (e.g., smoking cessation); or (6) have stated no need or desire to learn. *Many factors affect the client's ability and desire to learn, and his or her expectations of the learning process must be addressed if learning is to be successful.*[1,11]
- Assess the level of the client's capabilities and the possibilities of the situation. *May need to assist SO(s) or caregivers to learn by introducing one new idea, by building on previous information, by finding pictures to demonstrate an idea, etc., to adapt teaching to client's specific needs.*[6]

NURSING PRIORITY NO. 3 To assess the client's/SO's motivation:

- Identify motivating factors for the individual (e.g., client needs to stop smoking because of advanced lung cancer, client wants to lose weight because family member died of complications of obesity). *Motivation may be negative (e.g., smoking causes lung cancer) or positive (e.g., client wants to promote health/prevent disease). Provides information that can guide content specific to client's situation and motivations.*[3,12]
- Provide information relevant only to the situation. *Reducing the amount of information at any one given time helps to keep the client focused and prevents client from feeling overwhelmed.*[4]
- Provide positive reinforcement rather than negative reinforcers (e.g., criticism and threats). *Enhances cooperation and encourages continuation of efforts.*[5]

NURSING PRIORITY NO. 4 To establish priorities in conjunction with client:

- Determine client's most urgent need from both client's and nurse's viewpoints. *Identifies whether client and nurse are together in their thinking and provides a starting point for teaching and outcome planning for optimal success.*[6]
- Discuss client's perception of need. *Takes into account the client's personal desires/needs and values/beliefs, providing a basis for planning appropriate care.*[6]
- Differentiate "critical" content from "desirable" content. *Identifies information that must be learned now as well as content that could be addressed at a later time. Client's emotional state may preclude hearing much of what is presented, and by only providing what is essential, client may hear it.*[3]

 Acute Care   Collaborative   Community/ Home Care   Cultural

NURSING PRIORITY NO. 5 To determine the content to be included:

- Identify information that needs to be remembered (cognitive) at client's level of development and education. *Enhances possibility that information will be heard and understood.*[6]
- Identify information having to do with emotions, attitudes, and values (affective). *The affective learning domain addresses a learner's emotions toward learning experiences, and attitudes, interest, attention, awareness, and values are demonstrated by affective behaviors. Knowing the client's affective state enhances learning possibilities.*[7,12]
- Identify psychomotor skills that are necessary for learning. *Psychomotor learning involves both cognitive learning and muscular movement. The phases for learning these skills are cognitive (what), associative (how), and autonomous (practice to automaticity). Learners need to know what, why, and how they will learn. For example, if papers need to be typed, the psychomotor skill will be touch typing. The individual will learn touch typing finger placement and how to type smoothly and rhythmically.*[8]

NURSING PRIORITY NO. 6 To develop learner's objectives:

- State objectives clearly in learner's terms to meet learner's (not instructor's) needs. *Understanding why the material is important to the learner provides motivation to learn.*[8]
- Identify outcomes (results) to be achieved. *Understanding what the outcomes will be helps the client realize the importance of learning the material, providing the motivation necessary to learning.*[8]
- Recognize level of achievement, time factors, and short-term and long-term goals. *Learning progresses in stages. Stage 1: unconsciously unskilled where we don't know that we don't know. Stage 2: consciously unskilled, we know that we don't know and start to learn. Stage 3: consciously skilled, we know how to do it but need to think and work hard to do it. Stage 4: we become unconsciously skilled, where the new skills are easier and even seem natural.*[9]
- Include the affective goals (e.g., reduction of stress). *The learner's emotional behaviors affect the learning experience and need to be actively addressed for maximum effectiveness.*[7]

NURSING PRIORITY NO. 7 To identify teaching methods to be used:

- Determine client's/SO's method of accessing information and preferred learning mode (e.g., auditory, visual, kinesthetic; group classes, one-to-one instruction, online) and include in teaching plan. *Using multiple modes of instruction facilitates learning and enhances retention, especially when faced with a stressful situation, illness, or new treatment regimen.*[3,10]
- Involve the client/SO(s) by using age-appropriate materials tailored to client's interest and literacy skills (e.g., interactive programmed books, questions, dialogue, audio/visual materials). *Accesses familiar mental images at client's developmental level to help individual learn more effectively.*[3,12,13]
- Involve others who have same problems, needs, or concerns. *Group presentations and support groups provide role models and opportunity for sharing of information to enhance learning.*
- Use team and group teaching as appropriate.

NURSING PRIORITY NO. 8 To facilitate learning:

- Provide mutual goal-setting and learning contracts. *Clarifies expectations of teacher and learner.*
- Provide written information/guidelines and self-learning modules for client to refer to as necessary. *Reinforces learning process.*
- Pace and time learning sessions and learning activities to individual's needs. Involve and evaluate effectiveness of learning activities with client. *Client statements, questions, comments provide feedback about ability to grasp information being presented.*
- Provide an environment that is conducive to learning *to limit distractions and allow client to focus on the material presented.*

 Diagnostic Studies   Evidence Based Practice   Medications 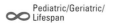 Pediatric/Geriatric/Lifespan

- Be aware of factors related to teacher in the situation (e.g., vocabulary, dress, style, knowledge of the subject, and ability to impart information effectively) *that may affect client's reaction to teacher or ability to learn from this individual.*
- Begin with information the client already knows and move to what the client does not know, progressing from simple to complex. *Can arouse interest and limit sense of being overwhelmed.*[12]
- Deal with the client's anxiety or other strong emotions. Present information out of sequence, if necessary, dealing first with material that is most anxiety producing *when the anxiety is interfering with the client's learning process.*
- Provide active role for client in learning process, including questions and discussion. *Promotes sense of control over situation.*
- Have client paraphrase content in own words, perform return demonstration, and explain how learning can be applied in own situation *to enhance internalization of material and to evaluate learning.*[3]
- Provide for feedback (positive reinforcement) and evaluation of learning and acquisition of skills. *Validates current level of understanding and identifies areas requiring follow-up.*[5]
- Be aware of informal teaching and role modeling that takes place on an ongoing basis. *Answering specific questions and reinforcing previous teaching during routine contacts or care enhances learning on a regular basis.*[1]
- Assist client to use information in all applicable areas (e.g., situational, environmental, personal). *Enhances learning to promote better understanding of situation or illness.*[1]

NURSING PRIORITY NO. 9   To promote wellness (Teaching/Discharge Considerations):

- Provide access information for contact person *to answer questions and validate information after discharge.*[1]
- Identify available community resources and support groups *to assist with problem-solving, provide role models, and support personal growth/change.*[4]
- Provide additional learning resources (e.g., bibliography, reliable Web sites, audio/visual media), as appropriate. *May assist with further learning and promote learning at own pace.*[7]

DOCUMENTATION FOCUS

Assessment/Reassessment
- Individual findings, learning style, and identified needs; presence of learning blocks (e.g., hostility, inappropriate behavior).

Planning
- Plan for learning, methods to be used, and who is involved in the planning.
- Teaching plan.

Implementation/Evaluation
- Responses of the client/SO(s) to the learning plan and actions performed.
- How the learning is demonstrated.
- Attainment or progress toward desired outcome(s).
- Modifications to plan of care.

Discharge Planning
- Additional learning and referral needs.

References

1. Bohny, B. A. (1997). A time for self-care: Role of the home healthcare nurse. *Home Healthc Nurse*, 15(4), 281–286.
2. Purnell, L. D. (2011). *Guide to Culturally Competent Health Care.* 2nd ed. Philadelphia: F. A. Davis.
3. Duffy, B. (1997). Using a creative teaching process with adult patients. *Home Healthc Nurse*, 15(2), 102–108.
4. Bartholomew, L. K. (2000). Watch, discover, think, and act: A model for patient education program development. *Patient Educ Couns*, 39(2–3), 269–280.
5. Lieb, S. (1991). Principles of adult learning. Retrieved March 2018 from https://petsalliance.org/sites/petsalliance.org/files/Lieb%201991%20Adult%20Learning%20Principles.pdf.

 Acute Care   Collaborative   Community/Home Care   Cultural

6. Townsend, M. C. (2011). *Psychiatric Mental Health Nursing: Concepts of Care in Evidence-Based Practice*. 7th ed. Philadelphia: F. A. Davis.

7. No author listed. (No date). Bloom's taxonomy of learning domains. The three types of learning. Retrieved April 2018 from http://www.nbna.org/files/Blooms%20Taxonomy%20of%20Learning.pdf.

8. Selwyn, N. (2013). *Education in a Digital World: Global Perspective*. New York: Routledge.

9. Adams, L. (No date). Learning a new skill is easier said than done. *Gordon Training International*. Retrieved April 2018 from http://www.gordontraining.com/free-workplace-articles/learning-a-new-skill-is-easier-said-than-done/.

10. McLeod, S. (2000, updated 2017). Kolb's learning styles and experiential learning model. *Simply Psychology*. Retrieved April 218 from https://simplypsychology.org/learning-kolb.html.

11. Maier-Lorentz, M. (2008). Transcultural nursing: Its importance in nursing practice. Retrieved April 2018 from http://www.redorbit.com/news/health/1372127/transcultural_nursing_its_importance_in_nursing_practice/l.

12. Anderson, N. R. (2006). The role of the home healthcare nurse in smoking cessation: Guidelines for successful intervention. *Home Healthc Nurse*, 24(7), 424–431.

13. Pieper, B., Sieggreen, M., Freeland, B. (2006). Discharge information needs of clients after surgery. *J Wound Ostomy Continence Nurs*, 33(3), 281–290.

readiness for enhanced Knowledge [Specify Level]

Taxonomy II: Perception/Cognition—Class 4 Cognition (00161) **[Diagnostic Division:** Teaching/Learning**],** Approved 2002; Revised 2013

DEFINITION: A pattern of cognitive information related to a specific topic, or its acquisition, which can be strengthened.

DEFINING CHARACTERISTICS

Subjective

Expresses desire to enhance learning

Sample Clinical Applications: As a health-seeking behavior, the patient may be healthy, or this diagnosis can occur in any clinical condition

DESIRED OUTCOMES/EVALUATION CRITERIA

Sample NOC linkages:

Knowledge: [specify—78 choices]: Extent of understanding conveyed about a specific disease process, its treatment, the promotion and protection of health, maintaining optimal health, etc.

Information Processing: Ability to acquire, organize, and use information

Client Satisfaction: Teaching: Extent of positive perception of instruction provided by nursing staff to improve knowledge, understanding, and participation in care

Client Will (Include Specific Time Frame)
• Exhibit responsibility for own learning by seeking answers to questions.
• Verify accuracy of informational resources.
• Verbalize understanding of information gained.
• Use information to develop individual plan to meet healthcare needs/goals.

ACTIONS/INTERVENTIONS

Sample NIC linkages:

Teaching: Individual: Planning, implementation, and evaluation of a teaching program designed to address a patient's particular needs

Learning Facilitation: Promoting the ability to process and comprehend information

Learning Readiness Enhancement: Improving the ability and willingness to receive information

 Diagnostic Studies
 Evidence Based Practice
 Medications
 Pediatric/Geriatric/Lifespan

NURSING PRIORITY NO. 1   To develop plan for learning:

* Verify client's level of knowledge about specific topic. *Provides opportunity to ensure accuracy and completeness of knowledge base for future learning.*[4]
* Determine motivation and expectation for learning. *Provides insight useful in developing goals and identifying information needs.*[4]
* Assist client to identify learning goals and measurable outcomes. *Helps to frame or focus content to be learned. Provides motivation for learning and a measure to evaluate learning process.*[5,8]
* Ascertain preferred methods of learning (e.g., auditory, visual, interactive, or "hands-on"). *Identifies best approaches for the individual to facilitate learning process.*[5]
* ∞⊕ Note personal factors (e.g., age and developmental level, gender, social and cultural influences, religion, life experiences, level of education) *that may impact learning style, choice of informational resources, willingness to take control of situation, accept responsibility for change.*[2]
* Determine challenges to learning, such as language barriers (e.g., client cannot read, speaks or understands language other than that of care provider, dyslexia), physical factors (e.g., sensory deficits such as vision or hearing impairments, aphasia), physical stability (e.g., acute illness, activity intolerance), or difficulty of material to be learned. *Identifies special needs to be addressed if learning is to be successful.*[6]

NURSING PRIORITY NO. 2   To facilitate learning:

* 🏠 Provide information in varied formats appropriate to client's learning style (e.g., audiotapes, print materials, videos, classes or seminars, online). *Use of multiple formats increases learning and retention of material.*[3]
* Provide information about additional or outside learning resources (e.g., bibliotherapy, pertinent Web sites). *Promotes ongoing learning at own pace.*[7]
* Discuss ways to verify accuracy of informational resources. *Encourages independent search for learning opportunities while reducing likelihood of acting on erroneous or unproven data that could be detrimental to client's well-being.*[4]
* ⊚ Identify available community resources and support groups. *Provides additional opportunities for role modeling, skill training, anticipatory problem-solving, etc.*[1]
* Be aware of and discuss informal teaching and role modeling that takes place on an ongoing basis. *Incongruencies in community or peer role models and support group feedback and print advertisements, popular music, and videos may exist, creating questions and potentially undermining learning process.*[4]

NURSING PRIORITY NO. 3.   To enhance optimum wellness:

* 🏠 Assist client to identify ways to integrate and use information in all applicable areas (e.g., situational, environmental, personal). *Ability to apply or use information increases desire to learn and retention of information.*[5]
* Encourage client to journal, keep a log, or graph as appropriate. *Provides opportunity for self-evaluation of effects of learning, such as better management of chronic condition, reduction of risk factors, and acquisition of new skills.*[6,9]

DOCUMENTATION FOCUS

Assessment/Reassessment
* Individual findings, learning style and identified needs, presence of challenges to learning.
* Motivation and expectations for learning.

Planning
* Plan for learning, methods to be used, and who is involved in the planning.
* Educational plan.

 Acute Care   Collaborative   Community/ Home Care   Cultural

Implementation/Evaluation

- Responses of the client/significant other(s) to the educational plan and actions performed.
- How the learning is demonstrated.
- Attainment or progress toward desired outcome(s).
- Modifications to lifestyle or treatment plan.

Discharge Planning

- Additional learning and referral needs.

References

1. Bohny, B. A. (1997). A time for self-care: Role of the home healthcare nurse. *Home Healthc Nurse*, 15(4), 281–286.
2. Purnell, L. D. (2011). *Guide to Culturally Competent Health Care*. 2nd ed. Philadelphia: F. A. Davis.
3. Duffy, B. (1997). Using a creative teaching process with adult patients. *Home Healthc Nurse*, 15(2), 102–108.
4. Bartholomew, L. K. (2000). Watch, discover, think, and act: A model for patient education program development. *Patient Educ Couns*, 39(2–3), 269–280.
5. Clark, D. (2000, updated 2014). Learning styles and preferences. Retrieved April 2018 from http://www.nwlink.com/~donclark/hrd/styles.html.
6. Townsend, M. C. (2011). *Psychiatric Mental Health Nursing: Concepts of Care in Evidence-Based Practice*. 7th ed. Philadelphia: F. A. Davis, 377–533.
7. No author listed. (No date). Bloom's taxonomy of learning domains. The three types of learning. Retrieved April 2018 from http://www.nbna.org/files/Blooms%20Taxonomy%20of%20Learning.pdf.
8. Selwyn, N. (2012). *Education in a Digital World: Global Perspective*. New York: Routledge.
9. Adams, L. (No date). Learning a new skill is easier said than done. *Gordon Training International*. Retrieved April 2018 from http://www.gordontraining.com/free-workplace-articles/learning-a-new-skill-is-easier-said-than-done/.

Latex Allergy Reaction

Taxonomy II: Safety/Protection—Class 5 Defensive Processes (00041) [**Diagnostic Division:** Safety], Approved 1998; Revised 2006, 2017

DEFINITION: A hypersensitive reaction to natural latex rubber products.

RELATED FACTORS

To Be Developed

DEFINING CHARACTERISTICS

Subjective

Life-Threatening Reactions Within 1 Hour of Exposure:
Chest tightness

Type IV Reactions Occurring ≥1 hour After Exposure:
Discomfort reaction to additives
Skin irritation
Gastrointestinal Characteristics: Abdominal pain; nausea
Orofacial Characteristics: Itching; nasal congestion
Generalized Characteristics: Generalized discomfort; total body warmth

Objective

Life-Threatening Reactions Within 1 Hour of Exposure:
Contact urticaria progressing to generalized symptoms
Edema [e.g., lips, throat, tongue, uvula]

(continues on page 516)

 Diagnostic Studies   Evidence Based Practice   Medications   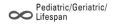 Pediatric/Geriatric/Lifespan

Latex Allergy Reaction (continued)

Dyspnea; wheezing; bronchospasm; respiratory arrest

Hypotension; syncope; myocardial infarction

Type IV Reactions Occurring ≥1 Hour After Exposure:

Eczema; skin irritation and/or redness

Orofacial Characteristics: Erythema; periorbital edema; rhinorrhea, tearing of the eyes

Generalized Characteristics: Skin flushing; generalized edema; restlessness

At Risk Population: Frequent exposure to latex product; history of latex reaction

History of allergy, or food allergy, or poinsettia plant allergy

History of asthma

History of surgery during infancy

Associated Condition: Hypersensitivity to natural latex rubber protein; multiple surgical procedures

Sample Clinical Applications: Multiple allergies, neural tube defects (e.g., spina bifida, myelomeningoceles), multiple surgeries at early age, chronic urological conditions (e.g., neurogenic bladder, exstrophy of bladder), spinal cord trauma

DESIRED OUTCOMES/EVALUATION CRITERIA

Sample NOC linkages:

Allergic Response: Localized: Severity of localized hypersensitive immune response to a specific environmental (exogenous) antigen

Allergic Response: Systemic: Severity of systemic hypersensitive immune response to a specific environmental (exogenous) antigen

Knowledge: Treatment Regimen: Extent of understanding conveyed about a specific treatment regimen

Client Will (Include Specific Time Frame)

• Be free of signs of hypersensitive response.

• Verbalize understanding of individual risks and responsibilities in avoiding exposure.

• Identify signs/symptoms requiring prompt intervention.

ACTIONS/INTERVENTIONS

Sample NIC linkages:

Latex Precautions: Reducing the risk of a systemic reaction to latex

Allergy Management: Identification, treatment, and prevention of allergic responses to food, medications, insect bites, contrast material, blood, or other substances

Environmental Management: Manipulation of the patient's surroundings for therapeutic benefit, sensory appeal, and psychological well-being

NURSING PRIORITY NO. 1　To assess contributing factors:

• Identify persons in high-risk categories such as (1) those with history of certain food allergies (e.g., banana, avocado, chestnut, kiwi, papaya, peach, nectarine); (2) prior allergies, asthma, and skin conditions (e.g., eczema and other dermatitis); (3) those occupationally exposed to latex products (e.g., healthcare workers, police, firefighters, emergency medical technicians [EMTs], food handlers, hairdressers, cleaning staff, factory workers in plants that manufacture latex-containing products); and (4) those with neural tube defects (e.g., spina bifida) or congenital urological conditions requiring frequent surgeries and/or catheterizations (e.g., exstrophy of the bladder). *Note: Studies have shown that while latex allergy is present in <1% of the general population, it is found in 8% to 17% of healthcare workers, and up to 68% of children with spina bifida.*[7,15,16]

 Acute Care　 Collaborative　 Community/Home Care　 Cultural

- Question client regarding latex allergy upon admission to healthcare facility, especially when procedures are anticipated (e.g., laboratory, emergency department, operating room, wound care management, 1-day surgery, dentist). *Basic safety information to help healthcare providers prevent/prepare for safe environment for client and themselves while providing care.*[2,4,7]
- Discuss history of exposure, e.g., client works in environment where latex is manufactured or latex gloves are used frequently, child was blowing up balloons (may be an acute reaction to the powder), use of condoms (may affect either partner), or individual requires frequent catheterizations. *Finding cause of reaction may be simple or complex but often requires diligent investigation and history-taking from multiple sources.*
- 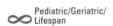Administer or note presence of positive skin-prick test, when performed. *Sensitive, specific, and rapid test but should be used with caution in persons with suspected sensitivity, as it carries risk of anaphylaxis.*[10]
- 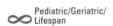Perform challenge or patch test, if appropriate, *to identify specific allergens in client with known type IV hypersensitivity. Note: Emergency department diagnosis and management depend on the history and physical examination as the following tests are not available in a useful time frame.*[10]
- 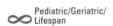Note response to radioallergosorbent test or enzyme-linked latex-specific IgE. *Performed to measure the quantity of IgE antibodies in serum after exposure to specific antigens and has generally replaced skin tests and provocation tests, which are inconvenient, often painful, and/or hazardous to the client. Note: These tests are useful in nonemergent evaluations.*[1,10,11]

NURSING PRIORITY NO. 2 To take measures to reduce/limit allergic response/avoid exposure to allergens:

- Ascertain client's current symptoms, noting rash, hives, and itching; red, teary eyes; and edema, diarrhea, nausea, and feeling of faintness. *Baseline for determining where the client is along a continuum of symptoms so that appropriate treatments can be initiated. Note: The most severe reactions tend to occur with latex proteins contacting internal tissues during invasive procedures and when they touch mucous membranes of the mouth, vagina, urethra, or rectum.*[7,9,12]
- Determine time since exposure (e.g., immediate or delayed onset such as 24–48 hr).
- Assess skin (usually hands but may be anywhere) for dry, crusty, hard bumps and horizontal cracks caused by irritation from chemicals used in/on the latex item (e.g., latex or powder used in latex gloves, condoms). *Dry, itchy rash (contact irritation) is the most common response and is not a true allergic reaction but can progress to a delayed type of allergic contact dermatitis with oozing blisters and spread in a way similar to poison ivy.*[2,12]
- Assist with treatment of contact dermatitis/type IV reaction:
  Wash affected skin with mild soap and water.
  Avoid latex gloves where possible; wear cotton glove liners where latex gloves must be used.
  Wash hands between glove changes and after each glove removal.
  Avoid powder, oil-based salves or lotions when using latex gloves. *Note: Powdered latex gloves are associated with higher amounts of aerosolized latex particles in the air. Those concerned with managing risks should minimize concentration of latex protein in the air in order to reduce respiratory and eye symptoms.*[5]
  Consider application of topical ointments such as corticosteroid, and antihistimine.
  Inform client that the most common cause is latex gloves but that many other products contain latex and could aggravate condition.
  Monitor closely for signs of systemic reactions (e.g., difficulty breathing or swallowing; wheezing; hoarseness; stridor; hypotension; tremors; chest pain; tachycardia; dysrhythmias; edema of face, eyelids, lips, tongue, and mucous membranes). *Type IV response can progress to type I anaphylaxis. A systematic review of studies found that a type I allergic reaction may be immediate in sensitized individuals and that acute treatment must be carried out in a latex-free environment.*[14]
  Note behavior such as agitation, restlessness, and expressions of fearfulness in the presence of above-listed symptoms. *Indicative of severe allergic response that can result in anaphylactic reaction and lead to respiratory or cardiac arrest.*[6]

Diagnostic Studies   Evidence Based Practice   Medications   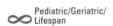Pediatric/Geriatric/Lifespan

Administer treatment, as appropriate, if severe or life-threatening reaction occurs:

Stop treatment or procedure, if needed.

Support airway and administer 100% oxygen or mechanical ventilation, if needed.

Administer emergency medications and treatments per protocol (e.g., antihistamines, epinephrine, corticosteroids, IV fluids).

- Educate care providers in ways to prevent inadvertent exposure (e.g., post latex precaution signs in client's room, document allergy to latex in chart, routinely monitor client's environment for latex-containing products and remove them promptly) and be prepared for emergency treatment measures should they be needed.
- Ascertain that latex-safe environment (e.g., surgical suite, hospital room) and products are available according to recommended facility guidelines and standards, including equipment and supplies (e.g., powder-free, low-protein latex products) and latex-free items (e.g., gloves, syringes, catheters, tubings, tape, thermometers, electrodes, oxygen cannulas, underpads, storage bags, diapers, feeding nipples), as appropriate.[2,9,10,13]
- Notify physicians, colleagues, and medical products suppliers of client's condition (e.g., pharmacy *so that medications can be prepared in latex-free environment,* home-care oxygen company *to provide latex-free cannulas). Users of latex gloves and purchasers should be aware that the risk of developing latex allergy is highest with the use of **powdered** latex gloves and that examination gloves may contain more latex allergen than surgical gloves.*[5]
- Encourage client to wear medical ID bracelet *to alert providers to condition if client is unresponsive.*[3,4,7]

NURSING PRIORITY NO. 3 To promote wellness (Teaching/Learning):

- Instruct in signs of reaction and emergency treatment needs. *Reactions range from skin irritation to anaphylaxis. Reaction may be gradual but progressive, affecting multiple body systems, or may be sudden, requiring lifesaving treatment. Allergy can result in chronic illness, disability, career loss, hardship, and death. There is no cure except complete avoidance of latex.*
- Emphasize the critical importance of taking immediate action for type I reaction *to limit life-threatening symptoms.*
- Demonstrate equipment and injection procedure and recommend client carry auto-injectable epinephrine *to provide timely emergency treatment, as needed.*
- Emphasize necessity of informing all new care providers of hypersensitivity *to reduce preventable exposures.*
- Instruct client/family/significant other (SO) that latex exposure occurs through contact with skin or mucous membrane, by inhalation, parenteral injection, or wound inoculation.
- Instruct client/SO to survey and routinely monitor environment for latex-containing products and replace as needed.
- Provide printed lists or Web sites for identifying common household products that may contain latex (e.g., carpet backing, hoses, rubber grip utensils, diapers, undergarments, shoes, toys, pacifiers, computer mouse pads, erasers, rubber bands, etc.) and where to obtain latex-free products and supplies.[4,7]
- Provide resource and assistance numbers for emergencies. *When allergy is suspected or the potential for allergy exists, protection must begin with identification and removal of possible sources of latex.*
- Provide work site review, where indicated, and recommendations to prevent exposure. *Latex allergy can be a disabling occupational disorder. Education about the problem promotes prevention of allergic reaction, facilitates timely intervention, and helps nurse to protect clients, latex-sensitive colleagues, and themselves.*[3,4]
- Recommend full medical work-up for client presenting with hand dermatitis, especially if job tasks include use of latex.[8]
- Contact suppliers to verify that latex-free equipment, products, and supplies are available, including (but not limited to) low-allergen or powder-free synthetic gloves, airways, masks, stethoscope tubings, IV tubing, tape, thermometers, urinary catheters, stomach and intestinal tubes, electrodes, oxygen cannulas, pencil erasers, wrist name bands, and rubber bands.[7]
- Ascertain that procedures are in place to identify and resolve problems with medical devices relevant to allergic reactions or glove performance.[4]

 Acute Care   Collaborative   Community/ Home Care   Cultural

- Advise client to be aware of potential for related food allergies (e.g., bananas, kiwis, melons, tomatoes, avocados, nuts). *These foods can trigger a latex-like allergic reaction because the proteins in them mimic latex proteins as they break down in the body.*
- Refer to resources, including, but not limited to, ALERT (Allergy to Latex Education & Resource Team, Inc.), Latex Allergy News, Spina Bifida Association, National Institute for Occupational Safety and Health, Kendall's Healthcare Products (Web site), and Hudson RCI (Web site), *for further information about common latex products in the home, latex-free products, and assistance.*

DOCUMENTATION FOCUS

Assessment/Reassessment

- Assessment findings including type and extent of symptoms.
- Pertinent history of contact with latex products and frequency of exposure.

Planning

- Plan of care and interventions and who is involved in planning.
- Teaching plan.

Implementation/Evaluation

- Response to interventions, teaching, and actions performed.
- Attainment or progress toward desired outcome(s).
- Modifications to plan of care.

Discharge Planning

- Discharge needs, specific referrals made, and additional resources available.

References

1. Cavanaugh, B. M. (2003). *Nurse's Manual of Diagnostic Tests.* 4th ed. Philadelphia, PA: F. A. Davis.
2. Hohler, S. (2015). Latex allergy: Protecting patients and staff. *OR Nurse 2015*, 9(1), 12–15.
3. National Institutes for Occupational Safety and Health (NIOSH). (Updated 2014). Latex allergy: A prevention guide. Retrieved April 2018 http://www.cdc.gov/niosh/docs/98-113/.
4. Sattler, B. (2001). Occupational and environmental risks in nursing. Retrieved April 2018 http://ana.nursingworld.org/mods/archive/mod312/cerm304.htm.
5. Nicholson, P. J. (2010). Evidence-based guidelines: Occupational contact dermatitis and urticaria. *Occup Med*, 60(502), 504.
6. Sommers, M. S., Johnson, S. A. (eds). (1997). Urticaria and angioedema. *Davis's Manual of Nursing Therapeutics for Diseases and Disorders*. Philadelphia, PA: F. A. Davis.
7. American Latex Allergy Association. (2018). Statistics. Retrieved April 2018 from http://latexallergyresources.org/statistics.
8. Worthington, K., Wilburn, S. (2001). Latex allergy: What's the facility's responsibility and what's yours? *Am J Nurs*, 101(7), 88.
9. Klotter, J. (2006). *Latex allergy prevention*. Townsend Letter for Doctors and Patients, May 1, 2006.
10. Behrman, A. J. (Updated 2016). Latex allergy. Retrieved April 2018 from http://emedicine.medscape.com/article/756632-overview.
11. Allergy testing. (Updated 2014). Article for Lab Tests Online (various pages). Retrieved April 2018 from http://labtestsonline.org/understanding/analytes/allergy/tab/test.
12. Gavin, M., Patti, P. J. (2009). Issues in latex allergy in children and adults receiving home healthcare. *Home Healthc Nurse*, 27(4), 231–239.
13. AORN Latex Guideline: 2004 standards, recommended practices, and guidelines. *AORN J*, 79(3), 653–672.
14. Hepner, D. L., Castells, M. C. (2003). Latex allergy: An update. *Anesth Analg*, 96(5 Suppl), 1219–1229.
15. Dorevitch, S., Forst, M. C. (2000). The occupational hazards of emergency physicians. *Am J Emerg Med*, 18(3), 300–311.
16. Galindo, M. J., et al. (2011). Latex allergy in primary care providers. *J Investig Allergol Clin Immunol*, 21(6), 459–465.

risk for Latex Allergy Reaction

Taxonomy II: Safety/Protection—Class 5 Defensive Processes (00042) [**Diagnostic Division:** Safety], Submitted 1998; Revised 2006, 2013, 2017

DEFINITION: Susceptible to a hypersensitivity to natural latex rubber products, which may compromise health.

RISK FACTORS
To Be Developed
At Risk Population: Frequent exposure to latex product; history of latex reaction
History of allergy, or food allergy, or poinsettia plant allergy
History of asthma
History of surgery during infancy
Associated Condition: Hypersensitivity to natural latex rubber protein; multiple surgical procedures
Sample Clinical Applications: Multiple allergies, neural tube defects (e.g., spina bifida, myelomeningoceles), multiple surgeries at early age, chronic urological conditions (e.g., neurogenic bladder, exstrophy of bladder), spinal cord trauma

DESIRED OUTCOMES/EVALUATION CRITERIA

Sample NOC linkages:
Allergic Response: Localized: Severity of localized hypersensitive immune response to a specific environmental (exogenous) antigen
Risk Control: Personal actions to understand, prevent, eliminate, or reduce modifiable health threats
Knowledge: Health Behavior: Extent of understanding conveyed about the promotion and protection of health

Client Will (Include Specific Time Frame)
• Identify and correct potential risk factors in the environment.
• Demonstrate appropriate lifestyle changes to reduce risk of exposure.
• Identify resources to assist in promoting a safe environment.
• Recognize need for and seek assistance to limit response or complications.

ACTIONS/INTERVENTIONS

Sample NIC linkages:
Latex Precautions: Reducing the risk of a systemic reaction to latex
Allergy Management: Identification, treatment, and prevention of allergic responses to food, medications, insect bites, contrast material, blood, or other substances
Risk Identification: Analysis of potential risk factors, determination of health risks, and prioritization of risk-reduction strategies for an individual or group

NURSING PRIORITY NO. 1   To assess causative/contributing factors:

• Identify persons in high-risk categories such as (1) those with history of certain food allergies (e.g., banana, avocado, chestnut, kiwi, papaya, peach, nectarine), (2) those with asthma or skin conditions (e.g., eczema), (3) those occupationally exposed to latex products (e.g., healthcare workers, police/firefighters, emergency medical technicians [EMTs], food handlers, hairdressers, cleaning staff, factory workers in plants that manufacture latex-containing products), and (4) those with neural tube defects (e.g., spina bifida) or congenital

 Acute Care   Collaborative   Community/ Home Care   Cultural

urological conditions requiring frequent surgeries and/or catheterizations (e.g., exstrophy of the bladder). *Most latex allergies are diagnosed by a detailed client history plus physical examination. Note: Studies have shown that while latex allergy is present in <1% of the general population, it is found in 8% to 17% of healthcare workers and in up to 68% of children with spina bifida.*[2,10–12] *Note: The most severe reactions tend to occur with latex proteins contacting internal tissues during invasive procedures and when they touch mucous membranes of the mouth, lungs, vagina, urethra, or rectum.*[2,5–7]

- Question client regarding latex allergy upon admission to each healthcare facility, especially when procedures are anticipated (e.g., new physician/healthcare provider, laboratory, emergency department, operating room, wound care management, 1-day surgery, dentist). *Current information indicates that natural latex is found in thousands of medical supplies; however, most manufacturers are now using synthetic latex for products, and new synthetic latex is under development. These products are associated with fewer allergic reactions among individuals who are sensitive to natural latex.*[1,2]

NURSING PRIORITY NO. 2 To assist in correcting factors that could lead to latex allergy:

- Ascertain that facilities have established policies and procedures. *Promotes awareness in the workplace to address safety and reduce risk to workers and clients.*[3]
- Create latex-safe environments in care setting (e.g., substitute nonlatex products, such as natural rubber gloves, polyvinyl chloride (PVC) IV tubing, latex-free tape, thermometers, electrodes, oxygen cannulas). *Reduces risk of exposure.*[8,9]
- Promote good skin care when latex gloves may be preferred/required for barrier protection (e.g., in specific disease conditions such as HIV or during surgery). Use powder-free gloves, change gloves frequently, and wash hands immediately after glove removal; refrain from use of oil-based hand cream. *Reduces dermal and respiratory exposure to latex proteins that bind to the powder in gloves.*[2,4]
- 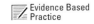 Discuss necessity of avoiding latex exposure. Recommend or assist high-risk client/family to survey environment and remove any medical or household products containing latex. *Avoidance of latex is the only way to prevent the allergic reaction.*[2]
- Provide worksite review, where indicated, and recommendations to prevent exposure. *Latex allergy can be a disabling occupational disorder. Education about the problem promotes prevention of allergic reaction, facilitates timely intervention, and helps nurse to protect clients, latex-sensitive colleagues, and themselves.*[1,4]

NURSING PRIORITY NO. 3 To promote wellness (Teaching/Discharge Considerations):

- 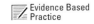 Instruct client/caregivers about types of potential reactions. *Reaction may be gradual and progressive (e.g., irritant contact rash with gloves); can be progressive, affecting multiple body systems; or may be sudden and anaphylactic, requiring lifesaving treatment.*[1,3]
- Identify measures to take if reactions occur and ways to avoid exposure to latex products *to reduce risk of injury and provide for prompt intervention.* (Refer to ND Latex Allergy Reaction.)
- Refer to allergist for testing as appropriate. *Testing may include the challenge test with latex gloves, a skin patch test, or a blood test for IgE.*
- Encourage client to wear medical ID bracelet/necklace and emphasize the importance of informing all new care providers of hypersensitivity *to reduce preventable exposures.*[1,4]
- Refer to resources (e.g., Latex Allergy News, National Institute for Occupational Safety and Health, Kendall's Healthcare Products [Web site], Hudson RCI [Web site]) *for further information about common latex products in the home, latex-free products, and assistance.*

DOCUMENTATION FOCUS

Assessment/Reassessment
- Assessment findings, pertinent history of contact with latex products, and frequency of exposure.

 Diagnostic Studies   Evidence Based Practice Medications Pediatric/Geriatric/Lifespan

Planning
- Plan of care and who is involved in planning.
- Teaching plan.

Implementation/Evaluation
- Response to interventions, teaching, and actions performed.
- Attainment or progress toward desired outcome(s).
- Modifications to plan of care.

Discharge Planning
- Long-term needs and who is responsible for actions to be taken.
- Specific referrals made.

References

1. Sattler, B. (2001). Occupational and environmental risks in nursing. Retrieved April 2018 from http://ana.nursingworld.org/mods/archive/mod312/cerm304.htm.
2. Lenehan, G. P. (2002). Latex allergy: Separating fact from fiction. *Nursing*, 32(3), 58–64.
3. Hohler, S. (2015). Latex allergy: Protecting patients and staff. *OR Nurse 2015*, 9(1), 12–15.
4. National Institutes for Occupational Safety and Health (NIOSH). (Updated 2014). Latex allergy: A prevention guide. Retrieved April 2018 from http://www.cdc.gov/niosh/docs/98-113/.
5. Klotter, J. (2006). Latex allergy prevention. *Townsend Letter for Doctors and Patients*, May 1.
6. Behrman, A. J. (Updated 2016). Latex allergy. Retrieved 2018 from http://emedicine.medscape.com/article/756632-overview.
7. Blahd, W. (Updated 2016). Are you allergic to latex? Retrieved April 2018 from www.webmd.com/allergies/guide/latex-allergies.
8. Association of Operating Room Nurses. (2006). Standards, recommended practices and guidelines. *AORN J*, 79(3), 199–214.
9. MoInlycke Health Care, US, LLC. (2006). Latex-safe is best gloving practice against latex allergy. *PR Newswire*. Retrieved April 2018 from http://www.prnewswire.com/news-releases/latex-safe-is-best-gloving-practice-against-latex-allergy-molnlycke-says-56008667.html.
10. American Latex Allergy Association. (2018). Statistics. Retrieved April 2018 from http://latexallergyresources.org/statistics.
11. Dorevitch, S., Forst, M. C. (2000). The occupational hazards of emergency physicians. *Am J Emerg Med*, 18(3), 300–311.
12. Galindo, M. J., Quirce, S., Garcia, O. L. (2011). Latex allergy in primary care providers. *J Investig Allergol Clin Immunol*, 21(6), 459–465.

sedentary Lifestyle

Taxonomy II: Health Promotion—Class 1 Health Awareness (00168) **[Diagnostic Division:** Activity/Rest], Approved 2004

DEFINITION: A habit of life that is characterized by a low physical activity level.

RELATED FACTORS
Insufficient interest in, motivation, or resources [e.g., time, money, companionship, facilities] for physical activity
Insufficient training for physical exercise
Insufficient knowledge of health benefits associated with physical exercise

DEFINING CHARACTERISTICS

Subjective
Preference for activity low in physical activity

Objective
Average daily physical activity is less than recommended for gender and age
Physical deconditioning

 Acute Care   Collaborative   Community/Home Care   Cultural

Sample Clinical Applications: Chronic or debilitating conditions (e.g., arthritis, multiple sclerosis [MS], chronic obstructive pulmonary disease [COPD], heart failure, paralysis), chronic pain, obesity, depression

DESIRED OUTCOMES/EVALUATION CRITERIA

Sample NOC linkages:
Knowledge: Prescribed Activity: Extent of understanding conveyed about physical activity by a health professional for a specific condition
Exercise Participation: Personal actions to perform a self-planned, structured, and repetitive regimen to maintain or advance the level of fitness and health

Client Will (Include Specific Time Frame)
• Verbalize understanding of importance of regular exercise to general well-being.
• Identify necessary precautions, safety concerns, and self-monitoring techniques.
• Formulate and implement realistic exercise program with gradual increase in activity.

ACTIONS/INTERVENTIONS

Sample NIC linkages:
Exercise Promotion: Facilitation of regular physical activity to maintain or advance to a higher level of fitness and health
Teaching: Prescribed Exercise: Preparing a patient to achieve or maintain a prescribed level of exercise
Self-Modification Assistance: Reinforcement of self-directed change initiated by the patient to achieve personally important goals

NURSING PRIORITY NO. 1 To assess precipitating/etiological factors:

• Identify client's specific condition(s) (e.g., obesity, depression, MS, arthritis, Parkinson's disease, surgery, hemiplegia or paraplegia, chronic pain, brain injury) *that may contribute to immobility or the onset and continuation of inactivity or sedentary lifestyle.*
• ∞ Assess client's age, developmental level, motor skills, ease and capability of movement, and posture and gait. *Determines type and intensity of needed interventions related to activity.*[1]
• Determine client's current weight and body mass index (BMI); note dietary habits. *If client is overweight and BMI is not in healthy range, a weight-loss program should be suggested along with exercise. Note: In general, BMI is considered a reliable measure of body fat for men and women. However, changes in body composition and stature that occur with aging can influence the reliability of BMI as a marker of body fat.*[8,12]
• Assess physical capabilities to participate in exercise/activities, noting attention span, physical limitations and tolerance, level of interest or desire, and safety needs. *Identifies barriers that need to be addressed.*[1,6]
• Review usual activities and work requirements/environment. *Absence of regular exercise and the presence of a stressful job with little physical exercise increases likelihood of deconditioning. Note: In 2008, the World Health Organization (WHO) reported that globally, around 31% of adults (aged 15 and over) were insufficiently active.*[7,8]
• Note emotional and behavioral responses to problems associated with a self- or condition-imposed sedentary lifestyle. *Feelings of disinterest, frustration, and powerlessness may impede attainment of goals.*[2]
• Determine family dynamics and support provided by family/friends. *Major lifestyle change may require support of others to achieve and maintain goals or client may be at increased risk of slipping back into "old" ways.*[8]
• Ascertain availability of resources (e.g., finances for gym membership, transportation, exercise facility or gym at work site, proximity of walking trail or bike path, safety of neighborhood for outdoor activity).

 Diagnostic Studies   Evidence Based Practice   Medications 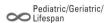 Pediatric/Geriatric/Lifespan

NURSING PRIORITY NO. 2   To motivate and stimulate client involvement:

- 🏠 Establish therapeutic relationship, acknowledging reality of situation and client's feelings. *Changing a life-long habit can be difficult, and client may feel discouraged with body and hopeless to turn situation into a positive experience.*[2]
- 🌐 Ascertain client's perception of current activity and exercise patterns, impact on life, and cultural expectations of client/others. *Helps to determine whether or not client perceives need for change and potential limitations in choices for activities.*[8]
- Discuss client's stated motivation for change. *Concerns of client/significant others (SOs) regarding threats to personal health/longevity or acceptance by teen peers may be sufficient to cause client to initiate change; however, client must want to change for himself or herself in order to sustain change.*[4,8]
- Review necessity for and benefits of regular exercise. *Research confirms that exercise has benefits for the whole body (e.g., can boost energy, enhance coordination, reduce muscle deterioration, improve circulation, lower blood pressure, produce healthier skin and a toned body, prolong youthful appearance). Regular exercise has also been found to boost cardiac fitness in both conditioned and out-of-shape individuals. Conversely, studies continue to demonstrate the prevalence of reduced physical activity. Sociocultural changes (e.g., increased reliance on automobiles and other modern conveniences) have reduced the need to be physically active. Computers and television have promoted a sedentary lifestyle for adults and children, whose opportunities for physical activity have been further diminished because of academic pressures, overscheduling, and safety concerns for out-of-doors play. Suburban living has produced long commutes to work, and technological advances have resulted in more people working in occupations that require no physical activity.*[4,13]
- Counsel client regarding individual health risks. *Focuses attention on own situation and helps prioritize needs, making change more manageable.*[8]
- Involve client, SO/parent, or caregiver in developing exercise plan and goals *to meet individual needs, desires, and available resources. Also increases commitment to program and successful attainment of goals.*
- Introduce activities at client's current level of functioning, progressing to more complex activities, as tolerated. *Reduces likelihood of overwhelming client at the beginning and maintains interest over time.*
- ∞ Recommend mix of age- and gender-appropriate activities or stimuli (e.g., movement classes, walking, hiking, jazzercise, swimming, biking, skating, bowling, golf, weight training). *Activities need to be personally meaningful for client to derive the most enjoyment and to sustain motivation to continue with program.*[2,6]
- Encourage change of scenery (indoors and outdoors where possible) and periodic changes in the personal environment when client is confined inside.

NURSING PRIORITY NO. 3   To promote optimal level of function and prevent exercise failure:

- 🏠 👥 Assist with treatment of underlying condition impacting participation in activities *to maximize function within limitations of situation.* Refer to dietitian for weight-loss program, as indicated.
- 👥 Collaborate with physical medicine specialist or occupational or physical therapist in providing active or passive range-of-motion exercises and isotonic muscle contractions. *Techniques such as gait training, strength training, and exercise to improve balance and coordination can be helpful in rehabilitating client.*[1]
- Schedule ample time to perform exercise activities balanced with adequate rest periods.[1]
- Provide for safety measures as indicated by individual situation, including environmental management and fall prevention. (Refer to ND risk for Falls.)
- Reevaluate ability/commitment periodically. *Changes in strength or endurance signal readiness for progression of activities or possibly to decrease exercise if overly fatigued. Wavering commitment may require change in types of activities and/or the addition of a workout buddy to reenergize involvement.*[2,5]
- Discuss discrepancies in planned and performed activities with client aware and unaware of observation. *Suggest methods for dealing with identified problems. May be necessary when client is using avoidance or controlling behavior or is not aware of own abilities due to anxiety or fear.*[2,5]

 Acute Care   Collaborative   Community/ Home Care   Cultural

NURSING PRIORITY NO. 4 To promote wellness (Teaching/Discharge Considerations):

- 🏠 Educate client/SO about benefits of physical activity as it relates to client's particular situation. *Many studies have shown the health benefits of physical activity in the setting of chronic illness (e.g., it increases function in arthritis, improves glycemic control in type 2 diabetes, and can enhance quality of life).*[10,11]
- Review components of physical fitness: (1) muscle strength and endurance, (2) flexibility, (3) body composition (muscle mass, percentage of body fat), and (4) cardiovascular health. *Fitness routines need to include all elements to attain maximized benefits and prevent deconditioning.*[4,5,7]
- Instruct in safety measures, as individually indicated (e.g., warm-up and cool-down activities; taking pulse before, during, and after activity; adequate intake of fluids, especially during hot weather or strenuous activity; wearing reflective clothing when jogging or reflectors on bicycle; locking wheelchair before transfers; judicious use of medications; supervision, as indicated).[1]
- Recommend keeping an activity or exercise log, including physical and psychological responses and changes in weight, endurance, and body mass. *Provides visual evidence of progress or goal attainment and encouragement to continue with program.*[2,6]
- Encourage client to involve self in exercise *as part of wellness management for the whole person.*[3,6]
- ∞ Encourage parents to set a positive example for children *by participating in exercise and engaging in an active lifestyle.*[3,6]
- Identify community resources, charity activities, and support groups. *Community walking/hiking trails, sports leagues, etc., provide free/low-cost options. Activities such as 5k walks for charity, participation in Special Olympics, or age-related competitive games provide goals to work toward. Note: Some individuals may prefer solitary activities; however, most individuals enjoy supportive companionship when exercising.*[3,4]
- Discuss alternatives for exercise program in changing circumstances (e.g., walking the mall during inclement weather, using exercise facilities at hotel when traveling, water aerobics at local swimming pool, joining a gym).
- Promote individual participation in community awareness of problem and discussion of solutions. *Physical inactivity (and associated diseases) is a major public health problem that affects large numbers of people in all regions of the world. Recognizing the problem and future consequences may empower the global community to develop effective measures to promote physical activity and improve public health.*[7]
- Promote community goals for increasing physical activity, such as school-based physical education; the Sports, Play, and Active Recreation for Kids program; a "buddy" system or contracting for specific physical activities; and the Physician-Based Assessment and Counseling for Exercise, *to address national concerns about obesity and major barriers to physical activity, such as time constraints, lack of training in physical activity, behavioral change methods, and lack of standard protocols.*[3,6,7,9]

DOCUMENTATION FOCUS

Assessment/Reassessment
- Individual findings, including level of function and ability to participate in specific or desired activities, motivation for change.

Planning
- Plan of care and who is involved in the planning.
- Teaching plan.

Implementation/Evaluation
- Responses to interventions, teaching, and actions performed.
- Attainment or progress toward desired outcome(s).
- Modifications to plan of care.

Discharge Planning
- Discharge and long-term needs, noting who is responsible for each action to be taken.
- Specific referrals made.
- Sources of and maintenance for assistive devices.

 Diagnostic Studies   Evidence Based Practice   Medications 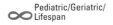 Pediatric/Geriatric/Lifespan

References

1. Boesch, C., Meyers, J., Habersaat, A. (2005). Maintenance of exercise capacity and physical activity patterns after cardiac rehabilitation. *J Cardiopulm Rehabil*, 25(1), 14–21.

2. Office of Behavioral and Social Sciences Research (OBSSR). (2006). The importance of behavioral and social sciences research to health: Health promotion and disease prevention. Bethesda, MD: OBSSR and the National Institutes of Health.

3. Wehling-Weepie, A. K., McCarthy, A. (2002). A healthy lifestyle program: Promoting child health in schools. *J School Nurs*, 18(6), 322–328.

4. Budd, G. M., Peterson, J. A. (2014). The obesity epidemic, part 1: Understanding the origins. *Am J Nurs*, 114(12), 40–46.

5. Lai, S. C., Cohen, M. N. (1999). Promoting lifestyle changes. *Am J Nurs*, 99(4), 63.

6. Fries, W. C. (2005). Family fitness across the generations. Retrieved April 2018 from http://www.medicinenet.com/script/main/art.asp?articlekey=56090.

7. World Health Organization. (2018). Physical inactivity: A global public health problem. Retrieved April 2018 from http://www.who.int/dietphysicalactivity/factsheet_inactivity/en/#.

8. Morantz, C., Torrey, B. (2004). Obesity and sedentary lifestyle guidelines. *Am Fam Physician*, 69(10), 2479–2480.

9. Task Force on Community Preventive Services—Independent Expert Panel. (2002). Recommendations to increase physical activities in communities. *Am J Prev Med*, 22(2 Suppl), 67–72.

10. Conn, V. S., et al. (2008). Physical activity interventions among adults with arthritis: Meta-analysis of outcomes. *Semin Arthritis Rheum*, 37(5), 307–316.

11. Conn, V. S., et al. (2007). Metabolic effects of interventions to increase physical exercise in adults with type 2 diabetes. *Diabetologia*, 50(5), 913–921.

12. Zamboni, M., et al. (2003). Body composition changes in stable-weight elderly subjects: The effect of sex. *Aging Clin Exp Res*, 15(4), 321–327.

13. Warburtin, D. E. R., Nicol, C. W., Bredin, S. S. D. (2006). Narrative review: Health benefits of physical activity: The evidence. *CMAJ*, 174(6), 801–809.

---

risk for impaired Liver Function

Taxonomy II: Nutrition—Class 4 Metabolism (0000178) **[Diagnostic Division:** Food/Fluid**],** Approved 2006; Revised 2008, 2013, 2017

DEFINITION: Susceptible to a decrease in liver function, which may compromise health.

RISK FACTORS

Substance misuse/[abuse]

Associated Condition: Human immunodeficiency virus (HIV) coinfection; viral infection
Pharmaceutical agent

Sample Clinical Applications: Hepatitis, HIV, substance abuse, drug overdose (acetaminophen), Epstein-Barr infection

DESIRED OUTCOMES/EVALUATION CRITERIA

Sample **NOC** linkages:

Knowledge: Disease Process: Extent of understanding conveyed about a specific disease process

Risk Control: Personal actions to understand, prevent, eliminate, or reduce modifiable health threats

Liver Function: Ability of the liver to manufacture, store, alter, and secrete substances essential for metabolism and other body functions

Client Will (Include Specific Time Frame)

• Verbalize understanding of individual risk factors that contribute to possibility of liver damage/failure.

• Demonstrate behaviors, lifestyle changes to reduce risk factors and protect self from injury.

• Be free of signs of liver failure as evidenced by liver function studies within normal range, and absence of jaundice, hepatic enlargement, or altered mental status.

 Acute Care   Collaborative   Community/Home Care   Cultural

ACTIONS/INTERVENTIONS

Sample NIC linkages:

Risk Identification: Analysis of potential risk factors, determination of health risk, and prioritization of risk reduction strategies for an individual or group

Infection Protection: Prevention and early detection of infection in a patient at risk

Substance Use Treatment: Care of patient and family members demonstrating dysfunction as a result of substance abuse or dependence

NURSING PRIORITY NO. 1 To identify individual risk factors/needs:

- Determine presence of disease condition(s), noting whether problem is acute (e.g., viral hepatitis, acetaminophen overdose) or chronic (e.g., alcoholic cirrhosis). *Influences choice of interventions.*
- Note client history of known/possible exposure to virus, bacteria, or toxins *that can damage liver:*[1–5,12,13]

  Works in high-risk occupation (e.g., performs tasks that involve contact with blood, blood-contaminated body fluids, other body fluids, or sharps). *Carries high risk for exposure to hepatitis B and C.*

  Injects drugs, especially if client shared a needle; received tattoo or piercing with an unsterile needle.

  Received blood or blood products prior to 1989.

  Ingested contaminated food or water or experienced poor sanitation practices by food service workers. *Poses risk for exposure to enteric viruses (hepatitis A and E).*

  Close contact (e.g., lives with or has sex with infected person or carrier; infant born to infected mother).

  Regular exposure to toxic chemicals (e.g., carbon tetrachloride cleaning agents, bug spray, paint fumes, tobacco smoke).

  Uses prescription drugs (e.g., sulfonamides, phenothiazines, isoniazid).

  Ingests certain herbal remedies or megadoses of vitamins.

  Uses alcohol with medications (including over-the-counter [OTC] medications).

  Consumes alcohol heavily and/or over long period of time.

  Ingested acetaminophen (accidentally, as may occur when client takes too large a dose or has several medications containing acetaminophen over time, or intentionally, as may occur with suicide attempt).

  Travels internationally to or emigrates from countries such as Africa, Southeast Asia, Korea, China, Vietnam, Eastern Europe, Mediterranean countries, or the Caribbean *(where hepatitis is endemic).*

- Review results of laboratory tests (e.g., liver function studies, such as hepatic function panel including alanine aminotransferase, alkaline phosphatase, aspartate aminotransferase; bilirubin, gamma-glutamyl transferase, lactic acid dehydrogenase, albumin, total protein and prothrombin time; drug levels, hepatitis screening tests and titers) and other diagnostic studies (e.g., ultrasonography, CT scanning, MRI imaging) *that indicate presence of hepatotoxic condition and need for medical treatment.*[6,15]

NURSING PRIORITY NO. 2 To assist client to reduce or correct individual risk factors:

- Assist with medical treatment of underlying condition (e.g., hepatitis, alcoholism, drug overdose) *to support organ function and minimize liver damage.*
- Educate client/significant other on way(s) to prevent exposure to or incidence of hepatitis infections and limit damage to liver:[4,9,17]

  Practice safer sex (e.g., avoid multiple-partner sex, wear condoms, avoid sex with partners known to be infected).

  Wash hands well after using the bathroom or changing soiled diapers.

  Avoid injecting drugs or sharing needles.

  Avoid sharing razors, toothbrushes, or nail clippers.

  Make sure needles and inks are sterile for tattooing and body piercing.

 Diagnostic Studies   Evidence Based Practice   Medications   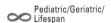 Pediatric/Geriatric/ Lifespan   **527**

Use proper precautions and appropriate protective equipment when working in high-risk occupations (e.g., healthcare, police and fire departments, emergency services, day-care services, chemical manufacturing) *where most at risk for inhalation of toxins or needlesticks or body fluid exposures.*

Avoid tap water and practice good hygiene and sanitation when traveling internationally.

Use harsh cleansers and aerosol products in well-ventilated room; wear mask and gloves, cover skin, and wash well afterward. *Chemicals can reach the liver through skin and destroy liver cells.*

Obtain vaccinations when appropriate. *Some hepatitis strains (e.g., A and B) are preventable, thus minimizing risk of liver damage.*

- Discuss safe use and concerns about client's medication regimen (e.g., acetaminophen, NSAIDs, herbal or vitamin supplements, phenobarbital, cholesterol-lowering drugs such as statins, certain antibiotics [e.g., sulfonamides, isonicotinyl hydrazine], certain cardiovascular drugs [e.g., amiodarone, hydralazine], certain antidepressants [e.g., tricyclics]) *known to cause hepatotoxicity, either alone or in combination or in overdose situation. Note: Many OTC and prescription medicines, even "natural" or herbal remedies, contain chemicals that can harm the liver over time. Very high doses of certain pain relievers (e.g., acetaminophen) can cause liver failure.*[6–9]

- Encourage client to read labels, especially when taking acetaminophen for pain, to determine strength of medication, note safe number of doses over 24 hr, and become familiar with "hidden" sources of acetaminophen (e.g., Nyquil, Vicodin). Limit alcohol intake *to avoid or reduce risk of liver damage. Note: Studies have demonstrated that alcoholic clients may develop severe, even fatal, toxic liver injury after ingestion of standard therapeutic doses of acetaminophen.*[5,13,14]

- Emphasize importance of responsible drinking (e.g., men should limit alcohol to no more than two drinks/day, and women, one drink/day) or avoid alcohol altogether when indicated (if client has any kind of liver disease) *to reduce incidence of cirrhosis and severity of liver damage or failure.*[4,11]

- Encourage smoking cessation. *The additives in cigarettes pose a challenge to the liver by reducing its ability to eliminate toxins.*[15]

- Encourage client with liver dysfunction to avoid fatty foods. *Fat interferes with normal function of liver cells and can cause additional damage and permanent scarring to liver cells when they can no longer regenerate.*[8]

- Refer to nutritionist, as indicated, for dietary needs, including calories, proteins, vitamins, and trace minerals *to promote healing and limit effects of deficiencies. Note: A balanced diet for liver health includes proteins, fruits, and vegetables and is low in cholesterol, fats, carbohydrates, and simple sugars.*[16,17]

- Discuss signs/symptoms (e.g., increased abdominal girth; rapid weight loss or gain; increased peripheral edema; dyspnea, fever; blood in stool or urine; excess bleeding of any kind; jaundice) *that warrant prompt notification of healthcare provider for evaluation and treatment of severe liver dysfunction and possible organ failure.*[9]

- Refer to specialist or liver treatment center, as indicated. *May be beneficial for client with chronic liver disease when decompensating, for client with hepatitis and other coexisting disease condition (e.g., HIV), or for client with intolerance to treatment due to side effects.*

NURSING PRIORITY NO. 3 To promote wellness (Teaching/Discharge Considerations):

- Emphasize importance of hand hygiene, use of bottled water, and avoidance of fresh produce and raw meat/seafood *if client is traveling to area where hepatitis A is endemic or food/waterborne illness is a risk.*[10]

- Instruct in measures including protection from blood or other body fluids and sharps safety, safer-sex practices, avoiding needle sharing, and body tattoos and piercings *to prevent occupational and nonoccupational exposures to hepatitis.*

- Discuss need for vaccination, as indicated (e.g., healthcare and public safety worker, children under 18, international traveler, recreational drug user, men who have sex with other men, client with clotting disorders or liver disease, anyone sharing household with an infected person) *to prevent exposure and transmission of blood or body fluid hepatitis and limit risk of liver injury.*[10]

- Discuss appropriateness of prophylaxis immunizations. *Although the best way to protect against hepatitis B and C infections is to prevent exposure to viruses, postexposure prophylaxis should be initiated promptly*

 Acute Care   Collaborative   Community/Home Care   Cultural

to prevent or limit severity of infection, especially in persons with close contact with infected individual or in client with compromised immune system.[11]

- Provide information regarding availability of gamma globulin, immune serum globulin, hepatitis B immune globulin, and HB vaccine (Recombivax HB, Engerix-B) through the health department or family physician.
- Emphasize necessity of follow-up care (in client with chronic liver disease) *to monitor liver function and effectiveness of interventions* and importance of adherence to therapeutic regimen *to prevent or minimize permanent liver damage.*
- Refer to community resources for immunizations/drug/alcohol treatment program, as indicated.

DOCUMENTATION FOCUS

Assessment/Reassessment
- Assessment findings, including individual risk factors.
- Results of laboratory tests and diagnostic studies.

Planning
- Plan of care and who is involved in planning.
- Teaching plan.

Implementation/Evaluation
- Response to interventions, teaching, and actions performed.
- Attainment or progress toward desired outcome(s).
- Modifications to plan of care.

Discharge Planning
- Long-term needs, plan for follow-up, and who is responsible for actions to be taken.
- Specific referrals made.

References

1. Bockhold, K. M. (2000). Who's afraid of hepatitis C? *Am J Nurs,* 100(5), 26–32.
2. Shovein, J. T., Camozo, R. J., Hyams, I. (2000). Hepatitis A: How benign is it? *Am J Nurs,* 100(3), 43–47.
3. National Digestive Diseases Information Clearinghouse (NDDIC). (Updated 2017). Hepatitis (Viral). *NIH Publication No. 03-4762.* Retrieved April 2018 from https://www.niddk.nih.gov/health-information/liver-disease/viral-hepatitis/all-content.
4. American Liver Foundation. (2017). The progression of liver disease (various pages). Retrieved April 2018 from http://www.liverfoundation.org/abouttheliver/info/progression/.
5. Lee, D. (Updated 2014, last reviewed 2016). Acetaminophen (Tylenol) liver damage. *MedicineNet.* Retrieved April 2018 from http://www.medicinenet.com/tylenol_liver_damage/article.htm.
6. American Association for Clinical Chemistry. (Updated 2018). Liver panel. *Lab Tests Online.* Retrieved April 2018 from http://labtestsonline.org/understanding/analytes/liver-panel/tab/glance/.
7. Nabili, S. T. (Updated 2014, last reviewed 2017). Liver blood tests. *MedicineNet.* Retrieved April 2018 from http://www.emedicinehealth.com/liver_blood_tests/article_em.htm.
8. Cormier, M. (2005). The role of hepatitis C support groups. *Gastroenterol Nurs,* 28(3 Suppl), S4–S9.
9. Whiteman, K., McCormick, C. (2005). When your patient is in liver failure. *Nursing,* 35(4), 58–63.
10. Durston, S. (2005). What you need to know about viral hepatitis. *Nursing,* 35(8), 36–41.
11. Kania, D. S., Scott, C. M. (2007). Postexposure prophylaxis considerations for occupational and nonoccupational exposures. *Adv Emerg Nurs J,* 29(1), 20–32.
12. Pozza, R., Hill, C., Heffner, A. M. (2017). Hepatitis C infection: Updates on treatment guidelines. *Nurse Pract,* 42(5), 14–23.
13. Heuman, D. M., Mihaus, A. A., Hung, P. D. (Updated 2017). Alcoholic hepatitis. Retrieved April 2018 from http://emedicine.medscape.com/article/170539-overview.
14. National Institutes of Health. (Updated 2018). Drug record: Acetaminophen. *LiverTox: Clinical and Research Information on Drug-Induced Liver Injury.* Retrieved April 2018 from https://livertox.nih.gov/Acetaminophen.htm#top.
15. El-Zayadi, A. R. (2006). Heavy smoking and liver. *World J Gastroenterol,* 12(38), 6089–6101.
16. O'Shea, R. S., Dasarathy, S., McCullough, R. S. (2010). Alcoholic liver disease. *Am J Gastroenterol,* 105(1), 14–32.
17. Holcomb, S. S. (2008). Caring for the patient with chronic hepatitis C. *Nursing,* 38(12), 32–37.

 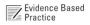

Diagnostic Studies Evidence Based Practice Medications Pediatric/Geriatric/Lifespan

risk for Loneliness

Taxonomy II: Comfort—Class 3 Social Comfort (00054) [**Diagnostic Division:** Social Interaction], Approved 1994; Revised 2006, 2013

DEFINITION: Susceptible to experiencing discomfort associated with a desire or need for more contact with others, which may compromise health.

RISK FACTORS

Affectional or emotional deprivation

Physical or social isolation

Sample Clinical Applications: Debilitating conditions (e.g., multiple sclerosis [MS], chronic obstructive pulmonary disease [COPD], renal failure), cancer, AIDS; major depression

DESIRED OUTCOMES/EVALUATION CRITERIA

Sample NOC linkages:

Loneliness Severity: Severity of emotional, social, or existential signs and symptoms of isolation

Social Involvement: Social interactions with persons, groups, or organizations

Client Will (Include Specific Time Frame)

• Identify individual difficulties and ways to address them.

• Engage in desired social activities.

• Report involvement in interactions or relationships that client views as meaningful.

Sample NOC linkages:

Knowledge: Parenting: Extent of understanding conveyed about provision of a nurturing and constructive environment for a child from 1 year through 17 years of age

Parent Will (Include Specific Time Frame)

• Provide infant/child with consistent and loving caregiving.

• Participate in programs for adolescents and families.

ACTIONS/INTERVENTIONS

Sample NIC linkages:

Socialization Enhancement: Facilitation of another person's ability to interact with others

Hope Inspiration: Enhancing the belief in one's capacity to initiate and sustain actions

Family Integrity Promotion: Promotion of family cohesion and unity

NURSING PRIORITY NO. 1   To identify causative/precipitating factors:

• Differentiate between ordinary loneliness and a state of constant sense of dysphoria. *This influences the type of and intensity of interventions.*[3]

• ∞ ☑ Note client's age and duration of problem—that is, situational (e.g., leaving home for college) or chronic. *Adolescents may experience lonely feelings related to the changes that are happening as they become adults. Elderly individuals incur multiple losses associated with aging, loss of spouse, decline in physical health, and changes in roles, thus intensifying feelings of loneliness.*[3,11]

 Acute Care   Collaborative   Community/ Home Care   Cultural

- Determine degree of distress, tension, anxiety, and restlessness present. Note history of frequent illnesses, accidents, and crises. *Identifies somatic complaints that can result from loneliness. Individuals under stress tend to have more illnesses and accidents related to inattention and anxiety.*[6]
- Note presence and proximity of family/significant others (SOs). *Loneliness may not be related to being alone, but knowing that family is available can help with planning care. Client may be estranged from other family members or they may not be willing to be involved with client.*[1,6]
- Discuss with client whether there is a person(s) in his or her life who is trustworthy and who will listen with empathy to the feelings that are expressed. *Identifying someone in the individual's life who can fill this role can help client talk about and understand feelings.*[1]
- Determine how individual perceives and deals with solitude. *Client may see being alone as positive, allowing time to pursue own interests, or may view solitude as sad and long for lost people, lifestyle pattern, or events.*[6,12]
- ∞ Review issues of separation from parents as a child or loss of SO(s)/spouse. *Early separation from parents often affects the individual as other losses occur throughout life, leading to feelings of inadequacy and inability to deal with current situation.*[6,12]
- Assess sleep and appetite disturbances and ability to concentrate. *Feelings of loneliness often accompany depression, and identifying whether client is adequately taking care of self is important to planning care.*[7]
- Note expressions of "yearning" for an emotional partnership. *For example, widows and widowers are particularly prone to feelings of loneliness. Going from being part of a couple to being alone is a difficult transition, and these feelings are indicative of a desire to return to the couple state.*[7]
- Assess feelings of loneliness in client who is receiving palliative/hospice care. *These individuals often feel alienated and lonely as they face the end of their life and may need additional socialization to help them feel valued.*[5]

NURSING PRIORITY NO. 2 To assist client to identify feelings and situations in which he or she experiences loneliness:

- 🏠 Establish therapeutic nurse-client relationship. *Provides a sense of connection with someone, thereby enabling client to feel free to talk about feelings of loneliness and current situation that is related to these feelings.*[1]
- Discuss individual concerns about feelings of loneliness and relationship between loneliness and lack of SOs. Note desire and willingness to change situation. *Motivation or lack thereof can facilitate or impede achieving desired outcomes. Often feelings of loneliness arise from underlying depression related to loss, thus affecting individual's coping abilities.*[7]
- Support expression of negative perceptions of others and whether client believes they are true. *Provides opportunity for client to clarify reality of situation and recognize own denial. Individual's view of the world is colored by feelings of loneliness and depression.*[1]
- Accept client's expressions of loneliness as a primary condition and not necessarily as a symptom of some underlying condition. *Provides a beginning point, which will allow the client to look at what loneliness means in life without having to search for deeper meaning.*[1,2]

NURSING PRIORITY NO. 3 To assist client to become involved:

- 🏠 Discuss reality versus perception of situation. Have client identify people with whom he or she interacts on a regular basis. *Provides opportunity for reality check and beginning to understand own feelings of loneliness related to what is happening in own life.*[2,12]
- ∞ Discuss importance of emotional bonding (attachment) between infants/young children, parents/caregivers, as appropriate. *Understanding the importance of attachment provides parents with information that will help them take measures to ensure that this bonding occurs.*[2]

- Involve in classes such as assertiveness, language and communication, and social skills. *Addressing individual needs will enhance socialization and provide client with the skills to become involved in social activities, thus promoting self-confidence and alleviating feelings of loneliness.*[3,8,10]
- Role-play situations that are new or are anxiety provoking for client. *Practicing new situations helps develop self-confidence and provides client with information about what to expect and how to deal with the unexpected in a positive manner.*[2]
- Discuss positive health habits, including personal hygiene, and exercise activity of client's choosing. *Improves feelings of self-esteem, thus enabling client to feel more confident in social situations.*[7]
- Identify individual strengths and areas of interest that client identifies and is willing to pursue. *Provides opportunities for involvement with others to develop new social skills.*[7,10]
- Encourage attendance at support groups (e.g., therapy, separation or grief, religious). *Participating in these activities can meet individual needs and help client begin to deal with feelings of loneliness.*[7]
- Help client establish plan for progressive involvement, beginning with a simple activity, such as calling an old friend or speaking to a neighbor, and then leading to more complicated interactions and activities. *Taking small steps promotes success, and confidence is gained as each step is taken, thus helping the client to be more involved and to resolve feelings of loneliness.*[7]
- Provide opportunities for interactions in a supportive environment (e.g., have client accompanied as in a "buddy system") during initial attempts to socialize. *Helps reduce stress, provides positive reinforcement, and facilitates successful outcome.*[7]

NURSING PRIORITY NO. 4 To promote wellness (Teaching/Discharge Considerations):

- Let client know that loneliness can be overcome. *While it is up to the individual to begin to feel good about self, hearing that loneliness doesn't have to be permanent, can provide hope in early days.*[4,12]
- Encourage involvement in special interest groups (e.g., computers, bird watchers) or charitable services (e.g., serving in a soup kitchen, youth groups, animal shelter). *Becoming involved with others takes focus off of self and own concerns, promotes feelings of self-worth, and encourages client to again be an active part of society.*[7]
- Suggest volunteering for church committee or choir, attending community events with friends and family, becoming involved in political issues or campaigns, or enrolling in classes at local college or continuing education programs, as able. *When client is willing to become involved in these kinds of activities, perception of loneliness fades into the background, and even though individual may still be lonely, the sense of loneliness is not so pervasive.*[7]
- Refer to appropriate counselors for help with relationships, social skills, or other identified needs. *May provide additional assistance to help client deal with feelings of loneliness and isolation.*[9]
- Refer to NDs Anxiety, Hopelessness, and Social Isolation for additional interventions, as appropriate.

DOCUMENTATION FOCUS

Assessment/Reassessment
- Assessment findings, including client's perception of problem, availability of resources or support systems.
- Client's desire and commitment to change.

Planning
- Plan of care and who is involved in planning.
- Teaching plan.

Implementation/Evaluation
- Response to interventions, teaching, and actions performed.
- Attainment or progress toward desired outcome(s).
- Modifications to plan of care.

 Acute Care   Collaborative   Community/ Home Care   Cultural

Discharge Planning
• Long-term needs, plan for follow-up, and who is responsible for actions to be taken.
• Specific referrals made.

References

1. Winch, G. (2014). 10 surprising facts about loneliness: Pangs that attack your body in ways you never expected. *Psychology Today*. Retrieved April 2018 from https://www.psychology today.com/us/blog/the-squeaky-wheel/201410/10-surprising-facts-about-loneliness.
2. No author listed. (2006). One is the loneliest number. *The Oprah Magazine*. Retrieved March 2015 from http://www.oprah.com/relationships/Loneliness-Research-How-Loneliness-Affects-Health-How-to-Help.
3. Herbert, W. (2007). The aging of loneliness. *We're Only Human*. Retrieved March 2015 from http://www.psychological science.org/onlyhuman/2007/08/aging-of-loneliness.cfm.
4. Burnett, P. (2009). Loneliness and low self-esteem. Retrieved March 2015 from http://ezinearticles.com/?Loneliness-and-Low-Self-Esteem&id=2499357.
5. Paice, J. (2002). Managing psychological conditions in pallia-tive care. *Am J Nurs*, 102(11), 36–43.
6. Hauge, S., Kirkevold, M. (2010). Older Norwegians' under-standing of loneliness. *Int J Qual Stud Health Well-Being*.

Retrieved April 2018 from http://www.ncbi.nlm.nih.gov/pmc/articles/PMC2879870/.
7. McAuley, E., et al. (2000). Social relations, physical activity, and well-being in older adults. *Prev Med*, 31(5), 608–617.
8. Acorn, S., Bampton, E. (1992). Patient's loneliness: A chal-lenge for rehabilitation nurses. *Rehabil Nurs*, 17(1), 22–25.
9. Davidson, L., Stayner, D. (1997). Loss, loneliness, and the desire for love: Perspectives on the social lives of people with schizophrenia. *Psychiatr Rehabil J*, 20(3), 3–12.
10. Finch, A. (No date). Fed up with feeling alone? Retrieved April 2018 from http://www.selfgrowth.com/articles/Finch3.html.
11. No author listed. (No date). Elderly perception of loneliness and ways of resolving it. *BoomersForever Web site*. Retrieved April 2018 from http://www.boomersforever.com/retire-loneliness.htm.
12. Seepersad, S., Choi, M., Shin, N. (2008). How does culture influence the degree of romantic loneliness and closeness. *J Psychol*, 142(2), 209–221.

risk for disturbed Maternal-Fetal Dyad

Taxonomy II: SexualityClass 3 Reproduction (00209) [**Diagnostic Division:** Safety], Approved 2008; Revised 2013, 2017

DEFINITION: Susceptible to disruption of the symbiotic maternal-fetal dyad as a result of comorbid or pregnancy-related conditions, which may compromise health.

RISK FACTORS
Inadequate prenatal care
Presence of abuse [e.g., physical, psychological, sexual]
Substance abuse
Associated Condition: Alteration in glucose metabolism; treatment regimen
Compromised fetal oxygen transport; pregnancy complication
Sample Clinical Applications: High-risk pregnancy, prenatal substance abuse, gestational hypertension, maternal diabetes mellitus, prenatal hemorrhage, prenatal infection, premature dilatation of cervix, abdom-inal trauma, domestic violence

DESIRED OUTCOMES/EVALUATION CRITERIA

Sample NOC linkages:
Maternal Status Antepartum: Extent to which maternal well-being is within normal limits from concep-tion to the onset of labor
Fetal Status Antepartum: Extent to which fetal signs are within normal limits from conception to the onset of labor
Prenatal Health Behavior: Personal actions to promote a healthy pregnancy and a healthy newborn

(continues on page 534)

 Diagnostic Studies
 Evidence Based Practice
 Medications
 Pediatric/Geriatric/Lifespan

risk for disturbed Maternal-Fetal Dyad (continued)

Client Will (Include Specific Time Frame)
- Verbalize understanding of individual risk factors or condition(s) that may impact pregnancy.
- Engage in necessary alterations in lifestyle and daily activities to manage risks.
- Participate in screening procedures as indicated.
- Identify signs/symptoms requiring medical evaluation or intervention.
- Display fetal growth within normal limits and carry pregnancy to term.

ACTIONS/INTERVENTIONS

Sample NIC linkages:

High-Risk Pregnancy Care: Identification and management of a high-risk pregnancy to promote healthy outcomes for mother and baby

Surveillance: Late Pregnancy: Purposeful and ongoing acquisition, interpretation, and synthesis of maternal-fetal data for treatment, observation, or admission

NURSING PRIORITY NO. 1   To identify individual risk/contributing factors:

- Review history of previous pregnancies for presence of complications, such as premature rupture of membranes (PROM), placenta previa, miscarriage or pregnancy losses due to premature dilation of the cervix, preterm labor and deliveries, previous birth defects, hyperemesis gravidarum, or repeated urinary tract or vaginal infections.[22,23]
- Obtain history about prenatal screening and amount and timing of care. *Prenatal screening can detect inherited and congenital abnormalities long before birth, providing opportunities for informed parental decisions, such as repair of abnormality in utero or helping mother understand a procedure. Lack of prenatal care or late prenatal care may be result of ignorance of or fear about pregnancy or the result of inadequate finances or other support and can place both mother and fetus at risk.*[9,23]
- Note conditions potentiating vascular changes and reduced placental circulation (e.g., diabetes, gestational hypertension, cardiac problems, smoking) or those that alter oxygen-carrying capacity (e.g., asthma, anemia, Rh incompatibility, hemorrhage). *Extent of maternal vascular involvement and reduction of oxygen-carrying capacity have a direct influence on uteroplacental circulation and gas exchange.*[8,10]
- 🖊 Note maternal age. *Maternal age above 35 years is associated with increased risk of placental separation or abruptio placentae, spontaneous abortions, preterm delivery or stillbirths, fetal chromosomal abnormalities and malformations, and intrauterine growth retardation (IUGR). The most common maternal complications in this age group are gestational hypertension and gestational diabetes. In pregnant adolescents (younger than 15) the most common high-risk conditions include gestational hypertension, anemia, labor dysfunction, cephalopelvic disproportion and low birth weight, and preterm delivery.*[2,5,8,11,14,23]
- 🖊 Ascertain current and past dietary patterns and practices. *Client may be malnourished, underweight or obese (weight less than 100 lb or greater than 200 lb), or may reveal preconception eating disorders that can have a negative impact on fetal organ development, especially brain tissue in the early weeks of pregnancy.*[1,3,15,23]
- Assess for severe, unremitting nausea and vomiting, especially when it persists after the first trimester. *Hyperemesis gravidarum places mother at risk for substantial weight loss and fluid and electrolyte imbalances and exposes the developing fetus to acidotic state and malnutrition. Development of hyperemesis gravidarum may require hospitalization.*[14,19,23]
- Note history of exposure to teratogenic agents and infectious diseases (e.g., tuberculosis, influenza, measles); high-risk occupations; exposure to toxic substances such as lead, organic solvents, and carbon monoxide; use of certain over-the-counter or prescription medications; and substance use or abuse (including illicit drugs and alcohol).[4,6,7,14,18]

 Acute Care   Collaborative   Community/Home Care   Cultural

- 🌐 Identify family or cultural influences in pregnancy. *Family history may include multiple births, congenital diseases, generational abuse, or lack of support or finances. Cultural background may identify health risks associated with nationality (e.g., sickle cell anemia in people of African descent or Tay-Sachs disease in people of Eastern European Jewish ancestry) or religious practices (e.g., exclusion of dairy products, no maternal immunizations for rubella), which can impact health of mother or fetal development.*[11,14]
- 🔬 Review laboratory studies. *Low hemoglobin suggests anemia, which is associated with hypoxia. Blood type and Rh group may reveal incompatibility risks and elevated serum glucose seen in gestational diabetes mellitus (GDM), elevated liver function studies suggest hypertensive liver involvement, and drop in platelet count may be associated with gestational hypertension and HELLP (hemolysis, elevated liver enzymes, and low platelet) syndrome. Nutritional studies may reveal decreased levels of serum proteins, electrolytes, minerals, and vitamins essential to maternal health and fetal development.*[8,9,15,23]
- 🔬 Review vaginal, cervical, or rectal cultures and serology results. *May reveal presence of sexually transmitted infections, a virus of the TORCH group (e.g., toxoplasmosis, other, rubella, cytomegalovirus, herpes simplex), or Listeria; identify active or carrier state of hepatitis, HIV.*[12,13,22]
- 🔬 Assist in screening for and identifying genetic or chromosomal disorders. *Disorders such as phenylketonuria or sickle cell anemia necessitate special treatment to prevent negative effects on fetal growth.*[11]
- Investigate current home situation. *May have history of unstable relationship or inadequate/lack of housing, which affects safety as well as general well-being.*[20]

NURSING PRIORITY NO. 2   To monitor maternal/fetal status:

- 📝 Weigh client and compare current weight with pregravid weight. Have client record weight between visits. *Underweight clients are at risk for anemia, inadequate protein/calorie intake, vitamin or mineral deficiencies, and gestational hypertension. Overweight women are at risk for possible changes in the cardiovascular system that create risks for development of gestational hypertension, GDM, and hyperinsulinemia of the fetus, resulting in macrosomia. Research indicates increased risk of fetal distress and cesarean delivery. A sudden weight gain of 2 or more pounds in a week may indicate gestational hypertension.*[3,8,15,23]
- Assess fetal heart rate (FHR), noting rate and regularity. Have client monitor fetal movement daily as indicated. *Tachycardia in a term infant may indicate a compensatory mechanism to reduced oxygen levels and/or presence of sepsis. A reduction in fetal activity occurs before bradycardia.*[23]
- 🔬 Test urine for presence of ketones. *Indicates inadequate glucose utilization and breakdown of fats for metabolic processes.*[10,23]
- 🔬 Provide information and assist with procedures as indicated, for example:[9,14,23]
  Amniocentesis: *May be performed for genetic purposes or to assess fetal lung maturity. Spectrophotometric analysis of the fluid may be done to detect bilirubin after 26 weeks gestation.*
  Ultrasonography: *Assesses gestational age of fetus and detects presence of multiples or fetal abnormalities. Locates placenta (and amniotic fluid pockets before amniocentesis, if performed), and monitors clients at risk for reduced/inadequate placental perfusion (such as adolescents; clients older than 35 years; clients with diabetes, gestational hypertension, cardiac/kidney disease, anemia, or respiratory disorders).*
  Biophysical profile: *Assesses fetal well-being through ultrasound evaluation to measure amniotic fluid index, FHR and nonstress test reactivity, fetal breathing movement, body movement (large limbs), and muscle tone (flexion and extension).*
  Contraction stress test (CST): *A positive CST with late decelerations indicates a high-risk client/fetus with possible reduced uteroplacental reserves.*
- Screen for abuse during pregnancy. *Prenatal abuse is correlated with a low maternal weight gain, infections, anemia, delay in seeking prenatal care until the third trimester, and preterm delivery.*[20]
- 📝 Screen for preterm uterine contractions, which may or may not be accompanied by cervical dilatation. *Occurs in 6% to 7% of all pregnancies and may result in delivery of a preterm infant if tocolytic management is not successful in reducing uterine contractility and irritability.*[21]

 Diagnostic Studies   Evidence Based Practice   Medications   Pediatric/Geriatric/Lifespan

NURSING PRIORITY NO. 3   To maintain or improve maternal and fetal well-being:

- Instruct client in reportable symptoms and monitor for unusual symptoms at each prenatal visit (e.g., vaginal bleeding, headache along with blurred vision and ankle swelling, faintness, persistent vomiting). *Provides opportunity for early intervention in event of developing complications.*[15,23]
- Assist in treatment of underlying medical condition(s) that have potential for causing maternal or fetal harm.[10]
- Assess perceived impact of complication on client and family members. Encourage verbalization of concerns. *Family stress often occurs in an uncomplicated pregnancy, and it is amplified in a high-risk pregnancy where concerns focus on the health of both the client and the fetus. Family is strengthened if all members have a chance to express fears openly and work cooperatively.*[23]
- Facilitate positive adaptation to situation through active listening, acceptance, and problem solving. *Helps in successful accomplishment of the psychological tasks of pregnancy, although the high-risk couple may remain ambivalent as a self-protective mechanism against possible loss of the pregnancy or fetal death.*[23]
- Develop dietary plan with client that provides necessary nutrients (calories, protein, vitamins, and minerals) *to create new tissue and to meet increased maternal metabolic needs.*[16,18]
- Promote fluid intake of at least 2 qt of noncaffeinated fluid per day. *Prevents dehydration, which may compromise optimal uterine and placental functioning and increase uterine irritability, which could potentiate premature labor.*
- Encourage client to participate in individually appropriate adaptations and self-care techniques, such as scheduling rest periods two to three times a day, avoiding overexertion or heavy lifting, or maintaining contact with family and daily life if bedrest is required. *Medical problems necessitating special therapy or restrictions at home or hospitalization significantly disrupt normal routines and cause stress. Preventive problem-solving promotes participation in own care and enhances self-confidence, sense of control, and client/couple satisfaction.*[23,25]
- Review medication regimen. *Prepregnancy treatment for chronic conditions may require alteration for maternal/fetal safety.*
- Review availability and use of resources. *Presence or absence of supportive resources can make the difference for the client and family in being able to manage the situation.*
- Administer Rh immune globulin (RhIgG) to client at 28 weeks gestation in Rh-negative clients with Rh-positive partners or following amniocentesis, if indicated. *RhIgG helps reduce incidence of maternal isoimmunization in nonsensitized mothers and helps prevent erythroblastosis fetalis and fetal red blood cell (RBC) hemolysis.*[23,24]
- Encourage modified or complete bedrest as indicated. *Activity level may need modification, depending on symptoms of uterine activity, cervical changes, or bleeding. Side-lying position increases renal and placental perfusion, which is effective in preventing supine hypotensive syndrome.*[23] *Note: Bedrest may result in generalized weakness, raising safety concerns when client is out of bed.*
- Provide supplemental oxygen as appropriate. *Increases the oxygen available for fetal uptake, especially in presence of severe anemia or sickle cell crisis or when maternal/fetal circulation is compromised.*
- Prepare for and assist with intrauterine fetal exchange transfusion as indicated by titers (Kleihauer-Betke test). *If excess fetal RBC hemolysis occurs, transfusion into fetal peritoneal cavity with Rh O-negative blood replaces hemolyzed RBCs when fetus is determined at risk of dying before 32 weeks gestation.*[24]

NURSING PRIORITY NO. 4   To promote wellness (Teaching/Discharge Considerations):

- Emphasize the normalcy of pregnancy, focus on pregnancy milestones, and count down to birth. *Avoids or limits perception of sick role and promotes sense of hope that modifications or restrictions serve a worthwhile purpose.*[23]
- Discuss implications of preexisting condition and possible impact on pregnancy. *Pregnancy may have no effect or may reduce or exacerbate severity of symptoms of chronic conditions. Repeat sickle cell crises predispose client and fetus to increased mortality and morbidity rates. Client with multiple sclerosis or spinal cord injury may have decreased ability to sense uterine contractions or presence of labor, necessitating closer monitoring.*[10]
- Provide information about risks of weight reduction during pregnancy and about nourishment needs of client and fetus. *Prenatal calorie restriction and resultant weight loss may result in nutrient deficiency or ketonemia, with negative effects on fetal central nervous system and possible IUGR.*[18]

 Acute Care   Collaborative   Community/ Home Care   Cultural

- Encourage smoking cessation, refer to community program or support group as indicated. *Severe adverse effects of smoking on the fetus may be reduced if mother quits smoking early in pregnancy, and pregnancy outcomes can still be improved if mother stops smoking as late as 32 weeks gestation.*[17]
- Help client/couple plan restructuring of roles or activities necessitated by complication of pregnancy. *Education, support, and assistance in maintenance of family integrity help foster growth of its individual members and reduce stress that the client may feel from her dependent role.*[23]
- Encourage client to demonstrate new behaviors or therapeutic techniques. *During pregnancy, control of condition may require specific modified or new behaviors. Demonstration allows accurate assessment of learning.*
- Recommend client assess uterine tone and presence of contractions for 1 hour once or twice a day as indicated *to monitor uterine irritability or early indication of premature labor.*[21]
- Encourage close monitoring of blood glucose levels, as appropriate. *Clients with type I or insulin-dependent diabetes mellitus generally need to check blood glucose levels 4 to 12 times/day because insulin needs may increase two to three times above pregravid baseline.*[10]
- Demonstrate technique and specific equipment used when FHR monitoring is done in the home setting. *Provides opportunity for more detailed information regarding fetal well-being in a less stressful environment. Enhances sense of active involvement.*
- Identify danger signals requiring immediate notification of healthcare provider (e.g., PROM, preterm labor, vaginal drainage or bleeding). *Recognizing risk situations encourages prompt evaluation and intervention, which may prevent or limit untoward outcomes.*[21,22]
- Review availability and use of resources. *Presence or absence of supportive resources can make the difference for the client and family in being able to manage the situation.*[22]
- Refer to community service agencies (e.g., visiting nurse, social service) or resources, such as Sidelines. *Community supports may be needed for ongoing assessment of medical problem, family status, coping behaviors, and financial stressors. Note: Sidelines is a national support group for high-risk pregnant women.*
- Refer for counseling if family does not sustain positive coping and growth. *May be necessary to promote growth and to prevent family disintegration.*

DOCUMENTATION FOCUS

Assessment/Reassessment
- Assessment findings, weight, signs of pregnancy, and safety concerns.
- Specific risk factors, comorbidities, and treatment regimen.
- Results of screening laboratory tests and diagnostic studies.
- Participation in prenatal care.
- Cultural beliefs and practices.

Planning
- Plan of care, specific interventions, and who is involved in the planning.
- Community resources for equipment or supplies.
- Specific referrals made.
- Teaching plan.

Implementation/Evaluation
- Client/fetal response to treatment and actions performed.
- Clients response to teaching provided.
- Attainment or progress toward desired outcome(s).
- Modifications to plan of care.

References

1. National Institute of Child Health and Human Development (NICHD). (Updated 2013, last reviewed 2017). What are the factors that put a pregnancy at risk? Retrieved April 2018 from https://www.nichd.nih.gov/health/topics/high-risk/conditioninfo/Pages/factors.aspx.

 Diagnostic Studies   Evidence Based Practice   Medications   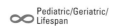 Pediatric/Geriatric/Lifespan

2. Cleary-Goldman, J., et al. (2005). Impact of maternal age on obstetric outcome. *Obstet Gynecol*, 105(5), 983–990.

3. Ehrenberg, H. M., et al. (2009). Maternal obesity, uterine activity, and the risk of spontaneous preterm birth. *Obstet Gynecol*, 113(1), 48–52.

4. No author listed. (Updated 2015). Surgeon Generals advisory on alcohol use in pregnancy. Retrieved April 2018 from http://come-over.to/FAS/SurGenAdvisory.htm.

5. Miller, D. A. (2005). Is advanced maternal age an independent risk factor for uteroplacental insufficiency? *Am J Obstet Gynecol*, 192(6), 1974–1982.

6. March of Dimes. (Last reviewed 2016). *Street drugs and during pregnancy.* Retrieved April 2018 from https://www.marchofdimes.org/pregnancy/street-drugs-and-pregnancy.aspx.

7. Acharya, K. S., Grotegut, C. A. (Updated 2017). Psychosocial and environmental pregnancy risks. Retrieved April 2018 from http://emedicine.medscape.com/article/259346-overview.

8. Carson, M. P., Gibson, P. (Updated 2017). Hypertension and pregnancy. Retrieved April 2018 from http://emedicine.medscape.com/article/261435-overview.

9. Prenatal screening and diagnostics (index page). (Updated 2013). *Yale Medical Group.* Retrieved December 2018 from https://www.yalemedicine.org/conditions/prenatal-screening-and-diagnostics/.

10. High-risk pregnancy: Pregnancy and medical conditions. *Yale Medical Group.* Retrieved December 2018 from https://www.yalemedicine.org/search/?q=high+risk+pregnancy+and+medical+conditions.

11. What are some factors that make a pregnancy high risk? *National Institutes of Health.* Retrieved December 2018 from https://www.nichd.nih.gov/health/topics/high-risk/conditioninfo/factors.

12. Centers for Disease Control and Prevention. (Updated 2016). *STDs and pregnancy. CDC fact sheet.* Retrieved April 2018 from http://www.cdc.gov/std/pregnancy/stdfact-pregnancy.htm.

13. U.S. Department of Health and Human Services. (2008, reviewed 2012). *HIV during pregnancy, labor and delivery, and after birth.* Retrieved April 2018 from http://permanent.access.gpo.gov/lps80129/perinatal_fs_en.pdf.

14. Springhouse Staff. (2008). Complications and high-risk conditions of the prenatal period. *Straight As in Maternal-Neonatal Nursing.* 2nd ed. Philadelphia, PA: Lippincott Williams & Wilkins.

15. Holloway, B., Moredich, C., Aduddell, K. (2006). *OB Peds Womens Health Notes: Nurse's Clinical Pocket Guide.* Philadelphia, PA: F. A. Davis.

16. RDAs for pregnant women. (2007). *Lippincott Manual of Nursing Practice Pocket Guides: Maternal-Neonatal Nursing.* Philadelphia, PA: Lippincott Williams & Wilkins.

17. Barclay, L., Vega, C. (2009). Severe adverse effects of smoking may be reversible if mothers quit early in pregnancy. Retrieved April 2018 from http://www.medscape.org/viewarticle/590543.

18. National Institute of Child Health and Human Development (NICHD). (Updated 2014, reviewed 2017). *What can I do to promote a healthy pregnancy?* Retrieved April 2018 from https://www.nichd.nih.gov/health/topics/preconceptioncare/conditioninfo/healthy-pregnancy.

19. Hyperemesis gravidarum. *American Pregnancy Association.* Retrieved December 2018 from http://americanpregnancy.org/pregnancy-complications/hyperemesis-gravidarum/.

20. Niolon, P. H., Kearns, M., Dills, J. (2017). Preventing intimate partner violence across the lifespan: A technical package of programs, policies, and practices. *National Center for Injury Prevention and Control, Centers for Disease Control and Prevention.* Retrieved April 2018 from https://www.cdc.gov/violenceprevention/pdf/ipv-technicalpackages.pdf.

21. Institute of Medicine. (2007). Preterm birth: Causes, consequences, and prevention. *Maternity and Pediatric Nursing.* Washington, D.C.: The National Academies Press.

22. Ross, M. G. (Updated 2017). Preterm labor. Retrieved April 2018 from http://emedicine.medscape.com/article/260998-overview.

23. Ricci, S. S., Kyle, T. (2008). *Maternity and Pediatric Nursing.* Philadelphia, PA: Lippincott Williams & Wilkins.

24. National Heart, Lung, and Blood Institute. (Updated 2011). *What is Rh incompatibility?* Retrieved April 2018 from http://www.nhlbi.nih.gov/health/health-topics/topics/rh.

25. Maloni, J. A., et al. (2002). Dysphoria among high-risk pregnant hospitalized women on bed rest: A longitudinal study. *Nurs Res*, 51(2), 92–99.

impaired Memory

Taxonomy II: Perception/Cognition—Class 4 Cognition (00131) [**Diagnostic Division:** Neurosensory], Approved 1994; Revised 2017

DEFINITION: Persistent inability to remember or recall bits of information or skills.

RELATED FACTORS
Alteration in fluid volume
[Substance use/abuse; effects of medications]

DEFINING CHARACTERISTICS

Subjective
Persistent inability to recall events or factual information

 Acute Care   Collaborative   Community/Home Care   Cultural

Objective

Persistent inability to recall if a behavior was performed; consistently forgets to perform a behavior at a scheduled time

Persistent inability to learn/retain new skills or information

Persistent inability to recall familiar names, words, or objects; inability to perform a previously learned skill

Persistent forgetfulness

Preserved capacity to perform daily activities independently

Associated Condition: Anemia, hypoxia, electrolyte imbalance, decrease in cardiac output

Brain injury, mild cognitive impairment, neurological impairment; Parkinson's disease

Sample Clinical Applications: Brain injury, stroke, dementia, Alzheimer's disease, hypoxia (e.g., chronic obstructive pulmonary disease [COPD], anemia, altitude sickness), alcohol intoxication or substance abuse

DESIRED OUTCOMES/EVALUATION CRITERIA

Sample **NOC** linkages:

Memory: Ability to cognitively retrieve and report previously stored information

Cognition: Ability to execute complex mental processes

Client Will (Include Specific Time Frame)

• Verbalize awareness of memory problems.

• Establish methods to help in remembering essential things when possible.

• Accept limitations of condition and use resources effectively.

ACTIONS/INTERVENTIONS

Sample **NIC** linkages:

Memory Training: Facilitation of memory

Environmental Management: Safety: Monitoring and manipulation of the physical environment to promote safety

NURSING PRIORITY NO. 1   To assess causative factor(s)/degree of impairment:

• Determine physical, biochemical, and environmental factors (e.g., systemic infections, brain injury, pulmonary disease with hypoxia, use of multiple medications, exposure to toxic substances; use or abuse of alcohol or other drugs, traumatic event, removal from known environment) *that may be related to changes in memory.*

• ∞ ⧉ Note client's age and potential for depression. *Depressive disorders are prevalent in older adults who report an inability to concentrate and poor memory; however, impairments can occur in depressed persons of any age. Note: The Centers for Disease Control and Prevention (CDC) (2017) reports that estimates of major depression in older people living in the community range from less than 1% to about 5%, but rise to 13.5% in those who require home healthcare and to 11.5% in older hospital patients.*[1,2,5–7,10]

• Note presence of stressful situation(s) and degree of anxiety. *Can increase client's confusion and disorganization, further interfering with attempts at recall. Stress may also accelerate memory decline in people whose cognitive function is already impaired.* (Refer to ND Anxiety for additional interventions as indicated.)

• ✑ Collaborate with medical and psychiatric providers *to evaluate extent of impairment to orientation, attention span, ability to follow directions, send/receive communication, and appropriateness of response.*

• ⟋ Assist with or review results of cognitive testing (e.g., Blessed Information-Memory-Concentration test, Clinical Dementia Rating Scale, Mini-Mental State Examination). *Although the etiology for some memory*

 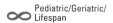

impairments may be obvious or established by client/significant other (SO)/caregiver report, a combination of tests may be needed to demonstrate that the client is below some cut-point on standardized memory tests that represents a significant change from the client's baseline to obtain a complete picture of the client's overall condition and prognosis.[3,6,7]

- Evaluate skill proficiency levels. *Evaluation may include many self-care activities (e.g., daily grooming, steps in preparing a meal, participating in a lifelong hobby, balancing a checkbook, driving ability) to determine level of independence or needed assistance.*[8]
- Ascertain how client/family views the problem (e.g., practical problems of client being able to take care of physical/grooming/toileting issues; forgetting to turn off the stove when cooking for self; client gets lost when driving, client has role and responsibility impairments related to loss of memory and concentration) *to determine significance and impact of problem and suggest direction of interventions, especially as relates to basic safety issues.*[1,8]

NURSING PRIORITY NO. 2   To maximize level of function:

- Assist with treatment of underlying conditions (e.g., electrolyte imbalances, infection, anemia, drug interactions/reaction to medications, alcohol or other drug intoxication, malnutrition, vitamin deficiencies, pain) *where treatment can improve memory processes.*
- Orient and reorient client, as needed. Introduce self with each client contact *to meet client's safety and comfort needs.* (Refer to NDs acute/chronic Confusion for additional interventions as appropriate.)
- Implement appropriate memory-retraining techniques (e.g., keeping calendars and to-do lists, memory cue games, mnemonic devices, computer programs for cognitive retraining) *to provide restorative or compensatory training. Note: One evidence-based review of clients with memory impairments associated with moderate to severe brain injury showed that "memory retraining programs appear effective, particularly for functional recovery although performance on specific tests of memory may or may not change."*[4,9]
- Assist in and instruct client and family in associate-learning tasks (e.g., practice sessions recalling personal information, reminiscing, locating a geographic location [stimulation therapy]). *Practice may improve performance and integrate new behaviors into the client's coping strategies.*
- Support and reinforce client's efforts to remember information or behavioral skills. *Can decrease anxiety levels and perhaps help with further memory recovery.*
- Encourage ventilation of feelings of frustration and helplessness. Refocus attention to areas of control and progress *to diminish feelings of powerlessness or hopelessness.*
- Provide for and emphasize importance of pacing learning activities and getting sufficient rest *to avoid fatigue and frustration that may further impair cognitive abilities.*[1]
- Monitor client's behavior and assist in use of stress-management techniques (e.g., music therapy, reading, television, games, socialization) *to reduce boredom and enhance enjoyment of life.*
- Structure teaching methods and interventions to client's level of functioning or potential for improvement.[5]
- Determine client's response to and effects of medications prescribed to improve attention, concentration, memory processes, and to lift spirits or modify emotional responses. *Medications used for cognitive enhancement can be effective (especially in the case of short-term impairments such as might occur following surgery or when client is being treated for infections or delirium), but long-term use and benefits need to be weighed against whether quality of life is improved when considering side effects and cost of drugs.*[3,6]

NURSING PRIORITY NO. 3   To promote wellness (Teaching/Discharge Considerations):

- Assist client/SO(s) to establish compensation strategies, such as menu planning with a shopping list, timely completion of tasks on a daily planner, and checklists at the front door to ascertain that lights and stove are off before leaving, *to improve functional lifestyle and safety.*[6]
- Instruct client and family/caregivers in memory involvement tasks, such as reminiscence and memory exercises *geared toward improving client's functional ability.*[6]

 Acute Care   Collaborative   Community/Home Care   Cultural

- Refer to or encourage follow-up with counselors, rehabilitation programs, job coaches, and social or financial support systems *to help deal with persistent or difficult problems.*
- Refer to rehabilitation services *that are matched to the needs, strengths, and capacities of individual and modified as needs change over time.*[4]
- Discuss and encourage safety interventions, as indicated (e.g., assistance with meal preparation, evaluation of driving abilities, cessation of tobacco use or its use only under supervision, removal of guns and other weapons) *to prevent injury to client/others.*
- Identify resources to meet individual needs (e.g., home-care assistant, Meals on Wheels, companion, short-term residential care), *thereby maximizing independence and general well-being.*

DOCUMENTATION FOCUS

Assessment/Reassessment
- Individual findings, testing results, and perceptions of significance of problem.
- Actual impact on lifestyle and independence.

Planning
- Plan of care and who is involved in planning process.
- Teaching plan.

Implementation/Evaluation
- Responses to interventions, teaching, and actions performed.
- Attainment or progress toward desired outcome(s).
- Modifications to plan of care.

Discharge Planning
- Long-term needs and who is responsible for actions to be taken.
- Specific referrals made.

References

1. Luo, L. (2008). Aging and memory: A cognitive approach. *Can J Psychiatry*, 53(6), 346–353.
2. Roussel, L. A. (1999). The aging neurological system. In Stanley, M., Beare P. G. (eds). *Gerontological Nursing: A Health Promotion/Protection Approach*. 2nd ed. Philadelphia: F. A. Davis.
3. Alzheimer's Association. (2015, updated 2018). Healthcare professionals and Alzheimer's (various pages). Retrieved April 2018 from http://www.alz.org/health-care-professionals/health-care-clinical-medical-resources.asp.
4. NIH Consensus Panel. (1999). Rehabilitation of persons with traumatic brain injury. *JAMA*, 8(10), 974–983.
5. Mayo Clinic Staff. (Updated 2017). Mild cognitive impairments (MCI). Retrieved April 2018 from http://www.mayoclinic.org/diseases-conditions/mild-cognitive-impairment/basics/definition/con-20026392.
6. Kirshner, H. S. (2015). *Confusional states and acute memory disorders*. Retrieved April 2018 from http://misc.medscape.com/pi/iphone/medscapeapp/html/A1135767-business.html.
7. Mehta, S., Herath, P. (Updated 2018). *Mild cognitive impairment*. Retrieved March 2018 from http://emedicine.medscape.com/article/1136393-overview.
8. Family Caregiver Alliance: National Center on Caregiving. (No date). Caring for adults with cognitive and memory impairments. Retrieved April 2018 from http://www.caregiver.org/caring-adults-cognitive-and-memory-impairment.
9. Teasell, R., et al. (2013). Evidence-based review of moderate to severe acquired brain injury: Executive summary. Retrieved November 2018 from https://www.abiebr.com/pdf/executive Summary.pdf.
10. Centers for Disease Control and Prevention (CDC). (2017). Depression is not a normal part of growing older. Retrieved November 2018 from https://www.cdc.gov/aging/mentalhealth/depression.htm.

Diagnostic Studies   Evidence Based Practice   Medications   Pediatric/Geriatric/Lifespan

risk for Metabolic Imbalance Syndrome

Taxonomy II: Nutrition—Class 4 Metabolism (00263) [**Diagnostic Division:** Food/Fluid], Approved 2016

DEFINITION: Susceptible to a toxic cluster of biochemical and physiological factors associated with the development of cardiovascular disease arising from obesity and type 2 diabetes, which may compromise health.

RISK FACTORS
Ineffective health maintenance; risk-prone health behavior; stress overload
Obesity; overweight; sedentary lifestyle
Risk for unstable blood glucose
At Risk Population: Age >30 years
Family history of diabetes mellitus, dyslipidemia, hypertension, obesity
Associated Condition: Excessive endogenous or exogenous glucocorticoids >25 g/dl; microalbuminuria >30 mg/dl; uric acid >7 mg/dl
Polycystic ovary syndrome; unstable blood pressure
Sample Clinical Applications: Diabetes mellitus, obesity, hypertension

DESIRED OUTCOMES/EVALUATION CRITERIA

Sample NOC linkages:
Risk Control: Cardiovascular Disease: Personal actions to understand, prevent, eliminate, or reduce the threat of cardiovascular disease
Metabolic Function: Ability of the metabolic system to regulate chemical transformations through anabolism and catabolism

Client Will (Include Specific Time Frame)
• Identify individual risk factors.
• Develop plan to address modifiable risks.
• Engage in lifestyle changes to support achieving health goals.
• Display diagnostic/lab studies within desired levels.

ACTIONS/INTERVENTIONS

Sample NIC linkages:
Risk Identification: Analysis of potential risk factors, determination of health status, and prioritization of risk reduction strategies for an individual or group
Teaching: Disease Process: Assisting the patient to understand information related to a specific disease process

NURSING PRIORITY NO. 1 To identify risk factors

• Obtain client history, including family, personal, and social history *to evaluate for diabetes; coronary, cerebral, and peripheral vascular disease; and family history of early heart disease and diabetes.*
• Identify client's associated risks (e.g., hypertension, large waistline [also known as central or abdominal obesity], high cholesterol and triglyceride and fasting blood glucose levels). *The National Heart Lung and Blood Institute (NHLBI) states three of the above risk factors existing together is known as "metabolic syndrome," also known by several other names, including "insulin resistance syndrome," "obesity syndrome," "syndrome x."*[1,2]
• Obtain client's weight and other anthropometric measurements, including waist circumference, as indicated. *Abdominal obesity is considered to be waist circumference of greater than 40 inches (men), and greater than 35 inches (women). Client with a abdominal obesity is typically obese or overweight. Note: In one recent*

 Acute Care   Collaborative   Community/ Home Care   Cultural

study of 734 participants, 250 (34%) participants were of normal weight, 247 (33.7%) were overweight, and 237 (32.3%) were obese. The study reported that in the normal weight, overweight, and obese groups, the prevalence of metabolic syndrome was 12.4%, 36.4%, and 61.6%, respectively.[2,6]

- Measure blood pressure using appropriately sized cuff and proper positioning (e.g., seated, legs uncrossed, feet flat on floor). *Blood pressure is determined to be elevated (systolic blood pressure [SPB] 120–129 and diastolic blood pressure [DBP] less than 80). Stage I hypertension = SBP 130–139 or DBP 80–89; Stage 2 hypertension = SBP 140 or DBP 90; Hypertensive crisis = SBP 180, or DBP 120.*[3]

- Review results of laboratory studies, i.e., cholesterol (including HDL and LDL), triglycerides, blood glucose. *There are typically abnormalities in these lab values when metabolic syndrome is suspected. Note: Current guidelines: triglycerides ≥150 mg/dL, or receiving drug therapy for hypertriglyceridemia; HDL cholesterol (so-called "good" cholesterol) <40 mg/dL (men) or <50 (women), or receiving drug therapy for reduced HDL-C; fasting glucose ≥100 mg/dL or receiving drug therapy for hyperglycemia.*[3]

- Determine use of available resources. *Inadequate use or lack of availability of support system impact treatment options and ability to achieve health goals.*

- Refer for/assist with treatment of underlying conditions (e.g., diabetes, obesity, hypertension).

NURSING PRIORITY NO. 2   To assist client to explore ways to reduce modifiable risk factors

- Discuss weight management/nutrition enhancement with client/SO:
  Recommend client make shifts in food choices (as individually able/desired), such as increasing vegetables (including legumes) and fruits, avocados, fish, and nuts, and reduce consumption of calories from fried foods, refined grains, and sugars, *to lower blood lipids, stabilize blood glucose, and reduce weight over time (e.g., 10%–20% reduction over a year). Note: A large body of research data suggests that traditional dietary habits unique to the Mediterranean region lower the incidence of chronic diseases and improve longevity.*[4,6,7]

  Identify reputable community or online weight loss groups *to provide ongoing support to achieve and maintain healthy weight.*

  Discuss management of hypertension:
  Discuss importance of routine blood pressure monitoring.
  Identify measuring devices available in home or community that provide accurate readings.
  Have client return to clinic (or other public places where BP machines are available) if unable to obtain equipment.
  Provide systolic and diastolic number limits (along with other possible symptoms) that should be reported to medical provider.
  Review medications if client is already on antihypertensives and determine if client is taking medications as prescribed. *Medications may be needed or adjusted to attain optimal BP control. Note: Studies have revealed that a lower risk of stroke and cardiovascular events is seen when systolic blood pressure levels are less than 140 mmHg and diastolic blood pressure is less than 90 mmHg.*[3]

  Discuss need for consistent exercise:
  Recommend exercise (that client might enjoy) and discuss ways to implement it. *Client may need to start with just minutes a day and increase gradually. Current guideline is for people to perform regular moderate-intensity physical activity for at least 30 minutes continuously at least 5 days per week (ideally, 7 days per week). It has been found, however, that maintaining long-term adherence is a challenge.*[5]

  Discuss management of other lifestyle factors (e.g., smoking, alcohol/other drugs, stress):
  Identify smoking cessation programs, alcohol/substance use support groups for client and family as appropriate. *Client may want/need assistance and or referrals for management of lifestyle conditions or factors that are negatively impacting health.*

- Refer to physician/other healthcare providers as needed *Client may need immediate or intermittent long-term follow-up for medications (e.g., antihypertensives, antiglycemics, statins) as well as for treatment of underlying conditions.*

- Refer to nutritionist *to develop dietary program reflecting client likes, physical activity level/usual energy expended, and personal resources.*

 Diagnostic Studies   Evidence Based Practice   Medications   Pediatric/Geriatric/Lifespan

- Collaborate with rehabilitation specialists *to develop appropriate exercise program and determine need for assistive devices to facilitate activity.*

NURSING PRIORITY NO. 3 To promote wellness (Teaching/Discharge Considerations):

- Determine most urgent need from client's/caregiver's and healthcare provider's viewpoints, *which may differ and require adjustments in teaching plan.*
- Teach home monitoring of blood pressure, where indicated, and obtain return demonstration of ability to take blood pressure (and medications) accurately.
- Elicit client's knowledge of reportable blood pressure measurements and symptoms and who to report to. *Provides opportunity for timely intervention.*
- Recommend obtaining accurate scale and recording weekly weight checks. *Provides visual reinforcement of progress, need for adjustment of interventions.*
- Review specifics and rationale for components of treatment plan. Ask client/SO if they have questions and/or if they are willing to adhere to plan. *Helps to identify areas of concern and need for further interventions.*
- Identify community resources to address home-care needs and financial issues *to support independence and accomplishment of healthcare goals.*

DOCUMENTATION FOCUS

Assessment/Reassessment
- Individual risk factors.
- Vital signs, weight.
- Results of lab studies.

Planning
- Client's healthcare goals.
- Plan of care and who is involved in planning.
- Teaching plan.

Implementation/Evaluation
- Client's response to interventions, teaching, and actions performed.
- Status and disposition at discharge.
- Attainment or progress toward desired outcome(s).
- Modifications to plan of care.

Discharge Planning
- Discharge considerations and who will be responsible for carrying out individual actions.
- Long-term needs and available resources.
- Specific referrals made.

References

1. National Heart Lung and Blood Institute (NHLBI). (No date). Metabolic syndrome. *National Institutes of Health.* Retrieved May 2018 from https://www.nhlbi.nih.gov/health-topics/metabolic-syndrome.
2. American Heart Association (AHA). (2016). Symptoms and diagnosis of metabolic syndrome (various pages). Retrieved May 2018 from https://www.heart.org/HEARTORG/Conditions/More/MetabolicSyndrome/Metabolic-Syndrome_UCM_002080_SubHomePage.jsp.
3. American College of Cardiology. (2017). New ACC/AHA high blood pressure guidelines lower definition of hypertension. Retrieved May 2018 from http://www.acc.org/latest-in-cardiology/articles/2017/11/08/11/47/mon-5pm-bp-guideline-aha-2017.
4. Wang, S. S. (Updated 2017). Metabolic syndrome. Retrieved May 2018 from https://emedicine.medscape.com/article/165124-overview.
5. Fappa, E., et al. (2008). Lifestyle intervention in the management of metabolic syndrome: Could we improve adherence issues? *Nutrition,* 23(3), 286–291.
6. Chang, S.-H., et al. (2008). Examining the links between lifestyle factors and metabolic syndrome. *Nutrition,* 23(3), 286–291.
7. Romagnolo, D. F., Selmin, O. I. (2017). Mediterranean diet and prevention of chronic diseases. *Nutr Today,* 52(5), 208–222.

 Acute Care   Collaborative   Community/Home Care   Cultural

impaired bed Mobility

Taxonomy II: Activity/Rest—Class 2 Activity/Exercise (00091) [**Diagnostic Division:** Safety], Approved 1998; Revised 2006, 2017

DEFINITION: Limitation of independent movement from one bed position to another.

RELATED FACTORS

Environmental barrier [e.g., bed size or type, equipment, restraints]
Insufficient knowledge of mobility strategies
Insufficient muscle strength; physical deconditioning; obesity
Pain

DEFINING CHARACTERISTICS

Objective
Impaired ability to: reposition self in bed, turn from side to side
Impaired ability to move between: prone and supine positions, sitting/long sitting and supine positions
Associated Condition: Alteration in cognitive functioning
Musculoskeletal or neuromuscular impairment
Pharmaceutical agent
Sample Clinical Applications: Paralysis (e.g., spinal cord injury [SCI], stroke), traumatic brain injury, neuromuscular disorders (e.g., amyotrophic lateral sclerosis [ALS]), major chest or back surgery, severe depression, dementia, catatonic schizophrenia

DESIRED OUTCOMES/EVALUATION CRITERIA

Sample NOC linkages:
Body Positioning: Self-Initiated: Personal actions to change own body position independently with or without assistive device
Coordinated Movement: Ability of muscles to work together voluntarily for purposeful movement
Immobility Consequences: Physiological: Severity of compromise in physiological functioning due to impaired physical mobility

Client/Caregiver Will (Include Specific Time Frame)
• Verbalize willingness to and participates in repositioning program.
• Verbalize understanding of situation or risk factors, individual therapeutic regimen, and safety measures.
• Demonstrate techniques or behaviors that enable safe repositioning.
• Maintain position of function and skin integrity as evidenced by absence of contractures, foot drop, decubitus, and other skin disorders.
• Maintain or increase strength and function of affected and/or compensatory body part.

ACTIONS/INTERVENTIONS

Sample NIC linkages:
Bed Rest Care: Promotion of comfort and safety and prevention of complications for a patient unable to get out of bed
Positioning: Deliberative placement of the patient or a body part to promote physiological and/or psychological well-being
Teaching: Prescribed Exercise: Preparing a patient to achieve or maintain a prescribed level of exercise

 Diagnostic Studies   Evidence Based Practice   Medications 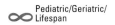 Pediatric/Geriatric/Lifespan

NURSING PRIORITY NO. 1   To identify causative/contributing factors:

- Determine diagnoses that contribute to current immobility (e.g., multiple sclerosis, arthritis, Parkinson's disease, hemi-/para- or tetraplegia; fractures [especially hip joint and long bone fractures], multiple trauma, head injury, burns) *to identify interventions specific to client's mobility impairment and needs.*
- Note individual factors (e.g., surgery, casts, amputation, traction, pain, advanced age, general weakness or debilitation, severe depression, dementia) *that can contribute to mobility problems.*
- Determine degree of perceptual or cognitive impairment or ability to follow directions. *Impairments related to age, acute or chronic conditions (including severe depression, dementia), trauma, surgery, or medications require alternative interventions or changes in plan of care. Note: Studies have shown that cognitive abilities are crucial to ongoing planning, decision making, and monitoring of one's own movements necessary for successful mobility.*[1,3,9]
- Review results of testing (e.g., Lower Extremity Functional Scale, Harris Hip Score; the self-paced walk, timed up-and-go tests) *to determine limitations in body activity, function, and structure.*[8]

NURSING PRIORITY NO. 2   To assess functional ability:

- Determine functional level classification 0 to 4 *(level 0 is full self-care, level I requires use of equipment or device, level II requires assistance or supervision of another person, level III requires assistance or supervision of another person and equipment or device, level IV is dependent and does not participate).*[12]
- Note emotional and behavioral responses to problems of immobility. *Can negatively affect self-concept and self-esteem, autonomy, and independence. Feelings of frustration and powerlessness may impede attainment of goals. Social, occupational, and relationship roles can change, leading to isolation, depression, and economic consequences.*[4,5]
- 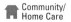 Note presence of complications related to immobility. *The effects of immobility are rarely confined to one body system and can include muscle wasting, contractures, pressure sores, constipation, aspiration pneumonia, etc. Studies have shown that as much as 5.5% of muscle strength can be lost each day of rest and immobility.*[1] *Other complications include changes in circulation and impairments of organ function affecting the whole person (e.g., cognition, immune system function, emotional state).* (Refer to ND risk for Disuse Syndrome for additional interventions.)

NURSING PRIORITY NO. 3   To promote optimal level of function and prevent complications:

- Assist with treatment of underlying condition(s) *to maximize potential for mobility and optimal function.*
- Ascertain that dependent client is placed in best bed for situation (e.g., properly functioning equipment, correct size and support surface) *to promote environmental, client, and caregiver safety.*[6]
- Instruct client/caregiver in bed capabilities (e.g., mobility functions and set positions), encouraging client to participate as much as possible, even if only to move head or run bed controls. *Promotes independence and purposeful movement.*
- Change client's position frequently, moving individual parts of the body (e.g., legs, arms, head), using appropriate support and proper body alignment. Encourage periodic changes in head of bed (if not contraindicated by conditions such as acute SCI), with client in supine and prone positions at intervals *to improve circulation and reduce tightening of muscles and joints, normalizing body tone and more closely simulating body positions individual would normally use.*[2]
- Instruct caregivers in methods of moving client relative to specific situations (e.g., turning side to side, or prone, or sitting) *to provide support for the client's body and to prevent injury to the lifter. Note: Positioning instructions and detailed sketches are available (e.g., Ossman)*[7] *on proper positions for certain conditions (e.g., paralyzed client) as well as the safe movement and positioning of body parts (e.g., rolling, bridging, scooting, sitting), which should become well known to caregivers in order to prevent injury to both the client and the caregivers.*

 Acute Care   Collaborative   Community/ Home Care   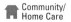 Cultural

- Place client in upright position at intervals, or out of bed into upright chair, if condition allows. *Being vertical has been shown to reduce the work of heart, improve circulation and lung ventilation, and may improve cognition and awareness.*[3]
- Use pressure-relieving devices (e.g., egg crate, alternating air pressure, or water mattress) and padding and positioning devices (e.g., foam wedge, pillows, hand rolls, etc., for bony prominences, feet, hands, elbows, head) *to prevent dermal injury or stress on tissues and reduce potential for disuse complications.*[3,6] Refer to ND risk for peripheral Neurovascular Dysfunction for additional interventions.
- Perform and encourage regular skin examination for reddened or excoriated areas. Use a pressure risk assessment scale (e.g., Braden, Norton) as appropriate. *A review of 33 studies revealed no decrease in pressure ulcer incidence that might be attributed to use of an assessment scale. However, the use of scales increased the intensity and effectiveness of prevention interventions.*[10]
- Provide frequent skin care (e.g., cleansing, moisturizing, gentle massage) *to reduce pressure on sensitive areas and prevent development of problems with skin or tissue integrity.* Refer to NDs impaired Skin Integrity; impaired Tissue Integrity.
- Provide or assist with daily range-of-motion interventions (active and passive) *to maintain joint mobility, improve circulation, and prevent contractures. Note: A random clinical trial found that regular exercising of joints prevented stiffness of knee tendons and improved joint function in clients on bedrest.*[11]
- Collaborate with rehabilitation team and physical or occupational therapists to create exercise and adaptive program designed specifically for client and to identify assistive devices (e.g., splints, braces, boots) and equipment (e.g., transfer board, sling, trapeze, hydraulic lift, specialty beds).
- Assist with activities of hygiene, feeding, and toileting, as indicated. Assist on and off bedpan and into sitting position (or use cardioposition bed or foot-egress bed) to facilitate elimination.
- Note change in strength to do more or less self-care (e.g., hygiene, feeding, toileting), *to promote psychological and physical benefits of self-care, and to adjust level of assistance as indicated.*
- Administer medication before activity as needed for pain relief *to permit maximal effort and involvement in activity.*
- Provide diversional activities (e.g., television, books, music, games, visiting) as appropriate *to decrease boredom and potential for depression.*
- Ensure telephone or call bell is within reach and client is able to activate surveillance alarm if provided. *Provides individually appropriate methods for client to communicate needs for assistance.*
- Refer to NDs Activity Intolerance, impaired physical Mobility, impaired wheelchair Mobility, risk for Disuse Syndrome, impaired Transfer Ability, and impaired Walking for additional interventions.

NURSING PRIORITY NO. 4   To promote wellness (Teaching/Discharge Considerations):

- Involve client/significant other in determining activity schedule. *Promotes commitment to plan, maximizing outcomes.*
- Instruct all caregivers in safety concerns regarding body mechanics, as well as client's required positions and exercises, *to prevent injury to both and to minimize potential for preventable complications.*
- Encourage continuation of regular exercise program *to maintain or enhance gains in strength and muscle control.*
- Obtain or identify sources for assistive devices. Demonstrate safe use and proper maintenance. *Promotes independence and enhances safety.*

DOCUMENTATION FOCUS

Assessment/Reassessment
- Individual findings, including level of function and ability to participate in specific or desired activities.

Planning
- Plan of care and who is involved in the planning.
- Teaching plan.

 Diagnostic Studies   Evidence Based Practice   Medications   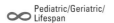 Pediatric/Geriatric/Lifespan

Implementation/Evaluation
- Responses to interventions, teaching, and actions performed.
- Attainment or progress toward desired outcome(s).
- Modification to plan of care.

Discharge Planning
- Discharge and long-range needs, noting who is responsible for each action to be taken.
- Specific referrals made.
- Sources of and maintenance for assistive devices.

References

1. Stanley, M. (1999). The aging musculoskeletal system. In Stanley, M., Beare, P. G. (eds). *Gerontological Nursing: A Health Promotion/Protection Approach.* 2nd ed. Philadelphia, PA: F. A. Davis.
2. Kumagai, K. A. S. (1998). Physical management of the neurologically involved client: Techniques for bed mobility and transfers. In Chin, P. A., et al. (eds). *Rehabilitation Nursing Practice.* New York, NY: McGraw-Hill.
3. Buchman, A. S., et al. (2011). Cognitive function is associated with the development of mobility impairments in community-dwelling elders. *Am J Geriatr Psychiatry*, 19(6), 571–580.
4. Crawford, A., Harris, H. (2016). Caring for adults with impaired physical mobility. *Nursing2018*, 46(12), 36–41.
5. Hogue, C. C. (1984). Falls and mobility late in life: An ecological model. *J Am Geriatr Soc*, 32, 858–861.
6. Dionne, M. (2005). This bed is just right. *Rehab Manag*, 18(1), 32–39.
7. Ossman, N., Campbell, M. (1995). *Adult Positions, Transitions, and Transfers: Reproducible Instruction Cards for Caregivers.* Tucson, AZ: Communication Skill Builders/Therapy Skill Builders.
8. Cibulka, N. T., et al. (2009). Hip pain and mobility deficits—Hip osteoarthritis: Clinical practice guidelines linked to the International Classification of Functioning Disability, and Health from the Orthopaedic Section of the American Physical Therapy Association. *J Orthop Sports Phys Ther*, 39(4), A1–A25.
9. Bakker, M., et al. (2006). Cerebral correlates of motor imagery of normal and precision gait. *Neuroimage*, 41, 998–1010.
10. Pancorbo-Hidalgo, P. L., Garcia-Fernandez, F. P., Lopez-Medina, I. M. (2006). Risk assessment scales for pressure ulcers prevention: A systematic review. *J Adv Nurs*, 54(1), 94–110.
11. Kubo, K., et al. (2004). Effects of resistance training during bed rest on the viscoelastic properties of tendon structures of tendon structures in the lower limb. *Scand J Med Sci Sports*, 14(5), 296–302.
12. Gordon, M. (2010). Functional levels code. *Manual of Nursing Diagnosis.* 12th ed. Sudbury, MA: Jones and Bartlett.

---

impaired physical Mobility

Taxonomy II: Activity/Rest—Class 2 Activity/Exercise (00085) [**Diagnostic Division:** Safety], Approved 1973; Revised 1998, 2013, 2017

DEFINITION: Limitation in independent, purposeful physical movement of the body or of one or more extremities.

RELATED FACTORS
Activity intolerance; decrease in endurance; reluctance to initiate movement; physical deconditioning; sedentary lifestyle

Alteration in metabolism; body mass index >75th age-appropriate percentile; malnutrition

Anxiety; depression

Cultural belief regarding acceptable activity

Decrease in muscle mass, control or strength; joint stiffness; contractures

Insufficient environmental support

Insufficient knowledge of value of physical activity

Pain

 Acute Care   Collaborative   Community/ Home Care   Cultural

DEFINING CHARACTERISTICS

Subjective
Discomfort

Objective
Alteration in gait; postural instability

Decrease in fine or gross motor skills; movement-induced tremor

Decrease in range of motion; difficulty turning

Decrease in reaction time; slowed or spastic movement; uncoordinated movement

Engages in substitutions for movement [e.g., attention to other's activities, controlling behavior, focus on preillness activity]

Exertional dyspnea

Associated Condition: Alteration in bone structure integrity; musculoskeletal or neuromuscular, or sensory-perceptual impairment; contractures

Alteration in cognitive functioning; developmental delay

Alteration in metabolism

Prescribed movement restrictions

Pharmaceutical agent

Sample Clinical Applications: Neuromuscular disorders (e.g., multiple sclerosis [MS], amyotrophic lateral sclerosis [ALS], Parkinson's disease), traumatic injuries (e.g., fractures, spinal cord or brain injuries), osteoarthritis, rheumatoid arthritis, severe depression

SUGGESTED FUNCTIONAL LEVEL CLASSIFICATION

0—Full self-care

I—Requires use of equipment or device

II—Requires assistance or supervision of another person

III—Requires assistance or supervision of another person and equipment or device

IV—Is dependent and does not participate[12]

DESIRED OUTCOMES/EVALUATION CRITERIA

Sample NOC linkages:

Mobility: Ability to move purposefully in own environment independently with or without assistive device

Immobility Consequences: Physiological: Severity of compromise in physiological functioning due to impaired physical mobility

Knowledge: Prescribed Activity: Extent of understanding conveyed about prescribed activity recommended by a health professional for a specific condition

Client Will (Include Specific Time Frame)
- Verbalize understanding of situation and individual treatment regimen and safety measures.
- Demonstrate techniques or behaviors that enable resumption of activities.
- Participate in activities of daily living (ADLs) and desired activities.
- Maintain position of function and skin integrity as evidenced by absence of contractures, footdrop, decubitus, etc.
- Maintain or increase strength and function of affected or compensatory body part.

(continues on page 550)

 Diagnostic Studies   Evidence Based Practice   Medications   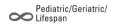 Pediatric/Geriatric/Lifespan

impaired physical Mobility (continued)

ACTIONS/INTERVENTIONS

Sample NIC linkages:

Exercise Therapy: Joint Mobility/Muscle Control: Use of active or passive body movement to maintain or restore joint flexibility/use of specific activity or exercise protocols to enhance or restore controlled body movement

Pain Management: Chronic: Alleviation or reduction of persistent pain that continues beyond the normal healing period, assumed to be 3 months, to a level that is acceptable to the patient

Traction/Immobilization Care: Management of a patient who has traction and/or a stabilizing device to immobilize and stabilize a body part

NURSING PRIORITY NO. 1   To identify causative/contributing factors:

- Determine diagnosis that contributes to immobility (e.g., MS, arthritis, Parkinson's disease, cardiopulmonary disorders, hemi/paraplegia, depression, developmental delays). *These conditions can cause physiological and psychological problems that can seriously impact physical, social, and economic well-being.*[1]
- Note factors affecting current situation (e.g., surgery, fractures, amputation, tubings [chest tube, Foley catheter, IVs, pumps], and potential time involved [e.g., few hours in bed after surgery versus serious trauma requiring long-term bedrest or debilitating disease limiting movement]). *Identifies potential impairments and determines type of interventions needed to provide for client's safety.*
- Assess client's developmental level, motor skills, ease and capability of movement, and posture and gait *to determine presence of characteristics of client's unique impairment and to guide choice of interventions.*[8]
- ∞ 📝 Note older client's general health status. *Hogue identified mobility as the most important functional ability that determines the degree of independence and healthcare needs among older persons.*[2] *While aging does not cause impaired mobility, per se, several predisposing factors in addition to age-related changes can lead to immobility (e.g., diminished body reserves of musculoskeletal system, chronic diseases, sedentary lifestyle, decreased ability to quickly and adequately correct movements affecting center of gravity). Thus, falls are a major source of morbidity and mortality for older persons.*[3,6,8]
- Evaluate for presence and degree of pain, listening to client's description about manner in which pain limits mobility *to determine if pain management can improve mobility.*[4]
- 🌐 📝 Ascertain client's perception of activity and exercise needs and impact of current situation. Identify cultural beliefs and expectations affecting recovery or response to long-term limitations. *Helps to determine client's expectations and beliefs related to activity and potential long-term effect of current immobility. Also identifies barriers that may be addressed (e.g., lack of safe place to exercise, focus on preillness or disability activity, controlling behavior, depression, cultural expectations, distorted body image).*[5]
- Assess nutritional status and client's report of energy level. *Deficiencies in nutrients and water, electrolytes, and minerals can negatively affect energy and activity tolerance.*
- 📝 Determine history of falls and relatedness to current situation. *Client may be restricting activity because of weakness or debilitation, actual injury during a fall, or from psychological distress (i.e., fear and anxiety) that can persist after a fall.*[6–8]

NURSING PRIORITY NO. 2   To assess functional ability:

- 📝 Determine degree of immobility in relation to 0–4 scale, noting muscle strength and tone, joint mobility, cardiovascular status, balance, and endurance. *Identifies strengths and deficits (e.g., ability to ambulate with or without assistive devices, inability to transfer safely from bed to wheelchair) and may provide information regarding potential for recovery (e.g., client with severe brain injury may have permanent limitations because*

 Acute Care   Collaborative   Community/ Home Care   Cultural

of impaired cognition affecting memory, judgment, problem solving, and motor planning, requiring more intensive inpatient and long-term care).[1,6]

- Determine degree of perceptual or cognitive impairment and ability to follow directions. *Impairments related to age, chronic or acute disease condition, trauma, surgery, or medications require alternative interventions or changes in plan of care.*[3]
- Observe movement when client is unaware of observation *to note any incongruency with reports of abilities.*
- Note emotional or behavioral responses to problems of immobility. *Can negatively affect self-concept and self-esteem, autonomy, and independence. Feelings of frustration and powerlessness may impede attainment of goals. Social, occupational, and relationship roles can change, leading to isolation, depression, and economic consequences.*[1,2]
- Determine presence of complications related to immobility. *The effects of immobility are rarely confined to one body system and can include muscle wasting, contractures, pressure sores, constipation, aspiration pneumonia, etc. Studies have shown that healthy individuals who were subjected to immobility experienced a 1.3% to 3% loss in muscle strength per day, and overall postural muscle strength decreased by 10% during 1 wk of bedrest.*[5,7] *Other complications include changes in circulation and impairments of organ function affecting the whole person (e.g., cognition, bone demineralization, venous pooling, thromboembolic phenomena, weakened immune system function).* (Refer to ND risk for Disuse Syndrome.)

NURSING PRIORITY NO. 3 To promote optimal level of function and prevent complications:

- 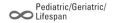 Assist with treatment of underlying condition(s) *to maximize potential for mobility and optimal function.*
- Discuss discrepancies in movement with client aware and unaware of observation and methods for dealing with identified problems. *May be necessary when client is using avoidance or controlling behavior or is not aware of own abilities due to anxiety or fear.*
- Assist with or encourage client to reposition self on a regular schedule as dictated by individual situation (including frequent shifting of weight when client is wheelchair-bound) *to enhance circulation to tissues and reduce risk of tissue ischemia.*
- Review and encourage use of proper body mechanics *to prevent injury to client and caregiver.*
- Demonstrate and assist with use of siderails, overhead trapeze, roller pads, and hydraulic lifts or chairs *for position changes and transfers.* Instruct in safe use of walker or cane *to facilitate safe ambulation.*
- Support affected body parts and joints using pillows or rolls, foot supports, shoes, gel pads, etc., *to maintain position of function and reduce risk of pressure ulcers.*
- Provide or recommend pressure-reducing mattress, such as egg crate, or pressure-relieving mattress, such as alternating air pressure or water. *Reduces tissue pressure and aids in maximizing cellular perfusion to prevent dermal injury.*
- Use padding and positioning devices (e.g., foam wedge, pillows, hand rolls) for bony prominences, feet, hands, elbows, head) *to prevent stress on tissues and reduce potential for disuse complications.*
- 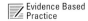 Collaborate with physical medicine specialist and occupational or physical therapists in providing range-of-motion exercise (active or passive), isotonic muscle contractions (e.g., flexion of ankles, push and pull exercises), assistive devices, and activities (e.g., early ambulation, transfers, stairs) *to limit or reduce effects and complications of immobility (e.g., contracture deformities, deep vein thromboses). Techniques such as gait training, strength training, and exercise to improve balance and coordination can be helpful in preventing complications and in rehabilitating client.*[11]
- Encourage client's participation in self-care activities and physical or occupational therapies as well as diversional and recreational activities. *Reduces sensory deprivation, enhances self-concept and sense of independence, and improves body strength and function.*
- Provide client with ample time to perform mobility-related tasks. Schedule activities with adequate rest periods during the day *to reduce fatigue and improve endurance and strength.*
- Avoid routinely assisting or doing for client those activities that client can do for self. *Caregivers can contribute to impaired mobility by being overprotective or helping too much.*

- Identify and encourage energy-conserving techniques for ADLs. *Limits fatigue, maximizing participation.*
- Provide for safety measures as indicated by individual situation, including environmental management and fall prevention. (Refer to ND risk for Falls.)
- Note change in strength to do more or less self-care (e.g., hygiene, feeding, toileting, therapies) *to promote psychological and physical benefits of self-care and to adjust level of assistance as indicated.*
- Administer medications before activity as needed for pain relief *to permit maximal effort and involvement in activity.*
- Perform and encourage regular skin examination and care *to reduce pressure on sensitive areas and to prevent development of problems with skin integrity.* (Refer to NDs risk for impaired Skin Integrity and risk for impaired Tissue Integrity for additional interventions.)
- Encourage adequate intake of fluids and nutritious foods. *Promotes well-being and maximizes energy production.*
- Refer to NDs Activity Intolerance, risk for Falls, impaired bed Mobility, impaired wheelchair Mobility, impaired Transfer Ability, impaired Sitting, impaired Standing, or impaired Walking for additional interventions.

NURSING PRIORITY NO. 4 To promote wellness (Teaching/Discharge Considerations):

- Encourage client's/significant other's (SO's) involvement in decision making as much as possible. *Enhances commitment to plan, optimizing outcomes.*
- Review importance and purpose of exercise *(e.g., increased cardiovascular and respiratory tolerance; improved flexibility, balance, and muscle strength and tone; enhanced sense of well-being).*
- Discuss safe ways that client can exercise. *Multiple options provide client choices and variety (e.g., walking around the block with companion or in a mall during bad air days, participating in a water aerobics class, attending regular rehab sessions).*
- Assist client/SO to learn safety measures as individually indicated. *May need instruction and to give return demonstration (e.g., use of heating pads, locking wheelchair before transfers, removal or securing of scatter or area rugs, judicious and accurate use of medications, supervised exercise).*
- Involve client and SO(s) in care, assisting them to learn ways of managing problems of immobility, especially when impairment is expected to be long term. *May need referral for support and community services to provide care, supervision, companionship, respite services, nutritional and ADL assistance, adaptive devices or changes to living environment, financial assistance, etc.*[8]
- Demonstrate use of standing aids and mobility devices (e.g., walkers, strollers, scooters, braces, prosthetics) and have client/care provider demonstrate knowledge about and safe use of device. Identify appropriate resources for obtaining and maintaining appliances or equipment. *Safe use of mobility aids promotes client's independence and enhances quality of life and safety for client and caregiver.*[9,10]

DOCUMENTATION FOCUS

Assessment/Reassessment
- Individual findings, including level of function and ability to participate in specific or desired activities.
- Use of assistive devices.

Planning
- Plan of care and who is involved in the planning.
- Teaching plan.

Implementation/Evaluation
- Responses to interventions, teaching, and actions performed.
- Attainment or progress toward desired outcome(s).
- Modifications to plan of care.

 Acute Care
 Collaborative
 Community/ Home Care
 Cultural

Discharge Planning
• Discharge and long-term needs, noting who is responsible for each action to be taken.
• Specific referrals made.
• Sources of and maintenance for assistive devices.

References

1. Crawford, A., Harris, H. (2016). Caring for adults with impaired physical mobility. *Nursing2018*, 46(12), 36–41.
2. Hogue, C. C. (1984). Falls and mobility late in life: An ecological model. *J Am Geriatr Soc*, 32, 858–861.
3. Rowe, J. W., Kahn, R. L. (1987). Human aging: Usual and successful. *Science*, 237, 143–149.
4. McCaffrey, M., Pasero, C. (1999). *Pain: Clinical Manual*. 2nd ed. St. Louis, MO: Mosby.
5. Pattillo, M. A., Stanley, M. (1999). The aging musculoskeletal system. In Stanley, M., Beare, P. G. (eds). *Gerontological Nursing: A Health Promotion/Protection Approach*. 2nd ed. Philadelphia, PA: F. A. Davis.
6. Tinetti, M. E., Williams, T. F., Mayewski, R. (1986). Fall risk index for elderly patients based on number of chronic disabilities. *Am J Med*, 80, 429–434.
7. Hopkins, R., et al. (2007). Transforming ICU culture to facilitate early mobility. *Crit Care Clin*, 23(1), 81–96.
8. Michael, K. M., Allen, J. K., Macko, R. F. (2006). Fatigue after stroke: Relationship to mobility, fitness, ambulatory activity, social support, and falls efficiency. *Rehabil Nurs*, 31(5), 210–217.
9. Becker, B. (2005). To stand or not to stand. *Rehab Manag*, 18(2), 28–34.
10. Dworak, P. A., Levy, A. (2005). Strolling along. *Rehab Manag*, 18(9), 26–31.
11. Ship, K. M. (2010). Gait disturbances in older age: The reasons are many and varied, but researchers agree that identifying the source and preserving mobility are primary concerns. *Duke Med Health News*, 16(8), 3–4.
12. Gordon, M. (2014). Functional levels code. *Manual of Nursing Diagnosis*. 13th ed. Burlington, MA: Jones and Bartlett.

---

impaired wheelchair Mobility

Taxonomy II: Activity/Rest—Class 2 Activity/Exercise (00089) [**Diagnostic Division:** Safety], Approved 1998; Revised 2006, 2017

DEFINITION: Limitation of independent operation of wheelchair within environment.

RELATED FACTORS
Alteration in mood
Decrease in endurance; insufficient muscle strength; physical deconditioning; obesity
Environmental barrier (e.g., stairs, inclines, uneven surfaces, obstacles, distance)
Insufficient knowledge of wheelchair use
Pain

DEFINING CHARACTERISTICS

Objective
Impaired ability to operate manual or power wheelchair on even or uneven surface; on an incline or decline; on curbs
[**Note:** Specify level of independence using a standardized functional scale, refer to ND impaired physical Mobility]
Associated Condition: Alteration in cognitive functioning; impaired vision
Musculoskeletal or neuromuscular impairment
Sample Clinical Applications: Neuromuscular disorders (e.g., multiple sclerosis [MS], amyotrophic lateral sclerosis [ALS]), paralysis (e.g., brain injury/stroke, spinal cord injury [SCI]), muscular dystrophy, cerebral palsy, fractures

(continues on page 554)

 Diagnostic Studies   Evidence Based Practice   Medications 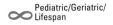 Pediatric/Geriatric/Lifespan

impaired wheelchair Mobility (continued)

DESIRED OUTCOMES/EVALUATION CRITERIA

Sample NOC linkage:

Ambulation: Wheelchair: Personal actions to move from place to place in a wheelchair

Coordinated Movement: Ability of muscles to work together voluntarily for purposeful movement

Client Will (Include Specific Time Frame)
- Move safely within environment, maximizing independence.
- Identify and use resources appropriately.

Sample NOC linkages:

Fall Prevention Behavior: Personal or family caregiver actions to minimize risk factors that might precipitate falls in the personal environment

Caregiver Will (Include Specific Time Frame)
- Provide safe mobility within environment and community

ACTIONS/INTERVENTIONS

Sample NIC linkages:

Positioning: Wheelchair: Placement of a patient in a properly selected wheelchair to enhance comfort, promote skin integrity, and foster independence

Exercise Therapy: Muscle Control: Use of specific activity or exercise protocols to enhance or restore controlled body movement

Self-Care Assistance: Transfer: Assisting a patient with limitation of independent movement to learn to change body location

---

NURSING PRIORITY NO. 1   To identify causative/contributing factors:

- Determine diagnosis that contributes to immobility (e.g., ALS, SCI, spastic cerebral palsy, brain injury) and client's functional level and individual abilities (e.g., 0–4 scale; see ND impaired physical Mobility).
- Identify factors in environments frequented by the client that contribute to inaccessibility (e.g., uneven floors or surfaces, lack of ramps, steep incline or decline, narrow doorways or spaces).
- Ascertain access to and appropriateness of public and/or private transportation.

NURSING PRIORITY NO. 2   To promote optimal level of function and prevent complications:

- 🏠 Determine that client's underlying physical, cognitive, and emotional impairment(s) (e.g., brain or spinal cord injury, fractures or other trauma; pain, depression, vision deficits) are treated or being managed *to maximize ability, desire, and motivation to participate in wheelchair activities.*[6]
- Ⓐ Collaborate with physical medicine or physical or occupational therapists in planning activities to improve client's ability to independently operate wheelchair within limits of tolerance and adjustment to various environments. *May require individual instruction and encouragement, strengthening exercises, assistance with various tasks, and close supervision.*
- ∞ Ascertain that wheelchair provides the base mobility to maximize function. *Wheelchair must be matched with client's age and size/body type; developmental level and diagnosis, or reason to use wheelchair; desired activities; and unique functional needs (e.g., proper seating and support for people in wheelchairs is critical to their ability to travel, work, participate in sports, learn at school, play, and interact*

 Acute Care   Collaborative   Community/ Home Care   Cultural

socially). If a spouse or family member will be assisting the person using the wheelchair then that person's needs may also need to be considered in the wheelchair selection.[1,10] *Correct seating is essential for prevention, correction, and compensation for postural changes in order to maintain client's comfort and function. Chair should provide for maximum reach, maneuverability, function, and center of gravity positioning and propulsion; should recline to change back contours, hip angles, and pelvic restrictions; should have back adjustment for changing trunk stability requirements; and should tilt for reposition, pressure relief, and comfort.*[1,2,7,8]

- Perform periodic assessments of client and wheelchair to monitor chair usage and function as well as changes in client's postural, behavioral, and functional status. *Helps to identify problems (e.g., abnormal wear patterns on the chair requiring mechanical adjustments/repair; loss of client's strength where power add-ons to the chair would improve mobility; or alternate methods of mobility that might be needed).*[2]
- Provide for or instruct client in safety while in a wheelchair (e.g., cushions, supports for all body parts, repositioning and transfer assistive devices, position and pressure relief products, feet and leg support, armrest choices, back and height adjustment).[2,7]
- Note surfaces client needs to negotiate and refer to appropriate sources for modifications (e.g., replacing carpet with tile; revising ramps that are too steep, narrow, or slippery). Clear pathways of obstructions.[2,10]
- Recommend and arrange for modifications to home, work, school, or recreational settings frequented by client. *Although most public buildings have certain adaptations in rooms and accesses, they are not always well constructed or in good working order. The client may need assistance in these settings and with requesting that appropriate alterations be carried out.*[9]
- Determine need for and capabilities of assistive persons. Provide training and support, as indicated. *Enhances safety for both client and caregiver.*
- Monitor client's use of joystick, sip and puff, sensitive mechanical switches, etc., *to provide necessary equipment if condition or capabilities change.*
- Monitor client for adverse effects of immobility (e.g., contractures, muscle atrophy, deep venous thrombosis, pressure ulcers). (Refer to NDs Disuse Syndrome and risk for peripheral Neurovascular Dysfunction for additional interventions.)

NURSING PRIORITY NO. 3 To promote wellness (Teaching/Discharge Considerations):

- Identify and refer to medical equipment suppliers *to customize client's wheelchair for size, proper seating angle, positioning aids, incline or decline stability, accessories (e.g., side guards, headrests, heel loops, brake extensions, tool packs), and electronics suited to client's ability (e.g., sip and puff, head movement, sensitive switches).*[6,8]
- Encourage client's/significant others' (SOs') involvement in decision making as much as possible. *Enhances sense of control and commitment to plan, thereby optimizing outcomes.*
- Involve client/SO(s) in care, assisting them in managing immobility problems. *Promotes independence in self-evaluation and self-care, including managing the type of wheelchair and other assistive devices best for client, how the user's needs and abilities change over time, and modifications that might be made (e.g., number and placement of ramps around the home; modifications to rooms, doors, and vehicles).*[3]
- Demonstrate, discuss, and provide information regarding wheelchair safety as individually appropriate, including safe transfers, dealing with uneven surfaces, ramps, and curbs; programming speed on power chairs; etc. Include information and refer for wheelchair preventative maintenance measures (e.g., for wheelchair locks, tires, axles, casters, metal parts, batteries) as indicated. *Wheelchair safety involves people and equipment and is a daily factor in the life of the client and caregivers. This includes not only acquiring the best chair but also maintenance of the chair and provision for obtaining relief when chair malfunctions. Many states have enacted wheelchair lemon laws that "mandate warranties to maintain assistive technology in proper working condition, to assure availability of appropriate loaner replacement chairs during repair time, and to encourage manufacturers and dealers to cooperatively pool assistive technology resources for loaner purposes to assure availability without undue burden."*[4]

 Diagnostic Studies   Evidence Based Practice   Medications   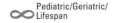 Pediatric/Geriatric/ Lifespan

- Refer to support groups relative to specific medical condition/disability and geared toward client's independence. Suggest involvement in political action group, as indicated. *Provides role modeling, assistance with problem-solving, and social change.*
- Identify community resources to provide ongoing support. *Persons with disabilities have the right to be self-determining and to achieve the quality of life each believes is personal best. This places as much emphasis on community regarding integration as on physical rehabilitation and functional capabilities.*[5]

DOCUMENTATION FOCUS

Assessment/Reassessment
- Individual findings, including level of function/ability to participate in specific/desired activities.
- Type of wheelchair and equipment needs.
- Environmental factors and problems.

Planning
- Plan of care and who is involved in the planning.
- Teaching plan.

Implementation/Evaluation
- Responses to interventions, teaching, and actions performed.

Discharge Planning
- Discharge and long-term needs, noting who is responsible for each action to be taken.
- Specific referrals made.
- Sources of and maintenance for assistive devices.

References

1. Rodby-Bousquet, E., Hagglund, C. (2010). Use of manual and powered wheelchair in children with cerebral palsy: A cross-sectional study. *BMC Pediatr.* Retrieved March 2018 from http://www.biomedcentral.com/1471-2431/10/59.
2. Rader, J., Jones, D., Miller, L. (No date). Individualizing wheelchair seating: For older adults. Part 1: A guide for caregivers. *Benedictine Institute for Long Term Care*. Retrieved March 2018 from http://primaris.org/sites/default/files/resources/Restraints%20and%20Falls/A%20Guide%20for%20Caregivers_Individualized%20Wheelchair%20Seating.pdf.
3. Mobility Advisor. (No date). Types of mobility ramps. Retrieved March 2018 from https://www.mobility-advisor.com/mobility-ramps.html.
4. Wisconsin Department of Health Services. (Updated 2016). Wisconsin's motorized wheelchair lemon law. Retrieved March 2018 from https://www.dhs.wisconsin.gov/disabilities/physical/lemonlaw.htm.
5. Scherer, M. (2002). *The Importance of Assistive Technology Outcomes*. Washington, DC: Institute for Matching Person & Technology.
6. Cohen, D. (2005). Optional but necessary. *Rehab Manag*, 18(10), 26–29.
7. Rosen, L. (2005). Sit on it. *Rehab Manag*, 18(2), 36–41.
8. Waugh, K. G. (2005). Measuring the right angle. *Rehab Manag*, 18(1), 40–49.
9. McCullagh, M. C. (2006). Home modification. *Am J Nurs*, 106(10), 54–63.
10. Department of Rehabilitation Science and Technology. (2006). Wheelchair selection: How to choose a new wheelchair. *Fact sheet from WheelchairNet*. Retrieved March 2018 from http://www.wheelchairnet.org/wcn_prodserv/consumers/selectwc.html.

 Acute Care   Collaborative   Community/Home Care   Cultural

impaired Mood Regulation

Taxonomy II: Coping/Stress Tolerance—Class 2 Coping Responses (00241) **[Diagnostic Division:** Ego Integrity], Approved 2013; Revised 2017

DEFINITION: A mental state characterized by shifts in mood or affect and which is comprised of a constellation of affective, cognitive, somatic and/or physiological manifestations varying from mild to severe.

RELATED FACTORS

Alteration in sleep pattern; appetite or weight change
Anxiety; hypervigilance
Loneliness; impaired social functioning; social isolation
Pain
Recurrent thoughts of death or suicide
Substance misuse/[abuse]

DEFINING CHARACTERISTICS

Subjective

Excessive self-awareness, guilt, self-blame
Hopelessness

Objective

Sad affect, withdrawal
Irritability; impaired concentration
Psychomotor agitation, retardation
Changes in verbal behavior; flight of thoughts; dysphoria; disinhibition
Influenced self-esteem
Associated Condition: Chronic illness; functional impairment; psychosis
Sample Clinical Applications: Depression, bipolar disorder, anxiety states, autism spectrum disorder

DESIRED OUTCOMES/EVALUATION CRITERIA

Sample NOC linkage:
Mood Equilibrium: Appropriate adjustment of prevailing emotional tone in response to circumstances

Client Will (Include Specific Time Frame)
• Acknowledge reality of mood problems/needs.
• Identify areas of concern.
• Participate in treatment program or therapy regimen.
• Maintain physical health as evidenced by adequate nutrition, weight within normal limits, and good sleep habits.

ACTIONS/INTERVENTIONS

Sample NIC linkage:
Mood Management: Providing for safety, stabilization, recovery, and maintenance of a person who is experiencing dysfunctionally depressed or elevated mood

 Diagnostic Studies   Evidence Based Practice   Medications   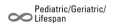 Pediatric/Geriatric/Lifespan

NURSING PRIORITY NO. 1   To assess causative/contributing factors:

- Determine specific reasons for client's mood swings/difficulties and specific manifestations. (Refer to Related Factors and Defining Characteristics.) *Allows for accurate planning of care for individual.*[1]
- Assess ability to understand current situation. *Mood disturbances are prevalent in many disorders and may affect individual's cognitive functioning and understanding of events.*[1]
- Review history and evaluate for underlying neurological disorders. *Presence of traumatic brain injuries, tumors, stroke, and autism may result in variations of mood and emotional processing deficits.*[1]
- Ascertain degree of depression individual is experiencing. *Impaired mood regulation is known to be a factor in vulnerability to depression.*[5]
- Identify behaviors that interfere with person's daily activities. *Being aware of behaviors, such as sleep or appetite disturbances, altered social activity, irritability, and impaired concentration, facilitates identification of treatment options for change.*[2]
- Determine availability and use of resources.

NURSING PRIORITY NO. 2   To assist client to regulate mood changes more effectively:

- Discuss how client perceives the current situation and how it is affecting emotions. *A negative outlook is associated with difficulty in cognitive control and emotional regulation strategies.*[5]
- Determine extent of rumination and reappraisal and expressive suppression. *As the individual goes over and over the negative thoughts, it is more difficult to effect cognitive control and depression can worsen.*[5]
- Encourage client to pay attention to emotional states and feelings and identify when they occur and record in a journal or notebook. *Awareness of one's emotions helps the individual to deal with them appropriately.*[3]
- Clarify meanings of feelings by checking meaning with client and providing feedback. *Validates and ensures accuracy of meaning of the communication.*[6]
- Discuss how negative thinking and rumination intensify depression. *It appears individual differences can affect the strategies the person uses to recover from a negative mood.*[5]
- Provide information regarding use of electroconvulsive therapy (ECT) as indicated. *It is not known exactly how this treatment helps; it is thought to alter brain chemistry and function that relieves depression in 80% to 90% of clients.*[8] *The client with severe depression that does not respond to medication may benefit from ECT along with psychotherapy.*[7]

NURSING PRIORITY NO. 3   To promote wellness (Teaching/Discharge Considerations):

- Involve client in cognitive/behavioral, mindfulness-based, or individual psychotherapy. *Having the client identify thinking patterns that result in depression allows the individual to recognize and avoid them, improving the ability to recover.*[5]
- Discuss the use of and administer medications as indicated. *Antidepressants can be useful in mood disorders and, along with psychotherapy, can help the client maintain usual activities.*[7]
- Involve client in group therapy. *Group discussions promote awareness of others who are experiencing similar difficulties and promote new ideas for dealing with own concerns.*[4]
- Encourage client to become involved in community activities. *Provides opportunity to develop social skills and interests outside of own concerns.*[5]

DOCUMENTATION FOCUS

Assessment/Reassessment
- Individual findings, including client's specific situation and impact on functioning/life.
- Description of negative thinking patterns.

Planning
- Treatment plan and individual responsibility for activities.
- Teaching plan.

 Acute Care   Collaborative   Community/ Home Care   Cultural

Implementation/Evaluation
• Client involvement and response to interventions, teaching and actions performed.
• Attainment or progress toward desired outcomes.
• Modification to plan of care.

Discharge Planning
• Specific referrals made and follow-up plan.

References

1. Brockmeyer, T., et al. (2012). Mood regulation expectancies and emotion avoidance in depression vulnerability. *Pers Individ Dif*, 53(3), 163–362.
2. Mazefsky, C. A., et al. (2013). The role of emotion regulation in autism spectrum disorder. *J Am Acad Child Adoles Psychiatry*, 52(7), 679–688.
3. van Eijndhoven, P., et al. (2013). Paralimbic cortical thickness in first-episode depression: Evidence for trait-related differences in mood regulation. *Am J Psychiatry*, 170, 1477–1486.
4. Hoppes, K. (2006). The application of mindfulness-based cognitive interventions in the treatment of co-occurring addictive and mood disorders. *CNS Spectr*, 11(11), 829–851.
5. Joormann, J., Gotlib, I. H. (2010). Emotion regulation in depression: Relation to cognitive inhibition. *Cogn Emot*, 24(2), 281–298.
6. Burns, D. D. (2008). *Feeling Good: The New Mood Therapy*. New York: Harper.
7. Marvel, C. L., Paradiso, S. (2004). Cognitive and neurological impairment in mood disorders. *Psychiatr Clin North Am*, 27(1), 19–viii.
8. Miller, M. C. (2013, updated 2017). Understanding depression: Special health report. Retrieved April 2018 from https://www.health.harvard.edu/mind-and-mood/understanding-depression.

Moral Distress

Taxonomy II: Life Principles—Class 3 Value/Belief/Action Congruence (00175) [**Diagnostic Division:** Ego Integrity], Approved 2006

DEFINITION: Response to the inability to carry out one's chosen ethical/moral decision/action.

RELATED FACTORS

Conflict among decision makers [e.g., client/family, healthcare providers, insurance payers, regulatory agencies]
Conflicting information available for moral or ethical decision making; cultural incongruences
Difficulty reaching treatment or end-of-life decisions
Time constraint for decision making

DEFINING CHARACTERISTICS

Subjective
Anguish about acting on one's moral choice
At Risk Population: Loss of autonomy
Physical distance of decision-making

DESIRED OUTCOMES/EVALUATION CRITERIA

Sample NOC linkages:
Decision-Making: Ability to make judgments and choose between two or more alternatives
Client Satisfaction: Protection of Rights: Extent of positive perception of a patient's legal and moral rights provided by nursing staff
Participation in Health Care Decisions: Personal involvement in selecting and evaluating health care options to achieve desired outcome

(continues on page 560)

 Diagnostic Studies   Evidence Based Practice   Medications   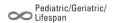 Pediatric/Geriatric/Lifespan

Moral Distress (continued)

Client Will (Include Specific Time Frame)
• Verbalize understanding of causes for conflict in own situation.
• Be aware of own moral values conflicting with desired or required course of action.
• Identify positive ways or actions necessary to deal with own self and situation.
• Express sense of satisfaction with or acceptance of resolution.

ACTIONS/INTERVENTIONS

Sample NIC linkages:
Values Clarification: Assisting another to clarify her/his own values in order to facilitate effective decision-making
Decision-Making Support: Providing information and support for a patient who is making a decision regarding health care
Mutual Goal-Setting: Collaborating with patient to identify and prioritize care goals, then developing a plan of care for achieving those goals

NURSING PRIORITY NO. 1 To identify cause/situation in which moral distress is occurring:

• Note situations or individuals at high risk for conflict. *For example, family members not agreeing on proper course of action for comatose loved one, parents faced with expectation of taking ventilator-dependent child home and effect on family as a whole;[8] and care providers discontinuing life support measures for preterm infant are likely to encounter some degree of distress with decision making but may be silent about their discomfort. Recognizing potential for moral distress allows for timely intervention and support for involved parties.*
• Determine client's perceptions and specific factors resulting in a sense of distress and all parties involved in situation. *Conflict may be personal or job related. Moral conflict centers around lessening the amount of harm suffered, with the involved individuals usually struggling with decisions such as what "can be done" to prevent, improve, or cure a medical condition or what "ought to be done" in a specific situation, often within financial constraints or scarcity of resources.[6]*
• Note use of sarcasm, avoidance, apathy, crying, reports of depression, or loss of meaning. *Individuals may not understand their feelings of uneasiness or distress or know that the emotional basis for moral distress is anger.[4]*
• Ascertain response of family/significant others (SOs) to client's situation/healthcare choices. *May provide clues to emotional or conflictual problems individual is experiencing.*
• Identify healthcare goals and expectations. *New treatment options and technology can prolong life or postpone death based on the individual's personal viewpoint, increasing the possibility of conflict with others, including healthcare providers.[2]*
• Ascertain cultural beliefs and values and degree of importance to client. *Cultural diversity may lead to disparate views and expectations between client, SO/family members, and healthcare providers. When tensions between conflicting values cannot be resolved, persons experience moral distress.[2]*
• Note attitudes and expressions of dissatisfaction of caregivers/staff. *Client may feel pressure or disapproval if own views are not congruent with expectations of those perceived to be more knowledgeable or in "authority." Furthermore, healthcare providers may themselves feel moral distress in carrying out or refraining from performing requested interventions.[7]*
• ⬛ Determine degree of emotional and physical distress (e.g., fatigue, headaches, forgetfulness, anger, guilt, resentment) individual(s) are experiencing and its impact on ability to function. *Moral distress can be very destructive, affecting one's ability to carry out daily tasks and care for self or others, and may lead to a crisis of faith.[5]*

 Acute Care   Collaborative   Community/Home Care   Cultural

- Assess sleep habits of involved parties. *Evidence suggests that sleep deprivation can harm a person's physical and emotional well-being, hindering the ability to integrate emotion and cognition to guide moral judgment.*[5]
- Perform or review results of moral distress test, such as the Moral Distress Assessment Questionnaire or the Moral Distress Scale, *to help measure degree of involvement and identify possible actions to improve situation.*[3,10]
- Note availability of family/friends/coworkers. *Provides support and encouragement for difficult situation.*[4]

NURSING PRIORITY NO. 2 To assist client/involved individuals to develop/effectively use problem-solving skills:

- Encourage involved individuals to recognize and name the experience, resulting in moral sensitivity. *Brings concerns out in the open so they can be dealt with.*[1]
- Provide time for nonjudgmental discussion of philosophical issues or questions about impact of conflict leading to moral questioning of current situation. *Moral issues have been discussed and studied for many years (e.g., philosophers, such as Piaget [1932] with his early work in developmental moral psychology, discussed what is the basis for moral reasoning). It is not possible to accurately read another's mind, and open discussion helps those involved in conflict to better understand the situation and begin to look at options.*[9]
- Use skills such as Active-listening, "I" messages, and problem-solving *to clarify feelings of anxiety and conflict. Helps to understand what the ethical dilemmas are that lead to moral distress (e.g., family members ignoring advanced directives of loved one, providing lifesaving care to a death row inmate, terminally ill individual requesting assistance to die, families living with the moral experience of caring for a ventilator-assisted child in the home).*[8]
- Provide privacy when discussing sensitive personal issues. *Shows regard and concern for individual's self-worth.*[2]
- Ascertain coping behaviors client has used successfully in the past that may be used in the current situation. *When encouraged, individuals can recall past situations where they had a positive experience and used successful coping skills.*[4]
- Identify role models (e.g., other individuals who have experienced similar problems in their lives). *Sharing of experiences and identifying options can be helpful to deal with current situation.*[1]
- Involve facility or local ethics committee or ethicist as appropriate *to educate, make recommendations, and facilitate mediation or resolution of conflicts.*[3]

NURSING PRIORITY NO. 3 To promote wellness (Teaching/Discharge Considerations):

- Engage all parties, as appropriate, in developing plan to address conflict. *Resolving one's moral distress requires making changes or compromises while preserving one's integrity and authenticity.*[4]
- Incorporate identified familial, religious, and cultural factors that have meaning for client. *Can provide comfort for the person.*[7]
- Refer to appropriate resources for support/guidance (e.g., pastoral care, counseling, organized support groups, classes) as indicated. *These resources can help client as they pursue the search for moral resolution.*[8]
- Assist individual to recognize that if she or he follows their moral decisions, they may clash with the legal system, and refer to appropriate resource for legal opinion/options.[3]
- Encourage the work organization to provide better support resources and structures. Discuss changes in the healthcare system that have resulted in more complex healthcare decisions. *The complexity of healthcare choices, expectations of clients/families, increasing costs or limitations in resources has resulted in increased pressures on healthcare providers and has led to ethics becoming a required component of clinical practice. Acknowledging reality of potential areas of conflict and providing proactive discussions for staff as well as support for involved individuals when making difficult decisions can decrease moral distress for staff and families.*[2,8]

DOCUMENTATION FOCUS

Assessment/Reassessment
- Individual findings, including nature of moral conflict, individuals involved in conflict.
- Physical and emotional responses to conflict.
- Individual cultural or religious beliefs and values, healthcare goals.
- Responses and involvement of family/SOs or coworkers.

Planning
- Plan of care and who is involved in planning.
- Teaching plan.

Implementation/Evaluation
- Responses to interventions and teaching.
- Effects of participation in classes or mediation activities.
- Attainment or progress toward desired outcome(s).
- Modifications to plan of care.

Discharge Planning
- Long-term needs and who is responsible for actions to be taken.
- Available resources.
- Specific referrals made.

References

1. Elpern, E. H., Covert, B., Kleinpell, R. (2005). Moral distress of staff nurses in a medical intensive care unit. *Am J Crit Care*, 14, 523–539.
2. Kalvemark, S., et al. (2004). Living with conflicts—Ethical dilemmas and moral distress in the health care system. *Soc Sci Med*, 58(6), 1075–1084.
3. Hanna, D. R. (2005). The lived experience of moral distress: Nurses who assisted with elective abortions. *Res Theory Nurs Pract*, 19(1), 95–124.
4. Cheshire, W. P. (2007). Grey matters when eloquence is inarticulate. *The Center for Bioethics and Human Dignity*. Retrieved April 2018 from http://cbhd.org/content/grey-matters-when-eloquence-inarticulate.
5. Kilgore, W. D., et al. (2006). The effects of 53 hours of sleep deprivation on moral judgment. *Sleep*, 30(3), 345–352.
6. Kopala, B., Burkhart, L. (2005). Ethical dilemma and moral distress: Proposed new NANDA diagnoses. *Int J Nurs Terminol Classif*, 16(1), 3–13.
7. Nichols, S. (2002). Mindreading and the core architecture of moral psychology. *Cognition*, 84, 221–236.
8. Carnevale, F. A., Alexander, E., Renneck, J. (2006). Daily living with distress and enrichment: The moral experience of families with ventilator-assisted children at home. *Pediatr*, 117(1), e48–e60.
9. Piaget, J. (1932). In Gabain, M. (ed.). *The Psychology of Moral Development: The Nature and Validity of Moral Stages*. (Translation published 1965). New York, NY: Free Press.
10. Corley, M. (1993). Moral distress of critical care nurses. *Am J Crit Care Nurs*, 4(4), 280–285.

---

impaired oral Mucous Membrane Integrity

Taxonomy II: Safety/Protection—Class 2 Physical Injury (00045) [**Diagnostic Division:** Food/Fluid], Approved 1982; Revised 1998, 2013, 2017

DEFINITION: Injury to the lips, soft tissue, buccal cavity, and/or oropharynx.

RELATED FACTORS
Alcohol consumption; smoking; stressors
Barrier to dental care or oral self-care; insufficient oral hygiene; insufficient knowledge of oral hygiene
Chemical injury agent
Decrease in salivation; dehydration; inadequate nutrition; malnutrition

 Acute Care
 Collaborative
 Community/Home Care
 Cultural

DEFINING CHARACTERISTICS

Subjective
Xerostomia
Oral pain or discomfort
Bad taste in mouth; decrease in taste sensation; difficulty eating or swallowing
Exposure to pathogen

Objective
Bleeding
Coated tongue; smooth atrophic or geographic tongue
Gingival or oral mucosal pallor
Stomatitis; hyperemia; macroplasia; vesicles; oral nodules or papules
White patches or plaques, spongy patches, or white curdlike exudate in mouth
Oral lesions or ulcers; fissures; bleeding; cheilitis; desquamation; mucosal denudation
Purulent oral-nasal drainage or exudates; enlarged tonsils
Oral edema
Halitosis
Gingival hyperplasia or recession, pocketing deeper than 4 mm [carious teeth]
Presence of mass [e.g., hemangiomas]
Difficulty speaking
At Risk Population: Economically disadvantaged
Associated Condition: Allergy; infection; Sjogren's syndrome; trauma; mechanical factors
Autoimmune, autosomal or behavioral disorder
Chemotherapy; radiation therapy; treatment regimen; nil per os (NPO) >24 hr
Cleft lip or palate; loss of oral support structure; oral trauma, surgical procedure
Decrease in hormone level in women; decrease in platelets; immunodeficiency or immunosuppression
Sample Clinical Applications: Oral trauma, cancer, chemo/radiation therapy, malnutrition, infection, oral surgery, cleft lip/palate, conditions requiring endotracheal (ET) intubation (e.g., brain injury, stroke, spinal cord injury [SCI], chronic obstructive pulmonary disease [COPD], acute respiratory distress syndrome, amyotrophic lateral sclerosis [ALS])

DESIRED OUTCOMES/EVALUATION CRITERIA

Sample NOC linkages:
Self-Care: Oral Hygiene: Personal actions to care for own mouth and teeth independently with or without assistive device
Tissue Integrity: Skin & Mucous Membranes: Structural intactness and normal physiological function of skin and mucous membranes

Client/Caregiver Will (Include Specific Time Frame)
• Verbalize understanding of causative factors.
• Identify specific interventions to promote healthy oral mucosa.
• Demonstrate techniques to restore and maintain integrity of oral mucosa.

Sample NOC linkages:
Oral Health: Condition of the mouth, teeth, gums, and tongue

(continues on page 564)

 Diagnostic Studies   Evidence Based Practice   Medications   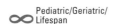 Pediatric/Geriatric/Lifespan

impaired oral Mucous Membrane Integrity (continued)

Client Will (Include Specific Time Frame)
• Report or demonstrate a decrease in signs/symptoms as noted in Defining Characteristics.

ACTIONS/INTERVENTIONS

Sample NIC linkages:
Oral Health Restoration: Promotion of healing for a patient who has an oral mucosa or dental lesion
Oral Health Maintenance: Maintenance and promotion of oral hygiene and dental health for the patient at risk for developing oral or dental lesions
Oral Health Promotion: Promotion of oral hygiene and dental care for a patient with normal oral and dental health

NURSING PRIORITY NO. 1   To identify causative/contributing factors affecting oral health:

• Perform oral screening or comprehensive assessment upon admission to facility using tool (e.g., Oral Health Assessment Tool for Long-Term Care), as indicated. *Use of standardized tool is beneficial in evaluating health of entire mouth including lips, tongue, gums, and other soft tissues, as well as condition of natural teeth or dentures, and status of oral hygiene.*[18]

• Note presence of systemic or local conditions (e.g., oral infections; dehydration, malnutrition, facial fractures, head or neck cancers or treatment including chemotherapy or radiation; AIDS, systemic lupus erythematosus, rheumatoid arthritis, Sjögren's syndrome, scleroderma, sarcoidosis, amyloidosis, hypothyroidism, diabetes) *that can affect health of buccal tissues. Note: Oral mucositis is a major complication of chemotherapy and/or radiation therapy.*[10,12,16]

• ∞ Note client's age and functional status upon admission to facility. *The very young, elderly, or any client with functional deficits (e.g., age-related dependency needs, cognitive or physical impairments, trauma, complex treatments) may require daily assistance with oral care.*[17]

• Determine if client is resistant to oral care. *Client with behavioral and/or communication difficulties (e.g., dementia, won't open mouth or is agitated or lethargic, doesn't understand instructions) may require special equipment, timing of efforts, and/or referral for professional services.*[17]

• Investigate reports of oral pain to determine possible source (e.g., oral lesion, gum disease, tooth abscess, ill-fitting dentures) *to identify needed interventions and reduce risk of complications such as systemic infection.*[1]

• Obtain history of client's medications *to identify those medications that can impact health of buccal tissues or cause immunosuppression that can impact oral health. Note: Many drugs (e.g., anticholinergics, antidepressants, anti-Parkinson drugs, antihistamines or decongestants, urinary antispastics, antipsychotics, diuretics, hypnotics, systemic bronchodilators, muscle relaxants, reserpine, laxatives, beta blockers, narcotics) can impair salivary function and promote xerostomia.*[3,8]

• ∞ Observe for abnormal lesions of mouth, tongue, and cheeks (e.g., white or red patches, ulcers). *White ulcerated spots may be canker sores, especially in children; white curd patches (thrush) are common in infants. Reddened, swollen bleeding gums may indicate infection, poor nutrition, or poor oral hygiene. A red tongue may be related to vitamin deficiencies.*[2,14] *Malignant lesions are more common in elderly than younger persons (especially if there is a history of smoking or alcohol use) or in persons who rarely visit a dentist.*[3,15]

• Note use of tobacco (including smokeless) and alcohol/other drugs [e.g., methamphetamines], *which may predispose gums and mucosa to effects of nutritional deficiencies, infection, cell damage, and cancer.*[10,12]

• Observe for chipped, sharp-edged teeth, or malpositioned teeth. Note fit of dentures or other prosthetic appliances when used. *Factors that increase the risk of injury to delicate tissues.*

 Acute Care   Collaborative   Community/Home Care   Cultural

- Determine problems with food and fluid intake (e.g., avoiding eating, reports change in taste, chews painstakingly, swallows numerous times for even small bites; insufficient fluid intake/dehydration; unexplained weight loss). *Malnutrition and dehydration are associated with problems with oral mucous membranes.*[6]
- Determine allergies to foods, drugs, or other substances *that may result in irritation of oral mucosa.*
- Review oral hygiene practices, noting frequency and type (e.g., brushing, flossing, water appliances). Inquire about client's professional dental care, regularity, and date of last dental examination.
- Evaluate client's ability to provide self-care and availability of necessary equipment and assistance. *Client's age (very young or elderly) impacts client's habits and lifestyle and ability to provide self-care, as well as current health issues (e.g., disease condition or treatment, weakness).*[4]

NURSING PRIORITY NO. 2   To correct identified/developing problems:

- Collaborate in treatment of underlying conditions (e.g., structural defects, infections) *that may correct or limit problem with oral tissues.*
- Inspect oral cavity routinely and recommend that client establish regular schedule of self-inspection, such as when performing oral care activities. *Can help with early identification and management of mucous membrane concerns.*
- Adjust medication regimen *to reduce use of drugs with potential for causing or exacerbating painful dry mouth.*
- Administer medications, as indicated (e.g., antibiotics, antifungal agents, including antimicrobial mouth rinse or spray) *to treat oral infections or reduce potential for bacterial overgrowth.*[8-10]
- Provide anesthetic lozenges or analgesics such as Stanford solution, viscous lidocaine (Xylocaine), mouthwash containing lidocaine, and sulfacrate slurry, as indicated *to provide protection and reduce oral discomfort or pain. Note: Pain of mucositis associated with anticancer therapies has been found to be controlled by mouthwashes containing lidocaine to coat the oral cavity.*[10,16]
- Discuss safe use of products used to treat xerostomia. *Artificial salivas mimic natural saliva to relieve soft tissue discomfort and are more effective and longer lasting than simple rinses but do not stimulate natural salivary gland production; cholinergic agonist preparations [e.g., pilocarpine, cevimeline] do stimulate saliva production). Note: Little research has been done regarding the causes for xerostomia, but one recent study showed that medication exposure was strongly associated with the incidence of the condition, with recent exposure to diuretics or daily aspirin strongly predicting it.*[13]
- Encourage use of tart, sour foods and drinks and chewing sugar-free gum or sucking hard candy to *stimulate saliva.*[11] Use citrus foods and liquids with caution *as they may irritate mucosa and increase pain.*
- Provide or encourage regular oral care (e.g., after meals and at bedtime) frequently for critically ill client. *Note: Oral care has been determined to be a nursing intervention that decreases colonization of oropharynx and saliva, thereby reducing the risk of ventilator-associated pneumonia (VAP) in the critically ill client:*[19]
  Use water; bland rinses or sodium bicarbonate solutions; and mucosal coating agents, lubricating agents, and topical anesthetics *for oral hydration or irrigation and treatment of mouth, gums, and mucous membrane surfaces.*[6,10,20]
  Avoid mouthwashes containing alcohol *(drying effect)* or hydrogen peroxide *(drying and foul tasting).*[5,13]
  Use soft-bristle brush or sponge/cotton-tip applicators to cleanse teeth and tongue. *Brushing the teeth is the most effective way to reduce plaque and manage periodontal disease.*[6]
  Floss gently or use a Waterpik *to remove food particles that promote bacterial growth and gum disease.*
  Use foam sticks where indicated *to swab mouth, tongue, and gums when client is intubated or has no teeth. Note: Chlorhexidine is also used in some critical care areas to decrease risk of VAP.*[21,22]
  Use lemon/glycerin swabs with caution. *Note: Although some end-of-life care discussions mention use of glycerin swabs, the issue appears to be controversial, with some sources stating that glycerin should not be used as it absorbs water and actually dries the oral cavity and can result in decreased salivary amylase, as well as erosion of tooth enamel.*[6,9,13]
  Provide or assist with denture care, as needed. *Evidence-based protocol for denture care states that dentures are to be removed and washed at least once daily, removed and rinsed after every meal, and kept in an appropriate solution at night.*[7]

 Diagnostic Studies   Evidence Based Practice   Medications   Pediatric/Geriatric/Lifespan

- Change position of ET tube or airway per facility protocol and as needed when client is on a ventilator *to minimize pressure on fragile tissues and improve access to all areas of oral cavity.*
- Suction oral cavity *if client cannot swallow secretions. Note: Saliva contains digestive enzymes that may be erosive to exposed tissues (such as might occur because of heavy drooling following radical neck surgery).*
- Use gentle low-intensity suctioning *to reduce risk of aspiration in intubated clients or those with decreased gag or swallow reflexes.*[8]
- Lubricate lips and provide commercially prepared oral lubricant solution, when indicated. Encourage use of chewing gum, hard candy, etc., *to stimulate flow of saliva to neutralize acids and limit bacterial growth.*[10]
- Encourage adequate fluids *to prevent dehydration and oral dryness and limit bacterial overgrowth.*[8]
- Suggest use of vaporizer or room humidifier *to increase humidity if client is mouth breather or ambient humidity is low.*[13]
- Implement diet modifications, as indicated:[10]
  Offer foods with adequate nutrients and vitamins to promote healing *when deficits are impairing health of oral tissues.*
  Avoid sharp, hard, coarse, spicy, salty, and acidic foods *that can irritate or damage fragile mucosa and existing ulcers.*
  Include bland, low-acid, high-protein foods (e.g., milkshakes, bananas, applesauce, mashed potatoes, cooked cereals, soft-boiled or scrambled eggs, cottage cheese, macaroni and cheese, pudding, custard, gelatin) *that are nutrient-dense and easy to eat.*
  Provide moderate-temperature foods and fluids, soft or pureed foods, popsicles, frozen yogurt or ice cream *that may be soothing to sensitive mucosa.*
  Drink liquids with meals and use gravies and sauces *to make food easier to swallow.*
  Avoid dry foods, such as crackers, cookies, and toast, or soften them with liquids before eating.[13]

NURSING PRIORITY NO. 3   To promote wellness (Teaching/Discharge Considerations):

- Recommend regular dental checkups and care, and episodic evaluation of oral health prior to certain medical treatments (e.g., chemotherapy, radiation) *to maintain oral health and reduce risks associated with impaired tissues.*[8]
- Review current oral hygiene concerns and provide informational resources including reliable Web sites about oral health *to reinforce learning and encourage proper care.*
- Promote general health and mental health habits *to prevent negative effects that altered immune response and/or neglect can exert on oral mucosa.*
- Provide nutritional information *to correct deficiencies, reduce mucosal inflammation or gum disease, and prevent dental caries.*
- ∞ Instruct parents in oral hygiene techniques and proper dental care for infants/children (e.g., safe use of pacifier, brushing of teeth and gums, avoidance of sweet drinks and candy, recognition and treatment of thrush). *Encourages early initiation of good oral health practices and timely intervention for treatable problems.*
- Discuss special mouth care required during and after illness or trauma or following surgical repair (e.g., cleft lip/palate, facial fractures, jaw surgery) *to facilitate healing.*
- Discuss and instruct caregiver(s) in special mouth care required during end-of-life care/hospice *to promote optimal comfort in client who has stopped eating or drinking, who has dry mouth, and who may not have sensation of thirst.*[23]
- Recommend avoiding alcohol and smoking or chewing tobacco, *which can contribute to mucosal inflammation and gum disease.*
- Discuss need for and demonstrate use of special appliances (e.g., power toothbrushes, dental water jets, flossing instruments, applicators) if indicated. *Enhances independence in self-care.*
- Identify community resources (e.g., low-cost dental clinics, smoking-cessation resources, cancer information services or support group, Meals on Wheels, supplemental nutrition program, home-care aide) *to meet individual needs.*

 Acute Care   Collaborative   Community/Home Care   Cultural

DOCUMENTATION FOCUS

Assessment/Reassessment
- Condition of oral mucous membranes, routine oral care habits and interferences.
- Availability of oral care equipment and products.
- Knowledge of proper oral hygiene and care.
- Availability and use of resources.

Planning
- Plan of care and who is involved in planning.
- Teaching plan.

Implementation/Evaluation
- Responses to interventions, teaching, and actions performed.
- Attainment or progress toward desired outcome(s).
- Modifications to plan of care.

Discharge Planning
- Long-term needs and who is responsible for actions to be taken.
- Specific referrals made, resources for special appliances.

References

1. Carl, W., Havens, J. (2000). The cancer patient with severe mucositis. *Cur Rev Pain*, 4(3), 197–202.
2. Engel, J. (2006). *Mosby's Pocket Guide to Pediatric Assessment*. 4th ed. St. Louis, MO: Mosby.
3. 123Dentist.com Staff. (2014). Are seniors more at risk for oral cancer? Retrieved April 2018 from https://www.123dentist.com/are-seniors-more-at-risk-for-oral-cancer/.
4. White, R. (2000). Nurse assessment of oral health: A review of practice and education. *Br J Nurs*, 9(5), 260–266.
5. Winslow, E. H. (1994). Don't use H_2O_2 for oral care. *Am J Nurse*, 94(3), 19.
6. Stiefel, K. A., et al. (2000). Improving oral hygiene for the seriously ill patient: Implementing research-based practice. *Medsurg Nurs*, 9(1), 40–46.
7. Curzio, J., McCowan, M. (2000). Getting research into practice: Developing oral hygiene standards. *Br J Nurs*, 9(7), 434–438.
8. Trieger, N. (2004). Oral care in the intensive care unit. *Am J Crit Care*, 13(1), 24.
9. Munro, C., Grap, M. J. (2004). Oral health and care in the intensive care unit: State of science. *Am J Crit Care*, 13(1), 25–33.
10. PDQ® Supportive and Palliative Care Editorial Board. (2014, updated 2016). PDQ oral complications of chemotherapy and head/neck radiation: Various sections. Retrieved April 2018 from https://www.cancer.gov/about-cancer/treatment/side-effects/mouth-throat/oral-complications-hp-pdq#section/_AboutThis_1.
11. Stegeman, C. A. (2005). Oral manifestations of diabetes. *Home Healthc Nurs*, 23(4), 233–240.
12. National Library of Medicine. (No date). Oral cavity cancer (Mouth cancer). Retrieved April 2018 from https://www.ncbi.nlm.nih.gov/pubmedhealth/PMHT0024374/.
13. Murray, T. W., Chalmers, J. M., Spenser, J. A. (2006). A longitudinal study of medication exposure and xerostomia among older people. *Gerodontology*, 23(4), 205–213.
14. Ranney, R. (1993). Classification of periodontal diseases. *Periodontology*, 2(1), 13–25.
15. Academy of Periodontology. (2006). Guidelines for the management of patients with periodontal diseases. *Academy Report*. Retrieved April 2018 from https://noveo.net/wp-content/uploads/2017/03/Guidelines-for-the-Management-of-Patients-With-Periodontal-Diseases-USA.pdf.
16. Li, E., Trovato, J. A. (2012). New developments in management of oral mucositis in patients with head and neck cancer or receiving targeted anticancer therapies. *Am J Health-Syst Pharm*, 69(12), 1031–1037.
17. Johnson, V. B., Chalmers, J. (2012). Oral hygiene care for functionally dependent and cognitively impaired older adults. *J Gerontol Nurs*, 38(11), 11–19.
18. University of Iowa College of Nursing, John A. Hartford Foundation Center of Geriatric Nursing Excellence - Academic Institution. (2002, revised 2011). Oral hygiene care for functionally dependent and cognitively impaired older adults. Revised guideline. Retrieved April 2018 from https://www.guidelinecentral.com/summaries/oral-hygiene-care-for-functionally-dependent-and-cognitively-impaired-older-adults/#.
19. Cutler, C., Davis, N. (2005). Improving oral care in patients receiving mechanical ventilation. *Am J Crit Care*, 14(5), 389–394.
20. Farris, C., McEnroe Petitte, D. (2013). Head, neck, and cancer update. *Home Healthcar Nurs*, 31(6), 322–328.
21. Feider, L. L., Mitchell, P., Bridges, E. (2010). Oral care practices for orally intubated critically ill adults. *Am J Crit Care*, 19(2), 175–183.

 Diagnostic Studies Evidence Based Practice Medications 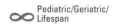 Pediatric/Geriatric/Lifespan

22. WebMD Drugs & Medications. (No date). Chlorhexidine gluconate mouthwash. Retrieved April 2018 from http://www.webmd.com/drugs/2/drug-5356/chlorhexidine-gluconate-mucous-membrane/details#uses.

23. Schwarz, J. K. (2014). Hospice care for patients who choose to hasten death by voluntarily stopping eating and drinking. *J Hosp Palliat Nurs*, 16(3), 126–131.

risk for impaired oral Mucous Membrane Integrity

Taxonomy II: Safety/Protection—Class 2 Physical Injury (00247) [**Diagnostic Division:** Food/Fluid], Approved 2013; Revised 2017

DEFINITION: Susceptible to injury to the lips, soft tissues, buccal cavity, and/or oropharynx, which may compromise health.

RISK FACTORS
Alcohol consumption; smoking; stressors
Barrier to dental care or oral self-care; insufficient oral hygiene; insufficient knowledge of oral hygiene
Chemical injury agent
Decrease in salivation; dehydration; inadequate nutrition; malnutrition
At Risk Population: Economically disadvantaged
Associated Condition: Allergy; infection; Sjogren's syndrome; trauma; mechanical factors
Autoimmune, autosomal or behavioral disorder
Chemotherapy; radiation therapy; treatment regimen; nil per os (NPO) >24 hours
Cleft lip or palate; loss of oral support structure; oral trauma, surgical procedure
Decrease in hormone level in women; decrease in platelets; immunodeficiency or immunosuppression

DESIRED OUTCOMES/EVALUATION CRITERIA

Sample NOC linkages:
Self-Care: Oral Hygiene: Personal actions to care for own mouth and teeth independently with or without assistive device
Tissue Integrity: Skin & Mucous Membranes: Structural intactness and normal physiological function of skin and mucous membranes

Client/Caregiver Will (Include Specific Time Frame)
• Verbalize understanding of causative factors.
• Identify specific interventions to promote healthy oral mucosa.
• Demonstrate techniques to maintain integrity of oral mucosa.

Sample NOC linkages:
• Client will be free of signs of mucosal irritation/injury.
Oral Health: Condition of the mouth, teeth, gums, and tongue

ACTIONS/INTERVENTIONS

Sample NIC linkages:
Oral Health Maintenance: Maintenance and promotion of oral hygiene and dental health for the patient at risk for developing oral or dental lesions
Oral Health Promotion: Promotion of oral hygiene and dental care for a patient with normal oral and dental health

 Acute Care Collaborative Community/Home Care Cultural

NURSING PRIORITY NO. 1 To identify factors/conditions that can affect oral health:

- Note presence of systemic or local conditions (e.g., oral infections; dehydration, malnutrition, facial fractures, head or neck cancers or treatment including chemotherapy or radiation; AIDS, systemic lupus erythematosus, rheumatoid arthritis, Sjögren's syndrome, scleroderma, sarcoidosis, amyloidosis, hypothyroidism, diabetes) *that can affect health of oral tissues. Note: Oral mucositis is a major complication of chemotherapy and/or radiation therapy.*[1,2,3]

- ∞ Note client's age and functional status. *The very young, the elderly client, or any client with functional deficits (e.g., age-related dependency needs, cognitive or physical impairments, trauma, complex treatments) may require daily assistance with oral care.*[4]

- Determine if client is resistant to oral care. *Client with behavioral and/or communication difficulties (e.g., dementia, won't open mouth or is agitated or lethargic, doesn't understand instructions) may require special equipment, timing of efforts, and/or referral for professional services.*[4]

- Obtain history of client's medications *to identify those medications that can impact health of buccal tissues or cause immunosuppression, which can impact oral health. Note: Many drugs (e.g., anticholinergics, antidepressants, anti-Parkinson drugs, antihistamines or decongestants, urinary antispastics, antipsychotics, diuretics, hypnotics, systemic bronchodilators, muscle relaxants, reserpine, laxatives, beta blockers, narcotics) can impair salivary function and promote xerostomia.*[5,6]

- Note use of tobacco (including smokeless) and alcohol/other drugs [e.g., methamphetamines], *which may predispose gums and mucosa to effects of nutritional deficiencies, infection, cell damage, and cancer.*[1,2]

- Observe for chipped, sharp-edged teeth, or malpositioned teeth. Note fit of dentures or other prosthetic appliances when used. *Factors that increase the risk of injury to delicate tissues.*

- Determine problems with food and fluid intake (e.g., avoiding eating, reports change in taste, chews painstakingly, swallows numerous times for even small bites; insufficient fluid intake/dehydration; unexplained weight loss). *Malnutrition and dehydration are associated with problems with oral mucous membranes.*[7]

- Determine allergies to foods, drugs, or other substances *that may result in irritation of oral mucosa.*

- ∞ Evaluate client's ability to provide self-care and availability of necessary equipment and assistance. *Client's age (very young or elderly) impacts client's habits and lifestyle, ability to provide self-care, and current health issues (e.g., disease condition or treatment, weakness).*[8]

NURSING PRIORITY NO. 2 To correct developing/potential problems:

- 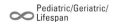 Collaborate in treatment of underlying conditions (e.g., structural defects, cancer, surgical/traumatic injuries) *that may impact oral tissues.*

- Inspect oral cavity routinely and recommend that client establish regular schedule of self-inspection, such as when performing oral care activities. *Can help with early identification and management of mucous membrane concerns.*

- **Refer to ND impaired oral Mucous Membrane Integrity, Nursing Priority No. 2 for interventions related to best practice nursing care to prevent oral complications.**

NURSING PRIORITY NO. 3 To promote wellness (Teaching/Discharge Considerations):[6–8]

- 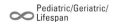 Recommend regular dental checkups and care and episodic evaluation of oral health prior to certain medical treatments (e.g., chemotherapy, radiation, total joint replacement) *to maintain oral health and reduce risks associated with impaired tissues.*

- Review current oral hygiene concerns and provide informational resources including reliable Web sites about oral health *to reinforce learning and encourage proper care.*

- Promote general health and mental health habits *to prevent negative effects that altered immune response and/or neglect can exert on oral mucosa.*

- Provide nutritional information *to correct deficiencies, reduce mucosal inflammation or gum disease, and prevent dental caries.*

 Diagnostic Studies   Evidence Based Practice   Medications ∞ Pediatric/Geriatric/Lifespan

- ∞ Instruct parents in oral hygiene techniques and proper dental care for infants/children (e.g., safe use of pacifier, brushing of teeth and gums, avoidance of sweet drinks and candy, recognition and treatment of thrush). *Encourages early initiation of good oral health practices and timely intervention for treatable problems.*
- Discuss need for and demonstrate use of special appliances (e.g., power toothbrushes, dental water jets, flossing instruments, applicators), if indicated. *Enhances independence and excellence in oral self-care.*
- Discuss special mouth care required during and after illness or trauma or following surgical repair (e.g., cleft lip/palate, facial fractures, jaw surgery) *to facilitate healing.*
- Recommend avoiding alcohol and smoking or chewing tobacco, *which can contribute to mucosal inflammation and gum disease.*
- Identify community resources (e.g., low-cost dental clinics, smoking-cessation resources, cancer information services or support group, Meals on Wheels, nutritional assistance program, home-care aide) *to meet individual needs.*

DOCUMENTATION FOCUS

Assessment/Reassessment
- Condition of oral mucous membranes, routine oral care habits and interferences.
- Availability of oral care equipment and products.
- Knowledge of proper oral hygiene and care.
- Availability and use of resources.

Planning
- Plan of care and who is involved in planning.
- Teaching plan.

Implementation/Evaluation
- Responses to interventions, teaching, and actions performed.
- Attainment or progress toward desired outcome(s).
- Modifications to plan of care.

Discharge Planning
- Long-term needs and who is responsible for actions to be taken.
- Specific referrals made, resources for special appliances.

References

1. PDQ Supportive and Palliative Care Editorial Board. (2014, updated 2016). PDQ oral complications of chemotherapy and head/neck radiation: Various sections. Retrieved April 2018 from https://www.cancer.gov/about-cancer/treatment/side-effects/mouth-throat/oral-complications-hp-pdq#section/_AboutThis_1.
2. National Library of Medicine. (No date). Oral cavity cancer (mouth cancer). Retrieved April 2018 from https://www.ncbi.nlm.nih.gov/pubmedhealth/PMHT0024374/.
3. Li, E., Trovato, J. A. (2012). New developments in management of oral mucositis in patients with head and neck cancer or receiving targeted anticancer therapies. *Am J Health Syst Pharm*, 69(12), 1031–1037.
4. Johnson, V. B., Chalmers, J. (2012). Oral hygiene care for functionally dependent and cognitively impaired older adults. *J Gerontol Nurs*, 38(11), 11–19.
5. 123Dentist Staff. (2014). Are seniors more at risk for oral cancer? Retrieved April 2018 from https://www.123dentist.com/are-seniors-more-at-risk-for-oral-cancer/.
6. Trieger, N. (2004). Oral care in the intensive care unit. *Am J Crit Care*, 13(1), 24.
7. Stiefel, K. A., et al. (2000). Improving oral hygiene for the seriously ill patient: Implementing research-based practice. *Medsurg Nurs*, 9(1), 40–46.
8. White, R. (2000). Nurse assessment of oral health: A review of practice and education. *Br J Nurs*, 9(5), 260–266.

 Acute Care   Collaborative Community/Home Care   Cultural

Nausea

Taxonomy II: Comfort—Class 1 Physical Comfort (00134) [**Diagnostic Division:** Food/Fluid], Approved 1998; Revised 2002, 2010, 2017

DEFINITION: A subjective phenomenon of an unpleasant feeling in the back of the throat and stomach, which may or may not result in vomiting.

RELATED FACTORS
Anxiety; fear
Exposure to toxin; noxious environmental stimuli; unpleasant visual stimuli
Noxious taste

DEFINING CHARACTERISTICS

Subjective
Nausea; sour taste

Objective
Aversion toward food
Increase in salivation
Increase in swallowing; gagging sensation
Associated Condition: Biochemical dysfunction [e.g., uremia, diabetic ketoacidosis]; pregnancy
Esophageal or pancreatic disease; liver or splenetic capsule stretch
Gastric distention; gastrointestinal irritation
Increase in intracranial pressure (ICP); meningitis
Intra-abdominal tumors; localized tumor [e.g., acoustic neuroma, brain tumor, bone metastasis]
Motion sickness; Ménière's disease; labyrinthitis
Psychological disorder
Treatment regimen
Sample Clinical Applications: Surgery, anesthesia, cancer, pregnancy, AIDS, gastritis, peptic ulcer disease, renal failure, brain injury, meningitis, panic disorders, phobias

DESIRED OUTCOMES/EVALUATION CRITERIA

Sample NOC linkages:
Nausea & Vomiting Severity: Severity of signs and symptoms of nausea, retching, and vomiting
Nausea & Vomiting Control: Personal actions to control nausea, retching, and vomiting symptoms
Nausea & Vomiting: Disruptive Effects: Severity of observed or reported disruptive effects of chronic nausea, retching, and vomiting on daily functioning

Client Will (Include Specific Time Frame)
- Be free of nausea.
- Manage chronic nausea, as evidenced by acceptable level of dietary intake.
- Maintain or regain weight, as appropriate.

ACTIONS/INTERVENTIONS

Sample NIC linkages:
Nausea Management: Prevention and alleviation of nausea
Vomiting Management: Prevention and alleviation of vomiting
Fluid Management: Promotion of fluid balance and prevention of complications resulting from abnormal or undesired fluid levels

 Diagnostic Studies   Evidence Based Practice   Medications   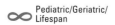 Pediatric/Geriatric/Lifespan

NURSING PRIORITY NO. 1 To determine causative/contributing factors:

- Assess for presence of conditions of the GI tract (e.g., peptic ulcer disease, bleeding into the stomach; cholecystitis, appendicitis, gastritis, constipation, intestinal blockage, ingestion of "problem" foods; food poisoning; excessive alcohol intake) *that may cause or exacerbate nausea.*
- Note systemic conditions that may result in nausea (e.g., pregnancy, cancer treatment, myocardial infarction, hepatitis, acid-base and metabolic disturbances, systemic infections; toxins, drug toxicity, migraine headache, presence of neurogenic causes—stimulation of the vestibular system, concussion, central nervous system trauma/tumor). *Helpful in determining appropriate interventions/need for treatment of underlying conditions.*
- Identify situations that client perceives as anxiety inducing, threatening, or distasteful (e.g., "this is nauseating") such as might occur if client is having multiple diagnostic studies or is facing surgery, anticipating chemotherapy that has previously induced nausea, or other stressful situations.[6]
- Note psychological factors, including those that are culturally determined (e.g., eating certain foods considered repulsive in one's culture, seeing or smelling something "gross"; eating disorders such as anorexia and bulimia).
- Determine if nausea is potentially self-limiting and/or mild (e.g., first trimester of pregnancy, 24-hr GI tract viral infection) or is severe and prolonged (e.g., advanced cancer with multiple medications accompanied by anorexia, constipation, imbalances of calcium/other electrolytes; certain cancer treatments; hyperemesis gravidarum). *Indicates potential degree of effect on fluid/electrolyte balance and nutritional status and determines type and intensity of interventions.*[3]
- Record food intake and changes in symptoms *to help identify food intolerances or eating disorders when nausea is chronic.*
- Note client age and developmental level. *Vomiting may occur along with nausea, especially in children (usually part of a short-lived viral infection). Nausea can occur with food intolerances, inner ear problems, pain, or medication reactions in any age client. Nausea in the elderly (in the absence of acute disease condition) may be associated with GI motility dysfunction or medications, pain, or end-or-life issues. Nausea in a female of childbearing age may indicate pregnancy or hormonal influences associated with menstruation, anorexia, or migraine headaches.*[5]
- Review medication regimen, especially in elderly client on multiple drugs. *Polypharmacy with drug interactions and side effects may cause or exacerbate nausea.*
- Review results of diagnostic studies. *Various studies may be done depending on the clinical suspicion of cause, such as blood tests (to check electrolytes, blood cell count), urinalysis (to check for dehydration and infection), and x-rays, ultrasound, or computed tomography (CT) scan to help identify or localize cause.*

NURSING PRIORITY NO. 2 To promote comfort and enhance intake:

- Collaborate with physician to treat underlying medical condition *when cause of nausea is known (e.g., infection, adverse side effect of medications, recent anesthesia, food allergies, GI reflux).*
- Administer and monitor response to medications used to treat underlying type of nausea (e.g., vestibular, bowel obstruction, dysmotility of gut, infection or inflammation, toxins, cancer treatments) *to determine effectiveness of treatment. Note: Targeting antiemetics to specific receptors associated with a certain type of nausea can optimize treatment. For example, receptors causing nausea in vestibular disorders and infection are cholinergic and histaminic. A targeted antiemetic drug class could be anticholinergic or antihistaminic such as promethazine [Phenergan]. Antiemetics must also be monitored for adverse side effects, such as oversedation with risk of aspiration.*[4,7]
- Select route of medication administration best suited to client's needs (i.e., oral, sublingual, injectable, rectal, transdermal).[6]
- Administer antiemetic on regular schedule before, during, and after administration of antineoplastic agents or radiation therapy as indicated. *Antiemetic agents may be administered prophylactically to prevent or limit severity of nausea and vomiting.*

 Acute Care   Collaborative   Community/ Home Care   Cultural

- Administer analgesics and/or antiemetics as scheduled *when postoperative pain is a factor in nausea and vomiting.*[1]
- Review pain control regimen for client experiencing nausea. *Converting to long-acting opioids or combination drugs may decrease stimulation of the chemotactic trigger zone, reducing the occurrence of narcotic-related nausea.*[4,7]
- Manage food and fluids:

  Have client try dry foods such as toast, crackers, or dry cereal before arising *when nausea occurs in the morning or throughout the day.*[7]

  ∞ Encourage client to begin with ice chips or sips/small amounts of fluids—4 to 8 oz for adult, 1 oz or less for child.[5]

  Advise client to drink liquids 30 min before or after meals instead of with meals.[7]

  Suggest sipping fluids slowly and using cool, clear liquids (e.g., water, ginger ale or lemon-lime soda, electrolyte drinks).

  Recommend avoiding milk and other dairy products (especially during acute episodes); overly sweet, fried, or fatty foods; and gas-forming vegetables (e.g., broccoli, cauliflower, cucumbers) *that may increase nausea and be more difficult to digest.*[3,5,7]

  Provide soft-bland diet and snacks high in carbohydrates with substitutions of preferred foods (including skinless chicken, rice, toast, pasta, potatoes) and fluids (including caffeine-free nondiet carbonated beverages, clear soup broth, nonacidic fruit juice, gelatin, sherbet, ices) *to reduce gastric acidity and improve nutrient intake.*[3,5,7]

  Instruct client to eat small meals spaced throughout the day rather than large meals *so stomach does not feel too full.*[3,7]

  Instruct client to eat and drink slowly, chewing food well *for easier digestion.*[7]

  Advise client to suck on ice cubes or tart or hard candies. *Keeps mucous membranes moist and can provide some fluid and nutrient intake.*

  Time chemotherapy doses *for least interference with food intake.*

  Monitor infusion rate of tube feeding, if present, *to prevent rapid administration that can cause gastric distention and produce nausea.*
- Manage environment *to reduce risk of nausea caused by noxious sights or smells:*

  Elevate head of bed or have client sit upright after meals *to promote digestion by gravity and eliminate feeling of fullness when that is causing nausea.*[7]

  Apply cool cloth to face and neck.

  Provide clean, pleasant-smelling, quiet environment and fresh air with fan or open window.

  Avoid offending odors (e.g., cooking smells, smoke, perfumes, mechanical emissions).[6,7]
- Implement nonpharmacological measures:

  Encourage slow, deep breathing *to promote relaxation.*

  Use such distraction techniques as guided imagery, music therapy, chatting with family/friends, and watching television *to refocus attention away from unpleasant sensations.*

  Provide frequent oral care *to cleanse mouth and minimize "bad tastes."*

  Avoid sudden changes in position or excessive motion; move to aisle seat on plane or front seat of car. Focus on distance and face forward when riding *to prevent or limit severity of nausea associated with motion sickness.*[5]
- Investigate use of electrical nerve stimulation or acupressure point therapy (e.g., elastic band worn around wrist with small, hard bump that presses against acupressure point). *Some individuals with chronic nausea or history of motion sickness report this to be helpful and without the sedative effect of medication.*[2]

NURSING PRIORITY NO. 3   To promote wellness (Teaching/Discharge Considerations):

- Review individual factors or triggers causing nausea and ways to avoid problem (e.g., identifying offending medications or foods). *Provides necessary information for client to manage own care. Note: Some individuals*

 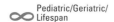

develop anticipatory nausea (a conditioned reflex) that recurs each time he or she encounters the situation that triggers the reflex.[7]

- Instruct in proper use, side effects, and adverse reactions of antiemetic medications. *Enhances client safety and effective management of condition.*
- Discuss appropriate use of over-the-counter medications and herbal products (e.g., Dramamine, antacids, antiflatulents, ginger) or the use of THC (Marinol).[5,7]
- Encourage use of nonpharmacological interventions. *Activities such as self-hypnosis, progressive muscle relaxation, biofeedback, guided imagery, and systemic desensitization promote relaxation, refocus client's attention, increase sense of control, and decrease feelings of helplessness.*[6]
- Advise client/significant other to prepare and freeze meals in advance, have someone else cook, or use microwave or oven instead of stove-top cooking for days when nausea is severe or cooking is impossible, as with chemotherapy/radiation therapy.[7]
- Suggest wearing loose-fitting clothing *to reduce pressure on abdomen if that is causing or exacerbating nausea.*[7]
- Recommend recording weight weekly, if appropriate, *to help monitor fluid and nutritional status.*
- Identify signs requiring immediate notification of healthcare provider (e.g., emesis appears bloody, black, or like coffee grounds; feeling faint) *to facilitate timely evaluation and intervention.*[7]
- Review signs of dehydration and emphasize importance of replacing fluids and/or electrolytes (with products such as Gatorade for adults or Pedialyte for children) if vomiting occurs, especially in young children or frail elderly. *Increases likelihood of preventing potentially serious complications.*[5]

DOCUMENTATION FOCUS

Assessment/Reassessment
- Individual findings, including individual factors causing nausea.
- Baseline periodic weight, vital signs.
- Specific client preferences for nutritional intake.

Planning
- Plan of care and who is involved in planning.
- Teaching plan.

Implementation/Evaluation
- Response to interventions, teaching, and actions performed.
- Response to medication.
- Attainment or progress toward desired outcome(s).
- Modifications to plan of care.

Discharge Planning
- Individual long-term needs, noting who is responsible for actions to be taken.
- Specific referrals made.

References

1. McCaffrey, R. (2007). Make POVN prevention a priority. *OR Nurse 2012*, 1(2), 39–45.
2. Kiefer, D. (2017). *Acupressure points and massage treatment*. Retrieved April 2018 from https://www.webmd.com/balance/guide/acupressure-points-and-massage-treatment#1.
3. The American Gastroenterological Association medical position statement: Nausea and vomiting. (2001). *Gastroenterology*, 120(1), 261–262.
4. Hallenbeck, J. (2003). Treatment of nausea and vomiting. *Palliative Care Perspectives*. New York: Oxford University Press.
5. Cunha, J. P. (2011, reviewed 2017). Vomiting and nausea. Retrieved April 2018 from http://www.emedicinehealth.com/vomiting_and_nausea/article_em.htm.
6. National Cancer Institute. (Updated 2017). Nausea and vomiting (PDQ®) summary. Retrieved April 2018 from http://www.cancer.gov/about-cancer/treatment/side-effects/nausea/nausea-pdq.
7. World Health Organization. (2004). Palliative care & symptom management: Nausea & vomiting. Retrieved April 2018 from http://www.who.int/hiv/pub/imai/genericpalliativecare082004.pdf.

 Acute Care   Collaborative   Community/Home Care   Cultural

Neonatal Abstinence Syndrome

Taxonomy II: Coping/Stress Tolerance—Class 3 Neurobehavorial Stress (00134) [**Diagnostic Division:** Safety], Approved 2016

DEFINITION: A constellation of withdrawal symptoms observed in newborns as a result of in-utero exposure to addicting substances or as a consequence of postnatal pharmacological pain management

RELATED FACTORS
To Be Developed

DEFINING CHARACTERISTICS

Objective
Disorganized infant behavior; neurobehavioral stress; risk for impaired attachment
Disturbed sleep pattern; impaired comfort
Risk for aspiration: ineffective infant feeding pattern
Diarrhea
Risk for imbalanced body temperature
Risk for impaired skin integrity
Risk for injury
At Risk Population: In-utero substance exposure secondary to maternal substance use
Iatrogenic substance exposure for pain control following a critical illness or surgery

DESIRED OUTCOMES/EVALUATION CRITERIA

Sample **NOC** linkages:
Substance Withdrawal Severity: Severity of signs and symptoms of withdrawal from addictive drugs, tobacco, alcohol
Newborn Adaptation: Adaptive response to the extrauterine environment by a physiologically mature newborn during the first 28 days of life

Infant Will (Include Specific Time Frame)
- Be free of adverse effects of substance withdrawal, e.g., irritability, tremors, vomiting, diarrhea, difficulty sleeping.
- Demonstrate feeding tolerance, appropriate weight gain, physiological stability with normal vital signs.
- Display neurobehavioral recovery as evidenced by reaching full alert state, responds to social stimuli, is consoled with appropriate measures.

Sample **NOC** linkages:
Drug Abuse Cessation Behavior: Personal actions to eliminate drug use that poses a threat to health
Family Participation in Professional Care: Capacity of a family to be involved in decision-making, care delivery, and evaluation of care provided by healthcare personnel

PARENT(S) Will (Include Specific Time Frame)
- Engage in behavior/lifestyle changes to eliminate substance use.
- Use available personal, professional, and community resources.
- Provide safe/growth promoting environment for child.

(continues on page 576)

 Diagnostic Studies   Evidence Based Practice   Medications   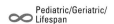 Pediatric/Geriatric/ Lifespan

Neonatal Abstinence Syndrome (continued)

ACTIONS/INTERVENTIONS

Sample NIC linkages:

Substance Use Treatment: Drug Withdrawal: Care of patient experiencing drug detoxification

Infant Care: Newborn: Provision of care to the infant during the transition from birth to extrauterine life and subsequent period of stabilization

NURSING PRIORITY NO. 1   To determine degree of impairment:

• Note maternal risks for fetal well-being including substance(s) used, dose, duration (especially last week before delivery), route; presence of infections. *Maternal IV drug use associated with increased risk of infections (e.g., HIV, hepatitis B, hepatitis C) requiring additional testing/surveillance and treatment. Note: Maternal self-report of substance use may understate fetal exposure by as much as 44%.*[3]

• Review maternal urine/drug screen. *Individual more likely to use more than one substance, complicating treatment. Use of opiates within 1 week of delivery causes withdrawal in over half of infants exposed prenatally. Exposure to amphetamines, cocaine, marijuana, and alcohol are associated with long-term problems. Note: Symptoms and timing of occurrence depend on type of substance(s) used and last dose.*[1,2]

• Note fetal status—full term or premature birth. *Preterm infants have lower risk for, or less severe, symptoms and tend to recover more quickly if no other complications present. Longer gestation with increased permeability of placental barrier can increase fetal exposure to drugs.*[2,4]

• Obtain urine and/or meconium samples for toxicology screen. *Urine sample reflects last several days of exposure while meconium is more sensitive with longer window of detection—from 20 weeks' gestation.*[1,5]

• Monitor for signs/symptoms of fetal abstinence syndrome (FAS), such as excessive high-pitched cry, problems with sleep, feeding difficulties, tremors, frequent yawning and sneezing, vomiting, and diarrhea. *Onset of symptoms reflecting dysregulation in central, autonomic, and gastrointestinal system function is varied based on substance(s) used, possibly appearing as early as 24 hr or delayed for 10 days, and require supportive interventions.*[2,4,5]

• Screen neonate at birth using standardized tool such as Finnegan Neonatal Abstinence Scoring form. Repeat evaluation every 3 to 4 hr when infant is awake. *Baseline used for comparison of subsequent tests with usually two or three consecutive scores of eight or above indicating need for pharmacological therapy. Scores assist in monitoring, titrating, and termination of therapy. Note: Scoring may not be useful in preterm infants as delayed CNS development impacts score.*[3,5]

NURSING PRIORITY NO. 2   To facilitate safe withdrawal from substance(s):

• Coordinate interdisciplinary team (e.g., neonatologist, pediatrician, nutritionist). *To address immediate needs of infant during withdrawal process.*[3]

• Encourage rooming in as appropriate. *Promotes attachment and greater maternal involvement in infant's care, improves breastfeeding outcomes, may reduce need for pharmacological therapy, and shortens length of hospital stay.*[3,5]

• Support breastfeeding efforts. Refer to lactation consultant as needed. *Confers immunological benefits to neonate, enhances bonding, and may lower Finnegan scores during first 9 days of life. Note: Not recommended in presence of HIV infection or presence of additional drug use except in maternal methadone therapy.*[3,4]

• Provide comfort measures based on individual needs: *Generally first option in treatment and may be sufficient in cases of mild withdrawal.*[1,3,5]

Swaddling in blanket *provides containment boundaries, enhances sleep.*

Kangaroo (skin-to-skin) care *may enhance neurophysiological organization.*

 Acute Care   Collaborative   Community/Home Care   Cultural

Gentle rocking of infant.

Lower light and noise levels *to minimize excess environmental stimuli.*

Frequent, demand feedings.

Pacifier for non-nutritive sucking.

Waterbed, but avoid oscillating bed.

Avoid unnecessary handling or awakening sleeping infant.

- Monitor vital signs, intake/output, weight. *Poor feeding efforts, vomiting, excessive diarrhea may result in dehydration.*
- Provide high-calorie (150–250 Kcal/kg/24 hr), small, more frequent feeding if infant not breastfeeding. *May be necessary to minimize weight loss, promote growth during significant withdrawal.*[3]
- Provide meticulous skin care. *Skin irritation from restlessness/agitation and excessive diarrhea requires careful cleaning and skin barrier creams to prevent breakdown.*
- Administer intravenous fluids (IV) as needed. *May be required to prevent dehydration or electrolyte imbalance.*[2]
- Administer medication(s) for withdrawal when supportive measures fail to improve or correct symptoms, withdrawal scores remain high, seizures develop, or presence of severe dehydration, vomiting and/or diarrhea:[3,5]
- Morphine (i.e., dilute tincture of opium)—administered orally, most commonly preferred medication for treatment of opioid withdrawal.
- Methadone—alternative to morphine and may shorten length of opioid withdrawal.
- Buprenorphine—may have shorter duration and hospital stay than treatment with oral morphine, approved for outpatient/post-discharge therapy due to characteristics of decreased respiratory and cardiovascular side effects.
- Phenobarbital—preferred for treatment of nonopiate and polydrug exposure.
- Clonidine—second-line treatment for symptoms refractory to opioid therapy.
- Wean from medication as indicated. *Once withdrawal scores decline and symptoms able to be managed by comfort measures, a modified protocol can be initiated to decrease pharmacological therapy. Note: Protocol can be extended for 3 weeks or more depending on infant's needs.*[4]

NURSING PRIORITY NO. 3   To promote optimal wellness (Teaching/Discharge Considerations):

- Interact with expand interdisciplinary team to include substance abuse counselor, social worker, child development specialist, etc. *Provides support for mother/family in preparation for discharge and future care needs of infant.*[3]
- Develop trusting relationship, project an accepting attitude about substance use. *Encourages maternal participation, provides client a sense of humanness, helping to decrease paranoia and distrust. (Client will be able to detect biased or condescending attitude of caregivers, negatively impacting relationship.)*[5]
- Determine parents' understanding of current situation. *Provides information about degree of denial, acceptance of personal responsibility and commitment to change.*
- Provide information to parents in multiple modes reviewing general infant care and long-term needs specific to substances used. *For example: Methadone exposure associated with increased motor rigidity and dysregulated motor patterns, can persist into toddlerhood and is associated with decreased attention span, impaired social responsibility with poor social engagement. Cocaine use can result in poor fetal growth, developmental delays, learning disabilities, and lower IQ.*[4,5]
- Stress importance/develop schedule for follow-up monitoring. *Necessary evaluations include neurodevelopmental assessments to monitor motor deficits, cognitive delays, or relative microcephaly; psychobehavioral assessments for hyperactivity, impulsivity, attention-deficit in preschool-aged child and behavioral problems in school-aged children; growth/nutritional assessment for short stature and failure to thrive.*[5]
- Perform home visit to determine safety of environment. *Optimum home environment required for global development and well-being of infant.*[5]
- Encourage continued involvement of mother in peer group therapy, individual/family counseling, drug recovery education programs. *Provides follow-up support to maintain mother's sobriety.*

 Diagnostic Studies   Evidence Based Practice   Medications   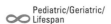 Pediatric/Geriatric/Lifespan

• Identify community/social assistance resources, e.g., safe housing, food pantry, licensed day care, transportation, medical care. *Provides for basic human needs of infant and family, enhances maternal coping abilities, decreases risk of relapse and possible abusive situation.*

DOCUMENTATION FOCUS

Assessment/Reassessment
• Individual findings including general health status or infant, comorbidities, signs/stage of withdrawal.
• Maternal substance(s) used, route, dose, frequency, last dose.
• Results of laboratory tests/diagnostic studies.
• Parent(s) attachment, involvement in care.

Planning
• Plan of care and who is involved in planning.
• Teaching plan.
• Plan for maternal sobriety.

Implementation/Evaluation
• Response to interventions, teaching, and actions performed.
• Attainment or progress toward desired outcomes.
• Modifications to plan.

Discharge Planning
• Long-term needs and who is responsible for actions to be taken.
• Specific referrals made.

References

1. Lee, K. G. (Reviewed 2017). Neonatal abstinence syndrome. May 2018 from https://medlineplus.gov/ency/article/007313.htm.
2. Stanford's Children's Hospital. (2018). Neonatal abstinence syndrome. June 2018 from http://www.stanfordchildrens.org/en/topic/default?id=neonatal-abstinence-syndrome-90-P02387.
3. Hamdan, A. H. (Updated 2017). Neonatal abstinence syndrome treatment & management. *Medscape*. June 2018 from https://emedicine.medscape.com/article/978763-treatment.
4. Logan, B. A., Brown, M. S., Hayes, M. J. (2013). Neonatal abstinence syndrome: Treatment and pediatric outcomes. *Clin Obstet Gynecol*, 56(1), 186–192.
5. Kocherlakota, P. (2014). Neonatal abstinence syndrome. *Pediatrics*, 134(2), 134–E547.

---

risk for peripheral Neurovascular Dysfunction

Taxonomy II: Safety/Protection—Class 2 Physical Injury (00086) **[Diagnostic Division:** Neurosensory**]**, Approved 1992; Revised 2013, 2017

DEFINITION: Susceptible to disruption in the circulation, sensation, and motion of an extremity, which may compromise health.

RISK FACTORS
To Be Developed
Associated Condition: Burn injury; trauma; vascular obstruction
Fracture; immobilization; orthopedic surgery
Mechanical compression [e.g., tourniquet, cane, cast, brace, dressing, restraint]
Sample Clinical Applications: Traumatic injuries, burns, joint replacement, laminectomy, deep vein thrombosis (DVT), peripheral vascular obstruction; compartment syndrome

 Acute Care   Collaborative   Community/Home Care   Cultural

DESIRED OUTCOMES/EVALUATION CRITERIA

Sample **NOC** linkages:

Tissue Perfusion: Peripheral: Adequacy of blood flow through the small vessels of the extremities to maintain tissue function

Neurological Status: Peripheral: Ability of the peripheral nervous system to transmit impulses to and from the central nervous system (CNS)

Risk Control: Personal actions to understand, prevent, eliminate, or reduce modifiable health threats

Client Will (Include Specific Time Frame)

- Maintain function as evidenced by sensation and movement within normal range for individual.
- Identify individual risk factors.
- Demonstrate and participate in behaviors and activities to prevent complications.
- Relate signs/symptoms that require medical reevaluation.

ACTIONS/INTERVENTIONS

Sample **NIC** linkages:

Peripheral Sensation Management: Prevention or minimization of injury or discomfort in the patient with altered sensation

Circulatory Care: Arterial [or] Venous Insufficiency: Promotion of arterial [or] venous circulation

NURSING PRIORITY NO. 1 To determine significance/degree of potential for compromise:

- Assess for individual risk factors: (1) trauma to extremity that causes internal tissue damage such as crush injuries, high-velocity and penetrating trauma, and fractures (especially long-bone fractures) with hemorrhage; (2) fluid accumulation into confined space (including IV infiltration, postoperative hematoma, circumferential burns); (3) long-term pressure on tissues, such as could occur from individual being trapped under collapsed structure; (4) external pressure on tissues (e.g., tight dressings, military anti-shock trousers, splints, casts, or restraints); and (5) presence of conditions affecting peripheral circulation, such as atherosclerosis, cardiovascular or cerebrovascular disease; diabetes, sickle cell disease, DVT, and coagulation disorders or use of anticoagulants *that potentiate risk of circulation disruption, insufficiency, and occlusion.*[1–3,6,10]
- Monitor for tissue bleeding and spread of hematoma *that can compress blood vessels and raise compartment pressures.*[1,2]
- Note position and location of casts, braces, traction apparatus, and use of restraints *to ascertain potential for pressure on tissues.*
- 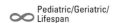 Review recent and current drug regimen, noting use of anticoagulants and vasoactive agents.

NURSING PRIORITY NO. 2 To assess for early signs of peripheral vascular impairment:

- Conduct a comprehensive upper or lower extremity assessment in at-risk client, including color, sensation, and functional ability. *Many individuals in this risk category are seen in the community healthcare setting for conditions not recognized as being related to peripheral vascular issues. However, early detection of circulatory issues may prevent the onset or severity of functional impairments associated with arterial or venous disorders of the extremities.*[6]
- Perform frequent neurovascular assessment in person immobilized for any reason (e.g., surgery, prolonged bedrest, diabetic neuropathy, fractures) or individuals with suspected neurovascular problems, noting differences in affected limb as compared with unaffected limb. Use the 6 Ps of assessment:[4]

Pain: Using 0 to 10 (or a similar pain scale), assess for presence, location, severity, and duration of pain. *Pain may be intermittent (e.g., intermittent claudication) or more constant (e.g., compartment syndrome or*

 Diagnostic Studies   Evidence Based Practice   Medications   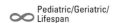 Pediatric/Geriatric/ Lifespan *arterial occlusion). Pain may range from muscle tension/tenderness and burning to severe pain. Pain may be present with active or passive movement, or at rest.*[2,5,6,8]

Pulses: Monitor presence (or absence) and quality of peripheral pulses (distal to injury or impairment) via palpation and/or Doppler. *Intact pulse usually indicates adequate circulation. However, occasionally a pulse may be palpated even though circulation is blocked by a soft clot; also, perfusion through larger arteries may continue after increased compartment pressure has collapsed the arteriole and venule circulation in the muscle.*[1,2,5,8]

Pallor: Evaluate skin temperature, capillary refill, and color changes to assess perfusion. *Pallor with cool, shiny, taut skin and slow venous refill is indicative of circulatory impairment. Cold, pale, bluish color with purpura indicates arterial insufficiency.*[5,6]

Paresthesia: Assess sensation (e.g., test peroneal nerve by pinch or pinprick in the dorsal web between first and second toe, and assess ability to dorsiflex toes in presence of leg fracture). *Changes in sensation cover a wide continuum and may include feeling of tingling, numbness, "pins and needles," burning, or diminished or absent sensation. Changes that might not be apparent to client could include loss of protective sensation in feet as determined by screening with tuning fork or percussion hammer. Sensation may be normal early in the presence of compartment syndrome because superficial circulation is not yet compromised.*[2,6,8,12]

Paralysis: Evaluate for range of motion. *Movement may be limited or absent because of tissue edema and nerve compression or because of nerve impingement such as would occur with spinal nerve compression.*[2,8]

Pressure: Evaluate by palpating the extremity. *Swelling or tightness may indicate obstruction, such as might occur with DVT, or compartment syndrome.*[11]

- ⬚ Assist with diagnostic studies (e.g., blood studies, Doppler, ultrasound, angiography, segmental arterial pressures, intracompartmental pressures, ankle-brachial index [ABI], transcutaneous oximetry) as indicated. *Numerous diagnostic tests may be needed if diagnosis is in doubt and in view of the multitude of medical and surgical conditions associated with peripheral vascular dysfunction.*[13]

NURSING PRIORITY NO. 3   To minimize edema formation/elevated tissue pressure:[1,3,5]

- Apply cold packs around injury/fracture site as indicated *to limit tissue swelling and hematoma formation.*
- Remove jewelry and constrictive clothing or other items from affected limb *to limit injury caused by swelling in injured tissues.*
- Elevate injured extremity(ies) unless contraindicated by confirmed presence of compartment syndrome *where elevation can actually impede arterial flow, decreasing perfusion.*[8]
- 🟦 Monitor for development of infiltration of IV fluids *to prevent excessive accumulation of fluids in tissues.*[8]
- Position extremity(ies) in proper alignment *to prevent nerve impingement and elevation of tissue pressures.*[8,9]
- Monitor skin and tissues around protective and corrective devices (e.g., dressings, splint, cast, traction devices) for proper application and function *to provide support and protection without causing undue pressure on tissues.*
- 🟢 Assist with or perform procedures (e.g., splitting cast, repositioning of restraints, continuous motion apparatus) *to release pressure and prevent permanent tissue damage or nerve injury.*
- 🟦 Observe position and location of supporting ring of traction splints or sling and readjust as indicated *to reduce pressure on tissues and risk of nerve impingement and improve blood flow.*
- 🟦 Avoid or limit use of restraints. Use padding and frequently evaluate extremity circulation, movement, and sensation when restraints are required.

NURSING PRIORITY NO. 4   To maximize circulation:[1–3,5,6]

- 🟦 Position all extremities in proper alignment and keep injured extremity in neutral position *to maximize circulation.*
- Provide or assist with range-of-motion exercises. Encourage client to routinely exercise digits and joints distal to injury *to enhance circulation.*

 Acute Care   Collaborative   Community/Home Care   Cultural

- Administer IV fluids and blood products as needed *to maintain circulating volume and reduce potential for ischemic tissue injury associated with loss of perfusion.*
- Monitor hemoglobin/hematocrit and coagulation studies if either clotting or bleeding into tissues is known or suspected or client is receiving anticoagulant therapy.[8,9]

NURSING PRIORITY NO. 5 Prevent/limit potential for complications:[1–3,5–7]

- Assist with treatment of underlying conditions *to reduce risks of complications.*
- Investigate sudden changes (e.g., changes in skin temperature or color, reports of pain that are extreme for type of injury, increased pain at rest or on passive movement of extremity, development of burning or tingling sensations, tense muscles, change in pulse quality distal to injury) *that are suggestive of compartment syndrome, requiring prompt intervention.*[1,2]
- Place limb in neutral position, avoiding elevation *to enhance circulation in compartment syndrome.*
- Report symptoms to physician at once *to provide for timely evaluation and intervention.*
- Assist with and encourage early ambulation *to help prevent DVT formation.*[9]
- Apply antiembolic hose or sequential compression devices as indicated.[9]
- Prepare for surgical intervention or other therapies (e.g., fibulectomy, fasciotomy, revascularization surgery, hyperbaric oxygen therapy) as indicated *to relieve increasing pressures and restore circulation.*[13]

NURSING PRIORITY NO. 6 To promote wellness (Teaching/Discharge Considerations):[1–3,5,6,9]

- Encourage good nutrition with adequate calories and micronutrients *to promote healing and reduce sluggishness of circulation.*
- Review proper body alignment of limbs (e.g., elevated or neutral position) as appropriate for individual situation.
- Instruct client and family in neurovascular findings to be reported to healthcare provider when indicated (e.g., client with new fractures in cast at home, client at risk for DVT) *to limit preventable complications through early intervention.*
- Promote benefits of walking and smoking cessation *to improve circulation.*
- Discuss necessity of avoiding constrictive clothing, sharp angulation of legs, crossing ankles or legs, and thermal or mechanical trauma, *especially if client has history of peripheral vascular insufficiency or is at risk for DVT.*[8,9]
- Demonstrate proper application and removal of antiembolic hose or sequential compression devices, as indicated.
- Review safe use of heat or cold therapy, especially if client has poor sensation in extremities *to avoid thermal injury.*
- Instruct client/SO(s) to check shoes and socks for proper fit and/or wrinkles *to reduce potential for foot problems associated with neuropathies.*
- Recommend continuation of prescribed exercise program *to maintain extremity circulation and strength.*
- Review proper use and monitoring of drug regimen and safety concerns associated with anticoagulant use *to ensure maximum benefit and avoid complications and bleeding problems.*
- Recommend regular follow-up with healthcare provider *to monitor status of condition, treatment efficacy, and to provide for timely intervention, when needed.*

DOCUMENTATION FOCUS

Assessment/Reassessment
- Specific risk factors, nature of injury to limb.
- Assessment findings, including comparison of affected and unaffected limb, characteristics of pain in involved area.
- Doppler or compartment pressure results.

 Diagnostic Studies   Evidence Based Practice   Medications   Pediatric/Geriatric/Lifespan

Planning
- Plan of care and who is involved in the planning.
- Teaching plan.

Implementation/Evaluation
- Response to interventions, teaching, and actions performed.
- Attainment or progress toward desired outcome(s).
- Modification of plan of care.

Discharge Planning
- Long-term needs, referrals, and who is responsible for actions to be taken.
- Specific referrals made.

References

1. Fort, C. W. (2003). How to combat 3 deadly trauma complications. *Nursing*, 33(5), 58–63.
2. Rasul, A. T. (Updated 2017). Acute compartment syndrome. Retrieved March 2018 from http://emedicine.medscape.com/article/307668-overview.
3. Bhimji, S. (Reviewed 2017). Peripheral vascular disease. Retrieved March 2018 from http://www.emedicinehealth.com/peripheral_vascular_disease/article_em.htm.
4. Ackley, B. J., Ladwig, G. B. (eds.). (2011). ND Risk for peripheral neurovascular dysfunction. *Nursing Diagnosis Handbook: A Guide to Planning Care*. 9th ed. St. Louis, MO: Mosby.
5. Dominguez, J. A., Lopez-Rowe, V. (Updated 2017). Peripheral arterial occlusive disease. Retrieved March 2018 from http://emedicine.medscape.com/article/460178-overview.
6. Bonham, P. A., et al. (2009). What's new in lower-extremity arterial disease? WOCN's 2008 Clinical Practice Guideline. *J Wound Ostomy Continence Nurs*, 36(1), 37–44.
7. Stephens, E. (Updated 2017). Peripheral vascular disease. Retrieved March 2018 from http://emedicine.medscape.com/article/761556-overview.
8. Heron Evans, M. R. (2006). Interventions for clients with musculoskeletal trauma. In Ignativicius, D. D., Workman, M. L. (eds.) *Medical-Surgical Nursing: Critical Thinking for Collaborative Care*. 5th ed. St. Louis, MO: Elsevier-Saunders.
9. Patel, K., Chun, L. J. (Updated 2017). Deep vein thrombosis (DVT). Retrieved March 2018 from http://emedicine.medscape.com/article/1911303-overview.
10. Dougherty, A. L., et al. (2009). Battlefield extremity injuries in Operation Iraqi Freedom. *Injury*, 40(7), 772–777.
11. Bucholz, R. W., Heckman, J. P., Court-Brown, C. M. (eds.). (2006). *Rockwood and Green's Fractures in Adults*. 6th ed. Philadelphia, PA: Lippincott, Williams & Wilkins.
12. Tesfaye, S., Boulton, A. J. M., Dyck, P. J. (2010). Diabetic neuropathies: Update on definitions, diagnostic criteria, estimation of severity, and treatments. *Diabetes Care*, 33(10), 2285–2293.
13. Berti-Hearn, L., Elliot, B. (2018). A closer look at lower extremity peripheral arterial disease. *Nursing*, 41(1), 34–41.

imbalanced Nutrition: less than body requirements

Taxonomy II: Nutrition—Class 1 Ingestion (00002) **[Diagnostic Division:** Food/Fluid], Approved 1975; Revised 2000; 2017

DEFINITION: Intake of nutrients insufficient to meet metabolic needs.

RELATED FACTORS
Insufficient dietary intake

DEFINING CHARACTERISTICS

Subjective
Insufficient interest in food; food aversion; alteration in taste sensation; perceived inability to ingest food
Satiety immediately upon ingesting food
Abdominal pain or cramping; sore buccal cavity
Insufficient information; misinformation; misconception

 Acute Care   Collaborative   Community/Home Care   Cultural

Objective

Body weight 20% or more below ideal weight range; insufficient muscle tone; [decreased subcutaneous fat or muscle mass]

Weight loss with adequate food intake

Food intake less than recommended daily allowances (RDA)

Hyperactive bowel sounds; diarrhea; steatorrhea

Weakness of muscles required for mastication or swallowing; insufficient muscle tone

Pale mucous membranes; capillary fragility

Excessive hair loss [or increased growth of hair on body (lanugo)]; [cessation of menses]

[Abnormal laboratory studies (e.g., decreased albumin, total proteins; iron deficiency; electrolyte imbalances)]

At Risk Population: Biological factors

Economically disadvantaged

Associated Condition: Inability to absorb nutrients; inability to ingest/digest food

Psychological disorder

Sample Clinical Applications: Cancer, AIDS, anorexia or bulimia nervosa, burns, facial trauma, brain injury, coma, stroke, Parkinson's disease, cleft lip/palate, anemia, dementia, Alzheimer's disease, major depression, schizophrenia

DESIRED OUTCOMES/EVALUATION CRITERIA

Sample **NOC** linkages:

Nutritional Status: Extent to which nutrients are ingested and absorbed to meet metabolic needs

Knowledge: Healthy Diet: Extent of understanding conveyed about a balanced nutritious diet

Weight Gain Behavior: Personal actions to gain weight following voluntary or involuntary significant weight loss

Client Will (Include Specific Time Frame)

• Demonstrate progressive weight gain toward goal.

• Display normalization of laboratory values and be free of signs of malnutrition as reflected in Defining Characteristics.

• Verbalize understanding of causative factors when known and necessary interventions.

• Demonstrate behaviors and lifestyle changes to regain or maintain appropriate weight.

ACTIONS/INTERVENTIONS

Sample **NIC** linkages:

Nutrition Management: Providing and promoting a balanced intake of nutrients

Weight-Gain Assistance: Facilitating gain of body weight

Eating Disorders Management: Prevention and treatment of severe diet restrictions and overexercising or binging and purging of foods and fluids

NURSING PRIORITY NO. 1 To assess causative/contributing factors:

• ∞ Identify client at risk for malnutrition (e.g., institutionalized elderly; client with chronic illness; child or adult living in poverty/low-income area; client with facial injuries or deformities; restrictive weight-loss program or surgical intervention; prolonged time of restricted intake, prior nutritional deficiencies; hypermetabolic states [e.g., hyperthyroidism, burns]; malabsorption syndromes).[2,9,10]

 Diagnostic Studies   Evidence Based Practice   Medications   Pediatric/Geriatric/Lifespan

- Obtain dietary history *to determine chronic problems and ongoing needs, such as:*
  Increased caloric requirements with difficulty ingesting sufficient calories (e.g., cancer, burns).
   Maturational or developmental issues (e.g., premature baby with sucking difficulties, child with lack of emotional stimulation, frail elderly living alone, hospitalized, or in nursing home). Note: A recent study confirms that almost 90% of elderly persons transitioning from acute care to a subacute facility are either malnourished or at risk of malnutrition.[2]
  Swallowing difficulties (e.g., stroke, Parkinson's disease, cerebral palsy, dementia [especially Alzheimer's disease]; other neuromuscular disorders).[2]
  Poor dentition (damaged or missing teeth, ill-fitting dentures, gum disease).
  Decreased absorption (e.g., lactose intolerance, Crohn's disease).
  Diminished desire or refusal to eat (e.g., anorexia nervosa, cirrhosis, pancreatitis, alcoholism, bipolar disorder, depression, chronic fatigue).[2,6]
  Treatment-related issues (e.g., chemotherapy, radiation, stomatitis, facial surgery, wired jaw).
  Personal or situational factors (e.g., inability to procure or prepare food, social isolation, grief, loss).[8]
- Assess pediatric concerns (e.g., changes in nutritional needs related to growth phase; congenital anomalies, including tracheoesophageal fistula, cleft lip/palate; metabolic or malabsorption problems, such as diabetes, phenylketonuria, cerebral palsy; chronic infections).[4]
- Determine lifestyle factors that may affect weight. *Socioeconomic resources, amount of money available for purchasing food, proximity of grocery store, and available storage space for food are all factors that may impact food choices and intake.*
- Evaluate impact of cultural, ethnic, and religious influences. *The nutritional balance of a diet is recognized by most cultures, with distinct theories of nutritional practices for health promotion and disease prevention. Foods are used for prevention or treatment of disease (e.g., client may believe in use of "hot" or "cold" foods to treat certain conditions or use low-fat, low-sodium foods to prevent heart disease). Certain foods may be thought to cause a disease condition (e.g., upset stomach caused from eating too many cold foods). Special diets or food preparation may be cultural or religious based (e.g., kosher preparation for Jewish client or eating no meat or meat by-products for vegetarian).[1]*
- Explore specific eating habits, the meaning of food to client (e.g., never eats breakfast, snacks throughout entire day, fasts for weight control, no time to eat properly), and individual food preferences and intolerances/aversions. *Identifies eating practices that may need to be corrected and provides insight into dietary interventions that may appeal to client.*
- Obtain history or review diary of daily portion (or calorie) intake and patterns and times of eating *to reveal recent changes in client's weight or appetite and to identify strengths and weaknesses in client's dietary habits.[2]*
- Assess client's knowledge of nutritional needs and ways client is meeting these needs. *Identifies teaching needs and/or helps guide choice of interventions.[2]*
- Note availability and use of financial resources and support systems. *These factors affect or determine ability to acquire, prepare, and store food. Lack of support or socialization may impact client's desire to eat.*
- Assess medication regimen, noting possible drug side effects or interactions, allergies, use of laxatives, and diuretics. *These factors may be affecting appetite, food intake, or absorption.[2,8]*
- Note client's ability to feed self or presence of interfering factors. *Difficulties such as paralysis, tremor, or injury to hands or arms with inability to grasp or lift utensils to mouth; cognitive impairments affecting coordination or remembering to eat; age; and/or developmental issues may require input of multiple providers and therapists to develop individualized plan of care.[2]*
- Auscultate for presence and character of bowel sounds *to determine ability and readiness of intestinal tract to handle digestive processes (e.g., hypermotility accompanies vomiting or diarrhea, while absence of bowel sounds may indicate bowel obstruction).*
- Determine psychological factors that may affect food choices. Perform psychological assessment as indicated *to assess body image and congruency with reality or to identify factors (e.g., dementia, severe depression) that may be interfering with client's appetite and food intake.[2]*

 Acute Care   Collaborative   Community/ Home Care   Cultural

- Note occurrence of amenorrhea, tooth decay, swollen salivary glands, or report of constant sore throat. *May be signs of eating disorder, such as bulimia, affecting eating patterns and requiring additional evaluation.*[5,6]
- Review usual activities and exercise program, noting repetitive activities (e.g., constant pacing) or inappropriate exercise (e.g., prolonged jogging). *Individuals with dementia may pace or be in constant motion, increasing energy needs. Clients who have eating disorders, such as anorexia or bulimia, may use obsessive activities as weight-control measures.*[6]

NURSING PRIORITY NO. 2   To evaluate degree of deficit:

- Assess current weight, compared to usual weight and norms for age and body size *to identify changes (e.g., sudden loss related to medical illness versus ongoing chronic depression with anorexia and weight loss; toddler with failure to meet growth expectations) that affect choice of intervention and help clarify expectations.*
- Obtain weights using same scale, same time of day, and same clothing as much as possible *to provide for accurate comparison to evaluate effectiveness of therapeutic regimen.*[2]
- ∞ Calculate growth percentiles in infants/children using growth chart *to identify deviations from the norm.*[4]
- ✎ Measure or calculate body fat, body water, and muscle mass (via triceps skinfold or other anthropometric measurements) or calculate body mass index (BMI) *to establish baseline parameters and assist in determining therapeutic goals. Note: BMI = weight (lb)/height (inches squared) × 703 according to the Centers for Disease Control and Prevention. Desirable adult BMI is 18.5 to 24.9. A BMI of 17 or below is considered severely underweight, or clinically anorexic.*[2,8,17]
- Observe for absence of subcutaneous fat or muscle wasting, loss of hair, fissuring of nails, delayed healing, gum bleeding, swollen abdomen, etc., that indicate protein-energy malnutrition.[9]
- ✎ ▨ Perform or review results of nutritional assessment using screening tools such as the Malnutrition Universal Screening Tool, the Veterans Affairs Nutrition Status Classification system, the screening tool developed by Brugler et al., or the Mini Nutritional Assessment (MNA). *Note: In 2006, Guigoz reported that the MNA had been used in 36 studies to assess the nutritional status of 8,596 hospitalized older adults worldwide; of these, 50% to 80% were classified as either at risk for malnourishment or malnourished.*[11–14]
- ✎ ▨ Review laboratory studies (e.g., serum albumin, prealbumin, transferrin, amino acid profile, iron, blood urea nitrogen, nitrogen balance studies, glucose, liver function, electrolytes, total lymphocyte count, indirect calorimetry). *Baseline screening may be done to determine whether more in-depth evaluation is needed. Note: Brugler et al. found that the characteristics that correlated best with malnutrition-related complications were occurrence of a wound, poor oral intake, malnutrition-related admission diagnosis, serum albumin value, hemoglobin value, and total lymphocyte count.*[2,14]

NURSING PRIORITY NO. 3   To establish a nutritional plan that meets individual needs:

- ⓐ Collaborate with interdisciplinary team *to set nutritional goals when client has specific dietary needs, malnutrition is profound, or long-term feeding problems exist.*[2,7,9]
- ⓐ Calculate client's energy and protein requirements using basal energy expenditure and the Harris-Benedict (or similar) formula. *The essential nutritional requirements include the needs for energy, protein, and hydration, along with vitamins and electrolytes. Various factors may be considered in choosing a useful formula, including age, sex, disease state, stress associated with current illness, body size (e.g., obesity), and activity (e.g., bedbound versus out of bed).*[15]
- Establish ongoing method of evaluating intake (e.g., calories/day, percent of food consumed at each feeding) *to assist in determining both amount of food taken and what food groups are consumed or left uneaten, to identify nutritional deficits.*[2]
- Discuss with client/significant other (SO) aspects of diet that can remain unchanged *to preserve those that are valuable or meaningful to individual, and enhance sense of control.* Negotiate with client aspects of diet that need to be changed, especially if eating or psychiatric disorder is limiting food intake.

 Diagnostic Studies   Evidence Based Practice   Medications   Pediatric/Geriatric/ Lifespan

NURSING PRIORITY NO. 4 To address specific underlying condition/treatment needs:

- Assist in treatments to correct or control underlying causative factors *to improve intake and utilization of nutrients:*[2,7]

  Administer oral antifungal agent *to treat cutaneous lesions of the mouth (e.g., candidiasis) that limit client's ability or desire for food.*

  Medicate for pain or nausea and manage drug side effects *to increase physical comfort and appetite.*

  Provide pureed foods, formula tube feedings, or parenteral nutrition infusions when indicated by client's condition (e.g., wired jaws or paralysis following stroke) and degree of malnutrition. *Enteral route is preferred when oral feeding is not appropriate. Recent evidence suggests a beneficial effect of implementation of early enteral nutrition (EN) in trauma patients, and there is no convincing evidence regarding any harmful effect. Early EN is defined as the provision of a standard EN formula via any feeding tube route within 24 hours of initial injury or ICU admission. The systemic contraindications for EN remain to be clarified. Early parenteral nutrition (PN) is not recommended.*[7,16]

  Consult occupational therapist *to identify appropriate assistive devices to facilitate independence in feeding and self-esteem.*

  Consult speech therapist *to develop specific exercises or activities to address swallowing difficulties related to neurological problems (e.g., stroke, amyotrophic lateral sclerosis).* (Refer to ND impaired Swallowing for additional interventions.)

  Refer for dental care *to correct missing teeth or poorly fitting dentures that affect client's ability to chew food or enjoy process of eating.*

  Develop or refer client to structured (behavioral modification) program for nutrition therapy, which may include documenting time/length of eating period, putting food in a blender, and tube feeding food not eaten. *These programs are used to change the maladaptive eating behaviors of clients with anorexia and bulimia and ensure adequate caloric intake. Because "control" is central to the etiology of these disorders, it is important to ensure that the client is perceived to be "in control."*[6]

  Recommend or support hospitalization for controlled environment, as indicated, in severe malnutrition or life-threatening situations.

NURSING PRIORITY NO. 5 To enhance dietary intake:

- Avoid or limit withholding of food (e.g., prolonged NPO for surgery) as much as possible and reinstitute oral feedings as early as possible *to reduce adverse effects of malnutrition.*
- Increase specific nutrients (e.g., protein, carbohydrates, fats, calories) as needed, providing client with preferred food and seasoning choices where possible *to enhance intake.*[9]
- Determine when client prefers or tolerates largest meal of the day. Maintain flexibility in timing of food intake *to promote sense of control and give client opportunity to eat when feeling more rested, less pain or nausea, family coming at mealtime, etc.*[2]
- Provide numerous small feedings as indicated; supplement with easily digested snacks *to reduce feeling of fullness that can accompany larger meals and to improve chances of increasing the amount of nutrients taken over 24-hr period.*[5]
- Promote adequate and timely fluid intake. *Fluid is essential to the digestive process and is often taken with meals. Fluids may need to be withheld before meals or with meals if interfering with food intake.*
- Encourage variety in food choices, varying textures and taste sensations (e.g., sweet, salty, fresh, methods of cooking) *to enhance food satisfaction and stimulate appetite.*[2]
- Offer and keep available to client finger foods and snacks *that are easy to self-feed.*
- Provide oral care before and after meals. *Reduces discomfort associated with nausea, vomiting, oral lesions, mucosal dryness, and halitosis, making eating easier or food more palatable.*
- Encourage use of lozenges, gum, hard candy, and beverages *to stimulate salivation when dryness is a factor.*
- Use alternative flavoring agents (e.g., lemon and herbs) *to enhance taste of foods, especially if salt is restricted.*

 Acute Care   Collaborative Community/ Home Care   Cultural

- Add nonfat milk powder to foods with a high liquid content (e.g., gravy, puddings, cooked cereal) and sugar or honey in beverages if carbohydrates are tolerated *to increase caloric value.*[2]
- Avoid foods that cause intolerances or increase gastric motility (e.g., gas-forming foods, hot or cold, spicy, caffeinated beverages, milk products, etc.) *to reduce postprandial discomfort that may discourage client from eating.*[3]
- Limit high-fat foods or fiber and bulk if indicated *because they may lead to early satiety.*
- Offer supplement drinks (or dispense in 2- to 4-oz portions several times/day). *Client may view this as a "medication" and thus will drink it, improving intake and energy level.*[2]
- Promote pleasant, relaxing environment, including socialization when possible. *Promotes focus on activity of eating, enhancing intake.*[2]
- Prevent or minimize unpleasant odors and sights or cooking odors. *Often have a negative effect on appetite or activate gag reflex.*
- 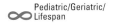Administer pharmaceutical agents as indicated. *Appetite stimulants and dietary supplements and digestive drugs or enzymes, vitamins and minerals (e.g., iron), antacids, anticholinergics, antiemetics, antidiarrheals, etc., may be used to enhance intake, improve digestion, and correct nutritional deficiencies.*[2]

NURSING PRIORITY NO. 6 To promote wellness (Teaching/Discharge Considerations):

- Discuss myths client/SO(s) may have about weight and weight gain *to address misconceptions and perhaps improve motivation for needed behavior changes.*
- Emphasize importance of well-balanced, nutritious intake. Provide nutritional information as indicated, taking into account client's age and developmental stage (e.g., toddler, teenager, pregnant woman, elderly person with chronic disease), physical health and activity tolerance, financial and socioeconomic factors, and client's/SO's potential for management of underlying conditions. *For example, older adults need same nutrients as younger adults but in smaller amounts and with attention to certain components, such as calcium, fiber, vitamins, protein, and water.*[3] *Infants/children require small meals and constant attention to needed nutrients for proper growth and development while dealing with child's food preferences and eating habits.*[4]
- Address financial issues and identify ways to meet dietary needs using nutrient-dense, low-budget foods.
- Involve SO(s) in treatment plan as much as possible *to provide ongoing support and increase likelihood of accomplishing dietary goals.*
- Consult with dietitian/nutritional support team as necessary *for long-term needs.*
- Involve client in developing behavior modification program appropriate to specific needs based on consistent, realistic weight gain goal. *Enhances commitment to change and likelihood of accomplishing desired outcomes.*[5,6]
- Provide positive regard, love, and acknowledgment of "voice within" guiding client with eating disorder. *These efforts encourage the client to recognize maladaptive eating patterns as defense mechanisms to ease the emotional pain and begin to resolve underlying issues and develop more adaptive coping strategies for dealing with stressful situations.*[6]
- Weigh as needed/prescribed and document results *to monitor effectiveness of dietary plan.*
- Develop regular exercise and stress-reduction programs. *Enhances general well-being, improves organ function/muscle tone, and increases appetite.*
- 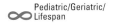Review medical regimen and provide information or assistance as necessary. Discuss drug side effects and potential interactions with other medications and over-the-counter drugs.
- Assist client to identify and access community resources such as nutrition assistance program, budget counseling, Meals on Wheels, community food banks, or other appropriate assistance programs.
- Refer for dental hygiene and professional care, counseling or psychiatric care, and family therapy as indicated.
- Provide and reinforce client teaching regarding preoperative and postoperative dietary needs when surgery is planned.
- Assist client/SO(s) to learn how to blenderize food or perform tube feeding when indicated. *Promotes independence in self-care and sense of some degree of control in a difficult situation.*
- Refer to home health resources *for initiation and supervision of home nutrition therapy when used.*

 Diagnostic Studies   Evidence Based Practice   Medications   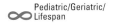 Pediatric/Geriatric/Lifespan

DOCUMENTATION FOCUS

Assessment/Reassessment
- Baseline and subsequent assessment findings to include signs/symptoms and laboratory diagnostic findings.
- Caloric and nutrient intake.
- Individual cultural or religious restrictions, personal preferences.
- Availability and use of resources.
- Personal understanding and perception of problem.

Planning
- Plan of care and who is involved in planning.
- Teaching plan.

Implementation/Evaluation
- Client's responses to interventions, teaching, and actions performed.
- Results of periodic weigh-in.
- Attainment or progress toward desired outcome(s).
- Modifications to plan of care.

Discharge Planning
- Long-term needs and who is responsible for actions to be taken.
- Specific referrals made.

References

1. Purnell, L. D. (2011). *Guide to Culturally Competent Health Care*. 2nd ed. Philadelphia, PA: F. A. Davis.
2. Sloane, P. D., et al. (2001). Nutritional issues in long term care. *J Am Med Dir Assoc*, 9(7), 476–485.
3. American Dietetic Association. (2005). Nutrition across the spectrum of aging. *J Am Diet Assoc*, 105(4), 616–633.
4. Engel, J. (2006). *Mosbys Pocket Guide to Pediatric Assessment*. 5th ed. St. Louis, MO: Mosby.
5. Smith, M., Robinson, L., Segal, J. (2015, updated 2018). Helping someone with an eating disorder. Retrieved April 2018 from http://www.helpguide.org/articles/eating-disorders/helping-someone-with-an-eating-disorder.htm.
6. Townsend, M. C. (2011). *Psychiatric Mental Health Nursing Concepts of Care in Evidence-Based Practice*. 7th ed. Philadelphia, PA: F. A. Davis.
7. Blaser, A. R. (2012). Update on enteral nutrition in trauma: Early enteral nutrition: Practical aspects. Retrieved April 2018 from https://www.nestlehealthscience.com/asset-library/documents/events/esicm%20trauma%20conference%20proceeding_final.pdf.
8. Hartford Institute for Geriatric Nursing. (2012). Nursing Standard of Practice Protocol: Assessment and management of mealtime difficulties. Retrieved April 2018 from https://consultgeri.org/geriatric-topics/mealtime-difficulties.
9. Scheinfeld, N. S., Lin, A., Mokashi, A. (2014, updated 2016). Protein-energy malnutrition. Retrieved April 2018 from http://emedicine.medscape.com/article/1104623-overview.
10. Sullivan, C. S., Logan, J., Kolasa, K. M. (2006). Medical nutrition therapy for the bariatric patient. *Nutr Today*, 41(5), 207–212.
11. DiMaria, R. A., Amelia, E. (2005). Nutrition in older adults: Intervention and assessment can curb the growing threat of malnutrition. *Am J Nurs*, 105(3), 40–50.
12. Guigoz, Y. (2006). The Mini Nutritional Assessment (MNA) review of the literature—What does it tell us? *J Nutr Health Aging*, 10(6), 466–485.
13. Malnutrition Advisory Group (No date). Malnutrition Universal Screening Tool (MUST). Retrieved April 2018 from http://www.bapen.org.uk/pdfs/must/must_full.pdf.
14. Brugler, L., et al. (2005). A simplified nutrition screen for hospitalized patients using readily available laboratory and patient information. *Nutrition*, 21(6), 650–658.
15. Dawodu, S. T., Scott, D. D., Chase, M. (2015). Nutritional management in the rehabilitation setting. Retrieved April 2018 from http://emedicine.medscape.com/article/318180-overview#a1.
16. Kirkland, L. L., Kashiwagi, D. T., Brantley, S. (2013). Nutrition in the hospitalized patient. *J Hosp Med*, 8(1), 52–58.
17. Centers for Disease Control and Prevention (CDC). (2017). About adult BMI. Retrieved April 2018 from https://www.cdc.gov/healthyweight/assessing/bmi/adult_bmi/index.html.

 Acute Care Collaborative Community/Home Care Cultural

readiness for enhanced Nutrition

Taxonomy II: Nutrition—Class 4 Metabolism (00163) [**Diagnostic Division:** Food/Fluid], Approved 2002; Revised 2013

DEFINITION: A pattern of nutrient intake, which can be strengthened.

DEFINING CHARACTERISTICS

Subjective
Expresses desire to enhance nutrition
Sample Clinical Applications: As a health-seeking behavior the client may be healthy, or this diagnosis can occur in any clinical condition

DESIRED OUTCOMES/EVALUATION CRITERIA

Sample NOC linkages:
Nutritional Status: Extent to which nutrients are ingested and absorbed to meet metabolic needs
Knowledge: Healthy Diet: Extent of understanding conveyed about a balanced nutritional diet
Weight Maintenance Behavior: Personal actions to maintain optimum body weight

Client Will (Include Specific Time Frame)
• Demonstrate behaviors to attain or maintain appropriate weight.
• Be free of signs of malnutrition.
• Be able to safely prepare and store foods.

ACTIONS/INTERVENTIONS

Sample NIC linkages:
Nutritional Counseling: Use of an interactive helping process focusing on the need for diet modification
Teaching: Prescribed Diet: Preparing a patient to correctly follow a prescribed diet
Weight Management: Facilitating maintenance of optimal body weight and percent body fat

NURSING PRIORITY NO. 1 To determine current nutritional status and eating patterns:

• Assess client's knowledge of current nutritional needs and ways client is meeting these needs. *Provides baseline for further teaching or interventions.*
• Assess eating patterns and food and fluid choices in relation to any health-risk factors and health goals. *Helps to identify specific strengths and weaknesses that can be addressed.*
• ∞ Verify that age-related and developmental needs are met. *These factors are constantly present throughout the lifespan, although differing for each age group. For example, older adults need the same nutrients as younger adults, but in smaller amounts and with attention to certain components, such as calcium, fiber, vitamins, protein, and water.[1] Infants/children require small meals and constant attention to needed nutrients for proper growth and development while dealing with child's food preferences and eating habits.[2]*
• 🌐 Evaluate influence of cultural and religious factors *to determine what client considers to be normal dietary practice as well as to identify food preferences and restrictions and eating patterns that can be strengthened or altered if indicated.[3]*
• Assess how client perceives food, food preparation, and the act of eating *to determine client's feeling and emotions regarding food (including the use of food for celebrations or as a reward) and self-image.*
• Ascertain occurrence of or potential for negative feedback from significant others (SOs). *May reveal control issues that could impact client's motivation for and commitment to change.*

 Diagnostic Studies   Evidence Based Practice   Medications   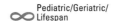 Pediatric/Geriatric/Lifespan

- Determine patterns of hunger and satiety. *Helps identify strengths and weaknesses in eating patterns and potential for change (e.g., person predisposed to weight gain may need a different time for a big meal than evening or may need teaching as to what foods reinforce feelings of satisfaction).*
- Assess client's ability to shop for, safely store, and prepare foods *to determine if health information or financial resources might be needed.*

NURSING PRIORITY NO. 2 To assist client/SO(s) to develop plan to meet individual needs:

- Determine motivation and expectation for change. *Motivation to improve and high expectations can encourage client to make changes that will improve his or her life. However, presence of unrealistic expectations may hamper efforts. Client may actually be satisfied with current nutritional state and eating behaviors or may be changing some aspect of food intake or preparation in response to new dietary information or change in health status.*
- Assist in obtaining or review results of individual testing (e.g., weight and height, body fat percent, lipids, glucose, complete blood count, total protein) *to determine that client is healthy and/or identify dietary changes that may be helpful in attaining health goals.*[5]
- Encourage client's beneficial eating patterns and habits (e.g., controlling portion size; eating regular meals; reducing high-fat, high-sugar, or fast-food intake; following specific dietary program; drinking water and healthy beverages). *Provides reinforcement and supports client's efforts to incorporate changes into lifestyle habits and continue with new behaviors.*[6]
- Provide instruction and reinforce information regarding special needs. *Client/SO may benefit from or desire assistance in learning new eating habits or following medically prescribed diets (e.g., very low calorie diet, tube feedings, diabetic or renal dialysis diet).*[4]
- Encourage the client to carefully read food labels, instructing in meaning of labeling, as indicated, *to assist client/SO in making healthful choices.*[6]
- Consult with or refer to nutritionist/physician, as indicated. *Client/SO may benefit from advice regarding specific nutrition or dietary issues or may require regular follow-up to determine that needs are being met when following a medically prescribed program.*
- Develop a system for self-monitoring *to provide a sense of control and enable the client to track own progress as well as to assist in making informed choices.*

NURSING PRIORITY NO. 3 To promote optimum wellness (Teaching/Discharge Considerations):

- Review individual risk factors and provide additional information or response to concerns. *Assists the client with motivation and decision making.*
- Provide bibliotherapy and help client/SO(s) identify and evaluate resources he or she can access. *Reinforces learning, allows client to progress at own pace, and encourages client to be responsible for own learning. When referencing the Internet and nontraditional or unproven resources, the individual must exercise some restraint and determine the reliability of the source and information before acting on it.*
- Encourage variety and moderation in dietary plan *to decrease boredom and encourage client in efforts to make healthy choices about eating and food.*
- Discuss use of nutritional supplements and over-the-counter and herbal products. *Confusion may exist regarding the need for and use of these products in a balanced dietary regimen.*
- Assist client to identify and access community resources when indicated. *May benefit from assistance, such as nutritional assistance program, budget counseling, Meals on Wheels, community food banks, and other assistance programs.*

DOCUMENTATION FOCUS

Assessment/Reassessment
- Baseline information, client's perception of need.
- Nutritional intake and metabolic needs.
- Motivation and expectations for change.

 Acute Care   Collaborative   Community/ Home Care   Cultural

Planning
- Plan of care, specific interventions, and who is involved in planning.
- Teaching plan.

Implementation/Evaluation
- Client's responses to interventions, teaching, and actions performed.
- Attainment or progress toward desired outcome(s).
- Modifications to plan of care.

Discharge Planning
- Long-term needs and actions to be taken.
- Support systems available, specific referrals made, and who is responsible for actions to be taken.

References

1. American Dietetic Association. (2005). Nutrition across the spectrum of aging. *J Am Diet Assoc*, 105(4), 616–633.
2. Caprio, S., et al. (2008). Influence of race, ethnicity, and culture on childhood obesity: Implications for prevention and treatment: A consensus statement of Shaping America's Health and the Obesity Society. *Diabetes Care*, 31(11), 2211–2221.
3. Purnell, L. D. (2011). *Guide to Culturally Competent Health Care*. 2nd ed. Philadelphia: F. A. Davis.
4. Pignone, M. P. (2003). Counseling to promote a healthy diet in adults: A summary of the evidence for the U.S. Preventive Services Task Force. *Am J Prev Med*, 24(1), 75–92.
5. Vogelzang, J. L. (2003). Making nutrition sense from OASIS. *Home Healthc Nurse*, 21(9), 592–600.
6. U.S. Department of Health and Human Services, Department of Agriculture. (2010). Dietary Guidelines for Americans, 2010 (various pages). Retrieved April 2018 from http://www.cnpp.usda.gov/DietaryGuidelines.htm.

Obesity

Taxonomy II: Nutrition—Class 1 Ingestion (00232) [**Diagnostic Division:** Food/Fluid], Approved 2013; Revised 2017

DEFINITION: A condition in which an individual accumulates abnormal or excessive fat for age and gender that exceeds overweight.

RELATED FACTORS
Average daily physical activity is less than recommended for gender and age; energy expenditure below energy intake based on standard assessment (e.g., WAVE [weight, activity, variety in diet, excess] assessment); sedentary behavior occurring for ≥2 hours/day

Consumption of sugar-sweetened beverages; frequent snacking; high frequency of restaurant or fried food; portion sizes larger than recommended; solid foods as major food source at <5 months of age

Disordered eating behaviors or perceptions; fear regarding lack of food supply

Excessive alcohol consumption

Shortened sleep time, sleep disorder

DEFINING CHARACTERISTICS

Objective

ADULT: Body mass index (BMI) of >30 kg/m^2

CHILD <2 years: Term not used with children this age

CHILD 2–18 years: Body mass index (BMI) >95th percentile or >30 kg/m^2 for age and gender

At Risk Population: Economically disadvantaged

(continues on page 592)

 Diagnostic Studies　 Evidence Based Practice　 Medications　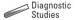 Pediatric/Geriatric/Lifespan

Obesity (continued)

Formula- or mixed-fed infants; overweight in infancy; rapid weight gain during infancy, including the first week, first 4 months, and first year; rapid weight gain during childhood

Premature pubarche

Heritability of interrelated factors; high disinhibition and restraint eating behavior score

Maternal diabetes mellitus, maternal smoking; paternal obesity

Associated Condition: Genetic disorder

Sample Clinical Applications: Bulimia nervosa, morbid obesity, diseases requiring long-term steroid use (e.g., chronic obstructive pulmonary disease [COPD]), conditions associated with immobility (e.g., stroke/paralysis, multiple sclerosis [MS], amputation), Alzheimer's disease, depression, developmental delay

DESIRED OUTCOMES/EVALUATION CRITERIA

Sample **NOC** linkages:

Weight Loss Behavior: Personal actions to lose weight through diet, exercise, and behavior modification

Knowledge: Diet: Extent of understanding conveyed about a balanced, nutritious diet

Nutritional Status: Extent to which nutrients are ingested and absorbed to meet metabolic needs

Weight: Body Mass: Extent to which body weight, muscle, and fat are congruent to height, frame, gender, and age

Client Will (Include Specific Time Frame)

• Verbalize a realistic self-concept or body image (congruent mental and physical picture of self).

• Participate in development of, and commit to, a personal weight loss program.

• Demonstrate appropriate changes in lifestyle and behaviors, including eating patterns, food quantity/quality, and exercise program.

• Attain desirable body weight with optimal maintenance of health.

ACTIONS/INTERVENTIONS

Sample **NIC** linkages:

Weight Reduction Assistance: Facilitating loss of weight and/or body fat

Nutrition Management: Providing and promoting a balanced intake of nutrients

Nutritional Counseling: Use of an interactive helping process focusing on the need for diet modification

NURSING PRIORITY NO. 1   To identify contributing factors/health status:

• ∞ 📝 Obtain weight history, noting if client has weight gain out of character for self or family, is or was obese child, or used to be much more physically active than is now *to identify trends. Note: Obesity is now the most prevalent nutritional disorder among children and adolescents in the United States (45% of all adults and approximately 18% of youths ages 2 to 19 years).*[1] *Being overweight during older childhood is highly predictive of adult obesity, especially if a parent is also obese.*[2]

• ∞ 📝 Assess risk and presence of factors or conditions associated with obesity (e.g., familial pattern of obesity; genetic disorders in children [e.g., Prader-Willi syndrome, Laurence-Moon-Biedls syndrome]; hypothyroidism; type 2 diabetes; reproductive dysfunction; menopause; chronic disorders, such as heart disease, kidney disease, chronic pain; food or other substance addictions; stressful or sedentary lifestyle; depression; use of certain medications such as steroids, birth control pills; physical disabilities or limitations; lack of socioeconomic resources for obtaining or preparing healthy foods) *to determine treatments and interventions that may be indicated in addition to weight management.*[2,3]

 Acute Care   Collaborative   Community/Home Care   Cultural

- Ascertain current and previous dieting history. *Client may report normal or excessive intake of food, but calories and intake of certain food groups (e.g., sweets and fats) are often underestimated. Client may report experimentation with numerous types of diets, repeated dieting efforts ("yo-yo" dieting) with varying results, or may never have attempted a weight-management program.*
- Assess client's knowledge of own body weight and nutritional needs and determine cultural expectations regarding size. *Although nutritional needs are not always understood, being overweight or having large body size may not be viewed negatively by individual because it is considered within relationship to family eating patterns and peer and cultural influences.[2] Ethnicity factors may influence the age of onset and the rapidity of weight gain. African American women and Hispanic women tend to experience weight gain earlier in life than Caucasians and Asians. Hispanic men tend to develop obesity earlier than African American and Caucasian men. Some cultures place importance on large body size (e.g., Samoan people or Cuban children).[3,4] Note: In 2017, a Centers for Disease Control and Prevention (CDC) report noted that in the United States (in most states examined) non-Hispanic black adults, almost half (48.4%) were considered to have obesity and about 12.4% were considered to have extreme obesity. Among Hispanic adults, 42.6% were considered to have obesity, and about 7% were considered to have extreme obesity.[5]*
- Identify familial and cultural influences regarding food. *People of many cultures place high importance on food and food-related events, while some cultures routinely observe fasting days (e.g., Arab, Greek, Irish, Jewish) that may be done for health or religious purposes.[4]*
- Ascertain how client perceives food and the act of eating. *Individual beliefs, values, and types of foods available influence what people eat, avoid, or alter. Client may be eating to satisfy an emotional need rather than physiological hunger, not only because food plays a significant role in socialization but also because food can offer comfort, sense of security, and acceptance.[3,4]*
- Assess dietary practices by means of diary covering 3 to 7 days. *Recall of foods and fluids ingested; times, patterns, and place of eating; whether alone or with other(s); and feelings before, during, and after eating can increase client's understanding of eating behavior and serve as the basis for dietary modifications.[6,7]*
- Identify problems with energy balance. *Studies indicate that few people can accurately estimate the number of calories they should consume in a day for a person their age, height, weight, and physical activity.[8] Note: Eating and physical activity patterns that are focused on consuming fewer calories, making informed food choices, and being physically active can help people attain and maintain a healthy weight, reduce their risk of chronic disease, and promote overall health. Note: For people who are overweight or obese, this will mean consuming fewer calories from both foods and beverages.[9]*
- Review daily activity and regular exercise program *for comparative baseline and to identify areas for modification. Note: The 2008 National Health Interview Survey showed that only 33% of American adults participated in leisure-time physical activity on a regular basis.[9]*
- Obtain anthropometric measurements *to determine presence and severity of obesity:*

  Calculate body mass index (BMI) *to estimate percentage of body fat. Note: The CDC has standardized BMI calculations, removing age and sex differences for adults with obesity being defined as 30 and above. Note: Obesity is also divided into classes. Class 3 obesity is sometimes categorized as "extreme" or "severe" obesity (may replace term morbid obesity) and is defined as BMI equal to or greater than 40.[13] The CDC has recommended that children (over age 2) and adolescents be considered obese if their BMI exceeds the 95th percentile on growth curves or exceeds 30 kg/m at any age. Note: Normal BMI in children changes as age and growth occurs and is also different between the sexes.[14]*

  Refer to ND Overweight for additional diagnostic studies information.
- Collaborate in assessment and interventions for client with disordered eating habits or eating perceptions:

  Obtain a comparative body drawing, having client draw self on wall with chalk and then standing against it and having actual body outline drawn to note difference between the two. *Determines whether client's view of self-body image is congruent with reality.*

  Ascertain occurrence of negative feedback from significant others (SOs). *May reveal control issues and impact motivation for change.*

 Diagnostic Studies   Evidence Based Practice   Medications   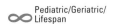 Pediatric/Geriatric/ Lifespan

Identify unhelpful eating behaviors (e.g., eating over sink; "gobbling, nibbling, or grazing") and address kinds of activities associated with eating (e.g., watching television or reading, being unmindful of eating or food) *that result in taking in too many calories as well as eliminating the joy of food because of failure to notice flavors or sensation of fullness or satiety.*[2]

NURSING PRIORITY NO. 2   To establish weight-reduction program:

- **Refer to ND Overweight, Nursing Priority 2 for interventions common to weight-loss programs.**
- Collaborate with nutritionist in addressing/implementing client's specific needs (e.g., what foods to incorporate or limit, how to identify nutrient-dense foods and beverages). *A healthy eating pattern limits intake of sodium, solid fats, added sugars, and refined grains and emphasizes nutrient-dense foods and beverages (e.g., vegetables, fruits, whole grains, fat-free or low-fat milk and milk products), seafood, lean meats and poultry, eggs, beans and peas, and nuts and seeds.*[9]
- Assist client in using technology to manage food choices. *Technology offers applications that can assist in monitoring dietary intake and food choices. Some calculate calories, providing immediate feedback and generating individualized reminders. The best applications include (1) a large database of foods with nutritional information for various serving sizes, (2) a bar scanner that allows users to add information about prepared foods to their database, (3) a calorie tracker that is easy to use, and (4) the ability to track other nutrients (e.g., carbohydrates, protein, calcium).*[6]
- Engage client and family in structured weight loss programs, as indicated. *Approaches to the treatment of severely obese individuals may include lifestyle modifications, physical activity, very controlled diets, and intensive psychiatric interventions, including individual, group, and family therapy.*[2] *Note: DeBar et al. recently reported that an intensive, group therapy approach was superior to standard, family-based therapy in achieving lifestyle changes (e.g., less consumption of fast foods) and in reducing the BMI of overweight adolescents.*[15]
- Refer to bariatric physician/surgeon, as indicated. *Evaluation for special measures may be needed (e.g., supervised fasting or bariatric surgery) for obese persons with comorbidities and for morbidly obese persons with BMI greater than 40. Currently there are several bariatric surgical procedures (e.g., gastric bypass [Roux-en-Y], laparoscopic adjustable gastric banding, biliopancreatic diversion [rare], vertical banded gastroplasty). At present, gastric bypass is the most successful procedure.*[16]

NURSING PRIORITY NO. 3   To promote wellness (Teaching/Discharge Considerations):

- **Refer to ND Overweight for related interventions.**

DOCUMENTATION FOCUS

Assessment/Reassessment
- Individual findings, including current weight, dietary pattern; perceptions of self, food, and eating; motivation for loss, support or feedback from SO(s).
- Results of laboratory and diagnostic testing.

Planning
- Plan of care, specific interventions, and who is involved in planning.
- Teaching plan.

Implementation/Evaluation
- Responses to interventions and actions performed.
- Attainment or progress toward desired outcome(s).
- Modifications to plan of care.

Discharge Planning
- Long-term needs and who is responsible for actions to be taken.
- Specific referrals made.

 Acute Care   Collaborative   Community/Home Care   Cultural

References

1. Rouen, P. A., Wallace, B.R. (2017). The 2015-2020 dietary guidelines: Overview and implications for nursing practice. *Home Healthc Now*, 35(2), 72–82.
2. Schwarz, S. M. (Updated 2017). Obesity in children. Retrieved April 2018 from http://emedicine.medscape.com/article/985333-overview.
3. Caprio, S., et al. (2008). Influence of race, ethnicity, and culture on childhood obesity: Implications for prevention and treatment: A consensus statement of Shaping America's Health and the Obesity Society. *Diabetes Care*, 31(11), 2211–2221.
4. Purnell, L. D., Paulanka, B. J. (1998). *Transcultural Health Care: A Culturally Competent Approach*. Philadelphia: F. A. Davis, 22.
5. National Institutes of Health (NIH); National Institute of Diabetes and Digestive and Kidney Diseases (NIDDK). (2013–2014). Prevalence of overweight and obesity. *Centers for Disease Control and Prevention (CDC)*. Retrieved April 2018 from https://www.niddk.nih.gov/health-information/health-statistics/overweight-obesity.
6. Budd, G. M., Peterson, J. A. (2015). The obesity epidemic, Part 2: Nursing assessment and intervention. *Am J Nurs*, 115(1), 38–46.
7. Fleury, J. (1991). Empowering potential: A theory of wellness motivation. *Nurs Res*, 40(5), 286–291.
8. International Food Information Council. (2012). Consumer attitudes towards food safety, nutrition, & health. *2012 Food & Health Survey*. Retrieved April 2018 from http://www.foodinsight.org/2012_Food_Health_Survey_Consumer_Attitudes_toward_Food_Safety_Nutrition_and_Health.
9. 2010 Dietary Guidelines Advisory Committee. (2010). Dietary guidelines for Americans (various pages). Retrieved April 2018 from http://www.health.gov/dietaryguidelines/dga2010/DietaryGuidelines2010.pdf.
10. Dawodu, S. T., Scott, D. D., Chase, M. (2015). *Nutrition management in the rehabilitation setting (various pages)*. Retrieved March 2018 from https://emedicine.medscape.com/article/318180-overview#a5.
11. Lab test: Insulin. (2014, modified 2018). *Lab Tests Online*. Retrieved April 2018 from http://labtestsonline.org/understanding/analytes/insulin/tab/test/.
12. Perry, B., Wang, Y. (2012). Appetite regulation and weight control: The role of gut hormones. *Nutr Diabetes*, 2(1), e26.
13. Centers for Disease Control and Prevention (CDC). (Updated 2016). About Adult BMI. Retrieved April 2018 from https://www.cdc.gov/obesity/adult/defining.html.
14. Centers for Disease Control and Prevention. (2014, updated 2015). About child and teen BMI. Retrieved April 2018 from http://www.cdc.gov/healthyweight/assessing/bmi/childrens_bmi/about_childrens_bmi.html.
15. DeBarr, L. L., et al. (2012). A primary care-based, multicomponent lifestyle intervention for overweight adolescent females. *Pediatrics*, 129(3), e611–e620.
16. Saber, A., Hale, K. L. (2014, reviewed 2017). Surgery in the treatment of obesity. Retrieved April 2018 from http://www.emedicinehealth.com/surgery_in_the_treatment_of_obesity/page5_em.htm#operative_procedures.

risk for Occupational Injury

Taxonomy II: Safety/Protection—Class 4 Environmental hazards (00265) **[Diagnostic Division:** Safety], Approved 2016

DEFINITION: Susceptible to sustain a work-related accident or illness, which may compromise health

RISK FACTORS

Individual: Excessive stress; psychological distress
Improper use of personal protective equipment
Inadequate role performance, or coping strategies, or time management
Insufficient knowledge; misinterpretation of information
Unsafe acts of overconfidence; unsafe acts of unhealthy negative habits
Environmental: Distraction from social relationships; labor relationships
Exposure to biological agents, or radiation, or teratogenic agents
Exposure to extremes of temperature, or vibration
Inadequate physical environment; lack of personal protective equipment
Night shift work rotating to day shift work; shift workload
Occupational burnout; physical workload

(continues on page 596)

 Diagnostic Studies   Evidence Based Practice   Medications 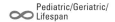 Pediatric/Geriatric/Lifespan

risk for Occupational Injury (continued)

Sample Clinical Applications: Any occupation and/or job setting has the potential for causing/aggravating injury

DESIRED OUTCOMES/EVALUATION CRITERIA

Sample NOC linkages:

Personal Safety Behavior: Personal actions to prevent unintentional physical injury to self

Risk Control: Environmental Hazards: Personal action to understand, prevent, eliminate, or reduce the threat of exposure to biological, chemical, physical, biochemical, or psychological hazards in personal environment

Physical Injury Severity: Severity of signs and symptoms of injuries to the body

Client Will (Include Specific Time Frame)

- Develop/engage in plan to address individual risk factors and safety hazards.
- Demonstrate proper body alignment to prevent injury when performing work-related activities.
- Conform to safety guidelines in the work place.
- Be free of injury.

ACTIONS/INTERVENTIONS

Sample NIC linkages:

Risk Identification: Analysis of potential risk factors, determination of health risks, and prioritization of risk-reduction strategies for an individual or group

Environmental Management: Worker Safety: Monitoring and manipulation of the worksite environment to promote safety and health of workers

NURSING PRIORITY NO. 1 To evaluate degree/source of risk inherent in work setting:

- Determine factors related to individual situation and extent of risk for injury/illness. *Influences scope and intensity of interventions to manage threats to safety, which are dynamic and constants in every life and situation.*[12]
- ∞ ▨ Note client's age, gender, developmental stage, decision-making ability, level of cognition and competence *to determine client's ability to recognize danger and to protect self. Note: Younger workers (14–24) are twice as likely to incur injuries than older workers, and women three times more likely than men, which may reflect client's ability or desire to protect self and influences choice of interventions or teaching.*[3]
- ▨ Ascertain client's history of injuries, medical conditions, and medications—prescribed, over-the-counter, vitamins and herbals. *Can impact client's ability to safely perform certain movements/activities and suggests possible choice of interventions. Note: Research suggests cannabis abuse can increase severity of/time away from work following injury.*[6]
- ▨ Evaluate visual, auditory, tactile, and kinesthetic perception. *Ability to correctly perceive and respond to one's environment greatly impacts worker's safety and well-being. Note: Blue-collar workers, older worker, and Hispanic workers have highest rates of uncorrected visual and/or hearing impairment, creating safety issues.*[7]
- Identify employment/job specifics (e.g., works with dangerous tools/machinery, electricity, explosives, hazardous chemicals, first responder, healthcare worker, computer data entry, works alone or above ground). *Aides in identifying risks and individual safety needs.*

 Acute Care Collaborative Community/Home Care Cultural

- Determine client's perception of individual safety and view of hazards in workplace, including exposure to violence. *Lack of knowledge of safety needs or appreciation of significance of individual hazards increases risk of injury.*[12] *Lack of focus on specific problem(s) can result in no change or may even result in increased injuries.*[4]
- Clarify client's awareness of Occupational Safety and Health Administration (OSHA) standards applicable to client. *Lack of awareness can limit client's ability to make best decisions to promote personal safety.*
- Observe client performing routine work activities. *Musculoskeletal injuries are estimated to account for 33% of all workplace injuries. Proper body mechanics is vital for safe lifting, bending, reaching, stooping, pushing/pulling, repetitive motions, etc. Note: Hospital workers experience injuries nearly three times the rate of professional and business services. Even physical therapists incur musculoskeletal injuries, especially low back, in spite of their knowledge of body mechanics.*[2,8,10]
- Evaluate workplace for environmental hazards and stressors (e.g., physical, biological, psychological, chemical, ergonomic) and their interrelationships. *May impair/negatively impact client's judgment and increase potential for injury. Furthermore, at a time of cost cutting and reorganization to sustain business profits/viability, organizational culture may deflect responsibility of occupational injuries onto the worker without adequately considering all factors contributing to the situation.*[5]

NURSING PRIORITY NO. 2   To assist client to reduce/correct individual risk factors:

- Review pertinent job-related safety regulations with client. *Provides information necessary for client to make informed decisions.*
- Develop plan with client to address individual needs and goals. *Being part of the solution increases likelihood of client commitment to the plan.*
- Identify facility/company resources available to decrease risk factors. *Solutions may be available at limited or no additional cost.*
- Modify work space as appropriate. *For example, for office worker consider ergonomic chair, elevated computer desk, head set/Bluetooth device, voice recognition computer program; industrial site might require better lighting, handrails on stairs, reflective paint marking floor step downs, containment barrier around chemical storage/mixing station, healthcare worker may need ceiling-mounted lifts to facilitate patient transfers, redesign of workstations with adjustable-height computer monitors.*[8]
- Instruct in safety techniques/procedures specific to client's situation, for example:[8,9]
  Wear appropriate protective gear—clothing/gowns, safety glasses/goggles, ear protectors, closed-toe/steel-toe footwear, gloves, mask/respirator, safety harness, helmet
  Avoid operating mechanical equipment/vehicle when using substances, including over-the-counter and prescription, that may impair functioning
  Adequate hydration/cooling in hot environments
  Use proper body mechanics, frequent change of work position
  Practice safe handling of sharps, double gloving during needlesticks, precautions with flammable materials, including oxygen
  Proper handling of biologic materials/body fluids, chemical spills
  Avoid mixing chemicals if possible; use in well-ventilated area
  Practice situational awareness or being aware of what is happening around self and recognizing unsafe situations
- Encourage client to read chemical labels or Material Safety Data Sheets (MSDS notebook) *to be aware of primary hazards, safe storage and handling.*
- Identify location of eye wash station/shower, first-aid kit and safe use of automated external defibrillator (AED).

NURSING PRIORITY NO. 3   To promote optimum safety and well-being:

- Stress importance of adherence to lunch/break policy and using vacation or personal time regularly. *Too often workers feel compelled to work through break time or postpone time away because of short staffing or to meet deadlines.*

 Diagnostic Studies   Evidence Based Practice   Medications   Pediatric/Geriatric/ Lifespan

- Refer to trainer or physical therapist for regular exercise program including focus on core strength/stability and flexibility. *Research suggests decreased core strength contributes to injuries of back and extremities.*[1]
- Encourage participation in wellness programs/monitoring of chronic conditions. *Stress management, weight loss, smoking cessation, and monitoring of long-term health issues such as hypertension and diabetes can help reduce illness and time away from work.*
- Recommend keeping vaccinations up to date and obtaining yearly flu shots and immunizations recommended for occupational risks. *Reduces risk of acquiring illness in workplace.*[8]
- Support modified or light-duty work options as indicated. *Provides time for recovery while keeping worker engaged and reducing sense of isolation.*
- Emphasize importance of reporting injuries/completing reports in timely manner. *While it is not unusual for minor injuries to go unreported, violence in the workplace is often accepted as "part of the job" and not reported but can cause significant psychological trauma and stress. Note: Workplace violence incidents requiring days off for worker to recuperate were four times more common in healthcare than in private industry.*[8,11]
- Obtain preventive screening/testing and initiate referrals to healthcare providers as appropriate. *Some chronic illnesses such as respiratory, some cancers, birth defects have long latencies between occupational exposure and clinical findings.*[7]

NURSING PRIORITY NO. 4 To promote safety in workplace:

- Identify applicable OSHA standards and workplace compliance with standards.
- Provide OSHA poster, copies of standards, and informational placards *to inform workers of their rights and responsibilities under OSHA.*
- Inform workers of hazardous substances to which they may be exposed.
- Use problem-solving framework such as Public Health Model *to systematically identify and prioritize problems or risks, identify interventions or develop new strategies to prevent injury/illness, implement activities, and evaluate and monitor results of interventions.*[4]
- Bring unsafe working conditions to employer's attention.
- Develop corrective plan with all parties involved. *Effectiveness of program requires commitment of management and participation of employees to analyze safety data and identify appropriate solutions.*[11]
- Initiate workplace health promotion programs based on identified health risk assessment (e.g., smoking cessation, weight loss, stress management).
- Provide incentives for meeting individual/group goals. *Rewards/bonuses for health and safety behaviors or number of injury-free days encourages continuation of efforts.*[8]
- Repair, replace, or correct unsafe equipment. Provide adaptive devices, e.g., step stool, handrails on moveable stairs, safety guard/shield on mechanical equipment.
- Provide protective devices such as locked external doors, gates at stairwells, emergency alarms/phone stations, metal detectors, trained security personnel.
- Initiate screening programs for environmental hazards, e.g., noise, pollutants, allergens, dust, asbestos, lead/other heavy metals, vapor intrusion, radon, diesel emissions.
- Collaborate with appropriate agencies, e.g., public health, Environmental Protection Agency, to improve environmental hazards.
- Develop plan for long-term monitoring of health risks and evaluation of risk-reduction strategies. *Provides evidence of effectiveness of interventions, possible need for revision. Information also adds to the body of knowledge in the field.*[4,10]

DOCUMENTATION FOCUS

Assessment/Reassessment
- Medical history including past injuries, current medications; sensory abilities.
- Client's awareness of safety needs, view of individual hazards in workplace.

 Acute Care   Collaborative   Community/Home Care   Cultural

- Specific requirements of client's job.
- Evaluation of workplace environmental hazards and stressors.

Planning
- Plan of care and who is involved in the planning including outside/public partners.
- Teaching plan.

Implementation/Evaluation
- Responses to interventions, teaching, and actions performed.
- Attainment or progress toward desired outcomes.
- Modifications to plan of care.

Discharge Planning
- Long-term needs and who is responsible for actions to be taken.
- Available resources, specific referrals made.

References

1. Peate, W. F., et al. (2007). Core strength: A new model for injury prediction and prevention. *J Occup Med Toxicol*, 2(3). Retrieved April 2018 from https://occup-med.biomedcentral.com/articles/10.1186/1745-6673-2-3.
2. Holder, N. L., et al. (1999). Cause, prevalence, and response to occupational musculoskeletal injuries reported by physical therapists and physical therapist assistants. *Phys Ther*, 79(7), 642–652.
3. Parish, M., et al. (2016). Factors associated with occupational injuries in seasonal young workers. *Occup Med*, 66(2), 164–167.
4. Stout, N. A., Linn, H. I. (2002). Occupational injury prevention research: Progress and priorities. *Inj Prev*, 8(4), iv9–iv14.
5. Woolford, M. H., et al. (2017). Missed opportunities to prevent workplace injuries and fatalities. *New Solutions: J Environ Occup Health Policy*, 7(1). Retrieved May 2018 from http://journals.sagepub.com/doi/full/10.1177/1048291117693389.
6. Khashaba, E., et al. (2017). Risk factors for non-fatal occupational injuries among construction workers: A case–control study. *Toxicol Ind Health*, 34(2), 83–89.
7. Utterback, D. F., et al. (2012). Occupational injuries, illnesses, and fatalities among workers in the services sector industries: 2003 to 2007. *J Occup Environ Med*, 54(1), 31–41.
8. Harolds, L., Hurst, H. (2016). Preventing workplace injuries among perinatal nurses. *Nurs Womens Health*, 20(1), 99–108.
9. Nelson, R. (2017). Nurses poorly protected from "second-hand exposure" to chemo. *Medscape Nurses*. Retrieved March 2018 https://www.medscape.com/viewarticle/879449.
10. No author (2013). Caring for our caregivers–Facts about hospital worker safety. *OSHA*. May 2018 from https://www.osha.gov/dsg/hospitals/documents/1.2_Factbook_508.pdf.
11. No author. (2015). Workplace violence in healthcare–Understanding the challenge. *OSHA*. May 2018 from https://www.osha.gov/dsg/hospitals/documents/1.2_Factbook_508.pdf.
12. Ebright, P. R., Patterson, E. S., Render, M. L. (2002). The "New Look" approach to patient safety: A guide for clinical specialist leadership. *Clin Nurs Spec*, 16(5), 247–253.

Overweight

Taxonomy II: Nutrition—Class 1 Ingestion (00233) [**Diagnostic Division:** Food/Fluid], Approved 2013; Revised 2017

DEFINITION: A condition in which an individual accumulates abnormal or excessive fat for age and gender.

RELATED FACTORS
Average daily physical activity is less than recommended for gender and age; energy expenditure below energy intake based on standard assessment (e.g., WAVE [weight, activity, variety in diet, excess] assessment); sedentary behavior occurring for ≥2 hours/day
Consumption of sugar-sweetened beverages; frequent snacking; high frequency of restaurant or fried food; portion sizes larger than recommended; solid foods as major food source at <5 months of age
Disordered eating behaviors or perceptions; fear regarding lack of food supply

(continues on page 600)

 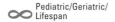

Overweight (continued)

Excessive alcohol consumption
Shortened sleep time, sleep disorder

DEFINING CHARACTERISTICS

Objective

ADULT: Body mass index (BMI) of >25 kg/m^2
CHILD <2 years: Weight-for-length >95th percentile
CHILD: 2–18 years: Body mass index (BMI) >85th percentile or >25 kg/m^2 for age and gender
At Risk Population: ADULT: Body mass index (BMI) approaching 25 kg/m^2
CHILD <2 years: Weight-for-length approaching 95th percentile
CHILD 2–18 years: Body mass index (BMI) approaching 85th percentile or 25 kg/m^2
Children with high body mass index (BMI), or who are crossing body mass index (BMI) percentiles upward
Economically disadvantaged
Formula- or mixed-fed infants; overweight in infancy; rapid weight gain during infancy, including the first week, first 4 months, and first year; rapid weight gain during childhood
Premature pubarche
Heritability of interrelated factors; high disinhibition and restraint eating behavior score
Maternal diabetes mellitus, maternal smoking; paternal obesity
Associated Conditions: Genetic disorder
Sample Clinical Applications: Bulimia nervosa, morbid obesity, diseases requiring long-term steroid use (e.g., chronic obstructive pulmonary disease [COPD]), conditions associated with immobility (e.g., stroke/paralysis, multiple sclerosis [MS], amputation), depression, developmental delay

DESIRED OUTCOMES/EVALUATION CRITERIA

Sample NOC linkages:

Weight Loss Behavior: Personal actions to lose weight through diet, exercise, and behavior modification
Knowledge: Healthy Diet: Extent of understanding conveyed about a balanced, nutritious diet
Nutritional Status: Extent to which nutrients are ingested and absorbed to meet metabolic needs
Weight: Body Mass: Extent to which body weight, muscle, and fat are congruent to height, frame, gender, and age

Client Will (Include Specific Time Frame)

- Verbalize a realistic self-concept or body image (congruent mental and physical picture of self).
- Participate in development of, and commit to, a personal weight-loss program.
- Demonstrate appropriate changes in lifestyle and behaviors, including eating patterns, food quantity/quality, and exercise program.
- Attain desirable body weight with optimal maintenance of health.

ACTIONS/INTERVENTIONS

Sample NIC linkages:

Weight Reduction Assistance: Facilitating loss of weight and/or body fat
Nutrition Management: Providing and promoting a balanced intake of nutrients
Nutritional Counseling: Use of an interactive process focusing on the need for diet modification

 Acute Care   Collaborative   Community/Home Care   Cultural

NURSING PRIORITY NO. 1 To identify contributing factors/health status:

- ∞ 📝 Obtain weight history, noting if client has weight gain out of character for self or family, is or was obese child, or used to be much more physically active than is now *to identify trends. Note: Unchecked weight gain can lead to obesity, which is now the most prevalent nutritional disorder among children and adolescents in the United States (45% of all adults and approximately 18% of youths ages 2 to 19 years).*[18] *Being overweight during older childhood is highly predictive of adult obesity, especially if a parent is also obese.*[1]

- Assess risk and presence of factors or conditions associated with obesity (e.g., familial pattern of obesity; decreased basal metabolic rate or hypothyroidism; type 2 diabetes; reproductive dysfunction; menopause; chronic disorders, such as heart disease, kidney disease, chronic pain; food or other substance addictions; stressful or sedentary lifestyle; depression; use of certain medications such as steroids, birth control pills; physical disabilities or limitations; lack of socioeconomic resources for obtaining or preparing healthy foods) *to determine treatments and interventions that may be indicated in addition to weight management.*[1,3]

- 🌐 Assess client's knowledge of own body weight and nutritional needs and determine cultural expectations regarding size. *Although nutritional needs are not always understood, being overweight or having large body size may not be viewed negatively by individual because it is considered within relationship to family eating patterns and peer and cultural influences.*[1] *Ethnicity factors may influence the age of onset and the rapidity of weight gain. African American women and Hispanic women tend to experience weight gain earlier in life than Caucasians and Asians. Hispanic men tend to develop obesity earlier than African American and Caucasian men. Some cultures place importance on large body size (e.g., Samoan people or Cuban children).*[2,3]

- 🌐 Identify familial and cultural influences regarding food. *People of many cultures place high importance on food and food-related events, while some cultures routinely observe fasting days (e.g., Arab, Greek, Irish, Jewish) that may be done for health or religious purposes.*[2]

- Ascertain how client perceives food and the act of eating. *Individual beliefs, values, and types of foods available influence what people eat, avoid, or alter. Client may be eating to satisfy an emotional need rather than physiological hunger, not only because food plays a significant role in socialization but also because food can offer comfort, sense of security, and acceptance.*[2,3]

- 💊 Evaluate client's routine medications. *Some medications can contribute to weight gain (e.g., cortisol and other glucocorticoids; sulfonylureas, tricyclic antidepressants, monoamine oxidase inhibitors; oral contraceptives; insulin [in excessive doses]; risperidone).*[6]

- 📝 Assess dietary practices by means of diary covering 3 to 7 days. *Recall of foods and fluids ingested; times, patterns, and place of eating; whether alone or with other(s); and feelings before, during, and after eating can increase client's understanding of eating behavior and serve as the basis for dietary modifications. Note: Few people can accurately estimate the number of calories they should consume in a day for a person their age, height, weight, and physical activity.*[4,7,19]

- Ascertain previous dieting history. *Client may report normal or excessive intake of food, but calories and intake of certain food groups (e.g., sweets and fats) are often underestimated. Client may report experimentation with numerous types of diets, repeated dieting efforts ("yo-yo" dieting) with varying results, or may never have attempted a weight-management program.*

- 🔄 Collaborate in assessment and interventions for client with disordered eating habits or eating perceptions: Obtain a comparative body drawing, having client draw self on wall with chalk and then standing against it and having actual body outline drawn to note difference between the two. *Determines whether client's view of self-body image is congruent with reality.*
  Ascertain occurrence of negative feedback from significant others (SOs). *May reveal control issues and impact motivation for change.*[1]

- 📝 Review daily activity and regular exercise program *for comparative baseline and to identify areas for modification. Note: The 2008 National Health Interview Survey showed that only 33% of American adults participated in leisure-time physical activity on a regular basis.*[8]

- ✏️ Review laboratory test results (e.g., complete blood count with differential, full lipid panel, fasting glucose, A_1C, insulin levels; thyroid, leptins; proteins, Mini-Nutritional Assessment) *that may reveal medical*

 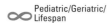

conditions associated with obesity and identify problems that may be treated with alterations in diet or medications.[5,10,20]

NURSING PRIORITY NO. 2 To determine weight-loss goals:

• Obtain anthropometric measurements *to determine presence and severity of obesity:* Calculate body mass index (BMI) *to estimate percentage of body fat. Note: The Centers for Disease Control and Prevention (CDC) has standardized BMI calculations, removing age and sex differences for adults, with overweight being defined as 25 to 29.9 kg/m²*[16,21] *The CDC has recommended that children (over age 2) and adolescents be considered overweight if the BMI exceeds the 85th percentile (and is less than the 95th percentile) on growth curves or exceeds 25 kg/m² at any age. Note: Normal BMI in children changes as age and growth occurs and is also different between the sexes.*[22]

Determine waist circumference (WC), if indicated. *Some studies support that WC is more closely linked to cardiovascular risk factors than BMI alone because a high WC can occur in persons with normal or near normal BMIs. These sources indicate high risk if WC is greater than 35 inches (for women) and greater than 40 inches (for men), even if BMI is greater than 25 but is accompanied by family history of cardiovascular disease or diabetes or exists in conjunction with two or more chronic health conditions.*[9]

Evaluate body fat, body water, and muscle mass via scale skin caliper measurements and scale weight (*direct* measurement), bioelectric impedance analysis, dual-energy x-ray absorptiometry, and hydrostatic weighing (*indirect* measurement) per facility protocol. *Note: The CDC does not recommend these methods of measuring body weight (over BMI) because "they are not always readily available, and they are either expensive or need highly trained personnel. Furthermore, many of these methods can be difficult to standardize across observers or machines, complicating comparisons across studies and time periods."*[9,21]

• Determine client's motivation for weight loss (e.g., for own satisfaction or self-esteem, to improve health status, to gain approval from another person). *Client is more likely to succeed and maintain desired weight when change is for self (e.g., acceptance of self "as is," general well-being) rather than to please others.*

• Discuss myths client/SO may have about weight and weight loss *to address misconceptions and possibly enhance motivation for needed behavior changes.*

NURSING PRIORITY NO. 3 To establish weight-reduction program:

• Obtain commitment or contract for weight loss. *Verbal agreement to goals or written contract formalizes the plan and may enhance efforts and maximize outcomes.*

• Involve SO(s) in treatment plan as much as possible *to provide ongoing support and increase likelihood of success.*

• Set realistic goals (short and long term) for weight loss. *Reasonable weight loss (1 to 2 lb/wk) has been shown to have more lasting effects than rapid weight loss, although sustaining motivation for small losses often makes it difficult for client to stick with a program. Note: A loss of 5% to 10% of total body weight can reduce many of the health risks associated with obesity in adults.*[1,12,13]

• Collaborate with physician and nutritionist *to develop and implement comprehensive weight-loss program that includes food, activity, behavior alteration, and support.*

• Calculate calorie requirements based on physical factors and activity. *While many weight-reduction programs focus on portion size and food components (e.g., low-fat, high-protein, low-glycemic foods), reducing calorie intake is essential for weight loss. Note: Decreasing calories by 500/day or expending 500 calories/day through exercise results in a weight loss of about 1 lb/wk.*[6]

• Provide information regarding specific nutritional needs. *Individual may be deficient in needed nutrients (e.g., proteins, vitamins, or minerals) or may eat too much of one food group (e.g., fats or carbohydrates) and not enough of another food group (e.g., vegetables).*[11,12] *Note: A recent CDC report revealed that between 2007 and 2010, children did not meet recommendations for the amount of fruit and vegetables they should eat, although fruit intake did increase, with fresh fruit replacing juices.*[23]

 Acute Care   Collaborative   Community/ Home Care   Cultural

- Discuss modifications to achieve healthy body weight:[8,12–16,19]

     Eat from each food group (fruits, vegetables, whole grains, lean meats, low-fat dairy, oils).

    Start with small changes, such as adding one more vegetable per day or introducing healthier versions of favorite foods.

    Choose "nutrient-dense" forms of foods that provide substantial amounts of fiber, vitamins, electrolytes, and minerals.

    Avoid saturated fats, trans fats, cholesterol, salt (sodium), and added sugars.

    Focus on portion sizes: calorie-dense foods (high in fat and/or sugar) should be eaten in smaller quantities, whereas high-fiber foods can be eaten in larger quantities.

    Discuss smart snacks (e.g., low-fat yogurt with fruit, nuts, apple slices with peanut butter, low-fat string cheese).

    Emphasize need for adequate fluid intake and taking fluids between meals rather than with meals to provide fluid while leaving more room for food intake at meals *to assist in digestive process and to quench thirst, which is often mistakenly identified as hunger.*
- Encourage involvement in planned activity program of client's choice and within physical abilities. Refer to formal exercise program, if desired. *Moderately increased physical activity for 30 to 45 min for 5 days/wk can expend an additional 1,500 to 2,000 calories/wk, supporting both loss of pounds and maintenance of lower weight.*[12,14] *Children should participate in vigorous physical activity throughout adolescence and limit time spent watching television and playing computer games to facilitate weight control.*[1]
- Recommend weighing only once/week, at the same time and wearing the same clothes, and graph it on chart. Measure and monitor body fat when possible *to track progress while focusing more on the idea of being health conscious and responsible than what scale may reveal.*
- Provide positive reinforcement and encouragement for efforts as well as actual weight loss. *Enhances commitment to program and enhances person's sense of self-worth.*
- Refer to bariatric physician/surgeon when indicated. *Evaluation for special measures may be needed (e.g., supervised fasting or bariatric surgery) for morbidly obese persons with BMI greater than 40.* Refer to ND Obesity for related interventions.

NURSING PRIORITY NO. 4 To promote wellness (Teaching/Discharge Considerations):

- Assist in and encourage periodic evaluation of nutritional status and alteration of dietary plan. *May be desired or needed for addressing special needs (e.g., diabetes mellitus, age considerations, very low calorie or fasting) and monitoring health status.*[17]
- Emphasize importance of avoiding fad diets *that may be harmful to health and often do not produce long-term positive results.*
- Identify and encourage finding ways to reduce tension when eating. *Promotes relaxation to permit focus on act of eating and awareness of satiety.*
- Identify unhelpful eating behaviors (e.g., eating over sink; "gobbling, nibbling, or grazing") and address kinds of activities associated with eating (e.g., watching television or reading, being unmindful of eating or food) *that result in taking in too many calories as well as eliminating the joy of food because of failure to notice flavors or sensation of fullness or satiety.*
- Review and discuss strategies to deal appropriately with stressful events *to avoid overeating as a means of coping.*
- Discuss importance of an occasional treat by planning for inclusion in diet *to avoid feelings of deprivation arising from self-denial.*
- Advise planning for special occasions (birthday or holidays) by reducing intake before event and/or eating "smart" *to redistribute or reduce calories and allow for participation in food events.*
- Discuss normalcy of ups and downs of weight loss: plateau, set point (at which weight is not being lost), hormonal influences, etc. *Prevents discouragement when progress stalls.*
- Encourage buying personal items and clothing *as reward for weight loss or other accomplishments.* Suggest disposing of "fat clothes" *to encourage positive attitude of permanent change and remove "safety valve" of having wardrobe available "just in case" weight is regained.*

- 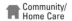 Review prescribed drug regimen (e.g., appetite suppressants, hormone therapy, vitamin and mineral supplements) *for benefits or adverse side effects and drug interactions.*
- Recommend reading labels of nonprescription diet aids if used. *Herbals containing diuretics or ma huang (product similar to ephedrine) may cause adverse side effects in vulnerable persons.*
- Encourage parents and school dieticians to model and offer good nutritional choices (e.g., offer vegetables, fruits, and lower-fat foods in daily meals and snacks) *to assist child in accepting healthy eating styles. Note: Studies have shown a high correlation between parents and children regarding patterns of food intake and food choices. Conversely, adult intake of fat has been shown to be higher when children under 17 are in the home (more pizza, cheese, processed food, junk food, and fast food).*[1,15]
- Refer to community support groups or psychotherapy, as indicated, *to provide role models and address issues of body image or self-worth.*
- Provide contact number for dietitian/nutritionist and/or audiovisual materials, bibliography, and reliable Internet sites for resources *to address ongoing nutrition needs and dietary changes.*
- Refer to NDs disturbed Body Image, ineffective Coping, and Obesity for additional interventions, as appropriate.

DOCUMENTATION FOCUS

Assessment/Reassessment
- Individual findings, including current weight, dietary pattern; perceptions of self, food, and eating; motivation for loss, support or feedback from SO(s).
- Results of laboratory and diagnostic testing.
- Results of interval weigh-ins.

Planning
- Plan of care, specific interventions, and who is involved in planning.
- Teaching plan.

Implementation/Evaluation
- Responses to interventions, weekly weight, and actions performed.
- Attainment or progress toward desired outcome(s).
- Modifications to plan of care.

Discharge Planning
- Long-term needs and who is responsible for actions to be taken.
- Specific referrals made.

References

1. Schwarz, S. M. (Updated 2017). *Obesity in children.* Retrieved April 2018 from http://emedicine.medscape.com/article/985333-overview.
2. Purnell, L. D., Paulanka, B. J. (1998). *Transcultural Health Care: A Culturally Competent Approach.* Philadelphia: F. A. Davis.
3. Caprio, S., et al. (2008). Influence of race, ethnicity, and culture on childhood obesity: Implications for prevention and treatment: A consensus statement of Shaping America's Health and the Obesity Society. *Diabetes Care,* 31(11), 2211–2221.
4. Fleury, J. (1991). Empowering potential: A theory of wellness motivation. *Nurs Res,* 40, 286–291.
5. Dawodu, S. T., Scott, D. D., Chase, M. (2015). *Nutrition management in the rehabilitation setting (various pages).* Retrieved April 2018 from https://emedicine.medscape.com/article/318180-overview#a5.
6. Galletta, G. M. (2014, reviewed 2017). *Obesity.* Retrieved April 2018 from http://www.emedicinehealth.com/obesity/page9_em.htm#surgery_for_obesity.
7. Lutz, C. A., Przytulski, K. R. (2010). *Nutrition and Diet Therapy.* 5th ed. Philadelphia: F. A. Davis.
8. U.S. Department of Health and Human Services, Department of Agriculture. The Dietary Guidelines for Americans 2010 (various parts). Retrieved April 2018 from http://www.health.gov/dietaryguidelines/dga2010/DietaryGuidelines2010.pdf.
9. Zhu, S., Wang, Z., Heska, S. (2002). Waist circumference and obesity-associated risk factors among whites in the third National Health and Nutrition Examination Survey: Clinical action thresholds. *Am J Clin Nutr,* 75(4), 743–749.
10. Lab test: Insulin. (2014, modified 2018). *Lab Tests Online.* Retrieved April 2018 from http://labtestsonline.org/understanding/analytes/insulin/tab/test/.

 Acute Care   Collaborative   Community/Home Care   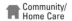 Cultural

11. Rippe, J. M., Hess, S. (1998). The role of physical activity in the prevention and management of obesity. *J Am Diet Assoc*, 10(2 Suppl), S31–S38.

12. Fruh, S. M. (2017). Obesity: Risk factors, complications, and strategies for sustainable long-term weight management. *J Am Assoc Nurse Pract*, 29(1 Suppl), S3–S14.

13. Wing, R., Phelan, S. (2005). Long-term weight loss maintenance. *Am J Clin Nutr*, 82(1 Suppl), 222S–225S.

14. Meadows, M. (2008). *Nutrition: Healthy eating*. Retrieved April 2018 from http://www.medicinenet.com/script/main/art .asp?articlekey=61982.

15. Laroche, H. H., Hofer, T. P., Davis, M. M. (2007). Adult fat intake associated with the presence of children in households: Findings from NHANES III. *J Am Board Fam Med*, 20(1), 9–15.

16. Hamdy, O., Uwaifo, G. I., Oral, E. A. (2012, updated 2018). Obesity. Retrieved April 2018 from http://emedicine.medscape .com/article/123702-overview.

17. Flegal, K. M., et al. (2001). Prevalence of overweight in U.S. children: Comparison of U.S. growth charts from the Centers for Disease Control and Prevention with other reference values for body mass index. *Am J Clin Nutr*, 73(6), 1086–1093.

18. Rouen, P. A., Wallace, B. R. (2017). The 2015-2020 dietary guidelines: Overview and implications for nursing practice. *Home Healthc Now*, 35(2), 72–82.

19. Budd, G. M., Peterson, J. A. (2015). The obesity epidemic, Part 2: Nursing assessment and intervention. *Am J Nurs*, 115(1), 38–46.

20. Perry, B., Wang, Y. (2012). Appetite regulation and weight control: The role of gut hormones. *Nutr Diabetes*, 2(1), e26.

21. Centers for Disease Control and Prevention (CDC). (Updated 2016). About BMI for adults. Retrieved April 2018 from https://www.cdc.gov/obesity/adult/defining.html.

22. Centers for Disease Control and Prevention (CDC). (2014, updated 2015). About child and teen BMI. Retrieved April 2018 from http://www.cdc.gov/healthyweight/assessing/bmi/ childrens_bmi/about_childrens_bmi.html.

23. Centers for Disease Control and Prevention (CDC). (2014). Progress on children eating more fruit, not vegetables. *CDC Vital Signs*. Retrieved April 2018 from http://www.cdc.gov/ vitalsigns/pdf/2014-08-vitalsigns.pdf.

risk for Overweight

Taxonomy II: Nutrition—Class 1 Ingestion (00234) [**Diagnostic Division:** Food/Fluid], Approved 2013; Revised 2017

DEFINITION: Susceptible abnormal or excessive fat accumulation for age and gender, which may compromise health.

RISK FACTORS

Average daily physical activity is less than recommended for gender and age; energy expenditure below energy intake based on standard assessment (e.g., WAVE [weight, activity, variety in diet, excess] assessment); sedentary behavior occurring for ≥2 hours/day

Consumption of sugar-sweetened beverages; frequent snacking; high frequency of restaurant or fried food; portion sizes larger than recommended; solid foods as major food source a <5 months of age

Disordered eating behaviors or perceptions; fear regarding lack of food supply

Excessive alcohol consumption

Shortened sleep time, sleep disorder

At Risk Population: ADULT: Body mass index (BMI) approaching 25 kg/m^2

CHILD <2 years: Weight-for-length approaching 95th percentile

CHILD 2–18 years: Body mass index (BMI) approaching 85th percentile or 25 kg/m^2

Children with high body mass index (BMI), or who are crossing body mass index (BMI) percentiles upward

Economically disadvantaged

Formula- or mixed-fed infants; overweight in infancy; rapid weight gain during infancy, including the first week, first 4 months, and first year; rapid weight gain during childhood

Premature pubarche

Heritability of interrelated factors; high disinhibition and restraint eating behavior score

Maternal diabetes mellitus, maternal smoking; paternal obesity

(continues on page 606)

 Diagnostic Studies   Evidence Based Practice   Medications   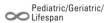 Pediatric/Geriatric/ Lifespan

risk for Overweight (continued)

Associated Condition: Genetic disorder

Sample Clinical Applications: Bulimia nervosa, diseases requiring long-term steroid use (e.g., chronic obstructive pulmonary disease [COPD]), conditions associated with immobility (e.g., stroke, paralysis, multiple sclerosis [MS], amputation), Alzheimer's disease, depression, developmental delay

DESIRED OUTCOMES/EVALUATION CRITERIA

Sample NOC **linkages:**

Weight Maintenance Behavior: Personal actions to maintain optimum body weight
Knowledge: Healthy Diet: Extent of understanding conveyed about a balanced, nutritious diet
Nutritional Status: Nutrient Intake: Nutrient intake to meet metabolic needs

Client/Caregiver Will (Include Specific Time Frame)
- Verbalize understanding of body and energy needs.
- Identify lifestyle and cultural factors that predispose to obesity.
- Demonstrate behaviors and lifestyle changes to reduce risk factors.
- Acknowledge responsibility for own actions and need to "act, not react" to stressful situations.

Sample NOC **linkages:**

Weight: Body Mass: Extent to which body weight, muscle, and fat are congruent to height, frame, gender, and age

Client Will (Include Specific Time Frame)
- Maintain weight at a satisfactory level for height, body build, age, and gender.

ACTIONS/INTERVENTIONS

Sample NIC **linkages:**

Weight Management: Facilitating maintenance of optimal body weight and percent body fat
Nutritional Counseling: Use of an interactive helping process focusing on the need for diet modification
Nutrition Management: Providing and promoting a balanced intake of nutrients

NURSING PRIORITY NO. 1   To assess potential factors for undesired weight gain:

- Note presence of factors or conditions that can contribute to weight gain or obesity (e.g., familial pattern of obesity; hypothyroidism; type 2 diabetes; pregnancy; menopause; chronic disorders [e.g., heart, kidney disease, chronic pain]; food, alcohol/other substance addictions; stressful and/or sedentary lifestyle; depression; use of certain medications [e.g., steroids, birth control pills, antipsychotics]; physical disabilities or limitations; lack of socioeconomic resources for obtaining or preparing healthy foods) *to determine treatment needs and possible behavioral changes for weight management.*[1]
- ∞ ⧄ Note client's particular situation and number/seriousness of risk factors *to help determine level of concern. For example, a high correlation exists between obesity in parents and children, which may reflect (in part) family patterns of food intake, exercise, selection of leisure activity (e.g., amount of television watching), family and cultural patterns of food selection. Also, family studies (e.g., twin and adoption) suggest genetic factors.*[2,3]
- ⊕ ⧄ Evaluate familial and cultural influences *that often place high importance on food and food-related events, groups that place importance on large body size, or frame of reference for "normal body weight"*

 Acute Care   Collaborative   Community/ Home Care   Cultural

higher than standard indicators (e.g., athletes such as football players or wrestlers; African American women, Samoan people, Cuban children).[2–4]

- Note client's age and activity level and exercise patterns *to identify areas where changes might be useful to prevent obesity and promote health. For example, older adults need same nutrients as younger adults but in smaller amounts and with attention to certain components, such as calcium, fiber, vitamins, protein, and water.*[5] *Infants/children require small meals and constant attention to needed nutrients for proper growth and development while dealing with child's food preferences and eating habits.*[6]

- Calculate growth percentiles in infants/children using growth chart specific to child's age and gender or BMI-for-age calculator if child is greater than 2 years old *to identify deviations from the norm.*[2,7]

- Review laboratory test results (e.g., complete blood count with differential, full lipid panel, fasting glucose, A₁C, insulin levels; thyroid, leptins; proteins, Mini-Nutritional Assessment) *that may reveal medical conditions associated with obesity and identify problems that may be treated with alterations in diet or medications.*[8–10]

- Assess eating patterns in relation to risk for obesity and disease conditions. *Food choices and amounts of certain food groups are known to impact health (in both children and adults) and cause or exacerbate disease conditions (e.g., heart disease, diabetes, hypertension, gallstones, colon cancer).*[1,11]

- Determine patterns of hunger and satiety. *Eating patterns often differ in those who are predisposed to weight gain and may include such factors as skipping meals (decreases the metabolic rate), fasting and binging (causes wide fluctuations in glucose and insulin), and eating or overeating in response to emotions (e.g., loneliness, anger, happiness).*

- Note history of dieting and kinds of diets used. *Client may have tried multiple diets with varying degrees of success in the past, but often has history of regaining weight ("yo-yo" dieting) or finding that diets are not desirable.*

- Determine whether binging or purging (bulimia) is a factor *to identify potential for eating disorder requiring in-depth intervention.*

- Identify personality characteristics (e.g., rigid thinking patterns, external locus of control, negative body image or self-concept, negative monologues [self-talk], dissatisfaction with life) *that are often associated with obesity and can impact choice and/or success of interventions.*

- Determine psychological significance of food to the client (e.g., derives love and comfort from food, uses food to escape deep unhappiness, eats when stressed or anxious).

- Listen to concerns and assess motivation to prevent weight gain. *If client's concerns regarding weight control are motivated for reasons other than personal well-being (e.g., partner's expectations or demands), the likelihood of success is decreased.*

NURSING PRIORITY NO. 2   To assist client to develop preventive program to avoid weight gain:

- Assess client's knowledge of nutritional needs and ways client is meeting these needs. *Provides baseline for further teaching and/or interventions.*

- Provide information, as indicated, on nutrition, taking into account client's age and developmental stage (e.g., toddler, teenager, pregnant woman, elderly person with chronic disease), physical health and activity tolerance, financial and socioeconomic factors, and client's/significant other's (SO's) potential for management of risk factors.

- Review and encourage client/caregiver to implement guidelines for achieving and maintaining healthy body weight:[2,12]

  Eat from each food group (fruits, vegetables, whole grains, lean meats, low-fat dairy, oils).

  Start with small changes, such as adding one more vegetable/day or introducing healthier versions of favorite foods.

  Choose "nutrient-dense" forms of foods that provide substantial amounts of fiber, vitamins, electrolytes, and minerals.

  Avoid saturated fats, trans fats, cholesterol, salt (sodium), and added sugars.

 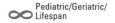

Focus on portion sizes: calorie-dense foods (high in fat and/or sugar) should be eaten in smaller quantities, whereas high-fiber foods can be eaten in larger quantities.

Discuss smart snacks (e.g., low-fat yogurt with fruit, nuts, apple slices with peanut butter, low-fat string cheese).

Review healthy eating patterns or habits (e.g., eating slowly and only when hungry, stopping when full, avoiding skipping meals, eating foods from every food group, using smaller plates, chewing food thoroughly, making healthy food choices even when eating fast food).

Encourage involvement in planned exercises of client's choice and within physical abilities. Refer to formal exercise program, if desired.

NURSING PRIORITY NO. 3   To promote wellness (Teaching/Discharge Considerations):

- Provide information about individual risk factors *to enhance decision making and support motivation.*
- Consult with nutritionist *to address client-specific issues (e.g., how to use food groups, how to read food labels and apply to self, how to help child avoid junk food, dietary restrictions that might be needed for certain chronic diseases such as kidney disease or diabetes).*
- Provide information to new mothers about nutrition for developing babies *to reduce potential for childhood obesity related to lack of knowledge.*
- Encourage parents and school dietitians to model and offer good nutritional choices (e.g., offer vegetables, fruits, and lower-fat foods in daily meals and snacks) *to assist child in accepting healthy food styles.*[2,12]
- Encourage the client to make a commitment to lead an active life, to manage food habits, and to develop a system for self-monitoring *to provide a sense of control and assist with making choices.*
- Provide bibliography including reliable Internet sites for resources *to reinforce learning, address ongoing nutrition needs, support informed decision making.*
- Refer to support groups and appropriate community resources for such things as food-buying assistance, cooking and food safety courses, and behavior modification as indicated. *Provides role models and assistance for making lifestyle changes.*

DOCUMENTATION FOCUS

Assessment/Reassessment
- Findings related to individual situation, risk factors, current caloric intake and dietary pattern; activity level.
- Baseline height and weight, growth percentile.
- Results of laboratory tests.
- Motivation to reduce risks or prevent weight problems.

Planning
- Plan of care and who is involved in the planning.
- Teaching plan.

Implementation/Evaluation
- Response to interventions, teaching, and actions performed.
- Attainment or progress toward desired outcome(s).
- Modifications to plan of care.

Discharge Planning
- Long-term needs, noting who is responsible for actions to be taken.
- Specific referrals made.

 Acute Care   Collaborative   Community/Home Care   Cultural

References

1. Galletta, G. M. (2014, reviewed 2017). *Obesity*. Retrieved April 2018 from http://www.emedicinehealth.com/obesity/page9_em.htm#surgery_for_obesity.

2. Schwarz, S. M. (2012, updated 2017). *Obesity in children*. Retrieved April 2018 from http://emedicine.medscape.com/article/985333-overview.

3. Purnell, L. D., Paulanka, B. J. (1998). *Transcultural Health Care: A Culturally Competent Approach*. Philadelphia: F. A. Davis.

4. Caprio, S., et al. (2008). Influence of race, ethnicity, and culture on childhood obesity: Implications for prevention and treatment: A consensus statement of Shaping America's Health and the Obesity Society. *Diabetes Care*, 31(11), 2211–2221.

5. American Dietetic Association. (2005). Nutrition across the spectrum of aging. *J Am Diet Assoc*, 105(4), 616s–633s.

6. Engel, J. (2006). *Mosby's Pocket Guide to Pediatric Assessment*. 5th ed. St. Louis, MO: Mosby.

7. Centers for Disease Control and Prevention (CDC). (2014, updated 2015). About child and teen BMI. Retrieved April 2018 from http://www.cdc.gov/healthyweight/assessing/bmi/childrens_bmi/about_childrens_bmi.html.

8. Dawodu, S. T., Scott, D. D., Chase, M. (2015). *Nutrition management in the rehabilitation setting (various pages)*. Retrieved April 2018 from https://emedicine.medscape.com/article/318180-overview#a5.

9. Lab test: Insulin. (2014, modified 2018). *Lab Tests Online*. Retrieved April 2018 from http://labtestsonline.org/understanding/analytes/insulin/tab/test/.

10. Perry, B., Wang, Y. (2012). Appetite regulation and weight control: The role of gut hormones. *Nutr Diabetes*, 2(1), e26.

11. Laroche, H. H., Hofer, T. P., Davis, M. M. (2007). Adult fat intake associated with the presence of children in households: Findings from NHANES IIIs. *J Am Board Fam Med*, 20(1), 9–15.

12. 2010 U.S. Department of Health and Human Services, Department of Agriculture. The Dietary Guidelines for Americans. (2010). Various parts. Retrieved April 2018 from http://www.health.gov/dietaryguidelines/dga2010/DietaryGuidelines2010.pdf.

---

acute Pain

Taxonomy II: Comfort—Class 1 Physical Comfort (00132) [**Diagnostic Division:** Pain/Discomfort], Approved 1986; Revised 2013

DEFINITION: Unpleasant sensory and emotional experience associated with actual or potential tissue damage or described in terms of such damage (International Association for the Study of Pain); sudden or slow onset of any intensity, from mild to severe, and with a duration of less than 3 months.

RELATED FACTORS

Biological injury agent [e.g., infection, ischemia, neoplasm]
Chemical injury agent
Physical injury agent [e.g., trauma, amputation, operative procedure, burn, heavy lifting, overtraining]

DEFINING CHARACTERISTICS

Subjective

Appetite change; hopelessness
Self-report of intensity using standardized pain scale [e.g., Wong-Baker FACES scale, visual analogue scale, numeric rating scale]
Self-report of pain characteristics using standardized pain instrument [e.g., McGill Pain Questionnaire, Brief Pain Inventory]
Proxy report of pain behavior/activity changes [e.g., family member, caregiver]

Objective

Change in physiological parameter [e.g., blood pressure, heart rate, respiratory rate, oxygen saturation]
Diaphoresis
Distraction behavior; expressive behavior

(continues on page 610)

 Diagnostic Studies   Evidence Based Practice   Medications   Pediatric/Geriatric/Lifespan

acute Pain (continued)

Evidence of pain using standardized pain behavior checklist for those unable to communicate verbally [e.g., Neonatal Infant Pain Scale, Pain Assessment Checklist for Seniors with Limited Ability to Communicate]

Facial expression of pain; pupil dilation

Guarding behavior; protective behavior; positioning to ease pain

Self-focused; narrowed focus

Sample Clinical Applications: Traumatic injuries, surgical procedures, infections, cancer, burns, skin lesions, gangrene, thrombophlebitis, pulmonary embolus, neuralgia

DESIRED OUTCOMES/EVALUATION CRITERIA

Sample NOC linkages:

Pain Level: Severity of observed or reported pain

Pain Control: Personal actions to eliminate or reduce pain

Pain: Adverse Psychological Response: Severity of observed or reported adverse cognitive and emotional responses to physical pain

Client Will (Include Specific Time Frame)

• Report pain is relieved or controlled.

• Follow prescribed pharmacological regimen.

• Verbalize methods that provide relief.

• Demonstrate use of relaxation skills and diversional activities as indicated for individual situation.

• Verbalize sense of control of response to acute situation and positive outlook for the future.

ACTIONS/INTERVENTIONS

Sample NIC linkages:

Pain Management: Acute Alleviation or reduction of pain to a level that is acceptable to the patient in the immediate healing period following tissue damage from an identifiable cause such as trauma, surgery, or injury

Analgesic Administration: Use of pharmacological agents to reduce or eliminate pain

Environmental Management: Comfort: Manipulation of the patient's surroundings for promotion of optimal comfort

NURSING PRIORITY NO. 1   To assess etiology/precipitating contributory factors:

• Note possible pathophysiological and psychological causes of pain (e.g., inflammation, tissue trauma, burns, fractures, surgery; infections, heart attack, angina; abdominal conditions [e.g., appendicitis, cholecystitis], grief, fear, anxiety, depression, personality disorders). *Acute pain is that which follows an injury, trauma, or procedure such as surgery or occurs suddenly with the onset of a painful condition (e.g., herniated disk, migraine headache, pancreatitis).*[4,11]

• Assess for potential types of pain that may be affecting client, i.e., nociceptive pain or neuropathic pain. *Can aid in understanding reason for severity of pain associated with client's condition and point toward needed interventions for pain management. Note: **Nociceptive** pain results from actual tissue damage or potentially tissue-damaging stimuli. Subsets of nociceptive pain include **somatic** (typically localized and usually stemming from muscle, joint, bone, or connective tissue) and **visceral** (caused from damage to thoracic, pelvic, or abdominal viscera [organs], with localized pain occurring from some obstruction, distension or ischemia).*

 Acute Care   Collaborative   Community/Home Care   Cultural

Neuropathic pain is a complex pain syndrome caused by a variety of problems with nerves or the processing of nerve impulses. Neuropathic pain can become chronic after a gradual onset, such as with diabetic neuropathy, or have an acute onset related to direct nerve injury, such as might occur with severe trauma, surgery, or certain types of cancer and chemotherapy.[4,9,11]

- ∞ 📝 Note client's age, developmental level, and current condition (e.g., infant/child; critically ill; ventilated, sedated, or cognitively impaired client) *affecting ability to report pain parameters or response to pain and pain management interventions.*[3,4,9,10,13–15]

- Determine history or presence of chronic conditions (e.g., multiple sclerosis, stroke, diabetes, depression) *that may also be associated with acute and chronic pain simultaneously, be associated with an exacerbation of pain symptoms, or interfere with accurate assessment of acute pain.*[3]

- 📝 Note anatomical location of surgical incisions or procedures. *This can influence the amount of postoperative pain experienced; for example, vertical or diagonal incisions are more painful than transverse or S-shaped. Presence of known and unknown complication(s) may make the pain more severe than anticipated.*[2,3,5]

- 🌐 Assess client's perceptions of pain, along with behaviors and cultural expectations regarding pain. *Client's perception of and expression of pain is influenced by age, developmental stage, underlying problem causing pain, cognitive, and behavioral and sociocultural factors.*[6]

- 💊 Note client's attitude toward pain and use of specific pain medications, including any history of substance abuse. *Client may have beliefs restricting use of medications, may have a high tolerance for drugs because of recent or current use, or may not be able to take pain medications at all if participating in a substance abuse recovery program.*

- Note client's locus of control (internal or external). *Individuals with external locus of control may take little or no responsibility for pain management.*

- 💊 Determine medications (e.g., skeletal muscle relaxants, antibiotics, antidepressants, anticoagulants), alcohol or other drugs currently being used, and any medication allergies *that may affect choice of analgesics.*[2,3]

- 👥 Collaborate with medical providers in pain assessment, including neurological and psychological factors (pain inventory, psychological interview) as appropriate when pain persists.

- ✒️ Assist with and review results of laboratory tests and diagnostic studies depending on results of history and physical examination.

NURSING PRIORITY NO. 2   To evaluate client's response to pain:

- 📝 Obtain client's/significant other's (SO's) assessment of pain to include location, characteristics, onset, duration, frequency, quality, and intensity. Identify precipitating or aggravating and relieving factors *in order to fully understand client's pain symptoms. Note: Experts agree that attempts should always be made to obtain self-reports of pain. When that is not possible, credible information can be received from another person who knows the client well (e.g., parent, spouse, caregiver).*[14] *Numerous studies have revealed that physicians and nurses need to be aware of their tendency to underestimate client's pain in early postoperative days.*[16]

- 📝 Perform pain assessment each time pain occurs. Document and investigate changes from previous reports and evaluate results of pain interventions *to demonstrate improvement in status or to identify worsening of underlying condition/developing complications.*[4,5,12]

- ∞ 📝 Accept client's description of pain. Be aware of the terminology client uses for pain experience (e.g., young child may say "owie" or "hurt"; elderly may say "it aches so bad"). *Pain is a subjective experience and cannot be felt by others.*[3,13] *Note: Some elderly clients experience a reduction in perception of pain or have difficulty localizing or describing pain, and pain may be manifested as a change in behavior (e.g., restlessness, loss of appetite, increased confusion or wandering, acting out, change in functional abilities).*[15]

- 🌐 Note cultural influences affecting pain response. *Verbal or behavioral cues may have no direct relationship to the degree of pain perceived (e.g., client may deny pain even when feeling uncomfortable, reactions can be stoic or exaggerated, reflecting cultural and familial norms). These factors affect client's and caregiver's attitudes and beliefs regarding the pain experience, expressions of pain, and expectations regarding pain management.*[6,10]

 Diagnostic Studies   Evidence Based Practice   Medications   Pediatric/Geriatric/Lifespan

- Observe nonverbal cues (e.g., how client walks, holds body, guarding behaviors; sleeplessness; grimacing facial expressions; distraction behaviors, narrowed focus; crying, poor feeding, lethargy in infants). Ask others who know client well (e.g., spouse, parent) to identify behaviors that may indicate pain in persons who cannot communicate verbally. *Helpful in recognizing presence of pain; however, cues not congruent with verbal reports indicate need for further evaluation.*[1-4,6]
- Assess for referred pain, as appropriate, *to help determine possibility of underlying condition or organ dysfunction causing pain to be perceived in area other than site of the problem.*[9]
- Monitor vital signs during episodes of pain. *Blood pressure, respiratory and heart rate are usually altered in acute pain.*[1-3]
- Ascertain client's knowledge of and expectations about pain management. *Provides baseline for interventions and teaching, provides opportunity to allay common fears and misconceptions (e.g., fears about addiction to opiates, belief that complete pain relief is possible in every situation) or to address expected side effects of analgesics (e.g., constipation).*
- Review client's previous experiences with pain and methods found either helpful or unhelpful for pain control in the past. *Useful in determining appropriate interventions.*
- Be aware of client's "Right to Treatment" *that includes prevention of or adequate relief from pain*[5] *and that failure to meet the standard of assessing for pain can be considered negligence. This means that the nurse is obligated to do everything within his/her professional capacity to relieve the pain when the client requests pain relief. Furthermore, professional standards require that nurses assess pain and reassess pain even when the client has not made a specific request.*[17]

NURSING PRIORITY NO. 3   To assist client to explore methods for alleviation/control of pain:

- Determine client's acceptable level of pain and pain control goal. *Client may not be 100% pain free but may feel that a "3" is a manageable level of discomfort, while another may require medication for pain at the same level because the experience is subjective.*[1-4,6]
- Determine factors in client's lifestyle (e.g., alcohol or other drug use or abuse) that can affect responses to analgesics and/or choice of interventions for pain management.[10]
- Note when pain occurs (e.g., only with ambulation, every night) *to medicate prophylactically as appropriate.*
- Collaborate in treatment of underlying condition or disease processes causing pain and proactive management of pain (e.g., epidural analgesia, nerve blockade for postoperative pain, surgical plication of a nerve, implantation of nerve stimulator).
- Work with client *to prevent rather than "chase" pain.* Use flow sheet to document pain, therapeutic interventions, response, and length of time before pain recurs. Instruct client to report pain as soon as it begins, *because timely intervention is more likely to be successful in alleviating pain.*[7]
- Encourage verbalization of feelings about the pain such as concern about tolerating pain, anxiety, and pessimistic thoughts *to evaluate coping abilities and to identify areas of additional concern.*[1,7]
- Review procedures and expectations and inform client when treatments will hurt. Discuss pain management methods that will be used *to reduce concerns of the unknown and muscle tension associated with anxiety or fear.*
- ∞ Use puppets or dolls for explanations and teaching, when indicated, *to demonstrate procedures for child and enhance understanding to reduce level of anxiety or fear.*
- Provide or promote nonpharmacological pain management, such as:
  a quiet environment and calm activities;
  comfort measures (e.g., back rub, change of position, use of heat or cold compresses);
  use of relaxation exercises (e.g., focused breathing, visualization, guided imagery);
  diversional or distraction activities, such as television and radio, socialization with others, and commercial or individualized tapes (e.g., "white" noise, music, instructional);

 Acute Care   Collaborative   Community/ Home Care   Cultural

∞ presence of parent during painful procedures *to comfort child;*

identification of ways to avoid or minimize pain *(e.g., splinting incision during cough, keeping body in good alignment and using proper body mechanics, and resting between activities can reduce occurrence of muscle tension or spasms or undue stress on incision).*

- Establish collaborative approach for pain management based on client's understanding about and acceptance of available treatment options. *Pharmacological management is based on client's symptomatology and mechanism of pain as well as tolerance for pain and for the various analgesics. Multimodal pain management may include pills, liquids, or suckers to take by mouth, skin patch, or suppository forms and injections, IV dosing, or patient-controlled analgesia (PCA), or regional analgesia (e.g., epidural and spinal blocking).*[3,7,9,10,12]

- Administer analgesics to maximal dosage as needed *to maintain "acceptable" level of comfort. The type of medication(s) ordered depends on the type and severity of pain (e.g., acetaminophen and NSAIDs are commonly used to treat mild to moderate pain, while opiates [e.g., morphine, oxycodone, fentanyl] are used to treat moderate to severe pain). Note: Various combinations of medications may be used at prescribed intervals.*[3,8]

- Notify physician/healthcare provider if regimen is inadequate to meet pain control goal. Assist client to prevent (rather than treat pain) and alter drug regimen based on individual needs. *Once established, pain is more difficult to suppress. Increasing dosage, changing medication, or using a stepped program (e.g., switching from injection to oral route, or lengthening time interval between doses) helps in self-management of pain.*[2,5]

- Evaluate and document client's response to analgesics and assist in transitioning or altering drug regimen based on individual needs and planned interventions *to limit adverse effects, reduce risk of drug dependence, and deal with barriers to adequate use of analgesics.*

- Evaluate for adverse medication effects (e.g., decrease in mental acuity, change in thought processes, confusion or delirium, urinary retention, severe nausea, vomiting, pruritus). *Intolerable symptoms that usually require change of medication(s).*[3,7,8]

- Demonstrate and monitor use of self-administration/PCA that involves client in plan *to administer own IV pain medication or bolus additional dose when on continual basis drip.*[3,7,8]

- Provide information and monitor use of site-specific medications (e.g., spinal, epidural, regional anesthesia) *that might be used for certain procedures such as back surgery, amputation, or labor and delivery.*[2,7,8]

- Instruct client in use of transcutaneous electrical stimulation unit when ordered.

NURSING PRIORITY NO. 4 To promote wellness (Teaching/Discharge Considerations):

- Acknowledge the pain experience and convey acceptance of client's response to pain. *Reduces defensive responses, promotes trust, and enhances cooperation with regimen.*
- Encourage adequate rest periods *to prevent fatigue that can impair ability to manage or cope with pain.*
- Review nonpharmacological measures for lessening pain. *Relaxation skills and techniques such as self-hypnosis, biofeedback, and therapeutic touch have no detrimental side effects.*
- Provide information and discuss pain management before planned procedures. *The primary concern of most clients/families is pain and discomfort following surgery or invasive procedure.*
- Encourage performance of individualized physical therapy/exercise program. *Promotes active role in preventing muscle spasms or contractures and enhances sense of control.*
- Discuss ways SO(s) can assist client with pain management. *Family members/SOs may provide assistance by transporting client to prevent walking long distances or by taking on client's strenuous chores, supporting timely pain control, encouraging eating nutritious meals to enhance wellness, and providing gentle massage to reduce muscle tension.*
- Identify specific signs/symptoms and changes in pain requiring evaluation by healthcare provider.

 Diagnostic Studies   Evidence Based Practice   Medications 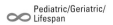 Pediatric/Geriatric/Lifespan

DOCUMENTATION FOCUS

Assessment/Reassessment
- Individual assessment findings, including client's description of response to pain, specifics of pain inventory, expectations of pain management, and acceptable level of pain.
- Locus of control and cultural beliefs affecting response to pain.
- Prior medication use; substance abuse.

Planning
- Plan of care and who is involved in planning.
- Teaching plan.

Implementation/Evaluation
- Response to interventions, teaching, and actions performed.
- Attainment or progress toward desired outcome(s).
- Modifications to plan of care.

Discharge Planning
- Long-term needs, noting who is responsible for actions to be taken.
- Specific referrals made.

References

1. Engel, J. (2006). *Mosby's Pocket Guide to Pediatric Assessment.* 5th ed. St. Louis, MO: Mosby.
2. Chou, R., Gordon, D. B., de Leon-Casasola, O. A. (2016). Guidelines on the management of postoperative pain: A Clinical Practice Guideline From the American Pain Society, the American Society of Regional Anesthesia and Pain Medicine, and the American Society of Anesthesiologists' Committee on Regional Anesthesia, Executive Committee, and Administrative Council. *J Pain,* 17(2), 131–157.
3. Ameres, M. J., Yeh, B. (Reviewed 2017). Pain after surgery. Retrieved April 2018 from http://www.emedicinehealth.com/pain_after_surgery/page2_em.htm.
4. Schroeder, D. L., et al. (2016). Enhancing nurses' pain assessment to improve patient satisfaction. *Orthop Nurs,* 35(2), 108–117.
5. U.S. Department of Health and Human Services. (2006). Clinical Practice Guideline for acute pain management: Operative or medical procedures and trauma. Honolulu, HI: University Press of the Pacific.
6. Narayan, M. C. (2010). Culture's effects on pain assessment and management. *Am J Nurs,* 110(4), 38–48.
7. Institute for Clinical Systems Improvement (ICSI). (Revised 2018). Low back pain: Adult acute and subacute. Retrieved April 2018 from https://www.icsi.org/guidelines__more/catalog_guidelines_and_more/catalog_guidelines/catalog_musculoskeletal_guidelines/low_back_pain/.
8. Cluett, J. (Updated 2018). Types of pain medicine. Retrieved April 2018 from http://orthopedics.about.com/od/medicati3/p/medications.htm.
9. Kiser-Larson, N. (2017). The experience of intense pain: Nursing management and interventions. *J Christ Nurs,* 34(2), 88–96.
10. Mann, A. R. (2006). Manage the power of pain. *Men in Nursing,* 1(4), 20–28.
11. D'Arcy, Y. (2007). Managing pain in a patient who's drug-dependent. *Nursing,* 37(3), 36–40.
12. Wheeler, M. S. (2006). Pain assessment and management in the patient with mild to moderate cognitive impairment. *Home Healthc Nurse,* 24(6), 354–359.
13. Hartjes, T. M., Meece, L., Horgas, A. L. (2016). Assessing and managing pain, agitation, and delirium in hospitalized older adults. *Am J Nurs,* 116(10), 38–46.
14. Herr, K., et al. (2006). Pain assessment in the nonverbal patient: Position statement with clinical practice recommendations. *Pain Manag Nurs,* 7(2), 44–52.
15. Kamel, H. K., et al. (2001). Utilizing pain assessment scales increases the frequency of diagnosing pain among elderly nursing home residents. *J Pain Symptom Manage,* 21(6), 450–455.
16. Rosenberger, P. H., et al. (2001). Shared decision making, preoperative expectations, and postoperative reality: Differences in physician and patient predictions and ratings of knee surgery outcomes. *Arthroscopy,* 21(5), 562–569.
17. O'Malley, P. (2005). The undertreatment of pain: Ethical and legal implications for the clinical nurse specialist. *Clin Nurs Spec,* 19(5), 236–237.

 Acute Care
 Collaborative
 Community/Home Care
 Cultural

chronic Pain and chronic Pain Syndrome [CPS]

Taxonomy II: Comfort—Class 1 Physical Comfort (00133) [Diagnostic Division: Pain/Discomfort], Approved 1986; Revised 1996, 2013, 2017

DEFINITION: chronic Pain: Unpleasant sensory and emotional experience arising from actual or potential tissue damage or described in terms of such damage (International Association for the Study of Pain); sudden or slow onset of any intensity, from mild to severe, constant or recurring without an anticipated or predictable end and a duration of greater than three (>3) months.

Taxonomy II: Comfort—Class 1 Physical Comfort (0000255) [Diagnostic Division: Pain/Discomfort], Approved 2013

DEFINITION: chronic Pain Syndrome: Recurrent or persistent pain that has lasted at least three months, and that significantly affects daily functioning or well-being.
[Author Note: Pain is a signal that something is wrong. Chronic pain may be recurrent and periodically disabling (e.g., migraine headaches, kidney stones, prostatitis) or may be unremitting. It is a complex entity, combining elements from many other NDs, such as risk for Disuse Syndrome; decreased Diversional Activity Engagement; disturbed Body Image; compromised family Coping; interrupted Family Processes; Powerlessness; Self-Care deficit (specify); sexual Dysfunction; Social Isolation]. The nurse is encouraged to refer to other NDs as indicated.

RELATED FACTORS (CHRONIC PAIN)
Alteration in sleep pattern
Emotional distress; fatigue; whole-body vibration
Nerve compression; prolonged computer use; repeated handling of heavy loads
Increase in body mass index; malnutrition
Ineffective sexuality pattern; social isolation
Injury agent

DEFINING CHARACTERISTICS

Subjective (chronic Pain)
Self-report of intensity using standardized pain scale [e.g., Wong-Baker FACES scale, visual analogue scale, numeric rating scale]
Self-report of pain characteristics using standardized pain instrument [e.g., McGill Pain Questionnaire, Brief Pain Inventory]
Alteration in ability to continue previous activities
Alteration in sleep pattern; anorexia
Proxy report of pain behavior/activity changes [e.g., family member, caregiver]
[Preoccupation with pain]

Subjective (chronic Pain Syndrome)
Anxiety, fear; stress overload
Constipation
Disturbed sleep pattern, fatigue; insomnia

Objective (chronic Pain)
Evidence of pain using standardized pain behavior checklist for those unable to communicate verbally [e.g., Neonatal Infant Pain Scale, Pain Assessment Checklist for Seniors with Limited Ability to Communicate]
Facial expression of pain; self-focused

(continues on page 616)

Diagnostic Studies   Evidence Based Practice   Medications   Pediatric/Geriatric/Lifespan

chronic Pain and chronic Pain Syndrome [CPS] (continued)

Objective (chronic Pain Syndrome)
Deficient knowledge
Impaired mood regulation; social isolation
Impaired physical mobility
Obesity
At Risk Population (Chronic Pain): Age >50 years; female gender
History of abuse; history of genital mutilation
History of over indebtedness; history of substance misuse/[abuse]
History of static work postures; history of vigorous exercise
Associated Condition (Chronic Pain): Chronic musculoskeletal condition; muscle injury; tumor infiltration
Contusion, crush injury; fracture; spinal cord injury
Genetic disorder; imbalance of neurotransmitters, neuromodulators, and receptors;
Immune disorder; impaired metabolic functioning; ischemic condition; prolonged increase in cortisol level
Post-trauma related condition
Sample Clinical Applications: Traumatic injuries, migraines, repetitive motion injury (carpal or cubital tunnel syndrome), osteoarthritis, rheumatoid arthritis; peripheral neuropathies in diabetes or AIDS, cancer, burns, endometriosis, neuralgia, gangrene

DESIRED OUTCOMES/EVALUATION CRITERIA

Sample NOC linkages:
Pain Control: Personal actions to eliminate or reduce pain
Pain: Disruptive Effects: Severity of observed or reported disruptive effects of chronic pain on daily functioning
Pain: Adverse Psychological Response: Severity of observed or reported adverse cognitive and emotional responses to physical pain

Client Will (Include Specific Time Frame)
• Verbalize and demonstrate (nonverbal cues) relief or control of pain or discomfort.
• Verbalize recognition of interpersonal and family dynamics, and reactions that affect the pain problem.
• Demonstrate or initiate behavioral modifications of lifestyle and appropriate use of therapeutic interventions.
• Verbalize increased sense of control and enhanced enjoyment of life.

Sample NOC linkage:
• **Family Coping:** Capacity of the family to manage stressors that tax family resources

Family/SO(s) Will (Include Specific Time Frame)
• Cooperate in pain management and rehabilitation programs. (Refer to ND readiness for enhanced family Coping.)

ACTIONS/INTERVENTIONS

Sample NIC linkages:
Pain Management: Chronic Alleviation or reduction of persistent pain that continues beyond the normal healing period, assumed to be three months, to a level that is acceptable to the patient

 Acute Care
 Collaborative
 Community/Home Care
 Cultural

Medication Management: Facilitation of safe and effective use of prescription and over-the-counter drugs

Relaxation Therapy: Use of techniques to encourage and elicit relaxation for the purpose of decreasing undesirable signs and symptoms such as pain, muscle tension, or anxiety

NURSING PRIORITY NO. 1 To assess etiology/precipitating factors:

- Identify contributing physical factors where known. *These factors associated with chronic pain and CPS appear to include (1) musculoskeletal disorders such as osteoarthritis, rheumatoid arthritis, and fibromyalgia; (2) back pain from various causes such as disc herniation, vertebral fractures, muscular strains/sprains, overuse syndromes such as tendonitis, and bursitis, as well as pelvic disorders; (3) neurological disorders, such as spinal/other conditions causing nerve impingement, and radiculopathies and neuropathies with direct or referred pain; (4) urological disorders such as bladder neoplasms, chronic urinary tract infections or stones, testicular torsion, prostatitis; (5) gastrointestinal disorders such as colitis, gastroesophageal reflux, inflammatory bowel disease, and pancreatitis; (6) reproductive/gynecological disorders including endometriosis, disorders of ovaries, prolapse, intrauterine contraceptive devices, etc.; and (7) miscellaneous/other causes including trauma (including childhood physical and sexual abuse), cardiovascular disease, peripheral vascular disease, and complications of medical treatments such as chemotherapy, radiation, or surgery.*[2,8]

- Evaluate for presence of/suspected psychological disorders. *Psychological factors may include (but are not limited to) depression, anxiety, somatization, posttraumatic stress disorders, substance abuse, compulsive sexual behaviors, eating disorders, and bipolar personality disorders. Testing may be indicated if organic cause of pain cannot be found, when psychological factors are known to exist, or when pain problems are prolonged and/or life-limiting.*[12]

- Assist in and/or review diagnostic testing, including physical (e.g., selected tests for identifying and/or monitoring suspected for known disease states; urine or blood toxicology for drug detoxification or therapy; imaging studies), neurological, and psychological evaluations (e.g., Minnesota Multiphasic Personality Inventory, pain inventory, psychological interview). *Note: While additional diagnostic studies may be indicated when advanced treatment of the client with CPS is initiated, care should be exercised in avoiding duplication of tests. This prevents unnecessary costs, as well as inadvertent reinforcement of client's psychological need for "something to be physically wrong."*[2]

- Evaluate emotional/psychological components of individual situation. *Individuals with certain psychological syndromes (e.g., major depression, somatization disorder, hypochondriasis) are prone to develop CPS. Note: The Institute for Chronic Pain reports that "it is a common and consistent finding in the research that, as a group, people with chronic pain tend to report much higher rates of having experienced trauma in their past, when compared to people without chronic pain. Thus the high rate of past trauma (e.g., combat, domestic violence, sexual assault, childhood neglect and physical/sexual abuse, terrorism) in people with chronic pain suggests a relationship to the development of chronic pain."*[2,6,12,16]

- Determine if client has history of physical or sexual abuse as a child. *A review of the literature shows that abuse in childhood is a strong predictor of depression and physical complaints, both expanded and unexplained, in adulthood.*[13,16]

- Evaluate client's pattern of coping and locus of control (internal or external). *Passive and avoidant behavioral patterns or lack of active engagement in self-management activities can contribute to diminished activity and perpetuation of chronic pain. Individuals with external locus of control may take little or no responsibility for pain management.*[13]

- Determine relevant cultural and spirituality factors affecting pain response. *Pain is accepted and expressed in different ways (e.g., moaning aloud or enduring in stoic silence); some may magnify symptoms to convince others of reality of pain or believe that suffering in silence helps atone for past wrongdoing.*[3] *A person with chronic pain who identifies himself or herself as a spiritual being may report the link to divine help as empowering him/her to use strategies for healing.*[14,15]

 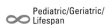

- ∞ 📝 Note gender and age of client. *There may be differences between women and men as to how they perceive and/or respond to pain. Pain in children, ethnic minorities, or cognitively impaired persons is often underestimated and undertreated. Recent studies are revealing large numbers of pediatric clients with chronic pain issues affecting academic attendance and function.[11] While the prevalence of chronically painful conditions (e.g., arthritis) and illnesses (e.g., cancers) is common in the elderly, they may be reluctant to report pain.[4,7]*
- 💊 Evaluate current and past analgesic or narcotic drug use and nonprescription drug use (including alcohol). *Provides clues to options to try or avoid and identifies need for changes in medication regimen, as well as possible need for detoxification program.*

NURSING PRIORITY NO. 2 To determine client response to chronic pain situation:

- 📝 Evaluate pain behavior, noting past and current pain experience, using pain rating scale or diary, and including functional effects and psychological factors. *Pain behaviors can include the same ones present in acute pain (e.g., crying, grimacing, withdrawal, narrowed focus), but may also include other behaviors (e.g., dramatization of complaints, depression, drug misuse). Pain complaints may be exaggerated because of client's perception that pain reports are not believed or because client believes caregivers are discounting reports of pain.[12]*
- 🅐 📝 Provide comprehensive assessment of pain problem, noting its duration, who has been consulted, and what therapies (including alternative/complementary) have been used. *The pathophysiology of chronic pain is multifactorial. If the condition causing the persistent pain is physiological and noncurable (e.g., terminal cancer), all diagnostics and treatments may have been exhausted and pain management becomes the primary goal. If medical treatments are ongoing for painful conditions (e.g., spinal stenosis, pancreatitis, endometriosis, arthritis), consultations with specialists may be helpful in finding curative or palliative treatments. If pain is present without a clear etiology or continues unabated, complex rehabilitation techniques may be required, incorporating physical, occupational, psychological, and recreational therapies.[1,2,12]*
- 📝 Note lifestyle effects of pain. *Major effects of chronic pain on the client's life can include depressed mood, fatigue, weight loss or gain, sleep disturbances, reduced activity and libido, excessive use of drugs and alcohol, dependent behavior, and disability seemingly out of proportion to impairment.[2,4,12]*
- 📝 Assess degree of personal maladjustment of the client such as isolationism, anger, irritability, loss of work time or employment, and school absenteeism. *Chronic pain reduces client's coping abilities and psychological well-being, often resulting in problems with relationships and life functioning.[11,12]*
- 📝 Determine issues of secondary gain for the client/significant others (SOs), such as financial or insurance compensation pending, legal or marital or family concerns, and school or work issues, *which may be present if there is marked discrepancy between claimed distress and objective findings or there is a lack of cooperation during evaluation and in complying with prescribed treatment.[5]*
- Note codependent components and enabling behaviors of caregivers/family members *that support continuation of the status quo and may interfere with progress in pain management or resolution of situation.*
- Note availability and use of personal and community resources. *Client/SO may need many things (e.g., equipment, financial resources, vocational training, respite services, placement in rehabilitation facility) in order to manage painful conditions and/or concerns or difficulties associated with condition.*
- 🏠 Make home visit when indicated, observing such factors as client's safety, equipment, adequate lighting, or family interactions, *to note impact of home environment on the client and to determine changes that might be useful in improving client's life (e.g., grab bars in bathrooms and hallways, wider doors, ramps, assistance with activities of daily living, housekeeping, yard work).*
- Acknowledge and assess pain matter-of-factly, avoiding undue expressions of concern, as well as expressions of disbelief about client's suffering. *Conveying an attitude of empathic understanding of client's disabling distress can have a beneficial impact on client's perception of health.*

NURSING PRIORITY NO. 3 To assist client to deal with pain:

- 🅐 Encourage participation in multidisciplinary pain management plan. *Comprehensive team may include physical medicine specialist; physical, occupational, recreational, and vocational therapists; and emotional or*

 Acute Care   Collaborative   Community/ Home Care   Cultural

behavioral therapists to address complex issues of unresolved pain issues, to set goals for pain relief, and to develop an individualized treatment and evaluation plan. Treatments could involve extended-relief oral pain medications or dermal patches, nerve-blocking injections or an implanted pump, and massage and other hands-on therapies, as well as counseling and home exercise programs.[8]

- Discuss pain management goals and review client expectations versus reality *because it may be that while pain cannot be completely resolved, it can be significantly reduced or managed to the degree that client can participate in desired or needed life activities, thus improving quality of life.*[8]
- Discuss the physiological dynamics of tension and anxiety and how this affects pain.
- Administer or encourage client use of analgesics, as indicated. *Medications may be available in pills, liquids, or suckers to take by mouth, and in injection, skin patch, and suppository forms. Different medications or combinations of drugs may be used such as opioids/narcotics, nonopioids, and adjuvant medications (e.g., muscle relaxants, anticonvulsants, antidepressants, serotonin and norepinephrine reuptake inhibitors) to manage persistent pain so that client may find relief and increase level of function.*[2,8,12] *Note: Studies support that people with intense pain can take very high doses of opioids without experiencing side effects. "Some people with intense pain receive such high doses that the same dose would be fatal if taken by someone who was not suffering from pain. In chronic pain that same high dose can control pain and still allow the person to be wide awake enough to do his or her activities of daily living."*[1]
- Provide consistent and sufficient medication for pain relief, tailored to the individual, especially in those who tend to be undermedicated (e.g., elderly, cognitively impaired, person with lifelong pain, those with terminal cancer). *Medications may need to be scheduled around the clock (not just administered "as needed"), doses titrated either up or down, and dose maximized to optimize pain relief while managing side effects.*[7]
- Recommend or employ nonpharmacological interventions, methods of pain control (e.g., heat or cold applications, progressive muscle relaxation, biofeedback, deep breathing, meditation, visualization or guided imagery, posture correction and muscle strengthening exercises, water therapy, electrical stimulation, massage, acupuncture, Therapeutic Touch) *to obtain comfort, improve healing, and decrease dependency on analgesics.*[9]
- Address medication misuse with client/SO and refer for appropriate counseling or interventions *when addiction is known or suspected to be interfering with client's well-being. Most people (if they don't already have a substance [drug or alcohol] abuse problem) don't become addicted to pain medications even when used on a long-term basis. These individuals will take the pain medications in order to go about the business of their lives. Addicts may misrepresent their pain levels and their activities in order to obtain pain medications or progressively higher doses of medications, and they require specialized evaluation and interventions.*[1,2,5]
- Assist family in developing a program of coping strategies (e.g., staying active even when modified activities are required, living a healthy lifestyle). *Positive reinforcement and encouraging client to use own control can aid in focusing energies on more productive activities.*[10]
- Encourage limiting attention to pain behaviors when appropriate (e.g., discussing pain for only a specified time; acknowledging "I'm sorry your pain returned today, but you need to go to school"; actively practicing relaxation or coping skills). *Reduces focus on pain, especially if client is highly dependent on pain for secondary gain issues or is addicted to medications.*[6]
- Encourage client to use positive affirmations (e.g., "I am healing," "I am relaxed," "I love this life"). Have client be aware of internal-external dialogue. Say "cancel" when negative thoughts develop. *Negative thinking can exacerbate feelings of hopelessness, and replacing those thoughts with positive ones can be helpful to pain management.*
- Encourage right-brain stimulation with activities such as love, laughter, and music. *These actions can release endorphins, enhancing sense of well-being.*
- Encourage use of subliminal tapes *to bypass logical part of the brain by reinforcing "I am becoming a more relaxed person" and "It is all right for me to relax."*
- Use tranquilizers, narcotics, and analgesics sparingly. *These drugs are physically and psychologically addicting and promote sleep disturbances, especially interference with deep rapid eye movement sleep. Client may need to be detoxified if many medications are currently used.*
- Be alert to changes in pain characteristics *that may indicate a new physical problem or developing complication.*

 Diagnostic Studies   Evidence Based Practice   Medications   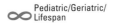 Pediatric/Geriatric/Lifespan

NURSING PRIORITY NO. 4 To promote wellness (Teaching/Discharge Considerations):

- Provide anticipatory guidance to client with condition in which pain is common and educate about when, where, and how to seek intervention or treatments.
- ∞ Discuss potential for developmental delays in child with chronic pain. Identify current level of function and review appropriate expectations for individual child.
- Instruct client/SO in medication administration, including use of patient-controlled analgesia pumps, as indicated. Review safe use of analgesics, including side effects requiring home management (e.g., constipation) or adverse effects requiring medical intervention (e.g., possible drug reactions). *Appropriate instruction in home management increases the accuracy and safety of medication administration.*
- Encourage and assist family member/SO(s) to learn home-care interventions. *Massage and other nonpharmacological pain management techniques benefit the client through reduction of pain level and sense that client is not alone/has support of SO.*
- Incorporate desired folk healthcare practices and beliefs into regimen whenever possible. *Has been shown to increase compliance with pain management treatment plan.*[12]
- Identify and discuss potential hazards of unproved or nonmedical therapies or remedies.
- Assist client and SO(s) to learn how to heal *by developing sense of internal control, by being responsible for own treatment, and by obtaining the information and tools to accomplish this.*
- Recommend that client and SO(s) take time for themselves. *Provides opportunity to reenergize and refocus on living/tasks at hand.*
- Address client's preferences and wishes for incurable pain or end-of-life pain management via advance directives *in order to assist family/SO in attending to client's needs.*[7]
- Identify community support groups and resources to meet individual needs (e.g., yard care, home maintenance, transportation). *Proper use of resources may reduce negative pattern of "overdoing" heavy activities and then spending several days in bed recuperating.*
- Refer for counseling (e.g., individual, family, marital therapy, parent effectiveness classes) as needed. *Presence of chronic pain affects all relationships and family dynamics.*
- Refer to NDs compromised family Coping and ineffective Coping.

DOCUMENTATION FOCUS

Assessment/Reassessment
- Individual findings, including duration of problem, specific contributing factors, previously and currently used interventions.
- Perception of pain, effects on lifestyle, and expectations of therapeutic regimen.
- Locus of control and cultural beliefs affecting response to pain.
- Family's/SO's response to client and support for change.
- Availability and use of resources.

Planning
- Plan of care and who is involved in planning.
- Teaching plan.

Implementation/Evaluation
- Responses to interventions, teaching, and actions performed.
- Attainment or progress toward desired outcome(s).
- Modifications to plan of care.

Discharge Planning
- Long-term needs and who is responsible for actions to be taken.
- Specific referrals made.

 Acute Care   Collaborative   Community/ Home Care   Cultural

References

1. Stoppler, M. C. (Reviewed 2017). Chronic pain. Retrieved April 2018 from http://www.emedicinehealth.com/chronic_pain/page10_em.htm.

2. Singh, M. K., Patel, J., Gallagher, R. M. (2012, updated 2018). Chronic pain syndrome. Retrieved April 2015 from http://emedicine.medscape.com/article/310834-overview.

3. Narayan, M. C. (2010). Culture's effects on pain assessment and management. *Am J Nurs*, 110(4), 38–48.

4. AGS Panel on Persistent Pain in Older Persons. (2002). The management of persistent pain in older persons. *J Am Geriatr Soc*, 50(6 Suppl), S205–S224.

5. Bienenfeld, D. (2010, updated 2017). Malingering. Retrieved April 2018 from http://emedicine.medscape.com/article/293206-overview.

6. Spratt, E. G., Ibeziako, P. I., DeMaso, D. (2012, updated 2014). Somatoform disorder. Retrieved April 2018 from http://emedicine.medscape.com/article/918628-overview.

7. American Medical Directors Association. (2009, updated 2012). Pain management in the long-term care setting. Retrieved April 2018 from https://www.guidelinecentral.com/summaries/pain-management-in-the-long-term-care-setting/#section-442.

8. Denenberg, R. S., Curtiss, C. P. (2016). Appropriate use of opioids in managing chronic pain. *Am J Nurs*, 116(7), 26–38.

9. Lark, S. (2005). The 21-day arthritis and pain miracle. *Lark Letter: A Woman's Guide to Optimal Health and Balance, Special Report*.

10. Warms, C. A., Marshal, J. M., Hoffman, A. J. (2006). There are a few things you did not ask about my pain: Writing in the margins of a survey questionnaire. *Rehabil Nurs*, 30(6), 248–256.

11. Parkins, J. M., Gfrorer, S. D. (2009). Chronic pain: The impact on academic, social, and emotional functioning. *National Association of School Psychologists: Communique*, 38(1), 24–25.

12. Institutes for Clinical Systems Improvement (ICSI). (2009, updated 2013). Assessment and management of chronic pain. Retrieved April 2018 from https://www.icsi.org/_asset/bw798b/ChronicPain.pdf.

13. Arnow, B. A. (2004). Relationships between childhood maltreatment, adult health and psychiatric outcomes, and medical utilization. *J Clin Psychiatry*, 65(12 Suppl), s10–s15.

14. Bordreaux, E. D., O'Hea, E., Chasuk, R. (2002). Spiritual role in healing, an alternative way of thinking. *Prim Care Clin Office Pract*, 29(2), 439–454.

15. Kiser-Larson, N. (2017). The experience of intense pain: Nursing management and interventions. *J Christ Nurs*, 34(2), 88–96.

16. Institute for Chronic Pain (ICP). (2012, updated 2017). Trauma. Retrieved April 2018 from http://www.instituteforchronicpain.org/understanding-chronic-pain/complications/trauma.

labor Pain

Taxonomy II: Comfort—Class 1 Physical Comfort (00256) **[Diagnostic Division:** Pain/Discomfort], Approved: 2013

DEFINITION: Sensory and emotional experience that varies from pleasant to unpleasant, associated with labor and childbirth.

RELATED FACTORS
To Be Developed

DEFINING CHARACTERISTICS

Subjective

Pain; uterine contraction; perineal pressure
Increase or decrease in appetite; nausea; vomiting
Alteration in urinary functioning, sleep pattern

Objective

Alteration in blood pressure/heart rate/respiratory rate
Distraction/expressive behavior; protective behavior; positioning to ease pain
Alteration in muscle tension; diaphoresis
Alteration in neuroendocrine functioning
Narrowed focus; self-focused; pupil dilation
Facial expression of pain

(continues on page 622)

 Diagnostic Studies   Evidence Based Practice   Medications 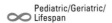 Pediatric/Geriatric/Lifespan

labor Pain (continued)

DESIRED OUTCOMES/EVALUATION CRITERIA

Sample **NOC** linkages:
Pain Control: Personal actions to eliminate or reduce pain
Client Satisfaction: Pain Management: Extent of positive perception of nursing care to relieve pain

Client Will (Include Specific Time Frame)
• Participate in decision making for pain management plan to include personal preferences and cultural beliefs.
• Engage in nonpharmacological measures to reduce discomfort/pain.
• Report pain at manageable level.

Partner/Labor Coach Will (Include Specific Time Frame)
• Participate in labor process, providing client's desired level of support.

ACTIONS/INTERVENTIONS

Sample **NIC** linkages:
Intrapartal Care: Monitoring and management of stages one and two of the birth process
Analgesic Administration: Intraspinal: Administration of pharmacologic agents into the epidural or intrathecal space to reduce or eliminate pain

NURSING PRIORITY NO. 1 To determine client's individual needs:

• Assess stage of labor; perform vaginal exam, noting nature and amount of vaginal show, cervical dilation, effacement, fetal station, and fetal descent. *Choice and timing of medication are affected by degree of dilation and contractile pattern.*[11]
• Note timing of initiation of prenatal care and participation in childbirth education classes. *Economic, emotional, and cultural concerns can limit the mother's access or involvement in preparation for labor, increasing her need for information and support during the labor and delivery process.*[1] *Also, research suggests classes and prenatal preparation may help decrease client's perception of pain.*[2]
• Evaluate degree of discomfort through verbal and nonverbal cues; note cultural influences on pain response. *Attitudes and reactions to pain are individual and based on past experiences, understanding of physiological changes, and familial/cultural expectations (e.g., the Filipino culture values stoicism and Chinese patients may refuse pain medication the first time it is offered).*[9,11]
• Ascertain presence of a birth plan, individual expectations, and cultural or religious beliefs affecting the labor and delivery process. *Birth plan provides information about client's childbirth preferences. Cultural influences may include how the laboring mother views pain management, as well as who attends the mother during the birth process (e.g., Hispanic and Asian women usually prefer their mothers be present, in Arab cultures the mother or sister of the baby's father is preferred). If cultural/religious preferences are not elicited, clients may not have the ability to follow their traditional practices, negatively impacting the birthing experience.*[9,11,12]
• Determine availability and preparation of support person(s). *Presence of a supportive partner, family/friend, or a doula can provide emotional support and enhance level of comfort, reducing analgesia. A doula provides labor coaching and support throughout the birthing process to both the mother and her partner.*[1,6]

 Acute Care   Collaborative   Community/Home Care   Cultural

NURSING PRIORITY NO. 2 To engage client in nonpharmacological pain management techniques:

- 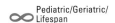Provide/encourage use of comfort measures (e.g., back/leg rubs, sacral pressure, back rest, mouth care, repositioning; cool, moist cloths to face and neck, hot compresses to perineum, abdomen; perineal care, linen changes). *Promotes relaxation and hygiene, enhancing feeling of well-being, and may reduce the need for analgesia or anesthesia. Position changes can also enhance circulation and reduce muscle tension.*[11]
- Assess client's desire for physical touch during contractions. *Touch may serve as a distraction, reduce anxiety, and provide encouragement, aiding in maintaining sense of control and reducing pain. Note: Remain respectful of client's preferences regarding touch.*[2]
- Coach use of appropriate breathing/relaxation techniques and abdominal effleurage based on stage of labor. *May block pain impulses within the cerebral cortex through conditioned responses and cutaneous stimulation and gives client a means of coping with and controlling the level of discomfort.*[11]
- Recommend client void every 1 to 2 hr. *Reduces bladder distention, which can increase discomfort and prolong labor.*[11]
- Review birth plan. Provide information about stage of labor and projected delivery, available analgesics, usual responses/side effects (client and fetal), and duration of analgesic effect in light of current situation. *Empowers client to make informed choice about means of pain control. Client may not be able to anticipate the degree of labor pain she will experience and may need to reevaluate her options as labor progresses. Note: Being able to move about and change positions at will can be important for some clients and impact their pain management choices.*[6,8]
- Assist with complementary therapies as indicated (e.g., acupressure/acupuncture, hypnosis, yoga). *Some clients and healthcare providers may prefer a trial of therapies theorized to stimulate/regulate contractions, reduce muscle tension, and mediate perception of pain before pursuing pharmacological interventions. For example, hypnosis may reduce fear, tension, and raise pain threshold, reducing need for analgesia. Research suggests acupressure may shorten labor time in addition to diminishing pain level.*[10] *Note: Differences in cultural and regional acceptance of these options as well as provider technique can impact the effectiveness of these interventions.*[1,2]
- Provide for a quiet environment that is adequately ventilated, dimly lit, and free of unnecessary personnel. Offer soothing music as appropriate. *Nondistracting environment provides optimal opportunity for rest and relaxation between contractions. Music may also reduce stress/anxiety, lift client's spirits, and decrease perception of pain.*[2]
- Discuss appropriateness/timing of hydrotherapy (shower, hot tub) as client desires. *Warm water during the first stage of labor stimulates the release of endorphins and relaxes muscles, enhancing circulation and tissue oxygenation with reduction in use of analgesia.*[1–3]
- Offer encouragement, provide information about labor progress, and provide positive reinforcement for client's/couple's efforts. *Provides emotional support, which can reduce fear, lower anxiety levels, and help minimize pain.*[11]

NURSING PRIORITY NO. 3 To provide more intensive pain management measures:

- 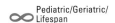Time and record the frequency, intensity, and duration of uterine contractile pattern per protocol. *Information necessary for choosing appropriate interventions and preventing or limiting undesired side effects of medication.*[11]
- Review birth plan, provide positive feedback for efforts to date, and be supportive of client's decisions regarding pain management. *Each labor and delivery experience is different and can challenge prenatal expectations. Changes in stated pain management preferences (e.g., unmedicated to medicated birth) can lead to client feeling disappointed or a failure at a life process. Acceptance and support from the nurse can enhance coping and promote a more positive birth experience.*[7]
- Administer analgesic, such as butorphanol tartrate (Stadol) or meperidine hydrochloride (Demerol), by IV during contractions or deep intramuscular (IM) if indicated during active phase of stage I labor. *IV route provides more rapid and equal absorption of analgesic, and IM route may require up to 45 min to reach*

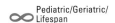

adequate plasma levels. Patient-controlled IV remifentanil provides better analgesia and patient satisfaction during the first and second stages of labor than other opioids but can cause serious maternal side effects. Effectiveness of opioids may be limited with the primary affect being sedation. Note: Administering IV drug during uterine contraction decreases amount of medication that immediately reaches fetus.[2,3,4]

- Monitor maternal vital signs and fetal heart rate (FHR) variability after drug administration. Note drug's effectiveness and the physiological response. *Narcotics can have a depressant effect on fetus, particularly when administered 2 to 3 hr before delivery.*[11]

- Provide safety measures (e.g., encourage client to move slowly, bed in low position, raise side rails) as indicated post-medication administration. *Regional block anesthesia produces vasomotor paralysis, so sudden movement may precipitate hypotension and risk for fall.*[11]

- Prepare for/assist with neuraxial anesthesia (i.e., epidural, spinal, combined spinal epidural, continuous epidural infusion, intermittent epidural bolus, client-controlled infusion epidural) using an indwelling catheter. *Research supports this method is the most effective in obtaining maternal pain relief once active labor is established. Note: Use of ultra-low-dose epidural is being promoted to achieve pain control without negative effect on client's ability to sense contractions and push effectively.*[2,5,11]

- Monitor FHR electronically and note decreased variability or bradycardia. *Decreased FHR variability is a common side effect of many anesthetics/analgesics. These side effects can begin 2 to 10 min after administration of anesthetic and may last for 5 to 10 min on occasion.*[11]

- Monitor level of block per protocol. *Migration of decreased sensation from belly button (dermatome T-10) to tip of breastbone (approximately T-6) increases risk of respiratory depression and profound hypotension.*[11]

- Turn client side to side periodically during continuous infusions. *Promotes even distribution of drug to prevent "one-sided" or unilateral block.*

- Inform client of onset of contractions as appropriate. *Client may "sleep" and/or encounter partial amnesia between contractions, impairing her ability to recognize contractions as they begin and her ability to initiate pain management techniques.*[11]

- Provide information about type of regional analgesia/anesthesia available at stage II specific to the delivery setting (e.g., local, pudendal block, lumbar epidural reinforcement, spinal block). *Although client is stressed, she still needs to be in control and make informed decisions regarding anesthesia.*

NURSING PRIORITY NO. 4   To support delivery process:

- Note perineal bulging or vaginal show. *Discomfort levels increase as cervix dilates, fetus descends, and small blood vessels rupture.*[11]

- Assist client in assuming optimal position for bearing down (e.g., squatting or lateral recumbent). *Proper positioning with relaxation of perineal tissue optimizes bearing-down efforts and facilitates labor progress, reducing discomfort.*[11]

- Assist with reinforcement of medication via indwelling lumbar epidural catheter when caput is visible. *Reduces discomfort associated with episiotomy, forceps application if needed, and fetal expulsion.*[11]

- Assist as needed with administration of local anesthetic just before episiotomy if performed. *Anesthetizes perineum tissue for incision/repair purposes.*[11]

DOCUMENTATION FOCUS

Assessment/Reassessment
- Stages of labor, results of vaginal exam, status of fetus/fetal monitoring.
- Client's degree of preparation and expectations for labor process.
- Choice of support person(s).

Planning
- Specifics of birth plan.
- Plan of care and who is involved in planning.

 Acute Care   Collaborative   Community/ Home Care   Cultural

Implementation/Evaluation
- Response to actions and interventions performed.
- Attainment or progress toward desired outcomes.

Discharge Planning
- Postpartal pain management choices.

References

1. Arendt, K. W., Tessmer-Tuck, J. A. (2013). Nonpharmacologic labor analgesia. *Clin Perinatol*, 40(3), 351–371.
2. Tournaire, M., Theau-Yonneau, A. (2007). Complementary and alternative approaches to pain relief during labor. *Evid Based Complement Alternat Med*, 4(4), 409–417.
3. Rooks, J. P. (2012). Labor pain management other than neuraxial: What do we know and where do we go next? *Birth*, 39(4), 318–322.
4. Tveit, T. O., et al. (2013). Efficacy and side effects of intravenous remifentanil patient-controlled analgesia used in a stepwise approach for labour: An observational study. *Int J Obstet Anesth*, 22(1), 19–25.
5. Gizzo, S., et al. (2014). Update on best available options in obstetrics anaesthesia: Perinatal outcomes, side effects and maternal satisfaction. *Arch Gynecol Obstet*, 290(1), 21–34.
6. Hardin, A. M., Buckner, E. B. (2004). Characteristics of a positive experience for women who have unmedicated childbirth. *J Perinat Educ*, 13(4), 10–16.
7. Carlton, T., Callister, L. C., Stoneman, E. (2005). Decision making in laboring women: Ethical issues for perinatal nurses. *J Perinat Neonatal Nurs*, 19(2), 145–154.
8. Lally, J. E., et al. (2014). Pain relief in labour: A qualitative study to determine how to support women to make decisions about pain relief in labour. *BMC Pregnancy Childbirth*. Retrieved April 2018 from http://www.biomedcentral.com/content/pdf/1471-2393-14-6.pdf.
9. Greene, M. J. (2007). Strategies for incorporating cultural competence into childbirth education curriculum. *J Perinat Educ*, 16(2), 33–37.
10. Akbarzadeh, M., et al. (2014). Comparison of the effects of maternal supportive care and acupressure (BL32 Acupoint) on pregnant women's pain intensity and delivery outcome. *J Pregnancy*. Retrieved April 2018 from http://dx.doi.org/10.1155/2014/129208.
11. Lowdermilk, D. L., Perry, S. E., Cashion, K. (2013). *Maternity Nursing*. 8th ed. Maryland Heights, MO: Mosby.
12. Ottani, P. A. (2002). When childbirth preparation isn't a cultural norm. *Int J Childbirth Educ*, 17(2), 12–16.

impaired Parenting

Taxonomy II: Role Relationships—Class 1 Caregiving Roles (00056) **[Diagnostic Division:** Social Interaction**]**, Approved 1998; Revised 1998, 2017

DEFINITION: Inability of the primary caretaker to create, maintain, or regain an environment that promotes the optimum growth and development of the child.

RELATED FACTORS
Infant or child
Prolonged separation from parent
Temperament conflicts with parental expectations
Parental
Alteration in sleep pattern; nonrestorative sleep pattern; sleep deprivation; depression
Conflict between partners; father or mother of child uninvolved; insufficient family cohesiveness
Insufficient or late-term prenatal care; insufficient resources, or access to resources
Failure to provide safe home environment; inability to put child's needs before own
Inadequate childcare arrangements; insufficient transportation
Ineffective communication skills or coping strategies; insufficient problem-solving skills
Insufficient parental role model; insufficient valuing of parenthood; insufficient social support

(continues on page 626)

 Diagnostic Studies
 Evidence Based Practice
 Medications
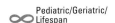 Pediatric/Geriatric/Lifespan

impaired Parenting (continued)

Insufficient response to infant cues; insufficient knowledge about child development or health maintenance or parenting skills

Low self-esteem, unrealistic expectations; role strain

Preference for physical punishment

DEFINING CHARACTERISTICS

Subjective

Parental Perceived inability to meet child's needs

Frustration with child; perceived role inadequacy

Objective

Infant or child

Frequent accidents or illness; failure to thrive

Low academic performance; delay in cognitive development

Impaired social functioning; behavior disorder [e.g., attention deficit, oppositional defiant]

History of trauma/abuse

Insufficient attachment behavior; diminished separation anxiety; runaway from home

Parental

Decrease in cuddling; inappropriate care-taking skills or childcare arrangements

Inconsistent care; neglects needs or inflexibility in meeting needs of child; decrease in ability to manage child; speaks negatively about child: rejection or abandonment of child

Failure to provide safe home environment; inappropriate stimulation

Inconsistent behavior management; hostile; punitive

At Risk Population: *Infant or child*

Prematurity; developmental delay

Gender other than desired

Difficult temperament

Parental

Change in family unit; relocation; single parent; young parental age

Insufficient cognitive readiness for parenting; unwanted or unplanned pregnancy

Closely spaced or high number of pregnancies; difficult birthing process; multiple births

Economically disadvantaged; low educational level; unemployment; work difficulty

History of abuse [physical, psychological, or sexual], or being abusive; history of substance misuse/ [abuse]; legal difficulties

History of mental illness

Associated Condition: *Infant or child*

Alteration in perceptual abilities; behavioral disorder

Chronic illness; disability condition

Parental

Alteration in cognitive functioning

Physical illness; disabling condition

Sample Clinical Applications: Prematurity, multiple births, genetic or congenital defects, chronic illness (parent/child), substance abuse, physical or psychological abuse, major depression, developmental delay, schizophrenia

 Acute Care   Collaborative   Community/ Home Care   Cultural

DESIRED OUTCOMES/EVALUATION CRITERIA

Sample **NOC** linkages:

Knowledge: Parenting: Extent of understanding conveyed about provision of a nurturing and constructive environment for a child from 1 year through 17 years of age

Parenting Performance: Parental actions to provide a child with a nurturing and constructive physical, emotional, and social environment

Child Development: [specify age]: Milestones of physical, cognitive, and psychosocial progression by [specific age]

Parent Will (Include Specific Time Frame)
- Verbalize realistic information and expectations of parenting role.
- Verbalize acceptance of the individual situation.
- Participate in appropriate classes, such as a parenting class.
- Identify own strengths, individual needs, and methods or resources to meet them.
- Demonstrate appropriate parenting behaviors.

ACTIONS/INTERVENTIONS

Sample **NIC** linkages:

Parenting Promotion: Providing parenting information, support, and coordination of comprehensive services to high-risk families

Family Integrity Promotion: Childbearing Family: Facilitation of the growth of individuals or families who are adding an infant to the family unit

Developmental Enhancement: Child [or] Adolescent: Facilitating or teaching parents/caregivers to facilitate the optimal gross motor, fine motor, language, cognitive, social, and emotional growth of preschool and school-age children. Facilitating optimal physical, cognitive, social, and emotional growth of individuals during the transition from childhood to adulthood

NURSING PRIORITY NO. 1   To assess causative/contributing factors:

- Note family constellation: two-parent, single, extended family, or child living with other relative such as grandparent/sibling. *Helps identify problem areas and strengths to formulate plans to change situation that is currently creating difficulties for the parents.*[3]
- Review type, severity, duration of problem and contribution of, as well as impact on, individual family members. *Affects choice of interventions; for example, when abuse is the problem, it is an act of commission, whereas neglect is considered an act of omission. These behaviors indicate the presence of problems with relationships and/or parenting skills and individual problems such as inability to deal with stressors, substance abuse, mental illness, cognitive limitations, or criminality.*[1]
- Note negative statements about child, signs of trauma/failure to thrive, and history of recurring accidents/illness. *May reflect physical or psychological abuse or neglect necessitating appropriate actions as legally and professionally indicated if child's safety is a concern. Note: Safety of child is paramount and needs to be dealt with immediately.*[5]
- Determine developmental stage of the family (e.g., new child, adolescent, child leaving or returning home). *These maturational crises bring changes in the family that can be stressful to parents and the family. Provides direction for improving parenting skills and family interactions.*[1]

 Diagnostic Studies   Evidence Based Practice   Medications   Pediatric/Geriatric/Lifespan

- Assess family relationships among individual members and with others, family boundaries, and needs of individual members. *These factors are critical to understanding individual family dynamics and developing strategies for change.*[3]
- Assess parenting skill level, taking into account the individual's intellectual, emotional, and physical strengths and weaknesses. *Parents with significant impairments may need more education or support. Ineffective parenting and unrealistic expectations contribute to problems of abuse and neglect. Understanding normal responses and progression of developmental milestones can help parents understand and cope with changes.*[1]
- Observe attachment behaviors between parental figure and child, recognizing cultural background. *Failure to bond effectively is thought to affect subsequent parent-child interaction. Behaviors such as eye-to-eye contact, use of en face position, and talking to the infant in a high-pitched voice are indicative of attachment behaviors in American culture but may not be appropriate in another culture.*[1,4]
- Note presence of factors in the child (e.g., birth defects, hyperactivity) that may be related to difficulties of parenting. *Unanticipated needs of the child may affect attachment and caretaking needs. Parents have an ideal of what is expected in a child, and when circumstances dictate otherwise, they may experience feelings of sadness and anger.*[1] Refer to ND complicated Grieving.
- Evaluate physical challenges or limitations of parent. *Presence of complicating factors (e.g., visual or hearing impairment, quadriplegia, severe depression, mental illness) may affect ability to care for a child and indicate need for additional planning to assist the parent.*[1]
- Determine presence and effectiveness of support systems, role models, extended family, and community resources available to the parent(s). *Lack of or ineffective use of support systems increases risk of continued inability to parent effectively.*[5]
- Note absence from home setting or lack of child supervision by parent. *Demands of working long hours, out of town, and multiple responsibilities, such as working and attending educational classes, will affect relationship between parent and child and ability to provide the care and nurturing necessary for children to grow and prosper.*[7]

NURSING PRIORITY NO. 2 To foster development of parenting skills:

- Create an environment in which relationships can be developed and needs of each individual met. *Learning is more effective when individuals feel safe and free to express feelings and concerns without fear of judgment.*[6,7]
- Make time for listening to concerns of the parent(s). *Listening conveys respect and acceptance, enabling parent(s) to openly discuss needs and desires regarding the situation and future plans.*[2]
- Emphasize positive aspects of the situation. *Maintaining a hopeful attitude toward the parent's capabilities and potential for improving the situation will help the parent to manage what is happening more effectively.*[1]
- Note staff attitudes toward parent/child and specific problem or disability. *The need for disabled parents to be seen as individuals and evaluated apart from a stereotype are crucial to helping individuals to cope with a difficult situation. Negative attitudes are detrimental to promoting positive outcomes.*[3]
- Encourage expression of feelings, such as helplessness, anger, and frustration. Set limits on unacceptable behaviors. *When feelings are expressed openly, they can be acknowledged and dealt with, enabling parent(s) to move forward in dealing with illness or situation. Individual may express anger by acting-out behaviors, which need to be restrained before damage is done to self, self-esteem, others, or environment.*[5,6]
- Acknowledge difficulty of situation and normalcy of feelings. *Individuals feel validated when difficulty is recognized, enhancing feelings of acceptance.*[1]
- Recognize stages of grieving process when the child is disabled or other than anticipated. *Expectation of a "normal" or desired child (e.g., having a girl instead of boy, child with a prominent birthmark or birth defect such as cleft palate) results in grieving for the loss of that expectation.*[1,8]
- Allow time for parents to express feelings and deal with the "loss." *Each person grieves at own pace, and allowing this time facilitates the process.*[8]
- Encourage attendance at skill classes, such as parent effectiveness. *Helps parents to develop communication and problem-solving techniques that promote positive relationships between parent and child.*[6,7]

 Acute Care   Collaborative   Community/Home Care   Cultural

• Emphasize parenting functions rather than mothering/fathering skills. *By virtue of gender, each person brings something to the parenting role; however, nurturing tasks can be done by both parents.*[1]

NURSING PRIORITY NO. 3 To promote wellness (Teaching/Discharge Considerations):

• Involve all available members of the family in learning. *Promotes understanding and effective communication when each individual has the same information and is able to ask questions and clarify what has been heard.*[2,5]
• Provide information appropriate to the situation, including time management, limit setting, and stress-reduction techniques. *Facilitates satisfactory implementation of plan and new behaviors.*[5]
• Discuss parental beliefs about child-rearing, punishment, and rewards. *Identifying these beliefs allows opportunity to provide new information regarding effective alternatives to spanking and/or yelling and what actions can be substituted for more effective parenting.*
• Develop support systems appropriate to the situation. *Extended family, friends, social worker, home-care services may be needed to help parents cope positively with what is happening.*[3]
• Assist parent to plan time and conserve energy in positive ways. *Enables individual to cope more effectively with difficulties as they arise.*[3]
• Encourage parents to identify positive outlets for meeting their own needs. *Going out for dinner or dating and making time for their own interests and each other promotes general well-being and helps reduce burnout.*[3,9]
• Refer to appropriate support or therapy groups as indicated. *Underlying issues may interfere with adaptation to situation, and additional support may help individuals to deal more effectively with them.*[5]
• Identify community resources (e.g., child-care services). *Will assist with individual needs to provide respite and support.*[2]
• Report and take necessary actions, as legally and professionally indicated, if child's safety is a concern. *Parents/caregivers who engage in corporal punishment as a technique to ensure desired behavior in a child are at risk for abusive behavior and increase the possibility of childhood depression.*[5]
• Refer to NDs ineffective Coping, compromised family Coping, risk for Violence [specify], Self-Esteem [specify], and interrupted Family Processes for additional interventions as appropriate.

DOCUMENTATION FOCUS

Assessment/Reassessment
• Individual findings, including parenting skill level, deviations from normal parenting expectations.
• Family makeup and developmental stages.
• Interactions between parent and child.
• Availability and use of support systems and community resources.

Planning
• Plan of care and who is involved in planning.
• Teaching plan.

Implementation/Evaluation
• Parent(s')/child's responses to interventions, teaching, and actions performed.
• Attainment or progress toward desired outcome(s).
• Modification to plan of care.

Discharge Planning
• Long-term needs and who is responsible for actions to be taken.
• Specific referrals made.

 Diagnostic Studies   Evidence Based Practice   Medications   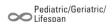 Pediatric/Geriatric/ Lifespan

References

1. Johnson, J. G., et al. (2006). Parenting behaviors associated with risk for personality disorder during adulthood. *Arch Gen Psychiatry*, 63(5), 579–587.
2. Gordon, T. (No date). Origins of the Gordon model. *Gordon Training International*. Retrieved April 2018 from http://www.gordontraining.com/thomas-gordon/origins-of-the-gordon-model/.
3. Riggio, R. E. (2011). How does your parenting style affect your kids? Retrieved April 2018 from https://www.psychologytoday.com/us/blog/cutting-edge-leadership/201410/how-does-your-parenting-style-affect-your-kids.
4. Ho, J., Birnham, C. (2010). Acculturation gaps in Vietnamese immigrant families: Impact on family relationships. *Int J Intercult Relat*, 34(1), 22–23.
5. Child Welfare Information Gateway. (Updated 2013). Long term consequences of child abuse and neglect. *U.S. Department of Health and Human Services*. Retrieved April 2018 from https://www.childwelfare.gov/pubpdfs/long_term_consequences.pdf.
6. Brhel, R. (2008). The age of gentle discipline. *The Attached Family*. Retrieved April 2018 from http://theattachedfamily.com/membersonly/?p=177.
7. Oswalt, A. (2008, updated 2015). Urie Bronfenbrenner and child development. Retrieved April 2018 from https://www.mentalhelp.net/articles/urie-bronfenbrenner-and-child-development/.
8. Neeld, E. H. (2003). *Seven Choices: Finding Daylight After Loss Shatters Your Life*. New York: Grand Central.
9. Adams, L. (2011). The language of love. *Gordon Training International*. Retrieved April 2018 from http://www.gordontraining.com/free-parenting-articles/the-language-of-love/.

readiness for enhanced Parenting

Taxonomy II: Role Relationships—Class 1 Caregiving Roles (00164) [**Diagnostic Division:** Social Interaction], Approved 2002; Revised 2013

DEFINITION: A pattern of providing an environment for children to nurture growth and development, which can be strengthened.

DEFINING CHARACTERISTICS

Subjective
Parent expresses desire to enhance parenting
Parent expresses desire to enhance emotional support of children/other dependent person
Children express desire to enhance home environment
Sample Clinical Applications: As a health-seeking behavior, the client/family may be healthy or this diagnosis can be associated with any clinical condition

DESIRED OUTCOMES/EVALUATION CRITERIA

Sample NOC linkages:
Parenting Performance: Parental actions to provide a child with a nurturing and constructive physical, emotional, and social environment
Knowledge: Parenting: Extent of understanding conveyed about provision of a nurturing and constructive environment for a child from 1 year through 17 years of age
Parenting: Psychosocial Safety: Parental actions to protect a child from social contacts that might cause harm or injury

Client Will (Include Specific Time Frame)
• Verbalize realistic information and expectations of parenting role.
• Identify own strengths, individual needs, and methods or resources to meet them.
• Participate in activities to enhance parenting skills.
• Demonstrate improved parenting behaviors.

 Acute Care Collaborative Community/Home Care Cultural

ACTIONS/INTERVENTIONS

Sample NIC **linkages:**

Parent Education: Childrearing Family: Assisting parents to understand and promote the physical, psychological, and social growth and development of their toddler, preschool, or school-age child/children

Parent Education: Adolescent: Assisting parents to understand and help their adolescent children

Parenting Promotion: Providing parenting information, support, and coordination of comprehensive services to high-risk families

NURSING PRIORITY NO. 1 To determine need/motivation for improvement:

- Ascertain motivation and expectations for change. *Motivation to improve and high expectations can encourage client to make changes that will improve skills. However, unrealistic expectations may hamper efforts.*
- Note family constellation, such as two-parent, single, extended family, or child living with other relative such as a grandparent/sibling, or relationship of dependent person (e.g., foster family). *Understanding makeup of the family provides information about needs to assist them in improving their family connections.*[1]
- ∞ Determine developmental stage of the family (e.g., new child, adolescent, child leaving or returning home, retirement). *These maturational crises bring changes in the family that can provide opportunity for enhancing parenting skills and improving family interactions.*
- Assess family relationships and identify needs of individual members, noting any special concerns that exist, such as birth defects, illness, and hyperactivity. *The family is a system, and when members make decisions to improve parenting skills, the changes affect all parts of the system. Identifying needs, special situations, and relationships can help to develop plans to bring about effective change.*[1]
- Assess parenting skill level, taking into account the individual's intellectual, emotional, and physical strengths and weaknesses. *Identifies areas of need for education, skill training, and information on which to base plan for enhancing parenting skills.*[2,4]
- ⊕ Observe attachment behaviors among parent(s) and child(ren), recognizing cultural background, which may influence expected behaviors. *Behaviors such as eye-to-eye contact, use of en face position, and talking to infant in high-pitched voice are indicative of attachment behaviors in American culture but may not be appropriate in another culture. Failure to bond is thought to affect subsequent parent-child interactions.*[3,4]
- Determine presence and effectiveness of support systems, role models, extended family, and community resources available to the parent(s). *Parents desiring to enhance abilities and improve family life can benefit by role models that help them strengthen own style of parenting.*[2,3]
- ⊕ Note cultural or religious influences on parenting, expectations of self/child, and sense of success or failure. *Expectations may vary with different cultures; for example, Arab Americans hold children to be sacred, but child-rearing is based on negative rather than positive reinforcements, and parents are stricter with girls than boys. These beliefs may interfere with ability to improve parenting skills when there is conflict between the two.*[3,4]

NURSING PRIORITY NO. 2 To foster development of parenting skills:

- Create an environment in which relationships can be strengthened and needs of each individual family member can be met. *A safe environment in which individuals can freely express their thoughts and feelings optimizes learning and positive interactions among family members, enhancing relationships.*[2,5]
- Make time for listening to concerns of the parent(s). *Promotes sense of importance and of being heard and identifies accurate information regarding needs of the family for enhancing relationships.*[2]
- Encourage expression of feelings, such as frustration and anger while setting limits on unacceptable behaviors. *Identification of feelings promotes understanding of self and enhances connections with others in the family. Unacceptable behaviors result in feelings of anger and diminished self-esteem and can lead to problems in family relationships.*[3]

 Diagnostic Studies   Evidence Based Practice   Medications   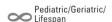 Pediatric/Geriatric/Lifespan

- Emphasize parenting functions rather than mothering/fathering skills. *By virtue of gender, each person brings something to the parenting role; however, nurturing tasks can be done by both parents, enhancing family relationships.*[5]
- Encourage attendance at skill classes, such as parent effectiveness training. *Assists in developing communication skills of active listening, "I" messages, and problem-solving techniques to improve family relationships and promote a win-win environment.*[2]

NURSING PRIORITY NO. 3 To promote optimum parenting skills/wellness:

- Involve all members of the family in learning. *The family system benefits from all members participating in learning new skills to enhance family relationships.*[1]
- Encourage parents to identify positive outlets for meeting their own needs. *Activities such as going out for dinner/dating and making time for their own interests and each other promotes general well-being, enhances family relationships, and improves family functioning.*[2]
- Provide information as indicated, including time management and stress-reduction techniques. *Learning about positive parenting skills and understanding growth and developmental expectations and ways to reduce stress and anxiety promotes individual's ability to deal with problems that may arise in the course of family relationships.*[1,6]
- Discuss current "family rules," identifying areas of needed change. *Rules may be imposed by adults rather than through a democratic process, involving all family members, leading to conflict and angry confrontations. Setting positive family rules with all family members participating can promote an effective, functional family.*[2,6]
- Discuss need for long-term planning and ways in which family can maintain desired positive relationships. *Each stage of life brings its own challenges, and understanding and preparing for each stage enables family members to move through them in positive ways, promoting family unity and resolving inevitable conflicts with win-win solutions.*[6]

DOCUMENTATION FOCUS

Assessment/Reassessment
- Individual findings, including parenting skill level, parenting expectations, family makeup, and developmental stages.
- Availability and use of support systems and community resources.
- Motivation and expectations for change.

Planning
- Plan for enhancement, who is involved in planning.

Implementation/Evaluation
- Family members' responses to interventions, teaching, and actions performed.
- Attainment or progress toward desired outcome(s).
- Modifications to plan.

Discharge Planning
- Long-term needs and who is responsible for actions to be taken.
- Modification to plan.

References

1. Families and Schools Together (FAST). (2018). Theoretical foundations (and other pages). Retrieved November 2018 from https://www.familiesandschools.org/why-fast-works/theoretical-foundations/.
2. Riesch, S. K., et al. (2010). Furthering the understanding of parent-child relationships: A nursing scholarship review series, Part 5: Parent-adolescent and teen parent-child relationships. *J Spec Pediatr Nurs*, 15(3), 182–201.
3. Watson, S. (Updated 2017). Understanding inappropriate behavior. Retrieved April 2018 from http://specialed.about.com/od/behavioremotional/a/behavsupport.htm.

 Acute Care   Collaborative   Community/ Home Care   Cultural

4. Institute of Public Care. (2008). What works in promoting good outcomes for children in need through enhanced parenting skills? *Social Services Improvement Agency, Wales*. Retrieved April 2018 from http://ipc.brookes.ac.uk/publications/pdf/What_Works_in_Promoting_Good_Outcomes_for_CIN_through_Parenting.pdf.
5. Bronte-Tinkew, J., Burkhauser, M., Metz, A. (2008). Elements of promising practice in teen fatherhood programs: Evidence-based and evidence-informed research findings on what works. *National Fatherhood Responsible Clearing House*. Retrieved April 2018 from http://www.lacdcfs.org/katiea/docs/EPP.pdf.
6. Duncan, L. G., Coatsworth, J. D., Greenberg, M. T. (2009). Pilot study to gauge acceptability of a mindfulness based, family-focused preventive intervention. *J Prim Prev*, 30(5), 605–618.

risk for impaired Parenting

Taxonomy II: Role Relationships—Class 1 Caregiving Roles (00057) **[Diagnostic Division:** Social Interaction], Approved 1978; Revised 1998; 2013, 2017

DEFINITION: Susceptible to primary caretaker difficulty in creating, maintaining, or regaining an environment that promotes the optimum growth and development of the child, which may compromise the well-being of the child.

RISK FACTORS
Infant or child
Prolonged separation from parent
Temperament conflicts with parental expectations
Parental
Alteration in sleep pattern; nonrestorative sleep pattern; sleep deprivation; depression
Conflict between partners; father or mother of child uninvolved; insufficient family cohesiveness
Insufficient or late-term prenatal care; insufficient resources, or access to resources
Failure to provide safe home environment; inability to put child's needs before own
Inadequate child-care arrangements; insufficient transportation
Ineffective communication skills or coping strategies; insufficient problem-solving skills
Insufficient parental role model; insufficient valuing of parenthood; insufficient social support
Insufficient response to infant cues; insufficient knowledge about child development or health maintenance or parenting skills
Low self-esteem, unrealistic expectations; role strain
Preference for physical punishment
At Risk Population: *Infant or child*
Prematurity; developmental delay
Gender other than desired
Difficult temperament
Parental
Change in family unit; relocation; single parent; young parental age
 Insufficient cognitive readiness for parenting; unwanted or unplanned pregnancy
Closely spaced or high number of pregnancies; difficult birthing process; multiple births
Economically disadvantaged; low educational level; unemployment; work difficulty
History of abuse [physical, psychological, or sexual], or being abusive; history of substance misuse/[abuse]; legal difficulties
History of mental illness
Associated Condition: *Infant or child*
Alteration in perceptual abilities; behavioral disorder
Chronic illness; disability condition

(continues on page 634)

 Diagnostic Studies   Evidence Based Practice   Medications 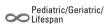 Pediatric/Geriatric/Lifespan

risk for impaired Parenting (continued)

Parental
Alteration in cognitive functioning
Physical illness; disabling condition
Sample Clinical Applications: Prematurity, multiple births, genetic or congenital defects, chronic illness (parent/child), substance abuse, physical or psychological abuse, major depression, developmental delay, schizophrenia

DESIRED OUTCOMES/EVALUATION CRITERIA

Sample **NOC** linkages:
Parenting Performance: Parental actions to provide a child a nurturing and constructive physical, emotional, and social environment
Knowledge: Parenting: Extent of understanding conveyed about provision of a nurturing and constructive environment for a child from 1 year through 17 years of age
Social Support: Reliable assistance from others

Client Will (Include Specific Time Frame)
• Verbalize awareness of individual risk factors.
• Identify own strengths, individual needs, and methods or resources to meet them.
• Demonstrate behavior or lifestyle changes to reduce potential for development of problem or reduce or eliminate effects of risk factors.
• Participate in activities, classes to promote growth.

ACTIONS/INTERVENTIONS

Sample **NIC** linkages:
Parenting Promotion: Providing parenting information, support, and coordination of comprehensive services to high-risk families
Parent Education: Childrearing Family: Assisting parents to understand and promote the physical, psychological, and social growth and development of their toddler, preschool, or school-aged child
Family Integrity Promotion: Promotion of family cohesion and unity

• **Refer to ND impaired Parenting for Actions/Interventions and Documentation Focus.**

disturbed Personal Identity

Taxonomy II: Self-Perception—Class 1 Self-Concept (00121) [**Diagnostic Division:** Ego Integrity], Approved 1978; Revised 2008, 2017

DEFINITION: Inability to maintain an integrated and complete perception of self.

RELATED FACTORS
Stages of growth, alteration in social role
Cultural incongruence; discrimination; perceived prejudice
Dysfunction in family processes

 Acute Care   Collaborative   Community/ Home Care   Cultural

Low self-esteem; manic states
Cult indoctrination

DEFINING CHARACTERISTICS

Subjective

Alteration in body image; delusional description of self
Fluctuating feeling about self; feelings of strangeness or emptiness
Confusion about goals, cultural values, or ideological values
Gender confusion
Inability to distinguish between internal and external stimuli

Objective

Inconsistent behavior
Ineffective relationships or role performance
Ineffective coping strategies
At Risk Population: Developmental transition; situational crisis
Exposure to toxic chemical
Associated Conditions: Dissociative identity disorder; psychiatric disorder
Organic brain disorder
Pharmaceutical agent
Sample Clinical Applications: Schizophrenia, dissociative disorders, borderline personality disorder, developmental delay, autism, gender identity conflict, dementia, traumatic injury (e.g., amputation, spinal cord injury [SCI], brain injury)

DESIRED OUTCOMES/EVALUATION CRITERIA

Sample NOC linkages:

Identity: Distinguish between self and non-self and characterize one's essence
Distorted Thought Self-Control: Self-restraint of disruption in perception, thought processes, and thought content
Anxiety Self-Control: Personal actions to eliminate or reduce feelings of apprehension, tension, or uneasiness from an unidentifiable source

Client Will (Include Specific Time Frame)

- Acknowledge threat to personal identity.
- Integrate threat in a healthy, positive manner (e.g., state anxiety is reduced, make plans for the future).
- Verbalize acceptance of changes that have occurred.
- State ability to identify and accept self (long-term outcome).

ACTIONS/INTERVENTIONS

Sample NIC linkages:

Self-Esteem Enhancement: Assisting a patient to increase his/her personal judgment of self-worth
Self-Awareness Enhancement: Assisting a patient to explore and understand his/her thoughts, feelings, motivations, and behaviors
Mood Management: Providing for safety, stabilization, recovery, and maintenance of a patient who is experiencing dysfunctionally depressed or elevated mood

 Diagnostic Studies   Evidence Based Practice   Medications   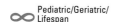 Pediatric/Geriatric/Lifespan

NURSING PRIORITY NO. 1 To assess causative/contributing factors:

- Ascertain client's perception of the extent of the threat to self and how client is handling the situation. *Many factors can affect an individual's self-image: illness (chronic or terminal), injuries, changes in body structure (amputation, spinal cord damage, burns), and client's view of what has happened will affect development of plan of care and interventions to be used.*[1,6]
- Determine speed of occurrence of threat. *An event (such as an accident or sudden diagnosis of diabetes or cancer) that has happened quickly may be more threatening.*[7]
- Ask client to define own body image. *Body image is the basis of personal identity, and client's perception will affect how changes are viewed, may prevent achievement of ideals and expectations, and have a negative effect.*[1]
- ∞ Note age of client. *An adolescent may struggle with the developmental task of personal/sexual identity, whereas an older person may have more difficulty accepting or dealing with a threat to identity, such as progressive loss of memory or aging body changes.*[3]
- Assess availability and use of support systems. Note response of family/significant others (SOs). *During stressful situations, support is essential for client to cope with changes that are occurring. Engaging family in choosing supportive interventions will help client and family members deal with situation or illness.*[3]
- ∞ Note withdrawn or automatic behavior, regression to earlier developmental stage, general behavioral disorganization, or display of self-mutilation behaviors in adolescent or adult and delayed development, preference for solitary play, and unusual display of self-stimulation in child. *Indicators of poor coping skills and need for specific interventions to help client develop sense of self and identity. Inability to identify self interferes with interactions with others.*[3]
- Be aware of physical signs of panic state (e.g., heart palpitations, trembling, shortness of breath, chest pressure or pain). *Presence of severe anxiety state may progress to panic when concerns seem overwhelming to client.* (Refer to ND Anxiety.)
- Determine presence of hallucinations or delusions or distortions of reality. *Indicators of presence of psychosis and need for immediate interventions to deal with inability to distinguish between self and non-self.*[1,3]

NURSING PRIORITY NO. 2 To assist client to manage/deal with threat:

- Make time to listen to client, encouraging appropriate expression of feelings, including anger and hostility. *Conveys a sense of confidence in client's ability to identify extent of threat, how it is affecting sense of identity, and how to deal with feelings in acceptable ways.*[7,8]
- 💊 Note use of alcohol or other drugs. *Individual may turn to these substances to relieve painful feelings, especially in the presence of fearful diagnoses (e.g., cancer, multiple sclerosis).*[8]
- Provide a calm environment. *Feelings of anxiety are contagious, and calm surroundings can help client to relax, maintain control, and be able to think more clearly about how illness or situation can be managed effectively.*[9]
- Use crisis intervention principles when indicated. *May be necessary to help client restore equilibrium when situation escalates.*[1]
- Discuss client's commitment to an identity. *Those who have made a strong commitment to an identity tend to be more comfortable with self and happier than those who have not.*[3]
- Assist client to develop strategies to cope with threat to identity. *Reduces anxiety, promotes self-awareness, and enhances self-esteem, enabling client to deal with threat more realistically.*[10]
- Engage client in activities appropriate to individual situation. *Using activities such as a mirror for visual feedback and tactile stimulation to reconnect with parts of the body (amputation, unilateral neglect) can help to identify self as an individual.*[2]
- Provide for simple decisions, concrete tasks, and calming activities. *Promotes sense of control and positive expectations to enable client to regain sense of self.*[3]
- Allow client to deal with situation in small steps. *May have difficulty coping with larger picture when in stress overload. Taking small steps promotes feelings of success and ability to manage illness or situation.*[9]

 Acute Care Collaborative Community/ Home Care Cultural

- Encourage client to develop and participate in an individualized exercise program. *While walking is an excellent beginning program, it is helpful to choose activities that client enjoys. Exercise releases endorphins, thereby reducing stress and anxiety, promoting a sense of well-being.*[1]
- Provide concrete assistance as needed. *Until basic-level needs, such as activities of daily living and food, are met, individual is unable to deal with higher-level needs. Once these needs are met, client can begin to deal with threat to identity.*[1]
- Take advantage of opportunities to promote growth. Realize that client will have difficulty learning while in a dissociative state. *Alterations in mental status can interfere with ability to process information, and new information can increase confusion and disorientation.*[3]
- Maintain reality orientation without confronting client's irrational beliefs. *Client may become defensive, blocking opportunity to look at other possibilities. Arguing does not change the perceptions and can interfere with or damage nurse-client relationship.*[1]
- Use humor judiciously when appropriate. *While humor can lift spirits and provide a moment of levity, it is important to note the mood or receptiveness of the client before using it.*[3]
- Discuss options for dealing with issues of gender identity. *Identification of client's concerns about role dysfunction or conflicting feelings about sexual identity will indicate need for therapies, possible gender-change surgery when client is a transsexual, or other available choices.*[2]
- Refer to NDs disturbed Body Image, Self-Esteem [specify], and Spiritual Distress.

NURSING PRIORITY NO. 3   To promote wellness (Teaching/Discharge Considerations):

- Provide accurate information about threat to and potential consequences for individual in current situation. *Fear and anxiety regarding the threat represented by the illness or situation can be potentiated by lack of knowledge, unknown consequences, and inaccurate beliefs. Accurate information can help client incorporate new knowledge into changed self-concept.*[7]
- Assist client and SO(s) to acknowledge and integrate threat into future planning. *A diagnosis, accident, etc., can require major life changes, such as wearing identification bracelet when prone to mental confusion, a new lifestyle to accommodate change of gender for transsexual client, or a diet and medication routine with the diagnosis of diabetes mellitus. Planning can help the client to make the changes required to move forward with new life.*[4,5]
- Refer to appropriate support groups. *May need additional assistance, such as day-care program, counseling or psychotherapy, gender identity, family or marriage counseling, or parenting classes.*[2]

DOCUMENTATION FOCUS

Assessment/Reassessment
- Findings, noting degree of impairment.
- Nature of and client's perception of the threat.

Planning
- Plan of care and who is involved in the planning.
- Teaching plan.

Implementation/Evaluation
- Client's response to interventions, teaching, and actions performed.
- Attainment or progress toward desired outcome(s).
- Modifications to plan of care.

Discharge Planning
- Long-term needs and who is responsible for actions to be taken.
- Specific referrals made.

 Diagnostic Studies   Evidence Based Practice   Medications   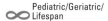 Pediatric/Geriatric/ Lifespan

References

1. Newell, R. (2002). Terminal illness and body image. *Nurs Times*, 98(14), 36–37.
2. Gillig, P. M. (2009). Dissociative identity disorder—A controversial diagnosis. *Psychiatry (Edgemont)*, 6(3), 24–29. Retrieved April 2018 from http://www.ncbi.nlm.nih.gov/pmc/articles/PMC2719457/.
3. Shaw, G. (2011). Coping with a life threatening illness—Palliative care: Improving life for patients and caregivers. Retrieved April 2018 from http://www.webmd.com/palliative-care/coping-with-a-life-threatening-illness.
4. Pinhas-Hamiel, O., et al. (1996). Increased incidence of non-insulin-dependent diabetes mellitus among adolescents. *J Pediatr*, 128(8), 608–615.
5. Deckelbaum, R. J., Williams, C. L. (2001). Childhood obesity: The health issue. *Obes Res*, 9(5), 239s–243s.
6. Badger, J. M. (2001). Burns: The psychological aspect. *Am J Nurs*, 101(11), 38–41.
7. Bartol, T. (2002). Putting a patient with diabetes in the driver's seat. *Nursing*, 32(2), 53–55.
8. Bruera, E., et al. (1995). The frequency of alcoholism among patients with pain due to terminal cancer. *J Pain Symptom Manage*, 10(8), 599–603.
9. Paice, J. (2002). Managing psychological conditions in palliative care. *Am J Nurs*, 102(11), 36–43.
10. Ghosh, S. (2015). Gender identity. Retrieved April 2018 from http://emedicine.medscape.com/article/917990-overview.

---

risk for disturbed Personal Identity

Taxonomy II: Self-Perception—Class 1 Self-Concept (00225) **[Diagnostic Division:** Ego Identity], Approved 2010; Revised 2013

DEFINITION: Susceptible to the inability to maintain an integrated and complete perception of self, which may compromise health.

RISK FACTORS

Stages of growth, alteration in social role
Cultural incongruence; discrimination; perceived prejudice
Dysfunction in family processes
Low self-esteem; manic states
Cult indoctrination
Stages of growth, alteration in social role
Cultural incongruence; discrimination; perceived prejudice
Dysfunction in family processes;
Low self-esteem; manic states
Cult indoctrination
At Risk Population: Developmental transition; situational crisis
Exposure to toxic chemical
Associated Condition: Dissociative identity disorder; psychiatric disorder
Organic brain disorder
Pharmaceutical agent
Sample Clinical Applications: Traumatic injury (e.g., amputation, spinal cord injury, traumatic brain injury), substance abuse, dementia, schizophrenia, borderline personality disorders, dissociative disorders, developmental delay, autism, gender identity conflict

DESIRED OUTCOMES/EVALUATION CRITERIA

Sample NOC linkages:
Personal Identity: Personal actions that distinguish self and non-self and characterize one's essence
Distorted Thought Self-Control: Self-restraint of disruption in perception, thought processes, and thought control
Anxiety Self-Control: Personal actions to eliminate or reduce feelings of apprehension, tension, or uneasiness from an unidentifiable source

 Acute Care Collaborative Community/Home Care Cultural

Client Will (Include Specific Time Frame)
- Acknowledge concern about potential threat to identity.
- Exhibit reality-based thinking with appropriate thought content.
- Integrate perceived threat in a healthy manner (e.g., accept self in current situation, look to the future).
- Use effective coping strategies to deal with situation/stressors.

ACTIONS/INTERVENTIONS

Sample NIC linkages:

Self-Awareness Enhancement: Assisting a patient to explore and understand his/her thoughts, feelings, motivations, and behaviors

Self-Esteem Enhancement: Assisting a patient to increase his/her personal judgment of self-worth

Coping Enhancement: Facilitation of cognitive and behavioral efforts to manage perceived stressors, changes, or threats that interfere with meeting life demands and roles

NURSING PRIORITY NO. 1   To assess risk/contributing factors:

- Ascertain client's perception of threat to self and how it is being dealt with. *Many factors can impinge on client's life and cause concern about possibility of changes that will make life different.*[1,5,12,13,15]
- Ask client to define own body image. *The basis of personal identity is body image, and perception of changes may affect client's view in a negative or positive manner.*[1,6,12,18]
- Determine whether issues of gender identity are a concern. *Client may have conflicting feelings about how to deal with realization he or she is homosexual or transsexual.*[10,12]
- ∞ Note age of individual. *Changes affect persons differently depending on their stage of life. The maturational changes of adolescence may generally be viewed as positive, while the older person may view aging changes in a negative way.*[2,12,13,15,17]
- Identify cultural affiliations/discontinuity. *Individuals belonging to subcultures or cults tend to come into conflict with the greater societal views affecting one's perception of self and perception of reality, often resulting in isolation from outside support groups and reluctance to engage in therapeutic interventions.*[12,19–21]
- Determine type and speed of changes that are imminent. *The diagnosis of a chronic illness, such as diabetes versus a terminal illness or a traumatic injury or disfiguring surgery that will change how life is lived, may be threatening, as the thought of how different life will be affects the individual.*[1,6,12,14,15]
- Note availability and use of support systems, including attitude of family/significant others. *Having a positive support system can help individual get through difficult situations/illness.*[3,4,6,14]
- Assess behaviors such as withdrawal, general behavioral disorganization, and delayed development. *Poor coping skills will affect how client deals with possibility of disturbance in personal identity by changes occurring in life.*[2,6,11,13]
- Discuss use of alcohol and other drugs. *Individuals often use these substances to avoid painful stressors.*[2,15]
- Note signs of anxiety. *Use of inadequate coping strategies to deal with changes affecting lifestyle may result in exacerbation of symptoms in anxious person. (Refer to ND Anxiety.)*
- Determine distortions of reality/symptoms of mental illness. *Requires more in-depth psychological counseling/medication to help client distinguish between self and non-self.*[2,11,12,15,18]

NURSING PRIORITY NO. 2   To assist client to manage/deal with stressors:

- Listen/Active-listen, making time to encourage client to express feelings, including anger and hostility. *Possibility of changes in life may affect sense of self and identity.*[6,7,9]

 Diagnostic Studies   Evidence Based Practice   Medications   Pediatric/Geriatric/ Lifespan

- Discuss client's concerns without confronting unreal ideas. *Irrational beliefs may interfere with ability to manage situation and maintain reality-based perception of self.*[2,6]
- Encourage client and family to maintain a calm environment and positive attitude. *Anxiety is contagious and can interfere with client's efforts to maintain control and deal with the situation.*[8,16]
- Help client to identify strategies to cope with current situation/possibility of threat. *Having a plan can reduce anxiety and promote self-esteem.*[2,3,14]
- Use humor when appropriate. *In an established nurse-client relationship, humor can be useful to help client look at reality of situation.*[16]
- Provide activities applicable for client's situation. *For example, viewing body part/using a mirror for visual feedback or tactile stimulation to reconnect with parts of the body (i.e., amputation) or participation in monitored social interactions helps client to confront fear and see self as an individual who is still worthwhile.*[1,18]
- Support client in making decisions and plans for the future. *Provides opportunity for client to feel in control and promotes positive expectations.*[3,14]
- Develop an individualized exercise program. *Releases endorphins, reducing stress and promoting a sense of well-being.*[5,22]
- Refer to NDs disturbed Body Image, Self-Esteem (specify), and Spiritual Distress for additional interventions as appropriate.

NURSING PRIORITY NO. 3   To promote wellness (Teaching/Discharge Considerations):

- Provide accurate information/resources for issues client is concerned about. *Worrying about what might happen is counterproductive to dealing with reality, and information can help to lessen anxiety, allowing individual to deal with current situation.*[3,4,7,18]
- Discuss potential changes in lifestyle that may occur with major diagnosis/accident. *Planning for these possibilities can enhance self-confidence and allow client to move forward with life.*[1,5,7,8]
- Refer to appropriate support groups. *Sharing concerns with others in group settings may help client to be realistic regarding concerns about effects of anticipated changes/life challenges.*[3,4,8,18]
- Explore community resources as appropriate. *Additional assistance such as day programs, individual/family counseling, and drug/alcohol-cessation programs can strengthen client's coping abilities and sense of control.*[4,12,23,24]

DOCUMENTATION FOCUS

Assessment/Reassessment
- Findings, noting concerns about possible changes in lifestyle, future expectations.
- Reality of potential threat.

Planning
- Plan of care and who is involved in the planning.
- Teaching plan.

Implementation/Evaluation
- Client's response to interventions, teaching, and actions performed.

Discharge Planning
- Long-term needs, and who is responsible for actions to be taken.
- Specific referrals made.

References

1. Newell, R. (2002). Terminal illness and body image. *Nurs Times*, 98(14), 36.
2. Gillig, P. M. (2009). Dissociative identity disorder—A controversial diagnosis. *Psychiatry (Edgmont)*, 6(3), 24–29.
3. Shaw, G. (2011). Coping with a life threatening illness. Palliative care: Improving life for patients and caregivers. Retrieved April 2018 from http://www.webmd.com/palliative-care/coping-with-a-life-threatening-illness.

 Acute Care   Collaborative   Community/Home Care   Cultural

4. Wheeler, S. K., Foster, J. (March 2013). Holistic healing: Putting patients in the driver's seat. *Minority Nurse*. Retrieved April 2018 from https://minoritynurse.com/holistic-healing-putting-patients-in-the-drivers-seat/.

5. Deckelbaum, R. J., Williams, C. L. (2001). Childhood obesity: The health issue. *Obes Res*, 9(5), S239–S243.

6. Smith, J. S., Smith, K. R., Rainey, S. L. (2006). The psychology of burn care. *J Trauma Nurs*, 13(3), 105–106.

7. Ulene, V. (May 23, 2011). Why are unhealthy people so reluctant to change their lifestyles? *LA Times*. Retrieved April 2018 from http://articles.latimes.com/2011/may/23/health/la-he-the-md-change-illness-20110523.

8. Marshal, C. (2012). Lifestyle changes due to chronic illness and how to deal with it. Retrieved April 2018 from https://msmeans.wordpress.com/2012/01/22/lifestyle-changes-due-to-chronic-illness-and-how-to-deal-with-it/.

9. Active listening: Hear what people are really saying. (No date). *Mind Tools*. Retrieved April 2018 from http://www.mindtools.com/CommSkll/ActiveListening.htm.

10. Ghosh, S. (2015). Gender identity. Retrieved April 2018 from http://emedicine.medscape.com/article/917990-overview.

11. Willkinson-Ryan, T., Westen, D. (2000). Identity disturbance in borderline personality disorder: An empirical investigation. *Am J Psychiatry*, 157(4), 528–541.

12. Daniels, R. (2003). *Nursing Fundamentals: Caring & Clinical Decision Making—Summary Chapter 43: Self-Concept*. Retrieved April 2018 from http://www.delmarlearning.com/companions/content/0766838366/students/ch43/summary.asp.

13. Boeree, G. (1997, 2006). Personality theories: Karen Horney. Retrieved April 2018 from webspace.ship.edu/cgboer/horney.html.

14. Breitenbach, M. (2006). Coping with serious illness: Letting change into your life. Retrieved April 2018 from ezinearticles.com/?coping-with-serious-illness-Letting-Change-into-your-Life&id=150109.

15. Gronley, M. (2018). What is depression. Retrieved April 2018 from http://psychiatristscottsdale.com/what-is-depression/.

16. Gronley, M. (No date). Health benefits of laughter. Retrieved April 2018 from http://psychiatristscottsdale.com/health-benefits-of-laughter/.

17. Berger, K. S. (2008). *The Developing Person Through the Life Span*. New York: Worth, 288–290.

18. Newell, R. (2002). The fear-avoidance model: Helping patients to cope with disfigurement. *Nurs Times*, 98(16), 38–39.

19. Langone, M. (1988). What is a cult? Adapted from Cults: Questions and answers. *International Cultic Studies Association (ICSA)*. Retrieved April 2018 from http://www.bibliotecapleyades.net/sociopolitica/esp_sociopol_mindcon27.htm.

20. Lalich, J., Langone, M. (2006). Characteristics associated with cult groups. In Lalich, J., Tobias, M. (eds). *Take Back Your Life: Recovering from Cults and Abusive Relationships*. 2nd ed., revised and expanded. Berkeley, CA: Bay Tree, 327–328.

21. Vedantam, S. (June 26, 2005). Patients' diversity is often discounted: Alternatives to mainstream medical treatment call for recognizing ethnic, social differences. *Washington Post*. Retrieved April 2018 from http://www.washingtonpost.com/wp-dyn/content/article/2005/06/25/AR2005062500982_pf.html.

22. Gronley, M. (No date). Effects of exercise on depression. Retrieved April 2018 from http://psychiatristscottsdale.com/effects-of-exercise-on-depression/.

23. Mays, G. P., Smith, S. A. (2011). Evidence links increases in public health spending to decline in preventable deaths. *Health Affairs*, 30(8), 1585–1593.

24. Griswold, K. S. (2012). Communities of solution: The Folsom Report revisited. *Ann Family Med*, 10(3), 250–260.

---

risk for Poisoning

Taxonomy II: Safety/Protection—Class 4 Environmental Hazards (00037) **[Diagnostic Division:** Safety**]**, Approved 1980; Revised 2006, 2013, 2017

DEFINITION: Susceptible to accidental exposure to, or ingestion of, drugs or dangerous products in sufficient doses that may compromise health.

RISK FACTORS
Internal

Emotional disturbance

Inadequate precautions against poisoning; inadequate knowledge of poisoning prevention

Inadequate knowledge of pharmacological agents; [narrow therapeutic margin of safety of specific pharmaceutical agents (e.g., therapeutic versus toxic level, half-life, method of uptake and degradation in body, adequacy of organ function)]

Occupational setting without adequate safeguards

Insufficient vision

External

Access to dangerous product

Access to pharmaceutical agent

(continues on page 642)

 Diagnostic Studies   Evidence Based Practice   Medications   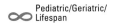 Pediatric/Geriatric/Lifespan

risk for Poisoning (continued)

Access to illicit drugs potentially contaminated by poisonous additives

[Use of multiple herbal supplements or megadosing]

Associated Condition: Alteration in cognitive function

Sample Clinical Applications: Substance abuse, dementia, cataracts, glaucoma, hepatitis, cirrhosis, renal failure, depression, suicidal ideation, developmental delay

DESIRED OUTCOMES/EVALUATION CRITERIA

Sample **NOC** linkages:

Risk Control: Drug Use: Personal actions to understand, prevent, eliminate, or reduce the threats to health associated with drug use

Knowledge: Medication: Extent of understanding conveyed about the safe use of medication

Safe Home Environment: Physical arrangements to minimize environmental factors that might cause physical injury in the home

Client/Caregiver Will (Include Specific Time Frame)

- Verbalize understanding of dangers of poisoning.
- Identify hazards that could lead to accidental poisoning.
- Correct external hazards as identified.
- Demonstrate necessary actions or lifestyle changes to promote safe environment.

ACTIONS/INTERVENTIONS

Sample **NIC** linkages:

Medication Management: Facilitation of safe and effective use of prescription and over-the-counter drugs

Environmental Management: Safety: Monitoring and manipulation of the physical environment to promote safety

NURSING PRIORITY NO. 1 To assess causative/contributing factors:

- Identify internal and external risk factors in client's environment, including presence of infants, young children, or frail elderly *(who are at risk for accidental poisoning)* and teenagers or young adults *(who are at risk for medication experimentation);* confused or chronically ill person on multiple medications; person with potential for suicidal action; person who partakes in illicit drug use/dealing (e.g., methamphetamines, opioids, cocaine, heroin); and person who manufactures drugs in home (e.g., methamphetamines).
- Note age and cognitive status of client and care providers *to identify individuals who could be at higher risk for accidental poisoning. Babies, toddlers, and preschoolers are at risk because they are curious, like to put things into their mouths, and aren't aware of what's safe to eat. Certain medications (e.g., calcium channel blockers, sulfonylureas, opiates, amphetamines, sodium channel blockers, and tricyclic antidepressants; drugs of abuse that are potentially fatal include opiates and all amphetamines [including methamphetamine and MDMA]) can kill a toddler with a single dose. While school-age children can recognize danger and are at lower risk of unintentional poisoning, they are at risk for inadvertent overdose when taking medications without adequate supervision or when taking medications belonging to another. Adolescents are at higher risk for experimentation due to natural inclination to take risks, peer pressure, and easy access to drugs. They are also at risk for suicide attempts (with overdose of medications, from illicit drug overdose or adverse reactions, alcohol toxicity).*[1,8,10] *Note: A 2013 U.S. study revealed that 67,000 children (most between the ages of 2 and 5 years) were treated in emergency departments for accidental ingestion of OTC or adult prescription drugs*

 Acute Care Collaborative Community/ Home Care Cultural

found in the home.[2] Elderly persons are at risk because of the higher number of prescription and OTC medications they consume (polypharmacy) and because of visual and cognitive impairments, which can cause them to forget what medications have been consumed and in what amounts they were taken. Elderly persons are also likely to share medications. In addition, the presence of nutritional deficits and renal or hepatic degeneration can reduce ability to detoxify drugs. Note: One large study showed that certain medication classes such as analgesics, anticoagulants, anticonvulsants, asthma therapies, psychotherapeutics, and some cardiovascular agents were associated with high hazard factors.[3,4]

- Assess mood, coping abilities, and personality styles (e.g., temperament, impulsive behavior, level of self-esteem) *that may result in carelessness and increased risk-taking without consideration of consequences or suicidal actions.* (Refer to ND risk for Suicide.)
- Determine client's allergies to medications and foods *in order to avoid exposure to substances causing potentially lethal reaction.*
- Ascertain client's knowledge and use of medications. *People may believe "if a little is good, a lot is better," placing them at risk for overdose and adverse drug effects or interactions. This belief pattern may also be responsible for client's use of multiple drugs at the same time (polypharmacy), which also can occur when multiple prescribers are unaware of each other or the client has multiple medical conditions requiring medications. Knowledge and use also affect the client's storage (e.g., may/may not use labeled bottles) and/or taking of medications that look alike (potentiating risk of overdose or adverse drug interactions). The elderly may unintentionally take the wrong medication at the wrong time or "double up," forgetting that they already took their daily dose of a prescription medicine.[13]*
- Determine specific drug hazards:
  - 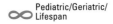Use of prescription, OTC medications, and culturally based home remedies. *These have potential for intentional and accidental overdose, as well as dangerous interactions. Drugs that are therapeutic in small doses may be deadly when taken in excess (e.g., beta blockers, warfarin, digoxin). One of the most common problems is inadvertent overdosage of acetaminophen (Tylenol), either by increased dosing or by taking it with a combination product also containing acetaminophen. Note: In 2013, the American Association of Poison Control Center reported that drug classes most frequently involved in toxic exposures in adults were analgesics (11.5%), sedatives/hypnotics/antipsychotics (5.9%), and antidepressants (4.2%). In children of 5 years or less, the drugs were analgesics (9.8%), and topical preparations (6.1%).[4,11]*
  - 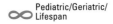Availability or regular use of vitamins and mineral and herbal supplements. *Vitamins (especially A and D) are toxic in large doses, and iron is especially harmful, often fatal to children.[10] Herbal drugs can be a source of poisoning (usually when taken long term) due to toxicity of individual ingredients or from contaminants (e.g., mercury, lead, arsenic).*
  - 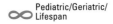Abuse of alcohol or other drugs (e.g., cocaine, methamphetamine, lysergic acid diethylamide, methadone). *Those who abuse street drugs are at high risk for overdose because the purity of these drugs is largely unknown. A person may be trying to get high but unwittingly take more drugs than his/her body can handle. These substances have potential for adverse reactions, cumulative effects with other substances, and risk for intentional and accidental overdose. Note: As little as 1 oz of alcohol or a single dose of many drugs of abuse can cause serious injury/death in a small child.[9,11]*
- Identify environmental hazards:

  Storage of household chemicals (e.g., oven, toilet bowl, or drain cleaners; dishwasher products; bleach; hydrogen peroxide; fluoride preparations; essential oils; furniture polish; lighter fluid; lamp oil; kerosene; paints; turpentine; rust remover; lubricant oils; bug sprays or powders; fertilizers) *are readily available toxins in various forms that are often improperly stored.[5–9]*

  Review client's home, employment, or work environment *for exposure to chemicals, including vapors and fumes.*

  Refer to ND risk for Contamination for environmental issues.
- Review results of laboratory tests and toxicology screening, as indicated. *Guides treatment when overdose or accidental poisoning is known or suspected.*

 Diagnostic Studies   Evidence Based Practice   Medications   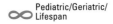 Pediatric/Geriatric/Lifespan   **643**

NURSING PRIORITY NO. 2   To assist in correcting factors that can lead to accidental poisoning:

- 🏠∞ 💊📝 Discuss medication safety with client/significant other (SO) according to individual needs:
Prevent accidental ingestion:[3-7,11]
Emphasize importance of supervising infant/child, frail elderly, or individuals with cognitive limitations.
Keep medicines and vitamins out of sight and reach of children or cognitively impaired persons.
Use child-resistant or tamper-resistant caps and lock medication cabinets.
Recap medication containers immediately after obtaining current dosage. Do not leave open container behind.
> *Note: Many accidental poisonings occur when parent/caregiver steps away for a moment and child gets into product that was left out.*
Code medicines for the visually impaired.
Tell client to turn on light if the room is dark and to put on glasses (if visually impaired) before taking or giving medications.
Refer to/administer children's medications as drugs, not candy, *to prevent confusion.*
Emphasize environmental safety regarding medications for all situations in which young child may be exposed (e.g., all rooms of the home, grandparents' home, day care, preschool).[8]
Discuss vitamin use (especially those containing iron) *that can be poisonous to children if taken in large doses or in small doses over time.*[8-10]
Prevent duplication/possible overdose:[3-7]
Review analgesic safety (e.g., acetaminophen is an ingredient in many OTC medications, and unintentional overdose can occur).[12]
Keep updated list of all medications (prescription, OTC, herbals, supplements) and review with healthcare providers when medications are changed, new ones are added, or new healthcare providers are consulted.
Keep prescription medication in original bottle with label. Do not mix with other medication or place in unmarked containers.
Have responsible SO(s)/home health nurse supervise medication regimen/prepare medications for the cognitively or visually impaired, or obtain prefilled medicine boxes from pharmacy.
Take prescription medications and OTC drugs as prescribed on label.
Do not adjust medication dosage.
Retain and read safety information that accompanies prescriptions about expected effects, nuisance side effects, reportable and adverse affects, and how to manage forgotten dose.
Prevent taking medications that interact with one another or OTC/herbals/other supplements in an undesired or dangerous manner:[3-7]
- Keep list of and reveal medication allergies, including type of reaction, to healthcare providers/pharmacist.
- Wear medical alert bracelet or necklace, as appropriate.
- Do not take outdated or expired medications. Do not save partial prescriptions to use another time.
- Encourage discarding outdated or unused drug safely (disposing in hazardous waste collection areas, not down drain or toilet).
- Do not take medications prescribed for another person.
- Avoid mixing alcohol with medications (potentiates effects of many drugs).
- 🔄 Coordinate care when multiple healthcare providers are involved *to limit number of prescriptions and dosage levels.*

NURSING PRIORITY NO. 3   To promote wellness (Teaching/Discharge Considerations):

- 🏠 Discuss general poison-prevention measures:[3-7]
∞ Encourage parent/caregiver to place safety stickers on dangerous products (drugs and chemicals) *to warn children of harmful contents.*
∞ Teach children about hazards of poisonous substances and to "ask first" before eating or drinking anything.
💊 Review drug side effects, potential interactions, and possibilities of misuse or overdosing (as with vitamin megadosing, etc.).[9]

    Acute Care   Collaborative   Community/Home Care   Cultural

∞ Discuss issues regarding drug use in home (e.g., alcohol, marijuana, heroin) *to provide opportunity to address potential for client's/SO's accidental overdose or accidental ingestion by children when drugs or drug paraphernalia are in the home.*[10]

- Provide list of emergency numbers (i.e., local or national poison control numbers, physician's office) to be placed by telephone *for use if poisoning occurs.*

- Instruct caregiver in event of poisoning, to have product container on hand when contacting emergency provider.

- Encourage client to obtain regular screening tests at prescribed intervals (e.g., prothrombin time/international normalized ratio for Coumadin; drug levels for Dilantin, digoxin; liver function studies when lipid-lowering agents [statins] are prescribed; renal and thyroid function and serum glucose levels for antimanics [lithium] use) *to ascertain that circulating blood levels are within therapeutic range and absence of adverse effects.*

- ∞ Ask healthcare provider/pharmacist about any considered medications if pregnant, nursing, or planning to become pregnant, *as some drugs are dangerous to fetus or nursing infant.*

- Refer substance abuser to detoxification programs, inpatient/outpatient rehabilitation, counseling, support groups, and psychotherapy.

- Encourage participation in community awareness and education programs (e.g., cardiopulmonary resuscitation and first aid class, home and workplace safety, hazardous materials disposal, access emergency medical personnel) *to assist individuals to identify and correct risk factors in environment and be prepared for emergency situation.*

DOCUMENTATION FOCUS

Assessment/Reassessment
- Identified risk factors noting internal and external concerns.
- Drug allergies or sensitivities.
- Current medications prescribed or available to individual, use of OTC medications, herbals or supplements, illicit drug use.

Planning
- Plan of care and who is involved in the planning.
- Teaching plan.

Implementation/Evaluation
- Response to interventions, teaching, and actions performed.
- Attainment or progress toward desired outcome(s).
- Modification to plan of care.

Discharge Planning
- Long-term needs and who is responsible for actions to be taken.
- Specific referrals made.

References

1. Food and Drug Administration. (2017). How the FDA can help solve the overdose crisis. Retrieved April 2018 from https://www.painnewsnetwork.org/stories/2017/10/4/how-the-fda-can-help-solve-the-overdose-crisis.
2. SafeKids Worldwide. (2013). An in-depth look at keeping young children safe around medications. Retrieved April 2018 from http://issuu.com/safekids/docs/2013-medication-safety-report/1?e=4874392/2095890.
3. Manno, M. S. (2006). Preventing adverse drug events. *Nursing*, 36(3), 56–61.
4. Hayes, B. D., Klein-Schwartz, W., Gonzales, L. F. (2009). Causes of therapeutic errors in older adults: Evaluation of National Poison Center data. *J Am Geriatr Soc*, 57(4), 653–658.
5. Stoppler, M. C. (Updated 2017). Poison proofing your home. Retrieved April 2018 from http://www.emedicinehealth.com/poison_proofing_your_home/article_em.htm.
6. Advance for Nurses. Patient Handouts. (No date). Keeping your children safe from accidental poisoning. Retrieved April 2018 from http://www.advanceweb.com/SharedResources/

 Diagnostic Studies   Evidence Based Practice   Medications   Pediatric/Geriatric/Lifespan

AdvanceforNurses/Resources/DownloadableResources/N6031405_p37Handout.pdf.

7. American Society of Health-System Pharmacists (ASHP). Preventing accidental poisoning. Retrieved April 2018 from http://www.safemedication.com/safemed/MedicationTipsTools/WhatYouShouldKnow/PreventingAccidentalPoisoning.aspx.

8. Lee, L. (2010). Home is where the hurt is? Child proofing your house. Retrieved April 2018 from http://childrenshospitalblog.org/home-is-where-the-hurt-is-tips-for-baby-proofing-your-house/.

9. Swierzewski, S. J. (2015). Prevention of poisoning. Retrieved April 2018 from http://www.healthcommunities.com/poisoning/prevention.shtml.

10. The Recommended Daily. (2012). The overdose risks of vitamins: Why proper dosage matters. Retrieved

April 2018 from https://smartypantsvitamins.com/the-overdose-risks-of-vitamins-why-proper-dosage-matters/.

11. Mowry, J. B., Spyker, D. A., Catilina, L. R. (2014). 2013 Annual Report of the American Association of Poison Control Centers' National Poison Data System (NPDS): 31st Annual Report. Retrieved April 2018 from https://www.readbyqxmd.com/read/25559822/2013-annual-report-of-the-american-association-of-poison-control-centers-national-poison-data-system-npds-31st-annual-report.

12. Smith, D. H. (2007). Managing acute acetaminophen toxicity. *Nursing*, 37(1), 58–63.

13. Zurakowski, T. (2009). The practicalities and pitfalls of polypharmacy. *Nurse Pract*, 34(4), 36–41.

risk for perioperative Positioning Injury

Taxonomy II: Safety/Protection—Class 2 Physical Injury (00087) [**Diagnostic Division:** Safety], Submitted 1994; Revised 2006, 2013, 2017

DEFINITION: Susceptible to inadvertent anatomical and physical changes as a result of posture or positioning equipment used during an invasive/surgical procedure, which may compromise health.

RISK FACTORS
Immobilization
Associated Condition: Disorientation; sensoriperceptual disturbance from anesthesia
Edema
Emaciation; obesity
Muscle weakness
Sample Clinical Applications: Operative procedures, arthritis, obesity, malnutrition, peripheral vascular disease

DESIRED OUTCOMES/EVALUATION CRITERIA

Sample NOC linkages:
Physical Injury Severity: Severity of signs and symptoms of injuries to the body
Risk Control: Personal actions to understand, prevent, eliminate, or reduce modifiable health threats
Tissue Perfusion: Peripheral: Adequacy of blood flow through the small vessels of the extremities to maintain tissue function

Client Will (Include Specific Time Frame)
• Be free of injury related to perioperative disorientation or altered consciousness.
• Be free of untoward skin and tissue injury or changes lasting beyond 24 to 48 hr postprocedure.

ACTIONS/INTERVENTIONS

Sample NIC linkages:
Positioning: Intraoperative: Placement of the patient or body part to promote surgical exposure while reducing the risk of discomfort and complications
Skin Surveillance: Collection and analysis of patient data to maintain skin and mucous membrane integrity
Circulatory Precautions: Protection of a localized area with limited perfusion

 Acute Care Collaborative Community/Home Care Cultural

NURSING PRIORITY NO. 1 To identify individual risk factors/needs:

- Consider anticipated type and length of procedure, type of anesthesia to be used, and customary required position (e.g., supine, lithotomy, prone, lateral, sitting) *to increase awareness of potential postoperative complications. Studies show consensus of clinical opinion that perioperative nerve injury is a significant issue and that safe and correct positioning is crucial to avoid causing peripheral neuropathy during the anesthetic and/ or surgical episode. Coppieters et al. suggest that there is evidence of several identifiable mechanisms that contribute to perioperative positioning injuries. These include stretch, traction, compression, generalized vascular ischemia, and metabolic derangement (e.g., diabetes and atherosclerosis).*[1,2,6,9,12]

- ∞ Review client's history, noting age, weight, height, nutritional status, physical limitations (e.g., prostheses, implants, range-of-motion restrictions) and preexisting conditions (vascular, respiratory, circulatory, neurological, immunocompromise). *These factors affect choice of position for the procedure (e.g., elderly person with no subcutaneous padding or severe arthritis). Presence of certain conditions can cause the risk of skin and tissue integrity problems during surgery (e.g., diabetes mellitus, hypertension and hypotension, tobacco use, obesity, presence of peripheral vascular disease, level of hydration, temperature of extremities).*[1,2,8,10,12]

- Evaluate and document client's preoperative reports of neurological, sensory, or motor deficits *for comparative baseline of perioperative and postoperative sensations.*

- Assess the individual's responses to preoperative sedation and medication, noting level of sedation or adverse effects (e.g., drop in blood pressure) and report to surgeon as indicated. *Hypotension is a common factor associated with nerve ischemia.*[3,12]

- Evaluate environmental conditions/safety issues surrounding the sedated client (e.g., client alone in holding area, side rails up on bed and cart, use of tourniquets and arm boards, need for local injections) *that predispose client to potential tissue injury.*[1,3,7,8]

NURSING PRIORITY NO. 2 To position client to provide protection for anatomic structures and to prevent injury:

- ✚ Stabilize and lock transport cart or bed when transferring client to and from operating room table. Provide body and limb support for client during transfers, using adequate numbers of personnel *to prevent client fall or shear and friction injuries, as well as to prevent injury to personnel.*[3,8,11]

- Position client, using sufficient staff, appropriate positioning equipment or devices, and padding *to provide protection for anatomic structures and to prevent injury:*[1–3,11]
  Keep head in neutral position (when client in supine position) and arm boards at less than a 90-degree angle and level with floor *to prevent neural injuries.*
  Maintain neck alignment and provide protection or padding for forehead, eyes, nose, chin, breasts, genitalia, knees, and feet *when client is in prone position.*
  Protect bony prominences and pressure points on dependent side (e.g., axillary roll for dependent axilla; lower leg flexed at hip, upper leg straight; padding between knees, ankles, and feet) *when client is in lateral position.*
  Place legs in stirrups simultaneously, adjusting stirrup height to client's legs, maintaining symmetrical position, and pad popliteal space as indicated *to reduce risk of peroneal and tibial nerve damage, prevent muscle strain, and reduce risk of hip dislocation when lithotomy position is used.*

- Check that positioning equipment is correct size for client, is firm and stable, and is adjusted accordingly.[2,11]

- Use gel pads or similar devices over the operating room bed. *Decreases pressure at any given point by redistributing overall pressure across a larger surface area.*[2,6]

- Limit use of pillows, blankets, molded foam devices, towels, and sheet rolls, *which may produce only a minimum of pressure reduction or contribute to friction injuries.*[2]

- Place safety straps strategically *to secure client for specific procedure. Avoid pressure on extremities when securing straps to limit possibility of compromising circulation and pressure injuries.*[11]

- Realign or maintain body alignment during procedure as needed. *Changes in position may expose or damage otherwise protected body tissue. The position change may be planned or imperceptible and may result from adding or deleting positioning devices, adjusting the procedure bed in some manner, or moving the client on the procedure bed.*[2,11]
- Apply and periodically reposition padding of pressure points/bony prominences (e.g., arms, shoulders, ankles) and neurovascular pressure points (e.g., breasts, knees, ears) *to maintain position of safety and prevent injury from prolonged pressure.*
- Protect body from contact with metal parts of the operating table, *which could produce electrical injury or burns.*[1,4]
- Position extremities to facilitate periodic evaluation of hands, fingers, and toes. *Prevents accidental trauma from moving table attachments and allows for repositioning of extremities to prevent neurovascular injuries from prolonged pressure. Extremities should not extend beyond the end of operating table to reduce risk of compression or stretch injury.*[8,11]
- Check peripheral pulses and skin color and temperature periodically *to monitor circulation.*
- Prevent pooling of prep and irrigating solutions and body fluids. *Pooling of liquids in areas of high pressure under client increases risk of pressure ulcer development and presents electrical hazard.*[5,6]
- Reposition slowly at transfer and in bed (especially halothane-anesthetized client) *to prevent severe drop in blood pressure, dizziness, or unsafe transfer.*
- Position client following extubation *to protect airway and facilitate respiratory effort.*
- Determine specific postoperative positioning guidelines (e.g., head of bed slightly elevated following spinal anesthesia *to prevent headache,* turn to unoperated side following pneumonectomy *to facilitate maximal respiratory effort).*[1]

NURSING PRIORITY NO. 3   To promote wellness (Teaching/Discharge Considerations):

- Maintain equipment in good working order *to identify potential hazards in the surgical suite and implement corrections as appropriate.*[6]
- Provide perioperative teaching relative to client safety issues (including not crossing legs during procedures performed under local or light anesthesia, postoperative needs or limitations, signs/symptoms requiring medical evaluation) *to reduce incidence of preventable complications.*
- Inform client and postoperative caregivers of expected or transient reactions (e.g., low backache, localized numbness, and reddening or skin indentations, which should quickly resolve) *to help them identify problems or concerns that require follow-up.*
- Assist with therapies and perform nursing actions, including skin care measures, application of elastic stockings, early mobilization *to enhance circulation and venous return, and to promote skin and tissue integrity.*
- Encourage and assist with frequent range-of-motion exercises *to prevent or reduce joint stiffness.*
- Refer to appropriate resources, as needed.

DOCUMENTATION FOCUS

Assessment/Reassessment
- Findings, including individual risk factors for problems in the perioperative setting and need to modify routine activities or positions.
- Periodic evaluation of monitoring activities.

Planning
- Plan of care and who is involved in planning.
- Teaching plan.

Implementation/Evaluation
- Response to interventions and actions performed.
- Attainment or progress toward desired outcome(s).
- Modifications to plan of care.

 Acute Care   Collaborative   Community/ Home Care   Cultural

Discharge Planning

• Long-term needs and who is responsible for actions to be taken.

References

1. Doenges, M. E., Moorhouse, M. F., Murr, A. C. (2010). Surgical intervention. *Nursing Care Plans: Guidelines for Individualizing Client Care Across the Life Span.* 8th ed. Philadelphia, PA: F. A. Davis.
2. Beckett, A. E. (2010). Are we doing enough to prevent patient injury caused by positioning for surgery? *J Perioper Pract,* 20(1), 160–163.
3. Knight, D. J. W., Mahajan, R. P. (2004). Patient positioning in anaesthesia. *Contin Educ Anaesth Crit Care Pain,* 4(5), 160–163.
4. Rothrock, J. (1996). *Perioperative Nursing Care Planning.* St. Louis, MO: Mosby.
5. Meeker, M., Rothrock, J. (1999). *Alexander's Care of the Patient in Surgery.* 11th ed. St. Louis, MO: Mosby.
6. Dagi, T. F., Schecter, W. (2008). Preparation of the operating room. *ACS Surgery: Principles and Practice Online.* Retrieved April 2018 from https://www.slideshare.net/medbookonline/acs0108-preparation-of-the-operating-room.
7. Dunn, D. (2005). Preventing perioperative complications in special populations. *Nursing,* 35(11), 36–43.
8. Dunn, D. (2006). Age-smart care: Preventing perioperative complications in older adults. *Nursing,* 4(3), 30–39.
9. Coppieters, M. W., van de Velde, M., Sappaerts, K. H. (2002). Positioning in anaesthesiology: Toward a better understanding of stretch-induced perioperative neuropathies. *Anesthesiology,* 97, 75–81.
10. Bale, E., Berrecloth, R. (2010). The obese patient. Anaesthetic issues: Airway and positioning. *J Periop Pract,* 8, 294–299.
11. Pirie, S. (2010). Patient care in the preoperative environment. *J Periop Pract,* 8, 294–299.
12. Welch, M. B., et al. (2009). Preoperative peripheral nerve injuries: A retrospective study of 380,680 cases during a 10-year period at a single institution. *Anesthesiology,* 111(3), 490–497.

Post-Trauma Syndrome

Taxonomy II: Coping/Stress Tolerance—Class 1 Post-Trauma Responses (00141) [**Diagnostic Division:** Ego Integrity], Submitted 1986; Revised 1998, 2010, 2017

DEFINITION: Sustained maladaptive response to a traumatic, overwhelming event.

RELATED FACTORS

Diminished ego strength; perceives event as traumatic; survivor role

Environment not conducive to needs; insufficient social support

Exaggerated sense of responsibility

Self-injurious behavior

DEFINING CHARACTERISTICS

Subjective

Intrusive thoughts or dreams; nightmares; flashbacks;

Heart palpitations; headache

Hopelessness; shame; guilt/[survival guilt; guilt about behavior required for survival]

Anxiety; fear; grieving; depression; horror

Reports feeling numb

Gastrointestinal irritation; [change in appetite]

Alteration in concentration

[Change in sleep; fatigue; loss of interest in usual activities, loss of feeling of intimacy or sexuality]

Objective

Alteration in mood; panic attacks

Hypervigilance; exaggerated startle response; irritability; neurosensory irritability

(continues on page 650)

 Diagnostic Studies   Evidence Based Practice   Medications   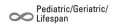 Pediatric/Geriatric/Lifespan

Post-Trauma Syndrome (continued)

Anger; rage; aggression
Avoidance behaviors; denial; repression; alienation
History of detachment; dissociative amnesia
Substance misuse/[abuse]; compulsive behavior; [poor impulse control]
Enuresis
[Difficulty with interpersonal relationships; dependence on others; work or school failure]
[Stages:
Acute: Begins within 6 months and does not last longer than 6 months
Chronic: Lasts more than 6 months
Delayed Onset: Period of latency of 6 months or more before onset of symptoms]
At Risk Population: Destruction of one's home; displacement from home
Event outside the range of usual human experience; history of being a prisoner of war; history of torture or criminal victimization
Duration of traumatic event
Exposure to disaster, war, or epidemic; exposure to event involving multiple deaths
History of abuse
Human service occupations
Serious accident; serious injury or threat to self or loved one
Witnessing mutilation or violent death
Sample Clinical Applications: Traumatic injuries, physical/psychological abuse, dissociative disorder

DESIRED OUTCOMES/EVALUATION CRITERIA

Sample NOC linkages:
Comfort Status: Psychospiritual: Psychospiritual ease related to self-concept, emotional well-being, source of inspiration, and meaning and purpose in one's life
Fear Self-Control: Personal actions to eliminate or reduce disabling feelings of apprehension, tension, or uneasiness from an identifiable source
Abuse Recovery: Emotional [or] Physical: Extent of healing of psychological/physical injuries due to abuse

Client Will (Include Specific Time Frame)
• Express own feelings and reactions, avoiding projection.
• Verbalize a positive self-image.
• Report reduced anxiety or fear when memories occur.
• Demonstrate ability to deal with emotional reactions in an individually appropriate manner.
• Demonstrate appropriate changes in behavior or lifestyle (e.g., share experiences with others, seek and get support from significant others [SOs] as needed, change in job or residence).
• Report absence of physical manifestations (e.g., pain, chronic fatigue).

ACTIONS/INTERVENTIONS

Sample NIC linkages:
Support System Enhancement: Facilitation of support to patient by family, friends, and community
Counseling: Use of an interactive helping process focusing on the needs, problems, or feelings of the patient and significant others to enhance or support coping, problem-solving, and interpersonal relationships
Anxiety Reduction: Minimizing apprehension, dread, foreboding, or uneasiness related to an unidentified source of anticipated danger

 Acute Care Collaborative Community/Home Care Cultural

NURSING PRIORITY NO. 1   To assess causative factor(s) and individual reaction:

Acute

- Observe for and elicit information about physical or psychological injury and note associated stress-related symptoms (e.g., numbness, headache, tightness in chest, nausea, pounding heart). *Anxiety is viewed as a normal reaction to a realistic danger or threat, and noting these factors can identify the severity of the anxiety the client is experiencing in the circumstances. In posttraumatic stress disorder (PTSD), this reaction is changed or damaged. People who have PTSD may feel stressed or frightened even when they're no longer in danger. Some factors that appear to increase the risk of PTSD are assaultive trauma or trauma that occurs at an early age.*[2,12]
- Identify such psychological responses as anger, shock, acute anxiety, confusion, and denial. Note laughter, crying, calm or agitated, excited (hysterical) behavior, as well as expressions of disbelief, guilt and/or self-blame, and labile emotions. *Indicators of severe response to trauma that client has experienced and need for specific interventions.*[7]
- Assess client's knowledge of and anxiety related to the situation. Note ongoing threat to self (e.g., contact with perpetrator and/or associates) or perception of others as threatening. *Client may be aware but speak as though the incident is related to someone else. Flashbacks may occur with the individual reliving the incident/event.*[7]
- Note occupation (e.g., police, fire, rescue, emergency department staff, corrections officer, mental health worker, disaster responders, soldier or support personnel in combat zone, as well as family members). *These occupations carry a high risk for constantly being involved in traumatic events and the potential for exacerbation of stress response and block to recovery. In addition, family members are subjected to the same trauma because they see the same events repeated on TV news channels and hear stories repeated by their loved one(s) who were directly involved.*[12]
- Identify social aspects of trauma or incident (e.g., disfigurement, chronic conditions or permanent disabilities, loss of home or community) *that affect ability to return to normal involvement in activities and work.*[7]
- Ascertain ethnic background, cultural and religious perceptions, and beliefs about the occurrence. *Client (or significant others) may believe occurrence is retribution from God or result of some indiscretion on client's part; client may in some way also blame self for the incident or occurrence. Individual's view of how he or she is coping may be influenced by cultural and community background, religious beliefs, and family influence.*[3,7]
- Determine degree of disorganization (e.g., task-oriented activity is not goal directed, organized, or effective; individual is overwhelmed by emotion much of the time). *Presence of persistent frightening thoughts and memories, reliving the event, feeling emotionally numb and unable to be close to friends and family members, and suffering from sleep and eating problems interfere with ability to manage daily living, work, and relationships with others.*[7,11]
- Identify whether incident has reactivated preexisting or coexisting situations (physical or psychological). *Traumas or difficulties in client's life and how they were dealt with will affect how the client views the current trauma.*[5]
- Determine disruptions in relationships (e.g., family, friends, coworkers, SOs). *Support persons may not know how to deal with client/situation and may be oversolicitous or withdraw; either of these actions will be counterproductive to client's ability to cope with situation.*[7]
- Note withdrawn behavior, use of denial, and use of chemical substances or impulsive behaviors (e.g., chain smoking, overeating). *Indicators of severity of anxiety and client's difficulty dealing with PTSD and need for interventions to address these behaviors.*[7]
- Be aware of signs of increasing anxiety (e.g., silence, stuttering, inability to sit still). *Increasing anxiety may indicate risk for violence or need for medication or other measures to decrease anxiety and help client manage feelings.*[7]
- Note verbal and nonverbal expressions of guilt or self-blame when client has survived trauma in which others died. Validate congruency of observations with verbalizations. *Sense of own responsibility (blame) and guilt about not having done something to prevent incident or not having been "good enough" to deserve survival are strong beliefs, especially in individuals who are influenced by background, religious, and cultural factors.*[1]

 Diagnostic Studies   Evidence Based Practice   Medications   Pediatric/Geriatric/Lifespan

- Assess signs and stage of grieving for self and others. *Identification and understanding of stages of grief assist with choice of interventions, plan of care, and movement toward resolution.*[1]
- Identify development of phobic reactions to ordinary articles (e.g., knives) and situations (e.g., walking in groups of people, strangers ringing doorbell). *These may trigger feelings from original trauma and need to be dealt with sensitively, accepting reality of feelings and stressing ability of client to deal with them.*[1]

Chronic (in addition to previous assessment)

- Evaluate continued somatic complaints. Investigate reports of new or changes in symptoms. *Reports of physical symptoms, such as gastric irritation, anorexia, insomnia, muscle tension, and headache may accompany disorganization and need further evaluation and interventions.*[1]
- Note manifestations of chronic pain or pain symptoms in excess of degree of physical injury. *Psychological responses may magnify or exacerbate physical symptoms, indicating need for interventions to help client deal with pain.*[5]
- Be aware of signs of severe or prolonged depression and note presence of flashbacks, intrusive memories, nightmares, panic attacks, and poor impulse control; problems with memory or concentration; thoughts and perceptions; and conflict, aggression, or rage. *Symptoms are not uncommon following a trauma of such magnitude, although client may feel that he or she is "going crazy."*[2,10]
- Assess degree of dysfunctional coping (including substance use or abuse, suicidal ideation) and consequences. *Identifies needs and depth of interventions required. Individuals display different levels of dysfunctional behavior in response to stress, and often the choice of chemical substances or substance abuse is a way of deadening the psychic pain.*[1]

NURSING PRIORITY NO. 2   To assist client to deal with situation that exists:

Acute

- Allow the client to work through own kind of adjustment. If the client is withdrawn or unwilling to talk, do not force the issue. *Each person is an individual and has own ways of coping. Being there and allowing client to choose own path conveys sense of confidence in ability to deal with situation.*
- Listen for expressions of fear of crowds or people. *May indicate continuing anxiety and difficulty reentering normal activities.*[7]
- ∞ Ascertain or monitor sleep pattern of children as well as adults. *Sleep disturbances or nightmares may develop, delaying resolution, impairing coping abilities, and interfering with return to desired lifestyle.*[5]
- Be aware of and assist client to use ego strengths in a positive way by acknowledging ability to handle what is happening. *Enhances self-concept and reduces sense of helplessness and powerlessness, thus enabling client to move on with life.*
- Encourage client to learn stress-management techniques, such as deep breathing, meditation, relaxation, and exercise. *Reduces stress, enhancing coping skills and helping to resolve situation.*[8]
- 🏠 Assist in dealing with practical concerns and effects of the incident, such as court appearances, altered relationships with SO(s), and employment problems. *In the period immediately following the traumatic incident, individual is in a state of numbness and shock. Thinking becomes difficult, and assistance with practical matters will help manage necessary activities for the person to move through this time.*
- 🌐 Identify employment and community resource groups. *Provides opportunity for ongoing support to deal with recurrent stressors as individual regroups and moves forward.*[9]
- 💊 Administer anti-anxiety or sedative and hypnotic medications with caution.

Chronic

- Continue listening to expressions of concern. *May have recurring symptoms, thus necessitating the need to continue talking about the incident.*[7]
- Permit free expression of feelings (may continue from the crisis phase). Do not rush client through expressions of feelings too quickly and refrain from providing false reassurances. *Client may believe pain or anguish is misunderstood and may be depressed. Statements such as "You don't understand" or "You weren't there" are a defense—a way of pushing others away—and need to be responded to with empathy and concern.*

 Acute Care   Collaborative   Community/ Home Care   Cultural

- Encourage client to talk out experience when ready, expressing feelings of fear, anger, loss, or grief. (Refer to NDs Grieving and complicated Grieving.) *Client may need to repeat story over and over and needs to be accepted and assured that feelings are normal for the unusual event experienced.*[7]
- Note whether feelings expressed appear congruent with events the client experienced. *Expressing feelings helps client recognize and identify them to enhance coping. Incongruency may indicate deeper conflict that can impede resolution.*[8]
- Encourage client to become aware and accepting of own feelings and reactions as being normal reactions in an abnormal situation. *There are no "bad" feelings, and awareness and acceptance enable client to deal with feelings once identified and move forward in recovery from traumatic event.*[4,11]
- Acknowledge reality of loss of self that existed before the incident. Assist client to move toward an acceptance of the potential for growth that exists within client. *Recognition that individual can never go back to being the person he or she was before the incident allows progress toward life as a different person.*[8]
- Continue to allow client to progress at own pace. *Taking own time to talk about what has happened and allowing feelings to be fully expressed aids in the healing process. If rushed, client may believe he or she is not accepted or understood.*[1]
- Give "permission" to express and deal with anger at the assailant or situation in acceptable ways. *Being free to express anger appropriately allows it to be dissipated so underlying feelings can be identified and dealt with, thus strengthening coping skills.*[1]
- Avoid prompting discussion of issues that cannot be resolved. Keep discussion on practical and emotional level rather than intellectualizing the experience. *When feelings (the experience) are intellectualized, uncomfortable insights and/or awareness are avoided by the use of rationalization, blocking resolution of feelings and impairing coping abilities.*[1]
- Provide for sensitive, trained counselors/therapists and engage in therapies, such as psychotherapy in conjunction with medications, implosive therapy (flooding), hypnosis, relaxation, Rolfing, memory work, cognitive restructuring, eye movement desensitization and reprocessing, and physical and occupational therapies. *Although it is not necessary for the helping person to have experienced the same kind of trauma as the client, sensitivity and listening skills are important to helping the client confront fears and learn new ways to cope with what has happened. Therapeutic use of desensitization techniques (flooding, implosive therapy) provides for extinction through exposure to the fear. Body work can alleviate muscle tension. Some techniques (Rolfing) help to bring blocked emotions to awareness as sensations of the traumatic event are reexperienced.*[7]
- Discuss use of psychotropic medication. *May be used to decrease anxiety, lift mood, aid in management of behavior, and ensure rest until client regains control of own self. Lithium may be used to reduce explosiveness; low-dose psychotropics may be used when loss of contact with reality is a problem.*[6]

NURSING PRIORITY NO. 3 To promote wellness (Teaching/Discharge Considerations):

- Assist client to identify and monitor feelings while therapy is occurring. *Promotes awareness and helps client know that control of feelings as they arise will help move beyond traumatic episode.*[7]
- Provide information about what reactions client may expect during each phase. Let client know these are common reactions and phrase in neutral terms of "You may or may not. . . ." *Knowledge of what may be experienced helps reduce fear of the unknown, thereby enabling client to manage reactions if they occur. Use of neutral terms lets client understand that not all reactions may occur in own situation.*
- Assist client to identify factors that may have created a vulnerable situation and that he or she may have power to change to protect self in the future. *While client is not responsible for event, may have unknowingly contributed to occurrence by his or her actions. Identifying those actions that are within client's power to change provides sense of control over seemingly uncontrollable situations.*[7]
- Avoid making value judgments. *Client may be judging self and caregiver needs to convey nonjudgmental stance to allow individual to deal with feelings of guilt and recrimination, accepting fact that he or she did the best client was capable of in the circumstances.*

 Diagnostic Studies   Evidence Based Practice   Medications   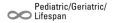 Pediatric/Geriatric/ Lifespan

- Discuss lifestyle changes client is contemplating and how they may contribute to recovery. *Client needs to evaluate appropriateness of plans and look at long-range consequences (e.g., moving away from effective support group) to make the best choice for the future.*[2]
- Assist with learning stress-management techniques. *Deep breathing, counting to 10 before reacting negatively or with violence, reviewing the situation, and reframing skills assist client in developing constructive ways to cope with feelings of powerlessness and to regain control of self. Reframing stressors or situation in other words or positive ideas can help client recognize and consider alternatives.*[2]
- Discuss drug regimen, potential side effects of prescribed medications, and necessity of prompt reporting of untoward effects.
- Discuss recognition of and ways to manage "anniversary reactions," reinforcing normalcy of recurrence of thoughts and feelings at this time. *Understanding that these feelings are to be expected and planning for them help client get through the anniversary of the event with the least difficulty.*
- Suggest support group for SO(s). *Family members may not understand client's reactions and need help with understanding them and learning how to deal with client in the most helpful manner.*[1]
- Encourage psychiatric consultation. *May need additional therapy if client is unable to maintain control, is violent or inconsolable, or does not seem to be making an adjustment. Participation in a group may be helpful.*[1]
- Refer for long-term family/marital counseling, if indicated. *Additional and ongoing support or therapy may be needed to help family resolve crisis and look at potential for growth. Client problems affect family members and other relationships, and further counseling may help resolve issues of enabling behavior and communication problems.*[9]
- Refer to NDs ineffective Coping, Grieving, complicated Grieving, and Powerlessness.

DOCUMENTATION FOCUS

Assessment/Reassessment
- Individual findings, noting current dysfunction and behavioral or emotional responses to the incident.
- Specifics of traumatic event.
- Reactions of family/SO(s).
- Cultural or religious beliefs and expectations.
- Availability and use of resources.

Planning
- Plan of care and who is involved in the planning.
- Teaching plan.

Implementation/Evaluation
- Responses to interventions, teaching, and actions performed.
- Emotional changes.
- Attainment or progress toward desired outcome(s).
- Modifications to plan of care.

Discharge Planning
- Long-term needs and who is responsible for actions to be taken.
- Specific referrals made.

References

1. Doenges, M., Townsend, M., Moorhouse, M. (1998). *Psychiatric Care Plans: Guidelines for Individualizing Care*. 3th ed. Philadelphia: F. A. Davis.
2. Townsend, M. (2003). *Psychiatric Mental Health Nursing: Concepts of Care*. 4th ed. Philadelphia: F. A. Davis.
3. Purnell, L. D. (2009). *Guide to Culturally Competent Health Care*. 2nd ed. Philadelphia: F. A. Davis.
4. Stuart, G. W. (2001). Anxiety responses and anxiety disorders. In Stuart, G. W., Laraia, M. T. (eds). *Principles and Practice of Psychiatric Nursing*. 7th ed. St. Louis, MO: Mosby.

 Acute Care   Collaborative   Community/Home Care   Cultural

5. Porth, C. M., Kunert, P. K. (2002). *Pathophysiology: Concepts of Altered Health States*. Philadelphia: J. B. Lippincott.
6. Townsend, M. (2001). *Nursing Diagnoses in Psychiatric Nursing: Care Plans and Psychotropic Medications*. 5th ed. Philadelphia: F. A. Davis.
7. National Institute of Mental Health. (2009, updated 2016). Anxiety disorders. NIH Publication No. 00-3879. Retrieved April 2018 from http://www.nimh.nih.gov/health/publications/anxiety-disorders/index.shtml?rf=53414.
8. Posttraumatic stress disorder—Part I. (June 1996). *Harvard Mental Health Letter*.
9. Posttraumatic stress disorder—Part II. (July 1996). *Harvard Mental Health Letter*.
10. Gore, T. A., Lucas, J. Z., Lubit, R. H. (Updated 2018). Posttraumatic stress disorder: Treatment and management. Retrieved April 2018 from http://emedicine.medscape.com/article/288154-treatment.
11. Lubit, R. (Updated 2016). Acute stress disorder. Retrieved April 2018 from http://emedicine.medscape.com/article/2192581-overview.
12. Breslau, N. (2009). The epidemiology of trauma, PTSD, and other posttrauma disorders. *Trauma Violence Abuse*, 10(3), 198–210.

risk for Post-Trauma Syndrome

Taxonomy II: Coping/Stress Tolerance—Class 1 Post-Trauma Responses (00145) [**Diagnostic Division:** Ego Integrity], Submitted 1986; Revised 1998, 2013, 2017

DEFINITION: Susceptible to sustained maladaptive response to a traumatic, overwhelming event, which may compromise health.

RISK FACTORS

Diminished ego strength; perceives event as traumatic; survivor role

Environment not conducive to needs; insufficient social support

Exaggerated sense of responsibility

Self-injurious behavior

At Risk Population: Destruction of one's home; displacement from home

Event outside the range of usual human experience; history of being a prisoner of war; history of torture or criminal victimization

Duration of traumatic event

Exposure to disaster, war, or epidemic; exposure to event involving multiple deaths

History of abuse

Human service occupations

Serious accident; serious injury or threat to self or loved one

Witnessing mutilation or violent death

Sample Clinical Applications: Traumatic injuries, physical/psychological abuse, dissociative disorder

DESIRED OUTCOMES/EVALUATION CRITERIA

Sample NOC linkages:

Fear Level: Severity of manifested apprehension, tension, or uneasiness arising from an identifiable source

Fear Self-Control: Personal actions to eliminate or reduce disabling feelings of apprehension, tension, or uneasiness from an identifiable source

Grief Resolution: Personal actions to adjust thoughts, feelings, and behaviors to actual or impending loss

Client Will (Include Specific Time Frame)
• Verbalize absence of disabling apprehension.
• Demonstrate ability to deal with emotional reactions in an individually appropriate manner.

(continues on page 656)

 Diagnostic Studies   Evidence Based Practice   Medications   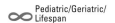 Pediatric/Geriatric/Lifespan

risk for Post-Trauma Syndrome (continued)

- Deal with practical aspects of situation (e.g., court appearances, temporary housing, funeral services, rebuilding life).
- Report relief or absence of physical manifestations (pain, nightmares, flashbacks, fatigue) associated with event.

ACTIONS/INTERVENTIONS

Sample NIC linkages:

Crisis Intervention: Use of short-term counseling to help the patient cope with a crisis and resume a state of functioning comparable to or better than the precrisis state

Coping Enhancement: Facilitation of cognitive and behavioral efforts to manage perceived stressors, changes, or threats which interfere with meeting life demands and roles

Support System Enhancement: Facilitation of support to patient by family, friends, and community

NURSING PRIORITY NO. 1   To assess contributing factors and individual reaction:

- Identify client who survived or witnessed traumatic event (e.g., airplane or motor vehicle crash, mass shooting, fire destroying home and lands, robbery at gunpoint, other violent act) *to recognize individual at high risk for posttrauma syndrome.*
- Note occupation (e.g., police, fire, emergency services personnel, rescue workers, disaster responders, soldiers and support personnel in combat areas, and family members). *Studies reveal a moderate to high percentage of posttraumatic stress disorder (PTSD) cases develop in these populations when they have been exposed to one or more traumatic incidents and their exposure lasts over longer periods of time (e.g., working a bomb site or plane crash).[10] In addition, family members are also at risk because they are subjected to the same trauma as they see the events repeated on TV news channels/hear stories repeated by their loved one(s) who were directly involved.*
- Assess client risk for developing PTSD using screening tool (e.g., Breslau Short Screening Scale or similar) should client report experiencing a traumatic event. *Short self-report questionnaire or other screening tool with simple "yes" or "no" responses may help with early identification of client at risk for posttrauma response. Recognizing symptoms and providing immediate treatment may prevent the development of PTSD.[12]*
- Assess client's knowledge of and anxiety related to potential for work-related trauma incident (e.g., shooting in line of duty or viewing body of murdered child); and number, duration, and intensity of recurring situations (e.g., emergency medical technician exposed to numerous on-the-job traumatic incidents; rescuers searching for victims of natural or human-caused disasters). *Having information about these situations enables individuals to think about and plan for eventualities so anxiety can be dealt with in a positive manner.[6]*
- Ascertain ethnic background and cultural or religious perceptions and beliefs about the occurrence. *Client may believe occurrence is retribution from God, the result of some indiscretion on his or her part, or in some way blame self for the incident or occurrence. Individual's view of how he or she is coping may be influenced by cultural background, religious beliefs, and family influence.[6]*
- Identify how client's experiences may affect current situation. *Individual who has had previous experiences with traumatic events (e.g., firefighter who deals with trauma on a regular basis or person who has been involved in a trauma herself or himself) may be more susceptible to PTSD and ineffective coping abilities.[1]*
- Listen for comments of guilt, humiliation, shame, or taking on responsibility (e.g., "I should have been more careful/gone back to get her"; "Don't call me a hero; I couldn't save my partner"; "My kids are the same age as the ones who died"). *Expressing guilt for actions that individual might have taken can lead to ruminations about lack of responsible behavior, leading to anxiety and PTSD.[7,10,11]*

 Acute Care   Collaborative   Community/ Home Care   Cultural

- Note verbal and nonverbal expressions of guilt or self-blame when client has survived trauma in which others died. *Sense of own responsibility (blame) and guilt about not having done something to prevent incident or not having been "good enough" to deserve surviving are strong beliefs, especially in individuals who are influenced by family background, religious, and cultural factors.*[1]
- Evaluate for life factors and stressors currently or recently occurring, such as displacement from home due to catastrophic event (e.g., illness or injury, fire, flood, violent storm, earthquake) happening to individual whose child is dying of cancer or who suffered abuse as a child. *Cumulative effects of multiple events can put the individual at higher risk for developing PTSD (acute added to delayed-onset reactions) and indicates need for preventive measures to be taken.*[3,10]
- Identify client's coping mechanisms. *Resolution of the posttrauma response is largely dependent on the coping skills the client has developed throughout own life and is able to bring to bear on current situation.*[3]
- Determine availability and usefulness of client's support systems, family, social, community, etc., being aware that family members themselves or community in general may also be at risk. *Having an effective available support system and talking with them about what is happening can help client and family members resolve feelings and move on with life in a positive manner.*[8]

NURSING PRIORITY NO. 2 To assist client to deal with situation that exists immediately post incident:

Postincident
- Provide a calm, safe environment. *Client can deal with disruption of life more effectively when surrounded by quiet and by knowing he or she is safe.*[9]
- Assist with documentation for police report, as indicated, and stay with the client. *Developing accurate chain of evidence (maintaining sequencing and collection of evidence) and labeling each specimen and storing and packaging it properly provides important evidence for possibility of future prosecution.*[1]
- Listen to and investigate physical complaints. *Physical injuries may have occurred during incident, which may be masked by emotional reactions and limit client's ability to recognize them. These need to be identified and differentiated from anxiety symptoms so appropriate treatment may be instituted.*[1]
- Identify supportive persons (e.g., loved ones, spiritual advisor or pastor). *Having unconditional support from loving and caring others can help the client cope with the situation and move on to live more fully.*[1]
- Remain with client, listen as client recounts incident and concerns—possibly repeatedly. If client does not want to talk, accept silence. *Establishes trust, thus providing psychological support and allowing client opportunity to vent emotions.*[3]
- Encourage expression of feelings and reinforce that feelings and reactions to trauma are common and not indicators of weakness or failure. Note whether feelings expressed appear congruent with events the client experienced. *Expressing feelings helps client recognize and identify them to enhance coping. Incongruency may indicate deeper conflict that can impede resolution.*[6]
- Help child to express feelings about event using techniques appropriate to developmental level (e.g., play for young child, stories or puppets for preschooler, peer group for adolescent). *Children are more likely to express in play what they may not be able to verbalize directly. Adolescents may benefit from groups, gaining knowledge, support, decreased sense of isolation, and improved coping skills.*[2]
- Assist with practical realities (e.g., temporary housing, money, notifications of family members, other needs). *Dealing with these issues is necessary and helps client remain connected to reality and maintain sense of control over daily living concerns.*[1]

NURSING PRIORITY NO. 3 To assist client to deal with situation that exists:
- Evaluate client's perceptions of events and personal significance (e.g., police officer who is also a parent and is investigating death of a child). *Individuals perceive events depending on their previous experiences, cultural and religious background, and family of origin and will respond to any given trauma based on these factors. Incidents that touch a person's own life will be more difficult to deal with and may have a deeper effect.*[2]

 Diagnostic Studies   Evidence Based Practice   Medications   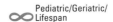 Pediatric/Geriatric/Lifespan

- Provide emotional and physical presence *to strengthen client's coping abilities. Spending time with the client promotes trust and provides an opportunity for client to think about what will help in the current situation.*[3]
- Observe for signs and symptoms of stress responses, such as nightmares, reliving an incident, poor appetite, irritability, numbness and crying, and family and relationship disruption. *These responses are normal in the early postincident time frame. If prolonged and persistent, the client may be experiencing PTSD.*[7]
- Identify and discuss client's strengths (e.g., very supportive family, usually copes well with stress) as well as vulnerabilities (e.g., client tends toward alcohol or other drugs for coping, client has witnessed a murder). *Knowing one's strengths and weaknesses helps client know what actions to take to cope with and prevent anxiety from becoming overwhelming.*[7]
- Discuss how individual coping mechanisms have worked in past traumatic events. *Awareness of previous successful experiences can help client remember coping skills that can be used to deal with current situation in a positive manner.*[3]

NURSING PRIORITY NO. 4 To promote wellness (Teaching/Discharge Considerations):

- Educate high-risk persons and families about signs/symptoms of posttrauma response, especially if it is likely to occur in their occupation or life. *Awareness allows individual to be proactive and seek support and timely intervention as needed.*
- Encourage client to identify and monitor feelings on an ongoing basis. *Promotes awareness of changes in ability to deal with stressors, allowing prompt intervention when necessary.*[4]
- Encourage learning stress-management techniques, such as deep breathing, meditation, relaxation, and exercise. *Reduces stress, enhancing coping skills and helping to resolve situation.*[5]
- Recommend participation in debriefing sessions that may be provided following major events. *Dealing with the stressor promptly may facilitate recovery from event and prevent exacerbation. Debriefing is being used by many organizations who regularly deal with traumatic events to prevent the development of PTSD, although issues about best timing of debriefing continue to be debated.*[3]
- Explain that posttraumatic symptoms can emerge months or sometimes years after a traumatic experience and that help or support can be obtained when needed or desired if client begins to experience intrusive memories or other symptoms.
- Encourage individual to develop a survivor mentality. *People often have it within their means to head off life-threatening situations and even survive the worst when they plan for emergencies and think ahead about ways to survive, such as taking food, water, and protective gear on a day hike in case you get lost, fall and break a bone, or in other ways have to spend more time than anticipated.*[9]
- Identify employment and community resource groups (e.g., Assistance Support and Self Help in Surviving Trauma, employee peer assistance programs, Red Cross or other survivor support services, Compassionate Friends). *Provides opportunity for ongoing support to deal with recurrent stressors as individual moves on with life.*[11]
- Refer for individual or family counseling, as indicated. *May need additional assistance to prevent continuation of anxiety and the onset of PTSD.*[6]

DOCUMENTATION FOCUS

Assessment/Reassessment
- Identified risk factors noting internal and external concerns.
- Client's perception of event and personal significance.
- Cultural or religious beliefs and expectations.

Planning
- Plan of care and who is involved in the planning.
- Teaching plan.

Implementation/Evaluation
- Response to interventions, teaching, and actions performed.
- Attainment or progress toward desired outcome(s).

 Acute Care   Collaborative   Community/ Home Care   Cultural

Discharge Planning
• Long-term needs and who is responsible for actions to be taken.
• Specific referrals made.

References

1. Doenges, M., Townsend, M., Moorhouse, M. (1998). *Psychiatric Care Plans: Guidelines for Individualizing Care*. 3th ed. Philadelphia: F. A. Davis.
2. American Psychological Association Act Against Violence Project. (No date). *When Children Experience Trauma: A Guide for Parents and Families*. Washington, DC: American Psychological Association.
3. Townsend, M. (2003). *Psychiatric Mental Health Nursing: Concepts of Care*. 4th ed. Philadelphia: F. A. Davis.
4. Stuart, G. W. (2001). Anxiety responses and anxiety disorders. In Stuart, G. W., Laraia, M. T. (eds). *Principles and Practice of Psychiatric Nursing*. 7th ed. St. Louis, MO: Mosby.
5. Porth, C. M., Kunert, P. K. (2002). *Pathophysiology: Concepts of Altered Health States*. Philadelphia: J. B. Lippincott.
6. National Institute of Mental Health. (2009, updated 2016). Anxiety disorders. *NIH Publication No. 02-3879*. Retrieved April 2018 from http://www.nimh.nih.gov/health/publications/anxiety-disorders/index.shtml?rf=53414.
7. Posttraumatic stress disorder—Part I. (June 1996). *Harvard Mental Health Letter*.
8. Posttraumatic stress disorder—Part II. (July 1996). *Harvard Mental Health Letter*.
9. Kamier, K. (2004). *Surviving the Extremes: A Doctor's Journey to the Limits of Human Endurance*. Boston: St. Martin's.
10. Davis, N. (2002, updated 2008). Job-related trauma and post traumatic stress disorder (PTSD). *[Brief summaries from] Multi-Sensory Trauma Processing, A Manual for Understanding and Treating PTSD and Job-Related Trauma*. Retrieved April 2018 from http://www.georgiadisaster.info/PublicSafety/PS07%20Importance%20of%20Psychological%20Health/PS07reactions_to_stress.pdf.
11. Galea, S., Nandi, A., Vlahov, D. (2005). The epidemiology of post-traumatic stress disorders after disasters. *Epidemiol Rev*, 27(1), 78–91.
12. Kimerling, R., et al. (2006). Brief report: Utility of a short screening scale for DSM-IV PTSD in primary care. *J Gen Intern Med*, 21(1), 65–67.

Powerlessness

Taxonomy II: Coping/Stress Tolerance—Class 2 Coping Responses (00125) [**Diagnostic Division:** Ego Integrity], Approved 1982; Revised 2010, 2017

DEFINITION: The lived experience of lack of control over a situation, including a perception that one's own actions do not significantly affect an outcome.

RELATED FACTORS
Anxiety, low self-self esteem; ineffective coping strategies
Caregiver role
Dysfunctional institutional environment
Insufficient knowledge to manage a situation
Insufficient social support; social marginalization; stigmatization
Pain

DEFINING CHARACTERISTICS

Subjective
Alienation; shame
Depression
Frustration about inability to perform previous activities; insufficient sense of control

---

Objective
Dependency
Inadequate participation in care

(continues on page 660)

 Diagnostic Studies   Evidence Based Practice   Medications   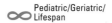 Pediatric/Geriatric/Lifespan

Powerlessness (continued)

At Risk Population: Economically disadvantaged
Associated Condition: Complex treatment regimen
Illness or progressive illness; unpredictably of illness trajectory
Sample Clinical Applications: Chronic or debilitating conditions (e.g., chronic obstructive pulmonary disease [COPD], multiple sclerosis [MS]), cancer, spinal cord injury [SCI], major depressive disorder, somatization disorders; posttraumatic stress; sexual assault

DESIRED OUTCOMES/EVALUATION CRITERIA

Sample **NOC** linkages:
Personal Autonomy: Personal actions of a competent individual to exercise governance in life decisions
Health Beliefs: Perceived Control: Personal conviction that one can influence a health outcome
Participation in Healthcare Decisions: Personal involvement in selecting and evaluating healthcare options to achieve desired outcomes

Client Will (Include Specific Time Frame)
• Express sense of control over the present situation and hopefulness about future outcome.
• Verbalize positive self-appraisal in current situation.
• Make choices related to and be involved in care.
• Identify areas over which individual has control.
• Acknowledge reality that some areas are beyond individual's control.

ACTIONS/INTERVENTIONS

Sample **NIC** linkages:
Self-Responsibility Facilitation: Encouraging a patient to assume more responsibility for own behavior
Health System Guidance: Facilitating a patient's location and use of appropriate health services
Decision-Making Support: Providing information and support for a person who is making a decision regarding healthcare

NURSING PRIORITY NO. 1 To assess causative/contributing factors:

• Identify situational circumstances (e.g., unfamiliar environment, immobility, diagnosis of terminal or chronic illness, lack of support system(s), lack of knowledge about situation) affecting the client at this time. *Knowing the specific situation of the client is essential to planning care and empowering the individual.*[4]
• Determine client's perception and knowledge of condition and treatment plan. *Identifying how client views and understands what is happening and what the plan of care entails is essential to begin to help client feel empowered.*[2]
• Ascertain client response to treatment regimen. Does client see reason(s) for and understand it is in the client's interest or is client compliant and helpless? *The manner in which the individual responds to the treatment indicates the depth of feelings of powerlessness and may interfere with progress.*[4]
• Identify client locus of control—internal (expressions of responsibility for self and ability to control outcomes—"I didn't quit smoking") or external (expressions of lack of control over self and environment—"Nothing ever works out"; "What bad luck to get lung cancer"). *Locus of control is a term used in reference to an individual's sense of mastery or control over events. Individuals view life change and stressful events differently. Those with internal locus of control tend to be more optimistic about their ability to deal with adversity even in the face of current difficulties. Individuals with external locus of control may attribute feelings of*

  Acute Care   Collaborative   Community/ Home Care   Cultural

powerlessness to an external source perceiving it as beyond his or her control and will look to others to solve problems and take care of them.[4,9]

- Note cultural or religious factors that may contribute to how client views self and is handling current situation. *One's values and beliefs may dictate gender roles and the individual's expectations of control, influencing the client's belief in ability to manage situation, participate in decision making, and direct own life.*[9,11]
- Assess degree of mastery client has exhibited in life. *How this individual has dealt with problems throughout life will help to understand feelings of powerlessness client is feeling during this crisis.*[4,5]
- Determine if there has been a change in relationships with significant others (SOs). *Conflict in relationships may be contributing to sense of powerlessness. Domestic violence situations often leave the individuals involved feeling powerless to change what is happening.*[4]
- Note availability/use of resources. *Client who has few options for assistance or who is not knowledgeable about how to use resources needs to be given information and assistance to know how and where to seek help.*[3]
- Investigate healthcare providers and personal caregiver practices to determine if they support client control and responsibility. *Caregivers who do for the client what he or she is able to do for own self diminish client's sense of control. When client is given as much control over self as possible, sense of power is regained.*[3]

NURSING PRIORITY NO. 2 To assess degree of powerlessness experienced by the client:

- Listen to statements client makes, such as "They don't care," "It won't make any difference," and "Are you kidding?"[2]
- Note expressions that indicate "giving up," such as "It won't do any good." *May indicate suicidal intent, indicating need for immediate evaluation and intervention.*[6]
- Note behavioral responses (verbal and nonverbal), including expressions of fear, interest or apathy, agitation, and withdrawal. *These responses can show depth of anxiety, feelings of powerlessness over what is happening, and indicate need for intervention to help client begin to look at situation with some sense of hope.*[6]
- Note lack of communication, flat affect, and lack of eye contact. *May indicate more severe state of mind, such as a psychotic episode, and need for immediate evaluation and treatment.*[4]
- Identify the use of manipulative behavior and reactions of client and caregivers. *Manipulation is used for management of powerlessness because of distrust of others, fear of intimacy, search for approval, and validation of sexuality.*[1,9]

NURSING PRIORITY NO. 3 To assist client to clarify needs relative to ability to meet them:

- Show concern for client as a person. *Communicates value of the individual, enhancing self-esteem.*[8]
- Active-listen client's perceptions and concerns and encourage questions. *Provides time for client to explore views and understand what is happening in order to come to some decisions about situation, enhancing sense of control.*[8,10]
- Accept expressions of feelings, including anger and hopelessness. *Communicates empathy and understanding of reality of those feelings and provides a point of discussion to move toward sense of control.*[4]
- Avoid arguing or using logic with hopeless client. *Client will not accept that anything can make a difference. Arguing denies client's reality and may impede client-nurse relationship.*[2]
- Deal with manipulative behavior by being straightforward and honest with your communication and letting client know that this is a better way to get needs met. *When client makes a commitment to stop using manipulation in life, steps can be taken to recognize the behaviors and feelings and begin to change them. Keeping a journal can help to identify these issues.*[9]
- Express hope for the client. *Although client may not accept expressions of hope, there is always hope of something, and when options are explored, client may begin to see there is hope.*[8]
- Identify strengths, assets, and past coping strategies that were successful. *Helps client to recognize own ability to deal with difficult situation, providing sense of power.*[5]
- Assist client to identify what he or she can do for self. Identify things the client can and cannot control. *Accomplishing something can provide a sense of control and helps client understand that there are things he*

Diagnostic Studies   Evidence Based Practice   Medications   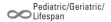Pediatric/Geriatric/Lifespan *or she can manage. Accepting that some things cannot be controlled helps client to stop wasting efforts and refocus energy.*[1]

- Encourage client to maintain a sense of perspective about the situation. *Discussing ways client can look at options and make decisions based on which will be best leads to the most effective solutions for situation.*[6]

NURSING PRIORITY NO. 4   To promote independence:

- Use client's locus of control to develop individual plan of care. *Tailoring care to the individual's ability will maximize effectiveness. For instance, client with internal control can take control of own care, and client with external control may need to begin with small tasks and add as tolerated, moving toward learning to take more control of care.*[6]
- Develop contract with client specifying goals agreed on. *When client is involved in planning, commitment to plan is enhanced, optimizing outcomes.*[2]
- Treat expressed decisions and desires with respect. Avoid critical parenting behaviors. *Listening to client and accepting what is said, no matter what the content, helps client hear own words and begin to process information and feelings. Comments that are heard as critical or condescending will block communication and growth.*[1,10]
- Provide client opportunities to control as many events as energy and restrictions of care permit. *Promotes sense of control over situation and helps client begin to feel more confident about own ability to manage what is happening.*[6,7]
- Discuss needs openly with client and set up agreed-on routines for meeting identified needs. *Minimizes use of manipulation. Manipulative behavior is often used to influence others to do what the person thinks he or she should do. Usually this results in defensiveness or outright rebellion against what is suggested, resulting in lack of trust and withdrawal on the part of the person being manipulated.*[9]
- Minimize rules and limit continuous observation to the degree that safety permits. *Provides sense of control for the client while maintaining a safe environment for the client.*[6]
- Support client efforts to develop realistic steps to put plan into action, reach goals, and maintain expectations. *Noting progress that is being made can provide a sense of control and diminish sense of powerlessness.*[6]
- Provide positive reinforcement for desired behaviors. *In behavioral therapy, the belief that when a behavior reinforces another behavior, the second behavior is called a "positive reinforcer," and the function is called "positive reinforcement." By providing this reinforcement, the desired behaviors are more likely to continue.*[4]
- Direct client's thoughts beyond present state to future when appropriate. *Focusing on possibilities in small steps can help the client see that there can be hope in small things each day.*[1,8]
- Schedule frequent and regular contacts to let client know someone is interested and available. *Communicates caring and concern for client and needs, reinforcing sense of worthiness.*
- Involve SO(s) in client care as desired or appropriate. *Personal involvement by supportive family members can help client see the possibilities for resolving problems related to feelings of powerlessness.*[6]

NURSING PRIORITY NO. 5   To promote wellness (Teaching/Discharge Considerations):

- Instruct in and encourage use of anxiety- and stress-reduction techniques. *Most individuals react to stress in predictable physiological and psychological ways. Feelings of powerlessness related to client's situation can be relieved by use of these techniques.*[5]
- Provide accurate verbal and written information about what is happening and discuss with client/SO(s). Repeat as often as necessary. *Providing information in different modalities allows better access and opportunity for increased understanding. People do not always hear every piece of information the first time it is presented because of anxiety and inattention, so repetition helps to fill in the missed information.*[6]
- Assist client to set realistic goals for the future. *Provides opportunity for client to decide what direction is desired and to gain confidence from completion of each goal.*[10]
- Assist client to learn and use assertive communication skills. *Practicing a new way of expressing thoughts and requests provides the client with a skill to achieve desires and improve relationships.*[10]

 Acute Care   Collaborative   Community/Home Care   Cultural

- 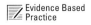 Facilitate return to a productive role in whatever capacity possible for the individual. Refer to occupational therapist or vocational counselor as indicated. *Feelings of powerlessness may result from inability to engage in or resume previous activities, and learning new ways to be productive enhances self-esteem and reduces feelings of powerlessness.*[6]
- Encourage client to think productively and positively and take responsibility for choosing own thoughts. *Negative thinking can result in feelings of powerlessness, and learning to use positive thinking can reverse this pattern, promoting feelings of control and self-worth.*[6]
- Model problem-solving process with client/SO(s). *Learning a problem-solving method that results in a win-win solution improves family relationships and promotes feelings of self-worth in those involved.*[10]
- Suggest client periodically review own needs and goals. *It is easy to become discouraged as time goes on, and reviewing, thinking about needs, and how previously set goals are relevant in the present helps to either renew those goals or develop new goals to meet current situation.*[6,8]
- Refer to support groups, counseling or therapy, etc., as indicated. *May need/desire additional assistance to resolve current problems, long-standing issues, or troubled relationships.*[4]

DOCUMENTATION FOCUS

Assessment/Reassessment
- Individual findings, noting degree of powerlessness, locus of control, individual's perception of the situation.
- Specific cultural or religious factors.
- Availability and use of support system and resources.

Planning
- Plan of care and who is involved in the planning.
- Teaching plan.

Implementation/Evaluation
- Responses to interventions, teaching, and actions performed.
- Specific goals and expectations.
- Attainment or progress toward desired outcome(s).
- Modifications to plan of care.

Discharge Planning
- Long-term needs and who is responsible for actions to be taken.
- Specific referrals made.

References

1. Hazrah, R. (2014). Manipulation: A symptom of powerlessness. Retrieved April 2018 from http://www.addictioncounselingleesburg.com/manipulation-symptom-powerlessness/.
2. Bradford Health. (No date). The power of admitting powerlessness. Retrieved April 2018 from https://bradfordhealth.com/power-admitting-powerlessness/.
3. Khleghi, K. (July 2012). Are you empowering or enabling? Retrieved April 2018 from https://www.psychologytoday.com/us/blog/the-anatomy-addiction/201207/are-you-empowering-or-enabling.
4. Blackwell, A. (2009). Five powerful ways to regain control of your life. Retrieved April 2018 from http://www.thebridgemaker.com/five-powerful-ways-to-regain-control-of-your-life-now/.
5. Messina, J. J. (2011). Accepting powerlessness. Retrieved April 2018 from http://www.coping.us/toolsforhandlingcontrol/eliminatemanipulation.html.
6. Beaumont, L. R. Developing the essential social skills to recognize, interpret and respond constructively to yourself and others. Retrieved April 2018 from http://emotionalcompetency.com/.
7. National Institute of Mental Health. (2002, updated 2016). Generalized anxiety disorder (GAD). Retrieved April 2018 from http://www.nimh.nih.gov/health/topics/generalized-anxiety-disorder-gad/index.shtml.
8. Neeld, E. H. (2003). Finding daylight after loss shatters your world. *Seven Choices*. New York: Grand Central Publishing.
9. Messina, J. J. (2010). Eliminating manipulation: Tools for handling control issues. Retrieved April 2018 from http://www.coping.us/toolsforhandlingcontrol/eliminatemanipulation.html.
10. Bolstadt, R., Hamblett, M. (1997). Win-win. Retrieved April 2018 from http://www.nlpca.com/DCweb/winwin.html.
11. Purnell, L. D. (2011). *Guide to Culturally Competent Health Care*. 2nd ed. Philadelphia: F. A. Davis.

 Diagnostic Studies   Evidence Based Practice   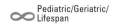 Medications   Pediatric/Geriatric/Lifespan

risk for Powerlessness

Taxonomy II: Coping/Stress Tolerance—Class 2 Coping Responses (00125) [**Diagnostic Division:** Ego Integrity], Approved 2000; Revised 2010; 2013

DEFINITION: Susceptible to the lived experience of lack of control over a situation, including a perception that one's actions do not significantly affect an outcome, which may compromise health.

RISK FACTORS
Anxiety, low self-esteem; ineffective coping strategies
Caregiver role
Dysfunctional institutional environment
Insufficient knowledge to manage a situation
Insufficient social support; social marginalization; stigmatization
Pain
At Risk Population: Economically disadvantaged
Associated Condition: Complex treatment regimen
Illness or progressive illness; unpredictably of illness trajectory
Sample Clinical Applications: New or unexpected diagnoses, chronic or debilitating conditions (e.g., chronic obstructive pulmonary disease [COPD], MS), cancer, SCI, major depressive disorder, somatization disorders

DESIRED OUTCOMES/EVALUATION CRITERIA

Sample NOC linkages:
Personal Autonomy: Personal actions of a competent individual to exercise governance in life decisions
Health Beliefs: Perceived Control: Personal conviction that one can influence a health outcome
Participation in Healthcare Decisions: Personal involvement in selecting and evaluating healthcare options to achieve desired outcome

Client Will (Include Specific Time Frame)
• Express sense of control over the present situation and hopefulness about future outcomes.
• Verbalize positive self-appraisal in current situation.
• Make choices related to and be involved in care.
• Identify areas over which individual has control.
• Acknowledge reality that some areas are beyond individual's control.

ACTIONS/INTERVENTIONS

Sample NIC linkages:
Self-Responsibility Facilitation: Encouraging a patient to assume more responsibility for own behavior
Health System Guidance: Facilitating a patient's location and use of appropriate health services
Decision-Making Support: Providing information and support for a person who is making a decision regarding healthcare

NURSING PRIORITY NO. 1 To assess causative/contributing risk factors:

• Identify situational circumstances (e.g., acute illness, sudden hospitalization, diagnosis of terminal or debilitating or chronic illness, very young or aging with decreased physical strength and mobility, lack of knowledge about illness, healthcare system). *Necessary information to develop individualized plan of care for client.*

 Acute Care   Collaborative   Community/ Home Care   Cultural

- Determine client's perception and knowledge of condition and proposed treatment plan. *Identifying how client views and understands what is happening and what the plan of care entails is essential to help client feel empowered.*[7]
- Identify client's locus of control—internal (expressions of responsibility for self and ability to control outcomes—"I didn't quit smoking") or external (expressions of lack of control over self and environment—"Nothing ever works out," "What bad luck to get lung cancer"). *Locus of control is a term used in reference to an individual's sense of mastery or control over events. Individuals view life change and stressful events differently. Those with internal locus of control tend to be more optimistic about their ability to deal with adversity even in the face of current difficulties. Individuals with external locus of control may attribute feelings of powerlessness to an external source, perceiving it as beyond his or her control, and will look to others to solve problems and take care of them.*[4,10]
- Note cultural or religious factors that may contribute to how client views self and is handling current situation. *One's values and beliefs may dictate gender roles and the individual's expectations of control, influencing the client's belief in ability to manage situation, participate in decision making, and direct own life.*[9,10]
- Assess client's self-esteem and degree of mastery client has exhibited in life situations. *Provides clues to client's ability to see self as in control and deal with current situation.*[7]
- Note availability and use of resources, relationship with significant other (SO)/family and degree of support provided to client. *Presence of support system and ability to use resources appropriately facilitates problem-solving, enhancing sense of control. Client who has few options for assistance or who is not knowledgeable about how to use resources needs to be given information and assistance to know how and where to seek help.*[3]
- Listen to statements client makes that might indicate feelings of possibility of loss of control (e.g., "They don't care," "It won't make a difference," "It won't do any good"). *Indicators of sense of powerlessness and hopelessness and need for specific interventions to provide sense of control over what is happening.*[4]
- Determine congruency of responses (verbal and nonverbal) and note expressions of fear, disinterest or apathy, or withdrawal. *These responses can show depth of anxiety over what is happening and indicate need for intervention to help client begin to look at situation with sense of hope.*[5]
- Be alert for signs of manipulative behavior and note reactions of client and caregivers. *Manipulation may be used for management of powerlessness because of fear and distrust.*[4,10]

NURSING PRIORITY NO. 2   To assist client to clarify needs and ability to meet them:

- Show concern for client as a person. Encourage questions. *Communicates value of the individual, enhancing self-esteem. Questions may reveal lack of information or concerns client may have.*[8]
- Make time to listen to client's perceptions of the situation as well as concerns. *Provides time for client to explore views and understand what is happening to come to some decisions about situation, enhancing sense of control.*[5]
- Accept expressions of feelings, including anger and reluctance to try to work things out. *Communicates unconditional regard for the client and encourages individual to think about options even though situation may be difficult.*[5]
- Express hope for client and encourage review of past experiences with successful strategies. *Provides an opportunity for person to remember and accept that he or she has managed difficult situations before and can apply these strategies in current situation.*[4]
- Assist client to identify what he or she can do to help self and what situations cannot be controlled. *Accomplishing something can provide a sense of control and helps client understand that there are things he or she can manage. Accepting that some things cannot be controlled helps client to stop wasting efforts and refocus energy.*[1,2]

NURSING PRIORITY NO. 3   To promote wellness (Teaching/Discharge Considerations):

- Encourage client to be active in own healthcare management and to take responsibility for choosing own actions and reactions. *Discussing ways client can look at options and make decisions based on which ones will be best lead to the most effective solutions for situation.*[6,7]

 Diagnostic Studies   Evidence Based Practice   Medications   Pediatric/Geriatric/Lifespan

- Involve client/SO(s) in planning process, using client's locus of control. *Tailoring care to the individual's ability will maximize effectiveness. For instance, client with internal control can take control of own care, and client with external control may need to begin with small tasks and add as tolerated, moving toward learning to take more control of care.*[6]
- Model problem-solving process with client and SOs. *Learning a problem-solving method that results in a win-win solution improves family relationships and promotes feelings of self-worth in those involved.*[8]
- Support client efforts to develop realistic steps to put plan into action, reach goals, and maintain expectations. *Noting progress that is being made can enhance sense of control.*[6]
- Provide accurate instructions in various modalities (e.g., verbal, written, audiovisual, Web sites) about what is happening and what realistically might happen. *Providing information in different formats allows better access and opportunity for increased understanding to support decision-making process.*[6]
- Identify resource books or classes for assertiveness training and stress reduction, as appropriate. *Reinforces learning and promotes self-paced review.*[8]
- Suggest client periodically review own needs and goals. *Reviewing needs and how previously set goals are relevant in the present helps to either renew those goals or develop new goals to meet current situation.*[5]
- Refer to support groups for chronic conditions or disability (e.g., Multiple Sclerosis Society, Easter Seals, Alzheimer's, Al-Anon) or counseling or therapy, as appropriate. *May need additional assistance to manage difficulties of current situation.*[4]

DOCUMENTATION FOCUS

Assessment/Reassessment
- Individual findings, noting potential for powerlessness, locus of control, individual's perception of the situation.
- Cultural values or religious beliefs.
- Locus of control.
- SO/family involvement and support.
- Availability and use of resources.

Planning
- Plan of care and who is involved in the planning.
- Teaching plan.

Implementation/Evaluation
- Responses to interventions, teaching, and actions performed.
- Specific goals and expectations.
- Attainment or progress toward desired outcomes.
- Modifications to plan of care.

Discharge Planning
- Long-term needs and who is responsible for actions to be taken.
- Specific referrals made.

References

1. Sandman, P. M. (1987; posted 2000). Explaining risks to non-experts: A communications challenge. Retrieved April 2018 from http://www.psandman.com/articles/nonexpt.htm.
2. Herbert, W. (2009). Try a little powerlessness: The pitfalls of self control. *Sci Am Mind*. Retrieved April 2018 from https://www.scientificamerican.com/article/try-a-little-powerlessness/.
3. U-M Depression Center Staff. (2011). Support systems. *DepressionToolkit.org*. Retrieved April 2018 from http://www.depressiontoolkit.org/download/Support_systems_facts_UMDC.pdf.
4. Messina, J. J. (2008). Letting go uncontrollables and unchangables. Retrieved April 2018 from http://www.trainingdimensions.net/tdArticles/Newsletter/May_2015/Letting%20Go%20Uncontrollables%20and%20Unchangables.pdf.
5. Barnett, C. (2016). Effects of natural disasters on children. Retrieved April 2018 from http://ggltrc.org/effects-of-natural-disasters-on-children/.
6. Levenson, S. (2014). Key health care decision making processes. Retrieved April 2018 from http://marylandmolst.org/

 Acute Care   Collaborative   Community/ Home Care   Cultural

docs/Health%20Care%20Decision%20Making,%20February%202014.pdf.

7. National Institute of Mental Health. (2009, updated 2016). *Anxiety disorders*. Retrieved April 2018 from http://www.nimh.nih.gov/health/topics/anxiety-disorders/index.shtml.

8. Matta, C. (2012). *The Stress Response: How Dialectical Behavior Therapy Can Free You from Needless Anxiety, Worry, Anger & Other Symptoms of Stress*. Oakland, CA: New Harbinger Publications, Inc.

9. Minority Nurse Staff. (2013). Culture, grief and bereavement: Applications for clinical practice. *Minority Nurse*. Retrieved April 2018 from https://minoritynurse.com/culture-grief-and-bereavement-applications-for-clinical-practice/.

10. Messina, J. J. (2010). Eliminating manipulation: Tools for handling control issues. Retrieved April 2018 from http://www.coping.us/toolsforhandlingcontrol/eliminatemanipulation.html.

readiness for enhanced Power

Taxonomy II: Coping/Stress Tolerance—Class 2 Coping Responses (00187) **[Diagnostic Division:** Ego Integrity**]**, Approved 2006; Revised 2013, 2017

DEFINITION: A pattern of participating knowingly in change for well-being, which can be strengthened.

DEFINING CHARACTERISTICS

Subjective

Expresses desire to enhance awareness of possible changes, or to enhance knowledge for participation in change, or to enhance identification of choices that can be made for change

Expresses desire to enhance independence with actions for change or involvement in change

Expresses desire to enhance participation in choices for daily living, or in choices for health

Expresses desire enhance power

Note: Even though power (a response) and empowerment (an intervention approach) are different concepts, the literature related to both concepts supports the defining characteristics of this diagnosis.

Sample Clinical Applications: Any acute or chronic condition, or healthy individual looking to change life/improve well-being

DESIRED OUTCOMES/EVALUATION CRITERIA

Sample NOC linkages:

Personal Autonomy: Personal actions of a competent individual to exercise governance in life decisions

Health Promoting Behavior: Personal actions to sustain or increase wellness

Health Beliefs: Perceived Control: Personal conviction that one can influence a health outcome

Client Will (Include Specific Time Frame)
- Verbalize knowledge of what changes he or she wants to make.
- Express awareness of own ability to be in charge of changes to be made.
- Participate in classes or group activities to learn new skills.
- State readiness to take power over own life.

ACTIONS/INTERVENTIONS

Sample NIC linkages:

Self-Modification Assistance: Reinforcement of self-directed change initiated by the patient to achieve personally important goals

Decision-Making Support: Providing information and support for a person who is making a decision regarding healthcare

Health System Guidance: Facilitating a patient's location and use of appropriate health services

 Diagnostic Studies
 Evidence Based Practice
 Medications
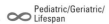 Pediatric/Geriatric/ Lifespan

NURSING PRIORITY NO. 1   To determine need/motivation for improvement:

- Determine current situation and circumstances that client is experiencing, leading to desire to improve life. *Provides information to help client with planning for enhancing life.*[8]
- Ascertain motivation and expectations for change. *Motivation to improve and high expectations can encourage client to make changes that will improve his or her life. However, unrealistic expectations or motivation to please someone else may hamper efforts.*[7]
- Identify emotional climate in which client and relationships live and work. *The emotional climate has a great impact between people. When a power differential exists in relationships, the atmosphere is largely determined by the person or people who have the power.*[4]
- Identify client locus of control: internal (expressions of responsibility for self and ability to control outcomes) or external (expressions of lack of control over self and environment). *Understanding locus of control can help client to work toward positive, internal control as he or she develops sense of ability to freely choose own actions.*[9]
- Determine cultural factors or religious beliefs influencing client's self-view. *These factors can be strong determinants in individual's ability to change and view self as powerful and may complicate growth process.*[9]
- Assess degree of mastery client has exhibited in his or her life. *Helps client to understand how he or she has functioned in the past, how that applies to current situation, and what is needed to improve.*
- Note presence of family/significant others that can or do act as support systems for client. *When family understands and supports client's desires and efforts, he or she is more likely to be successful.*
- Determine whether client knows or uses assertiveness skills. *Learning and enhancing these skills will help client to improve ability to take personal responsibility for own self and relationships with others.*[1,3,5,7]

NURSING PRIORITY NO. 2   To assist client to clarify needs relative to ability to improve feelings of power:

- Discuss how client is currently involved in creating change in life. *Provides a baseline to measure growth and suggests possibilities for change.*[8]
- Active-listen client's perceptions and beliefs about the concept of power. *Enables client to identify underlying feelings and thoughts about this issue and how power can be gained in his or her life.*[8]
- Identify strengths, assets, and past coping strategies that were successful. *These strategies can be built on to enhance feelings of control.*[6]
- Discuss the importance of assuming personal responsibility for life and relationships. *This requires one to be open to new ideas and experiences, different values, and beliefs and to be inquisitive.*[7]
- Assist client in identifying things client can and or cannot control. *Avoids wasting time on things that are not in the control of the client.*[8]
- Treat expressed desires and decisions with respect. Avoid critical parenting expressions. *Individual may express thoughts and opinions that are creative and out of the ordinary, and critical parenting responses such as "That's a dumb idea" can crush person's brainstorming.*[9]

NURSING PRIORITY NO. 3   To promote optimum wellness, enhancing power (Teaching/Discharge Considerations):

- Assist client to set realistic goals for the future. *Even though client is thinking creatively and brainstorming ideas, goals need to be planned step by step to reach the desired outcome.*[6]
- Provide accurate verbal and written information about client's concerns and life situation. *Reinforces learning and promotes self-paced review.*[8]
- Assist client to learn/use assertive communication skills. *These techniques require practice, but as the client becomes more proficient, they will help to develop relationships that are more effective.*[2,3]
- Use "I" messages instead of "You" messages. *"I" messages acknowledge ownership of what is said, whereas "You" messages suggest the other person is wrong or bad, fostering resentment and resistance instead of understanding and cooperation.*[8]

 Acute Care   Collaborative   Community/Home Care   Cultural

- Discuss importance of paying attention to nonverbal communication. *Messages are often confusing or misinterpreted when verbal and nonverbal communications are not congruent.*[9]
- Help client learn to problem-solve differences. *Problem-solving process allows for each person involved to have input and promotes win-win solutions.*[8]
- Instruct and encourage use of stress-reduction techniques. *Relaxation helps individual to function more effectively, thus enhancing feelings of power.*[9]
- 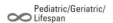 Refer to support groups or classes, as indicated, assertiveness training, effectiveness training for women; "Be Your Best" training program.*Provides role models and allows individuals to learn from one another, thereby promoting problem-solving and enhancing learning.*[7]

DOCUMENTATION FOCUS

Assessment/Reassessment
- Individual findings, noting determination to improve sense of power, locus of control.
- Motivation and expectations for change.
- Cultural or religious beliefs affecting self-view.
- Locus of control.

Planning
- Plan of care, specific interventions, and who is involved in planning.
- Teaching plan.

Implementation/Evaluation
- Client's responses to interventions, teaching, and actions performed.
- Attainment or progress toward desired outcome(s).
- Modifications to plan of care.

Discharge Planning
- Long-term needs and who is responsible for actions to be taken.
- Specific referrals made.

References

1. Edu Resource.com. (No date). Assertive behavior, characteristics of assertive behavior. Retrieved April 2018 from http://www.edu-resource.com/training-and-development/assertive-behavior.php.
2. Hopkins, L. (2005). Assertive communication: 6 Tips for effective use. Retrieved April 2018 from http://ezinearticles.com/?Assertive-Communication---6-Tips-For-Effective-Use&id=10259.
3. Dombeck, M. (2006). Setting boundaries appropriately: Assertiveness training. Retrieved April 2018 from http://www.mentalhelp.net/articles/setting-boundaries-appropriately-assertiveness-training/.
4. Adams, L. (No date). Climate—The emotional one, that is. Retrieved April 2018 from http://www.gordontraining.com/free-workplace-articles/climate-the-emotional-one-that-is/.
5. Adams, L. (No date). Being a leader doesn't make you one. Retrieved April 2018 from http://www.gordontraining.com/free-workplace-articles/being-a-leader-doesnt-make-you-one/.
6. No author. (No date). What is assertiveness and how to be assertive. *The Corner of Excellence*. Retrieved November 2018 from https://www.thecornerofexcellence.com/en/assertiveness-assertive/.
7. Gordon, T. (No date). Families need rules. Retrieved April 2018 from http://www.gordontraining.com/free-parenting-articles/families-need-rules/.
8. Clinebell, H. J. (1981). Growth resources in transactional analysis. *In Contemporary Growth Therapies*. Nashville, TN: Abingdon Press.
9. Thompson-Tormaschy, T. (2013, updated 2016). What's the big deal about "I"-Messages? Retrieved April 2018 from http://psychcentral.com/lib/2007/whats-the-big-deal-about-i-messages/.

 Diagnostic Studies   Evidence Based Practice   Medications 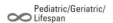 Pediatric/Geriatric/Lifespan

risk for Pressure Ulcer

Taxonomy II: Safety/Protection—Physical Injury 00249) [Diagnostic Division: Safety], Approved 2013, 2017

DEFINITION: Susceptible to localized injury to the skin and/or underlying tissue usually over a bony prominence as a result of pressure, or pressure in combination with shear (National Pressure Ulcer Advisory Panel [NPUAP, 2007]).

RISK FACTORS

Decrease in mobility; extended period of immobility on hard surface

Dehydration; inadequate nutrition; self-care deficit

Dry skin; scaly skin; skin moisture; use of linen with insufficient moisture wicking property

Hyperthermia

Incontinence

Insufficient caregiver knowledge of pressure ulcer prevention, or of modifiable factors

Pressure over bony prominence; shearing forces; surface friction

Smoking

At Risk Population: ADULT: Braden scale score of <17

American Society of Anesthesiologists (ASA) Physical Status classification score ≥1

CHILD: Braden Q Scale score of ≤15

Low score on Risk Assessment Pressure Sore (RAPS) scale; history of pressure ulcer

New York Heart Association (NYHA) Functional Classification ≥1

Extremes of age or weight; female gender

History of cerebral vascular accident; trauma;

Associated Condition: Alteration in cognitive functioning

Alteration in sensation; edema

Anemia; cardiovascular disease; decrease in tissue oxygenation or perfusion; impaired circulation

Elevated skin temperature by 1–2°C

Physical immobilization; hip fracture

Lymphopenia, decrease in serum albumin; reduced triceps skin fold thickness

Pharmaceutical agent

Sample Clinical Applications: Para/quadriplegia; diabetes mellitus; obesity; CVA, coma, dementia; amputation; burns; peripheral vascular disease, thrombophlebitis

DESIRED OUTCOMES/EVALUATION CRITERIA

Sample **NOC** linkages:

Tissue Integrity: Skin and Mucous Membranes: Structural intactness and normal physiological function of skin and mucous membranes

Risk Control: Personal actions to understand, prevent, eliminate, or reduce modifiable health threats

Immobility Consequences: Physiological: Severity of compromise in physiological functioning due to impaired physical mobility

Client Will (Include Specific Time Frame)

• Display and maintain healthy skin in risk areas (e.g., bony prominences, skin folds) during time in care facility.

• Participate in prevention measures and treatment program.

• Verbalize understanding of risk factors and when to contact healthcare provider.

• Demonstrate behaviors or lifestyle changes to improve circulation (e.g., engage in regular exercise, cessation of smoking, weight reduction, disease management).

 Acute Care Collaborative Community/ Home Care Cultural

Client/Caregiver Will (Include Specific Time Frame)
• Participate in prevention measures.

ACTIONS/INTERVENTIONS

Sample NIC linkages:

Skin Surveillance: Collection and analysis of patient data to maintain skin and mucous membrane integrity

Pressure Ulcer Prevention: Prevention of pressure ulcers for an individual at high risk for developing them

NURSING PRIORITY NO. 1 To assess risk and contributing factors:

• Identify presence of underlying condition that increases risk of pressure ulcer. *Skin integrity problems can be the result of (1) disease processes that affect circulation and perfusion of tissues (e.g., arteriosclerosis, venous insufficiency, hypertension, obesity, diabetes, malignant neoplasms), (2) medications (e.g., vasopressors, antidepressants; anticoagulants, corticosteroids, immunosuppressives, antineoplastics) that adversely affect or impair healing, (3) burns or radiation (can break down internal tissues as well as skin), and (4) nutrition and hydration (e.g., malnutrition deprives the body of protein and calories required for cell growth and repair, dehydration impairs transport of oxygen and nutrients).*[1–3]

• ✚ 📝 Evaluate client's risk for developing pressure injury upon admission to care, using NPUAP Pressure Injury Stages, Braden risk scale (or similar scale per facility policy) as listed above. *Using susceptibility factors of sensory perception, skin moisture, activity, mobility, nutritional status, friction, and shear potential, the client's risk can be quickly determined. Note: "Although the terms decubitus ulcer, pressure sore, and pressure ulcer have often been used interchangeably, the National Pressure Ulcer Advisory Panel (NPUAP) currently (2016) considers pressure injury the best term to use, given that open ulceration does not always occur."*[6,9–11,14]

• ∞ 📝 Determine client's age and developmental factors affecting skin/tissue health. *One of the structural differences in an infant's skin is that the skin cells are smaller and thinner than in an adult's skin, which can result in a weakened barrier to the environment. Infants are also predisposed to a dry, flaky, and impaired skin barrier.*[12] *However, studies have shown that similar to adult patients, acutely ill infants and children are at risk for pressure injury. The negative effect of immobility and physiological instability on a patient's skin does not discriminate on age or developmental level.*[13] *In older adults, there are often comorbid conditions (e.g., end-stage renal disease, diabetes, peripheral vascular impairment), as well as decreased epidermal regeneration; fewer sweat glands; and less subcutaneous fat, elastin, and collagen, causing skin to become thinner, drier, and less responsive to pain sensations.*[1,3–5]

• 📝 Note skin color discoloration (e.g., nonblanchable erythema; persistent red, blue, or purple hues) in pressure areas *suggestive of impaired tissue health. Note: It may be necessary in a darker-skinned individual to focus more on other evidence of pressure injury development, such as bogginess, induration, coolness, or increased warmth, as well as signs of skin discoloration.*[5]

• Note presence of compromised mobility, sensation, vision, hearing, or speech *that may impact client's self-care as relates to skin and pressure area care.*[3]

• Ascertain current medication regimen. *Individual may be receiving medications that contribute to development of pressure injuries or affect wound healing (e.g., NSAIDs, vasopressors, beta blockers, anticoagulants, inotropics, immunosuppressives, antineoplastics, some analgesics) and that can adversely affect the skin.*[16]

• ✏ Review laboratory results (e.g., hemoglobin/hematocrit, blood glucose, blood and/or wound culture and sensitivities for infectious agents [viral, bacterial, fungal], albumin, prealbumin, transferrin, protein) *to evaluate for potential risk factors or ability to heal. Note: Albumin less than 3.5 correlates to decreased wound healing and increased incidence of pressure ulcers.*[1,6,14]

 Diagnostic Studies   Evidence Based Practice   Medications 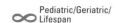 Pediatric/Geriatric/Lifespan

671

NURSING PRIORITY NO. 2   To maintain optimal skin/tissue integrity:[5,7,8,15]

- ⊞ ☑ Monitor for incontinence, changing diapers, briefs, padding, and bedding as needed. *Maintains skin that is clean, dry, and free of contaminants that can cause/exacerbate skin/tissue breakdown.*
- Develop regularly timed repositioning schedule for client with mobility and sensation impairments; encourage or assist with periodic weight shifts for client in chair *to reduce stress on pressure points and to promote circulation to tissues.*
- Use proper turning and transfer techniques and sufficient personnel when repositioning client. *Avoids movements that cause friction or shearing (e.g., pulling client with parallel force, dragging movements).*
- Use appropriate padding or pressure-reducing devices (e.g., egg crate, gel pads, heel rolls, or foam boots) or pressure-relieving devices (e.g., air or water mattress) when indicated *to reduce pressure on sensitive areas and enhance circulation.*
- ⊛ Participate in practices that prevent medical device related-pressure ulcers:
  Choose the correct size of medical device(s) (e.g., endotracheal tube [ET], other tubings, anti-embolism stocking, splints) to fit the individual.
  Remove or move the device daily to assess skin.
  Avoid placement of device(s) over sites of prior or existing pressure ulceration.
  ∞ Cushion and protect skin with cushioning in high-risk areas (e.g., nasal bridge, ears, sacrum, heels, occipital area of head in infants/small children).
  Educate other care providers about client's devices and interventions for prevention of skin breakdown.
- ⊛ Provide optimum nutrition (including adequate protein, lipids, calories, trace minerals, and multivitamins [e.g., A, C, D, E]) *to promote skin and tissue health and to maintain general well-being.* Refer to nutritionist as indicated.
- ⊛ Provide adequate hydration (e.g., oral, tube feeding, IV, ambient room humidity) *to reduce and replenish transepidermal water loss.*

NURSING PRIORITY NO. 3   To promote wellness (Teaching/Discharge Considerations):

- ⌂ Encourage regular inspection and monitoring of skin for changes or failure to heal. *Early detection and reporting to healthcare providers promotes timely evaluation and intervention.*
- Encourage good nutrition, adequate hydration, early and ongoing mobility, and range-of-motion and strengthening exercises *to enhance circulation and promote health of skin and other organs.*
- Discuss proper and safe use of equipment or appliances (e.g., heating pad, ostomy appliances, padding straps of braces).
- Encourage abstinence from smoking, *which causes vasoconstriction, impairing circulation.*

DOCUMENTATION FOCUS

Assessment/Reassessment
- Individual findings, including specific risk factors, status of skin, and ability to manage/direct own care.

Planning
- Plan of care and who is involved in planning.
- Teaching plan.

Implementation/Evaluation
- Responses to interventions, teaching, and actions performed.
- Attainment or progress toward desired outcome(s).
- Modifications to plan of care.

Discharge Planning
- Long-term needs and who is responsible for actions to be taken.
- Specific referrals made.

 Acute Care   Collaborative   Community/ Home Care   Cultural

References

1. Llewellyn, S. (2002). *Skin integrity and wound care (lecture materials)*. Chapel Hill, NC: Cape Fear Community College Nursing Program.
2. Colburn, L. (2001). Prevention for chronic wounds. In: Krasner, D., et al (eds). *Chronic Wound Care: A Clinical Source Book for Healthcare Professionals*. 2nd ed. Wayne, PA: HMP Communications.
3. LeBlanc, K., Baranoski, S. (2009). Prevention and management of skin tears. *Adv Skin Wound Care*, 22(7), 325–332.
4. Lund, C. H., Osborne, J. W., Culler, J. (2001). Neonatal skin care: Clinical outcomes of the AWHONN/NANN evidence-based clinical practice guideline. *J Neonatal Nurs*, 30(1), 30–40.
5. National Pressure Ulcer Advisory Panel. (2014). Prevention and treatment of pressure ulcers: Quick reference guide. Retrieved April 2015 from http://www.npuap.org/resources/educational-and-clinical-resources/prevention-and-treatment-of-pressure-ulcers-clinical-practice-guideline/.
6. Catania, K., et al. (2007). PUPPI: The pressure ulcer prevention protocol interventions. *Am J Nurs*, 107(4), 44–51.
7. Reddy, M., Gill, S. S., Rochan, P. A. (2006). Preventing pressure ulcers: A systematic review. *JAMA*, 296(8), 974–984.
8. Wadland, D. L. (2010). Maintaining skin integrity in the OR. *OR Nurse 2011*, 4(2), 26–32.
9. Stotts, N. A., Gunningberg, L. (2007). How to try this: Predicting pressure ulcer risk. *Am J Nurs*, 107(11), 40–48.
10. Pancorbo-Hildago, P. L., et al. (2006). Risk assessment scales for pressure ulcer prevention: A systematic review. *J Adv Nurs*, 54(1), 94–110.
11. Kottner, J., Dassen, T., Lopez-Medina, I. M. (2010). Pressure ulcer risk assessment in critical care: Interrater reliability and validity studies of the Braden and Waterlow scales and subjective ratings in two intensive care units. *Int J Nurs Stud*, 47(6), 671–677.
12. Blume-Peytavi, U., Hauser, M., Pathirana, D., et al. (2012). Skin care practices for newborns and infants: Review of the clinical evidence for best practices. *Pediatr Dermatol*, 29(1), 1–14.
13. Curley, M. A., et al. (2003). Predicting pressure ulcer risk in pediatric patients: The Braden Q Scale. *Nurs Res*, 52(1), 22–33.
14. Kinman, C. N. (2014, updated 2017). Pressure injuries (pressure ulcers) and wound care. Retrieved April 2018 from http://emedicine.medscape.com/article/190115-overview.
15. Schober-Flores, C. (2012). Pressure ulcers in the pediatric population. *JDNA*, 4(5), 295–306.
16. Scott, W. (2011). Medications that increase the risk of pressure ulcer development. Retrieved April 2018 from https://www.healthguideinfo.com/skin-disease/p113866/.

ineffective Protection

Taxonomy II: Health Promotion—Class 2 Health Management (00043) **[Diagnostic Division:** Safety**],** Approved 1990; Revised 2017

DEFINITION: Decrease in the ability to guard self from internal or external threats such as illness or injury.

RELATED FACTORS
Inadequate nutrition
Substance misuse/[abuse]

DEFINING CHARACTERISTICS

Subjective
Anorexia
Chilling
Itching
Insomnia; fatigue; weakness

Objective
Deficient immunity
Impaired healing; alteration in clotting
Maladaptive stress response
Alteration in perspiration
Dyspnea; coughing

(continues on page 674)

 Diagnostic Studies   Evidence Based Practice   Medications   Pediatric/Geriatric/Lifespan

ineffective Protection (continued)

Restlessness; immobility

Disorientation

Pressure ulcer

At Risk Population: Extremes of age

Associated Condition: Abnormal blood profile

Cancer, immune disorder

Pharmaceutical agent

Treatment regimen

Sample Clinical Applications: Cancer, AIDS, systemic lupus, substance abuse, tuberculosis, dementia, Alzheimer's disease, anorexia or bulimia nervosa, diabetes mellitus, thrombophlebitis, conditions requiring long-term steroid use (e.g., chronic obstructive pulmonary disease [COPD], asthma, renal failure), major surgery

Author Note: The purpose of this diagnosis seems to combine multiple NDs under a single heading for ease of planning care when a number of variables may be present. It is suggested that the user refer to specific NDs based on identified related factors and individual concerns for this client to find appropriate outcomes and interventions that are specifically tied to individual related factors that are present, such as the following:

Extremes of age: Includes concerns regarding body temperature or thermoregulation; memory or sensory-perceptual alterations; impaired mobility, risk for falls, sedentary lifestyle, or self-care deficits; risk for trauma, suffocation, or poisoning; and risk for skin or tissue integrity and fluid volume imbalances.

Inadequate nutrition: Brings up issues of nutrition and unstable blood glucose; risk for infection and delayed surgical recovery; impaired swallowing; impaired skin or tissue integrity; and trauma, problems with coping, and interrupted family processes.

Substance use/abuse: May be situational or chronic with problems ranging from impaired respirations, decreased cardiac output, impaired liver function, and fluid volume deficits to nutritional problems, infection, trauma, risk for self- or other-directed violence, and coping or family process difficulties.

Abnormal blood profile: Suggests possibility of fluid volume imbalances, decreased tissue perfusion, problems with oxygenation, activity intolerance, or risk for infection or injury.

Pharmaceutical agents, and treatment-related side effects or concerns: Includes ineffective tissue perfusion and activity intolerance; cardiovascular, respiratory, and elimination concerns; risk for infection, fluid volume imbalances, impaired skin or tissue integrity, and impaired liver function; pain, nutritional problems, fatigue, sleep difficulties, and ineffective health management; and emotional responses (e.g., anxiety, sorrow, grief, coping).

Sample NOC linkages:

Symptom Control: Personal actions to minimize perceived adverse changes in physical and emotional functioning

Blood Coagulation: Extent to which blood clots within normal period of time

Immune Status: Natural and acquired appropriately targeted resistance to internal and external antigens

---

Sample NIC linkages:

Postanesthesia Care: Monitoring and management of the patient who has recently undergone general or regional anesthesia

Bleeding Precautions: Reduction of stimuli that may induce bleeding or hemorrhage in at-risk patients

Infection Protection: Prevention and early detection of infection in a patient at risk

Surveillance: Purposeful and ongoing acquisition, interpretation, and synthesis of patient data for clinical decision making

***Author Note: It is suggested that the reader refer to specific NDs based on identified related factors or defining characteristics and individual client concerns to find appropriate assessments, outcomes, interventions, and documentation foci.**

 Acute Care   Collaborative   Community/ Home Care   Cultural

Rape-Trauma Syndrome

Taxonomy II: Coping/Stress Tolerance—Class 1 Post-Trauma Responses (000142) [**Diagnostic Division:** Ego Integrity], Approved 1980; Revised 1998, 2017

DEFINITION: Sustained maladaptive response to a forced, violent, sexual penetration against the victim's will and consent. [Rape is not a sexual crime but a crime of violence and is identified as sexual assault. Although attacks are most often directed toward women, men also may be victims.]

RELATED FACTORS
To Be Developed

DEFINING CHARACTERISTICS

Subjective
Embarrassment; humiliation; shame; guilt; self-blame
Helplessness; powerlessness
Shock; fear; anxiety; anger; thoughts of revenge
Nightmares; alteration in sleep pattern
Change in relationship(s); sexual dysfunction

Objective
Physical trauma; muscle tension/spasm
Confusion; disorganization; impaired decision making
Agitation; hyperalertness; aggression
Mood swings; perceived vulnerability; dependency; low self-esteem; depression
Substance misuse/[abuse]; history of suicide attempt
Denial; phobias; paranoia; dissociative identity disorder
At Risk Population: Rape

DESIRED OUTCOMES/EVALUATION CRITERIA

Sample NOC linkages:
Abuse Recovery: Sexual: Extent of healing of physical and psychological injuries due to sexual abuse or exploitation
Coping: Personal actions to manage stressors that tax an individual's resources

Client Will (Include Specific Time Frame)
- Report absence of physical complications, pain, and discomfort.
- Deal appropriately with emotional reactions as evidenced by behavior and expression of feelings.
- Verbalize a positive self-image.
- Verbalize recognition that incident was not of own doing.
- Identify behaviors or situations within own control that may reduce risk of recurrence.
- Deal with practical aspects (e.g., court appearances).
- Demonstrate appropriate changes in lifestyle (e.g., change in job, residence) that contribute to recovery or seek and obtain support from significant others (SOs), as needed.
- Interact with individuals or groups in desired and acceptable manner.

(continues on page 676)

 Diagnostic Studies Evidence Based Practice Medications 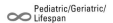 Pediatric/Geriatric/Lifespan

Rape-Trauma Syndrome (continued)

ACTIONS/INTERVENTIONS

Sample NIC linkages:

Rape-Trauma Treatment: Provision of emotional and physical support immediately following a reported rape

Crisis Intervention: Use of short-term counseling to help the patient cope with a crisis and resume a state of functioning comparable to or better than the precrisis state

Counseling: Use of an interactive helping process focusing on the needs, problems, or feelings of the patient and significant others to enhance or support coping, problem-solving, and interpersonal relationships

NURSING PRIORITY NO. 1 To assess trauma and individual reaction, noting length of time since occurrence of event:

- Observe for and elicit information about physical injury and assess stress-related symptoms such as numbness, headache, tightness in chest, nausea, pounding heart, etc. *Indicators of degree of and reaction to trauma experienced by the client, which may occur immediately and in the days or weeks following the attack.*[4]
- Identify psychological responses such as anger, shock, acute anxiety, confusion, and denial. Note laughter, crying, calm or agitated, excited (hysterical) behavior, and expressions of disbelief or self-blame. *Victim may exhibit expressed response pattern (compound reaction), displaying these feelings openly and freely as manifestations of experiencing the trauma of rape/sexual assault and the accompanying feelings of fear of death, violation, powerlessness, and helplessness. On the other hand, client may exhibit controlled (silent) response pattern with little or no emotion expressed. Any emotion is appropriate, as each person responds in own individual way; however, inappropriate behaviors or acting out may require intervention.*[3,4] Refer to NDs risk for self-/other-directed Violence.
- Note silence, stuttering, and inability to sit still. *May be signs of increasing anxiety, thus indicating need for further evaluation and intervention. Anxiety is suppressed and client does not talk about the trauma, resulting in an overwhelming emotional burden.*[3,4]
- Determine degree of disorganization. *Initially, the individual may be in shock and disbelief, which is a normal response to the incident. The person may respond by withdrawing and be unable to manage activities of daily living, especially when the incident was particularly brutal, requiring assistance and treatment to enable her or him to recover and move on.*[3,4]
- Identify whether incident has reactivated preexisting or co-existing situations (physical or psychological). *The presence of these factors can affect how the client views the current trauma. Previous traumatic incidents that have not been effectively resolved may compound the current incident.*[1]
- Ascertain cultural values or religious beliefs that may affect how client views incident, self, and expectations of significant other (SO)/family reaction. *Client may believe incident will bring shame on the family, blame self, or believe that family will blame client, thus affecting client's ability to reach out to others for support.*[6]
- Determine sexual orientation of the survivor. *Heterosexual men/boys may believe that they are now gay (after being sexually assaulted) and need to be assured that is not true. Gay, bisexual, or gay-identified may be targeted because of this. Healthcare providers may treat these individuals with suspicion, disregard, and disrespect, contributing to the survivor's sense of shame and guilt and making it more difficult to seek help.*[5]
- Determine disruptions in relationships (e.g., spouse/partner, family, friends, coworkers). *Many women find that they react to men in general in a different way, seeing them as reminders of the assault. Male survivors may withdraw entirely from sexual relations.*[5,7]
- Identify development of phobic reactions to ordinary articles (e.g., knives) and situations (e.g., walking in groups of people, strangers ringing doorbell). *These are manifestations of extreme anxiety, and client may need treatment to learn how to manage feelings.*[3,4]

 Acute Care   Collaborative   Community/ Home Care   Cultural

- Note degree of intrusive repetitive thoughts, sleep disturbances. *Survivor may notice disruptions in activities of daily living, reliving the attack, thoughts of recrimination, self-blame ("Why didn't I . . . ?"), and nightmares. Although these factors are distressing and upsetting, they are part of the normal healing process.*[3,4]
- Assess degree of dysfunctional coping. *Client may turn to use of alcohol or other drugs, have suicidal or homicidal ideation, or display marked change in sexual behavior in an attempt to cope with traumatic event.*[4]

NURSING PRIORITY NO. 2   To assist client to deal with situation that exists:

- Explore own feelings regarding rape/incest issue prior to interacting with the client. *Since the feelings related to these incidents are so pervasive, the individual involved in caregiving needs to recognize own biases to prevent imposing them on the client.*[1]

Acute phase/immediate care

- ✚∞ Stay with the client—do not leave child unattended. Listen but do not probe. Tell client you are sorry this has happened and that she or he is safe now. *During this phase, the client experiences a complete disruption of life as she or he has known it, and presence of caregiver may provide reassurance and sense of safety.*[2,4]
- 🚑 Involve rape or sexual assault response team or sexual assault nurse examiner when available. Provide a same-sex examiner when appropriate. *Presence of the response team trained to collect evidence appropriately and sensitively provides assurance to the survivor that she or he is being taken care of. Client may react to someone who is the sex of the attacker, and use of a same-sex examiner communicates sensitivity to her or his feelings at this difficult time.*[11]
- 🌐 Be sensitive to cultural factors that may affect specifics of examination process. *For example, in some cultures, women cannot be examined without a male family member present. These issues need to be considered when treating the survivor.*[6]
- ∞ Evaluate client as dictated by age, gender, and developmental level. *Age of the survivor is an important consideration in deciding plan of care and appropriate interventions. Note: While underreported, it is believed that 1 in 6 men are sexually assaulted and 1 in 6 boys will be sexually assaulted or abused before the age of 18.*[5,8]
- Assist with documentation of incident for law enforcement officers and child-protective services reports, explaining each step of the procedure. Maintain sequencing and collection of evidence (chain of evidence), label each specimen, and store and package properly. *It is crucial to provide accurate information to law enforcement for potential legal proceedings when perpetrator is charged.* Be careful to use nonjudgmental language. *Words can carry legal implications that may affect subsequent proceedings.*[1]
- Provide environment in which client can talk freely about feelings and fears. *Client needs to talk about the incident and concerns, such as issues of relationship with or response of SO(s), pregnancy, and sexually transmitted infections (STIs), so they may be dealt with in a positive manner.*[10]
- Provide information about emergency birth control and prophylactic treatment for STIs and assist with finding resources for follow-through. *Promotes client's peace of mind and opportunity to prevent these conditions.*[10]
- Provide psychological support by listening and remaining with client. If client does not want to talk, accept silence. *May indicate silent reaction or controlled style of dealing with the occurrence in which the individual contains his or her emotions, using all his or her energy to maintain composure.*[4]
- 🚑 Listen to and investigate physical complaints. Assist with medical treatments, as indicated. *Emotional reactions may limit client's ability to recognize physical injury.*[4]
- Assist with practical realities. *Client may be so emotionally distraught that she or he may not be able to attend to needs for such things as safe, temporary housing, money, or other issues that may need to be addressed. Assistance helps individual maintain contact with reality.*
- Determine client's ego strengths and help him or her use them in a positive way by acknowledging client's ability to handle what is happening. *Validation of belief that person can deal with what has happened and move forward with life promotes self-acceptance and helps client begin this process.*[6,9]
- Identify supportive persons for this individual. *Client needs to know she or he can go to a strong system of friends, family, or advocate who will respond with empathy.*[7]

 Diagnostic Studies   Evidence Based Practice   Medications   Pediatric/Geriatric/Lifespan

Postacute phase

• Allow the client to work through own kind of adjustment. Do not force issue if client is withdrawn or unwilling to talk (silent reaction). *Individuals react in many ways to the traumatic event of rape, and no response is abnormal. Factors that influence how the survivor deals with the situation are personality, support system, existing life problems and prior sexual victimization, relationship with the offender, degree of violence used, social and cultural influences, and ability to cope with stress.*[2,4]

• Listen for expressions of fear (e.g., of perpetrator returning, of being in crowds or being alone, etc.). *May reveal developing phobias needing evaluation and appropriate interventions and ongoing therapy.*[2,4]

• Discuss specific concerns and fears. Identify appropriate actions and provide information as indicated. *May need diagnostic testing for pregnancy, STIs, or other resources. Meeting these needs and providing information will help client begin the process of recovery.*[10]

• Include written instructions that are concise and clear regarding medical treatments, crisis support services, etc. Encourage return for follow-up. *Reinforces teaching and provides opportunity to deal with information at own pace. Follow-up appointment provides opportunity for determining how client is managing feelings and what needs may not have been met.*

Long-term phase

• Continue listening to expressions of concern. Note persistence of somatic complaints (e.g., nausea, anorexia, insomnia, muscle tension, headache). *May need to continue to talk about the assault. Repeating the story helps client to move on, but continued somatic concerns may indicate developing posttraumatic stress disorder.*[6,8]

• Permit free expression of feelings (may continue from the crisis phase). Refrain from rushing client through expressions of feelings too quickly and avoid reassuring inappropriately. *Client may believe pain and/or anguish is misunderstood, and depression may limit responses.*[1,6]

• Acknowledge reality of loss of self that existed before the incident. Assist client to move toward an acceptance of the potential for growth that exists within individual. *Following this traumatic event, the individual will not be able to go back to the person he or she was before. Life will always have the memory of what happened, and client needs to accept that reality and move on in the best way possible.*[2]

• Continue to allow client to progress at own pace. *The process of grieving is a very individual one, and each person needs to know that she or he can take whatever time needed to resolve feelings and move on with life.*[4] (Refer to ND Grieving for additional interventions.)

• Give "permission" to express and deal with anger at the perpetrator and situation in acceptable ways. Set limits on destructive behaviors. *Facilitates resolution of feelings without diminishing self-concept.*[6]

• Keep discussion on practical and emotional level rather than intellectualizing the experience. *When the person talks about the incident intellectually, instead of identifying and talking about feelings, client avoids dealing with the feelings, thus inhibiting recovery.*[1]

• Assist in dealing with ongoing concerns about and effects of the incident, such as court appearance, STI, relationship with SO(s), etc. *Depending on degree of disorganization, client will need help to deal with these practical and emotional issues.*

• Provide for sensitive, trained counselors, considering individual needs. *Male/female counselors may be best determined on an individual basis, as counselor's gender may be an issue for some clients, affecting ability to disclose and deal with feelings.*[1]

NURSING PRIORITY NO. 3 To promote wellness (Teaching/Discharge Considerations):

• Provide information about what reactions client may expect during each phase. Let client know these are common reactions and phrase in neutral terms of "You may or may not . . . experience, know, be aware of. . . ." *Such information helps client anticipate and deal with reactions if they are experienced. Note: Be aware that although male rape perpetrators are usually heterosexual, the male victim may be concerned about his own sexuality and may exhibit a homophobic response.*[1]

• Assist client to identify factors that may have created a vulnerable situation and that she or he may have power to change to protect self in the future. *While client needs to be assured that she or he is not to blame for*

 Acute Care   Collaborative   Community/ Home Care   Cultural

incident, the circumstances of the incident need to be assessed to identify factors that are within the individual's control to avoid a similar incident occurring.[6]

- Avoid making value judgments. *The survivor often blames self about the incident and agonizes over the circumstances; therefore, nonjudgmental language is very important to help the person accept that the fault is not hers or his.*[1,6]
- Discuss lifestyle changes client is contemplating and how they will contribute to recovery. *Helps client evaluate appropriateness of plans. In the anxiety of the moment, the individual may believe that changing residence, job, or other aspects of her or his environment will be healing. In reality, while this response is normal and represents an attempt to regain control over own life, these changes may not help and may make matters worse.*[4]
- Encourage psychiatric consultation if client is violent, inconsolable, or does not seem to be making an adjustment. Participation in a group may be helpful. *May need intensive professional help to come to terms with the assault.*[1,6]
- Refer to family or marital counseling, as indicated. *When relationships with family members are affected by the incident, counseling may be needed to resolve the issues.*[1,9]
- Refer to NDs Anxiety, ineffective Coping, Fear, Grieving, complicated Grieving, and Powerlessness, as appropriate.

DOCUMENTATION FOCUS

Assessment/Reassessment
- Individual findings, including nature of incident, individual reactions and fears, degree of trauma (physical and emotional), effects on lifestyle.
- Cultural or religious factors.
- Reactions of family/SO(s).
- Samples gathered for evidence and disposition or storage (chain of evidence).

Planning
- Plan of action and who is involved in planning.
- Teaching plan.

Implementation/Evaluation
- Responses to interventions, teaching, and actions performed.
- Attainment or progress toward desired outcome(s).
- Modifications to plan of care.

Discharge Planning
- Long-term needs and who is responsible for actions to be taken.
- Specific referrals made.

References

1. Townsend, M. C. (2010). *Essentials of Psychiatric Mental Health Nursing: Concepts of Care in Evidence-Based Practice.* 5th ed. Philadelphia: F. A. Davis.
2. Rape Crisis Staff. (No date). Phases of recovery. Retrieved April 2018 from http://rapecrisis.org.za/information-for-survivors/phases-of-recovery/.
3. Burgess, A. W., Holstrom, L. L. (2003). Dancing in the darkness. Retrieved April 2018 from http://www.dancinginthedarkness.com/articles.php?show=11&arc=83.
4. Rape Victim Advocates. (2010). Effects of sexual violence. Retrieved April 2018 from http://www.rapevictimadvocates.org/trauma.asp.
5. No author listed. (No date). Facts about male sexual abuse: FACT #5 – Sexual abuse does not determine sexual identity/orientation. Retrieved April 2018 from https://www.malesurvivor.org/fact-5/.
6. Hensley, L. G. (2002). Treatment for survivors of rape: Issues and interventions. *J Mental Health Counseling*, 24(4), 330–347.
7. Menna, A. (2004, update 2014). Rape trauma syndrome: The journey to healing belongs to everyone. Retrieved April 2018 from www.giftfromwithin.org/html/journey.html.
8. National Sexual Violence Resource Center. (2015). Statistics about sexual violence. Retrieved April 2018 from http://www.nsvrc.org/sites/default/files/publications_nsvrc_factsheet_media-packet_statistics-about-sexual-violence_0.pdf.
9. Lauer, T. M. (2006). Rape trauma syndrome in intimate relationships. *Family Therapy Magazine*, 5(1), 36–41.

 Diagnostic Studies   Evidence Based Practice   Medications   Pediatric/Geriatric/Lifespan

10. Rape, Abuse & Incest National Network (RAINN). (2018). After sexual assault (Receiving medical attention and various other pages). Retrieved April 2018 from https://rainn.org/articles/receiving-medical-attention.

11. The Advocates for Human Rights. (Updated 2009). Sexual assault response teams. Retrieved April 2018 from http://www.stopvaw.org/sexual_assault_response_teams.html.

ineffective Relationship

Taxonomy II: Role Relationships—Class 3 Role Performance (00223) [**Diagnostic Division:** Ego Integrity], Approved 2010; Revised 2017

DEFINITION: A pattern of mutual partnership that is insufficient to provide for each other's needs.

RELATED FACTORS
Stressors
Substance misuse/[abuse]
Unrealistic expectations
Ineffective communication skills

DEFINING CHARACTERISTICS

Subjective
Dissatisfaction with complementary relationship between partners
Dissatisfaction with physical or emotional need fulfillment between partners
Dissatisfaction with information or idea sharing between partners

Objective
Unsatisfying communication between partners
Insufficient balance in autonomy or collaboration between partners
Insufficient mutual respect between partners
Insufficient mutual support in daily activities between partners
Inadequate understanding of partner's compromised functioning
Delay in meeting of developmental goals appropriate for family life-cycle stage
Partner not identified as support person
At Risk Population: Developmental crisis
History of domestic abuse; incarceration of one partner
Associated Condition: Alteration in cognitive functioning in one partner
Sample Clinical Applications: Chronic conditions (e.g., MS, spinal cord injury, gastric bypass surgery, mental health problems, depression, anxiety, bipolar disorder, substance abuse, dementia), domestic violence

DESIRED OUTCOMES/EVALUATION CRITERIA

Sample NOC linkages:
Social Interaction Skills: Personal behaviors that promote effective relationships
Role Performance: Congruence of an individual's role behavior with role expectations
Social Involvement: Social interactions with persons, groups, or organizations

Client Will (Include Specific Time Frame)
• Verbalize a desire to improve relationship with partner.
• Acknowledge worth and value of partner as a key person.

 Acute Care
 Collaborative
 Community/ Home Care
 Cultural

- Seek information regarding physical and emotional needs of partner.
- Engage in effective communication skills for both partners.
- Participate in marital therapy sessions to learn ways to develop a satisfactory relationship.

ACTIONS/INTERVENTIONS

Sample **NIC** linkages:

Role Enhancement: Assisting a patient, significant other, and/or family to improve relationships by clarifying and supplementing specific role behaviors

Socialization Enhancement: Facilitation of another person's ability to interact with others

Conflict Mediation: Facilitation of a constructive dialogue between opposing parties with a goal of resolving disputes in a mutually acceptable manner

NURSING PRIORITY NO. 1   To assess current situation and determine needs:

- ∞ ▧ Determine makeup of family, length of relationship, and financial situation—parents/children, older/younger, and other members of household. *Stressors of family relationships within a household, difficulties with child-rearing, older adult needing care, and financial difficulties can strain the relationship between partners.*[2,3,7,8]
- Discuss individual's perception of own and other's needs and how partner sees own needs. *Identifies how each person sees situation and areas of agreement and disagreement, providing a basis for beginning plan of care.*[3,6]
- ▧ Determine each person's self-image and locus of control. *View of self as a positive or negative individual who is in control or controlled by others influences behavior and how partners react to each other.*[3,4,7,12]
- ▧ Assess emotional intelligence skills of each individual. *This is the ability to recognize and control one's own emotions and recognize the emotions of the other.*[1,7]
- 🌐 Investigate cultural factors that may be affecting relationship and contributing to conflict. *Roles from family of origin for each person may promote conflict when beliefs clash and neither is willing to change or even discuss thinking.*[3,4,12]
- Determine style of communication used by partners. *Poor communication is unclear and indirect leading to conflict, ineffective problem-solving, and poor emotional bonding in families with problems.*[1,3]
- ▧ Determine how family as a whole functions. *Personal and family history affects relationships between family members, and situational dynamics can create conflict as individuals take sides in disagreements, escalating the situation.*[3,4,7]
- Ascertain ways in which family members deal with conflict. *Conflict is inevitable in relationships, and partners need to identify whether how they deal with it is effective or ineffective.*[1,2,8]
- ▧ Identify concerns about sexual aspects of relationship from both partners' viewpoints. *Intimacy is an important part of a relationship, and if both individuals are avoiding that activity, they will need to discuss specific ways to resolve these problems.*[1,4,6,9]
- Note medical problems that may be affecting sexual relationship. *Conditions such as hysterectomy, prostatitis, breast cancer, and erectile dysfunction may cause partners to withdraw from one another.*[8,10]

NURSING PRIORITY NO. 2   To assist partners to resolve existing conflict:

- ▧ Maintain positive attitude toward partners and family members. *A safe environment allows individuals to speak freely, knowing they will not be judged for comments and opinions, so couple can get to the deeper roots of current situation.*[1,6,7]

- Discuss surface symptoms of dysfunctional relationships and the fact that these are not the problems that need to be dealt with. *Individuals are often not aware of underlying emotions that are influencing their behavior and continue to focus on surface issues.*[6]
- Explore each partner's emotional needs. *Unconscious desires to gain acceptance, recognition, and a sense of being cared about or valued are often motivators for relationships.*[6,7]
- Discuss and clarify nonverbal communication. *Partners need to be aware of and ask about the meaning of body language, tone of voice, and subtle movements that convey positive or negative messages. When these cues are misinterpreted, they can lead to misunderstandings.*[1,6]
- ▨ Assist partners/family to learn effective conflict resolution skills such as the win-win method. *Individuals have traditionally used ineffective means of solving conflict or avoided it altogether. Resolving to listen to each other's needs and agree on a mutually acceptable solution provides new ways to resolve problems and enhances relationship.*[5,11]
- Provide information about the Active-listening technique. *Avoids giving advice and encourages other person to find own solution, enhancing self-esteem.*[5]
- ▨ Have partners identify thoughts and feelings when starting a discussion with each other. *A system of thinking (a paradigm) forms the basis for how we look at and experience life and determines how we perceive our world, forming the basis for our reality, and exists below our level of conscience.*[11,12]
- ▨ Recommend individuals verify what they believe the other has said. *Allows speaker to correct misperception and respond more effectively.*[1,5,11,12]
- ▨ Have partners role-play a specific conflict that is a frequent issue. *Practicing how to defuse arguments and repair hurt feelings helps to identify other's feelings and use new skills for resolution.*[11]
- Encourage partners to maintain a calm demeanor. *Regardless of circumstances, staying focused enables individuals to think more rationally and come to a desired solution.*[5]
- Discuss sexual concerns and provide opportunity for questions. *Conflict in the relationship inevitability affects these concerns and providing information and discussing them can enhance intimacy.*[1,9]
- ▨ Promote nonblameful self-disclosure when having a discussion. *Not placing blame results in a more considerate and respectful resolution.*[7,11]

NURSING PRIORITY NO. 3 To promote optimal functioning (Teaching/Discharge Considerations):

- 🏠 Have partners acknowledge beliefs they have become aware of during therapy. *Unconscious thinking influences each person's view of the world in negative or positive ways.*[1,11]
- ▨ Encourage use of relaxation and mindfulness techniques. *Helps individuals to ease anxiety and learn to relate to each other in a calm manner.*[7]
- Discuss the use of humor and laughter in daily lives. *Helps to lighten difficult moments and provide opportunities to share fun moments.*[6]
- Recommend books and Web sites to provide additional information. *Encourages partners to seek and learn new ways to improve relationship.*[3]
- 👥 Refer to support groups and classes as indicated. *Parenting, assertiveness, and financial assistance will help partners learn new skills as needed.*[2,3,8,11]
- ▨ Include all family members in discussions, as indicated. *Promotes involvement, provides opportunities for communication and clarification of family dynamics, and enhances commitment to achieving goals.*[1,3,7]
- 👥 Refer to other physical/psychological resources, as needed. *May need further treatment to address pathology and help partners understand other's needs.*[2,6,8]

DOCUMENTATION FOCUS

Assessment/Reassessment
- Individual's perception of situation and self.
- Partner's views and expectations.
- How partners communicate and deal with conflict.

 Acute Care   Collaborative   Community/ Home Care   Cultural

Planning
- Plan of care and who is involved in planning.
- Teaching plan.

Implementation/Evaluation
- Response of partners to plan, interventions, and actions performed.
- Attainment or progress toward desired outcomes.

Discharge Planning
- Long-range plan and who is responsible for actions to be taken.
- Referrals made.

References

1. Peterson, R. (2009). Families first: Keys to successful family functioning: Communication. *Virginia Cooperative Extension.* Retrieved April 2018 from http://www.pubs.ext.vt.edu/350/350-092/350-092.html.
2. Pincus, D. (2018). Encouragement and empowerment for moms (with free parenting mantras!). *EmpoweringParents.com.* Retrieved April 2018 from https://www.empoweringparents.com/article/encouragement-and-empowerment-for-moms-with-free-parenting-mantras/.
3. Riesch, S. K., et al. (2010). Furthering the understanding of parent-child relationships: A nursing scholarship review series. Part 5: Parent-adolescent and teen parent-child relationships. *J Spec Pediatr Nurs*, 15(3), 182–201.
4. Fincham, F. D., Bradbury, T. N. (eds), (1990). *The Psychology of Marriage: Basic Issues & Applications.* New York: Guilford Press.
5. Scott, E. (Updated 2018). Conflict resolution skills for healthy relationships. Retrieved April 2018 from http://stress.about.com/od/relationships/a/conflict_res.htm.
6. Robinson, L., Smith, M., Segal, J. (Updated 2018). Relationship help: Building satisfying relationships that last. Retrieved April 2018 from https://www.helpguide.org/articles/relationships-communication/relationship-help.htm.
7. Duncan, L. G., Coatsworth, J. D., Greenberg, M. T. (2009). Pilot study to gauge acceptability of a mindfulness based, family-focused preventive intervention. *J Prim Prev*, 30(5), 605–618.
8. Stewart, C. (2008, updated 2017). Common traits of a dysfunctional family. *Everyday Health.* Retrieved April 2018 from https://www.everydayhealth.com/emotional-health/common-traits-dysfunctional-family/.
9. Nusbaum, M. R. H., et al. (2000). The high prevalence of concerns among women seeking routine gynecological care. *J Fam Pract*, 49(3), 229–232.
10. Vorvick, L. J. (2010). Sexual problems overview. Retrieved April 2018 from https://ufhealth.org/sexual-problems-overview.
11. Davidson, J., Wood, C. (Winter 2004). A conflict resolution model. *Theory Into Practice*, 43(1), 6–13.
12. Yolles, M. (1996). The systems paradigm. Retrieved April 2018 from http://www.academia.edu/175318/The_Systems_Paradigm_Paradigm.

readiness for enhanced Relationship

Taxonomy II: Role Relationships—Class 3 Role Performance (00207) [**Diagnostic Division:** Ego Integrity], Approved 2006; Revised 2013

DEFINITION: A pattern of mutual partnership to provide for each other's needs, which can be strengthened.

DEFINING CHARACTERISTICS

Subjective
Expresses desire to enhance:
Communication between partners
Satisfaction with information/idea sharing between partners
Emotional need fulfillment for each partner

(continues on page 684)

readiness for enhanced Relationship (continued)

Satisfaction with physical or emotional need fulfillment for each partner
Satisfaction with complementary relation between partners
Mutual respect between partners
Autonomy or collaboration between partners
Understanding of partners' functional deficit
Sample Clinical Applications: Applicable in any setting, not dependent on presence of pathology although may be useful in chronic physical conditions or mental health challenges

DESIRED OUTCOMES/EVALUATION CRITERIA

Sample **NOC** linkages:
Social Interaction Skills: Personal behaviors that promote effective relationships
Role Performance: Congruence of an individual's role behavior with role expectations
Social Involvement: Social interactions with persons, groups, or organizations

Client Will (Include Specific Time Frames)
• Verbalize a desire to learn more effective communication skills.
• Verbalize understanding of current relationship with partner.
• Seek information to improve emotional and physical needs of both partners.
• Talk with partner about circumstances that can be improved.
• Develop realistic plans to strengthen relationship.

ACTIONS/INTERVENTIONS

Sample **NIC** linkages:
Role Enhancement: Assisting a patient, significant other, and/or family to improve relationships by clarifying and supplementing specific role behaviors
Socialization Enhancement: Facilitation of another person's ability to interact with others

NURSING PRIORITY NO. 1   To assess current situation and determine needs:

• ∞ Determine makeup of family: parents/children, older/younger. *Life changes, such as developmental, situational, and health-illness, can affect the relationship between partners and require readjustment and thinking of ways to enhance situation.*[1]
• Discuss client's perception of needs and how partner sees desire to improve relationship. *Identifies thinking and whether both partners see the situation in the same way and individual expectations for change.*[4]
• Identify use of effective communication skills. *May need to improve understanding of words partners use in discussion of sensitive subjects.*[4]
• Help client to identify thoughts and feelings when starting a discussion with partner. *A system of thinking (referred to as a paradigm) forms the basis for how we look at and experience life and determines how we perceive our world, forms the basis for our reality, and exists below our level of conscience.*[4]
• Ask partners how they deal with conflict. *Since conflict is a normal, natural, and inevitable part of life, this needs to be acknowledged, and individuals need to learn how to deal with it effectively.*[4]
• Ascertain client's view of sexual aspects of relationship. *Changes that occur with aging or medical conditions, such as hysterectomy or erectile dysfunction, can affect the relationship and need specific interventions to resolve.*[2]
• ⊕ Identify cultural factors relating to individual's view of role in relationship. *Although changing, in the United States, men may typically take care of financial affairs and car and house repairs, while women may manage household and caregiving roles.*[1]

 Acute Care   Collaborative   Community/ Home Care   Cultural

- Discuss how family as a whole functions. *Interrelationships with members of the family, personal and family history, and situational dynamics can impact the functioning of the whole family.*[2]

NURSING PRIORITY NO. 2 To assist the client to enhance existing relationship:

- Maintain positive attitude toward client. *Promotes safe relationship in which client can feel free to speak openly and plan for a positive future.*[1]
- Have couple discuss paradigms that they have become aware of in own thinking that interfere with relationship. *These beliefs exist below our conscious mind, influencing our behavior and whether we see the world in negative or positive ways.*[4]
- Determine how each person views himself of herself as a positive or negative person. *One's self-image influences behavior and how he or she relates to others. When emotional needs are met, individuals relate to others in positive ways, while unmet needs result in low self-image and insecurity.*[5]
- Discuss the skills of emotional intelligence, which are important for maintaining positive relationships. *This is the ability to recognize and effectively control our own emotions and to recognize the emotions of others.*[6]
- Help couple to recognize that surface symptoms of dysfunctional relationships are not the problems that need to be dealt with. *Underlying emotions influence our behaviors, and individuals often are not aware of them and continue to deal with the superficial conflicts.*[6]
- Explore individual's emotional needs. *Relationships are often motivated by unconscious desires to gain acceptance, recognition, and a sense of being cared about or valued.*[5]
- Note client's awareness of nonverbal communications. *Body language, tone of voice, a roll of the eyes, or subtle movements convey strong messages, positive or negative, that need to be discussed and clarified.*[6]
- Discuss effective conflict-resolution skills. *People tend to be afraid of conflict because effective ways to deal with it have not been learned, and it often ends in a lose-lose situation.*[4]
- Encourage client to remain calm and focused regardless of circumstances. *Maintaining a calm demeanor helps individual to be able to think more clearly and be more rational in dealing with situation.*[6]
- Recommend cross-checking or verifying what listener believes speaker said. *Clarifies communication and allows speaker to respond or correct perception of listener as needed.*[5]
- Help partners to learn the win-win method of conflict resolution. *Although conflict can damage a relationship, learning to listen to each other's needs can assist partners to arrive at mutually acceptable solutions.*[4]
- Role-play ways to defuse arguments and repair injured feelings. *Provides a realistic situation wherein each person can identify own and partner's view and practice new ways of interacting.*[6]
- Provide open environment for partners to discuss sexual concerns and questions. *Problems may arise out of lack of information about these issues, and when individuals are comfortable with this knowledge, the relationship can be improved.*[2]
- Discuss nonblameful self-disclosure when having a dialogue. *Partners take turns talking about own needs and feelings without blaming the other, resulting in being able to find a solution in a climate of mutual consideration and respect.*[4]

NURSING PRIORITY NO. 3 To promote optimal relationship (Teaching/Discharge Considerations):

- Provide information for partners, using bibliotherapy and appropriate Web sites. *Promotes continuation of learning about how to enhance relationship.*[3]
- Encourage couple to use humor and playfulness in their relationship. *Sharing laughter and enjoying life helps to weather difficult times that may occur.*[6]
- Discuss the importance of being an empathic, understanding, and nonjudgmental listener when either partner has a problem. *The expectation that the partner will be willing to help by listening eases the anxiety of talking about major problems.*[5]
- Encourage use of the skill of Active-listening. *This avoids giving advice and helps other person to find own solution, enhancing self-esteem.*[4]

- Refer to support groups and classes on assertiveness and parenting, as indicated by individual needs.[3]
- Include family members in discussions as needed. *Knowing how the family relates as a whole will help improve relationships of partners as well as the other family members.*[3]
- Refer for care as indicated by psychological or physical problems of either individual. *May need further treatment and explanation to help partner understand these situations.*[1]

DOCUMENTATION FOCUS

Assessment/Reassessment
- Baseline information, individual's perception of situation and self.
- Reasons for desire to improve relationship and expectations for change.

Planning
- Plan of care and who is involved in planning.
- Teaching plan.

Implementation/Evaluation
- Response of partners to plan, interventions, and actions performed.
- Attainment or progress toward desired outcomes(s).

Discharge Planning
- Long-term plan and who is responsible for actions to be taken.

References

1. Perrone, L. M., Webb, L. K., Jackson, Z. V. (2007). Relationships between parental attachment, work and family roles and life satisfaction. *Career Dev Quart*, 55(3), 237–248.
2. Denberg, D. (1999). Factors that influence a couple's relationship. *Couple Therapy: An Information Guide*. Toronto, Canada: The Centre for Addiction and Mental Health.
3. Glass, J. S., Mann, M. A. (2004). Harmonious families: Using family counseling and adventure based learning opportunities to enhance growth. Retrieved April 2018 from http://www.shsu.edu/~piic/spring%202006/Glass.html.
4. Wilmot, W. W., Bergstrom, M. J. (2018). Relationship theories—Self-other relationship. *International Encyclopedia of Marriage and Family Therapy*. Retrieved April 2018 from https://www.encyclopedia.com/reference/encyclopedias-almanacs-transcripts-and-maps/relationship-theories-self-other-relationship.
5. Hollister, W. G., Edgerton, J. W. (1974). Teaching relationship building skills. *Am J Public Health*, 64(1), 41–46.
6. Robinson, L., Smith, M. A., Segal, J. (Updated 2018). Relationship help: Tips for building romantic relationships that last. Retrieved November 2015, 2018 from https://www.helpguide.org/articles/relationships-communication/relationship-help.htm.

---

risk for ineffective Relationship

Taxonomy II: Role Relationships—Class 3 Role Performance (00229) **[Diagnostic Division:** Ego Integrity**],** Approved 2010; Revised 2013, 2017

DEFINITION: Susceptible to developing a pattern that is insufficient for providing a mutual partnership to provide for each other's needs.

RISK FACTORS
Stressors
Substance misuse/[abuse]
Unrealistic expectations
Ineffective communication skills

 Acute Care   Collaborative   Community/Home Care   Cultural

At Risk Population: Developmental crisis
History of domestic abuse; incarceration of one partner
Associated Condition: Alteration in cognitive functioning in one partner
Sample Clinical Applications: Chronic conditions (e.g., MS, spinal cord injury, gastric bypass surgery, mental health problems, depression, anxiety, bipolar disorder, substance abuse, dementia/Alzheimer's), domestic violence

DESIRED OUTCOMES/EVALUATION CRITERIA

Sample **NOC** linkages:

Social Interaction Skills: Personal behaviors that promote effective relationships
Role Performance: Congruence of an individual's role behavior with role expectations
Social Involvement: Social interactions with persons, groups, or organizations

Client Will (Include Specific Time Frames)
• Verbalize desire to make changes to meet each other's needs as appropriate.
• Express a desire to improve communication skills.
• Develop realistic plans to improve relationship.

ACTIONS/INTERVENTIONS

Sample **NIC** linkages:

Counseling: Use of an interactive helping process focusing on the needs, problems, or feelings of the patient and significant others to enhance or support coping, problem-solving, and interpersonal relationships
Role Enhancement: Assisting a patient, significant other, and/or family to improve relationships by clarifying and supplementing specific role behaviors
Socialization Enhancement: Facilitation of another person's ability to interact with others

NURSING PRIORITY NO. 1   To assess current situation and determine needs:

• ∞ ▦ Determine makeup of family, length of relationship, and specific stressors. *Stressors of family—developmental issues, elderly parents needing assistance, financial difficulties, and domestic violence—strained relationships between partners.*[2,3,7,8]
• ▦ Identify how each partner sees own self-image and locus of control. *View of self as a positive or negative person who is in control or controlled by others influences how each relates to the other.*[3,4,7,8,12]
• Discuss needs of each partner and how each views the other's needs. *Identifies misperceptions and areas of disagreement to provide a basis of planning for change.*[1,3]
• Identify style of communication and understanding of nonverbal cues used by family members. *Poor communication and lack of understanding of what the other is saying, or inferring, leads to conflicts and lack of problem-solving.*[1,3]
• Determine how partners deal with conflict. *Many individuals try to avoid conflict instead of working to resolve it.*[5,6]
• 🌐 Identify cultural beliefs that affect how each person deals with daily activities in family. *Family of origin influences how individuals think roles are to be dealt with, and conflict arises if partners are not willing to discuss and change beliefs.*[3,4,12]

 Diagnostic Studies   Evidence Based Practice   Medications   Pediatric/Geriatric/Lifespan

- Identify medical problems/sexual concerns that may affect relationship. *Conditions such as prostate problems, breast cancer, hysterectomy, and erectile dysfunction can affect interactions between partners.*[4,8,10]
- Ascertain how couple deals with sexual aspects of their relationship. *When anger and conflict interfere with intimacy, couple may distant themselves from one another.*[1,4,6,9]
- Note how family as a whole functions. *Interactions among family members and situational dynamics provide information about need to improve relationships.*[3,7]

NURSING PRIORITY NO. 2   To assist couple to improve relationship:

- Maintain positive attitude in interactions with individuals. *Provides an environment in which clients feel comfortable and safe discussing problems openly.*[1,6,7]
- Promote discussion of awareness of individuals' beliefs and thoughts that may strain relationship. *Enables individuals to begin to discuss potential problem areas.*[3,6]
- Have client identify thoughts and feelings when starting a conversation with partner. *Individuals have a system of thinking that forms the basis for reality, determines how we see the world, and exists below the level of our consciousness.*[11]
- Discuss the skills of emotional intelligence. *The ability to recognize and control own emotions and recognize emotions of others is important to maintain healthy relationships.*[1,7]
- Explore each person's emotional needs. *Understanding that unconscious needs underlie desire to gain acceptance, recognition, and sense of being cared about or valued help client to deal more openly with these issues.*[6,7]
- Assist partners to understand effects of nonverbal language. *Lack of awareness of body language, tone of voice, and subtle movements can be misinterpreted and need to be discussed and clarified.*[1,6]
- Encourage couple to learn effective conflict-resolution skills. *Family may have used ineffective ways to deal with conflict, resulting in fighting and a lose-lose situation.*[5,11]
- Role-play a specific problem couple argues about, using the win-win method of resolution. *Practicing how to defuse arguments and repair hurt feelings helps to identify other's feelings and use new skills for resolution.*[11]
- Encourage partners to practice remaining calm and focused regardless of circumstances. *When issue has previously resulted in violence, remaining calm can help individuals think more clearly and be more rational in dealing with situation, avoiding further conflict.*[5]
- Have each person verify what he or she heard the other person say. *Provides the opportunity for the speaker to correct or acknowledge what was said.*[1,5,11]
- Discuss issues/provide information about sexual relationship. *Conflict inevitably affects intimacy, and couple may need to resolve issues around this part of their life.*[1,9]
- Discuss use of nonblameful self-disclosure during discussions with partner. *Promotes an atmosphere of respect and mutual consideration in which individuals can talk about feelings and resolve problems.*[7,11]

NURSING PRIORITY NO. 3   To promote optimal relationship between couple/family (Teaching/Discharge Considerations):

- Involve all family members in discussions, as indicated. *Encourages input from each member so he/she feels heard and views self as part of the solution.*[1,3,7,11]
- Encourage family members to use Active listening. *Avoids giving advice and allows others to find their own solution, enhancing self-esteem.*[1,5,11]
- Discuss appropriate use of humor and playfulness in daily interactions. *Helps family members to enjoy life and makes difficult issues easier to deal with.*[6]
- Encourage use of relaxation, mindfulness techniques. *Promotes calm manner and ability to deal with difficult issues more effectively.*[7]

 Acute Care   Collaborative   Community/Home Care   Cultural

- Recommend information sources, books, and Web sites as appropriate. *Provides additional resources to access information to assist couple in learning to deal with relationship/family issues.*[3]
- Identify community resources/support groups as appropriate. *Individuals who have successfully dealt with similar issues can provide role model for change and effective use of problem-solving skills.*[2,3,8,11]
- Refer to therapy as indicated. *May need further in-depth care to deal with individual physical/psychological problems.*[2,6,8,11]

DOCUMENTATION FOCUS

Assessment/Reassessment
- Individual's perception of situation and self.
- Partner's views and expectations.
- How partners communicate and deal with conflict.

Planning
- Plan of care and who is involved in planning.
- Teaching plan.

Implementation/Evaluation
- Response of partners to plan, interventions, and actions performed.
- Attainment or progress toward desired outcomes.

Discharge Planning
- Long-range plan and who is responsible for actions to be taken.
- Any referrals made.

References

1. Peterson, R. (2009). Families first: Keys to successful family functioning: Communication. *Virginia Cooperative Extension.* Retrieved April 2018 from http://www.pubs.ext.vt.edu/350/350-092/350-092.html.
2. Pincus, D. (2018). Encouragement and empowerment for moms (with free parenting mantras!). *EmpoweringParents.com.* Retrieved April 2018 from https://www.empoweringparents.com/article/encouragement-and-empowerment-for-moms-with-free-parenting-mantras/.
3. Riesch, S. K., et al. (2010). Furthering the understanding of parent-child relationships: A nursing scholarship review series. Part 5: Parent-adolescent and teen parent-child relationships. *J Spec Pediatr Nurs,* 15(3), 182–201.
4. Anderson, L. S., et al. (2010). Furthering the understanding of parent-child relationships: A nursing scholarship review series. Part 4: Parent-child relationships at risk. *J Spec Pediatr Nurs,* 15(2), 111–134.
5. Scott, E. (Updated 2018). Conflict resolution skills for healthy relationships. Retrieved April 2018 from http://stress.about.com/od/relationships/a/conflict_res.htm.
6. Robinson, L., Smith, M., Segal, J. (Updated 2018). Relationship help: Building satisfying relationships that last. Retrieved April 2018 from https://www.helpguide.org/articles/relationships-communication/relationship-help.htm.
7. Duncan, L. G., Coatsworth, J. D., Greenberg, M. T. (2009). Pilot study to gauge acceptability of a mindfulness based, family-focused preventive intervention. *J Prim Prev,* 30(5), 605–618.
8. Stewart, C. (2008, updated 2017). Common traits of a dysfunctional family. *Everyday Health.* Retrieved April 2018 from https://www.everydayhealth.com/emotional-health/common-traits-dysfunctional-family/.
9. Nusbaum, M. R. H., et al. (2000). The high prevalence of concerns among women seeking routine gynecological care. *J Fam Pract,* 49(3), 229–232.
10. Vorvick, L. J. (2010). Sexual problems overview. Retrieved April 2018 from https://ufhealth.org/sexual-problems-overview.
11. Davidson, J., Wood, C. (Winter 2004). A conflict resolution model. *Theory Into Practice,* 43(1), 6–13.
12. Yolles, M. (1996). The systems paradigm. Retrieved April 2018 from http://www.academia.edu/175318/The_Systems_Paradigm_Paradigm.

 Diagnostic Studies   Evidence Based Practice   Medications   Pediatric/Geriatric/Lifespan

impaired Religiosity

Taxonomy II: Life Principles—Class 3 Value/Belief/Action Congruence (00169) [**Diagnostic Division:** Ego Integrity], Approved 2004; Revised 2017

DEFINITION: Impaired ability to exercise reliance on beliefs and/or participate in rituals of a particular faith tradition.

RELATED FACTORS
Anxiety; depression
Cultural or environmental barrier to practicing religion; spiritual distress
Fear of death
Ineffective caregiver or coping strategies
Insecurity; insufficient social support or sociocultural interaction
Pain
Insufficient transportation

DEFINING CHARACTERISTICS

Subjective
Distress about separation from faith community
Desire to reconnect with previous belief pattern or customs
Questioning of religious belief patterns or customs
Difficulty adhering to prescribed religious beliefs and rituals [e.g., ceremonies, regulations, clothing, prayer, services, holiday observances]
At Risk Population: Aging; hospitalization;
Life transition; personal or spiritual crisis; end-of-life crisis
History of religious manipulation
Associated Condition: Illness
Sample Clinical Applications: Any acute or chronic condition, palliative care, end-of-life situation

DESIRED OUTCOMES/EVALUATION CRITERIA

Sample NOC linkages:
Spiritual Health: Connectedness with self, others, higher power, all life, nature, and the universe that transcends and empowers the self

Client Will (Include Specific Time Frame)
- Express ability to once again participate in beliefs and rituals of desired religion.
- Discuss beliefs and values about spiritual or religious issues.
- Attend religious or worship services of choice, as desired.
- Verbalize concerns about end-of-life issues and fear of death.

ACTIONS/INTERVENTIONS

Sample NIC linkages:
Spiritual Growth Facilitation: Facilitation of growth in patients' capacity to identify, connect with, and call upon the source of meaning, purpose, comfort, strength, and hope in their lives
Religious Ritual Enhancement: Facilitating participation in religious practices
Spiritual Support: Assisting the patient to feel balance and connection with a greater power

 Acute Care
 Collaborative
 Community/ Home Care
 Cultural

NURSING PRIORITY NO. 1   To assess causative/contributing factors:

- Determine client's usual religious and spiritual beliefs, values, and past spiritual commitment. *Provides a baseline for understanding current problem.*[5]
- Note client's/significant other's (SO's) reports and expressions of anger/concern, alienation from God, and sense of guilt or retribution. *Perception of guilt may cause spiritual crisis and suffering, resulting in rejection of religious beliefs or anger toward God.*[6]
- Determine sense of futility, feelings of hopelessness, and lack of motivation to help self. *Indicators that client may see no, or only limited, options or personal choices, and treatment needs to be directed at finding what happened in client's life to bring about these feelings.*[5]
- Assess extent of depression client may be experiencing. *Some studies suggest that a focus on religion may protect against depression.*[7]
- Note recent changes in negative behaviors (e.g., withdrawal from others or religious activities, dependence on alcohol or medications). *Lack of connectedness with self and others impairs ability to trust others or feel worthy of trust from others or God.*[6,7]
- Identify cultural values and expectations regarding religious beliefs or practices. *Individuals grow up in a family that instills a value system within them. As the person grows up, ideas, values, and expectations may change or be strengthened by new information, different questioning, and alternative viewpoints, which may affect current situation.*[3]
- Note socioeconomic status of individual/family. *Women who are poor may have high levels of personal religiosity yet participate less in organized religion because they may feel stigmatized by their situation (e.g., single mothers, those receiving public assistance, those engaging in a lifestyle that conflicts with church norms).*[2]

NURSING PRIORITY NO. 2   To assist client/SOs to deal with feelings/situation:

- Use therapeutic communication skills of reflection and active listening. *Communicates acceptance and enables client to find own solutions to concerns as situation is discussed and deeper meanings are discovered.*[4]
- Encourage expression of feelings about illness or condition or death. *As people age, they become more concerned about their own mortality, and others often see them as in poor health and as spiritual and religious. If they have been diagnosed with a long-term chronic or terminal illness, they may be feeling more angry and rejecting of God than seeking God's help.*[5,8]
- Discuss personal beliefs that may hinder participation in religious activities. *Provides opportunity for self-reflection, such as own worthiness and ability to forgive self for past decisions/life choices.*
- Discuss differences between grief and guilt and help client to identify and deal with each. Point out consequences of actions based on guilt. *Individuals often feel guilty about the "what if's" of life. "If only I had done this!" "If only I had paid more attention!" "If only I had made him go to the doctor!" Most of these guilty feelings are not based on reality, and when they are acted on, the individual does not get the release he or she seeks.*[5]
- Suggest use of journaling and reminiscence. *Promotes life review and can assist in clarifying values and ideas, recognizing and resolving feelings and situation.*[4]
- Encourage client to identify individuals who can provide needed support (e.g., spiritual advisor, parish nurse). *When client is seeking to restore reliance on religious beliefs, these providers can often be helpful.*[6]
- Review client's religious affiliation, associated rituals, and beliefs. *Helps client examine what was important in the past and may trigger some desire to reconnect with these previous beliefs.*[6]
- Provide opportunity for nonjudgmental discussion of philosophical issues related to religious belief patterns and customs. *Open communication can assist client to check reality of perceptions and identify personal options and willingness to resume desired activities.*[1]
- Discuss desire to continue or reconnect with previous belief patterns and customs and perceived barriers. *As client begins to think about current feelings of alienation from previous religious connections, these discussions can help to clarify and allow client to think about how these beliefs can be regained.*[5]

Diagnostic Studies   Evidence Based Practice   Medications   Pediatric/Geriatric/Lifespan

- Identify ways to strengthen spiritual or religious expression. *There are multiple options for enhancing participation in faith community (e.g., joining prayer or study group, volunteering time to community projects, singing in the choir, reading spiritual writings).*
- ▨ Involve client in refining healthcare goals and therapeutic regimen as appropriate. *Identifies role illness or condition is playing in current concerns about ability to participate and appropriateness of participating in desired religious activities.*[7]

NURSING PRIORITY NO. 3 To promote spiritual wellness (Teaching/Discharge Considerations):

- 🏠 Assist client to identify spiritual counselor who could be helpful (e.g., minister, priest, spiritual advisor who has qualifications or experience) in dealing with specific concerns of client. *Provides answers to spiritual questions, assists in the journey of self-discovery, and can help client learn to accept and forgive self.*[6]
- Provide privacy for meditation or prayer and performance of rituals, as appropriate. *Many individuals prefer to pray or meditate in private so they can concentrate without interruption or questions from others.*
- ▨ Explore alternatives or modifications of ritual based on setting and individual needs and limitations. *Individual may not be able to go to a church or temple, so providing another setting—chapel in the facility or quiet room with appropriate religious artifacts or material—can provide the setting desired.*[6]
- Provide bibliotherapy, including list of relevant resources and Web sites *for later reference, promoting self-paced learning and ongoing support.*[4]

DOCUMENTATION FOCUS

Assessment/Reassessment
- Individual findings, including nature of spiritual conflict, effects of participation in treatment regimen.
- Physical and emotional responses to conflict.

Planning
- Plan of care and who is involved in planning.
- Teaching plan.

Implementation/Evaluation
- Responses to interventions, teaching, and actions performed.
- Attainment or progress toward desired outcomes(s).
- Modifications to plan of care.

Discharge Planning
- Long-term needs and who is responsible for actions to be taken.
- Available resources, specific referrals made.

References

1. Smith, A. R. (2006). Using the synergy model to provide spiritual nursing care in cardiovascular settings. *Crit Care Nurs*, 26(2), 41–47.
2. Sullivan, S. (Updated 2015). Faith and poverty: Personal religiosity and organized religion in the lives of low-income urban mothers. Retrieved April 2018 from http://www.bc.edu/content/bc/centers/boisi/publicevents/s06/sullivan.html.
3. Ahrold, T. K., Meston, C. (2010). Ethnic differences in sexual attitudes among U.S. college students: Gender, acculturation, and religiosity. *Arch Sex Behav*, 39(1), 190–202.
4. Herbert, R. S., et al. (2001). Patient perspectives on spirituality and the patient-physician relationship. *J Gen Intern Med*, 16(10), 685–692.

5. McNamara, P., Durso, R., Brown, A. (2006). Religiosity in Parkinson's patients. *Neuropsychiatr Dis Treat*, 2(3), 341–348.
6. Ko, B., et al. (2007). Religious beliefs and quality of life in an American inner city haemodialysis population. *Nephrol Dial Transplant*, 22(10), 2985–2990.
7. Murray-Swank, A., et al. (2006). Religiosity, psychosocial adjustment, and subjective burden of persons who care for those with mental illness. *Psychiatr Serv*, 57(3), 361–365.
8. Mills, J. (1999). The ontology of religiosity: The oceanic feeling and the value of the lived experience. *Humanists*. Retrieved April 2018 from http://huumanists.org/publications/journal/ontology-religiosity-oceanic-feeling-and-value-lived-experience.

 Acute Care   Collaborative   Community/Home Care   Cultural

readiness for enhanced Religiosity

Taxonomy II: Life Principles—Class 3 Value/Belief/Action Congruence (00171) [**Diagnostic Division:** Ego Integrity], Approved 2004; Revised 2013

DEFINITION: A pattern of reliance on religious beliefs and/or participation in rituals of a particular faith tradition, which can be strengthened.

DEFINING CHARACTERISTICS

Subjective
Expresses desire to enhance belief patterns or religious customs used in the past
Expresses desire to enhance participation in religious experiences or practices [e.g., ceremonies, regulations, clothing, prayer, services, holiday observances]
Expresses desire to enhance religious options, use of religious materials
Expresses desire to enhance connection with religious leader
Expresses desire to enhance forgiveness
Sample Clinical Applications: As a health-seeking behavior, the client/family may be healthy, or this diagnosis can be associated with any clinical condition or life process

DESIRED OUTCOMES/EVALUATION CRITERIA

Sample NOC linkages:
Spiritual Health: Connectedness with self, others, higher power, all life, nature, and the universe that transcends and empowers the self

Client Will (Include Specific Time Frame)
• Acknowledge need to strengthen religious affiliations and continue or resume previously comforting rituals.
• Verbalize willingness to seek help to enhance desired religious beliefs.
• Become involved in spiritually based programs of own choice.
• Recognize the difference between belief patterns and customs that are helpful and those that may be harmful.

ACTIONS/INTERVENTIONS

Sample NIC linkages:
Spiritual Growth Facilitation: Facilitation of growth in patients' capacity to identify, connect with, and call upon the source of meaning, purpose, comfort, strength, and hope in their lives
Religious Ritual Enhancement: Facilitating participation in religious practices
Spiritual Support: Assisting the patient to feel balance and connection with a greater power

NURSING PRIORITY NO. 1 To determine spiritual state/motivation for growth:

• Determine client's current thinking about desire to learn more about religious beliefs and actions.
• Ascertain religious beliefs or cultural values of family of origin and climate in which client grew up. *Early religious training deeply affects children and is carried on into adulthood. Conflict between family's beliefs and client's current learning may need to be addressed.*[7]
• Identify cultural values and expectations regarding religious beliefs and/or practices. *Individuals grow up in a family that instills a value system within them. As the person grows up, ideas, values, and expectations may change or be strengthened by new information, different questioning, and alternative viewpoints.*[3]

 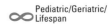

- Note socioeconomic status of individual/family. *Women who are economically disadvantaged may have high levels of personal religiosity, yet participate less in organized religion because they feel stigmatized by their situation (e.g., single mothers, those receiving public assistance, those engaging in a lifestyle that conflicts with church norms).*[2]
- Discuss client's spiritual commitment, beliefs, and values. *Enables examination of these issues and helps client learn more about self and what he or she desires/believes.*[7]
- Explore how spirituality and religious practices have affected client's life. *Some believe that the value of religiosity is the deepened sense of quality of life associated with practicing one's beliefs or tenets.*[8]
- Ascertain motivation and expectations for change. *The client's motivation needs to be for self and not for others, and client needs to understand own expectations to move forward with desire to improve status.*[4]

NURSING PRIORITY NO. 2 To assist client to integrate values and beliefs to strengthen sense of wholeness and achieve optimum balance in daily living:

- Establish nurse-client relationship in which dialogue can occur. *Client can feel safe in this relationship to say anything and know it will be accepted.*[5]
- Identify barriers and beliefs that may hinder growth or self-discovery. *Provides opportunity for self-reflection such as own worthiness and ability to forgive self for past decisions or life choices. Previous practices and beliefs may need to be considered and accepted or discarded in new search for religious beliefs.*[8]
- ⊕ Discuss cultural beliefs of family of origin and how they have influenced client's religious practices. *As client expands options for learning new or other religious beliefs and practices, these influences will provide information for comparing and contrasting new information.*[7]
- Explore connection of desire to strengthen belief patterns and customs to daily life. *Becoming aware of how these issues affect the individual's daily life can enhance ability to incorporate them into everything he or she does.*[1]
- Identify ways in which individual can develop a sense of harmony with self and others. *Client may have some beliefs that may or may not be shared with others, and discussing these can clarify understanding by each individual.*[1]

NURSING PRIORITY NO. 3 To enhance spiritual wellness (Teaching/Discharge Considerations):

- 🏠 Encourage client to seek out and experience different religious beliefs, services, and ceremonies, as desired. *Trying out different religions will give client more information to contrast and compare what will fit his or her belief system.*[6]
- Provide bibliotherapy or reading materials pertaining to spiritual issues. *Client may be interested in learning about new spiritual ideas, and finding resources that clarify thinking will help to develop own beliefs.*[4]
- Encourage client to engage in stress-reducing activities, such as meditation, relaxation exercises, or mindfulness (method of being in the moment). *Promotes general well-being and sense of control over self and ability to choose desired religious activities.*[5]
- Encourage participation in religious activities, worship or religious services, and prayer or study groups; volunteering in church choir or other needed duties; and reading/viewing religious materials and media. *Enhances client's knowledge and promotes connectedness with self, others, and/or higher power.*[4]
- Ⓐ Refer to community resources (e.g., pastor, parish nurse, religion classes, other support groups).

DOCUMENTATION FOCUS

Assessment/Reassessment

- Assessment findings, including client perception of needs and desire for growth.
- Motivation and expectations for change.

 Acute Care   Collaborative   Community/ Home Care ⊕ Cultural

Planning
• Plan for growth and who is involved in planning.

Implementation/Evaluation
• Response to activities, learning, and actions performed.
• Attainment or progress toward desired outcome(s).
• Modifications to plan.

Discharge Planning
• Long-term needs, expectations, and plan of action.
• Specific referrals made.

References

1. Burkhardt, L. (2005). A click away: Documenting spiritual care. *J Cardiovasc Nurs*, 22(1), 6–12.
2. Sullivan, S. (Updated 2015). Faith and poverty: Personal religiosity and organized religion in the lives of low-income urban mothers. Retrieved April 2018 from http://www.bc.edu/content/bc/centers/boisi/publicevents/s06/sullivan.html.
3. Lipson, J. G., Dibble, S. L., Minarik, P. A. (1999). *Culture & Nursing Care: A Pocket Guide*. San Francisco: UCSF Nursing Press.
4. Townsend, M. (2006). *Psychiatric Mental Health Nursing Concepts of Care*. 5th ed. Philadelphia: F. A. Davis.
5. Doenges, M. E., Moorhouse, M. F., Murr, A. C. (2014). *Nursing Care Plans: Guidelines for Individualizing Client Care Across the Life Span*. 9th ed. Philadelphia: F. A. Davis.
6. Doenges, M., Moorhouse, M., Murr, A. (2008). *Nurse's Pocket Guide: Diagnoses, Prioritized Interventions, and Rationales*. 11th ed. Philadelphia: F. A. Davis.
7. Murray-Swank, A., et al. (2006). Religiosity, psychosocial adjustment, and subjective burden of persons who care for those with mental illness. *Psychiatr Serv*, 57(3), 361–365.
8. Mills, J. (1999). The ontology of religiosity: The oceanic feeling and the value of the lived experience. *Humanists*. Retrieved April 2018 from http://humanists.org/publications/journal/ontology-religiosity-oceanic-feeling-and-value-lived-experience.

risk for impaired Religiosity

Taxonomy II: Life Principles—Class 3 Value/Belief/Action Congruence (00170) **[Diagnostic Division:** Ego Integrity**],** Approved 2004; Revised 2013, 2017

DEFINITION: Susceptible to an impaired ability to exercise reliance on religious beliefs and/or participate in rituals of a particular faith tradition, which may compromise health.

RISK FACTORS
Anxiety; depression
Cultural or environmental barrier to practicing religion; spiritual distress
Fear of death;
Ineffective caregiver or coping strategies
Insecurity; insufficient social support or sociocultural interaction
Pain
Insufficient transportation
At Risk Population: Aging; hospitalization;
Life transition; personal or spiritual crisis; end-of-life crisis
History of religious manipulation
Associated Condition: Illness
Sample Clinical Applications: Any acute or chronic condition, palliative care, end-of-life situation

(continues on page 696)

 Diagnostic Studies　 Evidence Based Practice　 Medications　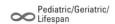 Pediatric/Geriatric/Lifespan

risk for impaired Religiosity (continued)

Sample NOC linkages:

Spiritual Health: Connectedness with self, others, higher power, all life, nature, and the universe that transcends and empowers the self

---

Client Will (Include Specific Time Frame)

- Express understanding of relation of situation or health status to thoughts and feelings of concern about ability to participate in desired religious activities.
- Seek solutions to individual factors that may interfere with reliance on religious beliefs or participation in religious rituals.
- Identify and use resources appropriately.

ACTIONS/INTERVENTIONS

Sample NIC linkages:

Religious Ritual Enhancement: Facilitating participation in religious practices

Spiritual Growth Facilitation: Facilitation of growth in patients' capacity to identify, connect with, and call upon the source of meaning, purpose, comfort, strength, and hope in their lives

Spiritual Support: Assisting the patient to feel balance and connection with a greater power

---

NURSING PRIORITY NO. 1 To assess causative/contributing factors:

- Ascertain current situation (e.g., illness, hospitalization, prognosis of death, depression, lack of support systems, financial concerns). *Identifies problems client is dealing with in the moment that may be affecting desire to be involved with religious activities.*[1]
- Note client's concerns, expressions of anger, and belief that illness or condition is result of lack of faith. *Individual may blame own self for what has happened and could reject religious beliefs and/or God.*
- Determine client's usual religious or spiritual beliefs and past or current involvement in specific church activities. *Provides an understanding of how client sees religion in own life before current disruption.*[1]
- Identify cultural values and expectations regarding religious beliefs and/or practices. *Individuals grow up in a family that instills a value system within them. As the person grows up, ideas, values, and expectations may change or be strengthened by new information, different questioning, and alternative viewpoints, which may affect current situation.*[3]
- Note quality of relationships with significant others and friends. *Individual may withdraw from others in relation to the stress of illness, pain, and suffering. Others may be encouraging client to rely on religious beliefs at a time when individual is questioning own beliefs in the current situation.*[1]
- Note socioeconomic status of individual/family. *Women who are poor may have high levels of personal religiosity, yet participate less in organized religion because they feel stigmatized by their situation (e.g., single mothers, those receiving public assistance, those engaging in a lifestyle that conflicts with church norms).*[2]
- Assess lack of transportation or environmental barriers to participation in desired religious activities. *These barriers can be realistic in the face of such issues as poor bus systems, inability of individual to get to bus stop (physical problems of walking or distance to the bus stop), or inability to drive a car.*[2]
- Ascertain substance use or abuse. *Individuals often turn to use of various substances in distress, and this can affect the ability to deal with problems in a positive manner.*[6]

NURSING PRIORITY NO. 2 To assist client to deal with feelings/situation:

- Develop nurse-client relationship. *Individual can express feelings and concerns freely when he or she feels safe to do so.*

 Acute Care   Collaborative   Community/Home Care   Cultural

- 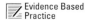 Discuss personal beliefs that may hinder participation in religious activities. *Provides opportunity for self-reflection such as own worthiness and ability to forgive self for past decisions or life choices.*[5]
- Use therapeutic communication skills of active listening, reflection, and "I" messages. *Helps client to find own solutions to problems/concerns and promotes sense of control.*[4]
- Have client identify and prioritize current and immediate needs. *Dealing with current needs is easier than trying to predict the future. Also, it is important to take care of basic needs before moving on to higher needs.*[4]
- Provide time for nonjudgmental discussion of individual's spiritual beliefs and fears about impact of current illness and/or treatment regimen. *Helps to clarify thoughts and promote ability to deal with stresses of what is happening.*
- Review with client past difficulties in life and coping skills that were used at that time. *Recalling problems with family, peers, and colleagues or individuals in position of authority can help client to remember how those were handled and how those skills could be used in current situation.*
- Encourage client to discuss feelings about death and end-of-life issues when illness or prognosis is grave. *People are often afraid to talk about the possibility of their own death for fear it will bring reality to self and upset family. Note: A 2015 study investigated whether spirituality/religiosity (S/R) plays an important role in the lives of cancer patients and in the work of health professionals who provide care for these patients. It was demonstrated that 94.1% of patients considered it important that health professionals addressed their spiritual beliefs, and 99.2% of patients relied on S/R to face cancer.*[1,8]

NURSING PRIORITY NO. 3 To promote wellness (Teaching/Discharge Considerations):

- Have client identify support systems available. *Individual will usually know who can provide the best support for him/her in present situation. Family may not be the most supportive if they don't want to accept the reality of client's illness or situation.*[5]
- Help client learn relaxation techniques, meditation, guided imagery, and mindfulness (living in the moment and enjoying it). *Learning to relax can help client to process information and make decisions in a more positive manner.*[4]
- Take the lead from the client in initiating participation in religious activities, prayer, and other activities. *Client may be vulnerable in current situation and needs to be allowed to decide own participation in these actions. Living and participating in desired religious activities will help client to understand the tenets of his or her choice.*[7]
- Refer to appropriate resources such as crisis counselor, governmental agencies, spiritual advisor (who has qualifications or experience dealing with specific problems such as death or dying process, relationship problems, substance abuse, suicide), hospice, psychotherapy, and Alcoholics or Narcotics Anonymous. *May require additional help to deal with current situation.*[4,6]

DOCUMENTATION FOCUS

Assessment/Reassessment
- Individual findings, including risk factors, nature of current distress.
- Physical and emotional response to distress.
- Access to and use of resources.

Planning
- Plan of care and who is involved in planning.
- Teaching plan.

Implementation/Evaluation
- Responses to interventions, teaching, and actions performed.
- Attainment or progress toward desired outcome(s).
- Modifications to plan of care.

Discharge Planning
- Long-term needs and who is responsible for actions to be taken.
- Available resources and specific referrals made.

References

1. Burkhardt, L. (2005). A click away: Documenting spiritual care. *J Cardiovasc Nurs*, 22(1), 6–12.
2. Sullivan, S. (Updated 2015). Faith and poverty: Personal religiosity and organized religion in the lives of low-income urban mothers. Retrieved April 2018 from http://www.bc.edu/content/bc/centers/boisi/publicevents/s06/sullivan.html.
3. Herbert, R. S., et al. (2001). Patient perspectives on spirituality and the patient-physician relationship. *J Gen Intern Med*, 16(10), 685–692.
4. Maslow, A. H. (1970). *Religions, Values, and Peak-Experiences*. New York: Penguin Books.
5. Wilkinson, M. L., Tanner, W. C. (1980). The influence of family size, interaction, and religiosity on family affection in a Mormon sample. *J Marriage Family*, 42(2), 297–304.
6. Murray-Swank, A., et al. (2006). Religiosity, psychosocial adjustment and subjective burden of persons who care for those with mental illness. *Psychiatr Serv*, 57(3), 361–365.
7. Mills, J. (1999). The ontology of religiosity: The oceanic feeling and the value of the lived experience. *Humanists*. Retrieved April 2018 from http://huumanists.org/publications/journal/ontology-religiosity-oceanic-feeling-and-value-lived-experience.
8. Goulart de Camargos, M., Paiva, C. E., Barroso, E. M. (2015). Understanding the differences between oncology patients and oncology health professionals concerning spirituality/religiosity. *Medicine*. Retrieved April 2018 from https://www.ncbi.nlm.nih.gov/pmc/articles/PMC5059012/.

Relocation Stress Syndrome

Taxonomy II: Coping/Stress Tolerance—Class 1 Post-Trauma Responses (00114) [**Diagnostic Division:** Ego Integrity], Approved1992; Revised 2000, 2017

DEFINITION: Physiological and/or psychosocial disturbance following transfer from one environment to another.

RELATED FACTORS

Move from one environment to another; significant environmental change
Ineffective coping strategies; impaired psychosocial functioning; powerlessness
Insufficient support system; insufficient predeparture counseling; unpredictability of experience
Social isolation; language barrier

DEFINING CHARACTERISTICS

Subjective

Anxiety [e.g., separation]; anger
Insecurity; worry; fear
Loneliness; depression
Unwillingness to move; concern about relocation
Alteration in sleep pattern

Objective

Increase in verbalization of needs; preoccupation
Pessimism; frustration
Increase in physical symptoms or illness
Withdrawal; aloneness; alienation
Loss of identity or self-worth; low self-esteem; dependency
At Risk Population: History of loss
Associated Condition: Compromised health status; impaired psychosocial functioning
Deficient mental competence
Sample Clinical Applications: Chronic conditions (e.g., multiple sclerosis [MS], asthma, cystic fibrosis), brain injury, stroke, dementia, schizophrenia, developmental delay, end-of-life/hospice care

 Acute Care
 Collaborative
 Community/ Home Care
 Cultural

DESIRED OUTCOMES/EVALUATION CRITERIA

Sample NOC linkages:

Psychosocial Adjustment: Life Change: Adaptive psychosocial response of an individual to a significant life change

Quality of Life: Extent of positive perception of current life circumstances

Coping: Personal actions to manage stressors that tax an individual's resources

Client Will (Include Specific Time Frame)

• Verbalize understanding of reason(s) for change.
• Demonstrate appropriate range of feelings and reduced fear.
• Participate in routine and special or social events, as able.
• Verbalize acceptance of situation.
• Experience no catastrophic event.

ACTIONS/INTERVENTIONS

Sample NIC linkages:

Relocation Stress Reduction: Assisting the individual to prepare for and cope with movement from one environment to another

Hope Inspiration: Enhancing the belief in one's capacity to initiate and sustain actions

Family Involvement Promotion: Facilitating participation of family members in the emotional and physical care of the patient

NURSING PRIORITY NO. 1   To assess degree of stress as perceived/experienced by client and determine issues of safety:

• Determine situation or cause for relocation (e.g., planned move for new job, change in marital status, deployment or returning from military duty, loss of home or community due to natural or human-caused disaster, deterioration in health status or ability to care for self, caregiver burnout, older parent being requested to move closer to adult child). *Although nursing and medical research is early and inconclusive in validating the defining characteristics of relocation stress syndrome as a nursing diagnosis,[1,7,12,13] the belief that stress associated with relocation can be extreme is widely accepted in society. The effects of relocation can be minimal and transient or very troubling and persistent.[14]*

• Note client's age, developmental level, and role in family. *Age and position in life cycle make a difference in the impact of issues involved in relocating. For example, children can be traumatized by transfer to new school and loss of friends and familiar surroundings. Note: One major reason that children are negatively affected by moves is that moves they are often precipitated by family problems (e.g., a divorce, death of a significant other; job loss).[2] Older persons may be affected by loss of their long-term home with its memories, neighborhood setting, and support persons.[8]*

• Identify cultural or religious concerns that may affect client's coping or impact social interactions and expectations. *Cultural norm may be that elders are cared for by family—not placed in a facility—causing client to feel abandoned, or individual may be required to defer to family decision maker and feel powerless in determining own destiny.[8]*

• Note ethnic ties and primary language spoken and read. *During times of stress, individuals may revert to language of childhood. This affects healthcare providers who must try to reduce the client's feelings of alienation or confusion while communicating with client of another primary language or client who is displaced from cultural attachments.[4]*

 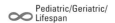

- Ascertain if client participated in the decision to relocate and perceptions about change(s) and expectations for the future. *A forced relocation is much more stressful than one that is desired. Also, client may be concerned that move/or placement will deplete savings or be fearful of being a burden on family members.*
- Determine involvement of family/significant others (SOs). Note availability and use of support systems and resources. Ascertain presence or absence of comprehensive information and planning (e.g., when and how move took place, if the environment for the client is similar or greatly changed). *These factors can greatly affect client's ability to adjust to change.*
- Note signs of increased stress in recently relocated client. *Client may report or demonstrate irritability, withdrawal, crying, moodiness, problems sleeping, or fatigue; "new" physical discomfort or pain (e.g., stomachaches, headaches, back pain); change in appetite; increased use of alcohol or other drugs; or greater susceptibility to colds.*[3,8,9]
- Observe behavior, noting presence of increasing anxiety, suspiciousness or paranoia, and defensiveness. Compare with SO's/staff's description of customary responses. *Relocation may temporarily exacerbate mental deterioration (cognitive inaccessibility) and impair communication (social inaccessibility).*
- Identify issues of safety that may be involved, such as difficulty adjusting to new environment (e.g., navigating streets or choosing correct bus; locating dining hall or bathroom in facility) or concerns of elopement or running away.

NURSING PRIORITY NO. 2 To assist client to deal with situation/changes:

- Collaborate in treatment of underlying conditions (e.g., chronic confusional states, brain injury, posttrauma rehabilitation), and physical stress symptoms *that are potentially exacerbating relocation stress or that may affect the length of time that relocation is required.*
- Begin relocation planning with client and SOs as early as possible. Provide support and advocate for client who is unable to participate in decisions. *Having a well-organized plan for move with support and advocacy may reduce anxiety.*[9,15]
- Encourage free expression of feelings about reason for relocation, including venting of anger; grief; loss of personal space, belongings, and friends; financial strains; powerlessness; etc. Acknowledge reality of situation and maintain hopeful attitude regarding move or change. *Bringing feelings out into the open helps clarify emotions and make feelings easier to deal with.*[6,9] Refer to NDs relating to client's particular situation (e.g., ineffective Coping, Grieving) for additional interventions.
- Anticipate variety of emotions and reactions. *May vary from insomnia and loss of appetite to becoming involved with alcohol or other drugs, exacerbation of health problems, onset of serious illness, or behavioral problems.*
- Identify strengths and successful coping behaviors the individual has used previously. *Incorporating these into problem-solving builds on past successes.*
- Encourage client to maintain contact with friends (e.g., telephone, letters, e-mail, video/audiotapes, arranged visits) *to reduce sense of isolation.*
- ∞ Provide client with information and list of local social groups, assistance organizations or community services (e.g., Welcome Wagon, senior citizens or teen clubs, churches, singles' groups, sports leagues) *to provide contacts for client to develop new relationships and learn more about the new setting.*[6]
- Obtain interpreter (where language differences exist) *to exchange information with the client/SO regarding residence or relocation wishes and to make helpful referrals.*[4]
- Refer to professionals (e.g., social worker, financial resources, mental healthcare provider, minister or spiritual advisor) if serious difficulties develop (e.g., depression, alcohol or other drug abuse, deteriorating behavior of child) *to assist client with special needs and/or persistent problems with adaptation.*[3,10]
- ∞ Take practical steps to alleviate stress for child. Encourage parents to walk with child to school or rehearse boarding the school bus, visit new classroom, contact friends child left behind, drive past places of interest to child, find a safe play place, unpack child's favorite toys, invite neighborhood children to a get-acquainted party, etc. *Helps child to maintain ties and develop new ones, thus reducing sense of loss and shifting focus to the future.*[2]

 Acute Care Collaborative Community/ Home Care Cultural

- Facilitate client's adjustment to new environment or facility:[5,8,9,11,16]

Determine client's usual schedule of activities and incorporate into facility routine, as possible. *Reinforces sense of importance of individual.*

Orient to surroundings and schedules and repeat directions, as needed.

Introduce to new staff members, roommate, and other residents. Encourage sharing of life story with others.

Provide clear, honest information about actions and events.

Provide consistency in daily routine; maintain same staff with client in new facility, as possible, during adjustment phase.

Address ways to preserve lifestyle (e.g., usual bath and bedtimes in new facility, involvement in church activities). *Helps reduce the sense of loss associated with move.*

Encourage individual/family to personalize area with pictures, own belongings, etc., as soon as possible. *Enhances sense of belonging, self-expression, and creation of personal space.*

Introduce socialization and diversional activities, such as meals with new acquaintances, art therapy, music, movies, etc. *Involvement increases opportunity to interact with others and form new friendships, thus decreasing isolation and stress reactions.*

Encourage hugging and use of touch unless client prefers to abstain from hugging or is paranoid or agitated at the moment. *Human connection reaffirms acceptance of individual.*

Place in private room, if appropriate, and include SO(s)/family in care activities, mealtime, etc. *Keeping client secluded may be needed under some circumstances (e.g., advanced Alzheimer's disease with fear or aggressive reactions) to decrease the client's stress reactions to new environment.*

Deal with aggressive behavior by imposing calm, firm limits. Control environment and protect others from client's disruptive behavior. *Promotes safety for client/others.*

Remain calm, place in a quiet environment, and provide a time-out *to prevent escalation of disruptive behaviors (e.g., panic state, violence).*

Anticipate and address feelings of distress and grieving in family/caregivers when placing loved one in a different environment (e.g., nursing home, foster care). *Support and referrals may be needed to help SOs in practical issues and adjustment.*

NURSING PRIORITY NO. 3 To enhance adjustment (Teaching/Discharge Considerations):

- Involve client in formulating goals and plan of care when possible. *Supports independence and commitment to achieving outcomes.*
- Encourage communication between client/family/SO *to provide mutual support and problem-solving opportunities.*[3]
- Discuss benefits of adequate nutrition, rest, and exercise *to maintain physical well-being and reduce adverse effects of stressful situation.*
- Instruct in anxiety- and stress-reduction activities (e.g., meditation, other relaxation techniques, exercise program, group socialization), as able, *to enhance psychological well-being and coping abilities.*
- Encourage participation in activities, hobbies, or personal interactions, as appropriate. *Promotes creative endeavors, stimulating the mind.*
- Identify community support or cultural or ethnic groups client can access.
- Support self-responsibility and coping strategies *to foster sense of control and self-worth.*

DOCUMENTATION FOCUS

Assessment/Reassessment
- Assessment findings, individual's perception of the situation and changes, specific behaviors.
- Cultural or religious concerns.
- Safety issues.

Planning
- Note plan of care, who is involved in planning, and who is responsible for proposed actions.
- Teaching plan.

 Diagnostic Studies   Evidence Based Practice   Medications   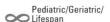 Pediatric/Geriatric/ Lifespan

Implementation/Evaluation
- Response to interventions (especially time-out or seclusion), teaching, and actions performed.
- Sentinel events.
- Attainment or progress toward desired outcome(s).
- Modifications to plan of care.

Discharge Planning
- Long-term needs and who is responsible for actions to be taken.
- Specific referrals made.

References

1. Mallick, M. J., Whipple, T. W. (2000). Validity of the nursing diagnosis of relocation stress syndrome. *Nurs Res*, 49(2), 97–100.
2. Chiaro, C. (2003). Preventing relocation stress, easing children's transition. Special report. *Colorado Springs Business Journal*.
3. Solomon, A. (2000). Relocation stress: The warning signs. Retrieved April 2018 from http://www.therapyinla.com/psych/psych0100.html.
4. Purnell, L. D., Paulanka, B. J. (1998). Purnell's model for cultural competence. *Transcultural Health Care: A Culturally Competent Approach*. Philadelphia: F. A. Davis, 11–14.
5. Nypaver, J. M., Titus, M., Brugler, C. J. (1996). Patient transfer to rehabilitation: Just another move? Relocation stress syndrome. *Rehabil Nurs*, 21(2), 94–97.
6. Puskar, K. R., Dvorsak, K. G. (1991). Relocation stress in adolescents: Helping teenagers cope with a moving dilemma. *Pediatr Nurs*, 17(3), 295–298.
7. Walker, C. A., Curry, L. C., Hogstel, M. O. (2007). Relocation stress syndrome in older adults transitioning from home to long term care facility: Myth or reality? *J Psychosoc Nurs Ment Health Serv*, 45(1), 38–45.
8. Mintz, T. G. (2005). Relocation stress syndrome in older adults. *Social Work Today*, 5(6), 38–45.
9. Novack, M. (2018). How to alleviate the stress of moving for older adults. *CaringHome*. Retrieved April 2018 from https://www.caring.com/articles/how-to-alleviate-the-stress-of-moving-for-older-adults.
10. Murphy, K. (2005). Anxiety: When is it too much? *Nursing Made Incredibly Easy!*, 3(5), 22–31.
11. Munhe, J. A., McCarty, S. (Updated 2017). Geriatric rehabilitation. Retrieved April 2018 from http://emedicine.medscape.com/article/318521-overview.
12. Capazuti, E., et al. (2006). Nursing home involuntary relocation: Clinical outcomes and perceptions of residents and families. *J Am Med Dir Assoc*, 7(8), 486–492.
13. Hodgson, N., et al. (2004). Biobehavioral correlates of relocation in the frail elderly: Salivary cortisol, affect, and cognitive function. *J Am Geriatr Soc*, 52(11), 1856–1862.
14. Hertz, J. E., et al. (2008). Early identification of relocation risk in older adults with critical illness. *Crit Care Quart*, 31(1), 59–64.
15. Talerico, K. A. (2004). Relocation to a long-term care facility: Working with patients and families before, during, and after. *J Psychosoc Nurs*, 42(3), 10–16.
16. Hertz, J. E., et al. (2007). Evidence-based guideline: Management of relocation in cognitively intact older adults. *J Geront Nurs*, 33(11), 12–18.

risk for Relocation Stress Syndrome

Taxonomy II: Coping/Stress Tolerance—Class 1 Post-Trauma Responses (00149) [**Diagnostic Division:** Ego Integrity], Approved 2000; Revised 2013, 2017

DEFINITION: Susceptible to physiological and/or psychosocial disturbance following transfer from one environment to another that may compromise health.

RISK FACTORS
Move from one environment to another; significant environmental change
Ineffective coping strategies; impaired psychosocial functioning; powerlessness
Insufficient support system; insufficient predeparture counseling; unpredictability of experience
Social isolation; language barrier
At Risk Population: History of loss
Associated Condition: Compromised health status; impaired psychosocial functioning
Deficient mental competence
Sample Clinical Applications: Chronic conditions (e.g., multiple sclerosis [MS], asthma, cystic fibrosis), brain injury, stroke, dementia, schizophrenia, developmental delay

 Acute Care   Collaborative   Community/Home Care   Cultural

DESIRED OUTCOMES/EVALUATION CRITERIA

Sample NOC linkages:
Psychosocial Adjustment: Life Change: Adaptive psychosocial responses of an individual to a significant life change
Quality of Life: Extent of positive perception of current life circumstances
Grief Resolution: Personal actions to adjust thoughts and behaviors to actual or impending loss

Client Will (Include Specific Time Frame)
- Verbalize understanding of reason(s) for change.
- Express feelings and concerns openly and appropriately.
- Experience no catastrophic event.

ACTIONS/INTERVENTIONS

Sample NIC linkages:
Discharge Planning: Preparation for moving a patient from one level of care to another within or outside the current healthcare agency
Relocation Stress Reduction: Assisting the individual to prepare for and cope with movement from one environment to another
Emotional Support: Provision of reassurance, acceptance, and encouragement during times of stress

NURSING PRIORITY NO. 1   To identify risk/contributing factors:

- Determine situation or cause for relocation (e.g., planned move for new job, deployment or returning from military duty, change in marital status, loss of home or community due to natural or human-caused disaster, deterioration in health status or ability to care for self, caregiver burnout, older parent being requested to move closer to adult child). *Although nursing research is early and inconclusive in validating the defining characteristics of relocation stress syndrome as a nursing diagnosis,[1,3,7,8] the belief that stress associated with relocation can be extreme is widely accepted in society. The effects of relocation can be minimal and transient or very troubling and persistent.[9]*
- ∞ Note client's age, developmental level, and role in family. *Age and position in life cycle make a difference in the impact of issues involved in relocating. For example, children can be traumatized by transfer to new school, loss of friends and familiar surroundings,[2] and older persons may be affected by loss of their long-term home with its memories, neighborhood setting, and support persons.[4]*
- Identify cultural and/or religious concerns that may affect client's coping or impact social interactions and expectations. *Cultural norm may be that elders are cared for by family—not placed in a facility—causing client to feel abandoned, or individual may be required to defer to family decision maker and feel powerless in determining own destiny.[4]*
- Note ethnic ties and primary language spoken and read. *During times of stress, individuals may lapse into language of childhood. This affects healthcare providers who must try to reduce client's feelings of alienation while communicating with client of another primary language or client who is displaced from cultural, familial attachments.[5]*
- Ascertain if client has participated in the decision to relocate, perceptions about change(s), and expectations for the future. *Decision may have been made without client's input or understanding of event or consequences, which can impact adjustment. A forced relocation is much more stressful than one that is desired. Client may be concerned that temporary placement will deplete savings or may be fearful of being a burden on family members and may have felt pressured to move.[4]*
- Note whether relocation will be temporary (e.g., extended care for rehabilitation therapies, moving in with family while house being repaired after fire) or long term or permanent (e.g., move from home of many years, placement in long-term care facility). *To some degree, a temporary relocation is usually easier to cope with*

than a permanent relocation. However, any anticipated disruption of the client's usual way of living is upsetting, and emotional responses aren't always congruent with the magnitude of the event.

- Determine involvement of family/significant others (SOs). Note availability and use of support systems and resources. Ascertain presence or absence of comprehensive information and planning (e.g., when and how move will take place, if the environment for the client will be similar or greatly changed). *These factors can greatly affect client's ability to cope with change.*

NURSING PRIORITY NO. 2   To prevent/minimize adverse response to change:

- Collaborate in treatment of underlying conditions (e.g., chronic confusional states, brain injury, posttrauma rehabilitation) and physical stress symptoms *that could exacerbate relocation stress or that affect length of time that relocation may be needed.*
- Provide information to client/SO as early in process as possible *to eliminate misconceptions and facilitate decision-making process. This can include obtaining audiovisual materials or Web sites about the new home, city, region, or country.*[5,6]
- ∞ Discuss relocation or move with child. *Information for child must be aimed at level of understanding and interest.*[2] *Child lacks ability to put problem into perspective, so minor mishap may seem catastrophic. Also, child is more vulnerable to stress because he or she has less control over environment than most adults.*[6]
- ∞ Avoid moving adolescent in middle of school year when possible. *Adolescent is vulnerable to emotional, social, and cognitive dysfunction because of the great importance of peer group and loss of friends and social standing caused by relocation.*[6]
- 🏠 Involve client in placement choices when possible (e.g., move to nursing home or adult foster care) *to provide client with some control over the situation.*
- 🏠 Encourage visit to new community, surroundings, or school before transfer when possible. *Provides opportunity to "get acquainted" with new situation, reducing fear of unknown.*
- 🏠 Suggest contact with someone (friend, family, business associate) who has been to or lived in new area where move is being planned *to absorb some of that person's experience and knowledge.*[5,6]
- Take practical steps to alleviate stress for child. Encourage parents to walk with child to school or rehearse boarding the school bus, visit new classroom, contact friends child left behind, drive past places of interest to child, find a safe play place, unpack child's favorite toys, invite neighborhood children to a get-acquainted party, etc. *Helps child to maintain ties and develop new ones, reducing sense of loss and shifting focus to the future.*[2]
- Encourage free expression of feelings about reason for relocation. Acknowledge reality of situation and maintain hopeful attitude regarding move or change. *Bringing feelings out into the open helps clarify emotion and make feelings easier to deal with.*[6]

NURSING PRIORITY NO. 3   To promote wellness (Teaching/Discharge Considerations):

- 🏠 Involve client in formulating goals and plan of care when possible. *Fosters sense of control and self-worth, supports independence and commitment to achieving outcomes.*
- Encourage client/SO to accept that relocation is an adjustment and that it takes time to adapt to new circumstances or environment.
- Instruct in anxiety- and stress-reduction activities (e.g., meditation, other relaxation techniques, exercise program, group socialization) as able *to enhance psychological well-being and coping abilities.*
- Provide client with information and list of organizations or community services (e.g., Welcome Wagon, senior citizens or teen clubs, churches, singles' groups, sports leagues) *to provide contacts for client to develop new relationships and learn more about the new setting.*[10]
- Discuss safety issues regarding new environment (e.g., how to navigate streets or choose correct bus, locate dining hall or bathroom in facility) and concerns of elopement or running away. *May help prevent adverse reactions.*
- Anticipate variety of emotions and reactions. *May vary from insomnia and loss of appetite to becoming involved with alcohol or other drugs, exacerbation of health problems, onset of serious illness, or behavioral problems. Awareness provides opportunity for timely intervention.*[6]
- Refer to ND Relocation Stress Syndrome for additional interventions.

 Acute Care   Collaborative   Community/Home Care   Cultural

DOCUMENTATION FOCUS

Assessment/Reassessment
- Assessment findings, individual's perception of the situation/changes, specific behaviors.
- Cultural or religious concerns.
- Safety issues.

Planning
- Note plan of care, who is involved in planning, and who is responsible for proposed actions.
- Teaching plan.

Implementation/Evaluation
- Response to interventions (especially time-out/seclusion), teaching, and actions performed.
- Sentinel events.
- Attainment or progress toward desired outcome(s).
- Modifications to plan of care.

Discharge Planning
- Long-term needs and who is responsible for actions to be taken.
- Specific referrals made.

References

1. Mallick, M. J., Whipple, T. W. (2000). Validity of the nursing diagnosis of relocation stress syndrome. *Nurs Res*, 49(2), 97–100.
2. Chiaro, C. (2003). Preventing relocation stress, easing children's transition. Special report. *Colorado Springs Business Journal*,
3. Walker, C. A., Curry, L. C., Hogstel, M. O. (2007). Relocation stress syndrome in older adults transitioning from home to long term care facility: Myth or reality? *J Psychosoc Nurs Ment Health Serv*, 45(1), 38–45.
4. Mintz, T. G. (2005). Relocation stress syndrome in older adults. *Social Work Today*, 5(6), 38.
5. Solomon, A. (2000). Relocation stress: The warning signs. Retrieved April 2018 from http://www.therapyinla.com/psych/psych0100.html.
6. Novack, M. (2018). How to alleviate the stress of moving for older adults. *CaringHome*. Retrieved April 2018 from
https://www.caring.com/articles/how-to-alleviate-the-stress-of-moving-for-older-adults.
7. Capazuti, E., et al. (2006). Nursing home involuntary relocation: Clinical outcomes and perceptions of residents and families. *J Am Med Dir Assoc*, 7(8), 486–492.
8. Hodgson, N., et al. (2004). Biobehavioral correlates of relocation in the frail elderly: Salivary cortisol, affect, and cognitive function. *J Am Geriatr Soc*, 52(11), 1856–1862.
9. Hertz, J. E., et al. (2008). Early identification of relocation risk in older adults with critical illness. *Crit Care Quart*, 31(1), 59–64.
10. Puskar, K. R., Dvorsak, K. G. (1991). Relocation stress in adolescents: Helping teenagers cope with a moving dilemma. *Pediatr Nurs*, 17(3), 295–298.

impaired Resilience

Taxonomy II: Coping/Stress Tolerance—Class 2 Coping Responses (00210) [**Diagnostic Division:** Ego Integrity], Approved 2008; Revised 2013, 2017

DEFINITION: Decreased ability to recover from perceived adverse or changing situations, through a dynamic process of adaptation.

RELATED FACTORS
Community violence
Disruption in family rituals or roles; inconsistent parenting
Disturbance in family dynamics; dysfunctional family processes; ineffective family adaptation
Inadequate or insufficient resources
Insufficient social support; perceived vulnerability
Multiple coexisting adverse situations; substance misuse/[abuse]

(continues on page 706)

 Diagnostic Studies Evidence Based Practice Medications 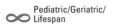 Pediatric/Geriatric/Lifespan

impaired Resilience (continued)

DEFINING CHARACTERISTICS

Subjective

Depression; guilt; shame

Impaired health status

Renewed elevation of distress

Decreased interest in academic or vocational activities

Objective

Ineffective coping skills; social isolation; low self-esteem

Ineffective integration or sense of control

At Risk Population: Chronicity of existing crisis; new crisis; demographics that increase chance of maladjustment

Economically disadvantaged; ethnic minority status; exposure to violence

Female gender; large family size

Low intellectual ability or maternal educational level

Parental mental illness

Associated Condition: Psychological disorder

Sample Clinical Applications: Substance abuse, mental health issues—depression, phobia, bipolar disorder, schizophrenia; chronic illness—renal failure, heart failure, cancer; debilitating conditions—multiple sclerosis (MS), Parkinson's disease, obesity; domestic abuse or violence

DESIRED OUTCOMES/EVALUATION CRITERIA

Sample NOC linkages:

Personal Resiliency: Positive adaptation and function of an individual following significant adversity or crisis

Hope: Optimism that is personally satisfying and life-supporting

Family Resiliency: Capacity of a family to positively adapt and function following significant adversity or crisis

Client Will (Include Specific Time Frame)

Acknowledge reality of current situation or crisis.

Express positive feelings about self and situation.

Seek appropriate resources to change circumstances that affect adaptation and resilience.

Be involved in programs to address problems presenting in life (e.g., substance abuse, low self-esteem, poverty).

ACTIONS/INTERVENTIONS

Sample NIC linkages:

Resiliency Promotion: Assisting individuals, families, and communities in development, use, and strengthening of protective factors to be used in coping with environmental and societal stressors

Hope Inspiration: Enhancing the belief in one's capacity to initiate and sustain actions

Family Mobilization: Utilization of family strengths to influence patient's health in a positive direction

 Acute Care Collaborative Community/ Home Care Cultural

NURSING PRIORITY NO. 1 To assess causative/contributing factors:

- Determine individuals involved, family, children, ages, and current circumstances. *Understanding the family makeup provides information that will guide choice of interventions.*[1]
- Note underlying stressors, health concerns, debilitating conditions, and mental health or behavioral issues, such as unemployment, poverty, diabetes, obesity, chronic obstructive pulmonary disease, Alzheimer's disease, and parental mental illness. *Provides information about situation to plan appropriate care.*[1,5]
- Identify locus of control. *Individuals with external locus of control are less likely to feel in control or rely on their own abilities or judgment to manage a situation.*[1,2,6]
- Determine client's education level, family dynamics, and parenting styles if relevant. *Drug use, violence, and poor impulse control affect ability of individual to develop resilience to adverse situations or crisis and may result in individual viewing self as a victim rather than a survivor.*[1,3]
- Note communication patterns within the family. *Skills learned within the family can make the difference between whether the individual develops low self-esteem or has positive feelings about self.*
- Identify maladaptive coping skills used by individual and in the family. *The use of food or drugs to deal with feelings, acting-out behaviors or violence, devaluing education or importance of learning new skills, and focusing on the negative in situations lead to members learning these methods of dealing with problems and difficulties that arise, resulting in lack of ability to adjust positively and learn attributes of resiliency.*[3]
- ∞ Note parental status including age and maturity. *Young parents may lack ability to deal with family responsibilities, financial concerns, and low socioeconomic factors.*[2,10]
- Ascertain stability of relationship, presence of separation or divorce. *Family members are vulnerable to breakup of the family unit and, depending on perception and circumstances, see it as causing long-term liability.*[4]
- Determine availability and use of resources, family, support groups, and financial. *Appropriate use can help individuals overcome and manage problems in their lives.*
- ⊕ Discuss religious and cultural beliefs held by the individual and family. *Including the members of the family in this discussion promotes the idea that they are partners in their healthcare and enables them to learn and have input into how these beliefs affect what they do. Knowing the role of the elements of culture in shaping and defining health behavior helps the family understand how this is important to them.*[5]

NURSING PRIORITY NO. 2 To assist client to improve skills to deal with adverse situations or crises:

- Encourage free expressions of feelings, including feelings of anger and hostility, setting limits on unacceptable behavior. *When feelings are verbalized, client begins to identify them and recognize how they affect personal behavior. Unacceptable behavior leads to feelings of shame and guilt if it is not controlled.*[1,2]
- Listen to client's concerns and acknowledge difficulty of adversity and making changes in situation. *Often, individuals who are feeling that life is difficult begin to doubt their ability to deal with circumstances and are not able to see positive outcomes. Being listened to provides opportunity for client to feel valued, capable, and like a survivor rather than a victim.*[3]
- Help client to assume responsibility for own life, to look at situation as a challenge rather than an obstacle, and to refrain from viewing crisis as insurmountable. *Resilience is not something that people have or do not have; it is learned and developed in people as they deal with adversities of life. Taking care of oneself keeps the mind ready to deal with adverse situations.*[3,6,9]
- Provide information at client's level of comprehension, being honest in explanations. *Provides data to assist in decision-making process and enhances client's cooperation in change process.*[1]
- Have client paraphrase information provided during teaching session. *Assures client's understanding and provides opportunity to correct misunderstandings.*[1]
- Promote parent involvement in developing a positive mind-set for fostering resilience in their children. *Parents are concerned that their children grow up to be competent adults. They can learn the parenting skills that promote optimal growth and resilience in their children for the problems they will face as grown-ups*[3,9]

 Diagnostic Studies   Evidence Based Practice   Medications   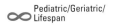 Pediatric/Geriatric/Lifespan

- Facilitate communication skills between client and family. *Sometimes, individuals who find themselves in difficult situations withdraw because they do not know what to do or say. Helping the client to learn new ways to interact will not only help him or her but also help family members learn effective ways of communicating.*[2,3,7]
- Focus on strengths of the individual as problems are being assessed and diagnosed. *Improving the future for the client is based on developing the capacity to deal successfully with the obstacles he or she meets in life.*[3]
- Encourage client/parents to model empathy with family members. *Empathy is an important interpersonal skill and a cornerstone of emotional intelligence.*[8] *Children learn empathy when parents are empathic with them.*[2,6]
- Discuss individual issues, such as obesity, substance use, poor impulse control, or violent behavior, providing information about the risks and helping client/parent understand how he or she can help family members develop habits that will promote physical and mental well-being. *For example, recent studies suggest that encouraging children to reduce sedentary behavior (e.g., watching TV, playing video games) can promote weight loss and reduce the intake of calorie-dense foods. Choosing enjoyable exercise and video games that provide for movement helps to improve feelings of satisfaction and sense of control.*[3,9]

NURSING PRIORITY NO. 3   To promote resilience (Teaching/Discharge Considerations):

- 🏠 Reinforce that client is responsible for self, for choices made, and actions taken. *The road to resilience is developed by the individual accepting that change is a part of living and beginning to live life more fully.*[3,9]
- 👥 Provide or identify learning opportunities specific to individual needs. *Activities such as assertiveness, regular exercise, and parenting classes can enhance knowledge and help develop a resilience mind-set.*[1,2,6]
- Discuss use of the problem-solving method to set mutually agreed-on goals. *As family accepts solutions that are acceptable to each member, their self-esteem is enhanced and individuals are more apt to follow through on decisions.*[2,3,10]
- Provide anticipatory guidance relevant to current situation and long-term expectations. *Client may have many issues to resolve, and planning ahead can help client make changes, have hope for the future, and have a sense of control over his or her life.*
- Encourage client/parents to take time for themselves. *They may believe they need to devote all their time to the family and feel guilty if they take time for themselves. This provides an opportunity for personal growth, and respite allows individuals to pursue own interests and return to tasks of life or parenting with renewed vigor.*[2]
- 👥 Refer to community resources as appropriate, such as social services, financial, domestic violence or elder abuse program, family therapy, divorce counseling, and special needs support services. *Appropriate support enhances ability to develop resilience in challenges client is dealing with.*[10]

DOCUMENTATION FOCUS

Assessment/Reassessment
- Findings, including specifics of individual situations or parental concerns, perceptions, expectations.
- Locus of control and cultural beliefs.

Planning
- Plan of care and who is involved in the planning.
- Teaching plan.

Implementation/Evaluation
- Response to interventions, teaching, and actions performed.
- Attainment or progress toward desired outcome(s).
- Modifications to plan of care.

Discharge Planning
- Long-term needs and who is responsible for actions to be taken.
- Specific referrals made.

 Acute Care   Collaborative   Community/Home Care   Cultural

References

1. Center on the Developing Child. (2015). The science of resilience. Retrieved April 2018 from https://developingchild.harvard.edu/resources/inbrief-the-science-of-resilience/.

2. No author. (No date). How resilient are you? *MindTools*. Retrieved December 2018 from https://www.mindtools.com/pages/article/resilience-quiz.htm.

3. Comas-Diaz, M., Luthar, S. S., Maddi, S. R. (No date). The road to resilience. *American Psychological Association Brochure*. Retrieved April 2018 from http://www.apa.org/helpcenter/road-resilience.aspx.

4. Eldar-Avidan, D., Haj-Yahia, M., Greenbaum, C. (2009). Divorce is a part of my life . . . resilience, survival, and vulnerability: Young adults' perception of the implications of parental divorce. *J Marital Fam Ther*, 35(1), 30–46.

5. Calamaro, C., Waite, R. (2008). Cultural proficiency, research, and evidence-based practice: Implications for the nurse practitioner. *J Pediatr Health Care*, 23(1), 69–72.

6. Adams, L. (No date). How do you deal with adversity?. *Gordon Training International*. Retrieved April 2018 from http://www.gordontraining.com/free-workplace-articles/how-do-you-deal-with-adversity/.

7. Brooks, R. L., Goldstein, S. (2006). Risk, resilience and futurists: Changing the lives of our children. *Education Horizons*, 9(3), 14–15.

8. National Institute for Mental Health Promotion and Youth Violence Prevention. (2009). Social and emotional learning and bullying prevention. Retrieved April 2018 from http://www.promoteprevent.org/sites/www.promoteprevent.org/files/resources/SELBullying(1).pdf.

9. Adams, L. (No date). Taking personal responsibility. *Gordon Training International*. Retrieved April 2018 from http://www.gordontraining.com/free-workplace-articles/taking-personal-responsibility/.

10. Bonanno, G., et al. (2007). What predicts psychological resilience after disaster? The role of demographics, resources, and life stress. *J Consult Clin Psychol*, 75(5), 671–682.

---

readiness for enhanced Resilience

Taxonomy II: Coping/Stress Tolerance—Class 2 Coping Responses (00212) [**Diagnostic Division:** Ego Integrity], Approved 2008; Revised 2013

DEFINITION: A pattern of ability to recover from perceived adverse or changing situations through a dynamic process of adaptation, which can be strengthened.

DEFINING CHARACTERISTICS

Subjective

Expresses desire to enhance:
- Communication skills, relationships with others
- Use of coping skills, conflict management strategies
- Resilience, self-esteem, positive outlook
- Involvement in activities, own responsibility for action, sense of control
- Goal-setting, progress toward goal
- Support system, available resources, use of resources
- Environmental safety

Sample Clinical Applications: Chronic health conditions (e.g., asthma, diabetes mellitus, arthritis, systemic lupus, multiple sclerosis [MS], AIDS); mental health concerns (e.g., depression, anxiety, bipolar disorder, attention deficit-hyperactivity disorder)

DESIRED OUTCOMES/EVALUATION CRITERIA

Sample NOC linkages:

Personal Resiliency: Positive adaptation and function of an individual following significant adversity or crisis

Hope: Optimism that is personally satisfying and life-supporting

(continues on page 710)

 Diagnostic Studies
 Evidence Based Practice
 Medications
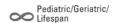 Pediatric/Geriatric/Lifespan

readiness for enhanced Resilience (continued)

Family Resiliency: Capacity of a family to positively adapt and function following significant adversity or crisis

Client Will (Include Specific Time Frame)
- Describe current situation accurately.
- Identify positive responses currently being used.
- Verbalize feelings congruent with behavior.
- Express desire to strengthen ability to deal with current situation or crisis.

ACTIONS/INTERVENTIONS

Sample **NIC** linkages:

Resiliency Promotion: Assisting individuals, families, and communities in development, use, and strengthening of protective factors to be used in coping with environmental and societal stressors

Hope Inspiration: Enhancing the belief in one's capacity to initiate and sustain actions

Family Mobilization: Utilization of family strengths to influence patient's health in a positive direction

NURSING PRIORITY NO. 1 To determine needs and desires for improvement:

- Evaluate client's perception and ability to provide a realistic view of the situation. *Provides information about how the client views the situation and specific expectations to aid in formulating plan of care.*[5]
- Determine client's coping abilities in current situation and expectations for change. *Client may be stressed to the point of having difficulty coping, recognizing need to improve ability to manage.*[4,6] *Motivation to improve and high expectations can encourage client to make changes that will improve his or her life. However, unrealistic expectations may hamper efforts.*
- Note client's verbal expressions indicating belief that he or she owns the responsibility for how to deal with adverse situation. *When client has internal locus of control, he or she accepts that life has its adversities and one needs to deal with them.*[3]
- Discuss religious and cultural beliefs held by the individual. *Knowing the role of the elements of culture and religion in shaping and defining health behaviors and expectations of client helps determine individual needs and possible options.*[1]
- Identify support systems available to client. *Having family and friends who are willing to listen as client works through problems can help to resolve them.*[5]

NURSING PRIORITY NO. 2 To assist client to enhance resilience to adverse situation:

- Active-listen and identify client's concerns about situation. *Reflecting client's statements helps to clarify what he or she is thinking and promotes accurate interpretation of reality.*[2]
- Determine previous methods of dealing with adversity. *Helps client to remember successful skills used in the past and see what might be helpful in current situation.*[3]
- Discuss desire to improve ability to handle adverse situations that arise throughout life. *The willingness to be open to change requires curiosity, listening to other's ideas and beliefs, and looking at new ways to do things.*[3]
- Discuss concept of what can be changed versus what cannot be changed. *Understanding that some things cannot be changed helps client to focus energies on those things that can be changed.*[2]
- Determine how client is dealing with activities of daily living. *While client may have some transient problems with sleeping or managing daily affairs, most people have the ability to function in a healthy manner over time.*[6]

 Acute Care   Collaborative   Community/Home Care   Cultural

- Help client to learn how to empathize with others. *Understanding own emotions as well as feelings of others enhances one's resiliency during stressful times.*[4]

NURSING PRIORITY NO. 3 To promote optimum growth and resiliency:

- Provide factual information and anticipatory guidance relevant to current situation and long-term expectations. *Planning ahead allows for problem-solving and review of options in a relaxed atmosphere, reinforcing sense of control and hope for the future.*[3]
- Review factors that might impact individual's response to stress. *Genetic influences, past experiences, and existing conditions can determine whether the client's response is adaptive or maladaptive and help individual to be resilient.*[3]
- Encourage client to maintain or establish good relationships with family and friends. *These connections are important, and accepting help and support from others enhances own coping and strengthens resilience.*[7]
- Help client to avoid seeing situation as insurmountable. *Catastrophic thinking locks individual into believing he or she has no control over outcome. While one cannot change the fact of the circumstances, how individual interprets and responds is within his or her control.*[7]
- Recommend setting realistic goals and doing something regularly, even if it is small. *Moving toward goals encourages a feeling of accomplishment and self-esteem.*[7]
- Encourage client to maintain a hopeful outlook, nurture a positive view of self, and take care of self. *Keeping a long-term perspective and paying attention to own needs help maintain and build resilience.*[7]
- Refer to classes and/or reading materials as appropriate. *Learning skills of meditation and assertiveness and engaging in enjoyable exercises help to foster resilience.*[3,7]

DOCUMENTATION FOCUS

Assessment/Reassessment
- Baseline information, including client's perception of situation, view of own ability to be resilient, and support systems available.
- Ways of dealing with previous life problems.
- Motivation and expectations for change.
- Cultural or religious influences.

Planning
- Plan of care and who is involved in planning.
- Teaching plan.

Implementation/Evaluation
- Responses to interventions, teaching, and actions performed.
- Attainment or progress toward desired outcomes(s).
- Modifications to plan.

Discharge Planning
- Long-term needs and who is responsible for actions to be taken.
- Specific referrals made.

References

1. Calamaro, C., Waite, R. (2008). Cultural proficiency, research, and evidence-based practice: Implications for the nurse practitioner. *J Pediatr Health Care*, 23(1), 69–72.
2. Adams, L. (No date). How do you deal with adversity?. Retrieved April 2018 from http://www.gordontraining.com/free-workplace-articles/how-do-you-deal-with-adversity/.
3. Brooks, R. (No date). The power to change your life: Ten keys to resilient living. Retrieved April 2018 from http://www.drrobertbrooks.com/wp/wp-content/uploads/2003/10/The-Power-to-Change-Your-Life-Ten-Keys-to-Resilient-Living.pdf.
4. Comas-Diaz, L., Luthar, S. S., Maddi, S. R. (No date). The road to resilience. Retrieved April 2018 from http://www.apa.org/helpcenter/road-resilience.aspx.

 Diagnostic Studies   Evidence Based Practice   Medications   Pediatric/Geriatric/Lifespan

5. Eldar-Avidan, D., Haj-Yahia, M., Greenbaum, C. (2009). Divorce is a part of my life…resilience, survival and vulnerability: Young adults' perception of the implications of parental divorce. *J Marital Fam Ther*, 35(1), 30–46.
6. McKeever, M. (2011). The brain and emotional intelligence: An interview with Daniel Goleman. *Learning & the Brain*. Retrieved November 2018 from https://www.learningandthebrain.com/blog/the-brain-and-emotional-intelligence-by-daniel-goleman/.
7. Adams, L. (No date). Taking personal responsibility. Retrieved April 2018 from http://www.gordontraining.com/free-workplace-articles/taking-personal-responsibility/.

risk for impaired Resilience

Taxonomy II: Coping/Stress Tolerance—Class 2 Coping Responses (00211) [**Diagnostic Division:** Ego Integrity], Approved 2008; Revised 2013, 2017

DEFINITION: Susceptible to decreased ability to recover from perceived adverse or changing situations, through a dynamic process of adaptation, which may compromise health.

RISK FACTORS

Community violence

Disruption in family rituals or roles; inconsistent parenting

Disturbance in family dynamics; dysfunctional family processes; ineffective family adaptation

Inadequate or insufficient resources

Insufficient social support; perceived vulnerability

Multiple coexisting adverse situations; substance misuse/[abuse]

At Risk Population: Chronicity of existing crisis; new crisis; demographics that increase chance of maladjustment

Economically disadvantaged; ethnic minority status; exposure to violence

Female gender; large family size

Low intellectual ability or maternal educational level

Parental mental illness

Associated Condition: Psychological disorder

Sample Clinical Applications: Chronic or debilitating illness (e.g., Alzheimer's disease, multiple sclerosis [MS], Parkinson's disease, Crohn's disease, diabetes, heart failure, cancer, renal failure); mental health issues (e.g., depression, anxiety)

DESIRED OUTCOMES/EVALUATION CRITERIA

Sample NOC linkages:

Personal Resiliency: Positive adaptation and function of an individual following significant adversity or crisis

Hope: Optimism that is personally satisfying and life supporting

Family Resiliency: Capacity of a family to positively adapt and function following significant adversity or crisis

---

Client Will (Include Specific Time Frame)

• Acknowledge reality of individual situation or crisis.
• Verbalize feelings associated with chronic situation.
• Verbalize awareness of own ability to deal with problems.
• Identify resources for assisting with chronic and new adverse occurrence.

 Acute Care   Collaborative   Community/Home Care   Cultural

ACTIONS/INTERVENTIONS

Sample NIC linkages:

Resiliency Promotion: Assisting individuals, families, and communities in development, use, and strengthening of protective factors to be used in coping with environmental and societal stressors

Hope Inspiration: Enhancing the belief in one's capacity to initiate and sustain actions

Family Mobilization: Utilization of family strengths to influence patient's health in a positive direction

NURSING PRIORITY NO. 1 To determine individual stressors/potential challenges:

- Note underlying stressors, health concerns, debilitating conditions, and mental health or behavioral issues, such as unemployment, pregnancy, diabetes, Alzheimer's disease, and anxiety disorder. *Provides information about situation to plan appropriate care.*[5]
- Determine alcohol or other drug use, smoking, sleeping, and eating habits. *Affects ability to cope with added stress of crises effectively and in a healthy manner.*[5]
- Assess functional capacity and how it affects client's ability to manage daily needs. *Presence of physical impairments may bring additional stress to adverse situation and unplanned new crisis.*[5]
- Evaluate client's ability to verbalize and understand current situation and impact of new crisis. *Informed choice cannot be made without a good understanding of reality of situation.*[5]
- Note speech and communication patterns. *Provides information about level of education and ability to understand situation and relate problems to caregiver(s).*[5]
- Determine locus of control. *Individuals with external locus of control are less likely to feel in control or rely on their own abilities or judgment to manage a situation and may wait for someone else, or luck, to change the circumstances and make life better.*[2,4,5]
- Evaluate client's current decision-making ability. *Crises affect individual's ability to think clearly and trust own ability to deal with situation.*[3]
- Ascertain stability of relationship, presence of separation or divorce, deteriorating health, or recent death of family member. *Family members are vulnerable to breakup of the family unit and, depending on perception and circumstances, may see it as causing long-term liability.*[3]

NURSING PRIORITY NO. 2 To assess coping skills and degree of resilience:

- Active-listen and identify client's perceptions of what has occurred as well as previous concerns. *Helps client to reflect back reality and distinguish between perceptions and actual events.*[2]
- Determine how adverse situation is affecting client's ability to deal with what is happening now. *When an unplanned situation occurs in addition to existing problems, it often results in decreased ability to maintain optimism.*[3,5,8]
- Determine how individual has dealt with problems in the past. *Having client remember these skills helps client to recognize what can be used to enhance current response or address future challenges.*[3,7]
- 🌐 Note cultural factors and religious beliefs that may affect situation. *Knowing how these factors shape and define health behavior and expectations of client/significant other (SO) helps determine individual needs and possible options.*[1]
- Determine availability and use of resources, family, support groups, and financial. *Appropriate use can help individuals continue to manage problems in their lives and plan for future needs.*

 Diagnostic Studies   Evidence Based Practice   Medications 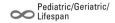 Pediatric/Geriatric/Lifespan

NURSING PRIORITY NO. 3 To assist client to deal with current/future situation:

- Ask client what name he or she prefers. *Acknowledging how client wants to be addressed provides sense of self, promoting esteem.*[5]
- Encourage free expressions of feelings, including feelings of anger and hostility, setting limits on unacceptable behavior. *When feelings are verbalized, client begins to identify them and recognize how they affect personal behavior. Unacceptable behavior leads to feelings of shame and guilt if it is not controlled.*[2,5]
- Allow client to react in own way without judgment by caregivers. Provide support and diversion as indicated. *Unconditional positive regard and support promote acceptance and help client to realize own ability to deal with situation.*[6]
- Listen to client's concerns and acknowledge difficulty of adversity and possible need to make changes. *Often, individuals who are feeling that life is difficult begin to doubt their ability to deal with circumstances. Being listened to provides opportunity for client to feel valued, capable, and like a survivor rather than a victim.*[8]
- Encourage communication with caregivers and SO(s). *Promotes effective interactions and common understanding of what is being said.*
- Provide reality orientation when necessary. *Depending on nature of crises, client may be disoriented by change in environment, serious diagnosis/treatment regimen, death of family member.*[5]
- Provide client with factual information and expected course of situation or crisis if known. *Knowledge helps to allay anxiety, enabling client to manage more effectively and begin to consider the possible resolution of the current situation.*[7]
- Focus on strengths of the individual as the problems are being assessed and diagnosed. *Treatment or intervention has often been based on a deficit model rather than a wellness approach. Improving the future for the client is based on strengthening the capacity to deal successfully with the obstacles he or she meets in life.*[6]

NURSING PRIORITY NO. 4 To promote optimum resiliency (Teaching/Discharge Considerations):

- 🏠 🌀 Provide or identify learning opportunities specific to individual needs. *Referral to activities, such as assertiveness training, regular exercise, parenting classes, can enhance knowledge and help develop a resilient mind-set.*[2,3,5]
- Encourage an attitude of realistic hope. *Client can accept that change is a part of living, and while some goals cannot be attained because of crisis or new circumstances, new goals can be developed and life can move forward.*[7]
- Support client in evaluating current lifestyle and changes that will need to be made. *Helps to put things in perspective and develop new plans gradually to avoid undue anxiety.*[9]
- Provide anticipatory guidance relevant to current situation and long-term expectations. *Client may have many issues to resolve, and planning ahead can help client make changes, have hope for the future, and have a sense of control over his or her life.*[3]
- 🌀 Determine need or desire for religious, spiritual counselor and make arrangements for visit. *Spiritual needs are part of being human, and providing the client an opportunity to discuss concerns about what has happened helps to build resilience to face future stressors.*[5]
- Reinforce importance of clients/SO(s) taking time for themselves. *They may believe they need to devote all their time to the family and feel guilty if they take time for themselves. This provides an opportunity for personal growth; respite allows individuals to pursue own interests and return to tasks of life with renewed vigor.*[2,9]
- 🌀 Refer to community resources as appropriate. *May need professional counseling, assistance with financial concerns, special needs support services, and child or parenting care in order to sustain move forward.*[2,5]

 Acute Care   Collaborative   Community/ Home Care   Cultural

DOCUMENTATION FOCUS

Assessment/Reassessment
- Assessment findings, including details of this client's situation or crisis, expectations.
- Client's degree of resiliency.

Planning
- Plan of care, and who is involved in planning.
- Teaching plan.

Implementation/Evaluation
- Response to interventions, teaching, and actions performed.
- Attainment or progress toward desired outcome(s).
- Modifications to plan of care.

Discharge Planning
- Long-term needs and who is responsible for actions to be taken.
- Support systems available, specific referrals made.

References

1. Calamaro, C., Waite, R. (2008). Cultural proficiency, research, and evidence-based practice: Implications for the nurse practitioner. *J Pediatr Health Care*, 23(1), 69–72.
2. Gordon, T. (No date). Origins of the Gordon model. Retrieved April 2018 from http://www.gordontraining.com/thomas-gordon/origins-of-the-gordon-model/.
3. Eldar-Avidan, D., Haj-Yahia, M., Greenbaum, C. (2009). Divorce is a part of my life . . . resilience, survival, and vulnerability: Young adults' perception of the implications of parental divorce. *J Marital Fam Ther*, 35(1), 30–46.
4. Adams, L. (No date). How do you deal with adversity? *Gordon Training International.* Retrieved April 2018 from http://www.gordontraining.com/free-workplace-articles/how-do-you-deal-with-adversity/.
5. Brooks, R., Goldstein, S. (2006). Risk, resilience and futurists: Changing the lives of our children. *Education Horizons*, 9(3), 14–15.
6. Center on the Developing Child. (2015). The science of resilience. Retrieved April 2018 from https://developingchild.harvard.edu/resources/inbrief-the-science-of-resilience/.
7. No author listed. (No date). How resilient are you? *MindTools.* Retrieved January 2019 from https://www.mindtools.com/pages/article/resilience-quiz.htm.
8. Graham, L. (No date). Resilience. *Sources for Recovering Resilience.* Retrieved April 2018 from http://lindagraham-mft.net/resources/published-articles/resilience/.
9. Mills, H., Dombeck, M. (2005). Resilience: Underlying attitudes and skills. *Mentalhelp.net.* Retrieved April 2018 from https://www.mentalhelp.net/articles/resilience-underlying-attitudes-and-skills/.

[acute/chronic] urinary Retention

Taxonomy II: Elimination and Exchange—Class 1 Urinary Function (00023) [**Diagnostic Division:** Elimination], Approved 1986; Revised 2017

DEFINITION: Inability to empty bladder completely.

RELATED FACTORS
To Be Developed

DEFINING CHARACTERISTICS

Subjective
Sensation of bladder fullness
Dribbling of urine
Small or frequent voiding; dysuria

(continues on page 716)

 Diagnostic Studies   Evidence Based Practice   Medications   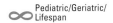 Pediatric/Geriatric/Lifespan

[acute/chronic] urinary Retention (continued)

Objective
Bladder distention
Absence of urinary output
Residual urine
Overflow incontinence
Associated Condition: Blockage in urinary tract; strong sphincter
High urethral pressure; reflex arc inhibition
Sample Clinical Applications: Benign prostatic hyperplasia (BPH), prostatitis, cancer, perineal surgery, birth trauma, urethral calculi, multiple sclerosis (MS), spinal cord compression, urinary tract infection (UTI), genital herpes

DESIRED OUTCOMES/EVALUATION CRITERIA

Sample **NOC** linkages:
Urinary Elimination: Collection and discharge of urine
Symptom Control: Personal actions to minimize perceived adverse changes in physical and emotional functioning
Knowledge: Acute Illness Management: Extent of understanding conveyed about a reversible illness, its treatment, and the prevention of complications

Client Will (Include Specific Time Frame)
• Verbalize understanding of causative factors and appropriate interventions for individual situation.
• Demonstrate techniques or behaviors to alleviate or prevent retention.
• Void in sufficient amounts with no palpable bladder distention, experience no postvoid residuals greater than 50 mL, and have no dribbling or overflow.

ACTIONS/INTERVENTIONS

Acute Retention
Sample **NIC** linkages:
Urinary Catheterization: Insertion of a catheter into the bladder for temporary or permanent drainage of urine
Urinary Retention Care: Assistance in relieving bladder distention

NURSING PRIORITY NO. 1   To assess causative/contributing factors:

• Note presence of pathological conditions, such as neurological injury or disease; kidney or bladder infection or stone formation; and reaction to medications, diagnostic dye, or anesthesia, *that can cause mechanical obstruction, nerve dysfunction, ineffective contraction, or decompensation of detrusor musculature, resulting in ineffective emptying of the bladder and urine retention.*[2]
• ∞ Note client's gender and age. *Retention is most common among men (young men due to renal calculi) and older men (where prostate abnormalities or urethral strictures cause outlet obstruction). In either gender, retention may be due to medications); neurogenic bladder such as occurs with diabetes, multiple sclerosis, Parkinson's disease; pelvic surgery; or any other condition resulting in bladder denervation.*[7,8,10]
• Investigate reports of sudden loss of ability to pass urine, great difficulty passing urine, pain with urination, blood in urine. *May indicate acute urinary retention due to UTI or outlet obstruction Note: Chronic urinary retention is typically painless and associated with increased volume of residual urine.*[2,8]

 Acute Care   Collaborative   Community/Home Care   Cultural

- Review results of lab tests, such as urinalysis for presence of red and white blood cells, nitrates, glucose, bacteria, and cultures, as indicated. Blood may be tested for infection, electrolyte imbalance, and (in men) prostate-specific antigen *to determine presence of treatable conditions.*
- Review medication regimen *for drugs that can cause or exacerbate retention (e.g., psychotropics, opiates, sedatives, alpha and beta blockers, anticholinergics, antihistamines, neuroleptics, anesthesia).*[2,8]
- Determine anxiety level. *Client may be too embarrassed to void in presence of others or talk about problem with care providers.*
- Examine for fecal impaction, pelvic or perineal surgical site swelling, postpartal edema, vaginal or rectal packing, enlarged prostate, or other "mechanical" factors *that may produce a blockage of the urethra.*
- Strain urine for presence of stones or calculi *that may be causing outlet obstruction or to note when treatments are being effective in stone breakup and removal.*[2]

NURSING PRIORITY NO. 2 To determine degree of interference/disability:

- Ascertain if client can empty bladder completely, partially, or not at all, in spite of urge to urinate. *Signs of urinary retention caused by (1) blockage of the urethra or (2) disruption of complex system of nerves that connects the urinary tract with the brain. In men, blockage is most commonly caused by enlargement of the prostate, cancer, stones, and urethral stricture. Causes that can occur in both genders include scar tissue, injury (as in car crash or fall), blood clots, infection, tumors, and stones (rare). Disruption of nerves or nerve transmission or interpretation of signals can be caused by injury (e.g., spinal cord injury [SCI] or tumor, herniated disk, stroke), pelvic infections, surgery, and certain medications.*[1,2]
- Determine if there has been any significant urine output in the previous 6 to 8 hr. *Small amount of urine may leak out of bladder but generally not enough to relieve symptoms.*
- Note recent amount and type of fluid intake. *Adequate fluid intake is necessary for production of healthy output. If client is not voiding in spite of adequate fluid intake, fluids may be restricted temporarily to prevent bladder overdistention until adequate urine flow is established.*
- Palpate height of the bladder. Ascertain whether client has sensation of bladder fullness and his or her level of discomfort. *Sensation and discomfort can vary depending on underlying cause of retention. Most people with acute retention also feel pain in lower abdomen (pelvis). Back pain, fever, and painful urination may be present with retention if the cause is urinary tract infection.*
- 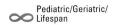Catheterize, or perform a bladder scan or ultrasound, for bladder residual after voiding *to determine presence and degree of urine retention.*[3]
- Review results of diagnostic tests. *Urine flow rate, bladder capacity, and postvoid residual scanning may be done. Ultrasound, computed tomography (CT) scan, intravenous pyelogram, and cystoscopy can help locate the source of obstruction (e.g., lower or upper tract). Lumbar spine radiographs, CT scan, or magnetic resonance imaging may be done when retention is thought to be due to an acute spinal problem (e.g., herniated disk, spinal cord disruption, infection).*[2,3]

NURSING PRIORITY NO. 3 To assist in treating/preventing retention:

- Assist in treatment to relieve mechanical obstruction (e.g., removal of blockage—vaginal packing, bowel impaction) or apply ice *to reduce perineal swelling.*
- Administer medications as indicated (e.g., antibiotics, stool softeners, pain relievers) *to treat underlying cause.*
- Provide privacy *to reduce retention caused by embarrassment or anxiety.*
- Assist client to sit upright on toilet or commode or stand *to provide functional position of voiding.*
- Encourage warm sitz bath or shower, voiding in tub or shower if need be. *Warm water stimulates bladder to relax and may facilitate voiding.*
- Use ice techniques or spirits of wintergreen, stroke inner thigh, and run water in sink or warm water over perineum if indicated *to stimulate reflex arc.*

- Instruct client with mild or moderate obstructive symptoms to "double void" by urinating, resting on toilet for 3 to 5 min, and then making a second attempt to urinate. *Promotes more efficient bladder evacuation by allowing the detrusor to contract initially and then rest and contract again.*[1]
- Drain bladder (using the appropriate catheter material and size) intermittently or catheterize with indwelling catheter *to resolve acute retention. Note: A variety of urethral catheters are available. Some have been developed specifically to lower the risk of catheter-associated infection, such as antiseptic or antibiotic impregnated catheters.*[9]
- Prepare for more intensive interventions (e.g., reconstructive surgery, lithotripsy, prostatectomy) as indicated *to remove source of obstruction, reconstruct sphincter, or provide for urinary diversion.*

NURSING PRIORITY NO. 4 To promote optimal elimination (Teaching/Discharge Considerations):

- Emphasize good voiding habits (e.g., four to six times/day). *Postponing or holding urination for prolonged periods can, over time, overstretch and weaken bladder muscles.*
- Encourage client to report problems immediately *so treatment can be instituted promptly.*
- Encourage adequate fluid intake, including use of acidifying fruit juices or ingestion of vitamin C or Mandelamine *to discourage bacterial growth and stone formation.*[8]
- Adjust fluid intake and timing if indicated, *to prevent bladder distention.*

Chronic Retention
Sample NIC linkages:
Urinary Retention Care: Assistance in relieving bladder distention
Urinary Catheterization: Intermittent: Regular periodic use of a catheter to empty the bladder

NURSING PRIORITY NO. 1 To assess causative/contributing factors:

- Review medical history for diagnoses, such as congenital defects, neurological disorders (e.g., MS, polio), prostatic hypertrophy or surgery, birth canal injury or scarring, and SCI with lower motor neuron injury or bladder stones, *that may cause detrusor-sphincter dyssynergia (loss of coordination between bladder contraction and external urinary sphincter relaxation), detrusor muscle atrophy, or chronic overdistention because of outlet obstruction.*[7,10]
- Determine presence of weak or absent sensory or motor impulses (as with cerebrovascular accidents, spinal injury, or diabetes) *that predispose client to compromised enervation or interpretation of sensory signals resulting in impaired urination.*[7]
- Assess client's medication regimen (e.g., psychotropic, antihistamines, atropine, belladonna) *to consult with primary care provider regarding client's continued use of drugs that are known to potentiate urinary retention.*

NURSING PRIORITY NO. 2 To determine degree of interference/disability:

- Ascertain effect of condition on functioning and lifestyle. *Chronic urinary retention can limit client's desired lifestyle (e.g., daily activities, social functioning) and can lead to chronic incontinence and life-threatening complications (e.g., intractable UTIs, kidney failure).*[4]
- Instruct client/significant other (SO) to maintain voiding log, noting dribbling and frequency and timing of voiding *to determine severity of condition.*[1]
- Determine presence and severity (0–10 scale) of bladder spasms, pelvic pain, and other discomforts.
- Assist with urodynamic testing (e.g., uroflowmetry *to assess urine speed and volume,* cystometrogram *to measure bladder pressure and volume,* bladder scan *to measure retention or postvoid residual, leak point pressure*).[2]

NURSING PRIORITY NO. 3 To assist in treating/preventing retention:

- Collaborate in treatment of underlying conditions (e.g., medications to treat BPH, reducing or eliminating medications responsible for retention, repairing perineal scarring or outlet obstruction), *which may correct or reduce severity of retention and associated overflow or total incontinence.*[10]

 Acute Care   Collaborative   Community/ Home Care 🌐 Cultural

- 🏠 Instruct client/SO in management of voiding problems as indicated:
  Attempt voiding in complete privacy *to reduce embarrassment and distractions.*
  Void on frequent, timed schedule *to maintain low bladder pressure and prevent overdistention of bladder.*
  Maintain consistent fluid intake *to wash out bacteria, avoid infections, and limit bladder stone formation.*[4]
  Adjust fluid amount and timing if indicated *to prevent bladder distention.*
- 🚫📋 Establish regular self-catheterization program, as indicated, *to prevent reflux and increased renal pressures and to improve client's quality of life (e.g., ability to participate in desired or needed activities and social interactions). Note: Clean intermittent catheterization is a treatment option for individuals who can urinate but cannot completely empty their bladder.*[4–6]
- 🚫 Perform and instruct client/SO in Credé's method (client or caregiver applies light pressure or tapping on the bladder) or Valsalva's maneuver (client tries to breathe out without letting air escape through the nose or mouth) if appropriate *to stimulate bladder emptying. Note: Client with SCI and spastic bladder may be able to "trigger" the bladder to contract and avoid having to use a catheter.*[7]
- 🚫 Consult with urologist and prepare for more intensive interventions (e.g., reconstructive surgery, lithotripsy, prostatectomy) as indicated *to remove source of obstruction, reconstruct sphincter, or provide for urinary diversion.*
- 🚫 Refer for consideration of advanced or research-based therapies (e.g., implanted sacral, tibial, or pelvic electrical stimulating device) *for long-term management of retention.*[4]

NURSING PRIORITY NO. 4   To promote optimum elimination (Teaching/Discharge Considerations):

- 🏠 Establish regular schedule for bladder emptying whether voiding or using catheter.
- Instruct SO/caregiver(s) in clean intermittent catheterization techniques *so that more than one individual is able to assist the client in care of elimination needs.*[9]
- Instruct client/SO in care when client has indwelling (urethral or suprapubic catheter) or urinary diversion device (e.g., clean technique, emptying and cleaning of leg bag or drainage bag; irrigation and replacement) *to promote self-care, enhance independence, and prevent complications.*[5]
- Emphasize need for adequate fluid intake, including use of acidifying fruit juices or ingestion of vitamin C or Mandelamine. *Maintains renal function, prevents infection and formation of bladder stones, and reduces risk of encrustation around indwelling catheter.*
- 💊 Discuss appropriate use of herbal products *such as saw palmetto to improve symptoms of BPH.*
- 🚫 Review signs/symptoms of complications *to promote timely contact with healthcare provider for evaluation and intervention.*

DOCUMENTATION FOCUS

Assessment/Reassessment
- Individual findings, including nature of problem, degree of impairment, and whether client is incontinent.

Planning
- Plan of care and who is involved in planning.
- Teaching plan.

Implementation/Evaluation
- Response to interventions.
- Attainment or progress toward desired outcome(s).
- Modifications to plan of care.

Discharge Planning
- Long-term needs and who is responsible for actions to be taken.
- Specific referrals made.

 Diagnostic Studies   Evidence Based Practice   Medications 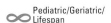 Pediatric/Geriatric/Lifespan

References

1. Gray, M. (2000). Urinary retention: Management in the acute care setting (part 2). *Am J Nurs*, 100(8), 36–44.
2. Newman, D. K. (2005). Assessment of the patient with an overactive bladder. *J Wound Ostomy Continence Nurs*, 32(3 Suppl), 5–10.
3. National Kidney and Urologic Diseases Information Clearinghouse. (Updated 2014). Urodynamic testing. Fact sheet. Retrieved May 2018 from http://kidney.niddk.nih.gov/KUDISEASES/pubs/urodynamic/index.aspx.
4. Santos, A., Hunt, M. (2005). Managing incontinence: Once a cause of isolation and embarrassment, incontinence does not have to limit quality of life. *Paraplegia News*, 59(11).
5. Herter, R., Kazer, M. W. (2010). Best practices in urinary catheter care. *Home Healthc Nurs*, 28(6), 342–349.
6. Doughty, D., Kisanga, J. (2010). Regulatory guidelines for bladder management in long-term care: Are you in compliance with F-Tag 315? *J Wound, Ostomy Cont Nurs*, 37(4), 399–411.
7. Shenot, P. J. (Updated 2016). Urinary retention (various pages). *The Merck Manual Professional Version*. Retrieved May 2018 from http://www.merckmanuals.com/professional/genitourinary-disorders/voiding-disorders/urinary-retention.
8. Selius, B. A., Subedi, R. (2008). Urinary retention in adults: Diagnosis and initial management. *Am Fam Physician*, 77(5), 643–650.
9. Smith, J. M. (2003). Indwelling catheter management: From habit-based to evidence-based practice. *J Wound, Ostomy Cont Nurs*, 49(12), 34–45.
10. Policastro, M. A., Sinert, R., Guerrero, P. (Updated 2016). Are your medications causing or increasing incontinence? Retrieved May 2018 from http://emedicine.medscape.com/article/778456-overview#showall.

parental Role Conflict

Taxonomy II: Role Relationships—Class 1 Role Performance (00064) [**Diagnostic Division:** Social Interaction], Approved 1988; Revised 2017

DEFINITION: Parental experience of role confusion and conflict in response to crisis.

RELATED FACTORS

Interruptions in family life due to home-care regimen [e.g., treatments, caregivers, lack of respite]
Intimidated by invasive modalities [e.g., intubation]; or by restrictive modalities [e.g., isolation]
Parent-child separation

DEFINING CHARACTERISTICS

Subjective

Perceived inadequacy to provide for child's needs
Concern about change in parental role; concern about family [e.g., functioning, communication, health]
Perceived loss of control over decisions relating to child
Guilt; frustration; anxiety; fear

Objective

Disruption in caregiver routines
Reluctance to participate in usual caregiver activities
At Risk Population: Change in marital status
Home care of child with special needs
Living in nontraditional setting
Sample Clinical Applications: Prematurity, genetic or congenital conditions, chronic illness (parent/child)

DESIRED OUTCOMES/EVALUATION CRITERIA

Sample NOC linkages:
Parenting Performance: Parental actions to provide a child a nurturing and constructive physical, emotional, and social environment

 Acute Care   Collaborative   Community/Home Care   Cultural

Role Performance: Congruence of an individual's role behavior with role expectations

Caregiver Lifestyle Disruption: Severity of disturbances in the lifestyle of a family member due to caregiving

Parent(s) Will (Include Specific Time Frame)
• Verbalize understanding of situation and expected parent's/child's role.
• Express feelings about child's illness or situation and effect on family life.
• Demonstrate appropriate behaviors concerning parenting role.
• Assume caretaking activities, as appropriate.
• Handle family disruptions effectively.

ACTIONS/INTERVENTIONS

Sample NIC **linkages:**

Parenting Promotion: Providing parenting information, support, and coordination of comprehensive services to high-risk families

Role Enhancement: Assisting a patient, significant other, and/or family to improve relationships by clarifying and supplementing specific role behaviors

Caregiver Support: Provision of the necessary information, advocacy, and support to facilitate primary patient care by someone other than a healthcare professional

NURSING PRIORITY NO. 1 To assess causative/contributory factors:

• Assess individual situation and parent's perception of and concern about what is happening and expectations of self as caregiver. *Identifies needs of the family to deal realistically with the current situation and what interventions are necessary to work toward identified goals.*[5]

• ∞Note parental status, including age and maturity, stability of relationship, single parent, and other responsibilities. *Young parents may lack the necessary maturity to deal with unexpected illness of infant or child. Single parent may feel overwhelmed in trying to balance work and caretaking responsibilities. Increasing numbers of elderly individuals who were expecting retirement and a simpler life are providing full-time care for young grandchildren whose parents are unavailable or unable to provide care.*[1]

• Ascertain parent's understanding of child's developmental stage and expectations for the future to identify misconceptions and strengths. *Parents often have no information regarding developmental stages and have unrealistic expectation of abilities of the child. Identifying what the parents know and providing information can help them deal more realistically with the situation.*[1]

• Note coping skills currently used by each individual as well as how problems have been dealt with in the past. *Provides basis for comparison and reference for client's coping abilities in current situation.*[1]

• ⚕Determine use of substances (e.g., alcohol, other drugs, including prescription medications). *May interfere with individual's ability to cope/problem-solve and manage current illness/situation and indicates need for additional interventions.*[8]

• ⊘Determine availability and use of resources, including extended family, support groups, and financial. *Factors that may affect ability to manage illness, unexpected expenses, caregiving activities, etc.*[1]

• ⬦Perform testing such as Parent-Child Relationship Inventory for further evaluation as indicated. *Provides information on which to develop plan of care and appropriate interventions.*[1]

• ⊕Determine cultural or religious influences on parenting expectations of self and child and sense of success or failure. *Parenting is one of the most important jobs individuals will have and one for which they are least prepared. Family of origin practices and beliefs will influence parenting style, and this information is crucial to developing a plan of care that meets their needs.*[4]

 Diagnostic Studies   Evidence Based Practice   Medications   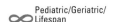 Pediatric/Geriatric/ Lifespan

NURSING PRIORITY NO. 2 To assist parents to deal with current crisis:

- Encourage free verbal expression of feelings (including negative feelings of anger and hostility), setting limits on inappropriate behavior. *Verbalization of feelings enables parent(s) to sift through situation and begin to deal with reality of what is happening. Inappropriate behavior is not helpful for dealing with the situation and will lead to feelings of guilt and low self-worth.*[2]
- Acknowledge difficulty of situation and normalcy of feeling overwhelmed and helpless. Encourage contact with parents who experienced similar situation with child and had positive outcome. *Parents feel listened to when feelings are acknowledged, and hearing how other parents have dealt with situation can give them hope.*[2]
- Provide information in an honest and forthright manner at level of understanding of the client, including technical information when appropriate. *Helping client understand what is happening corrects misconceptions and helps to make decisions that meet individual needs.*[3,12]
- Promote parental involvement in decision making and care as much as possible or desired. *When family members are involved in the process, it enhances their sense of control, and they are more likely to follow through on plans that are made.*[2]
- Encourage interaction and facilitate communication between parent(s) and child. *Sometimes people who find themselves in difficult or distressful situations tend to withdraw because they do not know what to do. Encouraging these interactions enables them to connect with one another to facilitate dealing with situation.*[2]
- Discuss problems of attachment disorder when diagnosed in an adopted child. *Children who have been adopted often suffer from problems of believing that they will not be loved, and parents need to learn reasons behind problems as well as skills to deal with them.*[9,10]
- Promote use of assertiveness and relaxation skills. *Providing information and helping individuals learn these skills will help them to deal more effectively with situation or crisis.*[6]
- Instruct parent in proper administration of medications and treatments as indicated. *May need to be involved in care, and knowing how to do these activities enhances their sense of control and comfort in their ability to handle situation.*[5]
- Provide for and encourage use of respite care and parent time off. *Parents may believe they are being "selfish" if they take time out for themselves and that they have to remain with the child. However, parents are important, children are important, and the family is important, and when parents take time for themselves, it enhances their emotional well-being and promotes ability to deal with ongoing situation.*[7,11]
- Help single parent distinguish between parental love and partner love. *New focus of parent's attention or love may result in neglect of relationship with child. Attention needs to be given to both individuals for the relationships to flourish.*[9]

NURSING PRIORITY NO. 3 To promote wellness (Teaching/Discharge Considerations):

- Provide anticipatory guidance relevant to the situation and long-term expectations of the illness. *Encourages making plans for future needs, provides feelings of hope, and promotes sense of control over difficult situation.*[12]
- Encourage parents to set realistic and mutually agreed-on goals. *As family members work together, they can feel empowered and more apt to follow through on decisions that they are involved in making.*[2]
- Discuss infant attachment behaviors such as breastfeeding on cue, cosleeping, and babywearing (carrying baby around on chest or back), as appropriate. *Dealing with ill child and home-care pressures can strain the bond between parent/child. Activities such as these encourage secure relationships.*
- Provide and identify learning opportunities specific to needs. *Activities such as parenting classes, information about equipment use, and methods of troubleshooting can enhance knowledge and ability to deal with situation.*[3,12]
- Refer to community resources, as appropriate (e.g., visiting nurse, respite care, social services, psychiatric care or family therapy, well-baby clinics, special needs support services). *Provides additional assistance as needed to handle individual situation or illness.*[5]
- Refer to ND impaired Parenting for additional interventions.

 Acute Care   Collaborative   Community/ Home Care   Cultural

DOCUMENTATION FOCUS

Assessment/Reassessment
• Findings, including specifics of individual situation, parental concerns, perceptions, expectations.

Planning
• Plan of care and who is involved in the planning.
• Teaching plan.

Implementation/Evaluation
• Parent's responses to interventions, teaching, and actions performed.
• Attainment or progress toward desired outcome(s).
• Modifications to plan of care.

Discharge Planning
• Long-term needs and who is responsible for each action to be taken.
• Specific referrals made.

References

1. Scott, E. (Updated 2018). Coping skills for parents and kids. Retrieved April 2018 from http://stress.about.com/od/parentingskills/a/coping_skills.htm.
2. McIntyre, L. L. (2008). Parent training for young children with developmental disabilities: Randomized control trial. *Am J Ment Retard*, 113(5), 356–368.
3. Colville, G., Darkins, J., Hesketh, J. (2009). The impact on parents of a child's admission to intensive care: Integration of qualitative findings from a cross-sectional study. *Intensive Crit Care Nurs*, 25(2), 72–79.
4. Purnell, L. D. (2011). *Guide to Culturally Competent Health Care*. 2nd ed. Philadelphia: F. A. Davis.
5. Power, N., Franck, L. (2008). Parent participation in the care of hospitalized children: A systematic review. *J Adv Nurs*, 62(6), 622–641.
6. Assertiveness skills. (1998). *Brain Injury Resource Center*. Retrieved April 2018 from http://www.headinjury.com/assertskills.html.
7. Major, D. A. (2001). Utilizing role theory to help employed parents cope with children's chronic illness. *Health Research Education*, 18(1), 45–57.
8. National Institute on Drug Abuse. (Updated 2015). Family checkup: Positive parenting prevents drug abuse (various sections). Retrieved April 2018 from https://www.drugabuse.gov/family-checkup/question-1-communication.
9. Pickhardt, C. (2002). Role conflict of the single parent. Retrieved April 2018 from http://www.carlpickhardt.com/page48.html.
10. Counseling Directory. (No date). Attachment disorder. Retrieved April 2018 from https://www.counselling-directory.org.uk/attachment-disorder.html.
11. Walant, K. (2000). When the going gets tough: A little self-care goes a long way. *Attachment Parenting International News*. Retrieved April 2018 from http://www.attachmentparenting.org/support/articles/artselfcare.php.
12. Berge, J. M., Holm, K. E. (2007). Boundary ambiguity in parents with chronically ill children: Integrating theory and research. *Family Relations*, 56(2), 123–134.

ineffective Role Performance

Taxonomy II: Role Relationships—Class 3 Role Performance (00055) [**Diagnostic Division:** Social Interaction], Approved 1978; Revised 1996, 1998, 2017

DEFINITION: A pattern of behavior and self-expression that does not match the environmental context, norms, and expectations.

[Note: There is a typology of roles, including sociopersonal (friendship, family, marital, parenting, community); home management; intimacy (sexuality, relationship building); leisure, exercise, and recreation; self-management; socialization (developmental transitions); community contributor; and religious, that can help to understand ineffective Role Performance.]

RELATED FACTORS
Alteration in body image
Conflict; stressors; domestic violence; substance misuse/[abuse]

(continues on page 724)

 Diagnostic Studies   Evidence Based Practice   Medications 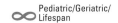 Pediatric/Geriatric/Lifespan

ineffective Role Performance (continued)

Depression; low self-esteem

Inadequate role model; insufficient role preparation; unrealistic role expectations

Insufficient support system, resources or rewards

Inappropriate linkage to the healthcare system

Pain

DEFINING CHARACTERISTICS

Subjective

Alteration in role perception; change in self-/other's perception of role

Change in usual pattern of responsibility or in capacity to resume role

Insufficient opportunity for role enactment

Role dissatisfaction; role denial

Discrimination; powerlessness

Objective

Insufficient knowledge of role requirements

Ineffective adaptation to change; inappropriate developmental expectations

Insufficient confidence, motivation, self-management, or skills

Ineffective coping strategies; ineffective role performance

Inadequate external support for role enactment

Role strain, conflict, confusion, or ambivalence [failure to assume role]

Uncertainty; anxiety; depression; pessimism

Domestic violence; harassment; system conflict

At Risk Population: Developmental level inappropriate for role expectation; young age

Economically disadvantaged; low educational level

High demands of job schedule

Associated Condition: Neurological defect; personality disorder

Physical illness; psychosis

Sample Clinical Applications: Chronic conditions (e.g., multiple sclerosis [MS], pain, chronic fatigue syndrome [CFS]), cancer, substance abuse, brain or spinal cord injury (SCI), major surgery, major depression, bipolar disorder, borderline personality disorder, schizophrenia

DESIRED OUTCOMES/EVALUATION CRITERIA

Sample NOC linkages:

Role Performance: Congruence of an individual's role behavior with role expectations

Coping: Personal actions to manage stressors that tax an individual's resources

Psychosocial Adjustment: Life Change: Adaptive psychosocial response of an individual to a significant life circumstance

Client Will (Include Specific Time Frame)

• Verbalize realistic perception and acceptance of self in changed role.

• Verbalize understanding of role expectations or obligations.

• Talk with family/significant others (SOs) about situation and changes that have occurred and limitations imposed.

• Develop realistic plans for adapting to new role or role changes.

 Acute Care   Collaborative   Community/ Home Care   Cultural

ACTIONS/INTERVENTIONS

Sample NIC **linkages:**

Role Enhancement: Assisting a patient, significant other, and/or family to improve relationships by clarifying and supplementing specific role behaviors

Normalization Promotion: Assisting parents and other family members of children with chronic illnesses or disabilities in providing normal life experiences for their children and families

Values Clarification: Assisting another to clarify her/his own values in order to facilitate effective decision making

NURSING PRIORITY NO. 1   To assess causative/contributing factors:

- Identify type of role dysfunction. *Life changes such as developmental (adolescent to adult), situational (husband to father, change in employment status, gender identity), and health-illness transitions can affect how client functions in usual role. This information is important to developing a plan of care and appropriate interventions and goals.*[1]
- Determine client role in family constellation. *How client has functioned in the past (i.e., husband/father, wife/ mother) provides a beginning point of reference for understanding changes that have occurred due to health alterations (mental or physical), lack of knowledge about role or role skills, lack of role model, or what other situation has occurred to bring about a role change.*[1]
- Identify how client sees self as a man/woman in usual lifestyle and role functioning. *Each person has a perception of self that is important to know to understand changes that may be occurring.*[1]
- Ascertain client's view of sexual functioning. *Changes (e.g., loss of childbearing ability following hysterectomy, erectile dysfunction following prostate surgery) can affect how client views self in role as male or female and may need specific interventions to resolve feelings of loss.*[1]
- Identify cultural factors relating to individual's gender roles. *Varies with the culture; for instance, for American Indians who are in matrilineal clans or band, women may make important decisions and male roles include rituals to protect family and community well-being. In Arab American families, men are expected to be responsible for financial affairs and women typically assume subordinate and caregiving roles.*[4]
- Determine client's perceptions and concerns about current situation. *May believe current role is more appropriate for the opposite sex (e.g., passive role of the "client" may be somewhat less threatening for women).*[2]
- Interview SO(s) regarding their perceptions and expectations. *The beliefs of the individuals directly involved with the client and the situation (e.g., parents bringing a new baby home from the hospital, adult child assuming responsibility for elder parent) are important to understanding the new roles the individuals are undertaking. Conflicts can arise when expectations vary from individual to individual.*[5]
- Determine client's socioeconomic status and linkage to the healthcare system. *People who are poor may not have healthcare insurance or access to care and perceive themselves as unworthy.*[1]
- Identify availability and use of resources. *Individual may be unaware or have difficulty accessing community support or assistance programs.*
- Investigate history of incidents of domestic violence in the family. Refer to psychiatric, protective, support, and legal services, as appropriate. *The roles of perpetrator and survivor are difficult to alter without intensive therapy. Neither individual in this situation sees self as worthy and both have poor self-esteem. The perpetrator does not get what he or she wants through the use of violence, and the survivor (the battered person) often believes she or he deserves this treatment.*[1,7]

NURSING PRIORITY NO. 2   To assist client to deal with existing situation:

- Discuss perceptions and significance of the situation as seen by client. *Provides opportunity to clarify any misperceptions and discuss changes client may have to make in regard to what has happened (e.g., loss of a limb, disfiguring surgery).*

 Diagnostic Studies   Evidence Based Practice   Medications   Pediatric/Geriatric/ Lifespan

- Maintain positive attitude toward the client. *Promotes safe relationship in which client can discuss changes that are occurring and plan for a positive future.*[1]
- Provide opportunities for client to exercise control over as much of situation as possible. *Enhances self-concept and promotes commitment to goals.*[1]
- Offer realistic assessment of situation and communicate hope. *Client may or may not accept reality, but opportunity to discuss issues and have a sense of hope can help client begin to accept reality.*[6]
- Discuss and assist the client/SO(s) to develop strategies for dealing with changes in role related to past transitions, cultural expectations, and value or belief challenges. *Helps those involved deal with differences between individuals (e.g., adolescent task of separation in which parents clash with child's choices).*[4,8]
- Acknowledge reality of situation related to role change and help client to express feelings of anger, sadness, grief, and depression. Encourage celebration of positive aspects of change and expressions of feelings. *Changes in role necessitated by illness, trauma, changes in family structure (new baby, child leaving home for college, elderly parent needing care), or any other circumstance result in a sense of loss and need to deal with the feelings that accompany the change.*[1,5]
- Provide open environment for client to discuss concerns about sexuality. *Embarrassment can block discussion of sensitive subject and potentially impede progress.* (Refer to NDs Sexual Dysfunction and ineffective Sexuality Pattern.)[7]
- Educate about role expectations using written and audiovisual materials. *Using different modalities enables client to review material at leisure and begin to incorporate information into own thinking.*
- Identify role model for the client. *Offers opportunity for client to observe how someone else functions in a role that is new to him or her.*[3]
- Use techniques of role rehearsal to practice new role. *Provides opportunity for the client to try and develop new skills to cope with anticipated changes.*[7]

NURSING PRIORITY NO. 3   To promote role enhancement (Teaching/Discharge Considerations):

- 🏠 Make information available (including bibliotherapy, appropriate Web sites) for client to learn about role expectations and demands that may occur. *Provides opportunity to be proactive in dealing with changes, such as classes to help new parent(s) learn about new roles and credible Web sites for additional information regarding individual's specific concerns.*[4]
- 💊 Discuss use of medication as appropriate. *Client may benefit from antidepressants to combat depression, or psychotropic medications may be required to address other mental health issues.*[1,7]
- Accept client in changed role. Encourage and give positive feedback for changes and goals achieved. *Provides reinforcement and facilitates continuation of efforts.*
- 👥 Refer to support groups, employment counselors, parent effectiveness classes, and counseling or psychotherapy, as indicated by individual need(s). *Provides ongoing support to sustain progress.*[6]
- Refer to NDs impaired Parenting and Self-Esteem [specify] as appropriate.

DOCUMENTATION FOCUS

Assessment/Reassessment
- Individual findings, including specifics of predisposing crises or situation, perception of role change.
- Cultural or religious factors.
- Expectations of SO(s).
- Availability and use of resources.

Planning
- Plan of care and who is involved in planning.
- Teaching plan.

Implementation/Evaluation
- Responses to interventions, teaching, and actions performed.
- Attainment or progress toward desired outcome(s).
- Modifications of plan of care.

 Acute Care   Collaborative   Community/ Home Care   Cultural

Discharge Planning
* Long-term needs and who is responsible for actions to be taken.
* Specific referrals made.

References

1. Karola, K. M. (1998). Family roles, alcoholism, and family dysfunction. *J Mental Health Counseling*, 20(3), 250–260.
2. Santuzzi, A. M., Metzger, P. L., Ruscher, J. B. (2006). Body image and expected future interactions. *Curr Res Soc Psychol*, 11(11), 153–171.
3. O'Hara, V. (No date). Stress and the role of perception. Retrieved April 2018 from http://stresscourse.tripod.com/id100.html.
4. Rideway, C. S., Correll, S. (2004). Unpacking the gender system: A theoretical perspective on gender beliefs and social relations. *Gender and Society*, 18(4), 510–531.
5. Gjerdingen, D., Center, B. A. (2003). First time parents prenatal to postnatal changes in health and the relation of postpartum

health to work and partner relationships. *J Am Board Fam Med*, 16(4), 304–311.
6. Rice, J., Hicks, P. B., Wiche, V. (2000). Life care planning: A role for social workers. *Soc Work Health Care*, 31(1), 85–94.
7. Collinson, T. (Updated 2017). Domestic violence and self-esteem: Low self-esteem linked to domestic violence. Retrieved April 2018 from http://womensissues.about.com/od/domestic violence/a/DomesticViolenceSelfEsteem.htm.
8. McLeod, S. (Updated 2017). The self-concept in psychology. *Simply Psychology*. Retrieved April 2018 from http://www.simplypsychology.org/self-concept.html.

caregiver Role Strain

Taxonomy II: Role Relationships—Class 1 Caregiving Roles (00061) [**Diagnostic Division:** Social Interaction], Approved 1992; Revised 1998, 2000; 2017

DEFINITION: Difficulty in fulfilling care responsibilities, expectations and/or behaviors for family or significant others.

RELATED FACTORS
Care Receiver
Condition inhibits conversation
Dependency; problematic behavior; substance misuse/[abuse]
Discharged home with significant needs; increase in care needs
Unpredictability of illness trajectory; unstable health condition
Caregiver
Physical conditions; not developmentally ready for caregiver role
Competing role commitments; insufficient fulfilment of self or others' expectations
Ineffective coping strategies; insufficient energy, privacy, or recreation
Inexperience with caregiving; insufficient knowledge about community resources
Stressors; substance misuse/[abuse]
Unrealistic self-expectations; insufficient emotional resilience; isolation
Caregiver–Care Receiver Relationship
Abusive or violent relationship; presence of abuse
Pattern of ineffective relationships; codependency
Unrealistic care receiver expectations
Caregiving Activities
Around-the-clock care responsibilities; insufficient time; change in nature or complexity of care activities
Excessive caregiving activities; extended duration of caregiving required
Inadequate physical environment or insufficient equipment for providing care; insufficient assistance or respite for caregiver
Recent discharge home with significant care needs; unpredictability of care situation

(continues on page 728)

 Diagnostic Studies   Evidence Based Practice   Medications   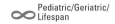 Pediatric/Geriatric/Lifespan

caregiver Role Strain (continued)

Family Processes
Family isolation; ineffective family adaptation; pattern of ineffective family coping
Pattern of family dysfunction; pattern of family dysfunction prior to the caregiving situation
Socioeconomic
Alienation; social isolation
Difficulty accessing assistance or support
Difficulty accessing/insufficient community resources
Insufficient transportation

DEFINING CHARACTERISTICS

Subjective
Caregiving Activities:
Apprehensiveness about: future ability to provide care or well-being of care receiver if unable to provide care; apprehensiveness about future health or institutionalization of care receiver
Caregiver Health Status: Physiological:
Fatigue; gastrointestinal distress; headache, rash, weight change
Hypertension; cardiovascular disease
Caregiver Health Status: Emotional:
Alteration in sleep pattern
Anger, emotional vacillation; depression; frustration, impatience; nervousness
Insufficient time to meet personal needs; stressors
Caregiver Health Status: Socioeconomic: Change in leisure activities; low work productivity; refusal of career advancement
Caregiver-Care Receiver Relationship:
Difficulty watching care receiver with illness
Grieving changes or uncertainty in relationship with care receiver
Family Processes: Concern about family members; family conflict

---

Objective
Caregiving Activities:
Difficulty performing or completing required tasks
Dysfunctional change in caregiving activities
Preoccupation with care routine
Caregiver Health Status: Physiological:
Cardiovascular disease; diabetes mellitus
Hypertension; weight change; rash
Caregiver Health Status: Emotional:
Anger, emotional vacillation; depression; frustration, impatience; nervousness
Ineffective coping strategies
Somatization
Caregiver Health Status: Socioeconomic: Low work productivity, refusal of career advancement; social isolation
Family Processes: Family conflict
At Risk Population: Care receiver's condition inhibits conversation
Developmental delay of caregiver or care receiver; prematurity
Female caregiver; partner of caregiver
Exposure to violence

 Acute Care   Collaborative   Community/ Home Care   Cultural

Associated Condition: Care Receiver
Alteration in cognitive functioning; psychiatric or psychological disorder
Chronic illness; illness severity
Congenital disorder
Caregiver
Alteration in cognitive functioning; psychological disorder
Health impairment
[Note: The presence of this problem may encompass other numerous problems/high-risk concerns, such as decreased Diversional Activity Engagement, Insomnia, Fatigue, Anxiety, ineffective Coping, compromised family Coping or disabled family Coping, Decisional Conflict, ineffective Denial, Grieving, Hopelessness, Powerlessness, Spiritual Distress, ineffective Health Maintenance, impaired Home Maintenance, Sexual Dysfunction or ineffective Sexuality Pattern, readiness for enhanced family Coping, interrupted Family Processes, and Social Isolation. Careful attention to data gathering will identify and clarify the client's specific needs, which can then be coordinated under this single diagnostic label.]

Sample Clinical Applications:
Chronic conditions (e.g., severe brain injury, spinal cord injury [SCI], severe developmental delay), progressive debilitating conditions (e.g., muscular dystrophy, multiple sclerosis [MS], dementia or Alzheimer's disease, end-stage chronic obstructive pulmonary disease [COPD], renal failure, renal dialysis), substance abuse, end-of-life care, psychiatric conditions (e.g., schizophrenia, personality disorders).

DESIRED OUTCOMES/EVALUATION CRITERIA

Sample **NOC** linkages:

Caregiver Role Endurance: Factors that promote family care provider's capacity to sustain caregiving over an extended period of time

Caregiver Stressors: Severity of biopsychosocial pressure on a family care provider caring for another over an extended period of time

Caregiver Well-Being: Extent of positive perception of primary care provider's health status

Caregiver Will (Include Specific Time Frame)
- Identify resources within self to deal with situation.
- Provide opportunity for care receiver to deal with situation in own way.
- Express more realistic understanding and expectations of the care receiver.
- Demonstrate behavior or lifestyle changes to cope with or resolve problematic factors.
- Report improved general well-being, ability to deal with situation.

ACTIONS/INTERVENTIONS

Sample **NIC** linkages:

Caregiver Support: Provision of the necessary information, advocacy, and support to facilitate primary patient care by someone other than a healthcare professional

Family Involvement Promotion: Facilitating participation of family members in the emotional and physical care of the patient

Parenting Promotion: Providing parenting information, support, and coordination of comprehensive services to high-risk families

NURSING PRIORITY NO. 1   To assess degree of impaired function:

- Inquire about and observe physical condition of care receiver and surroundings as appropriate. *Important to determine factors that may indicate problems that can interfere with ability to continue caregiving.*[4]

 Diagnostic Studies   Evidence Based Practice   Medications   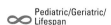 Pediatric/Geriatric/Lifespan

- Assess caregiver's current state of health and functioning (e.g., caregiver has multiple medical issues; is unable to get enough sleep, has poor nutritional intake, personal appearance and demeanor are indicating stress). *Provides basis for determining needs that indicate caregiver is having difficulty dealing with role.*[4]
- Determine use of medications/drugs (e.g., prescription, over-the-counter, or illicit drugs and/or alcohol). *Caregiver may turn to using these substances to deal with situation.*[1]
- Identify safety issues concerning caregiver and receiver. *The stress and anxiety of caregiving situations can lead to inattention, and by identifying these issues, an opportunity is provided to correct problems before injury occurs.*[1]
- Assess current actions of caregiver and how they are received by care receiver. *Caregiver may be trying to be helpful but is not perceived as helpful; may be too protective or may have unrealistic expectations of care receiver's abilities, which can lead to misunderstanding and conflict.*[4]
- Note choice and frequency of social involvement and recreational activities. *Caregiver needs to take time away from situation to maintain own sense of self and ability to continue in role.*[1]
- Determine use and effectiveness of resources and support systems. *May not be aware of what is available or may need help in using them to the best advantage.*[4]

NURSING PRIORITY NO. 2 To identify the causative/contributing factors relating to the impairment:

- ∞ Note presence of high-risk situations (e.g., elderly client with total care dependence on spouse; or caregiver with several small children, with one child requiring extensive assistance due to physical condition or developmental delays). *Such situations result in added stress (e.g., imposing unwanted role reversal, placing excessive demands on parenting skills).*[4]
- Determine current knowledge of the situation, noting misconceptions and lack of information. *May interfere with caregiver/care receiver's response to situation.*
- Identify relationship of caregiver to care receiver (e.g., spouse/lover, parent/child, sibling, friend). *Close relationships may make it more difficult to remain separate when caring for care receiver. Note: Younger-aged family caregivers are at increased risk for lower levels of hope and higher levels of caregiver strain.*[6]
- Determine quality of couple's relationship/presence of intimacy issues. *Disease/condition, caregiving activities, and possible change in role responsibilities may strain relationship, adding to sense of loss and unmet needs.*[3]
- Ascertain proximity of caregiver to care receiver. *Caregiver could be living in the home of care receiver (e.g., spouse or parent of disabled child) or could be adult child stopping by to check on elderly parent each day, providing support, food preparation, shopping, and assistance in emergencies. Note: There is added stress in maintaining own life and responsibilities when caregiver has to travel some distance to provide care.*[4,10]
- Note care receiver's physical and mental condition, as well as the complexity of therapeutic regimen. *Caregiving activities can be complex, requiring hands-on care, problem-solving skills, clinical judgment, and organizational and communication skills that can tax the caregiver, increasing likelihood of burnout.*[7,10]
- Determine caregiver's level of involvement in and preparedness for the responsibilities of caring for the client and anticipated length of care. *Information needed to develop plan of care that takes into consideration who will provide care, timing, and any other factors to maintain coverage for situation.*[4]
- Ascertain physical and emotional health, developmental level and abilities, and additional responsibilities of caregiver (e.g., job, raising family). *Provides clues to potential stressors and possible supportive interventions.*[10,11]
- Assess caregiver as appropriate, using tool such as Burden Interview, Herth Hope Index, Caregiver Reaction Assessment, or Caregiver Strain Index *to further determine caregiver's stressors and abilities, providing additional information to aid in planning.*[17,18]
- Identify individual cultural factors and impact on caregiver. *Helps clarify expectations of caregiver and receiver, family, and community. Many cultures, such as Native American and Cuban, believe strongly in keeping care receivers in the home and caring for them.*[5]
- Identify presence and degree of conflict between caregiver/care receiver/family. *Stressful situations can exacerbate underlying feelings of anger and resentment, resulting in difficulty managing caregiving needs.*[1]

 Acute Care Collaborative Community/ Home Care Cultural

- Determine pre-illness and current behaviors that may be interfering with the care or recovery of the care receiver. *Underlying personality of care receiver may create situation in which old conflicts interfere with current treatment regimen.*[1]
- Note codependency needs and enabling behaviors of caregiver. *These behaviors can interfere with competent caregiving and contribute to caregiver burnout.*[2]

NURSING PRIORITY NO. 3 To assist caregiver to identify feelings and begin to deal with problems:

- Establish a therapeutic relationship, conveying empathy and unconditional positive regard. *A compassionate approach blending the nurse's expertise in healthcare with the caregiver's firsthand knowledge of the care receiver can provide encouragement, especially in a long-term difficult situation.*[10,12]
- Acknowledge difficulty of the situation for the caregiver/family. *Research shows that the two greatest predictors of caregiver strain are poor health and the feeling that there is no choice but to take on additional responsibilities.*[10]
- Discuss caregiver's view of and concerns about situation. *Important to identify issues so planning and solutions can be developed.*[7]
- Encourage caregiver to acknowledge and express negative feelings. Discuss normalcy of the reactions without using false reassurance. *Individual needs to understand that all feelings are acceptable to be expressed and dealt with, but not acted on in the situation.*[1]
- Discuss caregiver's life goals, perceptions, and expectations of self. *Clarifies unrealistic thinking and identifies potential areas of flexibility or compromise.*[4]
- Discuss caregiver's perception of impact of and ability to handle role changes necessitated by situation. *May not initially realize the changes that will be encountered as situation develops, and it helps to identify and plan for changes before they arise.*

NURSING PRIORITY NO. 4 To enhance caregiver's ability to deal with current situation:

- Identify strengths of caregiver and care receiver. *Bringing these to the individual's awareness promotes positive thinking and helps with problem-solving to deal more effectively with circumstances.*[4]
- Discuss strategies to coordinate caregiving tasks and other responsibilities (e.g., employment, care of children/other dependents, housekeeping activities). *Managing these tasks will reduce the stress associated with performing the activities of daily living.*[1]
- Facilitate family conference to share information and develop plan for involvement in care activities as appropriate. *Involving everyone promotes sense of control and ownership of plan and willingness to follow through on responsibilities.*
- Identify classes or needed specialists (e.g., first aid and cardiopulmonary resuscitation classes, enterostomal specialist, physical therapist). *Provides information needed to manage tasks of caregiving more effectively, giving individuals more sense of control.*
- Determine need for and sources of additional resources (e.g., financial, legal, respite care, educational, social, spiritual). *Can help to resolve problems that arise in the course of caregiving that are out of the knowledge or abilities of the individual. Solving these issues can relieve caregiver of anxiety and concern.*[4,13]
- Provide information or demonstrate techniques for dealing with acting out, violent, or disoriented behavior. *Presence of dementia necessitates learning these techniques or skills to enhance safety of caregiver and receiver.*[1]
- Identify equipment needs and resources and appropriate adaptive aids. *Enhances the independence and safety of the care receiver and makes the task of caregiving easier.*
-   Provide contact person or case manager to partner with care provider(s) in coordinating care, providing physical and social support, and to assist with problem-solving as needed or desired. *As care receiver's condition declines or caregiving activities are prolonged/intensify, caregiver strain may escalate and psychological well-being of caregiver may decline. Ongoing support by health and social services promotes more effective caregiving and thereby lessens strain on caregiver.*[2,10,14]

 Diagnostic Studies   Evidence Based Practice   Medications   Pediatric/Geriatric/Lifespan

NURSING PRIORITY NO. 5 To promote wellness (Teaching/Discharge Considerations):

- Advocate for and assist caregiver to plan for and implement changes that may be necessary (e.g., home-care providers, adult day care, eventual placement in long-term care facility). *As caregiving tasks become more difficult, other options need to be considered, and planning ahead can promote acceptance of necessary changes.*[8,11,15]
- Encourage attention to own needs (e.g., eating and sleeping regularly, setting realistic goals, talking with trusted friend, periodic respite from caregiving), accepting own feelings, acknowledging frustrations and limitations, and being realistic about loved one's condition. *Supports and enhances caregiver's general well-being and coping ability.*[15,16]
- Review signs of burnout (e.g., emotional or physical exhaustion, changes in appetite and sleep, withdrawal from friends/family or life interests). *Recognition of developing problem allows for timely intervention.*
- Discuss and demonstrate stress management techniques and importance of self-nurturing (e.g., pursuing self-development interests, hobbies, social activities, spiritual enrichment). *Being involved in activities such as these can prevent caregiver burnout.*[4,15]
- Encourage involvement in caregiver support group. *Having others to share concerns and fears is therapeutic and provides ideas for different ways to manage problems, helping caregivers deal more effectively with the situation.*[1]
- Refer to classes or other therapies as indicated. *Provides additional information as needed.*
- Identify an available 12-step or other support/recovery program when indicated *to provide tools to deal with enabling or codependent behaviors that impair level of function. Provides a more structured environment to learn how to deal with problems of caregiving situation.*[1]
- Refer to counseling or psychotherapy as needed. *Intensive treatment may be needed in highly stressful situations.*
- Provide bibliotherapy of appropriate references and Web sites for self-paced learning and updated information and contact with other caregivers. *Further information can help individuals understand what is happening and manage more effectively.*[9]

DOCUMENTATION FOCUS

Assessment/Reassessment
- Assessment findings, functional level and degree of impairment, caregiver's understanding and perception of situation.
- Identified risk factors.

Planning
- Plan of care and individual responsibility for specific activities.
- Identification of inner resources, behavior or lifestyle changes to be made.
- Needed resources, including type and source of assistive devices and durable equipment.
- Teaching plan.

Implementation/Evaluation
- Caregiver's/receiver's response to interventions, teaching, and actions performed.
- Attainment or progress toward desired outcome(s).
- Modifications to plan of care.

Discharge Planning
- Plan for continuation or follow-through of needed changes.
- Referrals for assistance and evaluation.

References

1. Townsend, M. C. (2011). *Psychiatric Mental Health Nursing: Concepts of Care in Evidence-Based Practice.* 7th ed. Philadelphia: F. A. Davis.

2. Peters, M., et al. (2012). The impact of perceived lack of support provided by health and social care services to caregivers of people with motor neuron disease. *Amyotroph Lateral Scler,* 13(2), 223–228.

 Acute Care   Collaborative   Community/Home Care   Cultural

3. Harris, S. M., et al. (2011). A caregiver perspective of how Alzheimer's disease and related disorders affect couple intimacy. *Aging Ment Health*, 15(8), 950–960.

4. Newfield, S. A., et al. (2007). *Cox's Clinical Applications of Nursing Diagnosis: Adult, Child, Women's, Psychiatric, Geron- tic, and Home Health Considerations*. 5th ed. Philadelphia: F. A. Davis.

5. Purnell, L. D., Paulanka, B. J. (2008). *Transcultural Health Care—A Culturally Competent Approach*. 3rd ed. Philadelphia: F. A. Davis.

6. Lohve, V., Miaskowski, C., Rusteen, T. (2011). The relation- ship between hope and caregiver strain in family caregivers of parents with advanced cancer. *Cancer Nurs*, 35(2), 99–105.

7. Hareven, T. K. (ed.) (1995). *Aging and Generational Relations over the Life Course: A Historical and Cross-Cultural Perspec- tive*. New York: Walter De Gruyter.

8. Liken, M. A. (2001). Caregivers in crisis: Moving a relative with Alzheimer's to assisted living. *Clin Nurs Res*, 10(1), 53–69.

9. Liken, M. A. (2001). Experiences of family caregivers of a rela- tive with Alzheimer's disease. *J Psychosoc Nurs*, 39(12), 32–37.

10. Schumacher, K., Beck, C. A., Marren, J. M. (2006). Family caregivers: Caring for older adults, working with their families. *Am J Nurs*, 106(8), 40–49.

11. Weiss, B. (2005). When a family member requires your care. *RN*, 68(4), 63–65.

12. Raina, P., et al. (2005). The health and well-being of caregivers of children with cerebral palsy. *Pediatrics*, 115(6), e626–e636.

13. Spurlock, W. R. (2005). Spiritual well-being and caregiver bur- den in Alzheimer's caregivers. *Geriatr Nurs*, 26(3), 154–161.

14. Haigler, D. H., Bauer, L. J., Travis, S. S. (2006). "Caring for you, caring for me": A ten-year caregiver educational initia- tive of the Rosalynn Carter Institute for Human Development. *Health Soc Work*, 31(2), 149–152.

15. Beckerman, J. (Updated 2016). *Heart failure and caregiver burnout*. Retrieved April 2018 from http://www.webmd.com/ heart-disease/heart-failure/heart-failure-recognizing-burnout- caregiver.

16. Boyles, S. (2005). *Spouse caregivers most likely to be abusive*. Retrieved April 2018 from http://www.webmd.com/balance/ news/20050211/spouse-caregivers-most-likely-to-be-abusive.

17. Given, C. W., et al. (1992). The caregiver reaction assessment (CRA) for caregivers to persons with chronic physical and mental impairments. *Res Nurs Health*, 15, 271–283.

18. Zarit, S. H., Todd, P. A., Zarit, J. M. (1986). Subjective burden of husbands and wives as caregivers: A longitudinal study. *Gerontologist*, 26, 260–266.

risk for caregiver Role Strain

Taxonomy II: Role Relationships—Class 1 Caregiving Roles (00062) **[Diagnostic Division:** Social Interaction], Approved 1992; Revised 2010, 2013, 2017

DEFINITION: Susceptible to difficulty in fulfilling care responsibilities, expectations and/or behaviors for family or significant others, which may compromise health.

RISK FACTORS
Care Receiver
Dependency; problematic behavior; substance misuse/[abuse]
Discharged home with significant needs; increase in care needs
Unpredictability of illness trajectory; unstable health condition
Caregiver
Physical conditions; not developmentally ready for caregiver role
Competing role commitments; insufficient fulfillment of self or others' expectations
Ineffective coping strategies; insufficient energy, privacy, or recreation
Inexperience with caregiving; insufficient knowledge about community resources
Stressors; substance misuse/[abuse]
Unrealistic self-expectations; insufficient emotional resilience; isolation
Caregiver–Care Receiver Relationship
Abusive or violent relationship; presence of abuse
Pattern of ineffective relationships; codependency
Unrealistic care receiver expectations
Caregiving Activities
Around-the-clock care responsibilities; insufficient time; change in nature or complexity of care activities
Excessive caregiving activities; extended duration of caregiving required
Inadequate physical environment or insufficient equipment for providing care; insufficient assistance or respite for caregiver

(continues on page 734)

 Diagnostic Studies   Evidence Based Practice   Medications   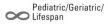 Pediatric/Geriatric/ Lifespan

risk for caregiver Role Strain (continued)

Recent discharge home with significant care needs; unpredictably of care situation

Family Processes

Family isolation; ineffective family adaptation; pattern of ineffective family coping

Pattern of family dysfunction; pattern of family dysfunction prior to the caregiving situation

Socioeconomic

Alienation or social isolation

Difficulty accessing assistance or support

Difficulty accessing/insufficient community resources

Insufficient transportation

At Risk Population: Care receiver's condition inhibits conversation

Developmental delay of caregiver or care receiver; prematurity

Female caregiver; partner of caregiver

Exposure to violence

Associated Condition: *Care Receiver*

Alteration in cognitive functioning; psychiatric or psychological disorder

Chronic illness; illness severity

Congenital disorder

Caregiver

Alteration in cognitive functioning; psychological disorder

Health impairment

[Note: The presence of this problem may encompass other numerous problems/high-risk concerns, such as decreased Diversional Activity Engagement, Insomnia, Fatigue, Anxiety, ineffective Coping, compromised family Coping or disabled family Coping, Decisional Conflict, ineffective Denial, Grieving, Hopelessness, Powerlessness, Spiritual Distress, ineffective Health Maintenance, impaired Home Maintenance, Sexual Dysfunction or ineffective Sexuality Pattern, readiness for enhanced family Coping, interrupted Family Processes, and Social Isolation. Careful attention to data gathering will identify and clarify the client's specific needs, which can then be coordinated under this single diagnostic label.]

Sample Clinical Applications: Chronic conditions (e.g., severe brain injury, spinal cord injury [SCI], severe developmental delay), progressive debilitating conditions (e.g., muscular dystrophy, multiple sclerosis [MS], dementia/Alzheimer's disease, end-stage chronic obstructive pulmonary disease [COPD], renal failure, renal dialysis), substance abuse, end-of-life care, psychiatric conditions (e.g., schizophrenia, personality disorders)

DESIRED OUTCOMES/EVALUATION CRITERIA

Sample NOC linkages:

Caregiver Home Care Readiness: Preparedness of a caregiver to assume responsibility for the healthcare of a family member in the home

Caregiver Stressors: Severity of biopsychosocial pressure on a family care provider caring for another over an extended period of time

Family Resiliency: Capacity of a family to positively adapt and function following a significant adversity or crisis

Caregiver Will (Include Specific Time Frame)

• Identify individual risk factors and appropriate interventions.

• Demonstrate or initiate behaviors or lifestyle changes to prevent development of impaired function.

• Use available resources appropriately.

• Report satisfaction with current situation.

 Acute Care Collaborative Community/ Home Care Cultural

ACTIONS/INTERVENTIONS

Sample **NIC** linkages:

Caregiver Support: Provision of the necessary information, advocacy, and support to facilitate primary patient care by someone other than a healthcare professional

Family Support: Promotion of family values, interests, and goals

Parenting Promotion: Providing parenting information, support, and coordination of comprehensive services to high-risk families

NURSING PRIORITY NO. 1 To assess factors affecting current situation:

- ∞ Note presence of high-risk situations (e.g., elderly client with total self-care dependence; having several small children, with one child requiring extensive assistance due to physical condition or developmental delays). *May necessitate role reversal resulting in added stress or places excessive demands on parenting skills. Identification of high-risk situations can help in planning and resolving problems before they can become unmanageable.*[4]

- Identify relationship and proximity of caregiver to care receiver (e.g., spouse/lover, parent/child, friend). *There is added stress in maintaining own life and responsibilities when caregiver has to travel some distance to provide care.*[11] *Close relationships may create problems of codependency and identification that can be counterproductive to caregiving. Note: A 2015 study by the National Alliance for Caregiving (NAC) reports "there are 43.5 million informal, unpaid caregivers in the United States. Over half (60%) are female and around 49 years old, although one in 10 are 75 years of age or older, and are caregiving without any additional unpaid help. The majority (34.2 million) provide care on average of 24.4 hours a week, 60% of caregivers have to cut back their work hours or take a leave of absence, and 42% of all caregivers perform care without any training or preparation."*[7] *Younger-aged family caregivers are at increased risk for lower levels of hope and higher levels of caregiver strain.*[2]

- Determine current knowledge of the situation, noting misconceptions and lack of information. *May interfere with caregiver/care receiver's response to situation.*

- Compare caregiver's and receiver's views of situation. *Different views need to be openly expressed so each person understands how other sees situation.*[1,3]

- Note complexity of therapeutic regimen and physical and mental status of care receiver to ascertain potential areas of need (e.g., teaching, direct care support, respite). *Knowledge of these factors is necessary for planning adequate care for the individual. Plans for additional help may be necessary to prevent caregiver role strain.*[1]

- Determine caregiver's level of responsibility, involvement in care, and anticipated length of care. *Information that may indicate level of stress that could be anticipated for the situation. Progressive debilitation taxes caregiver and may alter ability to meet client's and own needs.*[4]

- Identify individual cultural factors and impact on caregiver. *Helps clarify expectations of caregiver/receiver, family, and community. Many cultures, such as Native American and Cuban, believe strongly in keeping care receiver in the home and caring for them.*[5]

- Ascertain caregiver's physical and emotional health, developmental level and abilities, and additional responsibilities of caregiver (e.g., job, raising family). *Provides information indicative of ability of the individual to take on the task of caregiver, as well as clues to potential stressors and possible supportive interventions.*[11,12]

- Assess caregiver as appropriate, using tool such as Burden Interview, Herth Hope Index, Caregiver Reaction Assessment, or Caregiver Strain Index (not a comprehensive list) *to further determine caregiver's stressors and abilities providing additional information to aid in planning.*[6,7,9]

- Identify strengths and weaknesses of caregiver and care receiver. *Caregiver may not be aware of demands that will be expected. Knowing these factors helps to determine how to use them to advantage in planning and delivering care.*[9]

 Diagnostic Studies   Evidence Based Practice   Medications   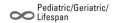 Pediatric/Geriatric/ Lifespan

- Note any codependency needs of caregiver and plan for dealing appropriately with them. *Can contribute to burnout unless identified and dealt with.*[15]
- Verify safety of caregiver/receiver. *Identifying and correcting unsafe situations is crucial so both individuals can be assured of safety in dealing with difficult situation.*[1,9]
- Determine available supports and resources currently used. *Helpful to identify if they are being used effectively.*[4]

NURSING PRIORITY NO. 2 To enhance caregiver's ability to deal with current situation:

- Establish a therapeutic relationship, conveying empathy and unconditional positive regard. *Promotes positive environment in which needs and concerns can be discussed and proactive solutions identified.*
- Discuss strategies to coordinate care and other responsibilities (e.g., employment, care of children/dependents, housekeeping activities). *Such planning can prevent chaos and resultant burnout.*[8]
- Facilitate family conference as appropriate to share information and develop plan for involvement in care activities. *When everyone is involved and listened to, each person is more likely to carry out his or her responsibilities.*[4]
- Refer to classes and/or specialists (e.g., first-aid and cardiopulmonary resuscitation classes, enterostomal specialist, physical therapist) for special training as indicated. *Additional information that can help individuals involved feel more competent and able to deal with situation more effectively.*[3]
- Identify additional resources, including financial, legal, and respite care. *Can help to resolve problems that arise in the course of caregiving that are outside of the knowledge or abilities of the individual. Solving these issues can relieve caregiver of associated anxiety and concern.*[1]
- Identify equipment needs and resources, and appropriate adaptive aids. *Enhances the independence and safety of the care receiver and reduces chances for untoward incidents.*[14]
- Identify contact person or case manager as needed to coordinate care, provide support, and assist with problem-solving. *Assistance with planning minimizes problems that could arise.*[10]
- Provide information or demonstrate techniques for dealing with acting out, violent, or disoriented behavior. *Planning ways to deal with these behaviors before they occur promotes safety and enhances positive outcomes.*[4]
- Assist caregiver to recognize codependent behaviors (i.e., doing things for others that others are able to do for themselves) and how these behaviors affect the situation. *Provides options for changing behaviors in ways that enhance the caregiving situation.*[15]

NURSING PRIORITY NO. 3 To promote wellness (Teaching/Discharge Considerations):

- Review signs of burnout (e.g., emotional or physical exhaustion, changes in appetite and sleep, withdrawal from friends/family or life interests). Note: In the NAC (2015) study, it was reported that 38% of caregivers relay high emotional stress, whereas 19% report high physical stress; 18% report high to very high financial stain. All of these needs, especially physical stress, are closely related to the complexity of the situation, such as number of hours of caregiving, caregiver age, and needs of the care recipient. *Recognition of developing problem allows for timely intervention.*[7,13]
- Discuss and demonstrate stress management techniques and importance of self-nurturing (e.g., meeting personal needs, pursuing self-development interests, hobbies, social activities, spiritual enrichment). *Improves or maintains quality of life for caregiver and may provide caregiver with options to protect self.*[6,13,14]
- Encourage involvement in caregiver or other specific support group(s). *Opportunity to be with others in similar situations and discussing different ways to handle problems help caregiver deal with difficult role in positive ways.*[1]
- Provide bibliotherapy of appropriate references and Web sites and encourage discussion of information. *Promotes retention of new information that can help caregiver manage more effectively.*[1]
- Advocate for and assist caregiver to plan for and implement changes that may become helpful or necessary for the care receiver. *Getting information and thinking about possibilities will help with decision making. These may include transportation, meal delivery, home healthcare services, home modification, and legal and financial counseling, as well as eventual placement in a long-term care facility and use of palliative or hospice*

 Acute Care   Collaborative   Community/Home Care   Cultural

services. As caregiving tasks at home become more difficult, other options need to be considered, and planning ahead can promote acceptance of necessary changes.[8,12,13]
- Identify an available 12-step/other recovery or support program when indicated to provide tools *to deal with codependent behaviors that impair level of function. Provides a more structured environment to learn how to deal with problems of caregiving situation in positive ways.*[3]
- Refer to counseling or psychotherapy as needed. *May need additional help to resolve issues that are interfering with caregiving responsibilities.*

DOCUMENTATION FOCUS

Assessment/Reassessment
- Identified risk factors and caregiver perceptions of situation.
- Reactions of care receiver/family.

Planning
- Treatment plan and individual responsibility for specific activities.
- Teaching plan.

Implementation/Evaluation
- Caregiver/receiver response to interventions, teaching, and actions performed.
- Attainment or progress toward desired outcome(s).
- Modifications to plan of care.

Discharge Planning
- Long-term needs and who is responsible for actions to be taken.
- Specific referrals provided for assistance and evaluation.

References

1. National Center on Elder Abuse. (2002). Preventing elder abuse by family caregivers. Retrieved April 2018 from https://ncea.acl.gov/resources/docs/archive/Preventing-EA-Family-Caregivers-Tech-2002.pdf.
2. Lohve, V., Miaskowski, C., Rusteen, T. (2011). The relationship between hope and caregiver strain in family caregivers of parents with advanced cancer. *Cancer Nurs*, 35(2), 99–105.
3. Townsend, M. C. (2011). *Psychiatric Mental Health Nursing: Concepts of Care in Evidence-Based Practice*. 6th ed. Philadelphia: F. A. Davis.
4. Newfield, S. A., et al. (2007). *Cox's Clinical Applications of Nursing Diagnosis: Adult, Child, Women's, Psychiatric, Gerontic, and Home Health Considerations*. 5th ed. Philadelphia: F. A. Davis.
5. Purnell, L. D., Paulanka, B. J. (2008). *Transcultural Health Care—A Culturally Competent Approach*. 3rd ed. Philadelphia: F. A. Davis.
6. Family Caregiver Alliance, Benjamin Rose Institute on Aging, & The Margaret Blenkner Research Institute. (2012). Selected Caregiver Assessment Measures: A Resource Inventory for Practitioners. 2nd ed. San Francisco, CA: Family Caregiver Alliance.
7. Grebeldinger, T .A., Buckley, K. M. (2016). You are not alone: Parish nurses bridge challenges for family caregivers. *J Christ Nurs*, 33(1), 50–56.
8. Liken, M. A. (2001). Caregivers in crisis: Moving a relative with Alzheimer's to assisted living. *Clin Nurs Res*, 10(1), 53–69.
9. Liken, M. A. (2001). (Not) a Hallmark holiday: Experiences of family caregivers of a relative with Alzheimer's disease. *J Psychosoc Nurs Ment Health Serv*, 39(12), 33–37.
10. Halper, J., Harris, C. J. (2003). *Multiple Sclerosis: Best Practices in Nursing Care*. Hackensack, NJ: International Organization of Multiple Sclerosis Nursing.
11. Schumacher, K., Beck, C. A., Marren, J. M. (2006). Family caregivers: Caring for older adults, working with their families. *Am J Nurs*, 106(8), 40–49.
12. Weiss, B. (2005). When a family member requires your care. *RN*, 68(4), 63–65.
13. Beckerman, J. (Updated 2016). *Heart failure and caregiver burnout*. Retrieved April 2018 from http://www.webmd.com/heart-disease/heart-failure/heart-failure-recognizing-burnout-caregiver.
14. Link, G., Hepburn, K. (2012, updated 2015). *Caregiver stress fact sheet*. Retrieved April 2018 from http://www.womenshealth.gov/publications/our-publications/fact-sheet/caregiver-stress.html?from=AtoZ.
15. O'Regan, M. K. (2007). *When caring becomes caretaking*. Retrieved April 2018 from http://ezinearticles.com/?When-Caring-Becomes-Caretaking&id=774141.

 Diagnostic Studies Evidence Based Practice Medications 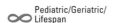 Pediatric/Geriatric/Lifespan

Self-Care Deficit: bathing, dressing, feeding, toileting

Taxonomy II: Activity/Rest—Class 5 Self-Care (Bathing 00108, Dressing 00109, Feeding 00102, Toileting 00110) [**Diagnostic Division:** Hygiene], Approved 1980; Nursing Diagnosis Extension and Classification Revision 1998, Bathing/Dressing/Toileting 2008; 2017

DEFINITION: Inability to independently perform or complete cleansing activities; put on or remove clothing; to eat; or to perform tasks associated with bowel and bladder elimination.

[Note: Self-Care also may be expanded to include the practices used by the client to promote health, the individual responsibility for self, and a way of thinking. Refer to NDs ineffective Health Maintenance and impaired Home Maintenance.]

RELATED FACTORS

Anxiety; decrease in motivation

Pain; weakness

Environmental barrier [mechanical restrictions such as cast, splint, traction, ventilator]

Impaired mobility; impaired ability to transfer

[Inability to perceive body part or spatial relationship]

DEFINING CHARACTERISTICS

Bathing Self-Care deficit

Impaired ability to: access bathroom [tub], gather bathing supplies, access water, regulate bathwater, wash or dry body

Dressing Self-Care deficit

Impaired ability to: choose clothing, gather clothing, pick up clothing, put clothing on upper or lower body, fasten clothing

Impaired ability to: put on/remove various items of clothing

Impaired ability to: use zipper or assistive device, maintain appearance

Feeding Self-Care deficit

Impaired ability to: prepare food, open containers

Impaired ability to: handle utensils, get food onto utensil, bring food to the mouth, use assistive device, pick up cup

Impaired ability to: manipulate food in mouth, chew food, swallow food or swallow sufficient amount of food, self-feed a complete meal or in an acceptable manner

Toileting Self-Care deficit

Impaired ability to: reach toilet, manipulate clothing for toileting, sit on or rise from toilet, complete toilet hygiene, flush toilet

Associated Condition: Alteration in cognitive functioning

Impaired ability to perceive body part or to spacial relationships; perceptual disorders

Neuromuscular; musculoskeletal impairment

Sample Clinical Applications: Arthritis, neuromuscular impairment (e.g., multiple sclerosis [MS], brain injury, stroke, Parkinson's disease, spinal cord injury [SCI]), chronic pain, chronic fatigue syndrome [CFS], depression, dementia, autism, developmental delay, end-of-life/hospice care

DESIRED OUTCOMES/EVALUATION CRITERIA

Sample **NOC** linkages:

Self-Care Status: Personal actions to perform basic personal care activities and instrumental activities of daily living

Self-Care: Bathing: Personal actions to cleanse own body independently with or without assistive device

 Acute Care Collaborative Community/Home Care Cultural

Self-Care: Dressing: Personal actions to dress self independently with or without assistive device
Self-Care: Eating: Personal actions to prepare and ingest food and fluid independently with or without assistive device
Self-Care: Toileting: Personal actions to toilet self independently with or without assistive device

Client Will (Include Specific Time Frame)
- Identify individual areas of weakness and needs.
- Verbalize knowledge of healthcare practices.
- Demonstrate techniques or lifestyle changes to meet self-care needs.
- Perform self-care activities within level of own ability.
- Identify personal and community resources that can provide assistance.

ACTIONS/INTERVENTIONS

Sample **NIC** linkages:
Self-Care Assistance: Assisting another to perform activities of daily living
Bathing: Cleaning of the body for the purposes of relaxation, cleanliness, and healing
Dressing: Choosing, putting on, and removing clothes for a person who cannot do this for self
Feeding: Providing nutritional intake for patient who is unable to feed self
Bowel [or] Urinary Elimination Management: Establishment and maintenance of a regular pattern of bowel elimination/maintenance of an optimum urinary elimination pattern

NURSING PRIORITY NO. 1   To identify causative/contributing factors:

- ∞ Determine age or developmental issues and existing conditions (e.g., heart or renal failure, SCI, malnutrition, pain, trauma, surgery) and cognitive or psychological factors (e.g., mental illness, brain injury, cerebrovascular accident, MS, Alzheimer's disease) affecting ability of individual to care for own needs. *Assists in setting realistic goals and creates baseline for evaluating effectiveness of interventions.*[1,8]
- Identify other etiological factors present, including language barriers, speech impairment, visual acuity, loss of visual or spatial orientation, hearing problem, and emotional instability or lability *that can both affect and be affected by self-care needs and deficits.* Refer to NDs impaired verbal Communication, Unilateral Neglect, and [disturbed Sensory Perception (specify)] for related interventions.
- 🥄 Review medication regimen *for possible effects on alertness and mentation, energy level, balance, and perception. Note: All prescribed and over-the-counter medications have the potential for side effects, adverse effects, and interactions that may be harmful to the client or affect client's ability to provide self-care.*
- Assess barriers to participation in regimen *that can limit use of resources or choice of options (e.g., lack of information, insufficient time for discussion, psychological or intimate family problems that may be difficult to share, fear of appearing stupid or ignorant, social or economic limitations, work or home environment problems).*

NURSING PRIORITY NO. 2   To assess degree of disability:

- Identify degree of individual impairment and functional level according to a functional scale as below:[16]
  0—Completely independent
  1—Requires use of equipment or device
  2—Requires help from another person for assistance, supervision, or teaching
  3—Requires help from another person and equipment device
  4—Dependent, does not participate in activity
- *Note: Many instruments have been developed to assess client's functional status. In the community healthcare setting, a more complex assessment may be used (e.g., Lawton and Brody's scale of Instrumental Activities of*

 Diagnostic Studies   Evidence Based Practice   Medications   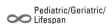 Pediatric/Geriatric/Lifespan

Daily Living) to determine client's self-care abilities (e.g., to communicate by phone, drive, cook, shop, balance a checkbook, manage multiple medical appointments or medications, etc.). In an acute or long-term care setting, the assessment may be confined to personal care (e.g., Katz Activities of Daily Living Scale). These instruments are used (1) to determine client's safety issues and care needs upon admission and (2) to ascertain changes in functional abilities and quality of life as a result of client's condition and treatment.[15,17]

- Note anticipated duration of disruption and intensity of care required. *A wide variety of factors can impact self-care, some of which may be (1) invariable or permanent (e.g., quadriplegia or advanced dementia), (2) temporary (e.g., fractures requiring immobilization, mild stroke with potential for good recovery), and (3) variable (e.g., person having episode of severe depression or episodes of relapsing-remitting type MS).*
- Assess cognitive functioning (e.g., memory, intelligence, concentration, ability to attend to task) *to determine client's ability to participate in care and potential to return to normal functioning or to learn/relearn tasks.*
- Determine individual strengths and skills of the client *to incorporate into plan of care, enhancing likelihood of achieving outcomes.*

NURSING PRIORITY NO. 3   To assist in correcting/dealing with deficit(s) **in general**:

- Collaborate in treatment of underlying conditions *to enhance client's capabilities and maximize rehabilitation potential.*
- Promote communication among all those involved in caring for or assisting the client. *Enhances coordination and continuity of care.*
- Active-listen client's/significant other's (SO's) concerns. *Exhibits regard for client's values and beliefs, clarifies barriers to participation in self-care, provides opportunity to work on problem-solving solutions, and provides encouragement and support.[8,10]*
- Provide accurate and relevant information regarding current and future needs *so that client can incorporate into self-care plans while minimizing problems (e.g., heightened anxiety, depression, resistance) often associated with change.[9]*
- Promote client/SO participation in problem identification and desired outcomes. *Can ease frustration of current loss of independence, enhancing recovery, optimizing outcomes, and supporting health promotion.[10]*
- Establish "contractual" partnership with client/SO(s) if appropriate or indicated for motivation or behavioral modification.
- Practice and promote short-term goal setting and achievement *to recognize that today's success is as important as any long-term goal, accept ability to do one thing at a time, and conceptualize self-care in a broader sense.*
- ∞ Instruct in or review appropriate skills necessary for self-care, using terms understandable to client (e.g., child, adult, cognitively impaired person) and with sensitivity to developmental needs for practice, repetition, or reluctance. *Individualized teaching best affords reinforcement of learning. Sensitivity to special needs attaches value to the client's needs.[1]*
- Encourage client to use vision and hearing aids as appropriate. *Improves reception and interpretation of sensory input to facilitate self-care.*
- Perform or assist with meeting client's needs when he or she is unable to meet own needs *(e.g., personal care assistance is part of nursing care and should not be neglected while promoting and integrating self-care independence).*
- Anticipate needs and begin with familiar, easily accomplished tasks *to encourage client and build on successes.*
- Cue client, as indicated. *A cognitively impaired or forgetful client can often successfully participate in many activities with cueing, which can enhance self-esteem and potentiate learning or relearning of self-care tasks.[1]*
- Maintain a supportive attitude and allow sufficient time for client *to accomplish tasks to fullest extent of ability.*
- Refrain from unnecessary conversation or interruptions *that divert focus from the task at hand and can contribute to client's level of frustration.*
- Avoid doing things for client that client can do for self, but provide assistance as needed. *Client may be fearful or dependent, and although assistance is helpful in preventing frustration (and sometimes easier for the caregivers in terms of their time), it is important for client to do as much as possible for self to regain or maintain self-esteem, reduce helplessness, and promote optimal recovery.*

 Acute Care   Collaborative   Community/ Home Care   Cultural

- Review coping skills (e.g., assertiveness, interpersonal relations, decision making, problem-solving, stigma management, time management) *that are useful in managing a wide range of stressful conditions.* Encourage client to ask for assistance as needed or desired.[9]
- Schedule activities *to conform to client's preferred schedule as much as possible (e.g., bathing at a relaxing time for client, rather than on a set routine).*
- Plan activities to prevent or accommodate fatigue and/or exacerbation of pain *to conserve energy and promote maximum participation in self-care.*
- Identify energy-saving behaviors *(e.g., sitting instead of standing when possible, organizing needs before beginning tasks).* Refer to NDs Activity Intolerance and Fatigue for additional interventions.
- Review medication needs (e.g., vitamins, nutritional supplements, pain reliever, antidepressants) *that may improve general well-being and ability to participate in self-care.*
- Arrange for home visit, as indicated, *to assess environmental concerns that can impact client's abilities to care for self in home. If necessary modifications are not feasible or cannot be made, client may require temporary or long-term relocation or regular home-care assistance.*
- Consult with rehabilitation professionals to identify and obtain assistive devices (e.g., modified eating utensils, modified clothing), mobility aids (e.g., rolling commode, shower chair), and home modification as necessary (e.g., adequate lighting; cutout under kitchen and bathroom sink; lowering cabinets and closet rods; handheld shower, raised toilet seat, grab bars for bathroom) *to optimize self-care efforts.*[1,8,10]
- Note availability and use of resources and supportive person(s) *to ascertain that client has means for sharing common concerns, needs, and wishes, as well as access to social support and approval (e.g., support group participants, family members, professionals).*[9]

NURSING PRIORITY NO. 4 To meet specific self-care needs:

Bathing deficit
- Ask client/SO for input on bathing habits or cultural bathing preferences. *Creates opportunities for client to (1) keep long-standing routines (e.g., bathing at bedtime to improve sleep) and (2) exercise control over situation. This enhances self-esteem, while respecting personal and cultural preferences.*[3]
- Bathe or assist client in bathing, providing for any or all hygiene needs as indicated. *Type of bath (e.g., bed bath, towel bath, tub bath, shower) and purpose (e.g., cleansing, removing odor, simply soothing agitation) is determined by individual need. Note: Bathing is a healing rite and should be a comforting experience that focuses on the client's needs, rather than being a routinely scheduled task.*[11]
- Obtain hygiene supplies (e.g., soap, toothpaste, toothbrush, mouthwash, lotion, shampoo, razor, towels) for specific activity to be performed and place in client's easy reach *to provide visual cues and facilitate completion of activity.*
- Ascertain that all safety equipment is in place and properly installed (e.g., grab bars, antislip strips, shower chair, hydraulic lift) and that client/caregiver(s) can safely operate equipment *to prevent injury to client and caregivers.*[4]
- Instruct client to request assistance when needed and place call device within easy reach *so client can summon help if bathing alone* or stay with client *as dictated by safety needs.*
- Provide for adequate warmth (e.g., covering client during bed bath or warming bathroom). *Certain individuals (especially infants, the elderly, very thin or debilitated persons) are prone to hypothermia and can experience evaporative cooling during and after bathing.*[5]
- Determine that client can perceive water temperature and adjust water temperature safely or that water is correct temperature for client's bath or shower *to prevent chilling or burns. This step requires that client is cognitively and physically able to perceive hot and cold and to adjust faucets safely; otherwise, adequate supervision must be provided at all times.*[5]
- Assist client in and out of shower or tub as indicated. *Needs are variable (e.g., client may need to get into tub before running water, may require a shower chair, may be independent with one fixture and not another), requiring assessment of individual situations.*

 Diagnostic Studies   Evidence Based Practice   Medications   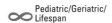 Pediatric/Geriatric/Lifespan

- Assist with or cue client to complete hygiene steps (e.g., oral care, lotion application, applying deodorant, washing and styling hair). *These steps may be completed at same or different time as bathing, but are usually part of a regular routine that is necessary for client's physical well-being and emotional or social comfort.*

Dressing deficit

- Ascertain that appropriate clothing is available. *Client may not have sufficient clothing, clothing may be inadequate for situation or weather conditions, or clothing may need to be modified for client's particular medical condition or physical limitations.*
- Assist client in choosing clothing or lay out clothing as indicated. *May be needed when client has cognitive, physical, or psychiatric conditions affecting ability to choose appropriate pieces of clothing or to maintain a satisfactory appearance.*[1]
- Dress client or assist with dressing, as indicated. *Client may need assistance in putting on or taking off items of clothing (e.g., shoes and socks, over-the-head shirt) or may require partial or complete assistance with fasteners (e.g., buttons, snaps, zippers, shoelaces).*
- Allow sufficient time for dressing and undressing *because tasks may be tiring, painful, and difficult to complete. Dressing may be done from seated position if balance is impaired.*
- Use adaptive clothing as indicated (e.g., clothing with front closure, wide sleeves and pant legs, Velcro or zipper closures). *These may be helpful for client with limited arm or leg movement or impaired fine motor skills or for cognitively impaired person who desires to dress self but cannot do so with regular clothing fasteners.*[12]
- Teach client to dress affected side first and then unaffected side (when client has paralysis or injury to one side of body) *to allow for easier manipulation of clothing.*[12]

Feeding deficit

- Assess client's need and ability to prepare and eat food as indicated (including shopping, cooking, cutting food, opening containers, managing environment, etc.). *Identifies specific assistance required.*[1,2,13,17]
- Assess for and alleviate pain where possible *to improve client's desire for food, and ability to eat/manage necessary tasks for food preparation and eating*
- Have client sitting upright (out of bed at table) as much as possible *Improves posture for eating and better digestion, and promotes idea that eating is a social activity*
- Arrange tray/table place setting to facilitate self-feeding (e.g., rearrange items for easy access; remove plate and cup covers; unwrap utensils; open packets; cut up food; butter bread. *to reduce client's frustration or apathy, and to promote ease of accessing food*
- Encourage food and fluid choices reflecting individual likes and abilities and that meet nutritional needs *to maximize food intake.*
- Ascertain that client can swallow safely, checking gag and swallow reflexes, as indicated. Refer to ND impaired Swallowing for related interventions.
- Provide food and fluid of appropriate consistency *to facilitate swallowing.* Cut food into bite-size pieces *to prevent overfilling mouth and reduce risk of choking.*
- Assist client to handle utensils or in guiding utensils to mouth. *May require specialized equipment (e.g., rocker knife, plate guard, built-up handles) to increase independence or assistance with movement of arms and hands.* Provide nutritious finger foods where possible, if the client wants to feed self but experiences difficulty managing utensils
- Assist client with small cup, glass, or bottle for liquids, using straw or adaptive lids as indicated, *to enhance fluid intake while reducing spills.*
- Allow client time for intake of sufficient food *for feeling satisfied or completing a meal.*
- Use verbal cueing and prompting (e.g., "pick up your spoon," "take a bite," "chew," "swallow"), where indicated. *May improve client's efforts when distraction, depression, or cognitive issues are interfering.*
- Remove distractions (e.g., turn off TV, avoid interruptions such as people entering or leaving the area where possible) *when manners might be offensive to others or client could be embarrassed.*
- Assist client with social graces when eating with others; provide privacy *when manners might be offensive to others or client could be embarrassed.*

 Acute Care   Collaborative   Community/ Home Care   Cultural

- Collaborate with nutritionist, speech-language pathologist, occupational therapist, or physician *for special diets, adaptive equipment, or feeding methods necessary to improve nutrition.*
- Feed client, allowing adequate time for chewing and swallowing, *when client is not able to obtain nutrition by self-feeding.* Avoid providing fluids until client has swallowed food and mouth is clear. *Prevents "washing down" foods, reducing risk of choking.*

Toileting deficit

- Provide mobility assistance to bathroom or commode or place on bedpan or offer urinal, as indicated. *Client might be impaired because of age, cognitive problems, weakness, or acute injury or illness, requiring a range of interventions from complete care to help with walking.*
- Direct or accompany cognitively impaired client to bathroom, as needed. *May need directions to the facilities or reminders to use the bathroom, etc.*[6]
- Observe for behaviors such as pacing, fidgeting, and holding crotch *that may be indicative of need for prompt toileting.*
- Provide privacy *to enhance self-esteem and improve ability to urinate or defecate.*[1]
- Assist with manipulation of clothing if needed, *to decrease incidence of functional incontinence caused by difficulty removing clothing/underwear.*[7]
- Observe need for and assist in obtaining modified clothing or fasteners *to assist client in manipulation of clothing, fostering independence in self-toileting.*
- Provide or assist with use of assistive equipment (e.g., raised toilet seat, support rails, spill-proof urinals, fracture pans, bedside commode) *to promote independence and safety in sitting down or arising from toilet or for aiding elimination when client unable to go to bathroom.*[14]
- Keep toilet paper or wipes and hand-washing items within client's easy reach *to enhance self-cleansing efforts.*
- Implement bowel or bladder training/retraining programs as indicated. *This may include developing a schedule for toileting and other interventions as seen in NDs bowel Incontinence, Constipation, urinary Incontinence [specify], and impaired Urinary Elimination.*

NURSING PRIORITY NO. 5 To promote optimal independence (Teaching/Discharge Considerations):

- Assist the client to become aware of rights and responsibilities in health and healthcare and to assess own health strengths—physical, emotional, and intellectual.
- Support client in making health-related decisions and assist in developing self-care practices and goals that promote health.
- Instruct in relaxation techniques (e.g., deep breathing, meditation, music, yoga) *to reduce frustration and enhance coping.*
- Provide for ongoing evaluation of self-care program *to note progress and identify changes in needs.*
- Modify program periodically *to accommodate changes in client's abilities. Assists client to adhere to plan of care to fullest extent.*
- Encourage keeping a journal *to note progress and identify factors affecting ability to perform self-care activities and to foster self-care and self-determination.*[9]
- Review safety concerns. Modify activities and environment *to reduce risk of injury and promote successful community functioning.*
- Refer to home-care provider, social services, physical or occupational therapy, speech-language pathologist, and rehabilitation and counseling resources as indicated.
- Arrange consult with community resources (e.g., Meals on Wheels, home care or visiting nurse service, senior services, nutritionist) *to provide long-term support and additional forms of assistance that may improve client's independence and self-care.*[1]
- Review instructions from other members of the healthcare team and provide written copy. *Provides clarification and reinforcement and opportunities for periodic review by client/caregivers.*
- Discuss respite or other care options with family. *Allows them free time away from the care situation to renew themselves and enhances coping abilities.* Refer to ND Caregiver Role Strain for related interventions.

 Diagnostic Studies   Evidence Based Practice   Medications   Pediatric/Geriatric/Lifespan

- Assist or support family with alternative placements as necessary. *Enhances likelihood of finding individually appropriate situation to meet client's needs.*
- Be available for discussion of feelings (e.g., grieving, anger, frustration). *Provides opportunity for client/family to get feelings out in the open, realize the feelings are normal, and begin to problem-solve solutions as indicated.*
- Refer to NDs ineffective Coping, compromised family Coping, risk for Disuse Syndrome, risk for Falls/Injury/Trauma, impaired physical Mobility, Powerlessness, and situational low Self-Esteem, as appropriate.

DOCUMENTATION FOCUS

Assessment/Reassessment
- Individual findings, functional level, and specifics of limitation(s).
- Needed resources and adaptive devices.
- Availability and use of community resources.
- Who is involved in care and provides assistance.

Planning
- Plan of care and who is involved in planning.
- Teaching plan.

Implementation/Evaluation
- Response to interventions, teaching, and actions performed.
- Attainment or progress toward desired outcome(s).
- Modifications of plan of care.

Discharge Planning
- Long-term needs and who is responsible for actions to be taken.
- Type of and source for assistive devices.
- Specific referrals made.

References

1. Newfield, S. A., et al. (2007). ND: Self Care Deficit (feeding, bathing-hygiene, dressing-grooming, toileting). *Cox's Clinical Applications of Nursing Diagnosis: Adult, Child, Women's, Psychiatric, Gerontic, and Home Health Considerations.* 5th ed. Philadelphia: F. A. Davis.
2. Amella, E. J., Lawrence, J. F. (2007). Eating and feeding issues in older adults with dementia: Part II: Interventions. Retrieved April 2018 from https://consultgeri.org/try-this/dementia/issue-d11.2.pdf.
3. Freeman, E. (1997). International perspectives on bathing. *J Gerontol Nurs*, 22(1), 40–44.
4. Schemm, R. L., Gitlin, L. N. (1998). How occupational therapists teach older patients to use bathing and dressing devices in rehabilitation. *Am J Occup Ther*, 52(4), 276–282.
5. Miller, M. (1997). Physically aggressive resident behavior during hygienic care. *J Gerontol Nurs*, 23(5), 24–39.
6. Sloane, P. (1995). Bathing the Alzheimer's patient in long term care: Results and recommendation from three studies. *Am J Alzheimer's Dis*, 10(4), 3–11.
7. Penn, C. (1996). Assessment of urinary incontinence. *J Gerontol Nurs*, 22, 8–19.
8. Baldwin, K. M. (2006). Stroke: It's a knock-out punch. *Nursing Made Incredibly Easy!* 4(2), 10–23.
9. Livneh, H., Antonak, R. F. (2005). Psychosocial adaptation to chronic illness and disability: A primer for counselors. *J Couns Dev*, 83(1), 12–20.
10. Singleton, J. K. (2000). Nurses' perspectives of encouraging client's care-of-self in a short-term rehabilitation unit within a long-term care facility. *Rehab Nurse*, 21(1), 23–30, 35.
11. Rasin, J., Barrick, A. L. (2004). Bathing persons with dementia. *Am J Nurs*, 104(3), 30–34.
12. Swann, J. (2008). Managing dressing problems in older adults in long-term care. *Nurs Resident Care*, 10(11), 564–567.
13. McCullough, K., et al. (2008). RN compliance with SLP dysphagia recommendations in acute care. *Top Geriatr Rehabil*, 23(4), 330–340.
14. Cohen, D. (2008). Providing an assist. *Rehab Manag*, 21(8), 16–19.
15. Graf, C. (2008). The Lawton Instrumental Activities of Daily Living Scale. *Am J Nurs*, 108(4), 52–62.
16. Gordon, M. (2010). Functional levels code. *Manual of Nursing Diagnosis*. 12th ed. Sudbury, MA: Jones and Bartlett.
17. Jenkins, J. B., McCoy, T. P. (2015). Symptom clusters, functional status, and quality of life in older adults with osteoarthritis. *Orthop Nurs*, 34(1), 36–42.

 Acute Care   Collaborative   Community/Home Care   Cultural

readiness for enhanced Self-Care

Taxonomy II: Activity/Rest—Class 5 Self-Care (00182) [**Diagnostic Division:** Teaching/Learning], Approved 2006; Revised 2013

DEFINITION: A pattern of performing activities for oneself to meet health-related goals, which can be strengthened.

DEFINING CHARACTERISTICS

Subjective
Expresses desire to enhance:
• Independence with life, health, personal development, or well-being
• Knowledge of self-care strategies
• Self-care

[Note: Based on the definition and defining characteristics of this ND, the focus appears to be broader than simply meeting routine basic activities of daily living (ADLs) and addresses independence in maintaining overall health, personal development, and general well-being.]

Sample Clinical Applications: Presence of chronic physical or psychological conditions, or any individual seeking improved well-being or independence in meeting own needs

DESIRED OUTCOMES/EVALUATION CRITERIA

Sample NOC linkages:

Self-Care Status: Ability to perform basic personal care activities and instrumental activities of daily living

Self-Care: Instrumental Activities of Daily Living (IADL): Ability to perform activities needed to function in the home or community independently with or without assistive device

Self-Direction of Care: Care recipient actions taken to direct others who assist with or perform physical tasks and personal healthcare

Client Will (Include Specific Time Frame)
• Maintain responsibility for planning and achieving self-care goals and general well-being.
• Demonstrate proactive management of chronic conditions, potential complications, or changes in capabilities.
• Identify and use resources appropriately.
• Remain free of preventable complications.

ACTIONS/INTERVENTIONS

Sample NIC linkages:

Self-Care Assistance: IADL: Assisting and instructing a person to perform instrumental activities of daily living (IADL) needed to function in the home or community

Self-Modification Assistance: Reinforcement of self-directed change initiated by the patient to achieve personally important goals

Self-Efficacy Enhancement: Strengthening an individual's confidence in his/her ability to perform a health behavior

 Diagnostic Studies   Evidence Based Practice   Medications   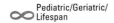 Pediatric/Geriatric/Lifespan

NURSING PRIORITY NO. 1 To determine current self-care status and motivation for improvement:

- Determine individual strengths and skills of the client *to incorporate into plan of care, enhancing likelihood of achieving outcomes. Note: Assessment might include use of an instrument to evaluate client's current functional status, in addition to client's self-report. In the community healthcare setting, a complex assessment tool may be used (e.g., Lawton and Brody's scale of IADL to determine client's self-care abilities [e.g., to communicate by phone, drive, cook, shop, balance a checkbook, manage medical appointments or medications, etc.]). In an acute-care (or emergent) setting, the assessment may be confined to personal care (e.g., Katz Activities of Daily Living Scale). These instruments are used to determine (1) client's safety issues and care needs upon entry into acute care and (2) to ascertain changes in functional abilities as a result of client's condition and treatment.*[4]
- Ascertain motivation and expectations for change. *Motivation to improve and high expectations can encourage client to make changes that will improve his or her life. However, unrealistic expectations may hamper efforts.*
- Note availability and use of resources and supportive person(s) *to ascertain that client has means for sharing common concerns, needs, and wishes, as well as has access to social support and approval (e.g., support group participants, family members, professionals).*[2]
- ∞ Determine age, developmental issues, and presence of medical conditions resulting in specific deficits (e.g., loss of visual or spatial orientation affecting driving, muscular weakness affecting fine motor coordination, peripheral neuropathy impairing sensory interpretation, fractured ankle affecting ability to transfer or ambulate) *that could impact potential for growth or interrupt client's ability to meet own needs.*[2,3]
- Assess for potential challenges to enhanced participation in self-care (e.g., language barrier with healthcare providers, lack of information, insufficient time for discussion; sudden or progressive change in health status, catastrophic events).

NURSING PRIORITY NO. 2 To assist client/significant other (SO) plan to meet individual needs:

- Discuss client's understanding of current situation *to determine areas that can be clarified or strengthened. When health changes occur, the ability to make necessary adaptations is influenced by a wide range of variables that include understanding the changes necessary, the readiness and motivation to change, and the motor and sensory abilities to execute those activities.*[5]
- Provide accurate and relevant information regarding current and future needs *so that client can incorporate into self-care plans while minimizing problems (e.g., stress, resistance) often associated with change.*[1]
- Promote client/SO participation in problem identification and decision making. *Optimizes outcomes and supports health promotion.*[3]
- Review coping skills (e.g., assertiveness, interpersonal relations, decision making, problem-solving, stigma management, time management) *that are useful in managing a wide range of stressful conditions.* Encourage client to ask for assistance, as needed or desired.[1]
- Active-listen client's/SO's concerns. *Exhibits regard for client's values and beliefs and provides opportunity to support positive responses and address questions or concerns.*[2]
- Encourage communication among those who are involved in the client's health promotion. *Periodic review provides clarification of issues, reinforcement of successful interventions, and possibility for early intervention, where needed, to manage chronic conditions.*

NURSING PRIORITY NO. 3 To promote optimum functioning (Teaching/Discharge Considerations):

- Assist client to set realistic goals for the future. *Enhances likelihood of success and commitment to behavioral changes.*
- Support client in making health-related decisions and pursuit of self-care practices that promote health *to foster self-esteem and support positive self-concept.*
- Identify reliable reference sources (including Web sites) regarding individual needs and strategies for self-care. *Reinforces learning and promotes self-paced review.*

 Acute Care   Collaborative   Community/Home Care   Cultural

- Provide for ongoing evaluation of self-care program *to identify progress and needed changes for continuation of health and adaptation in management of limiting conditions.*
- Review safety concerns and modification of medical therapies or activities and environment, as needed, *to prevent injury and enhance successful functioning.*
- Refer to home-care provider, social services, physical or occupational therapy, speech-language pathologist, rehabilitation, and counseling resources, as indicated or requested, *for education, assistance, and adaptive devices and modifications that may be desired.*
- Identify additional community resources (e.g., senior services, handicap transportation van for appointments, accessible and safe locations for social or sports activities, Meals on Wheels) *to obtain additional forms of assistance that may improve client's independence and self-care.*

DOCUMENTATION FOCUS

Assessment/Reassessment
- Individual findings, including strengths, health status, and any limitation(s).
- Availability and use of resources, support person(s), assistive devices.
- Motivation and expectations for change.

Planning
- Plan of care, specific interventions, and who is involved in planning.
- Teaching plan.

Implementation/Evaluation
- Client's responses to interventions, teaching, and actions performed.
- Attainment or progress toward desired outcome(s).
- Modifications to plan.

Discharge Planning
- Long-term needs and who is responsible for actions to be taken.
- Type of and source for assistive devices.
- Specific referrals made.

References

1. Livneh, H., Antonak, R. F. (2005). Psychosocial adaptation to chronic illness and disability: A primer for counselors. *J Couns Dev*, 83(1), 12–20.
2. Baldwin, K. M. (2006). Stroke: It's a knock-out punch. *Nursing Made Incredibly Easy!* 4(2), 10–23.
3. Singleton, J. K. (2000). Nurses' perspectives of encouraging client's care-of-self in a short-term rehabilitation unit within a long-term care facility. *Rehab Nurse*, 21(1), 23–30, 35.
4. McCullough, K., et al. (2008). RN compliance with SLP dysphagia recommendations in acute care. *Top Geriatr Rehabil*, 23(4), 330–340.
5. Boltz, M., Resnick, B., Galik, E. (2016). Preventing functional decline in the acute care setting. In Boltz, M. et al. (eds). *Evidence-Based Geriatric Nursing Protocols for Best Practice*. 5th ed. New York: Springer.

 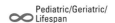

readiness for enhanced Self-Concept

Taxonomy II: Self-Perception—Class 1 Self-Concept (00167) [**Diagnostic Division:** Ego Integrity], Approved 2002; Revised 2013

DEFINITION: A pattern of perceptions or ideas about the self, which can be strengthened.

DEFINING CHARACTERISTICS

Subjective
Expresses:
• Desire to enhance self-concept, role performance
• Acceptance of strengths, limitations
• Confidence in abilities
• Satisfaction with thoughts about self, sense of worth
• Satisfaction with body image, personal identity

Objective
Actions congruent with verbal expressions
Sample Clinical Applications: As a health-seeking behavior, the client may be healthy or this diagnosis can occur in any clinical condition or life process

DESIRED OUTCOMES/EVALUATION CRITERIA

Sample **NOC** linkages:
Self-Esteem: Personal judgment of self-worth
Hope: Optimism that is personally satisfying and life-supporting
Personal Autonomy: Personal actions of a competent individual to exercise governance in life decisions

Client Will (Include Specific Time Frame)
• Verbalize understanding of own sense of self-worth.
• Participate in programs and activities to enhance self-esteem.
• Demonstrate behaviors or lifestyle changes to promote positive self-esteem.
• Participate in family, group, or community activities to enhance self-concept.

ACTIONS/INTERVENTIONS

Sample **NIC** linkages:
Self-Modification Assistance: Reinforcement of self-directed change initiated by the patient to achieve personally important goals
Self-Awareness Enhancement: Assisting a patient to explore and understand his/her thoughts, feelings, motivations, and behaviors
Self-Esteem Enhancement: Assisting a patient to increase his/her personal judgment of self-worth

NURSING PRIORITY NO. 1   To assess current situation and desire to enhance self-concept:

• Determine current status of individual's belief about self. *Self-concept consists of the physical self (body image), personal self (identity), and self-esteem, and information about client's current thinking about self provides a beginning for making changes to improve self.*[1,2]
• Determine availability and quality of family/significant other (SO) support. *Presence of supportive people who reflect positive attitudes regarding the individual promotes a positive sense of self.*[1]

 Acute Care   Collaborative   Community/ Home Care   Cultural

- Identify family dynamics, both present and past. *Self-esteem begins in early childhood and is influenced by the perceptions of how the individual is viewed by significant others. Provides information about family functioning that will help to develop plan of care for enhancing client's self-concept.*[1,2]
- Note willingness to seek assistance and motivation for change. *Individuals who have a sense of their own self-image and are willing to look at themselves realistically will be better able to achieve desired growth.*[1]
- 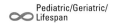Determine client's concept of self in relation to cultural or religious ideals and beliefs. *Culture and religion play a major role in view individual has of self in relation to self-worth.*[9]
- Observe nonverbal behaviors and note congruence with verbal expressions. Discuss cultural meanings of nonverbal communication. *Incongruence between verbal and nonverbal communication requires clarification. Interpretation of nonverbal expressions is culturally determined and needs to be identified to avoid misinterpretation.*[1,9]

NURSING PRIORITY NO. 2   To promote client sense of self-esteem:

- Develop therapeutic relationship. Be attentive, validate client's communication, maintain open communication, and use skills of active listening and "I" messages. *Promotes trusting situation in which client is free to be open and honest with self and others.*[2–4]
- Accept client's perceptions and view of current status. *Avoids threatening existing self-esteem and provides opportunity for client to develop realistic plan for improving self-concept.*[3]
- Be aware that people are not designed to be rational in their thinking. *Individuals must seek information—choosing to learn and to think rather than merely accepting/reacting—in order to have respect for self, facts, and honesty and to develop positive self-regard.*[7]
- Discuss client perception of self, confronting misconceptions and identifying negative self-talk. Address distortions in thinking, such as self-referencing (beliefs that others are focusing on individuals' weaknesses or limitations), filtering (focusing on negative and ignoring positive), and catastrophizing (expecting the worst outcomes). *Addressing these issues openly allows client to identify things that may negatively affect self-concept and provides an opportunity for change.*[7,8]
- Have client review current and past successes and strengths. *Emphasizes fact that client is and has been successful in many actions taken.*[1,8]
- Use positive "I" messages rather than praise. *Praise is a form of external control, coming from outside sources, whereas "I" messages allow the client to develop internal sense of self-worth.*[4,5]
- Discuss what behavior does for client (positive intention). Ask what options are available to the client/SO(s). *Encourages thinking about what inner motivations are and what actions can be taken to enhance self-esteem.*[3]
- Provide reinforcement for progress noted. *Positive words of encouragement support development of effective coping behaviors and promotes continuation of efforts and personal growth.*[6]
- Encourage client to progress at own rate. *Adaptation to a change in self-concept depends on its significance to the individual and disruption to lifestyle.*[3]
- Involve in activities or exercise program of choice and promote socialization. *Enhances sense of well-being and can help to energize client.*[6,8]

NURSING PRIORITY NO. 3   To promote enhanced sense of personal worth (Teaching/Discharge Considerations):

- 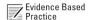Assist client to identify personally achievable goals. Provide positive feedback for verbal and behavioral indications of improved self-view. *Increases likelihood of success and commitment to change.*[3,6]
- Refer to vocational or employment counselor and educational resources, as appropriate. *Assists with improving development of social or vocational skills.*[3]
- Encourage participation in classes, activities, or hobbies that client enjoys or would like to experience. *Provides opportunity for learning new information or skills that can enhance feelings of success, improving self-concept.*[5]

- Reinforce that current decision to improve self-concept is ongoing. *Continued work and support are necessary to sustain behavior changes and personal growth.*[3,5]
- Discuss ways to develop optimism. *Optimism is a key ingredient in happiness and can be learned.*[7]
- Suggest enrolling in assertiveness training classes. *Promotes learning to assist with developing new skills of voice control, posture, eye contact, or expression of feelings in an assertive, rather than aggressive or passive, manner to promote self-esteem.*[3]
- Emphasize importance of grooming and personal hygiene and assist in developing skills to improve appearance and dress for success. *Looking your best improves sense of self-worth, and presenting a positive appearance enhances how others see you. While these things are important, having an adequate foundation for the experience of competence and worth is essential to maintaining one's self-concept.*[1,6]

DOCUMENTATION FOCUS

Assessment/Reassessment
- Individual findings, including evaluations of self and others, current and past successes.
- Interactions with others, family dynamics, lifestyle.
- Cultural or religious influences.
- Motivation for and willingness to change.

Planning
- Plan of care and who is involved in planning.
- Educational plan.

Implementation/Evaluation
- Responses to interventions, teaching, and actions performed.
- Attainment or progress toward desired outcome(s).
- Modifications to plan of care.

Discharge Planning
- Long-term needs and who is responsible for actions to be taken.
- Specific referrals made.

References

1. Purkey, W. W. (1988). An overview of self-concept theory for counselors. Retrieved April 2018 from http://www.ericdigests.org/pre-9211/self.htm.
2. Rohany, N., et al. (2011). Family functioning, self esteem, self concept and cognitive distortion among juvenile delinquents. *Social Sciences*, 6(3), 155–163.
3. Top, B. L., Chadwick, B. S., McClendon, R. J. (2003). Spirituality and self-worth: The role of religion in shaping teens' self-image. *The Religious Educator*, 4(2), 77–93.
4. Rogers, C., Farson, R. E. (No date). Active listening. Retrieved April 2018 from http://www.gordontraining.com/free-workplace-articles/active-listening/.
5. Gordon Training International. (No date). The power of the language of acceptance. Retrieved April 2018 from http://www.gordontraining.com/free-parenting-articles/the-power-of-the-language-of-acceptance/.
6. Branden, N. (2013). Answering misconceptions about self-esteem. Retrieved April 2018 from http://www.nathanielbranden.com/answering-misconceptions-about-self-esteem.
7. Goldhill, O. (2017). Humans weren't designed to be rational. Retrieved April 2018 from https://qz.com/922924/humans-werent-designed-to-be-rational-and-we-are-better-thinkers-for-it/.
8. Beland, N. (2005). How to be happy. *Women's Health*. Retrieved April 2018 from http://www.womenshealthmag.com/health/be-happy-happily-ever-after.
9. Purnell, J. D. (2011). *Guide to Culturally Competent Health Care*. 2nd ed. Philadelphia: F. A. Davis.

 Acute Care   Collaborative   Community/Home Care   Cultural

chronic low Self-Esteem

Taxonomy II: Self-Perception—Class 2 Self-Esteem (00119) [**Diagnostic Division:** Ego Integrity], Approved 1988; Revised 1996, 2008, 2017

DEFINITION: Negative evaluation and/or feelings about one's own capabilities lasting at least 3 months.

RELATED FACTORS
Cultural or spiritual incongruence
Inadequate affection received; receiving insufficient approval or inadequate respect from others
Inadequate belonging or group membership
Ineffective coping with loss

DEFINING CHARACTERISTICS

Subjective
Shame; guilt
Underestimates ability to deal with situation
Rejection of positive feedback

Objective
Hesitant to try new experiences
Repeatedly unsuccessful in life events
Exaggerates negative feedback about self
Overly conforming; dependent on others' opinions
Poor eye contact
Nonassertive or indecisive behavior; passivity
Excessive seeking of reassurance
At Risk Population: Exposure to traumatic situation
Pattern of failure; repeated negative reinforcement
Associated Condition: Psychiatric disorder
Sample Clinical Applications: Chronic health conditions, degenerative diseases, eating disorders, substance abuse, depressive disorders, personality disorders, pervasive developmental disorders

DESIRED OUTCOMES/EVALUATION CRITERIA

Sample NOC linkages:
Self-Esteem: Personal judgment of self-worth
Personal Autonomy: Personal actions of a competent individual to exercise governance in life decisions
Hope: Optimism that is personally satisfying and life-supporting

Client Will (Include Specific Time Frame)
• Verbalize understanding of negative evaluation of self and reasons for this problem.
• Participate in treatment program to promote change in self-evaluation.
• Demonstrate behaviors or lifestyle changes to promote positive self-image.
• Verbalize increased sense of self-worth in relation to current situation.
• Participate in family, group, or community activities to enhance change.

(continues on page 752)

 Diagnostic Studies
 Evidence Based Practice
 Medications
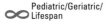 Pediatric/Geriatric/Lifespan

chronic low Self-Esteem (continued)

ACTIONS/INTERVENTIONS

Sample NIC linkages:

Self-Esteem Enhancement: Assisting a patient to increase his/her personal judgment of self-worth

Self-Awareness Enhancement: Assisting a patient to explore and understand his/her thoughts, feelings, motivations, and behaviors

Body Image Enhancement: Improving a patient's conscious and unconscious perceptions and attitudes toward his/her body

---

NURSING PRIORITY NO. 1   To assess causative/contributing factors:

• Determine factors in current situation that can exacerbate low self-esteem, noting age and developmental level of individual. *Identifying potentially aggravating occurrences (e.g., family crises, physical disfigurement from an accident or illness, feelings of abandonment by significant other [SO] resulting in social isolation) are important for developing plan of care and choosing appropriate interventions that help client develop a sense of self-worth.*[1]

• Assess content of negative self-talk. Note client's perceptions of how others view him or her. *Constant repetition of negative words and thoughts reinforce idea that individual is worthless and belief that others view him or her in a negative manner. Identifying these negative ruminations and bringing them to the client's awareness enables person to begin to replace them with positive thoughts.*[1]

• Note nonverbal behavior (e.g., nervous movements, lack of eye contact). *Incongruencies between verbal and nonverbal communication require clarification to ensure accuracy of interpretation.*[1,5]

• Determine availability and quality of family/SO(s) support. *Family is an important component of how an individual views self. The development of a positive sense of self depends on how the person relates to members of the family, as they are growing up and in the current situation.*[1,3]

• Identify family dynamics, present and past. *How family members interact affects an individual's development and sense of self-esteem. Whether family members are negative and nonsupportive, or positive and supportive, affects the needs of the client at this time.*[4]

• 🌐 Be alert to client's concept of self in relation to cultural and religious ideal(s). *Composition and structure of nuclear family influences individual's sense of who they are in relation to others in the family and in society. For example, Mexican American culture dictates that family comes first, the father is the authority in the family, and the behavior of the individual reflects on the entire family.*[9]

• 💊 Determine degree of participation and cooperation with therapeutic regimen. *Maintaining scheduled medications (e.g., antidepressants, antipsychotics) and other aspects of the plan of care requires ongoing evaluation and possible changes in regimen.*[1,2]

• Note willingness to seek assistance and motivation for change. *Determines client's degree of participation in adhering to therapeutic regimen.*[1,10]

NURSING PRIORITY NO. 2   To promote client's sense of self-esteem in dealing with situation:

• Develop therapeutic nurse/client relationship. Be attentive, validate client's communication, provide encouragement for efforts, maintain open communication, and use skills of active listening and "I" messages. *Promotes trusting environment in which client is free to be open and honest with self and therapist so current situation can be dealt with most effectively.*[1,4]

• Collaborate in addressing/presenting medical issues and safety concerns. *Client's self-esteem may be affected by physical changes of current medical situation. Changes in body, such as weight loss or gain, chronic illness, or amputation, will affect how client sees self as a person. Attitude may contribute to feelings of depression and lack of attention to personal safety requiring evaluation and assistance.*[1,3,7]

 Acute Care   Collaborative   Community/ Home Care   Cultural

- Accept client's perceptions or view of situation. Avoid threatening existing self-esteem. *Promotes trust and allows client to begin to look at options for improving self-esteem.*[2,8]
- Be aware that people are not designed to be rational in their thinking. *They must seek information—choosing to learn and to think rather than merely accepting or reacting—in order to have respect for self, facts, and honesty and to develop positive self-esteem.*[1,13]
- Discuss client perceptions of self related to what is happening; confront misconceptions and negative self-talk. Address distortions in thinking, such as self-referencing (belief that others are focusing on individual's weaknesses or limitations), filtering (focusing on negative and ignoring positive), and catastrophizing (expecting the worst outcomes). *Addressing these issues openly provides opportunity for change.*[1,3,10]
- Emphasize need to avoid comparing self with others. Encourage client to focus on aspects of self that can be valued. *Changing negative thinking can be effective in developing positive self-talk to enhance self-esteem.*[2,5]
- Have client review current and past successes and strengths. *Often in the depths of despair and sense of failure in current situation, individual forgets positive aspects of his or her life. Bringing them to mind can remind client of these successes, enhancing sense of self-esteem.*[3,4]
- Use positive "I" messages rather than praise. *Praise may be heard as manipulative and insincere and be rejected. Use of positive "I" messages communicates a feeling that is genuine and real and allows client to feel good about himself or herself, developing internal sense of self-esteem.*[4,5]
- Discuss what behavior does for client (positive intention) and what options are available to the client/SO(s). *Helping client begin to look at what rewards are gained from current actions and what actions might be taken to achieve the same rewards in a more positive way can provide a realistic and accurate self-appraisal, enhancing sense of competence and self-worth.*[1,3,10]
- Assist client to deal with sense of powerlessness. Refer to ND Powerlessness.
- Set limits on aggressive or problem behaviors such as acting out, suicide preoccupation, or rumination. Put self in client's place using empathy, not sympathy. *Preventing undesirable behavior prevents feelings of worthlessness. Suicidal thoughts need further evaluation and intervention. Use of empathy helps caregiver to understand client's feelings better.*[1,2]
- Give reinforcement for progress noted. *Positive words of encouragement promote continuation of efforts, supporting development of coping behaviors.*[2,4,10]
- Encourage client to progress at own rate. *Adaptation to a change in self-concept depends on its significance to individual, disruption to lifestyle, and length of crisis or condition.*[1,2,5]
- Assist client to recognize and cope with events, alterations, and sense of loss of control. *Incorporating changes accurately into self-concept enhances sense of self-worth.*[1,2,7]
- Involve in activities/exercise program and promote socialization. *Enhances sense of well-being and can help energize client.*[1,5]

NURSING PRIORITY NO. 3   To promote wellness (Teaching/Discharge Considerations):

- Discuss inaccuracies in self-perception with client/SO(s). *Enables client and SOs to begin to look at misperceptions and accept reality, and look at options for change to improve sense of self-worth.*[1,6,8]
- Model behaviors being taught, involving client in goal setting and decision making. *Facilitates client developing trust in his or her own unique strengths.*
- Prepare client for events or changes that are expected, when possible. *Providing time to adapt to changes allows client to prepare self and feel more confident in ability to manage the changes, enhancing sense of self-worth.*[1,2,7]
- Provide structure in daily routine and care activities. *Knowing what to expect promotes a sense of control and ability to deal with activities as they occur.*[1,2]
- Emphasize importance of grooming and personal hygiene. Assist in developing skills as indicated (e.g., makeup classes, dressing for success). *People feel better about themselves when they present a positive outer appearance.*[1,3,5]
- Assist client to identify goals that are personally achievable. Provide positive feedback for verbal and behavioral indications of improved self-view. *Increases likelihood of success and commitment to change.*[5,11]
- Refer to vocational or employment counselor and educational resources as appropriate. *Assists with development of social or vocational skills, promoting sense of competence and self-responsibility.*[1,2,5]

 Diagnostic Studies   Evidence Based Practice   Medications   Pediatric/Geriatric/ Lifespan

- Encourage participation in classes, activities, or hobbies that client enjoys or would like to experience. *Meaningful accomplishment, assuming self-responsibility, and participating in new activities engenders one's sense of competence and self-worth.*[8,12]
- Reinforce that this therapy is a brief encounter in overall life of the client/SO(s), with continued work and ongoing support being necessary to sustain behavior changes and personal growth. *Provides individual with information and encouragement to build on for the future.*[1,6,7]
- Refer to classes to assist with learning new skills (e.g., assertiveness training, positive self-image, communication skills). *These skills can help client develop a sense of competence through realistic and accurate self-appraisal promoting self-esteem.*[10]
- Refer to counseling or therapy and mental health or other special needs support groups as indicated. *May need additional intervention to develop needed changes.*[1,10,11]

DOCUMENTATION FOCUS

Assessment/Reassessment
- Individual findings, including early memories of negative evaluations (self and others), subsequent and precipitating failure events.
- Effects on interactions with others, family dynamics, lifestyle.
- Specific medical or safety issues.
- Cultural or religious factors.
- Motivation for and willingness to change.

Planning
- Plan of care and who is involved in planning.
- Teaching plan.

Implementation/Evaluation
- Responses to interventions, teaching, and actions performed.
- Attainment or progress toward desired outcome(s).
- Modifications to plan of care.

Discharge Planning
- Long-term needs and who is responsible for actions to be taken.
- Specific referrals made.

References

1. Townsend, M. C. (2006). *Psychiatric Mental Health Nursing Concepts of Care.* 5th ed. Philadelphia: F. A. Davis.
2. Doenges, M. E., Townsend, M. C., Moorhouse, M. F. (1998). *Psychiatric Care Plans: Guidelines for Individualizing Patient Care.* 3rd ed. Philadelphia: F. A. Davis.
3. Doenges, M. E., Moorhouse, M. F., Geissler-Murr, A. C. (2004). *Nurse's Pocket Guide: Diagnoses, Interventions, and Rationales.* 9th ed. Philadelphia: F. A. Davis.
4. Gordon, T. (2000). *Parent Effectiveness Training.* Updated ed. New York: Three River Press.
5. Branden, N. (2013). Answering misconceptions about self-esteem. Retrieved April 2018 from http://www.nathanielbranden.com/answering-misconceptions-about-self-esteem.
6. Vasconcellos, J., et al. (2014). In defense of self-esteem. Retrieved April 2018 from https://www.depressionforums.org/forums/topic/1341-in-defense-of-self-esteem/.
7. Battle, J. (1990). *Self-Esteem: The New Revolution.* Edmonton, Alberta, Canada: James Battle & Associates.
8. Reasoner, R. (No date). The true meaning of self-esteem. Retrieved April 2018 from https://brainmass.com/psychology/developmental-psychology/true-meaning-self-esteem-64869.
9. Purnell, J. D. (2011). *Guide to Culturally Competent Health Care.* Philadelphia: F. A. Davis.
10. Peden, A. R., et al. (2000). Reducing negative thinking and depressive symptoms in college women. *J Nurs Scholar,* 32(2), 145–151.
11. Seligman, M., et al. (1996). *The Optimistic Child.* New York: Houghton Mifflin.
12. Branden, N. (1995). *The Six Pillars of Self-Esteem.* New York: Bantam Book.
13. Goldhill, O. (2017). Humans weren't designed to be rational. Retrieved April 2018 from https://qz.com/922924/humans-werent-designed-to-be-rational-and-we-are-better-thinkers-for-it/.

 Acute Care   Collaborative   Community/Home Care   Cultural

risk for chronic low Self-Esteem

Taxonomy II: Self-Perception—Class 2 Self-Esteem (00224) [**Diagnostic Division:** Ego Integrity], Approved 2010; Revised 2013, 2017

DEFINITION: Susceptible to long-standing negative self-evaluating/feelings about self or self-capabilities, which may compromise health.

RISK FACTORS
Cultural or spiritual incongruence
Inadequate affection received; receiving insufficient approval or inadequate respect from others
Inadequate belonging or group membership
Ineffective coping with loss
At Risk Population: Exposure to traumatic situation
Pattern of failure; repeated negative reinforcement
Associated Condition: Psychiatric disorder
Sample Clinical Applications: Chronic health conditions, eating disorders, substance abuse, depression, personality/pervasive developmental disorders

DESIRED OUTCOMES/EVALUATION CRITERIA

Sample NOC linkages:
Self-Esteem: Personal judgment of self-worth
Coping: Personal actions to manage stressors that tax an individual's resources
Personal Resiliency: Positive adaptation and function of an individual following significant adversity or crisis

Client Will (Include Specific Time Frame)
• Acknowledge understanding of discrepancy between self and cultural/spiritual norms.
• Participate in therapy program to improve self-esteem.
• Demonstrate behaviors to change negative self-evaluation.
• Verbalize understanding of reason for failures and how to make changes for success.
• Participate in family, group, or community activities to enhance change.

ACTIONS/INTERVENTIONS

Sample NIC linkages:
Self-Esteem Enhancement: Assisting a patient to increase his/her personal judgment of self-worth
Coping Enhancement: Facilitation of cognitive and behavioral efforts to manage perceived stressors, changes, or threats that interfere with meeting life demands and roles
Socialization Enhancement: Facilitation of another person's ability to interact with others

NURSING PRIORITY NO. 1   To assess causative/contributing factors:

• ∞ Note age and developmental level of client and circumstances surrounding current situation. *Younger people may not have learned skills to deal with negative occurrences and/or rejection from others.*[2,15]
• Elicit client's perceptions of current situation. *Provides understanding of underlying/aggravating occurrences (e.g., family crisis, loss of employment, academic failure, physical disfigurement from an accident or illness, relationship problems/divorce with feelings of abandonment by significant other [SO] resulting in social*

 Diagnostic Studies   Evidence Based Practice   Medications   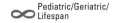 Pediatric/Geriatric/Lifespan *isolation) necessary for choosing interventions appropriate to assist client to address feelings and develop realistic sense of self-worth.*[1,15]

- Ascertain sense of control client perceives to have over self/situation. *Client's locus of control or the degree of control client believes he or she has may be a critical factor in ability to deal with current situation. Individuals with external locus of control tend to blame others for their problems rather than taking responsibility for their actions. As a result, they may feel helpless or powerless and look to others to solve problems and take care of them.*[3,14,15]
- Determine client's awareness of self-destructive behavior, acting out, aggression, and suicidal thoughts. *Choices individual makes result from low self-esteem and pleasing others and lead to feelings of worthlessness.*[1,8]
- Note content of negative self-talk and client's perception of how others see him or her. *As negative thoughts are repeated in one's head, they become the basis for believing that the individual is indeed worthless and others must agree with that conclusion.*[1,3]
- Observe nonverbal behavior (e.g., nervous movements, lack of eye contact) and how it relates to verbal statements. *Incongruencies between verbal and nonverbal need to be clarified to be sure perceived meaning of communication is accurate.*[10]
- Note religious and cultural factors that have influenced client. *Family of origin affects how one views self in relation to family members and others in society. For instance, Islamic families tend to be patriarchal, with the father exercising unmitigated power over female family members and making all decisions for them.*[5,8]
- Determine family makeup and whether they are available and supportive. *Support of family is essential to client's self-esteem. Predominant world view is determined by the time an individual is 5 years of age.*[3,15]
- Note family dynamics and how client interacts within the family. *Crucial to individual's development and self-esteem in a positive or negative way.*[8,15]
- 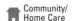 Evaluate current medication regimen noting client adherence. *Maintaining therapeutic regimen requires ongoing evaluation to determine efficacy or need for change. The client who is asymptomatic or depressed may not feel the need to take prescribed medications. Other factors can also impact client's willingness to follow therapeutic plan (e.g., complexity of regimen, poor quality of the client-provider relationship, issues of access to care).*[13,16]

NURSING PRIORITY NO. 2 To promote client's sense of self-esteem in dealing with changes in life:

- Establish therapeutic nurse/client relationship, maintaining open communication and using Active-listening and "I" messages. *Promotes a trusting environment in which client is free to talk about potential problems that may arise.*[9]
- Determine willingness to improve attitudes and sense of self. *Negative perceptions, sense of alienation, and lack of involvement in positive activities lead to sense of worthlessness. Making a commitment to change provides an opportunity to learn new ways to interact with others and choose activities that promote individual successes.*[1,8]
- Address possible situations that client may be facing. *Sense of loss, lack of involvement in group, traumatic event, and repeated failures in attempts to change situation may discourage client from wanting to try to make life better.*[1,15]
- Avoid challenging client's perception of events. *May threaten sense of self-esteem, limiting client's ability to check out perceptions and make own corrections.*[11]
- Reinforce that people are not necessarily rational in their thinking. *They must seek information, choosing to learn and to think, rather than merely accepting or reacting, in order to have respect for self and develop positive self-esteem.*[1,3,8,17]
- Discuss misperceptions and negative self-talk as well as distortions in thinking, such as self-referencing (belief that others are focusing on person's weaknesses or limitations), filtering (focusing on negative and ignoring positive), or catastrophizing (believing the worst will happen). *These issues keep individual believing in a negative, worthless view of self and need to be addressed before person can move on and improve life.*[1,3]

 Acute Care   Collaborative   Community/ Home Care   Cultural

- Discuss the problem of comparing self to others. Encourage client to focus on own positive aspects. *These actions will help individual to change negative thinking.*[1,3]
- List current and previous successes. *Focusing on these can help the client realize that failures can be overcome.*[1]
- Provide positive feedback, for verbal and behavioral indications of improved self-view, using "I" messages instead of praise. *Praise can be interpreted as insincere and manipulative and be rejected. Positive "I" messages convey a sense of acceptance and let the individual feel good about self, enhancing self-esteem and encouraging individual to continue efforts.*[9,12]
- Ask client to think about what behavior does (positive intention) in relation to low self-esteem, reluctance to join groups, and seeing self as less than others. *As individual thinks about this aspect of behavior, awareness of having a choice to change life may facilitate positive changes.*[3,8]
- Discuss feelings of powerlessness. *It is important to differentiate between what the client can control or change and what cannot be controlled. Inability of the client to make this distinction can cause client to feel defeated and increase sense of low self-esteem. Understanding that one is incapable of making everything right and perfect with all people, places, and things in life gives the individual the ability to retain the "locus of control."*[15] Refer to ND: Powerlessness.
- Contract with client/set limits on acting out and aggressive or self-destructive behaviors. *Aids in preventing negative behaviors that can result in/exacerbate feelings of worthlessness.*[7] Refer to NDs risk for other-/self-directed Violence and risk for Suicide for additional interventions.
- Encourage client to progress at own pace, providing reinforcement as progress is made. *Helps individual to value self and believe life changes can be made.*[1,8]
- Promote socialization and involvement in exercise and activity programs. *Helps individual to realize involvement with others can lead to positive feelings about self.*[4,6]

NURSING PRIORITY NO. 3   To promote wellness (Teaching/Discharge Considerations):

- 🏠 Involve client in goal setting and decision making. *Facilitates trust and belief that change can be made and life can improve.*[9]
- Encourage client to structure daily activities so routine becomes manageable. *Promotes a sense of control and belief in own abilities.*[6]
- Discuss importance of grooming and personal hygiene, involvement in classes (i.e., Dress for Success). *Others often judge an individual by the outward appearance presented, as well as individual's own positive appraisal and sense of confidence.*[10]
- Refer to educational resources and vocational or employment counselor as indicated. *Promotes future success, reinforcing self-worth.*[4,15]
- Identify/refer to support groups and classes, such as assertiveness, communication skills, and parenting as appropriate. *These skills can help client develop or strengthen a sense of competence through realistic and accurate self-appraisal, promoting self-esteem.*[4,6,12,15]
- Review importance of adherence to medication regimen when prescribed. *A number of factors influence client's decisions about taking medications, including awareness of illness, beliefs about treatment, and side effects of medication. While education increases client's understanding of his or her illness/situation and treatment, it does not always improve compliance. Interventions such as individual or group counseling or compliance therapy based on cognitive–behavioral techniques may be useful in supporting personal growth and commitment to change.*[13,16]

DOCUMENTATION FOCUS

Assessment/Reassessment
- Individual findings, noting risk factors, client's perceptions, interaction with others.
- Cultural values or religious beliefs, locus of control.
- Family support, availability, and use of resources.

 Diagnostic Studies   Evidence Based Practice   Medications   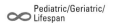 Pediatric/Geriatric/Lifespan

Planning
* Plan of care and who is involved in planning.
* Individual teaching plan.

Implementation/Evaluation
* Response to interventions, teaching, actions performed, and changes that may be indicated.
* Attainment or progress toward desired outcomes.
* Modification to plan of care.

Discharge Planning
* Long-term needs and goals and who is responsible for actions to be taken.
* Specific referrals made.

References

1. Mayo Clinic Staff. (Updated 2017). Self-esteem: Take steps to feel better about yourself. Retrieved April 2018 from http://www.mayoclinic.org/healthy-lifestyle/adult-health/in-depth/self-esteem/art-20045374.
2. Watson, S. (Updated 2017). Understand inappropriate behavior. Retrieved April 2018 from http://specialed.about.com/od/behavioremotional/a/behavsupport.htm.
3. Selvarajah, A. (No date). Self-esteem: The problem behind all problems. Retrieved April 2018 from http://www.selfgrowth.com/articles/selvarajah13.html.
4. Garcia, J., et al. (2010). Healthy eating, physical activity, and healthy weights guideline for public health in Ontario. Retrieved April 2018 from http://ocp.cancercare.on.ca/common/pages/UserFile.aspx?fileId=64413.
5. Alaoui, S. (2011). Women's status in Islam: The line between culture and religion. Retrieved April 2018 from http://prospectjournal.org/2011/02/22/womens-status-in-islam-the-line-between-culture-and-religion/.
6. National Institute for Health and Clinical Excellence (NICE). (2009, updated 2015). Occupational therapy interventions and physical activity interventions to promote the mental well being of older people in primary care and residential care. Retrieved April 2018 from http://arms.evidence.nhs.uk/resources/hub/1043082/attachment.
7. Webster, J. (Updated 2017). Behavior contracts to support good behavior: Explicit contracts can help students improve problem behavior. Retrieved April 2018 from http://specialed.about.com/od/behavioremotional/a/Behavior-Contracts-To-Support-Good-Behavior.htm.
8. Corey, G., Corey, M. S. (2010). *I Never Knew I Had a Choice—Explorations in Personal Growth*. 9th ed. Belmont, CA: Brooks/Cole.
9. McGreevey, M. (2006). *Patients as Partners: How to Involve Patients and Families in Their Own Care*. Oak Brook, IL: Joint Commission Resources.
10. Knapp, M. L., Hall, J. A. (2010). *Nonverbal Communication in Human Interaction*. 7th ed. Boston, MA: Wadsworth/Cengage Learning.
11. Taylor, S. E., Brown, J. D. (1988). Illusion and well-being: A social psychological perspective on mental health. *Psychol Bull*, 103(2), 193–210.
12. Bright Horizons Family Resources. (2012). Practicing positive parenting: The benefits of encouragement vs. praise. Retrieved April 2018 from http://www.brighthorizons.com/family-resources/e-family-news/2012-positive-parenting-encouragement-versus-praise/.
13. Gray, R., Wykes, T., Gournay, K. (2002). From compliance to concordance: A review of the literature on interventions to enhance compliance with antipsychotic medication. *J Psychiatr Ment Health Nurs*, 9(3), 277–284.
14. Judge, T. A. (2009). Core self-evaluations and work success. *Curr Dir Psychol Sci*, 18(1), 58–62.
15. Daniels, R. (2009). Self-concept. *Nursing Fundamentals: Caring & Clinical Decision Making*. 2nd ed. Clifton Park, NY: Delmar Cengage Learning.
16. Ho, P. M., Bryson, C. L., Rumsfield, J. S. (2009). Medication adherence—Its importance in cardiovascular outcomes. *Circulation*, 119(23), 3028–3035.
17. Goldhill, O. (2017). Humans weren't designed to be rational. Retrieved April 2018 from https://qz.com/922924/humans-werent-designed-to-be-rational-and-we-are-better-thinkers-for-it/.

 Acute Care Collaborative Community/ Home Care Cultural

risk for situational low Self-Esteem

Taxonomy II: Self-Perception—Class 2 Self-Esteem (00153) [**Diagnostic Division:** Ego Integrity], Approved 2000; Revised 2013, 2017

DEFINITION: Susceptible to developing a negative perception of self-worth in response to a current situation, which may compromise health.

RISK FACTORS

Alteration in body image or social role
Pattern of helplessness; history of rejection; inadequate recognition
Behavior inconsistent with values
Decrease in control over environment
Unrealistic expectations
At Risk Population: Developmental transition
History of: abandonment, abuse, loss, neglect, rejection
Pattern of failure
Associated Condition: Functional impairment
Physical illness
Sample Clinical Applications: Traumatic injuries, surgery, pregnancy, newly diagnosed conditions (e.g., diabetes mellitus, hypertension), adjustment disorders, substance use, stroke, dementia

DESIRED OUTCOMES/EVALUATION CRITERIA

Sample NOC linkages:
Self-Esteem: Personal judgment of self-worth
Psychosocial Adjustment: Life Change: Adaptive psychosocial response of an individual to a significant life circumstance
Abuse Recovery: Emotional: Extent of healing of psychological injuries due to abuse

Client Will (Include Specific Time Frame)
• Acknowledge factors that lead to possibility of feelings of low self-esteem.
• Verbalize view of self as a worthwhile, important person who functions well both interpersonally and occupationally.
• Demonstrate self-confidence by setting realistic goals and actively participating in life situation.

ACTIONS/INTERVENTIONS

Sample NIC linkages:
Self-Esteem Enhancement: Assisting a patient to increase his/her personal judgment of self-worth
Coping Enhancement: Facilitation of cognitive and behavioral efforts to manage perceived stressors, changes, or threats that interfere with meeting life demands and roles
Self-Awareness Enhancement: Assisting a patient to explore and understand his/her thoughts, feelings, motivations, and behaviors

NURSING PRIORITY NO. 1   To assess causative/contributing factors:

• Determine individual factors that may contribute to diminished self-esteem. *Proactive information allows identification of appropriate interventions to deal with current situation.*[1,2]

 Diagnostic Studies   Evidence Based Practice   Medications   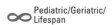 Pediatric/Geriatric/ Lifespan

- Identify basic sense of self-worth of client and image client has of self—existential, physical, and psychological. *The components of self-concept consist of the physical self or body image, the personal self or personal identity, and the self-esteem, with each aspect playing a role in the client's ability to deal with anticipated changes.*[1]
- Note client's perception of threat to self in current situation. *Perception is more important than reality of what is happening. Some individuals view a potentially severe situation as something easily handled, while others may view a minor problem with anxiety and catastrophizing.*[2,3]
- Ascertain sense of control client has (or perceives to have) over self and situation. *Individual with internal locus of control tends to perceive self in control of what is happening and will participate more actively in care and feel more sense of self-worth.*[7,8]
- Determine client awareness of own responsibility for dealing with situation, personal growth, etc. *Acceptance of responsibility for self enables client to feel more comfortable with treatment regimen and participate more fully, promoting self-esteem.*[1,9]
- Assess family/significant other (SO) dynamics and support of client. *How family interacts with one another affects not only the development of self-esteem but also the maintenance of a sense of self-worth when client is facing an illness or crisis. Dysfunctional interactions may be detrimental to client's ability to deal with what is happening.*[1,5]
- Verify client's concept of self in relation to cultural or religious ideals. *Culture and religion play a major role in view individual has of self in relation to self-worth. Illness may interfere with this view; for instance, males in Mexican American culture are seen as the head of the household, and giving up this role because of illness can diminish self-esteem.*[4] *Note: Recent studies support that self-esteem functions similarly across cultures.*[10]
- Assess negative attitudes and/or self-talk. *Contributes to view of situation as hopeless and/or difficult.*[3,6]
- Listen for or note self-destructive or suicidal thoughts or behaviors. *Indicates high level of stress and need for further evaluation and referral for mental health services.*[1,6] Refer to ND risk for Suicide as appropriate.
- Note nonverbal body language. *Incongruencies between verbal and nonverbal communications require clarification to ensure accuracy of interpretation.*[1]
- Identify previous adaptations to illness or disruptive events in life. *Provides information about how client handled those situations and may be predictive of current outcome.*[1]
- Determine availability and use of support systems. *Feeling hopeless and alone lowers client ability to manage care and concentrate on healing. Support systems can provide role modeling and the help needed to engender hope and enhance self-esteem.*[1]
- Note availability and use of resources to address specific need (e.g., rehabilitation services, home-care support, job placement). *Individual may be unaware or have difficulty accessing community supports or assistance programs.*

NURSING PRIORITY NO. 2 To assist client to deal with loss/change and maintain sense of positive self-esteem:

- Encourage expression of feelings and anxieties. *Facilitates grieving the loss.*
- Active-listen client's concerns without comment or judgment.
- Help client identify individual strengths and assets, reinforcing positive traits and self-view.
- Assist client to problem-solve situation and develop plan of action.
- Convey confidence in client's ability to cope with current situation.
- Mobilize appropriate support systems.

NURSING PRIORITY NO. 3 To promote wellness (Teaching/Discharge Considerations):

- Provide information to assist client in making desired changes. *Appropriate books, DVDs, or Internet resources allow client to learn at own pace.*

Acute Care   Collaborative   Community/ Home Care   Cultural

- Suggest participation in group or community activities or volunteer work *that can provide opportunity for success and positive feedback for accomplishments.*
- Involve significant others/extended family in treatment plan. *Increases likelihood they will provide appropriate support to client.*
- 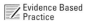 Promote attendance in therapy or support groups as indicated.

DOCUMENTATION FOCUS

Assessment/Reassessment
- Individual findings, including individual expressions of lack of self-esteem, effects on interactions with others, lifestyle.
- Underlying dynamics and duration (situational or situational exacerbating chronic).
- Cultural values or religious beliefs, locus of control.
- Family support, availability and use of resources.

Planning
- Plan of care and who is involved in planning.
- Teaching plan.

Implementation/Evaluation
- Responses to interventions, teaching, actions performed, and changes that may be indicated.
- Attainment or progress toward desired outcome(s).
- Modifications to plan of care.

Discharge Planning
- Long-term needs and goals, and who is responsible for actions to be taken.
- Specific referrals made.

References

1. Townsend, M. C. (2003). *Psychiatric Mental Health Nursing Concepts of Care*. 4th ed. Philadelphia: F. A. Davis.
2. Gross, S. J. (Reviewed 2016). How to raise your self esteem. *PsychCentral*. Retrieved April 2018 http://psychcentral.com/lib/how-to-raise-your-self-esteem/000737.
3. Reasoner, R. (No date). What is self-esteem? Retrieved April 2018 from https://brainmass.com/psychology/developmental-psychology/true-meaning-self-esteem-64869.
4. Purnell, L. D. (2011). *Guide to Culturally Competent Health Care*. 2nd ed. Philadelphia: F. A. Davis.
5. Pearson, A. B. (Updated 2010). Effective communication with children. Retrieved April 2018 from http://www.education.com/reference/article/effective-parent-child-communication/.
6. Adams, L. (No date). Working together with I-messages. *Gordon Training International*. Retrieved April 2018 from http://www.gordontraining.com/free-workplace-articles/working-together-with-i-messages/.
7. Peden, A. R., et al. (2000). Reducing negative thinking and depressive symptoms in college women. *J Nurs Scholarsh*, 32(2), 145–151.
8. Munson, P. J. (1991). Life's decisions—By chance or by choice? *Adapted from Winning Teachers, Teaching Winners*. Santa Cruz, CA: ETR Associates.
9. Vasconcellos, J., et al. (2004). In defense of self-esteem. Retrieved April 2018 from https://www.depressionforums.org/forums/topic/1341-in-defense-of-self-esteem/.
10. Brown, J. D., et al. (2009). Cultural similarities in self-esteem functioning. *Psychology*, 40(1), 140–157.

 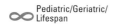

situational low Self-Esteem

Taxonomy II: Self-Perception—Class 2 Self-Esteem (00120) **[Diagnostic Division:** Ego Integrity**]**, Approved 1988; Revised 1996, 2000, 2017

DEFINITION: Development of a negative perception of self-worth in response to a current situation.

RELATED FACTORS
Alteration in body image or social role
Pattern of helplessness; history of rejection; inadequate recognition
Behavior inconsistent with values
Decrease in control over environment
Unrealistic expectations

DEFINING CHARACTERISTICS

Subjective
Helplessness; purposelessness
Underestimates ability to deal with situation

Objective
Situational challenge to self-worth
Self-negating verbalizations
Indecisive or nonassertive behavior
At Risk Population: Developmental transition
History of: abandonment, abuse, loss, neglect, rejection
Pattern of failure
Associated Condition: Functional impairment
Physical illness
Sample Clinical Applications: Traumatic injuries, surgery, pregnancy, newly diagnosed conditions (e.g., diabetes mellitus), adjustment disorders, substance use, stroke, dementia

DESIRED OUTCOMES/EVALUATION CRITERIA

Sample NOC linkages:
Self-Esteem: Personal judgment of self-worth
Psychosocial Adjustment: Life Change: Adaptive psychosocial response of an individual to a significant life circumstance
Personal Resiliency: Positive adaptation and function of an individual following significant adversity or crisis

Client Will (Include Specific Time Frame)
• Verbalize understanding of individual factors that precipitated current situation.
• Identify feelings and underlying dynamics for negative perception of self.
• Express positive self-appraisal.
• Demonstrate behaviors to restore positive self-image.
• Participate in treatment regimen or activities to correct factors that precipitated crisis.

 Acute Care   Collaborative   Community/ Home Care   Cultural

ACTIONS/INTERVENTIONS

Sample NIC linkages:

Self-Esteem Enhancement: Assisting a patient to increase his/her personal judgment of self-worth

Coping Enhancement: Facilitation of cognitive and behavioral efforts to manage perceived stressors, changes, or threats that interfere with meeting life demands and roles

Support System Enhancement: Facilitation of support to patient by family, friends, and community

NURSING PRIORITY NO. 1 To assess causative/contributing factors:

- Determine individual situation (e.g., family crisis, termination of a relationship, loss of employment, physical disfigurement) related to low self-esteem in the present circumstances. *Many factors are involved in a person's self-esteem, and this information is essential for planning accurate care.*[1]
- Identify basic sense of self-esteem of client; image client has of self—existential, physical, and psychological. *The components of self-concept consist of the physical self or body image, the personal self or personal identity, and the self-esteem. Each aspect plays a role in the client's ability to deal with current situation/crisis.*[1]
- Assess degree of threat and perception of client concerning crisis. *How individuals perceive themselves is based on the self-judgments they make. How the client sees the current situation in relation to ability to cope will affect his or her sense of self-worth and needs to be acknowledged and planned for to help client deal with feelings of low self-esteem.*[1,2]
- Ascertain sense of control client has (or perceives to have) over self and situation. *Client's locus of control or degree of control client believes or perceives he or she has may be a critical factor in ability to deal with current situation or crisis. Individuals with internal locus of control tend to be more optimistic about their ability to deal with adversity even in the face of current difficulties. Individuals with external locus of control will look to others to solve problems and take care of them.*[1-3]
- Determine client's awareness of own responsibility for dealing with situation, personal growth, etc. *These factors enhance the ability of the client to effectively manage situation in a positive manner.*[4]
- Assess family/significant other (SO) dynamics and support of client. *How family members interact affects an individual's development and sense of self-esteem. Effective interactions among family members usually lead to positive support for the client in current situation. Dysfunctional interactions may be detrimental to client's ability to deal with what is happening.*[2,3]
- Verify client's concept of self in relation to cultural and religious ideals. *Self-esteem is developed by many factors, including genetics and environment. Cultural and religious influences during the individual's life affect beliefs about self, measure of worth, and ability to deal with current situation or crisis.*[1,5] *Note: Recent studies support that self-esteem functions similarly across cultures.*[6]
- Determine past coping skills in relation to current episode. *Trust is built over time, and past experiences with failure or success will affect client's expectations regarding the eventual outcome of dealing with current illness or crisis.*[8,9]
- Assess negative attitudes or self-talk. *An individual who is feeling unimportant, incompetent, and not in control often is unconsciously saying negative things to himself or herself that contribute to a loss of self-esteem and an attitude of despair, affecting current situation.*[1,7]
- Note nonverbal body language. *Incongruencies between verbal or nonverbal communication require clarification to ensure accuracy of interpretation.*[1,2]
- Assess for self-destructive or suicidal thoughts or behavior. *Client who believes situation is hopeless often begins to consider suicide as an option.* Refer to ND risk for Suicide as appropriate.[1]
- Identify previous adaptations to illness or disruptive events in life. *May be predictive of current ability to deal with situation and suggest eventual outcome.*[1]

 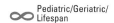

- 🏠 Note availability and use of resources to address specific need (e.g., rehabilitation services, home-care support, job placement). *Individual may be unaware or have difficulty accessing community supports or assistance programs.*

NURSING PRIORITY NO. 2   To assist client to deal with loss/change and recapture sense of positive self-esteem:

- 🔬 Assist with treatment of underlying condition when possible. *For example, cognitive restructuring and improved concentration in mild brain injury often result in restoration of positive self-esteem.*[1]
- Encourage expression of feelings, anxieties; facilitate grieving the loss. *As client expresses feelings and anxieties, he or she begins to deal with the realities of the current situation and the loss that occurs with the changes of illness.*[1] Refer to ND Grieving as appropriate.
- Active-listen to client's concerns or negative verbalizations without judgment. *Conveys a message of acceptance and confidence in client's ability to deal with whatever occurs.*
- 📝 Identify individual strengths, assets, and aspects of self that remain intact and can be valued. Reinforce positive traits, abilities, and self-view. *Client may not see these in the anxiety and hopelessness of the immediate situation, and reminding client of own positive attributes can help him or her recover hope and develop a positive attitude about situation.*[1,7]
- Help client identify own responsibility and control or lack of control in situation. *Accepting responsibility enables client to look realistically at what is under own control and what is not. When client stops expending energy on issues that cannot be controlled, energy is freed up to concentrate on more productive avenues.*[1,8]
- Assist client to problem-solve situation, developing a plan of action and setting goals to achieve desired outcome. *Personal involvement enhances commitment to plan, optimizing outcomes.*
- Convey confidence in client's ability to cope with current situation. *Validation helps client accept own ability to deal with what is happening.*[1]
- Mobilize support systems; identify individuals in similar circumstances. *Feeling hopeless and alone lowers client's ability to manage care and concentrate on healing. Support systems can provide role modeling and the help needed to engender hope and enhance self-esteem.*[1,3]
- 📝 Provide opportunity for client to practice alternative coping strategies, including progressive socialization opportunities. *Involvement with others provides client with situation in which new actions can be tried out and validated or discarded to enhance feelings of self-worth.*[1,3]
- Encourage use of visualization, guided imagery, and relaxation. *These strategies promote a positive sense of self and general well-being, enhancing client's coping ability.*[1]
- Provide feedback about client's self-negating remarks or behavior, using "I" messages. *Allows client to experience a different view. "I" messages are a nonjudgmental way to let individual understand how behavior is perceived by or affecting others and self.*
- Encourage involvement in decisions about care when possible. *Promotes sense of control over what is happening, enhancing feelings of self-worth.*[1,8]
- Give reinforcement for progress noted. *Positive words of encouragement promote continuation of efforts, supporting development of coping behaviors.*[10]

NURSING PRIORITY NO. 3   To promote wellness (Teaching/Discharge Considerations):

- 🏠 Assist client to identify personally achievable goals. *Increases likelihood of client's success and commitment to change.*[2,10]
- Encourage client to look to the future and set long-range goals for achieving necessary lifestyle changes. *Supports view that this is an ongoing process, providing client with hope for the future.*[1,3]
- Support independence in activities of daily living and mastery of therapeutic regimen. *Individuals who are confident are more secure and positive in self-appraisal.*[1,2]
- 🔬 Promote attendance in therapy or support group as indicated. *Provides opportunity to discuss own situation and hear how others are dealing with similar problems, promoting new ideas about own ability to deal with issues.*[1,9,10]

 Acute Care   Collaborative   Community/ Home Care   Cultural

- Involve extended family/SO(s) in treatment plan as appropriate. *Enhances their understanding of what client wishes to accomplish, increasing likelihood they will provide appropriate support to client.*[1]
- Provide information and bibliotherapy, including reliable Web sites as appropriate. *Reinforces learning, allowing client to progress at own pace. Promotes opportunity for making informed decisions and improving ability to deal with situation.*[1,7]
- 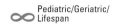 Refer to vocational or employment counselor and educational resources, as appropriate. *Assists with development of social or vocational skills, promoting sense of competence and self-responsibility.*[1,2]
- Suggest participation in group or community activities (e.g., assertiveness classes, volunteer work, support groups). *Provides opportunities for learning new information and being appreciated for contributions, enhancing sense of self-worth.*[1,2]
- Refer to counseling or therapy, mental health, or other special-needs support groups, as indicated. *May need additional support to deal with crisis.*[1,10]

DOCUMENTATION FOCUS

Assessment/Reassessment
- Individual findings, noting precipitating crisis, client's perceptions, effects on desired lifestyle/interaction with others.
- Cultural values or religious beliefs, locus of control.
- Family support, availability and use of resources.

Planning
- Plan of care and who is involved in planning.
- Teaching plan.

Implementation/Evaluation
- Responses to interventions, teaching, actions performed, and changes that may be indicated.
- Attainment or progress toward desired outcome(s).
- Modifications to plan of care.

Discharge Planning
- Long-term needs and goals and who is responsible for actions to be taken.
- Specific referrals made.

References

1. Townsend, M. C. (2003). *Psychiatric Mental Health Nursing Concepts of Care*. 4th ed. Philadelphia: F. A. Davis.
2. Reasoner, R. (No date). The true meaning of self-esteem. Retrieved April 2018 from https://brainmass.com/psychology/developmental-psychology/true-meaning-self-esteem-64869.
3. Murray, E., Murray, C. A., Murray, M. P. (No date). Two experiments examine induced anxiety, depression, anger and assertiveness that are contrasted with the conditions of relaxed music, role playing and silence and indicate their impacts on cognitions and the emotion of anxiety. Retrieved April 2018 from http://www.nssa.us/journals/2009-33-1/2009-33-1-12.htm.
4. Selvarajah, A. (2000). Self-esteem: The problem behind all problems. Retrieved April 2018 from http://www.selfgrowth.com/articles/selvarajah13.html.
5. Purnell, L. D. (2011). *Guide to Culturally Competent Health Care*. 2nd ed. Philadelphia: F. A. Davis.
6. Brown, J. D., et al. (2009). Cultural similarities in self-esteem functioning. *Psychology*, 40(1), 140–157.
7. Peden, A. R., et al. (2000). Reducing negative thinking and depressive symptoms in college women. *J Nurs Scholarsh*, 32(2), 145–151.
8. Munson, P. J. (1991). Life's decisions—By chance or by choice? *Adapted from Winning Teachers, Teaching Winners*. Santa Cruz, CA: ETR Associates.
9. Stepp, G. (2010). Helping children develop a positive sense of self. Retrieved April 2018 from http://www.vision.org/vision-media/family-relationships/children-and-self-esteem/34763.aspx.
10. Seligman, M., et al. (1996). *The Optimistic Child*. New York: Houghton Mifflin.

 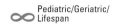

Self-Mutilation

Taxonomy II: Safety/Protection—Class 3 Violence (00151) [**Diagnostic Division:** Safety], Approved 2000; Revised 2017

DEFINITION: Deliberate self-injurious behavior causing tissue damage with the intent of causing nonfatal injury to attain relief of tension.

RELATED FACTORS

Absence of family confidant; disturbance in interpersonal relationships; feeling threatened with loss of significant relationship

Ineffective communication between parent and adolescent; eating disorder

Alteration in body image; low self-esteem

Dissociation; emotional disturbance; labile behavior

Irresistible urge for self-directed violence or to cut self

Impulsiveness; ineffective coping strategies; inability to express tension verbally; mounting tension that is intolerable; requires rapid stress reduction

Isolation from peers

Negative feeling [e.g., depression, rejection, self-hatred, separation anxiety, guilt]; perfectionism; loss of control over problem-solving situation

Pattern of inability to plan solutions or to see long-term consequences; use of manipulation to obtain nurturing relationship with others

Substance misuse/[abuse]

DEFINING CHARACTERISTICS

Subjective

Self-inflicted burn

Ingestion or inhalation of harmful substances or objects

Objective

Cuts or scratches on body

Picking at wound

Biting; abrading

Insertion of object(s) into body orifice(s)

Hitting

Severing or constricting a body part

At Risk Population:

Adolescence

Battered child; history of childhood abuse; history of self-directed violence; peers who self-mutilate

Childhood illness or surgery; developmental delay

Family divorce; family history of self-destructive behavior or substance abuse; violence between parental figures

Incarceration; living in nontraditional setting

Sexual identity crisis

Associated Condition: Autism

Borderline personality or character disorder; depersonalization

Psychotic disorder

Sample Clinical Applications: Borderline personality, dissociative disorders, bipolar disorder, developmental delay, autism, eating disorders, substance abuse, physical or psychological abuse, gender identity crisis

 Acute Care

 Collaborative

 Community/ Home Care

 Cultural

DESIRED OUTCOMES/EVALUATION CRITERIA

Sample NOC linkages:

Mutilation Self-Restraint: Personal actions to refrain from intentional self-inflicted injury (nonlethal)

Impulse Self-Control: Self-restraint of compulsive or impulsive behaviors

Distorted Thought Self-Control: Self-restraint of disruptions in perception, thought processes, and thought content

Client Will (Include Specific Time Frame)
- Verbalize understanding of reasons for occurrence of behavior.
- Identify precipitating factors and awareness of arousal state that occurs prior to incident.
- Express increased self-concept or self-esteem.
- Seeks help when feeling anxious and having thoughts of harming self.

ACTIONS/INTERVENTIONS

Sample NIC linkages:

Behavior Management: Self-Harm: Assisting the patient to decrease or eliminate self-mutilating or self-abusive behaviors

Environmental Management: Safety: Monitoring and manipulation of the physical environment to promote safety

Limit Setting: Establishing the parameters of desirable and acceptable patient behavior

NURSING PRIORITY NO. 1   To assess causative/contributing factors:

- Determine underlying dynamics of individual situation as listed in Related Factors. Note previous episodes of self-mutilation behavior. *Although some body piercing (e.g., ears, nose, lip, eyebrow) is generally accepted as decorative, piercing of multiple sites or industrial piercings are often an attempt to establish individuality, addressing issues of separation and belonging, but are not considered self-injury or self-mutilating behaviors.*[1,7]
- Identify previous history of self-mutilative behavior and relationship to stressful events. *Self-injury is considered an attempt to alter a mood state and/or an outlet for negative emotions such as anger and shame. Information about previous behavior and precipitating factors is important to understanding and planning care in current situation.*[1,7,9,11]
- Determine presence of inflexible, maladaptive personality traits that reflect personality or character disorder. *Identification of impulsive, unpredictable, or inappropriate behaviors; intense anger; or lack of control of anger is important for planning appropriate interventions and plan of care. Clients diagnosed as borderline personality disorder are often unstable and prone to self-injury and need a specific treatment plan to diminish these behaviors.*[1,9]
- Evaluate history of mental illness (e.g., borderline personality, identity disorder, bipolar disorder). *These illnesses may be the underlying cause of the self-injurious behavior.*[1,2,10]
- Note beliefs and cultural or religious practices that may be involved in choice of behavior. *Growing up in a family that did not allow feelings to be expressed, individual may believe that feelings are wrong or bad. Family dynamics may come out of religious or cultural expectations that support strict punishment for transgressions. Individuals may believe mental illness is the result of unacceptable actions, and feelings of guilt may lead to anxiety and subsequent self-injurious behaviors.*[4]
- Note use or abuse of addicting substances. *May be indicative of attempt to treat self and needs further evaluation and additional intervention.*[2,6,10]

- 🖊 Review laboratory findings (e.g., blood alcohol, polydrug screen, glucose, electrolyte levels). *Helpful for identifying drug use or medical problems that may be affecting behavior negatively.*[1]

NURSING PRIORITY NO. 2 To structure environment to maintain client safety:

- Assist client to identify feelings leading up to desire for self-mutilation. *Early recognition of recurring feelings provides opportunity to seek other ways of coping.*[5]
- 📝 Provide external controls or limit setting. *Reducing opportunities for client to self-mutilate can help client learn to stop the behavior.*[4,8]
- Encourage appropriate expression of feelings. *Helps client to identify feelings and promote understanding of what leads to development of tension and subsequent injurious behavior.*[2]
- ➕ Keep client in continuous staff view and do special observation checks during inpatient stay. *Promotes safety by recognizing escalating behaviors and providing timely intervention.*[2,5]
- 📝 Structure inpatient milieu to maintain positive, clear, open communication among staff and clients, with an understanding that "secrets are not tolerated" and will be confronted. *Prevents manipulative behavior, so client does not pit one staff member against another to fulfill own desires.*[1,4,5]
- 📝 Note feelings of healthcare providers/family, such as frustration, anger, defensiveness, and need to rescue. *Client may be manipulative, evoking defensiveness and conflict. These feelings need to be identified, recognized, and dealt with openly with staff/family and client.*[4]
- 🌐 Provide care for client's wounds when self-mutilation occurs in a matter-of-fact manner. Refrain from offering sympathy or additional attention. *A matter-of-fact approach can convey empathy and concern but not undue concern that could provide reinforcement for maladaptive behavior and encourage its repetition.*[2]
- 💊📝 Discuss use of medication, such as clozapine. *This medication has been shown to reduce acts of self-injurious behavior and help client maintain a more stable mood.*[3]
- 🌐 Develop schedule of or refer to alternative healthy, success-oriented activities. *Group or family therapy or groups such as Eating Disorders or a similar 12-step program based on individual needs; self-esteem activities, including positive affirmations; visiting with friends; and exercise help client to practice new behaviors in a supportive environment.*[7,11]

NURSING PRIORITY NO. 3 To promote movement toward positive changes:

- Encourage client involvement in formulating plan of care and developing goals for preventing undesired behavior. *Being involved in own decisions can help to reestablish ego boundaries and enhance commitment to goals, optimizing outcomes and enhancing self-esteem.*[2,5]
- 📝 Develop a contract between client and counselor to enable the client to stay physically safe, such as "I will not cut or harm myself for the next 24 hours." Renew contract on a regular basis and have both parties sign and date each contract. *Making a commitment in writing helps client to think before acting and can prevent new incidents of self-injury.*[4]
- Provide avenues of communication for times when client needs to talk. *Having an opportunity to discuss anxieties helps client to avoid cutting or damaging self.*[4,6]
- Assist client to learn assertive behavior. Include the use of effective communication skills, focusing on developing self-esteem by replacing negative self-talk with positive comments. *Low self-esteem is a factor in this behavior, and by learning new ways of expressing self, client can begin to feel better and deal with anxieties in a more positive manner.*[2,10]
- Choose interventions that help the client to reclaim power in own life (e.g., experiential and cognitive). *Beginning to think in a positive manner and then translating that into action provides reinforcement for using power to stop injurious behaviors and develop a more productive lifestyle.*[2]

NURSING PRIORITY NO. 4 To promote long-term safety (Teaching/Discharge Considerations):

- 🏠 Discuss commitment to safety and ways in which client will deal with precursors to undesired behavior. *Identifies specific precursors for individual and provides a plan for client to follow when anxiety becomes overwhelming.*[2,8,10]

 Acute Care   Collaborative   Community/ Home Care   Cultural

- Promote the use of healthy behaviors, identifying the consequences and outcomes of current actions. *As client develops a more positive attitude and accepts the idea that current actions are being destructive to desired life-style, new behaviors can help make needed changes.*[2]
- Identify support systems. *Knowing who client can turn to when anxiety becomes a problem helps to avoid injurious behavior.*[1]
- Discuss living arrangements when client is discharged from inpatient program. *May need assistance with transition to changes required to avoid recurrence of self-mutilating behaviors.*[2,10]
- 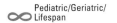 Involve family/significant other (SO) in planning for discharge and involve in group therapies as appropriate. *Promotes coordination and continuation of plan and commitment to goals.*[2,6]
- Discuss the role neurotransmitters play in predisposing individual to beginning this behavior. *It is believed that problems in the serotonin system may make the person more aggressive and impulsive, and when combined with a home where they have learned that feelings are bad or wrong, this leads to turning aggression on self.*[8]
- Provide information and discuss the use of medication as appropriate. *Antidepressant medications may be useful, but they need to be weighed against the potential for overdosing.*[1,3]
- Refer to NDs Anxiety, Self-Esteem (specify), and impaired Social Interaction.

DOCUMENTATION FOCUS

Assessment/Reassessment
- Individual findings, including risk factors present, underlying dynamics, prior episodes.
- Cultural or religious practices.
- Laboratory test results.
- Substance use or abuse.

Planning
- Plan of care and who is involved in planning.
- Teaching plan.

Implementation/Evaluation
- Response to interventions, teaching, and actions performed.
- Attainment or progress toward desired outcome(s).
- Modifications to plan of care.

Discharge Planning
- Long-term needs and who is responsible for actions to be taken.
- Community resources, referrals made.

References

1. No surname, Alexandra. (Updated 2014). Self-mutilation: The truth behind the shame. Retrieved April 2018 from http://www.healthyplace.com/eating-disorders/articles/self-mutilation-the-truth-behind-the-shame/.
2. Doenges, M. E., Townsend, M. C., Moorhouse, M. F. (1998). *Psychiatric Care Plans: Guidelines for Individualizing Care.* 3rd ed. Philadelphia: F. A. Davis.
3. Chengappa, K. N. (1999). Clozapine reduces severe self-mutilation and aggression in psychotic patients with borderline personality disorder. *J Clin Psychiatry,* 60(7), 477–484.
4. Clarke, L., Whittaker, M. (1998). Self-mutilation: Culture, contexts, and nursing responses. *J Clin Nurs,* 7(2), 129–137.
5. Dallam, S. J. (1997). The identification and management of self-mutilating patients in primary care. *Nurse Pract,* 22(5), 151–165.
6. Selekman, M. D. (2004). Adolescent self-harm: A growing epidemic. *Family Therapy Magazine,* 1(2), 34–40.
7. Cox, H. C., et al. (2002). *Clinical Applications of Nursing Diagnosis: Adult, Child, Women's, Psychiatric, Gerontic, and Home Health Considerations.* 4th ed. Philadelphia: F. A. Davis.
8. Martinson, D. (No date). Self-injury: Beyond the myths. Retrieved April 2018 from http://www.psyke.org/history/200003/selfinjury/secretshame03.html.
9. Davidson, T., Frey, R. (No date). Self-mutilation. *Encyclopedia of Children's Health.* Retrieved April 2018 from http://www.healthofchildren.com/S/Self-Mutilation.html.
10. Iannelli, V. (Updated 2018). Cutting and self-harm behaviors. *About.com Mental Health.* Retrieved April 2018 from http://mentalhealth.about.com/cs/familyresources/a/selfinjury.htm.
11. Brennan, D. (Updated 2018). Teens, cutting, and self-injury. Retrieved April 2018 from https://teens.webmd.com/cutting-self-injury#1.

 Diagnostic Studies   Evidence Based Practice   Medications   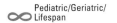 Pediatric/Geriatric/Lifespan

risk for Self-Mutilation

Taxonomy II: Safety/Protection—Class 3 Violence (00139) [Diagnostic Division: Safety], Approved 1992; Revised 2000, 2013, 2017

DEFINITION: Susceptible to deliberate self-injurious behavior causing tissue damage with the intent of causing nonfatal injury to attain relief of tension.

RISK FACTORS

Absence of family confidant; disturbance in interpersonal relationships; feeling threatened with loss of significant relationship

Ineffective communication between parent and adolescent; eating disorder

Alteration in body image; low self-esteem

Dissociation; emotional disturbance; labile behavior

Irresistible urge for self-directed violence or to cut self

Impulsiveness; ineffective coping strategies; inability to express tension verbally; mounting tension that is intolerable; requires rapid stress reduction

Isolation from peers

Negative feeling [e.g., depression, rejection, self-hatred, separation anxiety, guilt]; perfectionism; loss of control over problem-solving situation

Pattern of inability to plan solutions or to see long-term consequences; use of manipulation to obtain nurturing relationship with others

Substance misuse/[abuse]

At Risk Population:

Adolescence

Battered child; history of childhood abuse; history of self-directed violence; peers who self-mutilate

Childhood illness or surgery; developmental delay

Family divorce; family history of self-destructive behavior or substance abuse; violence between parental figures

Incarceration; living in nontraditional setting

Sexual identity crisis

Associated Condition: Autism

Borderline personality or character disorder; depersonalization

Psychotic disorder

Sample Clinical Applications: Borderline personality, dissociative disorders, bipolar disorder, developmental delay, autism, eating disorders, substance abuse, physical/psychological abuse, gender identity crisis

DESIRED OUTCOMES/EVALUATION CRITERIA

Sample NOC linkages:

Mutilation Self-Restraint: Personal actions to refrain from intentional self-inflicted injury (nonlethal)

Impulse Self-Control: Self-restraint of compulsive or impulsive behaviors

Distorted Thought Self-Control: Self-restraint of disruptions in perception, thought processes, and thought content

Client Will (Include Specific Time Frame)
• Verbalize understanding of reasons for occurrence of behavior.
• Identify precipitating factors and awareness of arousal state that occurs prior to incident.
• Express increased self-concept or self-esteem.

 Acute Care Collaborative Community/ Home Care Cultural

- Demonstrate self-control as evidenced by lessened (or absence of) episodes of self-mutilation.
- Engage in use of alternative methods for managing feelings and individuality.

ACTIONS/INTERVENTIONS

Sample **NIC** linkages:
Behavior Modification: Promotion of a behavior change
Calming Technique: Reducing anxiety in patient experiencing acute distress
Behavior Management: Self-Harm: Assisting the patient to decrease or eliminate self-mutilating or self-abusive behaviors

---

NURSING PRIORITY NO. 1   To assess causative/contributing factors:

- Determine underlying dynamics of individual situation as listed in Risk Factors. Note the presence of conditions that may interfere with ability to control own behavior (e.g., psychotic state, mental retardation, autism) *and may lead to incidents of self-injury.*[1]
- Assess for inflexible, maladaptive personality traits. *May reflect personality or character disorder (e.g., impulsive, unpredictable, inappropriate behaviors, intense anger or lack of control of anger) that may lead to self-mutilative behaviors.*[1]
- Evaluate history of mental illness (e.g., borderline personality, identity disorder, bipolar disorder). *These illnesses may be the underlying cause of the self-injurious behavior.*[1,2,10]
- Identify previous episodes of self-mutilating behavior (e.g., cutting, scratching, bruising). *Self-injury is considered an attempt to alter a mood state and/or an outlet for negative emotions such as anger and shame. Information about previous behavior and precipitating factors is important to understanding and planning care in current situation.*[1,7-9,11] *Although some body piercing (e.g., ears) is generally accepted as decorative, piercing of multiple sites or industrial piercings are often an attempt to establish individuality, addressing issues of separation and belonging, but are not considered as self-injury or self-mutilating behaviors.*[2]
- Note beliefs and cultural or religious practices that may be involved in choice of behavior. *Growing up in a family that did not allow feelings to be expressed, individual may believe that feelings are wrong or bad. Family dynamics may come out of religious or cultural expectations that support strict punishment for transgressions. Individuals may believe mental illness is the result of unacceptable actions, and feelings of guilt may lead to anxiety and subsequent self-injurious behaviors.*[4]
- Determine use or abuse of addictive substances, including alcohol. *Individuals often use these substances to self-medicate feelings of anxiety and may increase the risk of suicide by sixfold.*[2,8,10]
- Note degree of impairment in social and occupational functioning. *May dictate treatment setting (e.g., specific outpatient program or short-stay inpatient when client is experiencing extreme anxiety).*[1,5,9]
- Review laboratory findings (e.g., blood alcohol, polydrug screen, glucose, electrolyte levels). *Helpful for identifying drug use or medical problems that may be affecting behavior negatively.*[1]

NURSING PRIORITY NO. 2   To structure environment to maintain client safety:

- Assist client to identify feelings and behaviors that precede desire for self-mutilation. *Early recognition of recurring feelings provides client opportunity to seek other ways of coping, including asking for help.*[2,6]
- Provide external controls or limit-setting as indicated. *Decreases the opportunity to injure self and helps client think about reasons for actions and learn different ways to deal with them.*[1]
- Encourage client to recognize and appropriately express feelings verbally. *Learning to express feelings enables client not only to recognize them, but also to begin to find acceptable and appropriate ways to deal with them.*[6,7,11]

 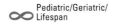

- Note feelings of healthcare providers/family, such as frustration, anger, defensiveness, distraction, despair and powerlessness, and need to rescue. *Client may be manipulating or splitting providers/family members, which evokes defensiveness and resultant conflict. These feelings need to be identified, recognized, and dealt with openly with staff/family and client.*[1]
- Refer to alternative healthy, success-oriented activities. *Groups such as Eating Disorders or a similar 12-step program based on individual needs; self-esteem activities, including positive affirmations; visiting with friends; and exercise can help client to practice new behaviors in a supportive environment.*[6]

NURSING PRIORITY NO. 3 To promote movement toward positive actions:

- 🏠 Encourage client involvement in formulating plan of care and developing goals for preventing undesired behavior. *Being involved in own decisions can help to reestablish ego boundaries and enhance commitment to goals, optimizing outcomes and enhancing self-esteem.*[2,5]
- Develop a contract between client and counselor to enable the client to stay physically safe, such as "I will not cut or harm myself for the next 24 hours." Renew contract on a regular basis, signed and dated by both parties. *Discussing the contract gets issues out in the open and conveys a sense of acceptance of the client, while placing some of the responsibility for safety on the client.*[1,2]
- Provide avenues of communication for times when client needs to talk. *Having an opportunity to discuss anxieties helps client to avoid cutting or damaging self.*[4,6]
- Choose interventions that help the client to reclaim power in own life (e.g., experiential and cognitive). *As client experiences new ways of interacting with others, he or she can begin to think more positively about self-worth and changing behaviors.*[2,10]
- 📝 Identify the consequences and outcomes of current actions (e.g., ask "Does this get you what you want?" or "How does this behavior help you achieve your goals?"). *Provides client with opportunity to look at own behaviors in a different way and begin to understand how they are harmful rather than helpful. Contrasting healthy behaviors versus current actions can help client decide to change them. Dialectic behavior therapy is effective in reducing injurious behavior, along with the use of medication.*[1,3,6]
- Assist client to learn assertive behavior rather than nonassertive or aggressive behavior. Include use of effective communication skills, focusing on developing self-esteem by replacing negative self-talk with positive comments. *By learning these new skills, client interacts with others and gets needs met in positive, acceptable ways, promoting self-worth and lessening anxiety and risk of injurious actions.*[1,8]
- Discuss with client/family normalcy of adolescent task of separation and ways of achieving. *Helps individual members understand these actions and begin to recognize the normal from those that are of concern and need intervention.*[1,6,9]
- 🩺 Involve client/family in group therapies as appropriate. *Group setting aids in promoting diffusion of anger and provides insight as to how negative, aggressive behavior affects others, making feedback easier to digest and understand.*[2]

NURSING PRIORITY NO. 4 To promote long-term safety (Teaching/Discharge Considerations):

- 🏠 Discuss commitment to safety and ways in which client will deal with precursors to undesired behavior. *Helps client verbalize anger and anxiety and understand how these feelings lead to desire to injure self and actions that can be taken to prevent this behavior.*[4,6]
- Mobilize support systems. *These individuals often come from abusive families, and unresolved feelings of abandonment remain in adulthood. Positive support by many people in their lives can help them begin to overcome these feelings.*[1,8,9]
- 🩺 Arrange for continued involvement in group therapy after discharge from program. *Remaining in this supportive environment can help client maintain new behaviors as he or she begins to increase responsibility for self and own action.*[2,10]
- 💊📝 Discuss and provide information about the use of medication as appropriate. *Antidepressant medications may be useful, but use needs to be weighed against potential for overdosing. Note: Medication may be tried for*

 Acute Care   Collaborative   Community/Home Care   Cultural

co-occurring disorders like depression or bipolar disorder. However, if the person has no co-occurring disorder, medications may be discouraged, as they can work to cover up feelings that a person has to work through in order to stop the self-harm behavior. Medications that stabilize moods, ease depression, and calm anxiety may be tried to reduce the urge to self-harm.[1,3,12]

- Refer to NDs Anxiety, Self-Esteem (specify), and impaired Social Interaction.

DOCUMENTATION FOCUS

Assessment/Reassessment
- Individual findings, including risk factors present, underlying dynamics, prior episodes.
- Cultural or religious practices.
- Laboratory test results.
- Substance use or abuse.

Planning
- Plan of care and who is involved in planning.
- Teaching plan.

Implementation/Evaluation
- Response to interventions, teaching, and actions performed.
- Attainment or progress toward desired outcome(s).
- Modifications to plan of care.

Discharge Planning
- Long-term needs and who is responsible for actions to be taken.
- Community resources, referrals made.

References

1. Townsend, M. C. (2006). *Psychiatric Mental Health Nursing Concepts of Care*. 4th ed. Philadelphia: F. A. Davis.
2. Doenges, M. E., Townsend, M. C., Moorhouse, M. F. (1998). *Psychiatric Care Plans: Guidelines for Individualizing Care*. 3rd ed. Philadelphia: F. A. Davis.
3. Chengappa, K. N., et al. (1999). Clozapine reduces severe self-mutilation and aggression in psychotic patients with borderline personality disorder. *J Clin Psychiatry*, 60(7), 477–484.
4. Clarke, L., Whittaker, M. (1998). Self-mutilation: Culture, contexts, and nursing responses. *J Clin Nurs*, 7(2), 129–137.
5. Dallam, S. J. (1997). The identification and management of self-mutilating patients in primary care. *Nurse Pract*, 22(5), 151–165.
6. Smith, M., Segal, J. (Updated 2018). Cutting and self-harm. *Helpguide.org*. Retrieved April 2018 from http://www.helpguide.org/articles/anxiety/cutting-and-self-harm.htm.
7. Selekman, M. D. (2004). Adolescent self-harm: A growing epidemic. *Family Therapy Magazine*, 1(2), 34–40.
8. Davidson, L., Frey, D. (No date). Self-mutilation. *Encyclopedia of Children's Health*. Retrieved April 2018 from http://www.healthofchildren.com/S/Self-Mutilation.html.
9. Simpson, C. (2001). Self-mutilation. Retrieved April 2018 from https://oxbowacademy.net/educationalarticles/self_mutilation/.
10. Bhandari, S. (Updated 2018). Mental health and self-injury. *WebMD*. Retrieved April 2018 from http://www.webmd.com/anxiety-panic/guide/self-injury.
11. Brennan, D. (Updated 2018). Teens, cutting, and self-injury. Retrieved April 2018 from https://teens.webmd.com/cutting-self-injury#1.
12. Croft (reviewer), H. (Updated 2016). Self-injury treatment: What are the treatments for self-harm? Retrieved April 2018 from https://www.healthyplace.com/abuse/self-injury/self-injury-treatment-what-are-the-treatments-for-self-harm/.

 Diagnostic Studies Evidence Based Practice Medications 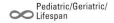 Pediatric/Geriatric/Lifespan

Self-Neglect

Taxonomy II: Activity/Rest—Class 5 Self-Care (00193) [**Diagnostic Division:** Hygiene], Approved 2008; Revised 2017

DEFINITION: A constellation of culturally framed behaviors involving one or more self-care activities in which there is a failure to maintain a socially accepted standard of health and well-being (Gibbons, Lauder, & Ludwick, 2006).

RELATED FACTORS
Deficient executive function
Fear of institutionalization
Inability to maintain control; stressors
Lifestyle choice; substance misuse/[abuse]

DEFINING CHARACTERISTICS

Objective
Insufficient personal or environmental hygiene
Nonadherence to health activity
Associated Condition: Alteration in cognitive functioning; learning disability
Frontal lobe dysfunction; Capgras syndrome
Malingering
Psychiatric or psychotic disorder
Sample Clinical Applications: Mental illness (as in related factors); terminal illness—cancer, amyotrophic lateral sclerosis (ALS); debilitating conditions—multiple sclerosis (MS), Parkinson's disease; alcohol/drug abuse

DESIRED OUTCOMES/EVALUATION CRITERIA

Sample NOC linkages:
Self-Care Status: Personal actions to perform basic personal care activities and instrumental activities of daily living (IADLs)
Health Promoting Behavior: Personal actions to sustain or increase wellness

Client Will (Include Specific Time Frame)
• Acknowledge difficulty maintaining hygiene practices.
• Demonstrate ability to manage lifestyle changes and medication regimen.
• Perform ADLs within level of own ability.

Caregiver Will (Include Specific Time Frame)
• Assist individual with personal and environmental hygiene as needed.
• Identify and assist client with medical, dental, and other healthcare appointments as indicated.

ACTIONS/INTERVENTIONS

Sample NIC linkages:
Self-Responsibility Facilitation: Encouraging a patient to assume more responsibility for own behavior
Self-Care Assistance: Assisting another to perform activities of daily living
Cultural Brokerage: The deliberate use of culturally competent strategies to bridge or mediate between the patient's culture and the biomedical healthcare system

 Acute Care   Collaborative   Community/Home Care   Cultural

NURSING PRIORITY NO. 1 To identify causative or precipitating factors:

- ∞ 📝 Determine existing health problems, age, developmental level, and cognitive psychological factors, including presence of delusions affecting ability to care for own needs. Use an appropriate screening instrument, such as the Elder Assessment Instrument. *A wide variety of impairments can cause a person to neglect hygiene needs, particularly aging, homelessness, and dementia. Neglect and elder abuse are underreported, and the use of a good tool can help identify its presence.*[2,3]

- 📝 Identify other problems that may interfere with ability to care for self. *A visual or hearing impairment, language barrier, and emotional instability or lability can create difficulties for individual to manage daily tasks.*[2,4]

- Note recent life events or changes in circumstances. *Losses (e.g., loved one, financial security, physical independence) can trigger or exacerbate self-neglect behaviors.*[4]

- Review circumstances of client illness, possible monetary rewards, and sympathy or attention from family. *On occasion, self-neglect may be malingering as an attempt to gain something from others or relinquish unwanted responsibilities.*

- 🔬 Perform mental status examination. *Mental illness (e.g., psychosis, depression, dementia) can affect individual's ability or desire to maintain self-care activities or care for home surroundings.*[5,11]

- 🔬📝 Review studies evaluating frontal lobe dysfunction and possibility of Diogenes syndrome. *These clients present with severe self-neglect and may have coexisting medical and psychiatric conditions.*[10,11]

- 📝 Assess economic situation and living arrangements. *May live alone or with family members who are not helpful, may be homeless, and may have little or no financial resources, resulting in inability or lack of concern about personal well-being.*[4]

- 📝 Determine availability and use of resources. *Depending on disability of client, agencies can work together to develop a plan to meet needs, noting whether individual is availing self of help.*[6]

- Interview significant other (SO)/family members to determine level of involvement and support. *Client may be exhibiting acting-out or paranoid behaviors, stressing caregivers who may not realize individual is unable to control self because of cognitive impairment.*[3]

NURSING PRIORITY NO. 2 To determine degree of impairment:

- Perform head-to-toe assessment, inspecting scalp and skin; noting personal hygiene, body odor, rashes, bruising, skin tears, lesions, burns, and presence of vermin; and inspecting oral cavity for gum disease, inflammation, lesions, loose or broken teeth, and fit of dentures. *Identifies specific needs and may reveal signs of trauma or abuse.*[1]

- 📝 Obtain weight. Perform nutritional assessment as indicated. *Neglecting oneself often includes not eating meals regularly or failing to eat nutritionally balanced foods. When alcoholism or drug abuse is a part of neglect, individual may be severely malnourished.*[1,3]

- 💊📝 Review medication regimen. *In addition to neglecting self-care activities, client will likely not pay attention to taking prescriptions as ordered, resulting in exacerbation of medical problem. Note: Some psychotropic medication may cause individual to "feel different" or not in control of self, resulting in reluctance to take drug.*[3]

- Determine willingness to change situation. *Depending on individual's situation (living alone, homeless, mental status), client may have difficulty committing to or be unwilling to change. May see change as a loss of independence.*[3,11]

NURSING PRIORITY NO. 3 To assist in correcting/dealing with situation:

- 🌐 Develop multidisciplinary team specific to individual needs, such as case manager, physician, dietitian, physical or occupational therapist, rehabilitation specialist, and social worker, *to review assessment data and develop a plan appropriate to the individual situation, making use of client's capabilities and maximizing potential.*[6,11]

 Diagnostic Studies   Evidence Based Practice   Medications   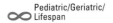 Pediatric/Geriatric/Lifespan

- Establish therapeutic relationship with client, as well as family if available and willing to be involved. *Promotes trust and encourages input into planning process.*[7,11]
- Identify specific priorities and goals of client/SOs. *Helps client to look at possibilities for dealing with difficult situation of no longer being able to maintain lifestyle and moving on to a new way of managing.*[6]
- Promote client/SOs participation in problem identification and decision making. *Enhances commitment to plan when individual has input and encourages participation, enhancing outcomes.*[7]
- Evaluate need for safety, balancing client's need for autonomy. *The ethical challenge of providing individual safety within the current laws for client's right to refuse care in face of self-neglect and self-destructive behaviors that can impact others as well as the client is difficult to manage.*[4,9]
- Perform home assessment, as indicated. *Determines safety issues, cleanliness, compulsive hoarding, and neglected property concerns, so plans can be made to take care of these matters if client is to remain in the home.*[7]
- Instruct in or review skills necessary for caring for self, using terms appropriate to client's level of understanding. *When individual is cognitively impaired or otherwise has difficulty processing information, instructions need to be simplified.*[5]
- Plan time for listening to client's/SOs' concerns. *Provides opportunity to determine whether plan is being followed and what the barriers to participation may be.*[7]
- Refer to NDs Self-Care deficit [specify], ineffective Health Maintenance, impaired Home Maintenance, and [disturbed Sensory Perception] for additional interventions as appropriate.

NURSING PRIORITY NO. 4 To promote wellness (Discharge/Evaluation Criteria):

- Establish remotivation or resocialization program when indicated. *Depending on where the client is residing, isolation may become a problem as individual withdraws from contact with others, and these programs may be helpful.*[2]
- Assist with setting up medication regimen. *Client may need help with arranging medications in specific ways to assure correct administration, especially in the presence of cognitive impairment.*[8]
- Discuss dietary needs and client's ability to provide nutritious meals. *May require support such as food stamps, community pantry, senior meal program, and Meals on Wheels.*[1]
- Provide for ongoing evaluation of self-care program. *Helps to identify whether client is managing effectively or whether cognitive functioning is deteriorating and a new plan needs to be developed.*[7]
- Evaluate for appropriateness of providing a companion animal. *Taking responsibility for another life and sharing unconditional love can provide purpose and motivation for client to take more interest in own situation.*[4]
- Refer to support services such as home care, day-care program, social services, food stamps, community clinic, physical or occupational therapy, and senior services as indicated. *Provides for long-term support to facilitate client's independence and general well-being.*[8]
- Investigate alternative placements as indicated. *Client may require group home, assisted living, or long-term care, and it is best to place in least restrictive environment capable of meeting client's needs.*[9]
- Discuss need for respite for family members. *Care of cognitively impaired member can be wearing, and time away allows for renewing oneself and enhancing ability to cope with continued care responsibilities.*[5]
- Refer for counseling as indicated. *Accurate mental health diagnoses may reveal the need for appropriate services: psychiatric, social, and home care.*[6]

DOCUMENTATION FOCUS

Assessment/Reassessment
- Individual findings, functional level and limitations, mental status.
- Personal safety issues.
- Needed resources, possible need for placement.

 Acute Care   Collaborative   Community/Home Care   Cultural

Planning
• Plan of care and who is involved in planning.
• Teaching plan.

Implementation/Evaluation
• Response to interventions, teaching, and actions performed.
• Attainment or progress toward desired outcomes.
• Modifications of plan of care.

Discharge Planning
• Long-term needs and who is responsible for actions to be taken.
• Type of assistance and resources needed.
• Specific referrals made.

References

1. Smith, S. M., et al. (2006). Nutritional status is altered in the self-neglecting elderly. *J Nutr*, 136(10), 2534–2541.
2. Abrams, R. C., et al. (2002). Predictors of self-neglect in community-dwelling elders. *Am J Psychiatry*, 159(10), 1724–1730.
3. Fulmer, T. (2003). Elder abuse and neglect assessment. *Gerontol Nurs*, 29(1), 8–9.
4. Dong, X., Simon, M., Mendes de Leon, C. (2009). Elder self-neglect and abuse and mortality risk in community dwelling populations. *JAMA*, 302(5), 517–526.
5. Brannon, G. E. (Updated 2016). History and mental status examination. *Medscape*. Retrieved April 2018 from http://emedicine.medscape.com/article/293402-overview.
6. Lauder, W., Anderson, I., Barclay, A. (2005). A framework for good practice in interagency interventions with cases of self-neglect. *J Psychiatr Ment Health Nurs*, 12(2), 192–198.
7. Lauder, W., Anderson, I., Barclay, A. (2005). Housing and self-neglect: The responses of health, social care and environmental health agencies. *J Interprof Care*, 19(4), 317–325.
8. Tierney, M., Charles, J., Naglie, G. (2004). Risk factors for harm in cognitively impaired seniors who live alone: A prospective study. *J Am Geriatr Soc*, 52(9), 1435–1441.
9. Nusbaum, N. (2004). Safety vs autonomy: Dilemmas and strategies in protection of vulnerable community dwelling elderly. *Ann Long-Term Care*, 12(5), 50–53.
10. Amanullah, S., Choi, N. (2016). Diogenes syndrome: What you need to know. Retrieved April 2018 from https://www.medicalnewstoday.com/articles/314595.php.
11. Braye, S., Orr, D., Preston-Shoot, M. (2011). Self-neglect and adult safeguarding: Findings from research. *Social Care Institute for Excellence*. Retrieved April 2018 from http://www.scie.org.uk/publications/reports/report46.pdf.

[disturbed Sensory Perception (specify: visual, auditory, kinesthetic, gustatory, tactile, olfactory)]

Taxonomy II: Perception/Cognition—Class 3 Sensation/Perception (00122) [**Diagnostic Division:** Neurosensory], Approved 1978; Revised 1980, 1998 (by small group work 1996); Retired 2012

DEFINITION: Change in the amount or patterning of incoming stimuli accompanied by a diminished, exaggerated, distorted, or impaired response to such stimuli.

RELATED FACTORS
Insufficient environmental stimuli: therapeutically restricted environments (e.g., isolation, intensive care, bedrest, traction, confining illnesses, incubator); socially restricted environment (e.g., institutionalization, homebound, aging, chronic/terminal illness, infant deprivation), stigmatized (e.g., mentally ill/developmentally delayed/handicapped)

Excessive environmental stimuli

Altered sensory reception/transmission/integration

Biochemical imbalances (e.g., elevated blood urea nitrogen [BUN], ammonia; hypoxia; electrolyte imbalance; drugs, e.g., stimulants or depressants, mind-altering drugs)

Psychological stress; sleep deprivation

(continues on page 778)

 Diagnostic Studies
 Evidence Based Practice
 Medications
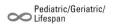 Pediatric/Geriatric/Lifespan

[disturbed Sensory Perception] (continued)

DEFINING CHARACTERISTICS

Subjective
Change in sensory acuity (e.g., photosensitivity, hypoesthesias or hyperesthesias, diminished or altered sense of taste, inability to tell position of body parts [proprioception])
Sensory distortions

Objective
Change in sensory acuity; or in usual response to stimuli
Change in behavior pattern; restlessness; irritability
Change in problem-solving abilities; poor concentration
Disorientation; hallucinations; illusions
Impaired communication
Motor incoordination, altered sense of balance, falls (e.g., Ménière's syndrome)
Sample Clinical Applications: Glaucoma/cataract/other visual impairments; brain tumor, stroke, traumatic injury, amputation, surgery, immobility, peripheral neuropathy (e.g., diabetes), substance abuse, schizophrenia, autism spectrum disorders, developmental delay

DESIRED OUTCOMES/EVALUATION CRITERIA

Sample NOC linkages:
Sensory Function: Extent to which an individual correctly senses skin stimulation, sounds, proprioception, taste and smell, and visual images
Distorted Thought Self-Control: Self-restraint of disruptions in perception, thought processes, and thought content
Risk Control: Hearing/Visual Impairments: Personal actions to understand, prevent, eliminate, or reduce threats to hearing [or] visual function

Client Will (Include Specific Time Frame)
• Regain or maintain usual level of cognition.
• Recognize and correct or compensate for sensory impairments.
• Verbalize awareness of sensory needs and presence of overload and/or deprivation.
• Identify and modify external factors that contribute to alterations in sensory or perceptual abilities.
• Use resources effectively and appropriately.
• Be free of injury.

ACTIONS/INTERVENTIONS

Sample NIC linkages:
Communication Enhancement: Hearing [or] Vision Deficit: Use of strategies augmenting communication capabilities for a person with diminished hearing [or] vision
Peripheral Sensation Management: Prevention or minimization of injury or discomfort in the patient with altered sensation
Hallucination [or] Delusion Management: Promoting the comfort, safety, and reality orientation of a patient experiencing hallucinations [or] false, fixed beliefs that have little or no basis in reality
Environmental Management: Manipulation of the patient's surroundings for therapeutic benefit, sensory appeal, and psychological well-being

 Acute Care   Collaborative   Community/ Home Care   Cultural

NURSING PRIORITY NO. 1   To assess causative/contributing factors:

- Identify client with condition that can affect sensing, interpreting, and communicating stimuli, as noted in Related Factors. *Specific clinical concerns (e.g., neurological disease or trauma, intensive care unit confinement, surgery, pain, biochemical imbalances, psychosis, substance abuse, toxemia) have the potential for altering one or more of the senses, with resultant change in the reception, sensitivity, or interpretation of sensory input.*[1]
- Be aware of current diagnosis or treatments *(e.g., glaucoma, surgery, immobility, recent stroke, diabetes, mental illness; drug toxicity or side effects [e.g., halos around lights, ringing in ears]; middle-ear disturbances [altered sense of balance]) that can cause or exacerbate sensory problems.*
- ∞ Note age and developmental stage. *Problems with sensory perception may be known to client/caregiver (e.g., child wearing hearing aid, elderly adult with known macular degeneration) where compensatory interventions are in place. Screening or evaluation may be required if sensory impairments are suspected but not obvious, as might occur when an infant is not progressing developmentally or an older individual has a gradual loss of sensory discrimination associated with aging, or sensory changes are associated with a sudden neurological event.*[2,3,8]
- Evaluate medication regimen and determine possible use or misuse of drugs (prescription, over the counter, illicit) *to identify effects, side effects, adverse effects, or drug interactions that may be causing or exacerbating sensory or perceptual problems.*
- 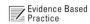 Review results of sensory and motor neurological testing and laboratory studies (e.g., cognitive testing or laboratory values, such as electrolytes, chemical profile, arterial blood gases, serum drug levels) *to note presence or possible cause of changes in response to sensory stimuli.*

NURSING PRIORITY NO. 2   To determine degree of impairment:

- Assess ability to speak, hear, interpret, and respond to simple commands *to obtain an overview of client's mental and cognitive status and ability to interpret stimuli.*
- Evaluate sensory awareness (e.g., hot and cold, dull or sharp, smell, taste, visual acuity and hearing, gait, mobility, location or function of body parts). *Screening can be done in clinic or facility and may identify problems requiring more extensive evaluation.*
- Determine response to touch and painful stimuli *to note whether response is appropriate to stimulus and whether it is immediate or delayed. The sense of touch is usually maintained throughout life and may become more important if other senses are diminished. Different types of touch or contact are associated with different meanings (including communication of ideas, information, emotion).*[3]
- Observe for behavioral responses (e.g., illusions, hallucinations, delusions; withdrawal, hostility, crying, inappropriate affect; confusion or disorientation) *that may indicate mental or emotional problems or chemical toxicity (as might occur with digoxin or other drug overdose or reaction) or be associated with brain or neurological trauma or infection.*
- Note inattention to body parts and segments of environment and lack of recognition of familiar objects or persons. *Loss of comprehension of auditory, visual, or other sensations may be indicative of unilateral neglect or inability to recognize and respond to environmental cues.*[9]
- Ascertain client's perception of problem or changes. Note significant other's (SO's) observations of changes that have occurred and client's responses to changes. *Client may or may not be aware of changes (e.g., diabetic with neuropathy may not realize he or she has lost discrimination for pain in feet, parents may notice child's problem with coordination or difficulty with words).*
- Refer to additional NDs Anxiety, acute/chronic Confusion, risk for Disuse Syndrome, Unilateral Neglect, as appropriate and based on findings.

NURSING PRIORITY NO. 3   To promote normalization of response to stimuli:

General interventions
- Note degree of alteration or involvement (single or multiple senses) *to determine scope and complexity of condition and needed interventions.*

 Diagnostic Studies   Evidence Based Practice   Medications   ∞ Pediatric/Geriatric/Lifespan

- Ascertain and validate client's perceptions. Listen to and respect client's expressions of deprivation *to assist in planning of appropriate care, to identify inconsistencies in reception and integration of stimuli, and to provide compassionate regard for client's feelings.*
- Provide means of communication as indicated by client's current situation.
- Document perceptual deficit in chart and code on wall in client's room, if needed, *so caregivers are aware of specific needs or limitations.*
- Avoid isolating client, physically or emotionally, *to prevent sensory deprivation and limit confusion.*
- Address client by name and have personnel wear name tags and reintroduce self, as needed, *to preserve client's sense of identity and orientation.*
- Reorient to time, place, and situation or events, as necessary, *to reduce confusion and provide sense of normalcy to client's daily life.*
- Explain procedures and activities, expected sensations, and outcomes. *Helpful in reducing anxiety associated with altered interpretation of environment.*
- Promote a stable environment with assignment of same personnel as much as possible *to promote continuity of care and limit confusion.*
- Provide appropriate sensory stimulation, including familiar smells and sounds, tactile stimulation with a variety of objects, and changing of light intensity and other cues (e.g., clocks, calendars).
- Eliminate extraneous noise or stimuli, including nonessential equipment, alarms, and audible monitor signals, when possible. *Reduces anxiety and exaggerated emotional responses or confusion associated with sensory overload.*
- Provide feedback *to assist client to separate reality from fantasy and altered perception.*
- Protect from bodily harm (e.g., falls, burns, positioning problems) *as client may not perceive pain or have impaired sense of position, thereby increasing the risk for falls.*
- Provide undisturbed rest and sleep periods *to reduce anxiety, agitation, or psychosis that can accompany sleep deprivation, particularly when client is confined to bed (e.g., intensive care unit).*
- Plan care with client/SO(s), as appropriate. *Enhances commitment to and continuation of plan, thus optimizing outcomes.*
- Encourage SO(s) to bring in familiar objects and to talk with and touch the client. *Client often can experience positive response to loved ones, thus enhancing recovery.*
- Ⓐ Collaborate with other healthcare team members in providing rehabilitative therapies and stimulating modalities (e.g., music therapy, sensory training, remotivation therapy) *to achieve maximal gains in function and psychosocial well-being.*[10]
- 💊∞ Limit and carefully monitor use of sedation, especially in older population *who are more sensitive to side effects.*
- Identify and encourage use of resources and prosthetic devices (e.g., hearing aids, computerized visual aid or glasses with a level plumb line for balance). *Useful for augmenting senses.*

Visual deficits
- Note particular vision problem (e.g., loss of visual field, change in depth perception, double vision, blindness) *that affects client's ability to perceive environment and learn or relearn motor skills.*[3]
- Speak to visually impaired or unresponsive client frequently, especially when first entering room or client's presence, *to provide auditory stimulation and prevent startle reflex. Note: A recent study on unconscious patients with brain injury supports the theory that sensory stimulation can enhance brain recovery.*[12]
- Approach from visually intact side, position objects to take advantage of intact visual field, and use eye patch, when needed, *to decrease sensory confusion when client has acute loss of vision or field of vision in one eye.*[3]
- Provide or encourage listening to music, radio, TV, talking books, and use of talking timepieces and computers, as appropriate.
- Supply adequate lighting for reading and activities.
- Place glasses or contacts where they can be easily found and encourage client to wear corrective lenses during waking hours.

 Acute Care   Collaborative   Community/ Home Care   Cultural

- Arrange bed, personal articles, and food trays to take advantage of functional vision. *Enhances independence and safety.*
- Describe food and placement, feeding or assisting client as necessary (e.g., cooking, cutting food, offering finger food, placing food in clock-position on plate) *when vision impairments could hinder nutritional intake or cause social discomfort.*
- Assist client with picking out clothing *if problems with color discrimination cause mismatching.*[3]
- Color-code doors and drawers to assist client with low vision *in locating belongings or a particular site (e.g., bathroom).*

Auditory deficits
- Determine if client reads lips and turn toward/face client, making sure you have his/her attention, and enunciating words clearly.
- Encourage client's use of hearing aid when one is available.
- Lower the pitch of the voice and speak in tone that does not include shouting *(which increases the pitch of the voice).*[3]
- Speak slowly and distinctly; use simple sentences. Rephrase sentences rather than repeating them. Avoid asking multiple questions at one time *to enhance client's comprehension and ability to respond.*[13]
- Use touch to get the client's attention, if needed.
- Be aware and careful of facial expressions.
- Pay attention to background noise and reduce it to a minimum when attempting conversation. *Background noise is often amplified, causing misinterpretation of conversation or inability to hear words, and often results in overstimulation of senses.*[3]
- Refer for periodic evaluation by audiologist *to note changes in acuity and determine if client might benefit from a hearing aid.*[3]

Kinesthetic and tactile deficits
- Encourage proper body positioning and alignment *to prevent muscle strain or injury.*
- Provide firm mattress or chair cushion *to maintain positioning and good posture.*
- Assist with or recommend periodic weight shifts *to enhance circulation and relieve tissue pressure, reducing risk of tissue damage.*
- Provide tactile stimulation as care is given and when communicating with or comforting client (respecting cultural and personal preferences). *Communicates presence and connection with other human being because touching is an important part of caring, and the need for touch is a deep psychological need. Note: The meaning people associate with touching is culturally determined to a great degree. Always consider a patient's culturally defined sense of modesty when giving nursing care. A recent research study concludes that nurses touch patients to perform clinical tasks, communicate caring, and ensure comfort. Nurses must exercise clinical judgment in deciding when, where, and how to touch patients. In providing the patient's perspective on intimate touch (e.g., bathing, catheterization, other sensitive procedures), participants said they want to know before intimate touch is provided, why it's necessary, and what it will involve.*[14,15]
- Be aware that older clients may be more desirous of touch than younger people *because they have lost loved ones, their appearance may not be as attractive as it once was, and the attitude of the public toward older adults does not encourage physical contact with them. Note: A recent study found that comfort touch improved the perceptions of self-esteem, well-being and social processes, health status, life satisfaction and self-actualization, faith or belief, and self-responsibility in institutionalized older female residents.*[3,16]
- Stimulate sense of touch (e.g., give client objects to touch, grasp; have client practice touching walls and other boundaries). *Aids in retraining sensory pathways to integrate reception and interpretation of stimuli.*
- Provide touch, using level of appropriate intensity (e.g., light, moderate, deep, strong), *depending on the need (e.g., light touch to get client's attention, stroking to convey love to infant).*[3,4]
- Teach client/SO to frequently inspect skin and extremities for redness, pressure points, bony deformities, or skin trauma *when client is unable to sense pain and is prone to tissue injury.*[5]

 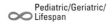

Taste and smell

- Note taste and smell dysfunction (loss or distortion of function) that may be associated with chronic conditions (e.g., cystic fibrosis, chronic sinusitis, hypothyroidism, multiple sclerosis, Alzheimer's disease, head trauma) or may suggest a new or developing problem (e.g., zinc deficiency, dental conditions, allergies).[6]
- Investigate reports of changes in tastes of foods (foods taste or smell odd), ability to salivate, or loss of appetite. *May reflect loss or distortion of smell and taste functions or side effects or interactions with medications.*[3,6,7]
- Encourage client to chew food well and to experiment with a variety of food colors, textures, and flavor enhancers *to maximize taste sensation.*[3,7]
- Discuss with client how he or she can check with others in observing for offensive or dangerous odors (e.g., body odor, spoiled foods, propane gas or smoke) *if sense of smell is diminished.*[3]
- Remove offensive odors from client's presence, especially *when client is immobile, debilitated, and/or suffering from oversensitivity to odors, nausea, or vomiting.*

NURSING PRIORITY NO. 4 To prevent injury/complications:

- Place call bell or other communication device within reach and verify that client knows where it is and how to use it.
- Provide safety measures (e.g., siderails or grab pole, bed in low position, adequate lighting, use of vision or hearing devices, assistance with walking, providing basic and specific information [e.g., "I am on your right side," "This water is hot," "Swallow now," "Stand up"]) *to protect client from injury or enhance client's ability to interpret stimuli.*[10]
- Monitor use of heating pads or lights and ice packs, the temperature of bath water, etc., *to reduce risk of thermal injury.*
- Position doors, rugs, and furniture so they are out of travel path and ambulate with assistance or strategically place grab bars *to aid in maintaining balance and reducing risk for falls.*
- Refer for evaluation of vocational abilities and driving skills. *Changes in sensory reception or integration may impair ability to perform complicated tasks, putting client and others at risk for injury.*
- Refer to NDs risk for Falls, risk for Thermal Injury, and risk for Trauma.

NURSING PRIORITY NO. 5 To promote optimal functioning (Teaching/Discharge Considerations):

- Provide explanations of and plan care with client, involving SO(s) as much as possible. *Enhances commitment to and continuation of plan, optimizing outcomes.*
- Review ways to prevent or limit exposure to conditions affecting sensory functions (e.g., how exposure to loud noise and toxins can impair hearing; early childhood screening for speech and language disorders; vaccines to prevent measles, mumps, and meningitis, once known to be major causes of hearing loss).[11]
- Assist client/SO(s) *to learn effective ways of coping with and managing sensory disturbances, anticipating safety needs according to client's sensory deficits and developmental level.*
- Demonstrate use and care of sensory prosthetic devices (e.g., assistive vision or hearing devices).
- Review home safety measures pertinent to deficits.
- Identify resources and community programs for acquiring and maintaining assistive devices.
- Discuss need for regular evaluation of drug regimen, noting possible toxic side effects or interactions of both prescription and OTC drugs. *Prompt recognition of side effects allows for timely intervention or change in drug regimen.*
- Promote meaningful socialization and diversional activities as able (e.g., TV/radio, conversation, large print or talking books). Refer to NDs decreased Diversional Activity Engagement and Social Isolation for related interventions.
- Refer to helping resources such as Society for the Blind, Self-Help for the Hard of Hearing, or local support groups, screening programs, etc., as indicated.
- Refer to additional NDs Anxiety, acute/chronic Confusion, and Unilateral Neglect as appropriate.

 Acute Care   Collaborative   Community/Home Care   Cultural

DOCUMENTATION FOCUS

Assessment/Reassessment
- Individual findings, noting specific deficit/associated symptoms, perceptions of client/SO(s).
- Safety issues.
- Assistive device needs.
- Availability and use of resources.

Planning
- Plan of care, including who is involved in planning.
- Teaching plan.

Implementation/Evaluation
- Responses to interventions, teaching, and actions performed.
- Attainment or progress toward desired outcome(s).
- Modifications to plan of care.

Discharge Planning
- Long-term needs and who is responsible for actions to be taken.
- Available resources; specific referrals made.

References

1. Newfield, S.A., et al. (2007). ND: Sensory Perception, disturbed. *Clinical Applications of Nursing Diagnosis: Adult, Child, Women's, Psychiatric, Gerontic, and Home Health Considerations.* 5th ed. Philadelphia: F. A. Davis.
2. Engel, J. (2002). *Pocket Guide to Pediatric Assessment.* 4th ed. St. Louis, MO: Mosby.
3. Gallman, L., Elfervig, L. S. (1999). The aging sensory system. In Stanley, M., Beare, P. G. (eds). *Gerontological Nursing: A Health Promotion/Protection Approach.* 2nd ed. Philadelphia: F. A. Davis.
4. D'Apolito, K., McGrath, J., O'Brien, A. (2000). Infant and family centered developmental care guidelines. *National Association of Neonatal Nurses Clinical Practice Guidelines.* 3rd ed. Des Plaines, IL: National Association of Neonatal Nurses.
5. American Diabetes Association. (2003). Preventative foot care in people with diabetes. *Diabetes Care,* 26(1 Suppl), 578–579.
6. Henkin, R. I. (Updated 2018). Taste and Smell Clinic research and clinical overview. Retrieved April 2018 from http://www.tasteandsmell.com/clinical.htm.
7. Leopold, D., Cairns, C. D., Holbrook, E. H. (Updated 2016). Disorders of taste and smell. Retrieved April 2018 from http://emedicine.medscape.com/article/861242-overview.
8. Whiteside, M. M., Wallhagen, M. I., Pettengill, E. (2006). Sensory impairment in older adults: Part 2: Vision loss. *Am J Nurs,* 106(11), 52–61.
9. Baldwin, K. M. (2006). Stroke: It's a knock-out punch. *Nursing Made Incredibly Easy!,* 4(2), 10–23.
10. Muche, J. A., McCarty, S. (Updated 2017). Geriatric rehabilitation. Retrieved April 2018 from http://emedicine.medscape.com/article/318521-overview.
11. National Institute on Deafness and Other Communication Disorders. (Updated 2010). Strategic plan: Plain language version FY 2003–2005. Retrieved April 2018 from http://www.nidcd.nih.gov/about/plans/strategic/pages/strategic03-05PL.aspx.
12. Urbenjaphol, P., Jitpanya, C., Khaoropthum, S. (2009). Effects of the sensory stimulation program on recovery in unconscious patients with traumatic brain injury. *J Neurosci Nurs,* 41(3), E10–E16.
13. Bagai, A., Thavendiranathan, P., Detsky, A. S. (2006). Does this patient have hearing impairment? *JAMA,* 295(4), 416–428.
14. Jonas, I. (Updated 2013). Understanding culture and transcultural nursing: Cultural diversity in nursing practice. Retrieved April 2018 from https://hubpages.com/education/What-is-Transcultural-Nursing.
15. O'Lynn, C., Krautscheid, L. (2011). How should I touch you? A qualitative study of attitudes on intimate touch in nursing care. *Am J Nurs,* 111(3), 24–31.
16. Butts, J. B. (2001). Outcomes of comfort touch in institutionalized elderly female residents. *Geriatr Nurs,* 22(4), 180–184.

 Diagnostic Studies   Evidence Based Practice   Medications 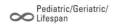 Pediatric/Geriatric/Lifespan

Sexual Dysfunction

Taxonomy II: Sexuality—Class 2 Sexual Function (00059) [**Diagnostic Division:** Sexuality], Approved 1980; Revised 2006, 2017

DEFINITION: A state in which an individual experiences a change in sexual function during the sexual response phases of desire, excitation, and/or orgasm, which is viewed as unsatisfying, unrewarding, or inadequate.

RELATED FACTORS
Inadequate role model
Absence of privacy
Misinformation or insufficient knowledge about sexual function
Vulnerability
Presence of abuse; psychosocial abuse
Value conflict

DEFINING CHARACTERISTICS

Subjective
Change in sexual role
Perceived sexual limitation
Alteration in sexual activity, excitation, or satisfaction; decrease in sexual desire
Undesired change in sexual function
Seeking confirmation of desirability
Change in self-interest/interest toward others
At Risk Population: Absence of significant other
Associated Condition: Alteration in body function or structure [e.g., due to pregnancy, medication, surgery, anomaly, disease, trauma, radiation, etc.]
Sample Clinical Applications: Arthritis, cancer, major surgery, heart disease, hypertension, diabetes mellitus, spinal cord injury (SCI), multiple sclerosis (MS), traumatic injury, pregnancy, childbirth, abuse, depression

DESIRED OUTCOMES/EVALUATION CRITERIA

Sample NOC linkages:
Sexual Functioning: Integration of physical, socioemotional, and intellectual aspects of sexual expression and performance
Physical Aging: Normal physical changes that occur with the natural aging process
Abuse Recovery: Sexual: Extent of healing of physical and psychological injuries due to sexual abuse or exploitation

Client Will (Include Specific Time Frame)
• Verbalize understanding of sexual anatomy, function, and alterations that may affect function.
• Verbalize understanding of individual reasons for sexual problems.
• Identify stressors in lifestyle that may contribute to the dysfunction.
• Identify satisfying, acceptable sexual practices and alternative ways of dealing with sexual expression.
• Discuss concerns about body image, sex role, desirability as a sexual partner with partner/significant other (SO).

 Acute Care   Collaborative   Community/Home Care   Cultural

ACTIONS/INTERVENTIONS

Sample NIC linkages:

Sexual Counseling: Use of an interactive process focusing on the need to make adjustments in sexual practice or to enhance coping with a sexual event or disorder

Teaching: Sexuality: Assisting individuals to understand physical and psychosocial dimensions of sexual growth and development

Values Clarification: Assisting another to clarify her/his own values in order to facilitate effective decision making

NURSING PRIORITY NO. 1   To assess causative/contributing factors:

- Perform a complete history and physical, including a sexual history, noting usual pattern of functioning, level of desire, and problems, such as rape or abuse. *Establishes a database from which an individualized plan of care can be formulated.*
- Note vocabulary and style of communication used by the individual/significant other (SO). *Maximizes communication and understanding of words and meaning in an area that individual may find difficult to discuss. Knowing that male and female brains are organized differently may help with recognizing different styles of communication.*[4]
- Have client describe problem in own words. *Sexual dysfunction is divided into four categories—sexual desire (decreased libido), arousal (erectile dysfunction [ED] or aversion or avoidance of sex), orgasm (delay, absence), and sexual pain disorders (dyspareunia, vaginismus).*[13,15] *Client's perception of the problem may differ from the care provider's, and plan of care needs to be based on client's perceptions for maximum effectiveness.*[1,9]
- Be alert to comments of client. *Sexual concerns are often disguised as humor, sarcasm, or off-hand remarks. Many people are uncomfortable talking about sexual issues but want to discuss them with care provider, so they use this method to bring up the subject. It is important for the caregiver to recognize and acknowledge client's concern.*[2,5]
- Determine importance of sex to individual/partner and client's motivation for change. *Both individuals may have differing levels of desire and expectations that may create conflict in relationship.*[3]
- Assess client's/SO's knowledge of sexual anatomy, function, and effects of current situation or condition (e.g., client's concern about penis size, failure with performance). *Basic knowledge is essential for understanding the problem and how it is affecting the individual. Lack of knowledge may impact client's understanding of situation and expectation for return to previous norm or change for the future.*[3,7]
- Determine preexisting problems or conditions (e.g., illness, surgery, trauma) that may affect current situation and perception of individual/SO. *Physical conditions (e.g., arthritis, MS, hypertension, diabetes mellitus, fatigue, presence of a colostomy, urinary incontinence) can directly affect sexual functioning, or individual can believe that condition precludes sexual activity, such as recent myocardial infarction or heart surgery.*[3,6,7,13,16,18]
- Identify stress factors in individual situation (e.g., marital or job stress, role conflicts). *Interpersonal problems (marital and relationship) and lack of trust and open communication between partners can contribute to difficulties. These factors may be producing enough anxiety to cause depression or other psychological reaction(s) that would cause physiological symptoms.*[5,11]
- Observe behavior and stage of grieving when related to body changes, loss of a body part, or change in function (e.g., pregnancy, obesity, amputation, mastectomy, hysterectomy, menopause). *A change in body image can affect how individual views body in many aspects, but particularly in the sensitive area of sexual functioning and indicates need for information and additional support.*[7,18]
- Discuss cultural values or religious beliefs and conflicts present. *Client may feel guilt or shame about sexual desires or difficulties because of family beliefs about sex and genital area of the body and how sexuality*

was communicated to the client as he or she was growing up or through religious teachings. Note: Research indicates that measurement of acculturation may reveal information about an individual's unique behavioral pattern that is not evident when focusing solely on ethnic group comparisons.[1,2,17]

- Explore with client the meaning of client's behavior. *Masturbation, for instance, may have many meanings or purposes, such as for relief of anxiety, sexual deprivation, pleasure, a nonverbal expression of need to talk, and a way of alienating.*[3] *Or, client's inhibitions may be diminished by changes in cognition.*[12]

- Review medication regimen and drug use (prescription, over the counter, illegal, alcohol) and cigarette use. *Antihypertensives may cause ED; monoamine oxidase inhibitors and tricyclics can cause erection or ejaculation problems and anorgasmia in women; selective serotonin reuptake inhibitor antidepressants can cause decreased libido or orgasm disorders; antihistamines may cause temporary vaginal dryness (dyspareunia); narcotics and alcohol produce ED and inhibit orgasm; and smoking creates vasoconstriction and may be a factor in ED. Evaluation of drug and individual response is important to determine accurate intervention.*[1,10,13,15]

- Review lab results (e.g., hormone levels, serum glucose, red blood cell count, drug levels). *Testing may reveal undiagnosed conditions, such as diabetes resulting in ED in men or anemia, affecting arousal. Inappropriate drug levels or hormone deficiencies—decreased estrogen in women and decreased testosterone in men and women—may result in decreased libido; and hypothyroidism may impair sexual arousal.*

- Assist with or review diagnostic studies to determine cause of ED. *More than half of the cases have a physical cause such as diabetes, vascular problems, etc.* Monitor penile tumescence during rapid eye movement sleep *to determine physical ability. Men are embarrassed to bring up the subject with their healthcare provider even when they are seeing him or her for other conditions; unless the provider specifically asks, the subject is not addressed.*[6,8,9,13]

- Assist with or review diagnostic studies for female sexual disorders (e.g., vaginal photoplethysmography *to assess vaginal blood flow and engorgement,* vaginal pH *to identify infection or diminished secretions,* and biothesiometer *to test sensitivity of clitoris and labia).*[16]

NURSING PRIORITY NO. 2   To assist client/SO(s) to deal with individual situation:

- Establish therapeutic nurse-client relationship. *Promotes treatment and facilitates sharing of sensitive information and feelings in a safe environment.*[1]

- Avoid making value judgments. *They do not help the client to cope with the situation. Nurse needs to be aware of and be in control of own feelings and response to client expressions and/or concerns. Client needs to be free to express concerns in whatever way is comfortable to individual.*[3] *Even clients with limited cognition have a right to engage in intimate behaviors.*[12]

- Assist with treatment of underlying medical conditions, including changes in medication regimen, weight management, cessation of smoking, etc. *Successful treatment/management of many conditions (e.g., cardiovascular, diabetes, arthritis) can improve sexual functioning. However, some treatments and medications also have deleterious affects on sexual abilities/desire.*[7,13–15]

- Collaborate with physical therapist/other specialist to identify mechanical aides that may be useful for clients with physical conditions/disabilities.

- Provide factual information about individual condition (e.g., premature ejaculation, female problems of dyspareunia; low sexual desire). *Accurate information helps client make informed decisions about own situation.*[2,8,15]

- Determine what client wants to know to tailor information to client needs. *Providing too much information may be overwhelming and result in client not remembering something that is essential. Information affecting client safety and consequences of actions may need to be reviewed or reinforced.*[1,7,9]

- Encourage and accept expressions of concern, anger, grief, and fear. *Individuals need to be free to express these feelings and be accepted so they can begin to deal with situation and move on in a positive way.*[6,13]

- Assist client to be aware and deal with stages of grieving for loss or change. *Sexual dysfunction is often a result of losses such as breast cancer treatment or prostate surgery and need to be addressed in the context of the whole. Healthcare providers need to be willing to help client understand grieving issues.*[2,7,11]

 Acute Care   Collaborative   Community/Home Care   Cultural

- Encourage client to share thoughts and concerns with partner and to clarify values or impact of condition on relationship. *Helps to identify issues in the relationship that may be related to the sexual dysfunction.*[3,11,15]
- Provide for or identify ways to obtain privacy to allow for sexual expression for individual or between partners without embarrassment or objections of others. *Often caregivers do not think about the importance of providing this basic need for couples, but in any setting, privacy may be difficult to provide unless it is thought about and planned for.*[6,12]
- Discuss client's rights regarding intimacy in residential or extended care settings with SO/family. Review appropriateness of home visits or provision for privacy for intimate contact. *Family members may not realize that the need for sexual expression is not limited by advancing age, declining cognition, or marital status, and they may be unaware that client has a right to engage in appropriate intimate behaviors.*[12]
- Assist client/SO(s) to problem-solve alternative ways of sexual expression. *When an illness or condition, such as arthritis or paraplegia, interferes with a couple's usual sexual activities, the couple needs to learn new ways to achieve satisfaction.*[3]
- Provide information about availability of corrective measures, including medications such as papaverine, sildenafil (Viagra), or vardenafil (Levitra) *for ED,* or lubricating gels, hormone creams, or possibly hormonal replacement therapy *for vaginal dryness and dyspareunia* as appropriate.[15,16]
- Provide information about availability of corrective measures such as reconstructive surgery (e.g., penile or breast implants), Eros Therapy (handheld device used to improve blood flow to clitoris and external labia to increase sensitivity of tissues), or behavioral therapies (e.g., self-stimulation, sensate focus exercises, Masters & Johnson treatment strategies), when indicated. *Sexual problems, such as ED, female orgasmic disorders, and female sexual arousal disorders, may respond to these interventions, providing more satisfactory sexual life.*[8,10,14–16]
- Refer to appropriate resources as need indicates (e.g., healthcare coworker with greater comfort level and/or knowledgeable clinical nurse specialist or professional sex therapist, family counseling). *Not all professionals are knowledgeable or comfortable dealing with sexual issues, and referrals to more appropriate resources can provide client/couple with accurate assistance.*[2,6,12]

NURSING PRIORITY NO. 3   To promote sexual wellness (Teaching/Discharge Considerations):

- Provide sex education and explanation of normal sexual functioning when necessary. *Many individuals are not knowledgeable about these areas, and often providing accurate information can help assuage anxiety about unknowns, such as normal changes of aging, or provide an accurate basis for understanding problems being experienced.*[6,15,16]
- Provide written material appropriate to individual needs. Include bibliotherapy and reliable Internet resources related to client's concerns. *Provides reinforcement for client to read and access at his or her leisure when ready to deal with sensitive materials.*[3,6,7]
- Encourage ongoing dialogue and take advantage of teachable moments. *Within a therapeutic relationship, comfort is achieved and individual is encouraged to ask questions and be receptive to continuing conversation about sexual issues.*[1,2]
- Demonstrate and assist client to learn relaxation or visualization techniques. *Stress is often a component of sexual dysfunction, and using these skills can help with resolution of problems.*[2,5]
- Identify resources for assistive devices/sexual "aids." *These aids can enhance sex life of couple and prevent or help with problems of dysfunction.*[3,6]
- Emphasize importance of engaging in regular self-examination as indicated (e.g., breast and testicular examinations). *Encourages client to participate in own health prevention activities, become more aware of potential problems, and become more comfortable with sexual self.*[3,5]
- Identify community resources for further assistance, such as Reach for Recovery, Can Surmount, and the Ostomy Association, *to provide role models and to problem-solve issues.*
- Refer for further professional assistance concerning relationship difficulties, low sexual desire, and other sexual concerns such as premature ejaculation, vaginismus, and painful intercourse. *May need additional or*

 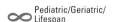

continuing support to deal with individual situation or associated depression. Note: Referral to counselor expert in trauma may be preferred to assist sexual abuse survivors to overcome sexual difficulties.[3,15]

DOCUMENTATION FOCUS

Assessment/Reassessment
- Individual findings, including nature of dysfunction, predisposing factors, perceived effect on sexuality and relationships.
- Cultural or religious factors, conflicts.
- Response of SO(s).
- Motivation for change.

Planning
- Plan of care and who is involved in planning.
- Teaching plan.

Implementation/Evaluation
- Response to interventions, teaching, and actions performed.
- Attainment or progress toward desired outcome(s).
- Modifications to plan of care.

Discharge Planning
- Long-term needs and who is responsible for actions to be taken.
- Community resources, specific referrals made.

References

1. Townsend, M. C. (2003). *Psychiatric Mental Health Nursing Concepts of Care*. 4th ed. Philadelphia: F. A. Davis.
2. Doenges, M. E., Townsend, M. C., Moorhouse, M. F. (1998). *Psychiatric Care Plans: Guidelines for Individualizing Care*. 3rd ed. Philadelphia: F. A. Davis.
3. Hyde, J., DeLamater, J. (2002). *Understanding Human Sexuality*. 7th ed. New York: McGraw-Hill.
4. Moir, A., Jessel, D. (1991). *Brain Sex: The Real Difference Between Men & Women*. New York: Dell.
5. Boston Women's Health Book Collective. (1998). *Our Bodies, Ourselves for the New Century*. 7th ed. Gloucester, MA: Peter Smith.
6. Harvard Medical School. (2010). *Sexuality in Midlife and Beyond: A Harvard Medical School Special Report*. Cambridge, MA: Harvard Health.
7. Stanley, M., Beare, P. G. (1999). *Gerontological Nursing*. 2nd ed. Philadelphia: F. A. Davis.
8. Carver, C. (1998). Premature ejaculation: A common and treatable concern. *J Am Psy Nurs Assoc*, 4(6), 199–204.
9. McEnany, G. (1998). Sexual dysfunction in the pharmacologic treatment of depression: When "don't ask, don't tell" is an unsuitable approach to care. *J Am Psy Nurs Assoc*, 4(1), 24–29.
10. Phillips, N. A. (2000). Female sexual dysfunction: Evaluation and treatment. *Am Family Phys*, 62(1), 127–136.
11. Phillips, R. L., Slaughter, R. (2000). Depression and sexual desire. *Am Family Phys*, 62(4), 782–786.
12. Sisk, J. (2009). Sexuality in nursing homes: Preserving rights, promoting well-being. Retrieved April 2018 from http://www.todaysgeriatricmedicine.com/news/septstory3.shtml.
13. Gaines, R. (2013). What are the root causes of erectile dysfunction? Retrieved April 2018 from https://www.aaghealth.com/blog/sexual-health-2/root-causes-erectile-dysfunction.
14. The Turek Clinic Staff. (Updated 2014). Male sexual health issues and treatment (various pages). Index page retrieved April 2018 from http://theturekclinic.com/services/male-mens-sexual-health/.
15. Swierzewski,, S. J. (Updated 2015). Sexual health overview. Retrieved April 2018 from http://www.healthcommunities.com/sexual-development/sexual-health-overview.shtml.
16. Stoppler, M. C. (2003, updated 2017). Female sexual problems. Retrieved April 2018 from http://www.emedicinehealth.com/female_sexual_problems/article_em.htm.
17. Brotto, L., Chik, H. M., Ryder, A. G. (2004). Acculturation and sexual function in Asian women. *Arch Sex Behav*, 34(6), 613–626.
18. Boyles, S. (2012). AHA: Sex safe for most heart patients. Retrieved April 2018 from http://www.webmd.com/heart-disease/news/20120119/aha-sex-safe-most-heart-patients.

Acute Care   Collaborative   Community/Home Care   Cultural

ineffective Sexuality Pattern

Taxonomy II: Sexuality—Class 2 Sexual Function (00065) [**Diagnostic Division:** Sexuality], Approved 1986; Revised 2006, 2017

DEFINITION: Expressions of concern regarding own sexuality.

RELATED FACTORS
Conflict about sexual orientation or variant preference
Fear of pregnancy or sexually transmitted infection
Impaired relationship with significant other; absence of privacy
Inadequate role model
Insufficient knowledge or skill deficit about alternatives related to sexuality

DEFINING CHARACTERISTICS

Subjective
Alteration in relationship with significant other (SO); change in sexual role
Alteration in/difficulty with sexual activity or behavior
Value conflict
At Risk Population: Absence of significant other
Sample Clinical Applications: Spinal cord injury (SCI), brain injury, stroke, sexually transmitted infection (STI), cancer, mastectomy, hysterectomy, menopause, prostatectomy, gender reassignment

DESIRED OUTCOMES/EVALUATION CRITERIA

Sample **NOC** linkages:
Sexual Identity: Acknowledgment and acceptance of own sexual identity
Child Development: Adolescence: Milestones of physical, cognitive, and psychosocial progression from 12 years through 17 years of age
Role Performance: Congruence of an individual's role behavior with role expectations

Client Will (Include Specific Time Frame)
• Verbalize understanding of sexual anatomy and function.
• Verbalize knowledge and understanding of sexual limitations, difficulties, or changes that have occurred.
• Verbalize acceptance of self in current (altered) condition.
• Demonstrate improved communication and relationship skills.
• Identify individually appropriate method of contraception.

ACTIONS/INTERVENTIONS

Sample **NIC** linkages:
Sexual Counseling: Use of an interactive process focusing on the need to make adjustments in sexual practice or to enhance coping with a sexual event or disorder
Teaching: Sexuality: Assisting individuals to understand physical and psychosocial dimensions of sexual growth and development
Teaching: Safe Sex: Providing instruction concerning sexual protection during sexual activity
Support System Enhancement: Facilitation of support to patient by family, friends, and community

NURSING PRIORITY NO. 1 To assess causative/contributing factors:

- Obtain complete physical and sexual history, as indicated, including perception of normal function. *Sexuality is multifaceted beginning with one's body, biological sex, and gender (biological, social, and legal status as girl/boy, woman/man).*
- Note use of vocabulary (assessing basic knowledge) and comments or concerns about sexual identity. *Components of sexual identity include one's gender identity (how one feels about his or her gender) as well as one's sexual orientation (straight, lesbian, gay, bisexual, transgendered).[12]*
- Determine importance of sexual activity and a description of the problem in the client's own words. Be alert to comments of client/significant other (SO) that may attempt to discount or mask significance of concerns. *Sexual concerns are often disguised as sarcasm, humor, or off-hand remarks.[1,2] Information about client's perception of the problem is essential to planning appropriate care to meet client's needs.*
- Note cultural values or religious beliefs and conflicts that may exist. Elicit impact of perceived problem on SO/family. *Individuals are enculturated as they grow up, and depending on particular family views and taboos, these factors may create conflicts regarding variant sexual practices with resultant feelings of shame and guilt.[8,14–16]*
- Assess stress factors in client's environment that might cause anxiety or psychological reactions. *Sexual variant behaviors, power issues involving SO, adult children, aging, employment, and loss of prowess related to illness or condition are often associated with stress in the client's life.[1,11]*
- Explore knowledge of effects of altered body function or limitations precipitated by illness or medical treatment of alternative sexual responses and expressions (e.g., reassignment procedure). *Client needs to understand when conditions, such as undescended testicle in young male, gender change, and mutilating cancer surgery, have an effect on sexuality.[10]*
- Review medication and substance use history (prescription medication, over-the-counter drugs, alcohol, illicit drugs). *Substance or prescription drug use may affect sexual functioning or be used to relieve anxiety of perceived sexually deviant behavior.[2,17]*
- Explore issues and fears associated with sex. *Possibility of pregnancy, acquiring STIs, trust and control issues, inflexible beliefs, preference confusion, and altered performance need to be addressed so they may be understood and resolved.[3,13]*
- Determine client's interpretation of the altered sexual activity or behavior. *May be a way of controlling partner, provide relief of anxiety or pleasure, or reflect a lack of partner. These behaviors, when related to body changes, including pregnancy, weight loss or gain, or loss of body part, may reflect a stage of grieving.[3,16]*
- ∞ Assess life-cycle issues, such as adolescence, young adulthood, menopause, and aging. *All people are sexual beings from birth to death. Stage of maturation/transition brings changes that affect sexual self and understanding of the normalcy can help individual grow with them.[7,16]*

NURSING PRIORITY NO. 2 To assist client/SO to deal with individual situation:

- Provide atmosphere in which discussion of sexual problems is permitted and encouraged. *Sense of trust and comfort enhances ability to discuss sensitive matters and begin to resolve issues.[5]*
- Avoid value judgments. *They do not help the client to cope with the situation. Nurse needs to be aware of and in control of own feelings and responses to the client's expressions and/or concerns.[9]*
- Provide information about individual situation, determining client needs and desires. *Lack of knowledge may contribute to current situation, and providing desired information conveys message of importance and self-responsibility.[3]*
- Encourage discussion of individual situation and open expression of feelings without judgment. *Sexuality includes feelings, attitudes, relationships, self-image, ideals, and behaviors, and influences how one experiences the world.[12] Talking about sexual practices, concerns about sexual identity, or sexual issues related to illness or condition provides opportunity for resolution.[1,2]*
- Provide specific suggestions about interventions directed toward the identified problems. *Being specific about actions client can take, such as alternate sexual positions when arthritis prevents movement, masturbation*

 Acute Care   Collaborative   Community/Home Care   Cultural

when no partner is available, use of condoms when infection is a concern, and positive discussion of normalcy of sexual behavior when identity is being questioned, can lead discussion in appropriate direction to begin to look for options or solutions.[3,5]

- Identify alternative forms of sexual expression that might be acceptable to both partners. *Being able to communicate satisfactorily with partner and identifying ways to achieve sexual satisfaction for both is important to the relationship.*[1,2]
- Discuss ways to manage individual devices or appliances. *Change in body image or medical condition may require the use of devices, such as an ostomy bag, breast prostheses, or a urinary collection device, that may affect how client views sexual activity. Providing information about ways to deal with these issues helps client to refocus attention on achieving satisfactory sexual experience.*[6,7]
- Discuss use of performance-enhancing medications, such as sildenafil (Viagra), vardenafil (Levitra), and tadalafil (Cialis). *Erectile dysfunction is a common occurrence as men age, and while frequently caused by an underlying physical condition or prescribed medication, psychological issues often accompany this problem. While an accurate diagnosis is necessary, there are many treatments available.*[2,3,17] *Prescription drugs are popular, but the individual needs to feel desire and be sexually stimulated for them to work.*[6]
- ∞ Determine concerns of older client regarding sexuality. *Myths abound regarding sexual activity as people grow older, and individual may believe he or she is no longer attractive or a satisfying sex life is no longer possible; accurate information can correct misperceptions.*[6,7]
- Provide anticipatory guidance about losses that are to be expected. *Surgical procedures resulting in a major change in body image, whether planned (as in transsexual surgery) or unplanned (as in emergency bowel resection with resultant colostomy or traumatic amputation), result in a loss of known self, which needs specific intervention to integrate change.*[3,9]
- Introduce client to individuals who have successfully managed a similar problem, when possible. *Provides a positive role model and support for problem-solving.*[9,18]

NURSING PRIORITY NO. 3 To promote wellness (Teaching/Discharge Considerations):

- 🏠 Provide factual information about problem(s) as identified by the client. *Specific facts about individual situation will provide client with knowledge needed to deal with what is happening, such as conflict with sexual orientation or variant preferences or impaired relationship with SO.*[9]
- Engage in ongoing dialogue with the client and SO(s) as situation permits. *As communication continues, new insights arise and understanding is enhanced.*[2,4]
- Discuss methods, effectiveness, and side effects of contraceptives if indicated. *Assists individual/couple to make an informed decision on a method that meets own values or religious beliefs and allows client to meet needs and desires to plan for and/or prevent pregnancy.*[1,5]
- Refer to community resources as indicated. *May need additional information and support that can be obtained at resources such as Planned Parenthood, gender identity clinic, social services, etc.*[9,14,18]
- Refer for intensive individual/group psychotherapy, which may be combined with couple/family and/or sex therapy, as appropriate.[18]
- Refer to NDs disturbed Body Image, low Self-Esteem (specify), and Sexual Dysfunction.

DOCUMENTATION FOCUS

Assessment/Reassessment
- Individual findings, including nature of concern, perceived difficulties, limitations or changes; specific needs or desires.
- Cultural or religious beliefs, conflicts.
- Response of SO(s).

Planning
- Plan of care and who is involved in the planning.
- Teaching plan.

 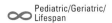

Implementation/Evaluation
- Response to interventions, teaching, and actions performed.
- Attainment or progress toward desired outcome(s).
- Modifications to plan of care.

Discharge Planning
- Long-term needs and teaching, and who is responsible for actions to be taken.
- Community resources, specific referrals made.

References
1. Townsend, M. C. (2015). *Psychiatric Mental Health Nursing Concepts of Care*. 9th ed. Philadelphia: F. A. Davis.
2. Doenges, M. E., Townsend, M. C., Moorhouse, M. F. (1998). *Psychiatric Care Plans: Guidelines for Individualizing Care*. 3rd ed. Philadelphia: F. A. Davis.
3. Hyde, J., DeLamater, J. (2002). *Understanding Human Sexuality*. 7th ed. New York: McGraw-Hill.
4. Moir, A., Jessel, D. (1991). *Brain Sex: The Real Difference Between Men & Women*. New York: Dell.
5. Hahn, C. (2017). 5 effective strategies to help you overcome sexual dysfunction. Retrieved April 2018 from https://www.anxiety.org/how-to-stop-anxiety-and-depression-from-causing-sexual-dysfunction.
6. Harvard Medical School. (2003). *Sexuality in Midlife and Beyond: A Special Health Report from Harvard Medical School*. Cambridge, MA: Harvard Health.
7. Stanley, M., Beare, P. G. (1999). *Gerontological Nursing*. 2nd ed. Philadelphia: F. A. Davis.
8. Johnson, R. (2003). Homosexuality: Nature or nurture. *AllPsych J*. Retrieved April 2018 from http://allpsych.com/journal/homosexuality.html.
9. Becker, J. V., Johnson, B. R. (2004). Sexual and gender identity disorders. In Hales, R. E., Yudofsky, S. C. (eds). *Essentials of Clinical Psychiatry*. 2nd ed. Washington, DC: American Psychiatric Press.
10. Ramirez, M., et al. (2009). Figuring out sex in a reconfigured body: Experiences of female colorectal cancer survivors with ostomies. *Women's Health*, 49(8), 608–624.
11. Meyer, I. H. (2003). Prejudice, social stress, and mental health in lesbian, gay, and bisexual populations: Conceptual issues and research evidenced. *Psychol Bull*, 129(5), 674–697.
12. Planned Parenthood. (2012, updated 2018). Sex & relationships (various pages). Retrieved April 2018 from http://www.plannedparenthood.org/learn/sexuality.
13. Montgomery, K. A. (2008). Sexual desire disorders. *Psychiatry*, 5(6), 674–697.
14. Bazemore, P. H., Wilson, W. H., Bigelow, D. A. (2012). Homosexuality. Retrieved April 2018 from http://www.socialvibes.net/socialvi/2012/05/09/homosexualitymedscape/.
15. American Psychological Association (APA). (2009). Resolution on appropriate affirmative responses to sexual orientation distress and change efforts: Research Summary. Retrieved April 2018 from http://www.apa.org/about/governance/council/policy/sexual-orientation.aspx.
16. Johnson, K. (1997). Human sexual motivation. Retrieved April 2018 from http://www.csun.edu/~vcpsy00h/students/sexmotiv.htm.
17. DeBlasio, C. J., Malcolm, J. B., Derweesh, I. H. (2009). Patterns of sexual and erectile dysfunction and response to treatment in patients receiving androgen deprivation therapy in prostate cancer. *BJU Int*, 102(1), 39–42.
18. Goldberg, J. (2014, updated 2016). When you don't feel at home with your gender. Retrieved April 2018 from http://www.webmd.com/mental-health/gender-dysphoria.

---

risk for Shock

Taxonomy II: Safety/Protection—Class 2 Physical Injury (00205) **[Diagnostic Division:** Circulation], Approved 2008; Revised 2013, 2017

DEFINITION: Susceptible to an inadequate blood flow to the body's tissues that may lead to life-threatening cellular dysfunction, which may compromise health.

RISK FACTORS
To Be Developed
Associated Condition: Hypotension
Hypovolemia
Hypoxemia, hypoxia
Infection, sepsis; systemic inflammatory response syndrome (SIRS)

 Acute Care Collaborative Community/ Home Care Cultural

Sample Clinical Applications: Gastrointestinal (GI) bleed, multiple trauma, disseminated intravascular coagulation (DIC); myocardial infarction, cardiomyopathy, malignant hypertension; pulmonary embolus, pneumothorax; spinal cord injury (SCI), anaphylaxis, sepsis

DESIRED OUTCOMES/EVALUATION CRITERIA

Sample NOC linkages:

Circulation Status: Unobstructed, unidirectional blood flow at appropriate pressure through large vessels of the systemic and pulmonary circuits

Blood Loss Severity: Severity of signs and symptoms of internal or external bleeding

Infection Severity: Severity of signs and symptoms of infection

Client Will (Include Specific Time Frame)

- Display hemodynamic stability as evidenced by vital signs within normal range for client and prompt capillary refill, adequate urinary output with normal specific gravity, and usual level of mentation.
- Verbalize understanding of disease process, risk factors, and treatment plan.
- Be afebrile and free of other signs of infection; achieve timely wound healing.

ACTIONS/INTERVENTIONS

Sample NIC linkages:

Shock Prevention: Detecting and treating a patient at risk for impending shock

Hypovolemia Management: Expansion of intravascular fluid volume in a patient who is volume depleted

Cardiac Care: Limitation of complications resulting from an imbalance between myocardial oxygen supply and demand for a patient with symptoms of impaired cardiac function

NURSING PRIORITY NO. 1   To assess causative/precipitating factors:

- Note possible medical diagnoses or disease processes that can result in one or more types of shock such as major trauma with heavy internal or external bleeding; heart failure; head or spinal cord injury; allergic reactions to insect stings, medications, or foods; pregnancy-related complications; and intra-abdominal infections, ruptured appendix, open wounds, or other conditions associated with sepsis.[1]
- Assess for history or presence of conditions leading to **hypovolemic shock,** such as trauma, surgery, inadequate clotting, and anticoagulant therapy; GI or other organ hemorrhage; prolonged vomiting and diarrhea; diabetes insipidus; and misuse of diuretics. *These conditions deplete the body's circulating blood volume and ability to maintain organ perfusion and function.*[1-3,10]
- Assess for conditions associated with **cardiogenic shock,** including myocardial infarction, cardiac arrest, lethal ventricular dysrhythmias, severe valvular dysfunction, cardiomyopathies, and malignant hypertension. *These conditions directly impair the heart muscle and its ability to pump.*[1-4,11]
- Assess for conditions associated with **obstructive shock,** including pulmonary embolus, aortic stenosis, cardiac tamponade, and tension pneumothorax. *In these conditions the heart itself may be healthy but cannot pump because of conditions outside the heart that prevent normal filling or adequate outflow.*[1-3]
- Assess for conditions associated with **distributive shock—neural induced,** including pain, anesthesia, and SCI or head injury, or **chemical induced,** including peritonitis, sepsis, burns, anaphylaxis, and hyperglycemia. *These situations result in loss of sympathetic tone, blood vessel dilation, pooling of venous blood, and increased capillary permeability with shifting of fluids.*[2,4]
- Monitor for persistent or heavy fluid loss, including wounds, drains, vomiting, gastrointestinal tube, and chest tube. Check all secretions and excretions for occult blood. Refer to NDs risk for Bleeding, deficient Fluid Volume, and risk for imbalanced Fluid Volume for additional interventions.[3,4]

 Diagnostic Studies   Evidence Based Practice   Medications   Pediatric/Geriatric/ Lifespan

- Inspect skin, noting presence of traumatic or surgical wounds, erythema, edema, tenderness, petechiae, and rashes or hives, *for evidence of hemorrhage, localized infections, or hypersensitivity reaction.*[5,7]
- Investigate reports of increased or sudden pain in wounds or body parts, *which could indicate ischemia or infection.*
- Be aware of invasive devices such as urinary and intravascular catheters, endotracheal tube, and implanted prosthetic devices *that potentiate risk for localized and systemic infections.*
- Assess vital signs and tissue and organ perfusion *for changes associated with shock states:*[1-11]

Heart rate and rhythm—noting progressive changes in heart rate *(reflecting an attempt to increase cardiac output)* and development of dysrhythmias *suggesting electrolyte imbalances and hypoxia.*

Respirations—noting rapid, shallow breathing, and use of accessory muscles *(in an attempt to increase vital capacity and compensate for metabolic acidosis associated with poor tissue perfusion and anaerobic metabolism)*, which can progress to respiratory failure.

Blood pressure—noting hypotension (systolic blood pressure 90 mmHg [or lower] lasting more than 30 min), postural hypotension, and narrowed pulse pressure. *May indicate hypovolemia and/or failure of cardiac pumping or compensatory mechanisms.*

Pulses and neck veins—noting rapid, weak, thready peripheral pulses and congested or flat neck veins. *Signs associated with changes in circulating volume, cardiac output, and progressive changes in vascular tone and/or capillary permeability.*

Temperature—higher than 100.4°F (38°C) or lower than 96.8°F (36°C). *Temperature changes in presence of elevated heart rate and respiratory rate along with mildly elevated white blood cells (WBCs) suggest SIRS, which can manifest in client without a documented infection, requiring prompt intervention to prevent progression to sepsis and septic shock.*[5,6]

State of consciousness and mentation—noting anxiety, restlessness, confusion, lethargy, or unresponsiveness. *Can occur because of changes in oxygenation, acid-base imbalances, and toxins associated with hypoperfusion. Depressed mentation accompanied by neck stiffness may reflect central nervous system infection.*

Skin color and moisture—noting overall flushing or pallor, bluish lips and fingernails and slow capillary refill, or cool or clammy skin. *Changes are associated with altered systemic circulation and hypoperfusion.*

Urine output—noting substantially decreased output. *One of the most sensitive indicators of change in circulating volume or poor perfusion.*

Urine characteristics—noting color and odor *suggestive of infection source.*

Bowel sounds—noting diminished or absent bowel sounds or other changes in GI function, such as vomiting, or change in color, amount, or frequency of stools, *reflecting hypoperfusion of GI tract.*

- Measure invasive hemodynamic parameters when available—central venous pressure, mean arterial pressure, and cardiac ouput—*to determine if intravascular fluid deficit or cardiac dysfunction exists.*
- Obtain specimens of wounds, drains, central lines, and blood for culture and sensitivity *to identify offending organisms and to direct antimicrobial therapies.*[8]
- Review lab data such as complete blood count with WBCs and differential; platelet numbers and function; other coagulation factors; tests for cardiac, renal, and hepatic function; pulse oximetry or arterial blood gases, serum lactate, and blood cultures; and urinalysis and urine cultures *to identify potential sources of shock and degree of organ involvement.*
- Review diagnostic studies such as x-ray and electrocardiogram, echocardiogram and angiography with ejection fraction, and computed tomography or magnetic resonance imaging scans and ultrasound *to determine presence of injuries or disorders that could cause or lead to shock conditions.*
- Refer to NDs ineffective peripheral Tissue Perfusion, risk for decreased cardiac Tissue Perfusion, risk for ineffective cerebral Tissue Perfusion, risk for ineffective Gastrointestinal Perfusion, as indicated.

NURSING PRIORITY NO. 2 To prevent/correct potential causes of shock:

- Collaborate in prompt treatment of underlying conditions, such as trauma, heart failure, and infections, and prepare for/assist with medical and surgical interventions *to maximize systemic circulation and tissue and organ perfusion.*

 Acute Care   Collaborative   Community/ Home Care   Cultural

- Administer oxygen by appropriate route (e.g., nasal prongs, mask, ventilator) *to maximize oxygenation of tissues.*
- Administer fluids, electrolytes, colloids, and blood or blood products, as indicated, *to rapidly restore or sustain circulating volume and electrolyte balance and prevent shock states associated with dehydration and hypovolemia.*[3,9,10]
- Administer medications as indicated (e.g., vasoactive drugs, cardiac glycosides, thrombolytics, anticoagulants, antimicrobials, analgesics) *to treat conditions and maximize organ function.*[4]
- Provide client care with infection-prevention interventions, such as diligent hand hygiene, aseptic wound care or dressing changes, isolation precautions, and early intervention in potential infectious condition *to reduce incidence or progression of infection.*[6,7]
- Provide nutrition by best means—oral, enteral, or parenteral feeding. Refer to nutritionist or dietitian *to provide foods rich in nutrients, vitamins, and minerals needed to promote healing and support immune system health.*

NURSING PRIORITY NO. 3 Promote wellness (Teaching/Discharge Considerations):[1,2,7,9]

- Instruct client/significant other in ways to prevent and/or manage underlying conditions that cause shock, including heart disease, injuries, dehydration, and infection.
- Identify reportable signs and symptoms, including unrelieved pain anywhere in body, unresolved bleeding, excessive fluid loss, persistent fever and chills, and change in skin color accompanied by chest pain, *for timely evaluation and intervention.*
- Emphasize need for recognition of substances that cause hypersensitivity or allergic reactions (e.g., insects, medicines, foods, latex) *to reduce risk of anaphylactic shock state.*
- Teach client purpose, dosage, schedule, precautions, and potential side effects of medications given to treat underlying conditions. *Enhances compliance with drug regimen, reducing individual risk.*
- Instruct in wound and skin care as indicated *to prevent infection and promote healing without complications.*
- Teach client/caregivers importance of good hand hygiene, clean environment, and avoiding crowds when ill, especially if client is immunocompromised.
- Reinforce importance of immunization against infections such as influenza and pneumonia, especially in client with chronic conditions.
- Encourage consumption of healthy diet, participation in regular exercise, and adequate rest *for healing and immune system support.*
- Recommend client at risk for hypersensitivity reactions wear medical alert device and maintain readily accessible emergency medication (e.g., Benadryl and/or Epi-pen).

DOCUMENTATION FOCUS

Assessment/Reassessment
- Individual risk factors such as blood loss, presence of infection.
- Assessment findings, including respiratory rate, character of breath sounds; heart rate and rhythm; temperature; frequency, amount, and appearance of secretions; presence of cyanosis; and mentation level.
- Results of laboratory tests and diagnostic studies.

Planning
- Plan of care, specific interventions, and who is involved in the planning.
- Teaching plan.

Implementation/Evaluation
- Client's responses to treatment, teaching, and actions performed.
- Attainment or progress toward desired outcome(s).
- Modifications to plan of care.

 Diagnostic Studies   Evidence Based Practice   Medications   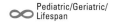 Pediatric/Geriatric/ Lifespan

Discharge Planning
- Long-term needs, identifying who is responsible for actions to be taken.
- Community resources for equipment and supplies post discharge.
- Specific referrals made.

References

1. Cunha, J. P. (Reviewed 2016). Medical shock. Retrieved April 2018 from http://www.medicinenet.com/shock/article.htm.
2. Workman, M. L. (2006). Interventions for clients with shock. In Workman, M. L. (ed). *Medical-Surgical Nursing: Critical Thinking for Collaborative Care*. 5th ed. St. Louis, MO: Elsevier Saunders.
3. Kolarik, M., Roberts, E. (2017). Permissive hypotension and trauma: Can fluid restriction reduce the incidence of ARDS? *J Trauma Nurs*, 24(1), 19–24.
4. Gorman, D., et al. (2008). Take a rapid treatment approach to cardiogenic shock. *Nurs Crit Care*, 3(4), 18–27.
5. Kalil, A., Bailey, L. L. (Updated 2018). Septic shock. Retrieved April 2018 from http://emedicine.medscape.com/article/168402-overview.
6. Nelson, D. P., et al. (2009). Recognizing sepsis in the adult patient. *Am J Nurs*, 109(3), 40–50.
7. Sommers, M. S., Johnson, S. A., Beery, T. A. (2007). *Diseases and Disorders: A Nursing Therapeutics Manual*. 3rd ed. Philadelphia: F. A. Davis.
8. Makic, M. B. F., Bridges, E. (2018). Managing sepsis and septic shock: Current guidelines and definitions. *Am J Nurs*, 118(2), 34–36.
9. Maier, R. V. (2005). Approach to the patient with shock. In Kasper, D. L., Harrison, T. R. (eds). *Harrison's Principles of Internal Medicine*. 16th ed. New York: McGraw-Hill.
10. Martin, N. D., Scantling, D. (2015). Hospital-acquired anemia: A contemporary review of etiologies and prevention strategies. *J Infus Nurs*, 38(8), 330–338.
11. Ren, X. (Mike), Lenneman, A. (Updated 2017). Cardiogenic shock. Retrieved April 2018 from http://emedicine.medscape.com/article/152191-overview.

impaired Sitting

Taxonomy II: Safety/Protection—Class 2 Activity/Exercise (000237) **[Diagnostic Division:** Safety], Approved 2013; Revised 2017

DEFINITION: Limitation of ability to independently and purposefully attain and/or maintain a rest position that is supported by the buttocks and thighs in which the torso is upright.

RELATED FACTORS
Insufficient endurance, energy or muscle strength
Malnutrition
Pain; self-imposed relief posture

DEFINING CHARACTERISTICS

Objective
Impaired ability to attain or maintain a balanced position of the torso; impaired ability to stress torso with body weight
Impaired ability to adjust position of one or both lower limbs on uneven surface
Impaired ability to flex or move both hips or knees
Associated Condition: Alteration in cognitive functioning; neurological or psychological disorder
Impaired metabolic functioning; sarcopenia
Orthopedic surgery; prescribed posture
Sample Clinical Applications: Neuromuscular disorders (e.g., multiple sclerosis [MS], amyotrophic lateral sclerosis [ALS], Parkinson's disease), traumatic injuries (e.g., fractures, spinal cord or brain injuries), rheumatoid arthritis, severe depression, dementia

 Acute Care   Collaborative   Community/Home Care   Cultural

DESIRED OUTCOMES/EVALUATION CRITERIA

Sample NOC linkages:
Knowledge: Body Mechanics: Extent of understanding conveyed about proper body alignment, balance, and coordinated movement
Balance: Ability to maintain body equilibrium
Body Mechanics Performance: Personal actions to maintain proper body alignment and to prevent musculoskeletal strain

Client Will (Include Specific Time Frame)
• Verbalize understanding of individual treatment regimen and safety measures.
• Attain and maintain sitting position that enables activities.
• Participate in activities of daily living (ADLs) and desired activities and prevent complications.

ACTIONS/INTERVENTIONS

Sample NIC linkages:
Positioning: Deliberative placement of the patient or a body part to promote physiological and/or psychological well-being
Exercise Therapy: Muscle Control: Use of specific activity or exercise protocols to enhance or restore controlled body movement
Body Mechanics Promotion: Facilitating the use of posture and movement in daily activities to prevent fatigue and musculoskeletal strain or injury

NURSING PRIORITY NO. 1   To identify causative/contributing factors:

• Determine diagnosis that contributes to sitting balance problems (e.g., MS, arthritis, Parkinson's disease, cardiopulmonary disorders, back pain conditions with client use of compensatory positions to reduce pain; traumatic brain injury, spinal cord injury with hemi/paraplegia; lower-limb injuries or amputations; psychiatric conditions including severe depression, dementias). *These conditions can cause postural impairments, muscular weakness, and inadequate range of motion. Sensory deficits may also be involved (e.g., impaired proprioception and/or visual processing, cognitive impairments). Note: Several studies have shown that sitting balance is a valid predictor for functional outcome in patients with stroke, paraplegia, and brain injury.*[1-6] *Sitting and standing balance are of major concern when assessing amputee's ability to maintain the center of gravity over the base of support. Both balance and coordination are required for weight shifting from one limb to another, thus improving the potential for an optimal gait.*[7]
• Note factors affecting current situation (e.g., surgery, fractures, amputation, tubings [chest tube, indwelling catheter, IVs, pumps]; potential time involved [e.g., few hours in bed after surgery versus serious trauma requiring long-term bedrest or debilitating disease or pain limiting movement]). *Identifies potential impairments and determines type of interventions needed to provide for client's safety.*
• ∞ Note older client's general health status. *Davis et al identified mobility as the most important functional ability that determines the degree of independence and healthcare-related quality of life (HRQol) among older persons.*[8] *While aging does not cause impaired mobility, per se, several aging-related changes can lead to immobility (e.g., sarcopenia with diminished endurance and core strength; impaired vision; loss of balance; decreased ability to quickly and adequately correct movements affecting center of gravity). Thus, falls are a major risk and source of morbidity and mortality.*[9-11]
• Assess nutritional and hydration status and client's report of energy level. *Deficiencies in nutrients and water, as well as electrolytes and minerals, can negatively affect energy and activity tolerance. Note: Research*

 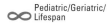

supports that the obese individual shows reduced seated functional reach abilities when compared to normal and overweight subjects.[12]

NURSING PRIORITY NO. 2 To assess functional ability:

• Determine functional status using a 0 to 4 scale, noting muscle strength and tone, joint mobility, cardiovascular status, balance, and endurance. *Identifies strengths and deficits (e.g., inability to sit upright, reach forward, or transfer safely from bed to wheelchair) and may provide information regarding potential for recovery (e.g., client with severe brain injury may have permanent limitations because of impaired cognition affecting memory, judgment, problem-solving, and motor planning).*[1,14]

• Determine degree of perceptual or cognitive impairment and ability to follow directions. *Impairments related to age, chronic or acute disease condition, trauma, surgery, or medications require alternative interventions or changes in plan of care.*

• Refer to physician and/or physical therapy specialists for special testing, as indicated. *May include many different functional tests (e.g., function in sitting test, balance performance monitor, Berger Balance Scale) to determine potential for improvement and direction for therapies.*[13]

NURSING PRIORITY NO. 3 To promote optimal level of function and prevent complications:

• Assist with treatment of underlying condition(s) *to maximize potential for optimal function.*

• Encourage client's participation in self-care activities and in physical or occupational therapies. *Improves body strength and function and enhances self-concept and sense of independence. Note: Sitting balance affects ADLs, including feeding, dressing, bathing, transfers, and mobility.*

• Support trunk and extremities when in seated position, using pillows or rolls, braces, shoes, gel pads, etc., *to maintain upright position and optimal internal organ function and to reduce risk of pressure ulcers.*

• Demonstrate and assist with use of assistive devices (e.g., side rails, overhead trapeze, roller pads, safety belt, hydraulic lifts, chairs) *for position changes and safe transfers.*

• Avoid routinely doing for client those activities that client can do for self. *Caregivers can contribute to deficits by being overprotective or helping too much.*

• Provide for safety measures as indicated by individual situation, including environmental management and fall prevention. (Refer to ND risk for Falls.)

• Note changes in ability to do more or less self-care (e.g., hygiene, feeding, toileting, therapies) *to promote psychological and physical benefits of self-care and to adjust level of assistance as indicated.*

• Collaborate with physical medicine specialist and occupational or physical therapists in providing range-of-motion exercise (active or passive), isotonic muscle contractions (e.g., sitting reach, push, and pull exercises), assistive devices, and activities.

• Administer pain medications before activity as needed *to promote maximal effort and involvement in activity.*

• Collaborate with nutritionist in providing nutritious foods and needed feeding assistance, maximizing client's abilities in ingesting and swallowing (upright position) *to optimize available energy for activities.*

• Refer to NDs Activity Intolerance, impaired bed Mobility, impaired physical Mobility, impaired Transfer Ability, impaired Standing, impaired wheelchair Mobility, and impaired Walking for additional interventions.

NURSING PRIORITY NO. 4 To promote wellness (Teaching/Discharge Considerations):

• Encourage client's/significant other's (SO's) involvement in decision making as much as possible. *Enhances commitment to plan, optimizing outcomes.*

• Demonstrate use of mobility devices (e.g., walkers, strollers, scooters, braces, prosthetics) and have client/caregiver demonstrate knowledge about and safe use of device. Identify appropriate resources for obtaining and maintaining appliances or equipment. *Safe use of mobility aides promotes client's independence and enhances quality of life and safety for client and caregiver.*

 Acute Care   Collaborative   Community/ Home Care   Cultural

- Discuss ways that client can exercise safely. *Options may be limited, but attending regular rehab sessions may provide best opportunity for improvement in function, including self-care, social independence, and recreation.*
- Involve client and SO(s) in care, assisting them to learn ways of managing problems of immobility and imbalanced sitting, especially when impairment is expected to be long term. Refer to support and community services as indicated *to provide care, supervision, companionship, respite services, nutritional and ADL assistance, adaptive devices or changes to living environment, financial assistance, etc.*

DOCUMENTATION FOCUS

Assessment/Reassessment
- Individual findings, including level of function and ability to participate in specific or desired activities.

Planning
- Plan of care and who is involved in the planning.
- Teaching plan.

Implementation/Evaluation
- Responses to interventions, teaching, and actions performed.
- Attainment or progress toward desired outcome(s).
- Modifications to plan of care.

Discharge Planning
- Discharge and long-term needs, noting who is responsible for each action to be taken.
- Specific referrals made.
- Sources of and maintenance for assistive devices.

References

1. Black, K., et al. (2000). Sitting balance following brain injury (does it predict outcome?). *Brain Inj*, 14(2), 141–152.
2. Wade, D. T., et al. (1984). Therapy after stroke: Amounts, determinants and effects. *Int Rehabil Med*, 6(3), 105–110.
3. Gorman, S. L., et al. (2010). Development and validation of the Function In Sitting Test in adults with acute stroke. *J Neurol Phys Ther*, 34(3), 150–160.
4. Juneja, G., Czyrny, J. J., Linn, R. T. (1998). Admission balance and outcomes of patients admitted for acute inpatient rehabilitation. *Arch Phys Med Rehabil*, 77(5), 388–393.
5. Feigen, L., et al. (1996). Sitting equilibrium 2 weeks after stroke can predict walking ability after six months. *Gerontology*, 42(6), 348–353.
6. Nixon, V. (1985). *Spinal Cord Injury: A Guide to Functional Outcomes in Physical Therapy Management*. Rockville, MD: Aspen.
7. Gaily, R. S., Clark, C. S. (2002). Physical therapy management of adult lower-limb amputees. *Atlas of Limb Prosthetics. Online Orthotics and Prosthetics Virtual Library*. Retrieved April 2018 from http://www.oandplibrary.org/alp/chap23-01.asp.
8. Davis, J. C., Bryan, S., Best, J. R. (2015). Mobility predicts change in older adults' health-related quality of life: Evidence from a Vancouver falls prevention prospective cohort study. *Health Qual Life Outcomes*, 13, 101–111.
9. Rowe, J. W., Kahn, R. L. (1987). Human aging: Usual and successful. *Science*, 237(4811), 143–149.
10. Tinetti, M. E., Williams, T. F., Mayewski, R. (1986). Fall risk index for elderly patients based on number of chronic disabilities. *Am J Med*, 80(3), 429–434.
11. Michael, K. M., Allen, J. K., Macko, R. F. (2006). Fatigue after stroke: Relationship to mobility, fitness, ambulatory activity, social support, and falls efficiency. *Rehabil Nurs*, 31(5), 210–217.
12. Kumareason, A., Pathrap, S., Anadh, V. (2012). Influence of body mass index on balance in sitting and standing. *JC PR*, 4(5), 22–27.
13. Gorman, S. L., Rivera, M., McCarthy, L. (2014). Reliability of the function in sitting test (FIST). *Rehabil Res Pract*. Retrieved April 2018 from http://www.hindawi.com/journals/rerp/2014/593280/.
14. Dworak, P. A., Levy, A. (2005). Strolling along. *Rehabil Manage*, 18(9), 26–31.
15. Gordon, M. (2009). Functional levels code. *Manual of Nursing Diagnosis*. 12th ed. Sudbury, MA: Jones and Bartlett.

 Diagnostic Studies   Evidence Based Practice   Medications 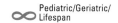 Pediatric/Geriatric/Lifespan

impaired Skin Integrity

Taxonomy II: Safety/Protection—Class 2 Physical Injury 00046) [**Diagnostic Division:** Safety], Approved 1975, Revised 1998, 2017

DEFINITION: Altered epidermis and/or dermis.

RELATED FACTORS

External
Chemical injury agent
Hypothermia; hyperthermia
Humidity; moisture; excretions; secretions
Extremes of age

Internal
Alteration in fluid volume
Inadequate nutrition
Psychogenic factor [e.g., obsessive compulsive disorder]

DEFINING CHARACTERISTICS

Subjective
 Pain; [itching, numbness of affected/surrounding area]

Objective
Alteration in skin integrity
Bleeding; hematoma, redness; localized area hot to touch
Foreign matter piercing skin
At Risk Population: Extremes of age
Associated Condition: Alteration in metabolism; hormonal change; immunodeficiency
Alteration in skin turgor, sensation, pigmentation
Arterial puncture; vascular trauma
Pharmaceutical agent; radiation therapy
Sample Clinical Applications: Anemias; arthritis; end-of-life conditions; contagious diseases, coronary artery disease; dementias; burns; diabetes mellitus, obesity; peripheral vascular disease, Raynaud's disease

DESIRED OUTCOMES/EVALUATION CRITERIA

Sample NOC linkages:
Tissue Integrity: Skin & Mucous Membranes: Structural intactness and normal physiological function of skin and mucous membranes
Wound Healing: Primary Intention: Extent of regeneration of cells and tissues following intentional closure
Wound Healing: Secondary Intention: Extent of regeneration of cells and tissues in an open wound

Client Will (Include Specific Time Frame)
• Display timely healing of skin lesions, wounds, or pressure sores without complication.
• Maintain optimal nutrition and physical well-being.
• Participate in prevention measures and treatment program.
• Verbalize feelings of increased self-esteem and ability to manage situation.

 Acute Care   Collaborative   Community/ Home Care   Cultural

ACTIONS/INTERVENTIONS

Sample NIC linkages:

Wound Care: Prevention of wound complications and promotion of wound healing

Incision Site Care: Cleansing, monitoring, and promotion of healing in a wound that is closed with sutures, clips, or staples

NURSING PRIORITY NO. 1   To assess causative/contributing factors:

- Identify underlying condition or pathology involved. *Skin integrity problems can be the result of (1) disease processes that affect circulation and perfusion of tissues (e.g., arteriosclerosis, venous insufficiency, hypertension, obesity, diabetes, malignant neoplasms); (2) conditions that can be associated with rashes (e.g., contagious diseases such as measles, chicken pox; infections such as methicillin-resistant Staphylococcus aureus, toxic shock syndrome; skin disorders such as eczema; disorders caused by spiders/insects such as Lyme disease, lice, bedbugs; contact dermatitis such as occurs with latex allergy, poison ivy; autoimmune disorders such as lupus; internal diseases such as liver disease, celiac disease, kidney failure, iron deficiency anemia, thyroid problems, and cancers, including leukemia and lymphoma); (3) medications that adversely affect skin or impair healing (e.g., anticoagulants, antibiotics, corticosteroids, immunosuppressives, antineoplastics); (4) burns or radiation (can break down internal tissues as well as skin); and (5) nutrition and hydration (e.g., malnutrition deprives the body of protein and calories required for cell growth and repair, dehydration impairs transport of oxygen and nutrients).*[1,2,5,12,19]
- Note: Disruption in skin integrity can be **intentional** (e.g., surgical incision) or **unintentional** (e.g., accidental trauma, drug effect, allergic reaction, rashes); and **open** (e.g., laceration, skin tears, penetrating wound, ulcerations) or **closed** (e.g., contusion, abrasion, rash).
- Evaluate client's health status in general terms. *Many factors (e.g., debilitation; immobility; use of restraints; extremes of age; mental status; dehydration or malnutrition; presence of chronic disease; occupational, treatment, and environmental hazards) can affect the ability of the skin to perform its functions (e.g., protection, sensation, movement and growth, chemical synthesis, immunity, thermoregulation and excretion).*[3,4]
- ∞ Determine client's age and developmental factors and ability to care for self. *Newborn/infant's skin is thin, provides ineffective thermal regulation, and nails are thin. Infant skin also has a higher absorption and deabsorption rate as compared with an adult's skin, which predisposes infants to a dry, flaky, and impaired skin barrier.[9] Babies and children are prone to skin rashes associated with viral, bacterial, and fungal infections and allergic reactions. In adolescence, hormones stimulate hair growth and sebaceous gland activity.[1,3,4,6] In adults, it takes longer to replenish epidermis cells, resulting in increased risk of skin cancers and infection. In older adults, there is decreased epidermal regeneration, fewer sweat glands, less subcutaneous fat, elastin, and collagen, causing skin to become thinner, drier, and less responsive to pain sensations.*[7,12]
- Evaluate client's skin care practices and hygiene issues. *Individual's skin may be oily, dry and scaly, or sensitive and is affected by bathing frequency (or lack of bathing), temperature of water, and types of soap and other cleansing agents. Incontinence (urinary or bowel) and ineffective hygiene can result in serious skin impairment and discomfort.*[17]
- Note presence of compromised mobility, sensation, vision, hearing, or speech *that may impact client's self-care as relates to skin care (e.g., diabetic with impaired vision probably cannot satisfactorily examine own feet).*[10,12]
- Ascertain allergy history. *Individual may be sensitive or allergic to substances (e.g., insects, grasses, medications, lotions, soaps, foods) that can adversely affect the skin.*
- Assess blood supply (e.g., capillary return time, color, warmth) and sensation of skin surfaces, pressure points, and broken or abraded skin areas on a regular basis *to provide comparative baseline and opportunity for timely intervention when problems are noted.*[3]

 Diagnostic Studies   Evidence Based Practice   Medications   ∞ Pediatric/Geriatric/Lifespan

- Note distribution and scarcity of hair *(e.g., loss of hair on lower legs may indicate peripheral vascular disease).* Refer to ND risk for Peripheral Neurovascular Dysfunction for additional interventions.[13]
- Calculate ankle-brachial index *to evaluate actual or potential for impairment of circulation to lower extremities. Result less than 0.9 indicates need for close monitoring or more aggressive intervention (e.g., tighter blood glucose and weight control in diabetic client).*[14]
- Determine treatment-related skin or tissue conditions (e.g., surgical incision, IV/invasive line insertion site, use of restraints). Assess surgical sites *for signs of infection (e.g., swelling, redness, pain);* assess IV site *for infiltration (e.g., swelling, erythema, coolness, pain; failure of infusion) or evidence of extravasation (e.g., blistering, blanching, skin sloughing).*[4] Evaluate skin surrounding restraints for abrasions, contusions, skin breaks, or skin color and temperature changes distal to restraints *suggesting impaired circulation.*
- Review lab results (e.g., hemoglobin/hematocrit, blood glucose, blood and/or wound culture, sensitivities for infectious agents [viral, bacterial, fungal], albumin, protein) *to evaluate causative factors or ability to heal. Note: Albumin less than 3.5 correlates to decreased wound healing and increased incidence of pressure ulcers.*[1,14,15]

NURSING PRIORITY NO. 2   To assess extent of involvement/injury:

- ∞ Obtain a complete history of current skin condition(s) (especially in children where recurrent rash or lesions are common), including age at onset, date of first episode, duration, original site, characteristics of lesions, and any changes that have occurred. *Common skin manifestations of sensitivity or allergies are hives, eczema, and contact dermatitis. Contagious rashes include measles, rubella, roseola, chickenpox, and scarlet fever. Bacterial, viral, and fungal infections can also cause skin problems (e.g., impetigo, cellulitis, cold sores, shingles, athlete's foot, candidiasis, diaper rashes).*[5,6,19]
- Perform routine skin inspections describing observed changes. Note color, temperature, surface changes, texture, and contours. Evaluate color changes in areas of least pigmentation (e.g., sclera, conjunctiva, nailbeds, buccal mucosa, tongue, palms, soles of feet). *Systematic inspection can identify improvement or changes for timely intervention.*

General wounds/lesions
- Describe rash or lesion, noting color, location, and significant characteristics (e.g., flat or raised rash, weeping or painful blisters, itching wheal) and surrounding information (e.g., exposure to contagious disease, reaction to medication, recent insect bite, ingrown toenail, sexually transmitted infection) *to assist in diagnosing problem and needed interventions.*
- Determine anatomic location and depth of skin or tissue injury or damage (e.g., epidermis, dermis, underlying issues) and describe (e.g., skin tear, partial or full-thickness burn) *to provide baseline and document changes.*[3,12]
- Utilize a skin integrity risk assessment tool (e.g., The International Skin Tear Advisory Panel (ISTAP) skin tears classification and risk assessment tool, or the Payne-Martin classification system) *to classify skin tears according to evidence-based practice guidelines.*[21]
- Photograph lesion(s) as appropriate *to document status and provide visual baseline for future comparisons.*
- Note character and color of drainage, when present (e.g., blood, bile, pus, stoma effluent), *which can cause or exacerbate skin irritation or excoriation.*

Pressure ulcers/decubitus
- Determine, document, and reassess periodically (1) dimensions and depth in centimeters; (2) exudates—color, odor, and amount; (3) margins—fixed or unfixed; (4) tunneling or tracts; and (5) evidence of necrosis (e.g., color gray to black), or healing (e.g., pink or red granulation tissue) *to establish comparative baseline and evaluate effectiveness of interventions.* Refer to ND risk for Pressure Ulcer for assessments and preventive interventions.[8,12,15]

NURSING PRIORITY NO. 3   To determine impact of condition:

- Determine if wound is acute (e.g., injury from surgery or trauma) or chronic (e.g., venous or arterial insufficiency), *which affects healing time and the client's emotional and physical responses. For example, an acute*

 Acute Care   Collaborative   Community/ Home Care   Cultural

and noninfected wound can heal in about 4 weeks, while a chronic wound often does not progress through phases of healing in an orderly or timely fashion.[8]

- Determine client's level of discomfort (e.g., can vary widely from minor itching or aching to deep pain with burns or excoriation associated with drainage) *to clarify intervention needs and priorities.*
- Ascertain attitudes of individual/significant others(s) about condition (e.g., cultural values, stigma). Obtain or review psychological assessment of client's emotional status, noting potential or sexual problems arising from presence of condition. *The healthy wholeness and beauty of skin impacts the client's body image and self-esteem. Lesions or wounds that disfigure can be especially devastating.*

NURSING PRIORITY NO. 4 To assist client with correcting/minimizing condition and achieving optimal healing:

- Practice and instruct client/caregiver(s) in scrupulous hand hygiene and clean or sterile technique *to reduce incidence of contamination or infection.*
- Provide optimum nutrition (including adequate protein, lipids, calories, trace minerals, and multivitamins [e.g., A, C, D, E]) *to promote skin health and healing and to maintain general good health.*
- Provide adequate hydration (e.g., oral, tube feeding, IV, ambient room humidity) *to reduce and replenish transepidermal water loss.*
- **Manage itching conditions:**[5,19,20]
  Cover itchy area, trim nails, and wear gloves at night.
  Apply cool, wet compresses.
  Take a lukewarm bath with baking soda, uncooked oatmeal, or colloidal oatmeal—a finely ground oatmeal made for the bathtub (e.g., Aveeno).
  Choose mild soaps without dyes or perfumes. Rinse the soap completely off body.
  Use a mild, unscented laundry detergent when washing clothes, towels, and bedding.
  Avoid substances that irritate skin or that cause an allergic reaction (e.g., nickel, jewelry, perfume or skin products containing fragrance).
  Encourage use of stress-management techniques (e.g., biofeedback, meditation, yoga).
- Apply high-quality moisturizing cream (e.g., Eurecin) or anti-itch creams (e.g., hydrocortisone cream, menthol, camphor, calamine) or topical anesthetics (e.g., lidocaine or benzocaine), concentrating on the areas where itching is most severe.
- Encourage client to verbalize feelings and discuss how or if condition affects self-concept. (Refer to NDs disturbed Body Image and situational low Self-Esteem.)
- Assist client to work through stages of grief and feelings associated with individual condition.
- Use touch, facial expressions, and tone of voice *to lend psychological support and acceptance of client.*
- Refer for counseling and/or behavior modification therapy, if indicated. *Client may need additional medical/psychological interventions if itching is severe, prolonged, or believed to be psychogenic in origin.*[20]
- **Promote wound healing:**[1,11–13,16]
  Keep surgical area(s) clean and dry, carefully dress wounds, support incision (e.g., use of Steri-Strips, splinting when coughing), and stimulate circulation to surrounding areas *to assist body's natural process of repair.*
  Consult with physician or wound specialist as indicated *to assist with developing plan of care for problematic or potentially serious wounds.*
  Assist with débridement or enzymatic therapy as indicated (e.g., burns, skin tears, severe pressure sores) *to remove nonviable, contaminated, or infected tissue.*[12,16]
  Use body temperature physiological solutions (e.g., isotonic saline) *to clean or irrigate wounds and prevent washout of electrolytes.*
  Cleanse wound with irrigation syringe or gauze squares, avoiding cotton balls or other products *that shed fibers.*
  Maintain appropriate moisture environment for particular wound (e.g., expose lesions or ulcer to air and light if excess moisture is impeding healing, use occlusive dressings to maintain a moist environment for autolytic débridement of wound) as indicated.[12,16]

 Diagnostic Studies   Evidence Based Practice   Medications   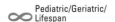 Pediatric/Geriatric/Lifespan

Use appropriate barrier dressings or wound coverings (e.g., semipermeable, occlusive, wet-to-damp, Duo-Derm, Tegaderm, hydrocolloid, hydrofiber or gel, hydropolymers), drainage appliances, and skin-protective agents for open or draining wounds and stomas *to protect wound and surrounding tissues from excoriating secretions or drainage and to promote wound healing.*[12,16]

Administer topical or systemic drugs as indicated *for individual situation.*

- **Prevent skin impairment:**[3–5,7,11,13,17,18]

Maintain or instruct in overall skin hygiene (e.g., shower instead of bathe, wash thoroughly, pat dry, gently massage with lotion or appropriate cream) *to provide barrier to infection, reduce risk of dermal trauma, improve circulation, and enhance comfort.*

Cleanse skin after toileting and incontinent or diaphoretic episodes *to restore normal skin pH and flora and limit potential for infection.*

Use proper turning and transfer techniques. Avoid movements *(e.g., pulling client with parallel force, dragging) that cause friction or shearing.*

Encourage early ambulation or mobilization. *Reduces risks associated with immobility.*

Develop regularly timed repositioning schedule for client with mobility and sensation impairments, using turn sheet as needed; encourage or assist with periodic weight shifts for client in chair *to reduce stress on pressure points and to promote circulation to tissues.*

Use appropriate padding or pressure-reducing devices (e.g., heel rolls, foam boots, egg crate, gel pads) or pressure-relieving devices (e.g., air or water mattress) when indicated *to reduce pressure on sensitive areas and enhance circulation to compromised tissues.*

Avoid or limit use of plastic material (e.g., rubber sheet, plastic-backed linen savers) and remove wet or wrinkled linens promptly. *Moisture potentiates skin breakdown and increases risk for infection.*

Remove adhesive products with care, removing on horizontal plane, and using mineral oil or Vaseline for softening, if needed, *to prevent abrasions or tearing of skin.*

Secure dressings with tape (e.g., elastic, paper tape, nonadherent dressings) or Montgomery straps when frequent dressing changes are required. Use stockinette, tubular or gauze wrap, or similar product instead of tape to secure dressings and drains *to limit dermal injury.*[12]

Apply hot and cold applications judiciously *to reduce risk of dermal injury in persons with circulatory and neurosensory impairments.*

Avoid use of latex products *when client has known or suspected sensitivity.* Refer to ND Latex Allergy Response.

NURSING PRIORITY NO. 5 To promote wellness (Teaching/Discharge Considerations):

- Discuss importance of skin and measures to maintain proper skin functioning. *The integumentary system is the largest multifunctional organ of the body and thus merits special care.*
- Review benefits of following medical regimen. *Enhances commitment to plan, optimizing outcomes.*
- Encourage regular inspection and monitoring of skin for changes or failure to heal. *Early detection and reporting to healthcare providers promotes timely evaluation and intervention.*
- Identify safety measures for client with persistent sensation impairments. *Proper care of skin and extremities during cold or hot weather (e.g., wearing gloves; clean, dry socks; properly fitting shoes or boots; face protection) reduces risk of injury.*[10,14]
- Encourage continued mobility, activity, and range of motion *to enhance circulation and promote health of skin and other organs.*
- Discuss avoidance of products containing perfumes, dyes, preservatives *(may cause dermatitis reactions)* or alcohol, povidone-iodine, and hydrogen peroxide *(may hinder wound healing).*
- Encourage restriction or abstinence from smoking, *which causes vasoconstriction.*
- Review measures *to avoid spread or reinfection of communicable conditions.*
- Discuss proper and safe use of equipment or appliances (e.g., heating pad, ostomy appliances, padding straps of braces).

 Acute Care   Collaborative   Community/ Home Care   Cultural

- Emphasize wisdom of limiting lengthy or unnecessary sun exposure, using high sun protection factor (SPF) sunblock and avoiding tanning beds.
- Assist client to learn stress reduction and alternate therapy techniques *to control feelings of helplessness and enhance coping ability.*
- Refer to dietitian or certified diabetes educator as appropriate *to manage general well-being, enhance healing, and reduce risk of recurrence of diabetic ulcers.*

DOCUMENTATION FOCUS

Assessment/Reassessment
- Characteristics of lesion(s) or condition, ulcer classification.
- Causative or contributing factors.
- Impact of condition.

Planning
- Plan of care and who is involved in planning.
- Teaching plan.

Implementation/Evaluation
- Responses to interventions, teaching, and actions performed.
- Attainment or progress toward desired outcome(s).
- Modifications to plan of care.

Discharge Planning
- Long-term needs and who is responsible for actions to be taken.
- Specific referrals made.

References

1. Llewellyn, S. (2002). *Skin integrity and wound care (lecture materials)*. Chapel Hill, NC: Cape Fear Community College Nursing Program.
2. Colburn, L. (2001). Prevention for chronic wounds. In Krasner, D., Rodeheaver, G., and Sibbald, R. G. (eds). *Chronic Wound Care: A Clinical Source Book for Healthcare Professionals.* 2nd ed. Wayne, PA: HMP Communications.
3. Calianno, C. (1999). Patient hygiene: Part 2. Skin care. Keeping the outside healthy. *Nursing*, 29(12), (1 Suppl) 1–13.
4. Lund, C. H., Osborne, J. W., Culler, J. (2001). Neonatal skin care: Clinical outcomes of the AWHONN/NANN evidence-based clinical practice guideline. *J Neonatal Nurs*, 30(1), 30–40.
5. WebMD staff. (No date). Skin problems & treatment guide. *Skin Problems & Treatments Health Center (index to various pages)*. Retrieved April 2018 from http://www.webmd.com/skin-problems-and-treatments/guide/default.htm.
6. Engel, J. (2002). *Pocket Guide to Pediatric Assessment*. 4th ed. St. Louis, MO: Mosby, 99–112.
7. Wiersema, L. A., Stanley, M. (1999). The aging integumentary system. In Stanley, M., Beare, P. G. (eds). *Gerontological Nursing: A Health Promotion/Protection Approach*. 2nd ed. Philadelphia: F. A. Davis.
8. Krasner, D., Rodeheaver, G., Sibbald, R. G. (2001). Advanced wound caring for a new millennium. In Krasner, D., Rodeheaver, G., Sibald, R. G. (eds). *Chronic Wound Care: A Clinical Source Book for Healthcare Professionals*. 2nd ed. Wayne, PA: HMP Communications.

9. Blume-Peytavi, U., Hauser, M., Stamatas, G. N. (2012). Skin care practices for newborns and infants: Review of the clinical evidence for best practices. *Pediatr Dermatol*, 29(1), 1–14.
10. American Diabetes Association. (2011). Standards of medical care in diabetes—2011: Foot care recommendations. *Diabetes Care*, 34(1 Suppl), S11–S61.
11. Reddy, M., Gill, S. S., Rochan, P. A. (2006). Preventing pressure ulcers: A systematic review. *JAMA*, 296(8), 974–984.
12. Baranoski, S., LeBlanc, K., Gloekner, M. (2016). Preventing, assessing, and managing skin tears: A clinical review. *Am J Nurs*, 116(11), 24–30.
13. Hess, C. (2002). *Clinical Guide to Wound Care*. 4th ed. Philadelphia: Lippincott Williams & Wilkins.
14. Carrington, A. L., et al. (2001). Peripheral vascular and nerve function associated with lower limb amputation in people with and without diabetes. *Clin Sci*, 101(3), 261–266.
15. Catania, K., et al. (2007). PUPPI: The pressure ulcer prevention protocol interventions. *Am J Nurs*, 107(4), 44–51.
16. Okan, K., Woo, K., Ayello, E. A. (2007). The role of moisture balance in wound healing. *Adv Skin Wound Care*, 20(1), 39–53.
17. Langemo, D., Hanson, D., Hunter, S. (2011). Incontinence and incontinence-associated dermatitis. *Adv Skin Wound Care*, 4(3), 126–140.
18. Wadland, D. L. (2010). Maintaining skin integrity in the OR. *OR Nurse*, 4(2), 26–32.

 Diagnostic Studies   Evidence Based Practice   Medications   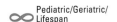 Pediatric/Geriatric/Lifespan

19. MayoClinic Staff. (2014, updated 2017). Itchy skin (pruritis) (various pages). Retrieved April; 2018 from http://www.mayoclinic.org/diseases-conditions/itchy-skin/basics/causes/con-20028460.

20. Hu, S. (2008). Psychogenic pruritus: A review. Retrieved April 2015 from http://www.vgrd.org/archive/cases/2008/pruritus/pruritus.html.

21. The International Skin Tear Advisory Panel (ISTAP). (No date). International Skin Tear Advisory Panel: Evidence based prediction, prevention, assessment, and management of skin tears. Retrieved November 2018 from http://www.skintears.org/education/tools/skin-tear-tool-kit/.

risk for impaired Skin Integrity

Taxonomy II: Safety/Protection—Class 2 Physical Injury 00247) [**Diagnostic Division:** Safety], Approved 1975; Revised 1998, 2010, 2013, 2017

DEFINITION: Susceptible to alteration in epidermis and/or dermis, which may compromise health.

RISK FACTORS

External
Chemical injury agent
Hypothermia; hyperthermia
Excretions; secretions; humidity; moisture

Internal
Alteration in fluid volume
Inadequate nutrition
Psychogenic factor [e.g., obsessive compulsive disorder]
At Risk Population: Extremes of age
Associated Condition: Alteration in metabolism; hormonal change; immunodeficiency
Alteration in skin turgor, sensation, pigmentation
Arterial puncture; vascular trauma
Pharmaceutical agent; radiation therapy
Sample Clinical Applications: AIDs; atherosclerosis, anemias; arthritis; coronary artery disease; dementias; amputation; Buerger's disease, burns; CVA; COPD; CHF; diabetes mellitus, obesity; peripheral vascular disease, Raynaud's disease, thrombophlebitis

DESIRED OUTCOMES/EVALUATION CRITERIA

Sample NOC linkages:
Risk Control: Personal actions to understand, prevent, eliminate, or reduce modifiable health threats
Immobility Consequences: Physiological: Severity of compromise in physiological functioning due to impaired physical mobility
Tissue Integrity: Skin & Mucous Membranes: Structural intactness and normal physiological function of skin and mucous membranes

Client Will (Include Specific Time Frame)
• Identify individual risk factors.
• Verbalize understanding of treatment or therapy regimen.
• Demonstrate behaviors or techniques to prevent skin breakdown.

 Acute Care   Collaborative   Community/Home Care   Cultural

ACTIONS/INTERVENTIONS

Sample **NIC** linkages:

Risk Identification: Analysis of potential risk factors, determination of health risks, and prioritization of risk reduction strategies for an individual or group

Skin Surveillance: Collection and analysis of patient data to maintain skin and mucous membrane integrity

Pressure Management: Minimizing pressure to body parts

NURSING PRIORITY NO. 1   To assess causative/contributing factors:

- Identify client with underlying conditions or problems that have potential for *skin integrity problems, such as (1) disease processes that affect circulation and perfusion of tissues (e.g., arteriosclerosis, venous insufficiency, hypertension, obesity, diabetes, malignant neoplasms), (2) medications (e.g., anticoagulants, corticosteroids, immunosuppressives, antineoplastics) that adversely affect or impair healing, (3) radiation (can break down internal tissues as well as skin), (4) nutrition and hydration (e.g., malnutrition deprives the body of protein and calories required for cell growth and repair, dehydration impairs transport of oxygen and nutrients), and (5) psychological stress and/or psychiatric conditions (e.g., skin excoriation is practiced to avoid increased anxiety or in reaction to a dreaded event, or may be elicited by an obsession). Disruption in skin integrity can be intentional (e.g., surgical incision) or unintentional (e.g., accidental trauma, drug effect, allergic reaction); and open (e.g., laceration, skin tears, penetrating wound, ulcerations) or closed (e.g., contusion, abrasion, rash).*[1–5,14]
- ✅ Note general health. *Many factors (e.g., debilitation; immobility; use of restraints; extremes of age; mental and psychiatric status; dehydration or malnutrition; presence of chronic disease; occupational, treatment, and environmental hazards) can affect the ability of the skin to perform its functions (e.g., protection, sensation, movement and growth, chemical synthesis, immunity, thermoregulation, and excretion).*[1,2,14]
- ∞ ✅ Determine client's age and developmental factors or ability to care for self. *Newborn/infant's skin is thin. Babies and children are prone to skin rashes associated with viral, bacterial, and fungal infections and allergic reactions. In adolescence, hormones stimulate hair growth and sebaceous gland activity. In adults, it takes longer to replenish epidermis cells, resulting in increased risk of skin cancers and infection. In older adults, there is decreased epidermal regeneration, fewer sweat glands, and less subcutaneous fat and elastin and collagen, causing skin to become thinner, drier, and less responsive to pain sensations.*[1,3,4,6–8]
- Evaluate client's skin care practices and hygiene issues. *Individual's skin may be sensitive or oily, dry, and scaly, and it is affected by bathing frequency (or lack of bathing), temperature of water, and types of soap and other cleansing agents. Incontinence (urinary or bowel) and ineffective hygiene can result in serious skin impairment and discomfort.*
- Note presence of compromised vision, sensation, hearing, or speech *that may impact client's self-care as relates to skin care (e.g., diabetic with impaired vision probably cannot satisfactorily examine own feet).*[9]
- Ascertain allergy history. *Individual may be sensitive or allergic to substances (e.g., insects, grasses, medications, lotions, soaps, foods) that can adversely affect the skin.*
- Assess blood supply (e.g., capillary return time, color, warmth) and sensation of skin surfaces or affected area on a regular basis *to provide comparative baseline and opportunity for timely intervention when problems are noted.*
- ✏️ ✅ Calculate ankle-brachial index *to evaluate actual or potential for impairment of circulation to lower extremities. Result less than 0.9 indicates need for close monitoring or more aggressive intervention (e.g., tighter blood glucose and weight control in diabetic client).*[10,11]
- ✏️ ✅ Review lab results (e.g., hemoglobin/hematocrit, blood glucose, albumin, protein) *to evaluate causative factors or ability to heal. Note: Albumin less than 3.5 correlates to decreased wound healing and increased incidence of pressure ulcers.*[12]

 Diagnostic Studies   ✅ Evidence Based Practice   💊 Medications   ∞ Pediatric/Geriatric/Lifespan

NURSING PRIORITY NO. 2 To maintain optimal skin integrity:[1,2,8]

- Perform routine skin inspections, assessing color, temperature, surface changes, texture, and contours. Evaluate color changes in areas of least pigmentation (e.g., sclera, conjunctiva, nailbeds, buccal mucosa, tongue, palms, soles of feet). Report potential problem areas (e.g., reddened/blanched areas, rashes) promptly. *Systematic inspection can identify developing problems and promotes early intervention, thus reducing likelihood of progression to skin breakdown.*[14]

- ∞Handle client gently (particularly infant, young child, elderly frail). *Epidermis of infants and very young children is thin and lacks subcutaneous depth that will develop with age. Skin of the older client is also thin, less elastic, and prone to injury, such as bruising and skin tears.*[2,5]

- Practice and instruct client/caregiver(s) in scrupulous hand hygiene and clean or sterile technique, as appropriate, *to reduce incidence of contamination or infection.*

- Maintain and instruct in overall good skin hygiene (e.g., shower instead of bath, wash thoroughly, pat dry, gently massage with lotion or appropriate cream) *to reduce risk of dermal trauma, improve circulation, and promote comfort.*

- Provide preventative skin care to incontinent client: Change continence pads or diapers frequently, cleanse perineal skin daily and after each incontinence episode, and apply skin protectant ointment *to minimize contact with irritants (urine, stool, excessive moisture).*[13]

- Cleanse skin after diaphoretic episodes *to maintain normal skin pH and flora and limit potential for infection.*

- Develop regularly timed repositioning schedule for client with mobility and sensation impairments, using turn sheet, as needed; encourage or assist with periodic weight shifts for client in chair *to reduce stress on pressure points and to promote circulation to tissues.*

- Use proper turning and transfer techniques. *Avoids movements that cause friction or shearing (e.g., pulling client with parallel force, dragging movements).*

- Pay special attention to bony prominences and other pressure points (e.g., heels, toes, elbows) when positioning client *to prevent pressure trauma and impaired circulation.*

- Provide foam, flotation, alternating pressure, or air mattress *to reduce or relieve pressure on skin, tissues, and lesions, decreasing tissue ischemia.*

- Use appropriate padding or pressure-reducing devices (e.g., egg crate, gel pads, heel rolls, or foam boots), when indicated, *to reduce pressure on sensitive areas and enhance circulation to compromised tissues.*

- Encourage ambulation. *Promotes circulation and reduces risks associated with immobility.*

- Provide for safety measures (e.g., assistive devices or sufficient personnel, grab bars, clear pathways, safe chairs, properly fitting hose and footwear, use of heating pads or lamps, restraints) during ambulation and other interventions *to reduce risk of dermal injury.*

- Avoid or limit use of plastic material (e.g., rubber sheet, plastic-backed linen savers) and remove wet or wrinkled linens promptly. *Moisture potentiates skin breakdown and increases risk for infection.*

- Use paper tape or a nonadherent dressing on frail skin and remove it gently, or use stockinette, tubular or gauze wrap, or other similar product instead of tape to secure dressings and drains *to limit dermal injury.*[5]

- Avoid use of latex products *when client has known or suspected sensitivity.* Refer to ND Latex Allergy Reaction.

- Apply hot and cold applications judiciously *to reduce risk of dermal injury in persons with circulatory and neurosensory impairments.*

- Provide adequate clothing or covers; protect from drafts *to prevent vasoconstriction and reduction of circulation to skin.*

- Keep bedclothes dry, use nonirritating materials, and keep bed free of wrinkles, crumbs, etc., *to prevent skin irritation.*

- Try colloidal bath, application of lotions, or careful use of ice pack *to decrease irritable itching.*

- Keep nails cut short, encouraging client *to refrain from scratching,* or suggest use of/obtain order for mittens (considered a restraint), if necessary, *to prevent dermal injury from scratching.*

- Refer to NDs impaired Skin Integrity and risk for Pressure Ulcer for additional interventions, as indicated.

 Acute Care   Collaborative   Community/ Home Care   Cultural

NURSING PRIORITY NO. 3 To promote healthy skin (Teaching/Discharge Considerations):

- Discuss importance of skin and measures to maintain proper skin functioning. *The integumentary system is the largest multifunctional organ of the body and thus merits special care.*
- Encourage regular inspection and monitoring of skin for changes and effective skin care in preventing skin problems. *Early detection and reporting to healthcare providers promotes timely evaluation and intervention.*
- Counsel diabetic and neurologically impaired client regarding the necessity of meticulous skin care, especially of lower extremities. *Healing of lower-extremity injuries tends to be more problematic in this population, resulting in increased incidence of amputation.*
- Avoid products containing perfumes, dyes, preservatives *(may cause dermatitis reactions)* or alcohol, povidone-iodine, and hydrogen peroxide *(may hinder healing).*
- Instruct in care of skin and extremities during cold or hot weather (e.g., wearing gloves, and clean, dry socks; properly fitting shoes or boots; face protection) *to reduce risk of tissue damage, especially in clients with impaired sensation.*
- Recommend elevation of lower extremities when sitting *to enhance venous return and reduce edema formation.*
- Encourage consistent exercise program (active or assistive) *to enhance circulation.*
- Discuss need for adequate nutritional intake (including adequate protein, lipids, calories, trace minerals, multivitamins) *to promote skin health and healing and to maintain general good health.*
- Determine fluid needs and sources for hydration (e.g., oral, tube feeding, ambient room humidity) *to reduce and replenish transepidermal water loss.*
- Encourage restriction or abstinence from smoking, *which can cause vasoconstriction.*
- Discuss importance of limiting lengthy or unnecessary sun exposure and avoiding use of tanning beds. Emphasize necessity of avoiding exposure to sunlight in specific conditions (e.g., systemic lupus, tetracycline or psychotropic drug use, radiation therapy) as well as potential for development of skin cancer.
- Advise use of high sun protection factor (SPF) sunblock or sunscreen, particularly on young child, client with fair skin (prone to burn), client using multiple medications, etc., *to limit skin damage (immediate and over time) associated with sun exposure.*

DOCUMENTATION FOCUS

Assessment/Reassessment
- Individual findings, including individual risk factors.

Planning
- Plan of care and who is involved in planning.
- Teaching plan.

Implementation/Evaluation
- Responses to interventions, teaching, and actions performed.
- Attainment or progress toward desired outcome(s).
- Modifications to plan of care.

Discharge Planning
- Long-term needs and who is responsible for actions to be taken.

References

1. Calianno, C. (2002). Patient hygiene, part 2—Skin care: Keeping the outside healthy. *Nursing*, 32(6), 1–13.
2. Lund, C. H., Osborne, J. W., Kuller, J. (2001). Neonatal skin care: Clinical outcomes of the AWHONN/NANN evidence-based clinical practice guideline. *J Neonatal Nurs*, 30(1), 30–40.
3. Llewellyn, S. (2002). *Skin integrity and wound care (lecture materials).* Chapel Hill, NC: Cape Fear Community College Nursing Program.
4. Colburn, L. (2001). Prevention for chronic wounds. In Krasner, D., Rodeheaver, G., and Sibbald, R. G. (eds). *Chronic Wound*

 Diagnostic Studies   Evidence Based Practice   Medications   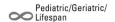 Pediatric/Geriatric/Lifespan

Care: A Clinical Source Book for Healthcare Professionals. 2nd ed. Wayne, PA: HMP Communications.

5. Baranoski, S., LeBlanc, K. (2016). Preventing, assessing, and managing skin tears: A clinical review. *Am J Nurs*, 116(11), 24–30.

6. McGovern, C. (2003, updated 2014). Skin, hair and nail assessment. Unit 2 (lecture materials). *Villanova University College of Nursing.* Retrieved April 2018 from http://www10.homepage.villanova.edu/marycarol.mcgovern/2104/SkinHair-Nail2.htm.

7. Engel, J. (2002). *Pocket Guide to Pediatric Assessment.* 4th ed. St. Louis, MO: Mosby.

8. Wiersema, L. A., Stanley, M. (1999). The aging integumentary system. In Stanley, M., Beare, P. G. (eds). *Gerontological Nursing: A Health Promotion/Protection Approach.* 2nd ed. Philadelphia: F. A. Davis.

9. American Diabetes Association. (2011). Standards of medical care in diabetes—2011: Foot care recommendations. *Diabetes Care,* 34(1 Suppl), S11–S61.

10. Murabito, J. M., et al. (2003). The ankle-brachial index in the elderly and risk of stroke, coronary disease and death. *Arch Intern Med,* 163(16), 1939–1942.

11. Carrington, A. L., et al. (2001). Peripheral vascular and nerve function associated with lower limb amputation in people with and without diabetes. *Clin Sci,* 101(3), 261–266.

12. Catania, K., et al. (2007). PUPPI: The pressure ulcer prevention protocol interventions. *Am J Nurs,* 107(4), 44–51.

13. Gray, M., et al. (2007). Incontinence-associated dermatitis: A consensus. *J Wound Ostomy Continence Nurs,* 34(1), 45–54.

14. Hu, S. (2008). Psychogenic pruritus: A review. Retrieved April 2018 from http://www.vgrd.org/archive/cases/2008/pruritus/pruritus.html.

Sleep Deprivation

Taxonomy II: Activity/Rest—Class 1 Sleep/Rest (00096) **[Diagnostic Division:** Activity/Rest], Approved 1998; Revised 2017

DEFINITION: Prolonged periods of time without sustained natural, periodic suspension of relative consciousness that provides rest.

RELATED FACTORS

Age-related sleep stage shifts; nonrestorative sleep pattern; sustained inadequate sleep hygiene; sustained circadian asynchrony

Average daily physical activity is less than recommended for gender and age

Environmental barrier; overstimulating environment

Late day confusion

Prolonged discomfort

Sleep terror; sleep walking

DEFINING CHARACTERISTICS

Subjective

Decrease in functional ability

Malaise; lethargy; fatigue

Anxiety

Perceptual disorders; heightened sensitivity to pain

Objective

Restlessness; irritability

Alteration in concentration; decrease in reaction time

Drowsiness; listlessness; apathy

Fleeting nystagmus; hand tremors

Confusion; transient paranoia; agitation; combativeness; hallucinations

At Risk Population: Familial sleep paralysis

Associated Condition: Conditions with periodic limb movement; nightmares

Dementia

Idiopathic central nervous system hypersomnolence; narcolepsy

 Acute Care   Collaborative   Community/Home Care   Cultural

Sleep apnea; sleep-related enuresis; sleep-related erections
Treatment regimen
Sample Clinical Applications: Chronic obstructive pulmonary disease (COPD), heart failure (nocturia), chronic pain, sleep apnea, pregnancy, postpartum, colic, dementia, Alzheimer's disease, anxiety disorders, posttraumatic stress disorder

DESIRED OUTCOMES/EVALUATION CRITERIA

Sample NOC linkages:
Sleep: Natural periodic suspension of consciousness during which the body is restored
Rest: Quantity and pattern of diminished activity for mental and physical rejuvenation
Pain Control: Personal actions to eliminate or reduce pain

Client Will (Include Specific Time Frame)
• Identify individually appropriate interventions to promote sleep.
• Verbalize understanding of sleep disorder.
• Adjust lifestyle to accommodate chronobiological rhythms.
• Report improvement in sleep and rest pattern.

Sample NOC linkages:
• **Family Coping:** Capacity of the family to manage stressors that tax family resources

Family Will (Include Specific Time Frame)
• Deal appropriately with parasomnias.

ACTIONS/INTERVENTIONS

Sample NIC linkages:
Sleep Enhancement: Facilitation of regular sleep/wake cycles
Anxiety Reduction: Minimizing apprehension, dread, foreboding, or uneasiness related to an unidentified source or anticipated danger
Environmental Management: Comfort: Manipulation of the patient's surroundings for promotion of optimal comfort

NURSING PRIORITY NO. 1   To assess causative/contributing factors:

• ∞ ▨ Note client's age and developmental stage. *The average adult requires 7 to 8 hours of sleep, although recent research indicates that the average total hours of sleep have decreased to less than 7 hours per night over the last few decades.[17] Teenagers require about 9 hours, and infants require about 16 hours. Pregnant women and new mothers, while needing more sleep, usually are sleep deprived. Studies show that sleep disorders occur in 35% to 45% of children 2 to 18 years of age,[13,17] and adolescents and young adults don't get enough sleep, have irregular sleep patterns, and are at risk for problem sleepiness.[2] Menopausal women often report interrupted sleep because of hot flashes or hormonal influences, and older people tend to sleep fewer hours and report less restful sleep and need for more sleep.[1–5,12,13]*
• Determine presence of physical or psychological stressors. *These include multiple, varying factors, such as night-shift work hours or rotating shifts; pain (acute and chronic), current or recent illness, and hospitalization, especially in intensive care unit; death of a spouse or loss of a job; new baby in the home and inadequate sleep-promoting behaviors; etc.*

 Diagnostic Studies   Evidence Based Practice   Medications   Pediatric/Geriatric/Lifespan

- Note presence of diagnoses *that are known to affect sleep (e.g., mental confusion or dementias, certain brain infections [e.g., encephalitis], brain injury, narcolepsy; chronic pain; obsessive/compulsive disorder, anxiety, depression, other major psychological disorders; drug or alcohol abuse; restless leg syndrome; sleep-induced respiratory disorders—sleep-disordered breathing, obstructive sleep apnea, childhood snoring with sleep apnea).*[4,5,19]
- Evaluate medication regimen for products affecting sleep. *Diet pills or other stimulants, sedatives, antidepressants, antihypertensives, diuretics, narcotics, agents with anticholinergic effects,* and need for medications requiring nighttime dosing *can inhibit getting to sleep or remaining asleep.*[6,7,16]
- Note environmental factors *affecting sleep (e.g., unfamiliar or uncomfortable sleep environment, excessive noise and light, frequent checking of vital signs, uncomfortable temperature, roommate irritations or actions— snoring, watching television late at night) that impair falling or staying asleep. Note: Clients in critical care units are known to experience lack of sleep or frequent disruptions, often compounding their illness.*[7]
- Determine presence of parasomnias: nightmares or terrors, sleepwalking or talking, or other complex behaviors during sleep. *May occur at any age, with as many as 30% of children (peak age 4 to 8 years) having a sleep disorder at some time.*[16] Note reports of terror, brief periods of paralysis, and sense of body being disconnected from the brain. *Occurrence of sleep paralysis, though not widely recognized in the United States, has been well documented elsewhere and may result in feelings of fear and reluctance to go to sleep. May require more extensive evaluation for serious sleep disorders.*[8,14]

NURSING PRIORITY NO. 2   To assess degree of impairment:

- Assess client's usual sleep patterns and current sleep disturbance, relying on client's/significant other's (SO's) report of problem. Incorporate screening information into in-depth sleep diary or testing if needed. *Usual sleep patterns are individual, but sleep loss has been shown to be the most common complaint reported in primary care settings;*[3,9] *therefore, screening for the problem should be routine. Data collected from a comprehensive assessment is needed to determine etiology of challenging sleep disturbances, including the stage of sleep that is impaired.*[7]
- Ascertain quality of sleep for bed partner/family members. *Loud irregular snoring (sleep apnea), periodic nightmares or sleep terrors, sleep talking, sleepwalking, or involuntary muscle activity can interfere with sleep of bed partner/entire family.*[16]
- Determine client's sleep expectations. *Individual may have faulty beliefs or attitudes about sleep and unrealistic sleep expectations (e.g., "I must get 8 hours of sleep every night, or I can't accomplish anything").*[9]
- Ascertain duration of current problem and effect on life and functional ability. *Client may not get enough sleep and not realize that life functioning is being impaired (e.g., can't concentrate in school, falls asleep when stopped at a light while driving).*[9]
- Listen to subjective reports of sleep quality (e.g., "short, interrupted") and response from lack of good sleep (feeling foggy, sleepy, and woozy; fighting sleep; fatigue). *Helps clarify client's perception of sleep quantity and quality and response to inadequate sleep.*[9]
- ∞ Observe for physical signs of fatigue. *Client may display restlessness, irritability, disorientation, frequent yawning, and/or other changes in mood, behavior, or performance (e.g., inability to tolerate stress, problems with concentration or learning). Fatigue, daytime sleepiness, and functional impairment have been reported as significant problems in teens and the elderly.*[2,3,9,12,16,20]
- Determine interventions client has tried to date. *Helps identify appropriate options and may reveal additional interventions that can be attempted.*
- Distinguish client's beneficial bedtime habits from detrimental ones *(e.g., drinking milk in the late evening [instead of coffee], restricting fluid intake, avoiding stimulating exercise, watching TV in bed, eliminating afternoon naps).*
- Instruct client and/or bed partner to keep a sleep-wake log *to document symptoms and identify factors that are interfering with sleep.*
- Obtain a chronological chart *to determine client's peak performance and sleep rhythms.*

 Acute Care   Collaborative   Community/ Home Care   Cultural

- Investigate anxious feelings *to help determine basis and appropriate anxiety-reduction techniques or behavioral therapy needs.*[16,20]

NURSING PRIORITY NO. 3 To assist client to establish optimal sleep pattern:[1,3,6,7,9–11,17,20]

- Review medications being taken and their effect on sleep, suggesting modifications in regimen *if medications are found to be interfering.*
- Encourage client to restrict caffeine and other stimulating substances from late-afternoon and evening intake. Recommend avoidance of bedtime alcohol. *Alcohol and some medications can produce immediate sleep followed by early awakening or difficulty remaining asleep.*
- Avoid eating large evening or late-night meals.
- Recommend light bedtime snack (protein, simple carbohydrate, low fat) and/or glass of warm milk for individuals who feel hungry, ingested 15 to 30 min before retiring. *Sense of fullness and satiety can encourage sleep.*
- Limit evening fluid intake if nocturia is present *to reduce need for nighttime elimination.*
- Promote adequate physical exercise activity during day, finishing workout at least 3 hr before bedtime. *Enhances expenditure of energy and release of tension so that client feels ready for sleep or rest. Note: Rigorous exercise close to bedtime can delay onset of sleep.*
- Suggest abstaining from daytime naps or napping in the morning *to improve ability to fall asleep at night.*
- Recommend quiet relaxing activities prior to bedtime such as reading, listening to soothing music, and meditation to *reduce stimulation and promote relaxation.*
- ∞ Discuss or implement effective age-appropriate bedtime rituals (e.g., going to bed at same time each night, brushing teeth, reading, drinking warm milk, rocking, story reading, cuddling, favorite blanket or toy) *to enhance client's ability to fall asleep, reinforce that bed is a place to sleep, and promote sense of security for child.*
- Provide back massage or other therapeutic touching activities, as appropriate. *Touch can be relaxing and emotionally pleasing, given that the client has SO's undivided attention for a few moments.*
- Provide calm, quiet environment for client, *to manage controllable sleep-disrupting factors (e.g., reduce noise and talking, dim lights, shut room door, adjust room temperature as needed, silence or reduce volume on phones, beepers, alarms, television, radios).*
- Administer pain medication first *to make sure client is pain-free* and then sedatives or other sleep medications *(so that hypnotic will be more effective)* when indicated, noting client's response. Time pain medications for peak effect and duration *to reduce need for redosing during prime sleep hours.*
- Discuss appropriate use of benzodiazepines when indicated. *May be useful in some clients for reducing risk of injury associated with sleepwalking or for management of severe sleep terrors. When possible, avoid use of longer-acting benzodiazepines in the elderly, as they are associated with prolonged sedation and increased risk of falls.*[16,20]
- Instruct client to get out of bed, leave bedroom, and engage in relaxing activities *if unable to fall asleep* and not return to bed until feeling sleepy.
- Recommend and instruct client in relaxation techniques (e.g., visualization, breathing, yoga).
- Refer for biofeedback, cognitive therapy, etc., *when measures that are more intensive are needed or desired to cope with stressors and promote relaxation.*
- Collaborate with healthcare team for evaluation and treatment of more serious sleep problems (e.g., obstructive sleep apnea, narcolepsy, sleep paralysis, bed-wetting, nocturnal leg cramps, restless leg syndrome).[13–16]
- Refer to physician and/or sleep specialist for evaluation and management of obstructive sleep apnea, such as medical or surgical treatment of obesity, medications and/or structural surgery (e.g., alteration of facial structures, removal of tonsils and adenoids in children),[15] or apnea/oxygenation therapy (continuous positive airway pressure, such as Respironics), *when sleep apnea is severe as documented by sleep-disorder studies.*[21]

 Diagnostic Studies   Evidence Based Practice   Medications   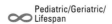 Pediatric/Geriatric/Lifespan

NURSING PRIORITY NO. 4 To promote wellness (Teaching/Discharge Considerations):

- 🏠 🥄 Review possibility of next-day drowsiness or "rebound" insomnia and temporary memory loss *that may be associated with sleep disorders and prescription sleep medications.*
- 🥄 Discuss short-term use and appropriateness of over-the-counter sleep medications or herbal supplements. Note possible side effects and drug interactions.
- ∞ Identify appropriate safety precautions (e.g., securing doors, windows, and stairways; placing client bedroom on first floor) and attach audible alarm to bedroom door *to alert parents when child is sleepwalking.*[16]
- 🔄 Refer to support group or counselor *to help deal with psychological stressors (e.g., grief, sorrow, chronic pain).* (Refer to NDs Grieving, chronic Sorrow, and chronic Pain.)
- 🔄 Encourage family counseling as indicated *to help deal with concerns arising from parasomnias (e.g., sleep talking, sleepwalking, night terrors).*
- 🔄 Refer to sleep specialist for sleep studies *when problem is unresponsive to customary interventions.*

DOCUMENTATION FOCUS

Assessment/Reassessment
- Assessment findings, including specifics of sleep pattern (current and past) and effects on lifestyle/level of functioning.
- Medications used, interventions tried, previous therapies.
- Family history of similar problem.
- Effects of sleep disturbance on SO/family.

Planning
- Plan of care and who is involved in planning.
- Teaching plan.

Implementation/Evaluation
- Client's response to interventions, teaching, and actions performed.
- Attainment or progress toward desired outcome(s).
- Modifications to plan of care.

Discharge Planning
- Long-term needs and who is responsible for actions to be taken.
- Specific referrals made.

References

1. Mindell, J. (1997). *Sleeping Through the Night: How Infants, Toddlers, and Their Parents Can Get a Good Night's Sleep.* New York: HarperCollins.
2. National Sleep Foundation. (2000). Adolescent sleep needs and patterns: Research report and resource guide. Booklet retrieved April 2018 from http://sleepfoundation.org/sites/default/files/sleep_and_teens_report1.pdf.
3. National Sleep Foundation. (No date). Do women need more sleep than men? Retrieved April 2018 from http://www.sleepfoundation.org/alert/do-women-need-more-sleep-men.
4. Sateia, M. J., et al. (2000). Evaluation of chronic insomnia: An American Academy of Sleep Medicine review. *Sleep*, 23(2), 243–308.
5. Subcommittee on Obstructive Sleep Apnea Syndrome, American Academy of Pediatrics Section on Pediatric Pulmonology. (2002). Clinical practice guideline: Diagnosis and management of childhood obstructive sleep apnea syndrome. *Pediatrics*, 109(4), 704–712.
6. Barroso, J. (2002). HIV-related fatigue: Nursing interventions to help patients manage. *Am J Nurs*, 102(5), 83–86.
7. Honkus, V. L. (2003). Sleep deprivation in critical care units. *Crit Care Nurs Quart*, 26(3), 179–191.
8. Russo, M. B., Shaikh, S. (Reviewed 2017). Sleep: Understanding the basics. Retrieved April 2018 from http://www.emedicine-health.com/sleep_understanding_the_basics/article_em.htm.
9. Cochran, H. (2003). Diagnose and treat primary insomnia. *Nurse Pract*, 28(9), 13–27.
10. Pronitis-Ruotolo, D. (2001). Surviving the night shift: Making Zeitgeber work for you. *Am J Nurs*, 101(7), 63–68.
11. Cmiel, C. A. (2004). Noise control: A nursing team's approach to sleep promotion. *Am J Nurs*, 104(2), 40–48.

 Acute Care   Collaborative   Community/Home Care   Cultural

12. National Agricultural Safety Database. (No date). Sleep deprivation: Cause and consequences. Fact sheet for Nebraska Rural Health and Safety Coalition. Retrieved April 2018 from http://nasdonline.org/document/871/d000705/sleep-deprivation-causes-and-consequences.html.

13. Neuspiel, D. R., Stubbs, E. H. (Updated 2015). Nightmare Disorder. Retrieved April 2018 from http://emedicine.medscape.com/article/914428-overview.

14. Blahd, D. (2014, reviewed 2016). Sleep disorders and parasomnias. Retrieved April 2018 from http://www.webmd.com/sleep-disorders/guide/parasomnias.

15. Garcia, J., Wills, L. (2002). Sleep disorders in children and teens: Helping patients and their families get some sleep. *Postgrad Med*, 107(3), 161–188.

16. Schenck, C. H., Mahowald, M. W. (2002). Parasomnias: Managing bizarre sleep-related behavior disorders. *Postgrad Med*, 107(3), 145–160.

17. Shiel, W. C. (2014, reviewed 2016). Sleep disorders: Insomnia, sleep apnea, and more: Slideshow. Retrieved April 2018 from http://www.medicinenet.com/sleep_disorders_pictures_slideshow/article.htm.

18. Aldabal, L., Bahammam, A. S. (2011). Metabolic, endocrine, and immune consequences of sleep deprivation. *Open Respir Med J*, 5, 31–43.

19. Cole, M. G., Dependukuri, N. (2003). Risk factors for depression among the elderly community subjects: A systematic review and meta-analysis. *Am J Psychiatr*, 160(6), 1147–1156.

20. Townsend-Roccichelli, J., Sandford, J. T., VandelWaa, E. (2010). Managing sleep disorders in the elderly. *Am J Primary Health*, 35(5), 30–37.

21. Barthlen, G. M. (2002). Sleep disorders: Obstructive sleep apnea, restless leg syndrome, and insomnia in geriatric patients. *Geriatrics*, 57(11), 34–39.

disturbed Sleep Pattern

Taxonomy II: Activity/Rest—Class 1 Sleep/Rest (00198) [**Diagnostic Division:** Activity/Rest], Approved 1980; Revised 1998, 2006

DEFINITION: Time-limited awakenings due to external factors.

RELATED FACTORS

Environmental barrier [e.g., ambient temperature/humidity, daylight/darkness exposure, ambient noise, unfamiliar setting]; immobilization

Nonrestorative sleep pattern [e.g., due to caregiver responsibilities, parenting practices, sleep partner]

Insufficient privacy; disruption caused by sleep partner

DEFINING CHARACTERISTICS

Subjective

Difficulty in daily functioning

Difficulty initiating sleep or maintaining sleep state; unintentional awakening

Feeling unrested; dissatisfaction with sleep

Sample Clinical Applications: Hospitalized or long-term care client, ill family member

DESIRED OUTCOMES/EVALUATION CRITERIA

Sample NOC linkages:

Sleep: Natural periodic suspension of consciousness during which the body is restored

Comfort Status: Environment: Environmental ease, comfort, and safety of surroundings

Client Will (Include Specific Time Frame)

• Report improved sleep.

• Report increased sense of well-being and feeling rested.

• Identify individually appropriate interventions to promote sleep.

(continues on page 816)

 Diagnostic Studies   Evidence Based Practice   Medications   Pediatric/Geriatric/Lifespan

disturbed Sleep Pattern (continued)

ACTIONS/INTERVENTIONS

Sample NIC linkages:

Sleep Enhancement: Facilitation of regular sleep/wake cycles

Environmental Management: Comfort: Manipulation of the patient's surroundings for promotion of optimal comfort

NURSING PRIORITY NO. 1 To assess causative/contributing factors:

- Identify presence of factors known to interfere with sleep, including current illness or hospitalization, new baby or sick family member in home, etc. *Sleep problems can arise from internal and external factors and may require assessment over time to differentiate specific cause(s). Note: Unresolved long-term disturbances in sleep are thought to be associated with dysfunction of the immune system, interference with wound healing, neurological and behavioral changes, and significant impairment of quality of life.*[1,10] Refer to ND Sleep Deprivation.

- Ascertain presence of short-term alteration in sleep patterns, such as can occur with travel (jet-lag), sharing bed with new sleep partner, fighting with family member, crisis at work, loss of job, or death in family. *Helps identify circumstances that are known to interrupt sleep acutely but do not necessarily represent long-term conditions. These situations may require short-term interventions but are often resolved over time.*[2]

- Note environmental factors, such as unfamiliar or uncomfortable room, excessive noise and light, uncomfortable temperature, frequent medical and monitoring interventions, and roommate actions (e.g., snoring, watching television late at night, wanting to talk). *These factors can reduce client's ability to rest and sleep at a time when more rest is needed. Note: Clients in critical care units are known to experience lack of sleep or frequent disruptions, often compounding their illness.*[3,5]

NURSING PRIORITY NO. 2 To evaluate sleep and degree of dysfunction:

- Assess client's usual sleep patterns and compare with current sleep disturbance, relying on client's/significant other's report of problem *to ascertain intensity and duration of problems.*

- Listen to reports of sleep quality (e.g., "short, interrupted") and response from lack of good sleep (e.g., feeling foggy, sleepy, and woozy; fighting sleep; fatigue). *Helps clarify client's perception of sleep quantity and quality and response to inadequate sleep.*[4]

- Determine client's sleep expectations. *Individual may have faulty beliefs or attitudes about sleep and/or unrealistic sleep expectations (e.g., "I must get 8 hours of sleep every night, or I can't accomplish anything").*[4]

- Observe for physical signs of fatigue (e.g., restlessness, hand tremors, thick speech, drooping eyes, inattention, lack of interest in activities).

- Incorporate screening information into in-depth sleep diary or testing if needed. *Information collected from a comprehensive assessment may be needed to evaluate the type and etiology of sleep disturbance and identify useful treatment options.*[4,5]

NURSING PRIORITY NO. 3 To assist client to establish optimal sleep/rest patterns:

- Manage environment for hospitalized client:[1,3,5–7]

  Adjust ambient lighting *to maintain daytime light and nighttime dark.*

  Provide privacy as indicated, such as requesting visitors to leave, closing room door, "quiet, patient sleeping" sign, etc.

  Encourage usual bedtime activities such as washing face and hands and brushing teeth.

 Acute Care   Collaborative   Community/Home Care   Cultural

Provide bedtime care such as straightening bed sheets, changing damp linens or gown, and back massage *to promote physical comfort.*

 Offer or provide sleep aids such as earplugs, eyemasks, if desired. *Note: One small study found that use of these aids prolonged client sleep time.*[11]

Turn on soft music, calm TV program, or quiet environment, as client prefers, *to enhance relaxation.*

 Minimize sleep-disrupting factors (e.g., shut room door; adjust room temperature as needed; reduce talking and other disturbing noises such as phones, beepers, alarms). *Studies show that use of these interventions can promote readiness for sleep and improve sleep duration and quality.*[5,8]

Perform monitoring and care activities without waking client whenever possible. *Allows for longer periods of uninterrupted sleep, especially during night.*

Avoid or limit use of physical restraints in accordance with client's needs and facility policy.

- Refer to physician or sleep specialist as indicated *for specific interventions and/or therapies, including medications and biofeedback.*
- Refer to NDs Insomnia and Sleep Deprivation for related interventions and rationale.

NURSING PRIORITY NO. 4 — To promote optimal sleep (Teaching/Discharge Considerations):

- Assure client that occasional sleeplessness should not threaten health and that resolving time-limited situation can restore healthful sleep. *Knowledge that occasional insomnia is universal and usually not harmful may promote relaxation and relief from worry, which can perpetuate the problem.*[9]
- Problem-solve immediate needs. *Short-term solutions (e.g., sleeping in different rooms if partner's illness is keeping client awake, acquiring a fan if sleeping quarters are too warm, getting a substitute to provide care to ill family member so client can get a good night's rest) may be needed until client adjusts to situation or crisis is resolved, with resulting return to more usual sleep pattern.*
- Encourage appropriate indoor light settings during day and night, especially exposure to bright light or sunlight in the morning; avoidance of daytime napping as appropriate for age and situation; and being active during day and more passive in evening. *Helps in promotion of normal sleep-wake patterns.*[6,9]
- Encourage use of aids to block out light and sound, such as sleep mask, room-darkening shades, earplugs, and white noise.[7]
- Discuss use and appropriateness of over-the-counter sleep medications or herbal supplements *to provide assistance in falling and staying asleep.*

DOCUMENTATION FOCUS

Assessment/Reassessment
- Assessment findings, including specifics of sleep pattern (current and past) and effects on lifestyle and level of functioning.
- Specific interventions, medications, or previously tried therapies.

Planning
- Plan of care and who is involved in planning.
- Teaching plan.

Implementation/Evaluation
- Response to interventions, teaching, and actions performed.
- Attainment or progress toward desired outcome(s).
- Modifications to plan of care.

Discharge Planning
- Long-term needs and who is responsible for actions to be taken.
- Available resources, specific referrals made.

 Diagnostic Studies   Evidence Based Practice   Medications   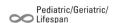 Pediatric/Geriatric/Lifespan

References

1. Weinhouse, G. L., Schwab, R. J. (2006). Sleep in the critically ill patient. *Sleep*, 29(5), 707–716.
2. Schutte-Rodin, S., et al. (2008). Clinical guideline for the evaluation and management of chronic insomnia in adults. *J Clin Sleep Med*, 4(5), 487–504.
3. Patel, M., et al. (2008). Sleep in the intensive care setting. *Crit Care Nurs Q*, 31(4), 309–318.
4. Cochran, H. (2003). Diagnose and treat primary insomnia. *Nurse Pract*, 28(9), 13–27.
5. Fontana, C. J., Pittigilo, L. I. (2007). Sleep deprivation among critical care patients. *Crit Care Nurs Q*, 33(1), 75–81.
6. Cole, C., Richards, K. (2007). Sleep disruption in older adults. *Am J Nurs*, 107(5), 40–49.
7. Floyd, J. A. (2008). Sleep enhancement. In Ackley, B. J., et al. (eds). *Evidence-Based Nursing Care Guidelines:* *Medical-Surgical Interventions*. St. Louis, MO: Mosby Elsevier.
8. Olson, D. M., et al. (2001). Quiet time: A nursing intervention to promote sleep in neurocritical care units. *Am J Crit Care*, 10(2), 74–78.
9. National Institute of Neurological Disorders and Stroke. (Updated 2017). Brain basics. Understanding sleep. Retrieved April 2018 from http://www.ninds.nih.gov/disorders/brain_basics/understanding_sleep.htm.
10. Aldabal, L., Bahammam, A. S. (2011). Metabolic, endocrine, and immune consequences of sleep deprivation. *Open Respir Med J*, 5, 31–43.
11. Richard, A., et al. (2007). Earplugs and eye masks: Do they improve critical care patients' sleep? *Nurs Crit Care*, 12(6), 278–286.

readiness for enhanced Sleep

Taxonomy II: Activity/Rest—Class 1 Sleep/Rest (00165) [**Diagnostic Division:** Activity/Rest], Approved 2002; Revised 2013

DEFINITION: A pattern of natural, periodic suspension of relative consciousness to provide rest and sustain a desired lifestyle, which can be strengthened.

DEFINING CHARACTERISTICS

Subjective
Expresses desire to enhance sleep
Sample Clinical Applications: Postoperative recovery, chronic pain, pregnancy—prenatal/postpartal period, sleep apnea

DESIRED OUTCOMES/EVALUATION CRITERIA

Sample NOC linkages:
Sleep: Natural periodic suspension of consciousness during which the body is restored
Rest: Quantity and pattern of diminished activity for mental and physical rejuvenation
Comfort Status: Environmental: Environmental ease, comfort, and safety of surroundings

Client Will (Include Specific Time Frame)
• Identify individually appropriate interventions to promote sleep.
• Verbalize feeling rested after sleep.
• Adjust lifestyle to accommodate routines that promote sleep.

ACTIONS/INTERVENTIONS

Sample NIC linkages:
Sleep Enhancement: Facilitation of regular sleep/wake cycles
Relaxation Therapy: Use of techniques to encourage and elicit relaxation for the purpose of decreasing undesirable signs and symptoms such as pain, muscle tension, or anxiety
Environmental Management: Manipulation of the patient's surroundings for therapeutic benefit, sensory appeal, and psychological well-being

 Acute Care   Collaborative   Community/Home Care   Cultural

NURSING PRIORITY NO. 1 To determine motivation for continued improvement:

- Listen to client's reports of sleep quantity and quality. Determine client's perception of adequate sleep. *Reveals client's experience and expectations regarding sleep. Provides opportunity to address misconceptions or unrealistic expectations and plan for interventions.*
- Observe or obtain feedback from client/significant other(s) regarding usual bedtime, number of hours of sleep, and time of arising *to determine usual sleep pattern and provide comparative baseline for improvements.*
- Ascertain motivation and expectation for change. *Motivation to improve and high expectations can encourage client to make changes that will improve his or her life. However, unrealistic expectations may hamper efforts.*
- Note client report of potential for alteration of habitual sleep time (e.g., change of work pattern or rotating shifts) or change in normal bedtime (e.g., hospitalization). *Helps identify circumstances that are known to interrupt sleep patterns and that could disrupt the person's biological rhythms.*[1,6]

NURSING PRIORITY NO. 2 To assist client to enhance sleep/rest:

- Review client's usual bedtime rituals, routines, and sleep environment needs. *Provides information on client's management of the situation and identifies areas that might be modified when the need arises.*
- ∞ Discuss or implement effective age-appropriate bedtime rituals for infant/child (e.g., rocking, story reading, cuddling, favorite blanket or toy). *Rituals can enhance ability to fall asleep, reinforce that bed is a place to sleep, and promote sense of security for child.*[2]
- Provide quiet environment and comfort measures (e.g., back rub, washing hands and face, cleaning and straightening sheets) for client in facility. *Promotes relaxation and readiness for sleep.*
- Arrange care *to provide for uninterrupted periods for rest.* Explain necessity of disturbances for monitoring vital signs or other care when client is hospitalized. Do as much care as possible during night without waking client. *Allows for longer periods of uninterrupted sleep, especially during night.*
- Suggest limiting fluid intake in evening if nocturia or bed-wetting is a problem *to reduce need for nighttime elimination.*
- Provide instruction in use of necessary equipment. *Client may use oxygen or continuous positive airway pressure (CPAP) system to improve sleep/rest in presence of hypoxia or sleep apnea.*
- Discuss dietary matters, such as limiting chocolate, heavy meals, caffeine, or alcoholic beverages prior to bedtime, *which are substances known to impair falling or staying asleep. Use of alcohol at bedtime may help individual fall asleep, but ensuing sleep is then fragmented.*[7]
- Explore or implement use of warm bath, intake of light protein snack before bedtime, comfortable room temperature, soothing music, or favorite calming television show. *Nonpharmaceutical aids can enhance falling asleep without the undesired side effects associated with medications.*
- Investigate use of sleep mask, darkening shades or curtains, earplugs, and low-level background (white) noise in situations *where sleep might not come easily or be disturbed by environmental factors.*
- Recommend continuing same schedule for sleep throughout week—including days off. *Maintaining sleep pattern helps sustain biological rhythms.*

NURSING PRIORITY NO. 3 To promote optimum sleep:

- Assure client that occasional sleeplessness should not threaten health. *Knowledge that occasional insomnia is universal and usually not harmful may promote relaxation and relief from worry.*[3]
- Encourage regular exercise during the day *to aid in stress control and release of energy. Note: Exercise at bedtime may stimulate rather than relax client and may actually interfere with sleep.*[5]
- Assist to develop individual program of relaxation (e.g., biofeedback, self-hypnosis, visualization, progressive muscle relaxation). *Reduces sympathetic response and stress to aid in inducing sleep.*[4]
- Address sleep management techniques that may be useful during stressful conditions or lifestyle changes (e.g., pregnancy, new baby, menopause, medical procedures, new job, moving, change in relationship, grief).
- Recommend periodic review of medications. *Many prescription and over-the-counter (OTC) drugs can disrupt sleep.*

 Diagnostic Studies   Evidence Based Practice   Medications   Pediatric/Geriatric/ Lifespan

- 💊 Advise using prescription or OTC sleep medications sparingly. *These medications, while useful for promoting sleep in the short term, can interfere with rapid eye movement sleep.*

DOCUMENTATION FOCUS

Assessment/Reassessment
- Assessment findings, including specifics of sleep pattern and effects on lifestyle/level of functioning.
- Any medications used, interventions tried, previous therapies.
- Motivation and expectations for change.

Planning
- Plan of care and who is involved in planning.
- Teaching plan.

Implementation/Evaluation
- Client's response to interventions, teaching, and actions performed.
- Attainment or progress toward desired outcome(s).
- Modifications to plan of care.

Discharge Planning
- Long-term needs and who is responsible for actions to be taken.
- Specific referrals made.

References

1. Cochran, H. (2003). Diagnose and treat primary insomnia. *Nurse Pract*, 28(9), 13–27.
2. Mindell, J. (1997). *Sleeping Through the Night: How Infants, Toddlers, and Their Parents Can Get a Good Night's Sleep.* New York: HarperCollins.
3. National Institute of Neurological Disorders and Stroke. (Updated 2017). Brain basics: Understanding sleep (various pages). Retrieved April 2018 from http://www.ninds.nih.gov/disorders/brain_basics/understanding_sleep.htm.
4. Cox, H. C., et al. (2002). ND: Sleep Pattern, disturbed. *Clinical Applications of Nursing Diagnosis: Adult, Child, Women's,* *Psychiatric, Gerontic, and Home Health Considerations.* 4th ed. Philadelphia: F. A. Davis.
5. Grandjean, C. K., Gibbons, S. W. (2000). Assessing ambulatory geriatric sleep complaints. *Nurse Pract: Am J Prim Health Care*, 25(9), 25–35.
6. Pronitis-Ruotolo, D. (2001). Surviving the night shift: Making Zeitgeber work for you. *Am J Nurs*, 101(7), 63–68.
7. National Sleep Foundation. (No date). Sleep hygiene. Retrieved April 2018 from http://www.sleepfoundation.org/article/ask-the-expert/sleep-hygiene.

impaired Social Interaction

Taxonomy II: Role Relationships—Class 3 Role Performance (00052) **[Diagnostic Division:** Social Interaction**]**, Approved 1986; Revised 2017

DEFINITION: Insufficient or excessive quantity or ineffective quality of social exchange.

RELATED FACTORS
Insufficient knowledge about ways to enhance mutuality
Insufficient skills to enhance mutuality
Communication barrier
Disturbance in self-concept
Impaired mobility
Therapeutic isolation
Sociocultural dissonance

 Acute Care   Collaborative   Community/Home Care   Cultural

Environmental barrier
Disturbance in thought processes

DEFINING CHARACTERISTICS

Subjective
Discomfort in social situations
Dissatisfaction with social engagement [e.g., belonging, caring, interest, shared history]
Family reports change in interaction

Objective
Impaired social functioning
Dysfunctional interaction with others
At Risk Population: Absence of significant other
Associated Condition: Therapeutic isolation
Sample Clinical Applications: Brain injury, stroke, cancer, neuromuscular disease (e.g., multiple sclerosis [MS]), cerebral palsy, substance abuse, Alzheimer's disease, schizophrenia, autism

DESIRED OUTCOMES/EVALUATION CRITERIA

Sample NOC linkages:
Social Interaction Skills: Personal behaviors that promote effective relationships
Child Development: (specify Middle Childhood or Adolescence): Milestones of physical, cognitive, and psychosocial progression from [6–11 or 12–17] years of age
Social Involvement: Social interactions with persons, groups, or organizations

Client Will (Include Specific Time Frame)
• Verbalize awareness of factors causing or promoting impaired social interactions.
• Identify feelings that lead to poor social interactions.
• Express desire or be involved in achieving positive changes in social behaviors and interpersonal relationships.
• Give self positive reinforcement for changes that are achieved.
• Develop effective social support system; use available resources appropriately.

ACTIONS/INTERVENTIONS

Sample NIC linkages:
Socialization Enhancement: Facilitation of another person's ability to interact with others
Behavior Modification: Social Skills: Assisting the patient to develop or improve interpersonal social skills
Complex Relationship Building: Establishing a therapeutic relationship with a patient to promote insight and behavioral change

NURSING PRIORITY NO. 1   To assess causative/contributing factors:

• Review social history with client/significant others (SOs) and go back far enough in time to note when changes in social behavior or patterns of relating occurred or began. *For example, loss or long-term illness of loved one; failed relationships; loss of occupation, financial, or political (power) position; change in status in family hierarchy (job loss, aging, illness); and poor coping or adjustment to developmental stage of life, as with marriage, birth or adoption of child, or children leaving home, are situations that may affect quality of social exchange.*[1]

 Diagnostic Studies   Evidence Based Practice   Medications   Pediatric/Geriatric/Lifespan

- Ascertain ethnic, cultural, or religious implications for the client. *These factors can dictate choice of behaviors and may even script interactions with others. Client may perceive behaviors as normal because of belief system or may have conflict regarding behaviors that are not accepted by larger society, such as homosexuality or gender identity disorder.*[1,5,6]
- Review medical history, noting stressors of physical or long-term illness/chronic conditions (e.g., stroke, cancer, MS, head injury, Alzheimer's disease), mental illness (e.g., schizophrenia), medications, substance use, debilitating accidents, learning disabilities (e.g., sensory integration difficulties, autism spectrum disorder, Asperger's disorder), and emotional disabilities. *Conditions such as these can isolate individual who feels disconnected from others, resulting in difficulty relating in social situations. Note: Evidence indicates that loneliness heightens sensitivity to social threats and can impair executive functioning, sleep, and mental and physical well-being.*[3,4,11]
- Note presence of visual or hearing impairments. *Individuals with these conditions may find communication barriers are increased, social interaction is affected, and interventions need to be designed to promote involvement with others in positive ways.*[1,3]
- ∞ Determine family patterns of relating and social behaviors. Explore possible family scripting of behavioral expectations in the children and how the client was affected. *Parents are important in teaching their children social skills (e.g., sharing, taking turns, allowing others to talk without interrupting). Family may not have effective patterns of relating to others, and the child learns these skills in this setting. Often child reflects family expectations rather than own desires, which may result in conforming or rebellious behaviors.*[2,6,10]
- Observe client while relating to family/SO(s) and note observations of prevalent patterns. *Identification of patterns will help with plan for change.*[2]
- Encourage client to verbalize feeling of discomfort about social situations. Note any causative factors, recurring precipitating patterns, and barriers to using support systems. *Identifies areas of concern and suggests possible ways to learn new skills.*[2]

NURSING PRIORITY NO. 2   To assess degree of impairment:

- Encourage client to verbalize perceptions of reasons for problems. Active listen, noting indications of hopelessness, powerlessness, fear, anxiety, grief, anger, feeling unloved or unlovable, problems with sexual identity, and hate (directed or not). *These feelings arise from the anxiety that comes with the need to participate with others in social situations and can interfere with work, friendships, and life in general.*[5,7]
- Observe and describe social and interpersonal behaviors in objective terms, noting speech patterns and body language (1) in the therapeutic setting and (2) in normal areas of daily functioning (if possible), including family, job, and social or entertainment settings. *Provides information about extent of anxiety client experiences in different settings and suggests possible interventions.*[5,7]
- Determine client's use of coping skills and defense mechanisms. *Symptoms associated with social anxiety affect ability to be involved in social situations, making client's life miserable and seriously interfering with work, friendships, and family life.*[5,7]
- Evaluate possibility of client being the victim of or using destructive behaviors against self or others. (Refer to ND risk for other-directed/self-directed Violence.) *Problems of poor communication lead to frustration and anger, leaving the individual with few coping skills, and may result in destructive behaviors.*[1,2,10]
- Interview family, SO(s), friends, spiritual leaders, coworkers, as appropriate. *Obtaining observations of client's behavioral changes from others associated with the individual provides a broader view of actual problems and how behavior affects client's life/others.*[5]

NURSING PRIORITY NO. 3   To assist client/SO(s) to recognize/make positive changes in impaired social and interpersonal interactions:

- Establish therapeutic relationship using positive regard for the person, Active listening, and providing safe environment for self-disclosure. *Client who is having difficulty interacting in social situations needs to feel comfortable and accepted before he or she is willing to talk about self and concerns.*[1,2]

 Acute Care   Collaborative   Community/Home Care   Cultural

- Have client list behaviors that cause discomfort. *Anxiety usually has physical symptoms (e.g., a racing heart, dry mouth, shaky voice, blushing, sweating, nausea), and once it is recognized, client can choose to begin treatment to change.*[5,7]
- Have family/SO(s) list client's behaviors that are causing discomfort for them. *Anxiety is contagious, and by identifying specific behaviors, all members of the family can begin to deal appropriately with them so they are diminished.*[5,7]
- Review negative behaviors observed previously by caregivers, coworkers, etc. *Others may see behaviors and the problems associated with them, such as unwillingness to participate in necessary activities (eating in a public place, interviewing for a job) and may provide additional information needed to develop an appropriate plan of care.*[1]
- Compare lists and validate reality of perceptions. Help client prioritize those behaviors needing change. *Each individual may have a different view of what constitutes a problem, and by comparing lists, each person hears how others view the problems, enabling the client/family to identify behaviors or concerns to be dealt with.*[1,7]
- Explore with client and role-play means of making agreed-on changes in social interactions or behaviors (as determined earlier). *Client needs to learn social skills if he or she has never learned the elements of interacting with others in social settings. Role-playing one-on-one is less threatening and can help individual identify with another and practice new social skills.*[5]
- Role-play random social situations in therapeutically controlled environment with "safe" therapy group. Have group note behaviors, both positive and negative, and discuss these and any changes needed. *Having client participate in a controlled group environment provides opportunities to try out different behaviors in a built-in social setting where members can make friends and provide mutual advice and comfort.*[1,5]
- Role-play changes and discuss impact. Include family/SO(s) as indicated. *Provides opportunity for person to recognize changes in feelings and behavior and enhances comfort with new behaviors.*[4]
- Provide positive reinforcement for improvement in social behaviors and interactions. *Encourages continuation of desired behaviors and efforts for change.*[5]
- 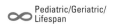 Participate in multidisciplinary client-centered conferences *to evaluate progress.* Involve everyone associated with client's care, family members, SO(s), and therapy group. *These conferences have the advantage of providing information from and to each participant in an atmosphere of trust where questions can be asked, decisions can be made, and goals for the future can be agreed on.*[1]
- Work with the client to alleviate underlying negative self-concepts *because they often impede positive social interactions. By replacing negative thoughts with positive messages, client can reduce anxiety and develop a positive sense of self-esteem. While this is not an easy process, the rewards are great when client is willing to practice consistently.*[2]
- Involve neurologically impaired client in individual or group interactions as situation allows. *Individual may not be able to interact appropriately because of disabilities, but involvement in the group provides an opportunity to practice and relearn skills to enable reintegration into social situations.*[1,8]
- 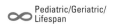 Refer for family therapy as indicated. *Social behaviors and interpersonal relationships involve more than the individual, and family may need additional help to resolve ongoing family problems.*[1,2]

NURSING PRIORITY NO. 4 To promote wellness (Teaching/Discharge Considerations):

- Encourage client to keep a daily journal in which social interactions of each day can be reviewed and the comfort or discomfort experienced noted with possible causes or precipitating factors. *Helps client to identify specific problem areas and begin to choose to take responsibility for own behavior(s).*[5,7]
- Assist the client to develop positive social skills through practice of skills in real social situations accompanied by a support person. Provide positive feedback with the use of "I" messages during interactions with client. *Cognitive and behavioral methods can help individuals overcome fears with the help of a trusted person. "I" messages convey a positive message, individual does not feel criticized, and he or she is encouraged to continue new thinking and behaviors.*[1,5]
- Discuss the use of medications when indicated and monitor for effectiveness and side effects. *Several kinds of drugs have been found to be effective in the treatment of social anxiety problems; selective serotonin*

 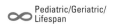

reuptake inhibitors (SSRIs), such as paroxetine (Paxil) and sertraline (Zoloft), are often the first choice. Anti-anxiety drugs, such as clonazepam (Klonopin), buspirone (BusPar), and alprazolam (Xanax), can reduce anxiety and may be used alone or in conjunction with SSRIs. Propranolol (Inderal) has been found to be useful for performance anxiety, and when taken an hour before the scheduled event, may suppress the physical symptoms of anxiety.[5,7]

- Seek community programs for client involvement that promote positive behaviors the client is striving to achieve. *Encouraging reading materials, attending classes, community support groups, and lectures for self-help can help to alleviate negative self-concepts that lead to impaired social interactions.*[2,5]
- Involve in a music-based program, if available. *There is a direct correlation between the musical portion of the brain and the language area, and the use of these programs may result in better communication skills. Music has been used to calm, to enable feelings of safety, and to reduce the social distance between people.*[9]
- Encourage ongoing family or individual therapy as long as it is promoting growth and positive change. Be alert to possibility of therapy being used as a crutch. *While therapy groups can be useful, individuals can become dependent on the process and not move on to managing on their own.*[1]
- Provide for occasional follow-up for reinforcement of positive behaviors after professional relationship has ended. *Change is difficult and identifying problems that may arise during these contacts can enhance maintenance and enable client/family to continue to progress.*[2]
- Refer to psychiatric clinical nurse specialist when indicated. *May need additional assistance to promote long-term change.*[1]

DOCUMENTATION FOCUS

Assessment/Reassessment
- Individual findings, including factors affecting interactions, nature of social exchanges, specifics of individual behaviors, and type of learning disability present.
- Cultural or religious beliefs and expectations.
- Perceptions and response of others.

Planning
- Plan of care and who is involved in the planning.
- Teaching plan.

Implementation/Evaluation
- Responses to interventions, teaching, and actions performed.
- Attainment or progress toward desired outcome(s).
- Modifications to plan of care.

Discharge Planning
- Long-term needs and who is responsible for actions to be taken.
- Community resources, specific referrals made.

References

1. Townsend, M. C. (2003). *Psychiatric Mental Health Nursing Concepts of Care*. 4th ed. Philadelphia: F. A. Davis.
2. Doenges, M. E., Townsend, M. C., Moorhouse, M. F. (1998). *Psychiatric Care Plans: Guidelines for Individualizing Care*. 3rd ed. Philadelphia: F. A. Davis.
3. Cox, H., et al. (2002). *Clinical Applications of Nursing Diagnosis: Adult, Child, Women's, Psychiatric, Gerontic, and Home Health Considerations*. 4th ed. Philadelphia: F. A. Davis.
4. Holly, U. A. (2007). Social isolation: A practical guide for nurses assisting clients with chronic illness. *Rehab Nurs*, 32(2), 51–56.
5. No author listed. (2003). Beyond shyness and stage fright: Social anxiety disorder. *Harv Ment Health Lett*, 20(3), 1–4.
6. Purnell, L. D. (2011). *Guide to Culturally Competent Health Care*. 2nd ed. Philadelphia: F. A. Davis.
7. Frey, R. J. (2012). Generalized anxiety disorder. *Encyclopedia of Mental Disorders*. Retrieved April 2018 from http://www.minddisorders.com/Flu-Inv/Generalized-anxiety-disorder.html.
8. Beck, T. J., Bellis, T. J. (2007). (Central) auditory processing disorders: Overview and amplifications. *Hear J*, 60(5), 44–47.

 Acute Care   Collaborative   Community/Home Care   Cultural

9. Life Change Health Institute. (2016). Music therapy & trauma: Insights from the Polyvagal Theory. Retrieved April 2018 from http://a.advancedbrain.com/tlp/the_listening_program.jsp.
10. Olsen, G., Fuller, M. L. (Updated 2010). Family interactions patterns: Bullying and victimization in children. Retrieved April 2018 from http://www.education.com/reference/article/family-interaction-patterns-bullying/.
11. Cacioppo, J. T., Cacioppo, S. (2014). Social relationships and health: The toxic effects of perceived social isolation. *Soc Personal Psychol Compass*, 8(2), 58–72.

Social Isolation

Taxonomy II: Comfort—Class 3 Social Comfort (00053) [**Diagnostic Division:** Social Interaction], Approved 1982; Revised 2017

DEFINITION: Aloneness experienced by the individual and perceived as imposed by others and as a negative or threatening state.

RELATED FACTORS

Difficulty establishing relationships; inability to engage in satisfying personal relationships
Insufficient personal resources (e.g., poor achievement, poor insight, affect unavailable and poorly controlled)
Developmentally inappropriate interests; social behavior incongruent with norms; values incongruent with cultural norms

DEFINING CHARACTERISTICS

Subjective

Aloneness imposed by others
Insecurity in public; desires to be alone
Inability to meet expectations of others; purposelessness
Developmentally inappropriate interests; values incongruent with cultural norms
Feeling different from others

Objective

Absence of support system; history of rejection
Sad or flat affect; withdrawn; poor eye contact
Disabling condition; illness
Developmental delay
Preoccupation with own thoughts; repetitive or meaningless actions; hostility
Cultural incongruence; member of a subculture
Associated Condition: Alteration in wellness or mental status or physical appearance
Sample Clinical Applications: Traumatic injuries, facial scarring/acne, chemotherapy, AIDS, dementia, major depression, conduct disorder, developmental delay, paranoid disorders, schizophrenia

DESIRED OUTCOMES/EVALUATION CRITERIA

Sample NOC linkages:
Social Involvement: Social interactions with persons, groups, or organizations
Loneliness Severity: Severity of emotional, social, or existential signs and symptoms of isolation
Social Support: Reliable assistance from others

Client Will (Include Specific Time Frame)
• Identify causes and actions to correct isolation.
• Verbalize willingness to be involved with others.

(continues on page 826)

 Diagnostic Studies   Evidence Based Practice   Medications   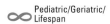 Pediatric/Geriatric/Lifespan

Social Isolation (continued)

- Participate in activities or programs at level of ability or desire.
- Express increased sense of self-worth.

ACTIONS/INTERVENTIONS

Sample NIC linkages:

Socialization Enhancement: Facilitation of another person's ability to interact with others

Behavior Management: Social Skills: Assisting the patient to develop or improve interpersonal social skills

Visitation Facilitation: Promoting beneficial visits by family and friends

NURSING PRIORITY NO. 1 To assess causative/contributing factors:

- Determine presence of factors as listed in Related Factors and other concerns (e.g., elderly, female, adolescent, ethnic or racial minority, economically or educationally disadvantaged, hearing or visually impaired). *Identifying individual factors allows for developing an accurate plan of care for the client.*[5]
- Perform physical exam, paying particular attention to any illnesses. *Individuals who are isolated appear to be susceptible to health problems, especially coronary heart disease, although little is understood about why that is.*[10]
- Note onset of physical or mental illness and whether recovery is anticipated or condition is chronic or progressive. *Individual may withdraw from activities because of concern about how others view changes that occur due to illness, concern with own thoughts, and alterations in physical appearance or mental status. Anticipated length of illness may dictate choice of interventions.*[1,4]
- Identify blocks to social contacts. *Reluctance to engage in social activities may be the result of problems such as physical immobility, sensory deficits, housebound for any reason, incontinence, financial constraints, and/or transportation difficulties. Individual may be afraid of what others might think of her or him, be concerned with embarrassing self, or not having money or means of transportation for desired activities.*[1]
- Ascertain implications of cultural values or religious beliefs for the client *that may dictate choice of behaviors and may even script interactions with others. Client may perceive behaviors as normal because of belief system or may have conflict regarding behaviors that may be unacceptable to the larger society, such as homosexuality or gender identity disorder.*[1,5,6]
- Assess factors in client's life that may contribute to sense of helplessness. *Losses, such as a spouse, parent, or other, or presence of chronic pain or other disabling conditions may cause individual to withdraw, desire to be alone, and refuse to participate in therapeutic activities.*[1,3]
- Listen to comments of client regarding sense of isolation. Differentiate isolation from solitude and loneliness *that may be acceptable or by choice. Provides clues to what client is thinking and feeling about current situation. Client who chooses to be alone and is satisfied may not need further intervention. Note: Research indicates that perceived social isolation is a risk factor for, and may contribute to, poorer overall cognitive performance, faster cognitive decline, poorer executive functioning, increased negativity, and heightened sensitivity to social threats. These differences impact on emotions, decisions, behaviors, and interpersonal interactions.*[3,5,11,12]
- Assess client's feelings about self, sense of ability to control situation, sense of hope, and coping skills. *If client is isolating self because of negative feelings, lack of hope, etc., measures to promote self-esteem will need to be taken.*
- Identify support systems available to the client, including presence of/relationship with extended family. *People with social anxiety often do not have support systems because of their withdrawal from contact with others. Often the family of origin may be anxious and does not provide the encouragement and support needed by a*

 Acute Care   Collaborative   Community/Home Care   Cultural

temperamentally inhibited child or may be too helpful, enabling client to withdraw further. It is difficult for these individuals to ask for help because they are afraid to meet new people and often find support only when they seek help for other conditions, such as depression.[4,9]

- Identify behavior response of isolation. *Individual may display behaviors such as excessive sleeping or day-dreaming, which also may potentiate isolation.*[7,10]
- 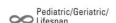Note drug use (prescription and illicit). *Individual may begin to use drugs such as alcohol or cocaine to control anxiety in social situations.*[7]
- Review history and elicit information about traumatic events that may have occurred. (Refer to ND Post-Trauma Syndrome.) *While little is known about the origins of social anxiety disorders, clients who have experienced a traumatic event may withdraw from contact and suffer from anxiety when faced with having to deal with social situations.*[1,5]

NURSING PRIORITY NO. 2 To alleviate conditions that contribute to client's sense of isolation:

- Establish therapeutic nurse-client relationship. *Promotes trust and acceptance, allowing client to feel safe and free to discuss sensitive matters without being judged.*[2]
- Spend time interacting with client and identify other resources available. *Getting to know client and identifying concerns about being involved in activities with others can lead to appropriate interventions. Other people such as volunteers, social workers, and chaplains may be able to spend time with client, enhancing circle of trusted people.*[4]
- Develop plan of action with client. Look at available resources; support risk-taking behaviors, financial planning, appropriate medical and self-care, etc. *Helping client to learn how to manage these issues of daily living can increase self-confidence and help individual to feel more comfortable in social settings.*[5]
- Introduce client to those with similar or shared interests and other supportive people. *Provides role models and encourages getting to know others who share feelings of anxiety, providing an opportunity to develop social skills and learn some ways of problem-solving to deal with anxiety.*[2,5]
- Promote participation in recreational or special interest activities in setting that client views as safe. *These activities have the advantage of providing physical and mental stimulation for client who feels isolated and anxious in social settings.*[2,9]
- Provide positive reinforcement when client makes move(s) toward other(s). *Acknowledges and encourages continuation of efforts, helping client toward independence.*[1,7]
- Identify foreign language resources for client who speaks another language. *A professional interpreter is important to ensure accuracy of interpretation; newspapers and radio programming in appropriate foreign language help client feel connected with own community.*[6,8]
- Assist client to problem-solve solutions to short-term or imposed isolation. *Condition may require individual to be isolated from others for his or her and/or others' protection, and working together to decide how to manage loneliness can promote successful outcome.*[1,3]
- Encourage open visitation when possible and/or telephone or computer contacts. *Maintains involvement with others, promoting social involvement, especially when client is unable to go out to activities.*[3]
- Provide environmental stimuli when client is confined. *Open curtains in room, display pictures of family or views of nature, promote television and radio listening, and provide Internet access to help client feel less isolated.*[3]
- 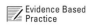Provide for placement in sheltered community when necessary. *The individual who is mentally impaired may be unable to learn to participate in society and display socially acceptable behaviors and will benefit from an environment that offers structure and assistance.*[3]

NURSING PRIORITY NO. 3 To promote wellness (Teaching/Discharge Considerations):

- Assist client to learn social skills as needed. *Enhancing problem-solving, communication, social skills, and learning skills to manage activities of daily living will improve sense of self-esteem.*[4]
- Encourage and assist client to enroll in classes as appropriate. *Assertiveness, vocational, and sex education classes may provide skills to improve ability to engage more effectively in social situations.*[5]

Diagnostic Studies   Evidence Based Practice   Medications   Pediatric/Geriatric/Lifespan

- Involve children and adolescents in age-appropriate programs or activities, as indicated. *Promotes socialization skills and peer contact to enable young person to learn by interacting with others.*[5]
- Help client differentiate between isolation and loneliness or aloneness and discuss how to avoid slipping into an undesired state. *Time for the individual to be alone is important to the maintenance of mental health, but the sadness created by isolation and loneliness needs different interventions.*[2,11]
- Involve client in programs directed to correction and prevention of identified causes of problem. *Activities such as senior citizen services, daily telephone contact, house sharing, pets, day-care centers, and church resources can help individual move out of isolation and become involved in life.*[5,10]
- Discuss use of medications, as indicated. *Prescribed medications, such as selective serotonin reuptake inhibitors, can be very effective in treating social disorders.*[3,7]
- Refer to counselor or therapist, as appropriate. *Facilitates grief work, promotes relationship building, and provides opportunity to work toward improvement of individual issues affecting social interactions.*[1]

DOCUMENTATION FOCUS

Assessment/Reassessment
- Individual findings, including precipitating factors, effect on lifestyle, relationships, and functioning.
- Client's perception of situation.
- Cultural or religious factors.
- Availability and use of resources and support systems.

Planning
- Plan of care and who is involved in planning.
- Teaching plan.

Implementation/Evaluation
- Responses to intervention, teaching, and actions performed.
- Attainment or progress toward desired outcome(s).
- Modifications to plan of care.

Discharge Planning
- Long-term needs and who is responsible for actions to be taken.
- Available resources, specific referrals made.

References

1. Robinson, L., et al. (Updated 2018). Emotional and psychological trauma: Symptoms, treatment and recovery. *HelpGuide.org.* Retrieved April 2018 from http://www.helpguide.org/articles/ptsd-trauma/emotional-and-psychological-trauma.htm.
2. Doenges, M. E., Townsend, M. C., Moorhouse, M. F. (1998). *Psychiatric Care Plans: Guidelines for Individualizing Care.* 3rd ed. Philadelphia: F. A. Davis.
3. Cox, H., et al. (2002). *Clinical Applications of Nursing Diagnosis: Adult, Child, Women's, Psychiatric, Gerontic, and Home Health Considerations.* 4th ed. Philadelphia: F. A. Davis.
4. Drew, N. (1991). Combating the social isolation of chronic mental illness. *J Psychosoc Nurs,* 29(6), 14–17.
5. No author listed. (2003). Beyond shyness and stage fright: Social anxiety disorder. *HarvMen Health Lett,* 20(4), 1–4.
6. Purnell, L. D. (2011). *Guide to Culturally Competent Health Care.* Philadelphia: F. A. Davis.
7. Frey, R. J. (No date). Generalized anxiety disorder. *Encyclopedia of Mental Disorders.* Retrieved April 2018 from http://www.minddisorders.com/Flu-Inv/Generalized-anxiety-disorder.html.
8. Andrulis, D. P. (2002). What a Difference an Interpreter Can Make: Health Care Experiences of Uninsured with Limited English Proficiency. *The Access Project.* Boston: Brandeis University.
9. McPherson, M., Smith-Lovin, L., Brashears, M. (2006). Social isolation in America: Changes in core discussion networks over two decades. *Am Sociol Rev,* 71(3), 353–375.
10. House, J. (2001). Social isolation kills, but how and why? *Psychosom Med,* 63(2), 273–274.
11. No author listed. (Updated 2015). Isolation. *GoodTherapy.org.* Retrieved April 2015 from http://www.goodtherapy.org/therapy-for-isolation.html.
12. Cacioppo, J. T., Hawkley, L. C. (2009). Perceived social isolation and cognition. *Trends Cogn Sci,* 13(10), 447–454.

 Acute Care Collaborative Community/Home Care Cultural

chronic Sorrow

Taxonomy II: Coping/Stress Tolerance—Class 2 Coping Responses (00137) [**Diagnostic Division:** Ego Integrity], Approved 1998; Revised 2017

DEFINITION: Cyclical, recurring, and potentially progressive pattern of pervasive sadness experienced (by a parent, caregiver, individual with chronic illness or disability) in response to continual loss, throughout the trajectory of an illness or disability.

RELATED FACTORS
Crises in illness or disability management
Missed opportunities or milestones

DEFINING CHARACTERISTICS

Subjective
Overwhelming negative feelings
Sadness
Feelings that interfere with well-being
Sample Clinical Applications: Cancer, multiple sclerosis (MS), Parkinson's disease, AIDS, amyotrophic lateral sclerosis (ALS), prematurity, genetic or congenital defects, infertility, dementia, Alzheimer's disease, bipolar disorder, schizophrenia, developmental delay

DESIRED OUTCOMES/EVALUATION CRITERIA

Sample NOC linkages:
Depression Level: Severity of melancholic mood and loss of interest in life events
Depression Self-Control: Personal actions to minimize melancholy and maintain interest in life events
Hope: Optimism that is personally satisfying and life supporting

Client Will (Include Specific Time Frame)
• Acknowledge presence and impact of sorrow.
• Demonstrate progress in dealing with loss(es) as evidenced by recognizing positive aspects of situation.
• Participate in work and/or self-care activities of daily living (ADLs) as able.
• Verbalize a sense of progress toward resolution of sorrow and hope for the future.

ACTIONS/INTERVENTIONS

Sample NIC linkages:
Mood Management: Providing for safety, stabilization, recovery, and maintenance of a patient who is experiencing depressed or elevated mood
Grief Work Facilitation: Assistance with the resolution of a significant loss
Hope Inspiration: Enhancing the belief in one's capacity to initiate and sustain actions

NURSING PRIORITY NO. 1 To assess causative/contributing factors and effect on life:

• Determine current or recent events or conditions contributing to client's state of mind (e.g., death of loved one, chronic physical or mental illness or disability). *Individual information is necessary when formulating a plan of care to address appropriate issues.*

 Diagnostic Studies   Evidence Based Practice   Medications   Pediatric/Geriatric/Lifespan

- Note cues of sadness. *Expressions of feelings of loss, such as sighing, faraway looks, unkempt appearance, inattention to conversation, and refusing food, can be indicators of sorrow that is not being dealt with. Note: Chronic sorrow may be cyclical—at times deepening versus times of feeling somewhat better.*[4,5]
- Be aware of use of avoidance behaviors. *Anger, withdrawal, and denial are part of the grieving process and may be used to avoid dealing with the reality of what has happened. However, in a situation that is unchangeable, such as a developmentally disabled child or a child with diabetes, sorrow is seen as a normal response and will continue to be a factor even as the family copes with the condition.*[5,7]
- Identify cultural values or religious beliefs and possible conflicts. *Expressions of sorrow are influenced by these beliefs and may result in conflicts. For instance, the Hispanic culture believes genetic defects are the will of God, but individual may be angry at God because of occurrence. Or, individual/family may have difficulty living up to the expectations of others (e.g., "God does not give us more than we can handle").*[6]
- ∞ Ascertain response of family/SOs to client's situation and support provided. *Parents who have chronically ill children or premature babies, adults who have multiple sclerosis, and elderly caregivers of spouses with dementia may continue to have feelings of sorrow even though they seem to be managing fairly well; due to cyclic nature of sorrow, they will require ongoing support/assistance from others to cope.*[4,7,11]
- Determine level of functioning and ability to care for self/others. Assess needs of family/SO. *Individual who is coping with chronic illness (e.g., Parkinson's disease, MS, HIV/AIDS) may exhibit chronic sorrow related to the illness, fear of death, poverty, and isolation associated with these conditions, which may lead to difficulty managing ADLs for self or meeting needs of family.*[2,3,11]
- Refer to NDs caregiver Role Strain, ineffective Coping, and complicated Grieving, as appropriate.

NURSING PRIORITY NO. 2   To assist client to move through sorrow:

- Encourage verbalization about situation. Active-listen feelings and be available for support and assistance. *Helpful in beginning resolution and acceptance. Individuals involved, client, and caregivers benefit from being able to talk freely about the situation. Active listening conveys a message of acceptance and helps individual come to own resolution.*[1,5]
- Encourage expression of anger, fear, or anxiety. (Refer to appropriate NDs.) *Individual needs to deal with these feelings before she or he can move forward.*[1]
- Acknowledge reality of feelings of guilt or blame, including hostility toward spiritual power. (Refer to ND Spiritual Distress.) *It was once believed that grief had an end stage, but research has shown that individuals with chronic conditions, such as diabetes mellitus, MS, and disabling conditions, continue to experience chronic sorrow and lifelong recurring sadness. Understanding this can help individual accept that these feelings are real, and when they are validated, they can be dealt with.*[4,5,10]
- Provide comfort and availability as well as caring for physical needs. *The way healthcare professionals respond to families is important to helping them cope with the situation as physical care is given.*[5,9,11]
- Discuss ways individual has dealt with past losses and reinforce use of previously effective coping skills. *As client begins to look at how they have handled previous situations, effective coping skills can be recalled and applied to current situation.*[2,9]
- Instruct in and encourage use of visualization and relaxation skills. *Learning these stress-management skills can help the individual relax, enhancing ability to deal with feelings of sorrow regarding the long-term situation.*[5,8]
- Discuss use of medication when depression is interfering with ability to manage life. *Client may benefit from the short-term use of an antidepressant medication to help deal with situation.*[1]
- Assist SOs to cope with client response. *Family/SO may not be dysfunctional, but may be intolerant and lack understanding of individual responses to long-term illness. Grief is unique to each individual and may not always follow a particular course to resolution that is understood by all.*[4,5,11]
- Include family/SO in setting realistic goals for meeting individual needs. *Inclusion of all family members ensures they all have the same information and are all working toward effective coping strategies.*[4,5]

  Acute Care   Collaborative   Community/ Home Care   Cultural

NURSING PRIORITY NO. 3 To promote wellness (Teaching/Discharge Considerations):

- 🏠 Discuss healthy ways of dealing with difficult situations. *Providing information about effective communication skills, understanding condition they are dealing with, and expectations of the course of the illness or condition can promote personal growth and lead to a positive outcome for the family.*[7,8]
- 🌐 Have client identify familial, religious, and cultural factors that have meaning for him or her. *May help bring loss or distressing situation into perspective and promote grief or sorrow resolution.*[6]
- Encourage involvement in usual activities, exercise, and socialization within limits of physical and psychological state. *Energy is restored and individuals can go on with their lives when they are willing and able to continue activities.*[5,7]
- Introduce concept of mindfulness (living in the moment) and encourage client to recognize and embrace moments of joy in own life. *Promotes feelings of capability and belief that this moment can be dealt with or enjoyed.*[4,8]
- 👥 Refer to other resources (e.g., pastoral care, counseling, psychotherapy, respite care providers, support groups). *Provides additional help when needed to resolve situation, continue grief work, and move on with life.*[11]

DOCUMENTATION FOCUS

Assessment/Reassessment
- Individual findings, including nature of sorrow, effects on participation in treatment regimen.
- Physical and emotional response to conflict, expressions of sadness.
- Cultural or religious issues and conflicts.
- Reactions of family/SO.

Planning
- Plan of care and who is involved in planning.
- Teaching plan.

Implementation/Evaluation
- Response to interventions, teaching, and actions performed.
- Attainment or progress toward desired outcome(s).
- Modifications to plan of care.

Discharge Planning
- Long-term needs and who is responsible for actions to be taken.
- Available resources, specific referrals made.

References

1. Doenges, M. E., Moorhouse, M. F., Murr, A. C. (2010). *Nurse's Pocket Guide Diagnoses: Interventions and Rationales.* 12th ed. Philadelphia: F. A. Davis.
2. Lindgren, C. L. (1996). Chronic sorrow in persons with Parkinson's and their spouse caregivers. *Sch Inq Nurs Pract,* 10(4), 351–366.
3. Lichtensten, B., Laska, M. K., Clair, J. M. (2002). Chronic sorrow in the HIV-positive patient: Issues of race, gender, and social support. *AIDS Patient Care STDs,* 16(1), 27–38.
4. Kearney, P. (2003, updated 2010). Chronic grief (or is it periodic grief?). *Lecture materials, Indiana University.* Retrieved April 2018 from http://www.indiana.edu/~famlygrf/units/chronic.html.
5. Lowes, L., Lyne, P. (2000). Chronic sorrow in parents of children with newly diagnosed diabetes: A review of the literature and discussion of the implications for nursing practice. *J Adv Nurs,* 32(1), 41–48.
6. Lipson, J. G., Dibble, S. L., Minarik, P. A. (1996). *Culture & Nursing Care: A Pocket Guide.* San Francisco: UCSF Nursing Press.
7. Mallow, G. E., Bechtel, G. A. (1999). Chronic sorrow: The experience of parents with children who are developmentally disabled. *J Psychosoc Nurs,* 17(7), 31–43.
8. Kabat-Zinn, J. (1994). *Wherever You Go, There You Are.* New York: Hyperion.
9. Kearney, P. M., Griffin, T. (2001). Between joy and sorrow: Being a parent of a child with a developmental disability. *J Adv Nurs,* 34(5), 582–592.
10. Hobdell, E. (2004). Chronic sorrow and depression in parents of children with neural tube defects. *J Neurosci Nurs,* 36(2), 82–94.
11. Gordon, J. (2009). An evidence-based approach supporting parents dealing with chronic sorrow. *Pediatr Nurs,* 35(2), 115–119.

 Diagnostic Studies
 Evidence Based Practice
 Medications
 Pediatric/Geriatric/Lifespan

Spiritual Distress

Taxonomy II: Life Principles—Class 3 Value/Belief/Action Congruence (00066) [Diagnostic Division: Ego Integrity], Approved 1978; Revised 2002, 2013, 2017

DEFINITION: A state of suffering related to the impaired ability to experience and integrate meaning in life through connections with self, others, the world, or a superior being.

RELATED FACTORS
Anxiety; depression
Barrier to experiencing love; ineffective relationships; loneliness; low self-esteem
Change in religious ritual or spiritual practice; cultural conflict
Environmental change
Inability to forgive; perception of having unfinished business
Increasing dependence on another; self-alienation; separation from support system
Pain
Social alienation; sociocultural deprivation
Substance misuse/[abuse]

DEFINING CHARACTERISTICS

Subjective
Anxiety, fear
Fatigue; insomnia
Questioning identity; questioning meaning of suffering or life
Connections to self:
Anger; guilt; insufficient courage
Decrease in serenity
Feeling of being unloved; inadequate acceptance
Connections with others:
Alienation
Connections with art, music, literature, nature:
Disinterest in nature or reading spiritual literature
Connections with power greater than self:
Anger toward power greater than self
Feeling abandoned; hopelessness; perceived suffering
Inability to pray or participate in religious activities, or to experience the transcendent

Objective
Crying
Connections to self:
Ineffective coping strategies; perceived insufficient meaning in life
Connections with others:
Refuses to interact with significant others or spiritual leader
Separation from support system
Connections with art, music, literature, nature:
Decrease in expression of previous pattern of creativity
Connections with power greater than self:
Inability for introspection; sudden change in spiritual practice; request for a spiritual leader
At Risk Population: Aging; birth of a child
Death of a significant other; exposure to death; loss

 Acute Care   Collaborative   Community/Home Care   Cultural

Life transition; unexpected life event; receiving bad news

Exposure to natural disaster

Increasing dependence on another

Associated Condition: Actively dying; imminent death

Illness; physical illness; chronic illness

Loss of a body part, or function of a body part

Treatment regimen

Sample Clinical Applications: Chronic conditions (e.g., cancer, AIDS, traumatic brain injury vegetative state, infertility); fetal demise, risk for Sudden Infant Death (SIDS); death of child; traumatic event with fatal outcome or severe disabilities

DESIRED OUTCOMES/EVALUATION CRITERIA

Sample **NOC** linkages:

Spiritual Health: Connectedness with self, others, higher power, all life, nature, and the universe that transcends and empowers the self

Hope: Optimism that is personally satisfying and life supporting

Psychosocial Adjustment: Life Change: Adaptive psychosocial response of an individual to a significant life circumstance

Client Will (Include Specific Time Frame)

• Verbalize increased sense of connectedness and hope for future.

• Demonstrate ability to help self and participate in care.

• Participate in activities with others, actively seek relationships.

• Discuss beliefs and values about spiritual issues.

• Verbalize acceptance of self as not deserving illness or situation: "No one is to blame."

ACTIONS/INTERVENTIONS

Sample **NIC** linkages:

Spiritual Support: Assisting the patient to feel balance and connection with a greater power

Hope Inspiration: Enhancing the belief in one's capacity to initiate and sustain actions

Grief Work Facilitation: Assistance with the resolution of a significant loss

NURSING PRIORITY NO. 1 To assess causative/contributing factors:

• Determine client's religious and spiritual orientation, current involvement, and presence of conflicts. *Identification of individual spiritual beliefs and practices that may affect client care, or create conflict between beliefs and treatment, provides for more accurate interventions.*[1]

• Listen to client's/SO's reports or expressions of concern, anger, alienation from God, belief that illness or situation is a punishment for wrongdoing, etc. *Indicates depth of grieving process and possible need for spiritual advisor or other resource to address client's belief system if desired.*[2]

• Assess for influence of cultural beliefs and spiritual values that affect individual in this situation. *Circumstances of illness or situation may conflict with client's view of self, cultural background, and distress over values. For instance, many Hispanics are Catholic with strong beliefs in the relationship between illness and religious practices.*[5]

• Note recent changes in behavior (e.g., withdrawal from others and creative or religious activities, dependence on alcohol or medications). *Helpful in determining severity and duration of situation and possible need for additional referrals such as substance withdrawal.*[7,11]

 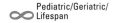

- Assess sense of self-concept and worth and ability to enter into loving relationships. *Lack of connectedness with self or others impairs client's ability to trust others or feel worthy of trust from others, leading to difficulties in relationships with others.*[1,7]
- Observe behavior indicative of poor relationships with others (e.g., manipulative, nontrusting, demanding). *Manipulation is used for management of client's sense of powerlessness because of distrust of others, interfering with relationships with others.*[3,6]
- Determine support systems available to client/SO(s) and how they are used. *Provides insight to client's willingness to pursue outside resources.*[4]
- Determine sense of futility, feelings of hopelessness and helplessness, and lack of motivation to help self. *Indicators that client may see no, or only limited, options, alternatives, or personal choices available; that client lacks energy to deal with situation; and that further evaluation is needed.*
- 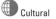 Note expressions of inability to find meaning in life and/or reason for living. Evaluate suicidal ideation *to refer for mental health evaluation and intervention as indicated. Crisis of the spirit or loss of will to live places client at increased risk for inattention to personal well-being and possible harm to self.*[1,7]

NURSING PRIORITY NO. 2   To assist client/SO(s) to deal with feelings/situation:

- Develop therapeutic nurse-client relationship. Ascertain client's views as to how care provider(s) can be most helpful. Convey acceptance of client's spiritual beliefs and concerns. *Promotes trust and comfort, encouraging client to be open about sensitive matters.*[6]
- Establish environment that promotes free expression of feelings and concerns. *Provides opportunity for client to explore own thoughts and make appropriate decisions regarding spiritual issues.*[4]
- Provide calm, peaceful setting when possible. *Promotes relaxation and enhances opportunity for reflection on situation/discussions with others and meditation.*[3]
- Encourage life review by client. Support client in finding a reason for living. *Promotes sense of hope and willingness to continue efforts to improve situation.*[3]
- Be aware of influence of care provider's own belief system. *It is still possible to be helpful to client while remaining neutral and not espousing own beliefs because client's beliefs and needs are what is important.*[6]
- Identify inappropriate coping behaviors currently being used and associated consequences and discuss with client. *Recognizing negative consequences of actions may enhance desire to change.*[2]
- Set limits on acting-out behavior that is inappropriate/destructive. *Promotes safety for client/others and helps prevent loss of self-esteem.*[2,7]
- Ascertain past successes and coping behaviors. *Helps to determine approaches used previously that may be effective in dealing with current situation, providing encouragement.*[6]
- Problem-solve solutions and identify areas for compromise. *May be useful in resolving conflicts that arise from feelings of anxiety regarding questioning of beliefs and current illness or situation.*[3]
- Assist in developing coping skills *to deal with stressors of illness and necessary changes in lifestyle.*[7,9]

NURSING PRIORITY NO. 3   To facilitate setting goals and moving forward:

- Use therapeutic communication skills of reflection and active-listening. *Conveys message of competence and helps client find own solutions to concerns.*[7]
- Involve client in refining healthcare goals and therapeutic regimen as appropriate. *Promotes feelings of control over what is happening, enhancing commitment to plan and optimizing outcomes.*[3]
- Encourage client/family to ask questions. *Demonstrates support for individual's willingness to learn.*
- Discuss difference between grief and guilt and help client to identify and deal with each. Point out consequences of actions based on guilt. *Aids client in assuming responsibility for own actions and avoids acting out of false guilt.*[6]
- Identify role models (e.g., individual experiencing similar situation). *Provides opportunities for sharing of experiences and hope and identifying new options to deal with situation.*[7]

 Acute Care   Collaborative   Community/ Home Care   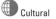 Cultural

- Assist client to learn use of meditation, mindfulness, and prayer, if desired. *Provides avenue for learning forgiveness to heal past hurts and developing a sense of peace.*[3,8]
- Provide information that anger with God is a normal part of the grieving process. *Realizing these feelings are not unusual can reduce sense of guilt, encourage open expression, and facilitate resolution of grief.*[3,7,11]
- Provide time and privacy to engage in spiritual growth or religious activities as desired (e.g., prayer, meditation, scripture reading, listening to music). *Allows client to focus on self and seek connectedness with spiritual beliefs and values.*[6]
- Encourage and facilitate outings to neighborhood park or nature walks. *Sunshine, fresh air, and activity can stimulate release of endorphins, promoting sense of well-being and encouraging connection with nature.*[6]
- ∞ Provide play therapy for child that encompasses spiritual data. *Interactive pleasurable activity promotes open discussion and enhances retention of information. Child will act out feelings in play therapy easier than talking. Provides opportunity for child to practice what has been learned and for therapist to evaluate child's progress.*[3]
- ∞ Abide by parents' wishes in discussing and implementing child's spiritual support. *Limits confusion for child and prevents conflict of values and beliefs.*[3]
- Refer to appropriate resources (e.g., pastoral or parish nurse or religious counselor, crisis counselor, hospice; psychotherapy; Alcoholics or Narcotics Anonymous). *Useful in dealing with immediate situation and identifying long-term resources for support to help foster sense of connectedness.*[7,8]
- Refer to NDs ineffective Coping, Powerlessness, Self-Esteem (specify), Social Isolation, and risk for Suicide for additional interventions as indicated.

NURSING PRIORITY NO. 4 To promote spiritual well-being (Teaching/Discharge Considerations):

- Make time for nonjudgmental discussion of philosophical issues or questions about spiritual impact of illness or situation and/or treatment regimen. *Open communication can assist client in reality checks of perceptions and help to identify personal options.*[6]
- Assist client to develop long-term goals for dealing with future and illness situation. *Involvement in planning for desired outcomes enhances commitment to goal, optimizing outcomes.*[7]
- Suggest use of journaling. *Provides opportunity to write feelings and happenings; reviewing them over time can assist in clarifying values and ideas, recognizing and resolving feelings or situation.*[6,10]
- Assist client to identify SO(s)/others who could provide support as needed. *Ongoing support is important to enhance sense of connectedness and continue progress toward goals.*[6]
- Identify spiritual resources that could be helpful (e.g., contact spiritual advisor who has qualifications or experience in dealing with specific problems such as death/dying, relationship problems, substance abuse, suicide). *Provides answers to spiritual questions, assists in the journey of self-discovery, and can help client learn to accept and forgive self.*[6]

DOCUMENTATION FOCUS

Assessment/Reassessment
- Individual findings, including nature of spiritual conflict, and effects of participation in treatment regimen.
- Physical and emotional responses to conflict.

Planning
- Plan of care and who is involved in planning.
- Teaching plan.

Implementation/Evaluation
- Responses to interventions, teaching, and actions performed.
- Attainment or progress toward desired outcome(s).
- Modifications to plan of care.

 Diagnostic Studies   Evidence Based Practice   Medications ∞ Pediatric/Geriatric/Lifespan

Discharge Planning
• Long-term needs and who is responsible for actions to be taken.
• Available resources, specific referrals made.

References

1. Slade, M. (2010). Mental illness and well-being: The central importance of positive psychology and recovery approaches. *BMC Health Serv Res*, 10, 26.
2. Koenig, H. G. (2013). Meeting the emotional and spiritual needs of patients. *Satisfaction Snapshot*. Retrieved April 2018 from http://www.pressganey.com.au/snapshots/2013/Meeting%20the%20Emotional%20and%20Spiritual%20Needs%20of%20Patients.pdf.
3. Baldacchino, D., Draper, P. (2001). Spiritual coping strategies: A review of the nursing research literature. *J Adv Nurs*, 34(6), 833–841.
4. Cox, H., et al. (2002). *Clinical Applications of Nursing Diagnosis*. 4th ed. Philadelphia: F. A. Davis.
5. Ludwik, R., Silva, M. C. (2000). Ethics: Nursing around the world: Cultural values and ethical conflicts. *Online J Issues Nurs*. Retrieved April 2018 from http://www.nursingworld.org/MainMenuCategories/ANAMarketplace/ANAPeriodicals/OJIN/Columns/Ethics/CulturalValuesandEthicalConflicts.html.
6. Ross, L. A. (1994). Spiritual aspects of nursing. *J Adv Nurs*, 19(3), 439–447.
7. Townsend, M. C. (2003). *Psychiatric Mental Health Nursing Concepts of Care*. 4th ed. Philadelphia: F. A. Davis.
8. Hospital and Palliative Nurses Association (HPNA). (2015). HPNA Position Paper: Spiritual care. Retrieved April 2018 from http://hpna.advancingexpertcare.org/wp-content/uploads/2015/08/Spiritual-Care.pdf.
9. Post, B. C., et al. (2013). Religion and spirituality in group counseling: Beliefs and practices of university counseling center counselors. *The Journal for Specialists in Group Work*, 38(4), 264–284.
10. Johnson, C. V., Hayes, J. A. (2003). Troubled spirits: Prevalence and predictors of religious and spiritual concerns among university students and counseling center clients. *J Couns Psychol*, 50(4), 409–419.
11. Sack, D. (Updated 2015). Grieving the addiction. Retrieved April 2018 from http://www.networktherapy.com/DonnaHunter/default.asp?pid=1534.

---

risk for Spiritual Distress

Taxonomy II: Life Principles—Class 3 Value/Belief/Action Congruence (00067) [**Diagnostic Division:** Ego Integrity], Approved 1998; Revised 2013, 2017

DEFINITION: Susceptible to an impaired ability to experience and integrate meaning and purpose in life through connectedness within self, others, literature, nature, and/or a power greater than oneself, which may compromise health.

RISK FACTORS
Anxiety; depression
Barrier to experiencing love; ineffective relationships; loneliness; low self-esteem
Change in religious ritual or spiritual practice; cultural conflict
Environmental change
Inability to forgive; perception of having unfinished business
Increasing dependence on another; self-alienation; separation form support system
Pain
Social alienation; sociocultural deprivation
Substance misuse/[abuse]
At Risk Population: Aging; birth of a child
Death of a significant other; exposure to death; loss
Life transition; unexpected life event; receiving bad news
Exposure to natural disaster
Increasing dependence on another
Associated Condition: Actively dying; imminent death
Illness; physical illness; chronic illness

 Acute Care   Collaborative   Community/Home Care   Cultural

Loss of a body part, or function of a body part

Treatment regimen

Sample Clinical Applications: Chronic conditions (e.g., cancer, AIDS, traumatic brain injury vegetative state) infertility; terminal conditions (e.g., end-stage renal disease, lung cancer); fetal demise, risk for Sudden Infant Death (SIDS); death of spouse or child; traumatic event with fatal outcome or severe disabilities

DESIRED OUTCOMES/EVALUATION CRITERIA

Sample **NOC** linkages:

Spiritual Health: Connectedness with self, others, higher power, all life, nature, and the universe that transcends and empowers the self

Hope: Optimism that is personally satisfying and life supporting

Psychosocial Adjustment: Life Change: Adaptive psychosocial response of an individual to a significant life circumstance

Client Will (Include Specific Time Frame)

- Identify meaning and purpose in own life that reinforces hope, peace, and contentment.
- Verbalize acceptance of self as being worthy, not deserving of illness or situation, and so forth.
- Identify and use resources appropriately.

ACTIONS/INTERVENTIONS

Sample **NIC** linkages:

Spiritual Support: Assisting the patient to feel balance and connection with a greater power

Coping Enhancement: Facilitation of cognitive and behavioral efforts to manage perceived stressors, changes, or threats that interfere with meeting life demands and roles

Grief Work Facilitation: Assistance with the resolution of a significant loss

NURSING PRIORITY NO. 1 To assess causative/contributing factors:

- Ascertain current situation (e.g., natural disaster, death of a spouse, personal injustice). *Identification of circumstances that put the individual at risk for loss of connectedness with spiritual beliefs is essential to plan for appropriate interventions.*
- Listen to client's/significant other's (SO's) expressions of anger or concern, belief that illness or situation is a punishment for wrongdoing, etc. *Identifies need for client to talk about and be listened to in regard to concerns about potential loss of control over his or her life.*[3,6]
- Note reason for living and whether it is directly related to situation. *Tragic occurrences, such as home and business washed away in a flood or lost in a fire, parent whose only child is terminally ill, or loss of a spouse, can cause individual to question previous beliefs.*[1,3]
- Determine client's religious or spiritual orientation, current involvement, and presence of conflicts, especially in current circumstances. *Client may be a member of a religious organization, and whether he or she is active or whether conflicts have risen in relation to current illness or situation will indicate need for assistance from spiritual advisor, pastor, or other resource client would accept.*[1,8,11]
- Assess sense of self-concept, worth, and ability to enter into loving relationships. *Lack of connectedness with self and others impairs client's ability to trust others or feel worthy of trust from others.*[1,7]
- Observe behavior indicative of poor relationships with others. *Client may be manipulative, nontrusting, and demanding because of distrust of self and others, which can interfere with relationships with others, indicating a need for learning positive ways to interact with others.*[2,4]

 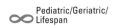

- Determine support systems available to, and used by, client/SO(s). *Provides insight into individual's willingness to pursue outside resources.*[6,10]
- Ascertain substance use or abuse. *Complicates situation, affects ability to deal with problems in a positive manner, and identifies need for referral to appropriate treatment programs.*[4,9,11]
- Assess for influence of cultural beliefs and spiritual values that affect individual in this situation. *Circumstances of illness or situation may conflict with client's view of self, cultural background, and distress over values. For instance, many Hispanics are Catholic with strong beliefs in the relationship of illness and religious practices.*[5]

NURSING PRIORITY NO. 2   To assist client/SO(s) to deal with feelings/situation:

- Establish environment that promotes free expression of feelings and concerns. *Provides opportunity for client to explore own thoughts and make appropriate decisions regarding spiritual issues and conflicts.*[6,7,10,12]
- Use therapeutic communication skills of reflection and Active listening. *Communicates confidence in client's ability to find own solutions to concerns.*[7]
- Have client identify and prioritize current or immediate needs. *Helps client focus on what needs to be done and identifies manageable steps to take to achieve goals.*
- Make time for nonjudgmental discussion of philosophical issues or questions about spiritual impact of illness or situation and/or treatment regimen. *Open communication can assist client to make reality checks of perceptions and begin to identify personal options.*[6,12]
- Discuss difference between grief and guilt and help client to identify and deal with each. *Helps client to assume responsibility for own actions, become aware of the consequences of acting out of false guilt.*
- Review coping skills used and their effectiveness in current situation. *Identifies strengths to incorporate into plan and techniques needing revision.*
- Identify role model (e.g., individual experiencing similar situation or disease). *Sharing of experiences and hope provides opportunity for client to look at options as modeled by others and to begin to deal with reality.*[7]
- Provide play therapy for child that encompasses spiritual data. *Interactive pleasurable activity promotes open discussion and enhances retention of information. Child will act out feelings in play therapy easier than talking. Provides opportunity for child to practice what has been learned and for therapist to evaluate child's progress.*[3]
- Abide by parents' wishes in discussing and implementing child's spiritual support. *Limits confusion for child and prevents conflict of values and beliefs.*[3]
- Refer to appropriate resources (e.g., crisis counselor, governmental agencies; pastoral or parish nurse or spiritual advisor who has qualifications or experience dealing with specific problems such as death/dying, relationship problems, substance abuse, suicide; hospice; psychotherapy; Alcoholics or Narcotics Anonymous). *Useful in dealing with immediate situation and identifying long-term resources for support to help foster sense of connectedness.*[7,8,12]

NURSING PRIORITY NO. 3   To promote spiritual well-being (Teaching/Discharge Considerations):

- Role-play new coping techniques. *Provides opportunity to practice and enhances integration of new skills or necessary lifestyle changes.*[4]
- Assist client to learn use of meditation, mindfulness, and prayer, if desired. *Provides avenue for learning forgiveness to heal past hurts and developing a sense of peace.*[3,8]
- Suggest use of journaling. *Provides opportunity to write feelings and happenings; reviewing them over time can assist in clarifying values and ideas and recognizing and resolving feelings or situation.*[6,9]
- Encourage individual to become involved in cultural activities of his or her choosing. *Art, music, plays, and other cultural activities provide a means of connecting with self and others.*
- Discuss possibilities of taking classes and becoming involved in discussion groups or community programs.
- Assist client to identify SO(s) and individuals/support groups who could provide ongoing support. *Having sufficient support can help client maintain spiritual resolve.*[6]

Acute Care   Collaborative   Community/ Home Care   Cultural

- 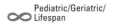 Discuss benefit of family counseling as appropriate. *Issues of this nature (e.g., situational losses, natural disasters, difficult relationships) affect family dynamics, and family may find it useful to discuss and resolve problems they are experiencing.*[7]

DOCUMENTATION FOCUS

Assessment/Reassessment
- Individual findings, including risk factors, nature of current distress.
- Physical and emotional responses to distress.
- Access to and use of resources.

Planning
- Plan of care and who is involved in planning.
- Teaching plan.

Implementation/Evaluation
- Responses to interventions, teaching, and actions performed.
- Attainment or progress toward desired outcome(s).
- Modifications to plan of care.

Discharge Planning
- Long-term needs and who is responsible for actions to be taken.
- Available resources, specific referrals made.

References

1. Slade, M. (2010). Mental illness and well-being: The central importance of positive psychology and recovery approaches. *BMC Health Serv Res*, 10, 26.
2. Koenig, H. G. (2013). Meeting the emotional and spiritual needs of patients. *Satisfaction Snapshot*. Retrieved April 2018 from http://www.pressganey.com.au/snapshots/2013/Meeting%20the%20Emotional%20and%20Spiritual%20Needs%20of%20Patients.pdf.
3. Baldacchino, D., Draper, P. (2001). Spiritual coping strategies: A review of the nursing research literature. *J Adv Nurs*, 34(6), 833–841.
4. Cox, H. C., et al. (2002). *Clinical Applications of Nursing Diagnosis: Adult, Child, Women's, Psychiatric, Gerontic, and Home Health Considerations*. 4th ed. Philadelphia: F. A. Davis.
5. Ludwik, R., Silva, M. C. (2000). Ethics: Nursing around the world: Cultural values and ethical conflicts. *Online J Issues Nurs*. Retrieved April 2018 from http://www.nursingworld.org/MainMenuCategories/ANAMarketplace/ANAPeriodicals/OJIN/Columns/Ethics/CulturalValuesandEthicalConflicts.html.
6. Conte, M. (No date). Spirituality in nursing. Retrieved April 2018 from https://www.spiritual-healing-for-you.com/spirituality-in-nursing.html.
7. Townsend, M. C. (2003). *Psychiatric Mental Health Nursing Concepts of Care*. 4th ed. Philadelphia: F. A. Davis.
8. Hospital and Palliative Nurses Association (HPNA). (Updated 2015). HPNA Position Paper: Spiritual care. Retrieved April 2018 from http://hpna.advancingexpertcare.org/wp-content/uploads/2015/08/Spiritual-Care.pdf.
9. Post, B. C., et al. (2013). Religion and spirituality in group counseling: Beliefs and practices of university counseling center counselors. *The Journal for Specialists in Group Work*, 38(4), 264–284.
10. Johnson, C. V., Hayes, J. A. (2003). Troubled spirits: Prevalence and predictors of religious and spiritual concerns among university students and counseling center clients. *J Couns Psychol*, 50, 409–419.
11. Leigh, J., Bowen, S., Mariatt, G. A. (2005). Spirituality, mindfulness and substance abuse. *Addict Behav*, 30(7), 1335–1341.
12. Smith, A. (2006). Using the Synergy Model to provide spiritual nursing care in critical care settings. *Crit Care Nurs*, 26(4), 41–47.

 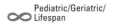

readiness for enhanced Spiritual Well-Being

Taxonomy II: Life Principles—Class 2 Beliefs (00068) [**Diagnostic Division:** Ego Integrity], Approved 1994; Revised 2002, 2013

DEFINITION: A pattern of experiencing and integrating meaning and purpose in life through connectedness with self, others, art, music, literature, nature, and/or a power greater than oneself, which can be strengthened.

DEFINING CHARACTERISTICS

Subjective

Connections to self:

Expresses desire to enhance: acceptance, surrender, coping, courage, self-forgiveness, hope, joy, love, serenity (e.g., peace), meaning or purpose in life, satisfaction with philosophy of life

Expresses desire to enhance meditative practice

Connections with others:

Expresses desire to enhance interaction with significant other/spiritual leaders, service to others

Expresses desire to enhance forgiveness from others

Connections with art, music, literature, and nature:

Expresses desire to enhance creative energy (e.g., writing, poetry, music), spiritual reading, time outdoors

Connections with powers greater than self:

Expresses desire to enhance participation in religious activity, prayerfulness, reverence, mystical experiences

Sample Clinical Applications: As a health-seeking behavior, the client may be healthy or this diagnosis can occur in any clinical condition

DESIRED OUTCOMES/EVALUATION CRITERIA

Sample NOC linkages:

Spiritual Health: Connectedness with self, others, higher power, all life, nature, and the universe that transcends and empowers the self

Hope: Optimism that is personally satisfying and life supporting

Quality of Life: Extent of positive perception of current life circumstances

Client Will (Include Specific Time Frame)

- Acknowledge the stabilizing and strengthening forces in own life needed for balance and well-being of the whole person.
- Identify meaning and purpose in own life, which reinforces hope, peace, and contentment.
- Verbalize a sense of peace or contentment and comfort of spirit.
- Demonstrate behavior congruent with verbalizations that lend support and strength for daily living.

ACTIONS/INTERVENTIONS

Sample NIC linkages:

Spiritual Growth Facilitation: Facilitation of growth in patients' capacity to identify, connect with, and call upon the source of meaning, purpose, comfort, strength, and hope in their lives

Religious Ritual Enhancement: Facilitating participation in religious practices

Meditation Facilitation: Facilitating a relaxed internal state of expanded awareness in the present moment by concentrating focus on a sound, object, visual image, the breath, or moment

 Acute Care

 Collaborative

 Community/ Home Care

 Cultural

NURSING PRIORITY NO. 1 To determine spiritual state/motivation for growth:

- Ascertain client's perception of current state or degree of connectedness and expectations. *Provides insight as to where client is currently and specific hopes for the future.*[1]
- Ascertain motivation and expectations for change. *Motivation to improve and high expectations can encourage client to make changes that will improve his or her life. However, unrealistic expectations may hamper efforts.*
- Review spiritual or religious history, activities, rituals, and frequency of participation. *Determines basis to build on for growth or change.*[1]
- 🌐 Determine influence of cultural beliefs or values. *Most individuals are strongly influenced by the spiritual or religious orientation of their family of origin, which can be a major determinate for client's choice of activities and receptiveness to various options.*[5]
- Determine relational values of support systems to client's spiritual centeredness. *The client's family may have differing beliefs from those espoused by the individual, which may be a source of conflict for the client. Comfort can be gained when family and friends share client's beliefs and support the search for spiritual knowledge.*[2]
- Explore meaning or interpretation and relationship of spirituality, life and death, and illness to life's journey. *This information helps client strengthen personal belief system, enabling him or her to move forward and live life to the fullest.*[2,3]
- Clarify the meaning of client's spiritual beliefs or religious practice and rituals to daily living. *Discussing these issues allows client to explore spiritual needs and decide what fits own view of the world to enhance life.*[6]
- Explore ways that spirituality or religious practices have affected client's life and given meaning and value to daily living. Note consequences as well as benefits. *Promotes understanding and appreciation of the difference between spirituality and religion and how each can be used to enhance client's journey of self-discovery.*[3]
- Discuss life's or God's plan (when this is the person's belief) for the individual. *Helpful in determining individual goals and choosing specific options.*[2]

NURSING PRIORITY NO. 2 To assist client to integrate values and beliefs to achieve a sense of wholeness and optimum balance in daily living:

- Explore ways beliefs give meaning and value to daily living. *As client develops understanding of these issues, he or she will provide support for dealing with current and future concerns.*[4]
- Clarify reality and appropriateness of client's self-perceptions and expectations. *Necessary to provide firm foundation for growth. Unrealistic ideas can impede desired improvement.*[2]
- Discuss the importance and value of connections to client's daily life. *The contacts that one has with others sustain the feeling of belonging and connection and promote feelings of wholeness and well-being.*[4,6]
- 🏠 Identify ways to achieve connectedness or harmony with self, others, nature, and/or a higher power (e.g., meditation, prayer, talking or sharing self with others; being out in nature, gardening, walking; attending religious activities). *This is a highly individual and personal decision, and no action is too trivial to be considered.*[4]

NURSING PRIORITY NO. 3 To enhance optimum spirituality:

- 🏠 Encourage client to take time to be introspective in the search for peace and harmony. *Finding peace within oneself will carry over to relationships with others and own outlook on life.*[1]
- Discuss use of relaxation or meditative activities (e.g., yoga, tai chi, prayer). *Helpful in promoting general well-being and sense of connectedness with self, nature, and/or spiritual power.*[4,6]
- Suggest attendance or involvement in dream-sharing group *to develop and enhance learning of the characteristics of spiritual awareness and facilitate the individual's growth.*[1]
- Identify ways for spiritual or religious expression. *There are multiple options for enhancing spirituality through connectedness with self/others (e.g., volunteering time to community projects, mentoring, singing in the choir, painting, spiritual writings).*[3,4]
- Encourage participation in desired religious activities and contact with minister or spiritual advisor. *Validating one's beliefs in an external way can provide support and strengthen the inner self.*[1,3]

 Diagnostic Studies   Evidence Based Practice   Medications   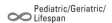 Pediatric/Geriatric/Lifespan

- Discuss and role-play, as necessary, ways to deal with alternative view or conflict that may occur with family/SO(s)/society or cultural group. *Provides opportunity to try out different behaviors in a safe environment and be prepared for potentialities.*[3]
- Provide bibliotherapy, list of relevant resources (e.g., study groups, parish nurse, poetry society), and reliable Web sites *for later reference, self-paced learning, and ongoing support.*[3]

DOCUMENTATION FOCUS

Assessment/Reassessment
- Assessment findings, including client perception of needs and desire for growth.
- Cultural values or religious beliefs.
- Motivation and expectations for change.

Planning
- Plan for growth and who is involved in planning.

Implementation/Evaluation
- Response to activities, learning, and actions performed.
- Attainment or progress toward desired outcome(s).
- Modifications to plan.

Discharge Planning
- Long-term needs, expectations, and plan of action.
- Specific referrals made.

References

1. Slade, M. (2010). Mental illness and well-being: The central importance of positive psychology and recovery approaches. *BMC Health Serv Res*, 10–26.
2. Koenig, H. G. (2013). Meeting the emotional and spiritual needs of patients. *Satisfaction Snapshot.* Retrieved April 2018 from http://www.pressganey.com.au/snapshots/2013/Meeting%20the%20Emotional%20and%20Spiritual%20Needs%20of%20Patients.pdf.
3. Baldacchino, D., Draper, P. (2001). Spiritual coping strategies: A review of the nursing research literature. *J Adv Nurs*, 34(6), 833–841.
4. Cox, H., et al. (2002). *Clinical Applications of Nursing Diagnosis*. 4th ed. Philadelphia: F. A. Davis.
5. Caplan, M. (2011). Psychology and Spirituality: One path or two? Retrieved April 2018 from http://www.huffingtonpost.com/mariana-caplan-phd/spirituality-and-psychology_b_941242.html.
6. Ross, L. A. (1994). Spiritual aspects of nursing. *J Adv Nurs*, 19(3), 439–447.

impaired Standing

Taxonomy II: Safety/Protection—Class 2 Activity/Exercise (00238) [**Diagnostic Division:** Safety], Approved 2013; Revised 2017

DEFINITION: Limitation of ability to independently and purposefully attain and/or maintain the body in an upright position from feet to head.

RELATED FACTORS
Emotional disturbance
Malnutrition; obesity
Insufficient endurance or energy; insufficient muscle strength
Pain
Self-imposed relief posture

 Acute Care Collaborative Community/Home Care Cultural

DEFINING CHARACTERISTICS

Objective

Impaired ability to adjust position of one or both lower limbs on uneven surface

Impaired ability to attain or maintain a balanced position of the torso; impaired ability to stress torso with body weight

Impaired ability to flex or extend one or both hips

Inability to flex or extend one or both knees

Associated Condition: Circulatory perfusion disorder; impaired metabolic functioning; neurological disorder; sarcopenia

Injury to lower extremity; surgical procedure

Prescribed posture

Sample Clinical Applications: Neuromuscular disorders (e.g., multiple sclerosis [MS], amyotrophic lateral sclerosis [ALS], Parkinson's disease), traumatic injuries (e.g., lower extremity fractures, spinal cord or brain injuries), osteoarthritis, rheumatoid arthritis, hip or knee joint replacement; severe depression, dementia

DESIRED OUTCOMES/EVALUATION CRITERIA

Sample NOC linkages:

Knowledge: Body Mechanics: Extent of understanding conveyed about proper body alignment, balance and coordinated movement

Balance: Ability to maintain body equilibrium

Body Mechanics Performance: Personal actions to maintain proper body alignment and to prevent musculoskeletal strain

Client Will (Include Specific Time Frame)

• Verbalize understanding of individual treatment regimen and safety measures.

• Attain and maintain position of standing function that enables activities and prevents complications.

• Participate in activities of daily living (ADLs) and desired activities.

ACTIONS/INTERVENTIONS

Sample NIC linkages:

Exercise Therapy: Muscle Control: Use of specific activity or exercise protocols to enhance or restore controlled body movement

Body Mechanics Promotion: Facilitating the use of posture and movement in daily activities to prevent fatigue and musculoskeletal strain or injury

NURSING PRIORITY NO. 1   To identify causative/contributing factors:

• Determine diagnosis that contributes to difficulty with standing balance (e.g., stroke, other neurological disorders [e.g., MS, Parkinson's disease; traumatic brain injury, spinal cord injury with hemi/paraplegia]; vestibular disorders/vertigo; osteoarthritis, rheumatoid arthritis, degenerative joint disease; back pain conditions; lower-limb amputations; psychiatric conditions including severe depression, dementias). *Impaired standing balance has a detrimental effect on a person's functional ability and increases the risk of falling. These conditions can cause postural and balance impairments, muscular weakness, and inadequate range of motion. Sensory deficits may also be involved (e.g., impaired proprioception and/or visual processing, cognitive impairments). For example, sitting and standing balance are major concerns in an amputee's ability to*

 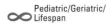

maintain the center of gravity over the base of support. Both balance and coordination are required for weight shifting from one limb to another, thus improving the potential for an optimal gait.[1] In persons with chronic neck pain, one study suggested that lack of proprioceptive inhibition of nociceptors at the dorsal horn of the spinal cord would result in suboccipital muscle atrophy and a loss of standing balance.[2] Dizziness and/or unsteadiness and episodes of loss of balance are not infrequent complaints of persons with persistent whiplash-associated disorders.[3]

- ∞ 📝 Assess client's mental status, noting age, developmental stage, and presence or potential for cognitive dysfunction (e.g., traumatic brain injury, stroke, dementia, extremes of age). *Several studies have suggested that seemingly automatic postural tasks (such as standing balance and walking) require some attention and cognitive processing.[4,5]*
- Determine fall risk, noting factors that may be present. *Fall risk is high in clients with certain conditions (e.g., advanced age or debilitating disease; vision and hearing loss, diminished depth perception; decreased sensation in feet, artificial joints; trauma to lower extremity; amputation, other surgery or immobilizer; presence of severe vertigo with postural sway; generalized or specific leg weakness; reaching upward, forward, or laterally outside of standing balance position).*
- 📝 Encourage sitting before attempting standing, when indicated (e.g., supine client with low blood pressure or dehydration, vertigo, first attempt to get up after long period on bedrest). *Longer sitting pause times might improve postural stability after rising from a supine position. One study suggested that longer sitting pause times may also provide improved adaptability to dimly lit environments.[6]*

NURSING PRIORITY NO. 2   To assess functional ability:

- Determine functional status using a 0–4 scale, noting muscle strength and tone, joint mobility, cardiovascular status, balance, and endurance. *Identifies strengths and deficits (e.g., unable to stand without assistance, but can maintain standing position once attained; standing balance improved as vertigo diminishes; standing improves with pain management and nutrition measures, etc.) and may provide information regarding potential for recovery (e.g., client with severe brain injury may have permanent limitations because of impaired cognition affecting memory, judgment, problem-solving, and motor planning).[7,8]*
- Determine degree of perceptual or cognitive impairment and ability to follow directions. *Impairments, which may be related to age, chronic or acute disease condition, trauma, surgery, or medications, can necessitate alternative interventions or changes in plan of care.*
- 🔵 📝 Refer to physician and/or physical therapy specialists, as indicated, *to determine potential for improvement and direction for therapies. May include many different functional and lab tests (e.g., sitting to standing, tolerance, muscle strength and movement, posture and balance monitor, American Spinal Injury Association Impairment Scale, Berger Balance Scale, Functional Independence Measure, electrophysiological and clinical measures of neuropathy).[9,10]*
- Note: Studies have shown that people with the earliest stage of impaired glucose tolerance exhibit deficits in standing balance and trunk position sense, highlighting the importance of early screening for diabetes.[11]

NURSING PRIORITY NO. 3   To promote optimal level of function and prevent complications:

- 🔵 Assist with treatment of underlying condition(s) *to maximize potential for optimal function.*
- 🔵 📝 Assist with/refer for rehabilitation therapies and techniques for implementing standing activities. *Various modalities may be used to gain physiological benefits from standing or modified standing therapy. For example, "standing" can be accomplished in a variety of positions with proper support (e.g., a prone-position with blanket under the abdomen), which helps preserve joint range of motion and improves muscle flexibility, weight-bearing ability, and bowel and bladder function even when person is not upright.[12] Note: Research found that a "Standing Strong" program was effective at improving strength, balance, and function, as well as at reducing falls in older adults. This program combines strength training with balance-specific exercises to target the muscular system as well as the three major sensory control systems that control balance.[13]*

 Acute Care   Collaborative   Community/ Home Care   Cultural

- Provide for safety measures as indicated by individual situation, including environmental management and fall prevention. (Refer to ND risk for Falls.)
- Encourage client's participation in self-care activities and in physical or occupational therapies. *Improves body strength and function and enhances self-concept and sense of independence.*
- Administer pain medications before activity as needed *to permit maximal effort and involvement in activity.*
- Collaborate with nutritionist in providing nutritious foods and needed feeding assistance, maximizing client's abilities in ingesting and swallowing (upright position) *to optimize available energy for activities.*
- Demonstrate and assist with use of assistive devices (e.g., siderails, overhead trapeze, roller pads, safety belt, hydraulic lifts, chairs) *for position changes and safe transfers.*
- Refer to NDs Activity Intolerance, impaired bed Mobility, impaired physical Mobility, impaired wheelchair Mobility, impaired Transfer Ability, impaired Sitting, and impaired Walking for additional interventions.

NURSING PRIORITY NO. 4 To promote wellness (Teaching/Discharge Considerations):

- Encourage client's/significant other's involvement in decision making as much as possible. *Enhances commitment to plan, optimizing outcomes.*
- Demonstrate use of mobility devices (e.g., walkers, strollers, scooters, braces, prosthetics) and have client/ caregiver demonstrate knowledge about and safe use of device. Identify appropriate resources for obtaining and maintaining appliances or equipment. *Safe use of mobility aides promotes client's independence and enhances quality of life and safety for client and caregiver.*
- Refer to support and community services as indicated *to provide care, supervision, companionship, respite services, nutritional and ADL assistance, adaptive devices or changes to living environment, financial assistance, etc.*

DOCUMENTATION FOCUS

Assessment/Reassessment
- Individual findings, including level of function and ability to participate in specific or desired activities.

Planning
- Plan of care and who is involved in the planning.
- Teaching plan.

Implementation/Evaluation
- Responses to interventions, teaching, and actions performed.
- Attainment or progress toward desired outcome(s).
- Modifications to plan of care.

Discharge Planning
- Discharge and long-term needs, noting who is responsible for each action to be taken.
- Specific referrals made.
- Sources of and maintenance for assistive devices.

References

1. Gaily, R. S., Clark, C. S. (No date). Physical therapy management of adult lower-limb amputees. *Atlas of Limb Prosthetics. Chapter 23. Physical therapy management of adult lower-limb amputees. Orthotics and Prosthetics Virtual Library.* Retrieved April 2018 from http://www.oandplibrary.org/alp/chap23-01.asp.
2. McPartland, J. M., Brodeur, R. R., Hallgren, R. C. (1997). Chronic neck pain, standing balance, and suboccipital muscle atrophy: A pilot study. *J Manipulative Physiol Ther*, 20(1), 24–29.
3. Treleaven, J., Jull, G., LowChoy, N. (2005). Standing balance in persistent whiplash: A comparison between subjects with and without dizziness. *J Rehabil Med*, 37(4), 224–229.
4. Rogers, M. E., Page, P. (2010). Standing Strong: A program to improve strength and balance in older adults. Retrieved April 2018 from http://www.standingstrongprogram.com/wp-content/uploads/2009/05/Standing-Strong-Guide-2010.pdf.
5. Cooper, R., Kuh, P., Hardy, R. (2010). Objectively measured physical capability levels and mortality: Systematic review and meta-analysis. *BMJ*. Retrieved April 2018 from http://www.bmj.com/content/341/BMJ.c4467.full.
6. Johnson, E. G., Meltzer, J. D. (2012). Effect of sitting pause times on postural stability after supine-to-standing transfer in dimly lit environments. *Geriatr Phys Ther*, 35(1), 15–19.

 Diagnostic Studies   Evidence Based Practice   Medications   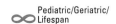 Pediatric/Geriatric/Lifespan

7. Black, K., et al. (2000). Sitting balance following brain injury (does it predict outcome?). *Brain Inj*, 14(2), 141–152.

8. Dworak, P. A., Levy, A. (2005). Strolling along. *Rehabil Manage*, 18(9), 26–31.

9. Gorman, S. L., Rivera, M., McCarthy, L. (2014). Reliability of the function in sitting test (FIST). *Rehabilitation Research and Practice.* Retrieved April 2018 from http://www.hindawi.com/journals/rerp/2014/593280/.

10. McKinley, W., Kulcarni, U., Pai, A. B. (2013, updated 2017). Functional outcomes per level of spinal cord injury. Retrieved April 2018 from http://emedicine.medscape.com/article/322604-overview#a1.

11. Goldberg, A., Russell, J. W., Alexander, B. B. (2008). Standing balance and trunk position sense in impaired glucose tolerance (IGT)-related peripheral neuropathy. *J Neurol Sci*, 270(1–2), 165–171.

12. Zwick, D., Dunn, M. (2007). Integrating Iyengar yoga into rehabilitation. *Nursing*, 37(10 Suppl: Therapy Insider), 10–12.

13. Page, P. (2010). Standing Strong. Bringing evidence to practice for a community-based fall prevention exercise program. *Topics Geriatric Rehabil*, 26(4), 335–352.

14. Gordon, M. (2009). Functional levels code. *Manual of Nursing Diagnosis*. 12th ed. Sudbury, MA: Jones and Bartlett.

Stress Overload

Taxonomy II: Coping/Stress Tolerance—Class 2 Coping Responses (00177) [**Diagnostic Division:** Ego Integrity], Approved 2006

DEFINITION: Excessive amounts and types of demands that require action.

RELATED FACTORS
Insufficient resources (e.g., financial, social, knowledge)
Stressors; repeated stressors

DEFINING CHARACTERISTICS

Subjective
Impaired functioning, decision making
Feeling of pressure; increase in impatience or anger
Negative impact from stress [e.g., physical symptoms, psychological distress, feeling sick]
Excessive stress; tension

Objective
Increase in anger behavior
Sample Clinical Applications: Chronic illness (e.g., multiple sclerosis [MS], diabetes, Parkinson's disease), terminal illness (e.g., ovarian cancer, amyotrophic lateral sclerosis [ALS]), abusive situations, bipolar disorder, depression, social phobia

DESIRED OUTCOMES/EVALUATION CRITERIA

Sample **NOC** linkages:
Stress Level: Severity of manifested physical or mental tension resulting from factors that alter an existing equilibrium
Anxiety Self-Control: Personal actions to eliminate or reduce feelings of apprehension, tension, or uneasiness from an unidentifiable source
Leisure Participation: Use of relaxing, interesting, and enjoyable activities to promote well-being

Client Will (Include Specific Time Frame)
• Assess current situation accurately.
• Identify ineffective stress-management behaviors and consequences.

 Acute Care Collaborative Community/Home Care Cultural

- Meet psychological needs as evidenced by appropriate expression of feelings, identification of options, and use of resources.
- Verbalize or demonstrate reduced stress reaction.

ACTIONS/INTERVENTIONS

Sample NIC linkages:

Emotional Support: Provision of reassurance, acceptance, and encouragement during times of stress

Coping Enhancement: Facilitation of cognitive and behavioral efforts to manage perceived stressors, changes, or threats that interfere with meeting life demands and roles

Resiliency Promotion: Assisting individuals, families, and communities in development, use, and strengthening of protective factors to be used in coping with environmental and societal stressors

NURSING PRIORITY NO. 1 To identify causative/precipitating factors and degree of impairment:

- Ascertain what tragic or difficult events have occurred (e.g., family violence, death of loved one; separation from living partner/parent; change in financial status or living conditions; chronic or terminal illness, workplace stress, loss of job or retirement; major trauma; catastrophic natural or human-caused event) over remote and recent past *to assist in determining number, duration, and intensity of difficult events causing perception of overwhelming stress.*
- ∞ Ascertain other life events (e.g., job promotion, moving to different home, change such as getting married, having a new baby or adding other new family member, child leaving home, adult children returning home, elder parent requiring care, traveling, spending holidays with relatives) that have occurred over recent months. *All such changes, even when desired, can be stressful and can evoke stress reactions.*[2]
- Evaluate client's report of physical or emotional problems (e.g., fatigue, aches and pains, irritable bowel, skin rashes, frequent colds, sleeplessness, crying spells, anger, feeling overwhelmed or numb, compulsive behaviors) *that can be representing body's response to stress.*[1]
- Determine client's/significant other's (SO's) understanding of events, noting differences in viewpoints.
- ∞ Note client's gender, age, and developmental level of functioning. *Although everyone experiences stress and stressors, women, children, young adults, divorced or separated persons, and people in roles or occupations requiring constant multitasking tend to have higher stress-related symptoms. Multiple stressors can weaken immune system and tax physical and emotional coping mechanisms of persons of any age, but particularly the elderly.*[1–3,9]
- 🌐 Note cultural values or religious beliefs *that may affect client's expectation for self in dealing with situation, ability to ask for help from others, and expectations placed on client by SO/family.*[7]
- Identify client locus of control: internal (expressions of responsibility for self and ability to control outcomes—"I didn't quit smoking") or external (expressions of lack of control over self and environment—"Nothing ever works out"). *Knowing client's locus of control will help in developing a plan of care reflecting client's ability to realistically make changes that will help to manage stress better.*
- Assess emotional responses and coping mechanisms being used.
- Determine stress feelings and self-talk client is engaging in. *Negative self-talk, all-or-nothing or pessimistic thinking, exaggeration, and unrealistic expectations will contribute to stress overload.*[2]
- Assess degree of mastery client has exhibited in life. *Passive individual may have more difficulty being assertive and standing up for rights.*
- Determine presence or absence and nature of resources (e.g., whether family/SO are supportive, lack money, problems with relationship or social functioning).
- Note change in relationships with SO(s). *Conflict in the family, loss of a family member, divorce can result in a change in support client is accustomed to and impair ability to manage situation.*

 Diagnostic Studies   Evidence Based Practice   Medications   Pediatric/Geriatric/ Lifespan

- Evaluate stress level using appropriate tool (e.g., Stress & Depression, Self-Assessment Tool) to help identify areas of most distress. *While most stress seems to come from disastrous events in individual's life, positive events can also be stressful.*
- Review lab results to identify physiological conditions (e.g., thyroid or other hormone imbalance, anemia, unstable glucose levels, kidney or liver disease) *that may be causing or exacerbating stress.*[1]

NURSING PRIORITY NO. 2   To assist client to deal with current situation:

- Discuss situation or condition in simple, concise manner. *May help client to express emotions, grasp situation, and feel more in control.*
- Active-listen concerns and provide empathetic presence, using talk and silence as needed.
- Deal with the immediate issues first (e.g., treatment of physical injury, meet safety needs, removal from traumatic or violent environment).
- Collaborate in treatment of underlying conditions (e.g., traumatic injury, chronic or terminal illness, hormone imbalance, depression and other psychiatric disorders).[1]
- Provide or encourage restful environment where possible.
- Assist client in determining whether or not he or she can change stressor or response. *May help client to sort out things over which he or she has control and determine responses that can be modified in order to view life through a more holistic lens.*
- Allow client to react in own way without judgment. Provide support and diversion as indicated.
- Help client to focus on strengths, to set limits on acting-out behaviors, and to learn ways to express emotions in an acceptable manner. *Promotes internal locus of control, enabling client to maintain self-concept and feel more positive about self.*
- Discuss benefits of a "Stop Doing" in place of a "To Do" list. *May help client identify and take action regarding energy drainers (e.g., internalizing others' criticism, fragmented boundaries, power struggles, unprotected personal time) in order to make room for what energizes and brings him/her closer to achieving goals.*[9]
- Address use of ineffective or dangerous coping mechanisms (e.g., substance use or abuse, self-/other-directed violence) and refer for counseling as indicated.

NURSING PRIORITY NO. 3   To promote wellness (Teaching/Discharge Considerations):

- Use client's locus of control to develop individual plan of care (e.g., for client with internal control, encourage client to take control of own care; for those with external control, begin with small tasks and add as tolerated).[4]
- Incorporate strengths, assets, and past coping strategies that were successful for client. *Reinforces that client is able to deal with difficult situations.*
- Encourage strengthening of positive SO/family routines and interactions *that support and provide assistance in managing stress.*[5]
- Provide information about stress and exhaustion phase, which occurs when person is experiencing chronic or unresolved stress. *Release of cortisol can contribute to reduction in immune function, resulting in physical illness, mental disability, and life dysfunction.*
- Review stress management and coping skills that client can use:[1,2,4–6]

    Practice behaviors that may help *reduce negative consequences*—change thinking by focusing on positives, reframing thoughts, and changing lifestyle.

    Learn to read own body signs (e.g., shakiness, irritability, sleep disturbances, fatigue).

    Take a step back and reduce obligations, simplify life, and learn to say no *to reduce sense of being overwhelmed.*

    Practice exchanging stresses (i.e., when a new stress comes into play, eliminate or postpone another stress) *to keep total stress level below overstress level.*

    Seek help or assistance in meeting obligations and delegate tasks as appropriate.

    Learn to control and redirect anger.

    Develop and practice positive self-esteem skills.

 Acute Care   Collaborative   Community/ Home Care   Cultural

Rest, sleep, and exercise on regular schedule or set times *to recuperate and rejuvenate self. Note: A recent study found that physically fit women in their mid-60s had essentially the same response to stress as a group of unfit women in their late 20s.*[8]

Postpone changes in living situation (e.g., moving, remodeling) if possible.

Participate in self-help actions (e.g., deep breathing and other relaxation exercises, spend time alone, get involved in recreation or desired activity, plan something fun, develop humor) *to actively relax.*

Eliminate possible food or environmental allergens and toxins.

Eat nutritious meals; avoid junk food and excessive sugars.

Avoid excessive caffeine, alcohol or other drugs, and nicotine *to balance body chemicals and support general health.*

Take a multivitamin, mineral, and/or trace element preparation.

Develop spiritual self (e.g., meditate or pray; block negative thoughts; learn to give and take, speak and listen, forgive and move on).

Interact socially, reach out, and nurture self and others *to reduce loneliness or sense of isolation.*

- Review proper medication use *to manage exacerbating conditions (e.g., depression, mood disorders).*
- Identify community resources (e.g., vocational counseling; educational programs; child or elder care; Women, Infants, and Children program or food stamps; home or respite care) *that can help client manage lifestyle and environmental stress.*
- Refer for therapy, as indicated (e.g., medical treatment, psychological counseling; hypnosis, massage, biofeedback).

DOCUMENTATION FOCUS

Assessment/Reassessment

- Individual findings, noting specific stressors, individual's perception of the situation, locus of control.
- Specific cultural or religious factors.
- Availability and use of support systems and resources.

Planning

- Plan of care and who is involved in planning.
- Teaching plan.

Implementation/Evaluation

- Responses to interventions, teaching, and actions performed.
- Attainment or progress toward desired outcome(s).
- Modifications to plan of care.

Discharge Planning

- Long-term needs and who is responsible for actions to be taken.
- Specific referrals made.

References

1. Burns, S. L., Burns, K. (1997–2018). The medical basis of stress, depression, anxiety, sleep problems and drug use. Retrieved April 2018 from http://www.teachhealth.com/.
2. Klimes Institute. (No date). Stress relief. Retrieved April 2018 from http://cecourses.org/preventive-care/stress-relief/.
3. Woolston, C. (Updated 2018). Aging and stress. Retrieved April 2018 from http://consumer.healthday.com/encyclopedia/aging-1/age-health-news-7/aging-and-stress-645997.html.
4. Donatelle, R. (2003). Managing stress: Coping with life's challenges. *Health: The Basics.* 5th ed. San Francisco: Benjamin Cummings.
5. Beckett, C. (2000). *Family theory as a framework for assessment.* Retrieved April 2018 from http://jan.ucc.nau.edu/~nur350-c/class/2_family/theory/lesson2-1-3.html.
6. Harvard Medical School. (2007). *Stress Control: Techniques for Preventing and Easing Stress.* Boston: Harvard Health.
7. Lipson, J. G., Dibble, S. L., Minarik, P. A. (1996). *Culture & Nursing Care: A Pocket Guide.* San Francisco: UCSF Nursing Press.
8. Traustadottir, T., et al. (2005). The HPA axis response to stress in women: Effects of aging and fitness. *Psychoneuroendocrinology,* 30(4), 392–402.
9. Martinuzzi, B. (2009–2018). The breaking point. Retrieved April 2018 from http://www.mindtools.com/pages/article/newTCS_93.htm.

 Diagnostic Studies   Evidence Based Practice   Medications   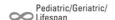 Pediatric/Geriatric/Lifespan

risk for Sudden infant Death

Taxonomy II: Safety/Protection—Class 2 Physical Injury (00156) [**Diagnostic Division:** Safety], Approved 2002; Revised 2013, 2017

DEFINITION: Susceptible to unpredicted death of an infant.

RISK FACTORS

Delay in or insufficient prenatal care
Infant placed in the prone or side-lying position to sleep
Infant less than 4 months placed in sitting devices for routine sleep
Soft sleep surface; soft, loose items placed near infant
Infant overheating or overwrapping
Exposure to second hand smoke
At Risk Population: African American or Native American ethnicity; male gender
Age 2–4 months
Infant not breast-fed exclusively or fed with expressed breast milk
Low birth weight; prematurity
Maternal smoking during pregnancy; prenatal or postnatal exposure to alcohol or illicit drug
Young parental age
Associated Condition: Cold weather
Sample Clinical Applications: Any child during first year of life

DESIRED OUTCOMES/EVALUATION CRITERIA

Sample NOC linkages:
Risk Control: Personal actions to understand, prevent, eliminate, or reduce modifiable health threats
Knowledge: Infant Care: Extent of understanding conveyed about caring for a baby from birth to first birthday

Parent/Caregiver Will (Include Specific Time Frame)
• Verbalize knowledge of modifiable factors.
• Make changes in environment to prevent death occurring from other factors.
• Follow medically recommended regimen for prenatal and postnatal care.

ACTIONS/INTERVENTIONS

Sample NIC linkages:
Risk Identification: Analysis of potential risk factors, determination of health risks, and prioritization of risk-reduction strategies for an individual or group
Teaching: Infant Safety [specify age 0–12 months]: Instruction on safety during first year of life

NURSING PRIORITY NO. 1 To assess causative/contributing factors:

• ▨ Identify individual risk factors pertaining to situation, noting presence of Risk Factors, as listed above. *Determines modifiable or potentially modifiable factors that can be addressed. Note: According to the Centers for Disease Control and Prevention (CDC, 2018), "(1) risk for Sudden Infant Death (SIDS), (2) accidental suffocation in a sleeping environment, and (3) other deaths from unknown causes fall under the umbrella of sudden unexpected infant deaths (SUIDs). In 2016, there were about 1,500 deaths due to SIDS, 1,200 deaths due to unknown causes, and about 900 deaths due to accidental suffocation and strangulation in bed."*[1,7,9–11]

 Acute Care   Collaborative   Community/ Home Care   Cultural

- Determine ethnicity and cultural background of family. *Although the overall rate of SUIDS in the United States declined between 1990 and 2015, disparities in risk factors and SUIDs rates remain. The CDC/ National Vital statistics system reports (2017) that SUID rates for American Indian/Alaska Native and non-Hispanic black infants were more than twice those of non-Hispanic white infants. SUIDs rates were lowest among Hispanic and Asian/Pacific Islander infants.*[7–9,12]

- Note whether mother smoked during pregnancy or is currently smoking. *Many risk factors for SIDS also apply to non-SIDS deaths as well, and smoking is known to negatively affect the fetus prenatally as well as the infant after birth. It has been reported that if both parents smoke, baby's SIDS risk is 3.5 times greater than if neither parent smokes. If mother smokes, but father doesn't, baby's risk is 2 times greater. If father smokes, but mother doesn't, baby's risk is 1.5 times greater.*[1,2,12]

- Assess extent of prenatal care, how early it was begun, and extent to which mother followed recommended care measures. *Prenatal care is important for all pregnancies to afford the optimal opportunity for all infants to have a healthy start to life.*[2–4]

- Determine client's knowledge of premature labor and actions to be taken in the event they occur. *Prompt action can prevent early delivery and the complications of prematurity.*[4]

- Note use of tobacco, alcohol or other drugs (including prescribed medications) during and after pregnancy. *"Alcohol is one of the most widely abused substances during pregnancy, and its effects on fetal development and infant outcomes have been well studied. Illicit drug use during pregnancy has been associated with a variety of adverse effects, though more research is needed to draw causal connections."*[5,12]

NURSING PRIORITY NO. 2 To promote use of activities to minimize risk of SIDS:

- Emphasize importance of placing infant on his or her back to sleep, both at nighttime and naptime. *Research confirms that fewer babies die of SIDS when they sleep on their backs, not on their tummies or sides.*[6,8,15]

- Advise all formal child-care providers, as well as grandparents, babysitters, neighbors, or anyone who will have responsibility for the care of the child during sleep, to maintain safe sleeping position in own sleeping place with head and face uncovered. *The recommendation is to always place the infant on the back until he or she can roll over; then repositioning is not required.*[1,2,4,6,7,15]

- Encourage parents to schedule "tummy time" only while infant is awake. *This activity promotes strengthening of back and neck muscles while parents are close and baby is not sleeping.*[1]

- Encourage well-baby checkups and immunizations. *Keeping babies healthy prevents problems that could put the infant at risk for SIDS. Immunizing infants prevents many illnesses that can be life-threatening.*[1,4,10]

- Encourage breastfeeding, if possible. *Breastfeeding has many advantages (immunological, nutritional, psychosocial), promoting a healthy infant. While this does not preclude the occurrence of SIDS, healthy babies are less prone to many illnesses and health problems. Note: One meta-analysis of 18 studies shows that breastfeeding to any extent and of any duration is protective against SIDS.*[1,4,13,15]

- Suggest providing pacifier at nap time and bedtime, refraining from placing around neck or attaching to clothing *due to risk of strangulation. Specific mechanism of action is unclear but studies demonstrate decreased incidence of SIDS with pacifier use.*[15]

- Discuss issues of bed-sharing. *Some of the many concerns include accidental entrapment under a sleeping adult or suffocation by becoming wedged in a couch or cushioned chair. There are also concerns about accidental death from suffocation when the mother smokes, has recently consumed alcohol, is fatigued, the infant is covered by a blanket or quilt, or there are multiple bed-sharers. Also, studies show that the odds of SIDS is 16 times greater if babies who bed-share are also exposed to secondhand smoke. Research suggests that infants in this setting have more difficulty rousing from sleep, perhaps because smoke exposure changes serotonin pathways of the brain.*[6,13,14]

- Note cultural beliefs about bed-sharing. *Studies show that bed-sharing is growing across all populations in the United States. Bed-sharing is more common among breastfed infants, young unmarried mothers, low-income families where multiple people share a bed, or those from a minority group. Additional study is needed to better understand bed-sharing practices and associated risks and benefits.*[6,14]

• Recommend infant share room with parents for at least first 6 months. *Studies suggest that sleeping in parents' room but on a separate surface can reduce incidence of SIDS by up to 50%.*[15]

NURSING PRIORITY NO. 3 To promote wellness (Teaching/Discharge Considerations):

• Discuss known facts about SIDS with parents. *SIDS is not preventable, although research indicates that SIDS deaths have reduced since back-sleeping position policy was implemented. The cause is determined only after autopsy and can only be determined after ruling out other causes. SIDS is not the same as suffocation, is not caused by vomiting or choking, is not caused by immunizations, is not contagious, is not the cause of every unexpected infant death, and is not the result of child neglect or abuse.*[1,2,7]

• Recommend attention to factors below that may help in reducing risk:

Avoid overdressing or overheating infants during sleep. *Baby should be kept warm, but not too warm. Too many layers of clothing or blankets can overheat the infant. Room temperature that is comfortable for an adult will be comfortable for the baby. Note: Infants who were dressed in two or more layers of clothes as they slept had six times the risk of SIDS as those dressed in fewer layers.*[1,4,15]

Place infant on a firm mattress in an approved crib. *Avoiding soft mattresses, sofas, cushions, waterbeds, and other soft surfaces, while not known to prevent SIDS, will minimize chance of suffocation.*[1,2,15]

Remove crib bumper pads, stuffed toys, fluffy and loose bedding from sleep area, making sure baby's head and face are not covered during sleep. *Minimizes possibility of entrapment and suffocation.*[1,2,15]

Verify that day-care center/provider(s) are trained in observation and modifying risk factors (e.g., sleeping position) *to reduce risk of death while infant in their care.*

Discourage excessive checking of the infant. *Since there is nothing that can currently be done (beyond proper sleep positioning) to reduce the occurrence of SIDS, excessive checking only tires the parents and creates an atmosphere of tension and anxiety.*[1,2]

• Discuss the use of apnea monitors, if appropriate. *Apnea monitors are not recommended to prevent SIDS but may be used to monitor other medical problems. Only a small percentage of infants who died of SIDS were known to have prolonged apnea episodes, and monitors are also not medically recommended for subsequent siblings.*[1,2,15]

• Recommend contacting public health nurse for visit to new mother at least once or twice following discharge. *These early visitation programs have demonstrated an improvement in infant safety outcomes.*[4]

• Refer parents to local SIDS programs and resources for learning (e.g., National SIDS/Infant Death Resource Center and similar Web sites). *Provides reassurance and information for self-paced learning.*[1]

• Encourage consultation with primary care provider if baby shows any signs of illness or behaviors that concern parent. *Promotes timely evaluation and intervention for treatable problems.*[1]

DOCUMENTATION FOCUS

Assessment/Reassessment
• Baseline findings, degree of parental anxiety or concern.
• History of infant deaths within family.

Planning
• Plan of care, specific interventions, and who is involved in planning.
• Teaching plan.

Implementation/Evaluation
• Parent's responses to interventions, teaching, and actions performed.
• Attainment or progress toward desired outcome(s).
• Modifications to plan of care.

 Acute Care   Collaborative   Community/Home Care   Cultural

Discharge Planning
* Long-term needs and actions to be taken.
* Support systems available, specific referrals made, and who is responsible for actions to be taken.

References

1. Angel Eyes (The Colorado SIDS Program). (2013). Infant sleep safety. Retrieved April 2018 from http://www.slideshare.net/425AngelEyes/infant-sleep-safety-understanding-risks-and-exploring-safety-measures.
2. Continuing Education Program on SIDS Risk Reduction. (2005). *U.S. Department of Health and Human Services, National Institutes of Health.*
3. Phillips, C. R. (1996). *Family-Centered Maternity and Newborn Care.* 4th ed. St. Louis, MO: Mosby.
4. London, M. L., et al. (2003). *Maternal & Child Nursing.* 3rd ed. Upper Saddle River, NJ: Prentice Hall.
5. National Institute on Drug Abuse (NIDA). (Updated 2011). Prenatal exposure to drugs of abuse—May 2011: A research update from the National Institute on Drug Abuse. Retrieved April 2018 from https://www.drugabuse.gov/sites/default/files/prenatal.pdf.
6. SIDS and Kids. (2015). Safe sleeping. Index page retrieved April 2018 from https://rednose.com.au/resources/education.
7. Centers for Disease Control and Prevention (CDC). (Updated 2018). Sudden unexpected infant deaths and sudden infant death syndrome (various pages). Retrieved November 2018 from https://www.cdc.gov/sids/data.htm.
8. American Academy of Pediatrics. (2005). Policy Statement: The changing concept of sudden infant death syndrome: Diagnostic coding shifts, controversies regarding the sleeping environment, and new variations to consider in reducing risk. *Pediatrics*, 116(5), 1245–1255.
9. Center for Disease Control and prevention/National Vital Statistics System (CDC/NCHS), Period Linked Birth/Infant Death Data. (2017). Sudden unexpected infant death by race/ethnicity, 2011–2014. Retrieved April 2018 from http://www.cdc.gov/sids/data.htm.
10. Leiter, J. C., Bohm, I. (2007). Mechanisms of pathogenesis in the sudden infant death syndrome. *Resp Physiol Neurobiol*, 159(2), 127–138.
11. Pharoah, P. O., Platt, M. J. (2007). Sudden infant death syndrome in twins and singletons. *Twin Res Hum Gen*, 10(4), 644–648.
12. AskDrSears. (2018). 4 Ways smoking increases the risk of SIDS. Retrieved April 2018 from https://www.askdrsears.com/topics/parenting/child-rearing-and-development/bringing-baby-home/how-smoking-harms-babies/4-ways.
13. Hauck, F. R., et al. (2011). Breastfeeding and reduced risk of sudden infant death syndrome: A meta-analysis. *Pediatrics*, 128(1), 103–110.
14. Horsley, T., et al. (2007). Benefits and harms associated with the practice of bed sharing. *Arch Pediatr Adolesc Med*, 161(3), 237–245.
15. American Academy of Pediatrics. (2016). SIDS and other sleep-related infant deaths: Updated 2016 recommendations for a safe infant sleeping environment. Retrieved April 2018 from http://pediatrics.aappublications.org/content/early/2016/10/20/peds.2016-2938.

risk for Suffocation

Taxonomy II: Safety/Protection—Class 2 Physical Injury (00036) **[Diagnostic Division:** Safety**],** Approved 1980; Revised 2013, 2017

DEFINITION: Susceptible to inadequate air availability for inhalation, which may compromise health.

RISK FACTORS
Access to empty refrigerator/freezer; low strung clothesline
Eating large mouthfuls [or pieces] of food; small object in airway
Gas leak; unvented fuel-burning heater; vehicle running in closed garage; smoking in bed
Pacifier around infant's neck; propped bottle in infant's crib
Playing with plastic bag; soft underlayment [loose items placed near infant]
Unattended in water
Associated Condition: Alteration in cognitive functioning; impaired motor functioning
Face/neck disease or injury; alteration in olfactory function
Emotional disturbance
Insufficient knowledge of safety precautions

(continues on page 854)

 Diagnostic Studies   Evidence Based Practice   Medications   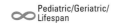 Pediatric/Geriatric/Lifespan

risk for Suffocation (continued)

Sample Clinical Applications: Substance use or abuse, spinal cord injury, crushing chest injury, obesity, near-drowning, burn or inhalation injury, sleep apnea, seizure disorder

DESIRED OUTCOMES/EVALUATION CRITERIA

Sample **NOC** linkages:
Risk Control: Aspiration: Personal actions to understand and prevent the passage of fluid and solid particles into the lung

Client/Caregiver Will (Include Specific Time Frame)
• Verbalize knowledge of hazards in the environment.
• Identify interventions appropriate to situation.
• Correct hazardous situations to prevent or reduce risk of suffocation.
• Demonstrate cardiopulmonary resuscitation (CPR) skills and how to access emergency assistance.

ACTIONS/INTERVENTIONS

Sample **NIC** linkages:
Airway Management: Facilitation of patency of air passages
Aspiration Precautions: Prevention or minimization of risk factors in the patient at risk for aspiration
Teaching: Infant Safety [specify months of age]: Instruction on safety during first year of life

NURSING PRIORITY NO. 1   To assess causative/contributing factors:

• Determine client's/significant other's (SO's) knowledge of individual safety concerns and environmental hazards present *to identify misconceptions and educational needs. Suffocation can be caused by (1) spasm of airway (e.g., food or water going down wrong way, irritant gases, asthma); (2) airway obstruction (e.g., foreign body, tongue falling back in unconscious person, swelling of tissues from burn injury or allergic reaction); (3) airway compression (e.g., tying rope or band tightly around neck, hanging, throttling, smothering); (4) conditions affecting the respiratory mechanism (e.g., epilepsy, tetanus, rabies, nerve diseases causing paralysis of chest wall or diaphragm); (5) conditions affecting respiratory center in brain (e.g., electric shock; stroke or other brain trauma; medications such as morphine, barbiturates); and (6) compression of the chest (e.g., crushing as might occur with cave-in, motor vehicle crash, pressure in a massive crowd).*[1,5,6]
• Identify level of concern or awareness and motivation of client/SOs to correct safety hazards and improve individual situation. *Lack of commitment may limit willingness to make changes, placing dependent individuals at risk.*
• ∞ Determine age, developmental level, and mentation (e.g., infant/young child, frail elder, person with developmental delay, altered level of consciousness, or cognitive impairments or dementia) *to identify individuals unable to be responsible for or protect self.*
• Assess neurological status and note history of conditions, such as stroke, cerebral palsy, multiple sclerosis, and amyotrophic lateral sclerosis, *that have potential to compromise airway or affect ability to swallow.*
• ⚕ Determine presence of seizure disorder, noting use of antiepileptics and how well condition is controlled. *Seizure activity (and especially status epileptics) is a major risk factor for respiratory inhibition or arrest, particularly when consciousness is impaired.*[10]
• Note reports of sleep disturbance and daytime fatigue. *May be indicative of sleep apnea (airway obstruction), requiring referral for evaluation.* Refer to NDs Insomnia and Sleep Deprivation.

 Acute Care   Collaborative   Community/ Home Care   Cultural

- 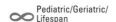 Review medication regimen *to note potential for oversedation and respiratory failure (e.g., central nervous system depressants, analgesics, sedatives, antidepressants).*
- Assess for allergies to medications, foods, and environmental factors *that could result in severe reaction or anaphylaxis resulting in respiratory arrest.*
- Be alert to and carefully monitor those individuals who are severely depressed, mentally ill, or aggressive and in restraints. *These individuals could be at risk for suicide by suffocation (e.g., inhaled carbon monoxide or death by strangling or hanging).*[2] Refer to ND risk for Suicide.
- Note signs of respiratory distress (e.g., cough, stridor, wheezing, increased work of breathing) *that could indicate swelling or obstruction of airways.*[3] Refer to NDs ineffective Airway Clearance, risk for Aspiration, ineffective Breathing Pattern, and impaired spontaneous Ventilation, as appropriate, for additional interventions.

NURSING PRIORITY NO. 2   To reverse/correct contributing factors:

- Discuss with client/SO(s) identified environmental or work-related safety hazards and problem-solve methods for resolution (e.g., need for smoke and carbon monoxide alarms, vents for household heater, clean chimney, properly strung clothesline, proper venting of machinery exhaust, monitoring of stored chemicals, bracing trench walls when digging).
- Protect airway at all times, especially if client unable to protect self:[2,5,8]

  Use proper positioning, suctioning, and use of airway adjuncts, as indicated, *for comatose or cognitively impaired individual or client with swallowing impairment or obstructive sleep apnea.*

  Provide seizure precautions and antiseizure medication, as indicated.

  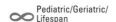 Administer medications when client is sitting or standing upright and can swallow without difficulty.

  Emphasize importance of chewing carefully, taking small amounts of food, and using caution *to prevent aspiration when talking or drinking while eating.*

  Provide diet modifications as indicated by specific needs (e.g., developmental level; presence/degree of swallowing disability, impaired cognition) *to reduce risk of aspiration.*

  Avoid physical and mechanical restraints, including vest or waist restraint, siderails, and choke holds. *Can increase client's agitation, causing struggle to escape and resulting in entrapment of head and hanging.*

- Emphasize with client/SO the importance of getting help when beginning to choke or feel respiratory distress (e.g., staying with people instead of leaving table, making gestures across throat, making sure someone recognizes the emergency) *in order to provide timely intervention such as abdominal thrusts and calling 911.*
- Avoid idling automobile (or using fuel-burning heaters) in closed or unvented spaces.
- Emphasize importance of periodic evaluation and repair of gas appliances, furnace, and automobile exhaust system *to prevent exposure to carbon monoxide.*
- Review child protective measures:[2,4,7,8]

  Place infant in supine position for sleep. Refer to ND risk for Sudden Infant Death.

  Do not prop baby bottles in infant crib.

  Attach pacifier to clothing—not around neck; remove bib before putting baby in bed.

  Store or dispose of plastic bags (e.g., shopping, garbage, dry cleaning, shipping) out of reach of infants/young children.

  Avoid use of plastic mattress or crib covers.

  Avoid placing infant to sleep on soft surfaces (e.g., beanbag chair, basket with soft sides, soft pillow or comforter, waterbed) *that baby can sink into or be unable to free face.*

  Use a crib with slats that are no more than 2 3/8 in. apart *so that baby cannot get head trapped or slip body through slats.*

  Refrain from bedsharing with infant/young child *to prevent accidental smothering.*

  Provide constant supervision of young children in bathtub, swimming pool, other bodies of water.

  Make certain that blind and curtain cords, drawstrings on clothing, etc., are out of reach of small children *to prevent accidental hanging.*

Prevent young child/impaired individual from putting objects in mouth (e.g., food such as chunks of raw vegetables, nuts and seeds, popcorn, hot dogs; toy parts; buttons; balloons; small balls/marbles; button-type batteries; refrigerator magnets; coins) *that can get lodged in airway and cause choking.*

Lock or remove lid or door of chests, trunks, old refrigerators or freezers *to prevent child from being trapped in airless environment.*

NURSING PRIORITY NO. 3 To promote wellness (Teaching/Discharge Considerations):

- Review safety factors identified in individual situation and methods for remediation.
- Develop plan with client/caregiver for long-range management of situation to avoid risks. *Enhances commitment to plan, optimizing outcomes.*
- Discuss possibility of choking resulting from relaxation of throat muscle and impaired judgment *when combining drinking alcohol with eating.*
- Involve family members in learning and practicing rescue techniques (e.g., treating of choking or breathing problems, CPR) *to deal with emergency situations (especially when at-home client is at risk on a regular basis).*
- Encourage individuals to read package labels and identify and remove safety hazards, such as toys with small parts, and monitor Web sites for product recalls.
- Promote water and swimming pool safety, vigilance, and use of approved flotation equipment, fencing and locked gates, alarm system, etc.
- Discuss fire safety and concerns regarding use of heaters; household gas appliances; and old, discarded appliances. Encourage home fire safety drills yearly.
- Promote public education in techniques for clearing blocked airways (e.g., Heimlich maneuver, CPR).
- Collaborate in community public health education regarding hazards for children (e.g., appropriate toy size for young child; discussing dangers of "huffing" [inhalants] and playing choking or hanging games with preteens; how to spot potential for depression and risk of suicidal gestures in adolescent) *to reduce potential for accidental or intentional suffocation.*[9]

DOCUMENTATION FOCUS

Assessment/Reassessment
- Individual risk factors, including individual's cognitive status and level of knowledge.
- Level of concern and motivation for change.
- Equipment or airway adjunct needs.

Planning
- Plan of care and who is involved in planning.
- Teaching plan.

Implementation/Evaluation
- Responses to interventions, teaching, and actions performed.
- Attainment or progress toward desired outcome(s).
- Modifications to plan of care.

Discharge Planning
- Long-term needs, appropriate preventive measures, and who is responsible for actions to be taken.
- Specific referrals made.

References

1. WebHealthCentre. (2015). Suffocation and artificial respiration. Retrieved April 2018 from http://www.webhealthcentre.com/HealthyLiving/first_aid_suffoc.aspx.
2. Masters, K. J., et al. (2001). Summary of the practice parameter for the prevention and management of aggressive behavior in child and adolescent psychiatric institutions with special reference to seclusion and restraint. *J Am Acad Child Adolesc Psychiatry*, 40(11), 1356–1358.
3. Kline, A. (2003). Pinpointing the cause of pediatric respiratory distress. *Nursing*, 33(9), 58–63.

 Acute Care   Collaborative   Community/Home Care   Cultural

4. Task Force on Infant Sleep Position and Sudden Infant Death Syndrome. (2000). Changing concepts of sudden infant death syndrome: Implications for infant sleeping environment and sleep position. *Pediatrics*, 105(3), 650–656.
5. Green, P. M. (1993). High risk for suffocation. In McFarland, G. K., McFarlane, E. A. (eds). *Nursing Diagnosis and Interventions*. St. Louis, MO: Mosby.
6. Suffocation/choking. (Updated 2013). *Fact Sheet for Manitoba Healthy Schools*. Retrieved April 2018 from http://www.gov .mb.ca/healthyschools/topics/safety.html.
7. healthychildren.org. (2015). Choking prevention. Retrieved April 2018 from http://www.kidsource.com/safety/prevent .choke.html.
8. Gupta, R. C. (Reviewed 2016). Household safety: Preventing suffocation. Retrieved April 2018 from http://kidshealth.org/ parent/firstaid_safe/home/safety_suffocation.html.
9. Urkin, J., Merrick, J. (2006). The choking game or suffocation roulette in adolescence. *Int J Adolesc Med Health*, 18(2), 207–208.
10. Ko, D. Y. (Updated 2018). Epilepsy and seizures. Retrieved April 2018 from http://emedicine.medscape.com/ article/1184846-overview.

risk for Suicide

Taxonomy II: Safety/Protection—Class 3 Violence (00150) [**Diagnostic Division:** Safety], Approved 2000; Revised 2013, 2017

DEFINITION: Susceptible to self-inflicted, life-threatening injury.

RISK FACTORS

Behavioral
Purchase of a gun; stockpiling medication
Making or changing a will; giving away possessions
Sudden euphoric recovery from major depression
Marked changes in behavior, attitude, or school performance

Psychological
Substance misuse/[abuse]
Guilt

Situational
Access to weapon
Loss of autonomy or independence

Social
Loss of significant relationship; disruptive family life; insufficient social support; social isolation
Grieving, loneliness
Hopelessness; helplessness
Disciplinary problems; legal difficulty
Cluster suicides

Verbal
Threat of killing self; reports desire to die

Other
Chronic pain

At Risk Population: Family history of suicide; history of suicide attempt
Adolescence; adolescents living in nontraditional settings; relocation
Caucasian or Native American ethnicity; male gender; homosexual youth
Older adults; retired; divorced status; widowed
Economically disadvantaged
Living alone; institutionalization
History of childhood abuse

(continues on page 858)

 Diagnostic Studies   Evidence Based Practice   Medications   Pediatric/Geriatric/Lifespan

risk for Suicide (continued)

Associated Condition: Physical illness; terminal illness
Psychiatric disorder
Sample Clinical Applications: Acute or chronic brain syndrome, hormonal imbalances (e.g., premenstrual syndrome [PMS], postpartum psychosis), substance use or abuse, chronic or terminal illness (e.g., amyotrophic lateral sclerosis [ALS], cancer), major depression, schizophrenia, bipolar disorder, panic state

DESIRED OUTCOMES/EVALUATION CRITERIA

Sample **NOC** linkages:
Suicide Self-Restraint: Personal actions to refrain from gestures and attempts at killing self
Coping: Personal actions to manage stressors that tax an individual's resources
Hope: Optimism that is personally satisfying and life supporting

Client Will (Include Specific Time Frame)
• Acknowledge difficulties perceived in current situation.
• Identify current factors that can be dealt with.
• Be involved in planning course of action to correct existing problems.
• Make decision that suicide is not the answer to perceived or real problems.

ACTIONS/INTERVENTIONS

Sample **NIC** linkages:
Suicide Prevention: Reducing the risk for self-inflicted harm with intent to end life
Behavior Management: Self-Harm: Assisting the patient to decrease or eliminate self-mutilating or self-abusive behaviors
Patient Contracting: Negotiating an agreement with an individual that reinforces a specific behavior change

NURSING PRIORITY NO. 1 To assess causative/contributing factors and degree of risk:

• ☑ Note behaviors indicative of intent. *Individual may not make statements of intent, but gestures (e.g., threats, giving away possessions), presence of means (e.g., guns), previous attempts, and presence of hallucinations or delusions may provide clues to intent.*[3,6,11]
• Ask directly if person is thinking of acting on thoughts or feelings to determine intent. *Most individuals want someone to see what desperate straits they are in, and by bringing the issue into the open, discussion can begin and plans made to keep the person safe.*[3,7]
• ⓐ ☑ Identify degree of risk or potential for suicide and seriousness of threat. *Information may be obtained from client or SO interviews, or over time in the course of care. Most people who are contemplating suicide send a variety of signals indicating their intent, and recognizing these warning signs allows for immediate intervention. Note: The Centers of Disease Control and Prevention (CDC) reported in 2013 that suicide remains a significant threat in the U.S. population with over 41,000 deaths and over 494,000 self-inflicted injuries treated in emergency departments that year. A 2013 Veterans Administration report estimated that 18–22 veterans died each day based on 2010 data.*[4,14–16]
• ☑ Use a risk scale (where available) to prioritize client risk according to severity of threat and availability of means. *Several risk scales may be used (e.g., Beck's Scale for Suicide Ideation, Linehan's Reasons for Living Inventory, Cole's self-administered adaptation of Linehan's structured interview called the Suicidal Behaviors Questionnaire) to assist in evaluating the severity of risk. Note: In recent years there have been "several*

 Acute Care   Collaborative   Community/ Home Care   Cultural

significant changes in how mental health professionals think about, and work with patients who are suicidal. Major modifications include (not a complete listing) (1) acknowledgment that 'traditional' suicide risk factors contribute little to clinicians' suicide prediction and prevention efforts; (2) ongoing clinical encounters and monitoring, including use of comprehensive suicide assessment interviewing protocols; and (3) asking client direct questions about suicide ideation when interviewing."[4,14]

- Note withdrawal from usual activities and lack of social interactions. *These are classic behaviors of the individual who is feeling depressed and sad and may be having negative thoughts of worthlessness.*[6]
- Identify what losses client has experienced, and meaning of those losses. *Unresolved issues may be contributing to thoughts of hopelessness, feelings of despair, and suicidal ideation.*[3,6]
- ∞ 🖾 Note age and gender. *While women may attempt suicide more frequently, men usually succeed more often. Risk of suicide is greater in teens and the elderly, but there is a rising awareness of risk in early childhood. Note: The CDC reported in 2013 that suicide was the second leading cause of death for young people ages 15 to 34 in the United States.*[4,8,10,15]
- 🌐 🖾 Determine cultural or religious beliefs that may be affecting client's thinking about life and death. *Family of origin and culture in which individual grew up influence attitudes toward taking one's own life. Note: A recent study showed that after other factors were controlled, greater moral objections to suicide and lower aggression level in religiously affiliated subjects seemed to function as protective factors against suicide attempts.*[2,4,10]
- Identify conditions such as acute or chronic brain syndrome, epilepsy, panic state, and hormonal imbalance (e.g., PMS, mental illness, postpartum or drug-induced psychosis). *These conditions may interfere with ability to control own behavior leading to impulsive actions that may put client at risk.*[1,4,10,13]
- ✐ Review lab results (e.g., blood alcohol, serum glucose, arterial blood gases, electrolytes, renal function tests). *Identifies factors that may affect reasoning ability, interfering with ability to think clearly about issues that are leading to thoughts of suicide.*[1,3,5]
- Assess physical complaints. *Sleeping difficulties and lack of appetite can be indicators of depression and suicidal ideation, requiring further evaluation.*[3,4]
- 🖾 Review family history for suicidal behavior. *Individual risk is increased when other family members have committed suicide or exhibited symptoms of depression. Studies have shown a possible genetic link toward suicidal behavior.*[12]
- Assess coping behaviors presently used. *Client's current negative thinking may preclude looking at positive behaviors that have been used in the past that would help in the current situation. Client may believe there is no alternative except suicide.*[6,7]
- Ascertain presence of significant others (SOs)/friends available for support. *Individuals who have positive support systems on whom they can rely during a crisis situation are less likely to commit suicide and are more apt to return to a successful life.*[3]
- 💊 Determine drug use or "self-medication." *The use of drugs and alcohol, especially the combination of alcohol and barbiturates, increases the risk of suicide.*[4]
- Note history of disciplinary problems or involvement with judicial system. *Feelings of despair over problems with the legal system and lack of hope about outcome can lead to belief that the only solution is suicide.*[3,10]

NURSING PRIORITY NO. 2   To assist client to accept responsibility for own behavior and prevent suicide:

- Develop therapeutic nurse-client relationship, providing a consistent care provider. *Promotes sense of trust, allowing individual to discuss feelings openly. Collaborating with the client to better understand the problem affirms the client's ability to solve the current situation.*[3,6]
- Maintain straightforward communication. *By being direct and honest and acknowledging need for attention, care provider can avoid reinforcing manipulative behavior.*[6]
- Explain concern for safety and willingness to help client stay safe. *Clients often believe their concerns will not be taken seriously, and stating clearly that they will be listened to sends a clear message of support and caring.*[6]

 Diagnostic Studies   Evidence Based Practice   Medications   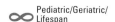 Pediatric/Geriatric/Lifespan

- Encourage expression of feelings and make time to listen to concerns. *Acknowledges reality of feelings and that they are okay. Helps individual sort out thinking and begin to develop understanding of situation.*[3,6]
- Give permission to express angry feelings in acceptable ways and let client know someone will be available to assist in maintaining control. *Promotes acceptance and sense of safety while client is regaining own control.*[3,4]
- Acknowledge reality of suicide as an option. Discuss consequences of actions if they follow through on intent. Ask how it will help individual to resolve problems. *Can help client to focus on consequences of actions and begin to discuss the possibility of other options.*[5,7]
- Help client identify more appropriate solutions/behaviors. *Alternative activities, such as exercise, can lessen sense of anxiety and associated physical manifestations.*[3]
- Maintain observation of client and check environment for hazards that could be used to commit suicide. Do not leave client alone if expressing "I'm going to kill myself." Do not promise to keep client's suicidal thoughts a secret. *Increases client safety and may reduce risk of impulsive behavior.*[11]
- Discuss medication regimen in general and note use of antidepressant medications, especially when there may be a significant organic component to the suicidal ideation. *Certain medications have been shown to increase risk of suicidal ideation or suicide, including (and not limited to) antidepressants, anticonvulsants, pain medications, and smoking-cessation medications. While the use of medications may be helpful in the short term, there are some drawbacks, namely, the length of time it takes for most medications to take effect and the potential for giving a client a means of suicide because of the possibility of a lethal overdose.*[4,6,9,10]
- Reevaluate potential for suicide periodically at key times (e.g., mood changes, increasing withdrawal), as well as when client is feeling better and planning for discharge becomes active. *The highest risk is when the client has both suicidal ideation and sufficient energy with which to act.*[5,6]

NURSING PRIORITY NO. 3 To assist client to plan course of action to correct/deal with existing situation:

- Gear interventions to individual involved. *Age, relationships, and current situation determine what is needed to help client deal with feelings of despair and hopelessness.*[6,10]
- Negotiate contract with client regarding willingness not to do anything lethal for a stated period of time. Specify what care provider will be responsible for and what client responsibilities are. *Making a contract in which the individual agrees to stay alive for a specified period of time, from Day 1 through the entire course of treatment, and which is written and signed by each party may help the client to follow through with therapy to find reason for living. Although there is little research on the effectiveness of these contracts, they are frequently used.*[6]
- Specify alternative actions necessary if client is unwilling to negotiate contract. *Client may be willing to agree to other actions (i.e., calling therapist if feelings are overwhelming) even though he or she is not willing to commit to a contract.*[6]
- Provide directions for actions client can take, avoiding negative statements such as "do nots." *Providing opportunity for client to have control over circumstances can promote a positive attitude and give client some hope for the future.*[3,5]

NURSING PRIORITY NO. 4 To promote wellness (Teaching/Discharge Considerations):

- Promote development of internal control. *Helping the client look at new ways to deal with problems can provide a sense of own ability to solve problems, improve situation, and hope for the future.*[3]
- Assist with learning problem-solving, assertiveness training, and social skills. *By learning these new skills, client can begin to feel more confidence in own ability to handle problems that arise and deal with the current situation.*[3,5]
- Engage in physical activity programs. *Promotes release of endorphins and feelings of self-worth, improving sense of well-being and giving client hope.*[3]
- Determine nutritional needs and help client to plan for meeting them. *Enhances general well-being and energy level.*[1,10]

 Acute Care   Collaborative   Community/Home Care   Cultural

- Review use of antidepressants, noting that it takes 4 to 8 weeks for effects of medication to be observed, and different medications may need to be tried to obtain maximum benefit. Stress importance of continuing medication after symptoms of depression resolve to reduce risk of relapse. *Antidepressants can be effective in quick relief of suffering in severe cases of depression. Studies have shown that cognitive behavior therapy has prevented relapse in 70% more cases than have drugs. In a sample of older adults with depression, the combination of medication and interpersonal psychotherapy was more effective than either alone.*[10,17]
- Involve family/SO in planning. *Improves understanding and support when family knows the facts and has a part in planning for rehabilitation efforts for the client.*[1,5]
- Refer to formal resources as indicated. *May need assistance with referrals to individual, group, or marital psychotherapy; substance abuse treatment program; or social services when situation involves mental illness or family disorganization.*[5,10,11]

DOCUMENTATION FOCUS

Assessment/Reassessment
- Individual findings, including nature of concern (e.g., suicidal or behavioral risk factors and level of impulse control, plan of action and means to carry out plan).
- Client's perception of situation, motivation for change.
- Cultural or religious beliefs influencing attitudes about life and suicide.
- Availability of family and other support systems.

Planning
- Plan of care and who is involved in the planning.
- Details of contract regarding suicidal ideation or plans.
- Teaching plan.

Implementation/Evaluation
- Actions taken to promote safety.
- Response to interventions, teaching, and actions performed.
- Attainment or progress toward desired outcome(s).
- Modifications to plan of care.

Discharge Planning
- Long-term needs and who is responsible for actions to be taken.
- Available resources, specific referrals made.

References

1. Brian, K., et al. (2017). Major physical health conditions and risk of suicide. *Am J Prev Med*, 53(3), 308–315.
2. Dervic, K., Oquendo, M. A., Grunebaum, M. F. (2004). Religious affiliation and suicide attempt. *Am J Psychiatry*, 161(12), 2303–2308.
3. Townsend, M. C. (2003). *Psychiatric Mental Health Nursing Concepts of Care*. 4th ed. Philadelphia: F. A. Davis.
4. Soreff, S. (Updated 2017). Suicide. *Medscape*. Retrieved April 2018 from http://emedicine.medscape.com/article/2013085-overview.
5. Doenges, M., Townsend, M., Moorhouse, M. (1998). *Psychiatric Care Plans: Guidelines for Individualizing Care*. 3rd ed. Philadelphia: F. A. Davis.
6. Jurich, A. P. (2003). The nature of suicide. *Clinical Update (insert in Family Therapy Magazine)*, 3(6), 1–8.
7. Firestone, L. (No date). Suicide: What therapists need to know. *American Psychological Association*. Retrieved April 2018 from https://www.apa.org/education/ce/suicide.pdf.
8. Whetstone, L., Morrissey, S. (2007). Children at risk: The association between perceived weight status and suicidal thoughts and attempts in middle school youth. *J School Health*, 77(2), 59–66.
9. Sherman, C. (2002). Antisuicidal effect of psychotropics remains uncertain. *Clin Psychiatry News*. Retrieved April 2018 from 308 http://www.baumhedlundlaw.com/media/ssri/paxil/FDAHearing/ANTISUICIDAL%20EFFECT%20REMAINS%20UNCERTAIN.pdf.
10. National Institute of Mental Health. (2016). Older adults: Depression & suicide facts. *NIH Publication No. QF 16-7697 (reprints authorized)*. Retrieved April 2018 from https://www.scribd.com/document/370433727/Older-Adults-and-Depression-NIMH-Brochure.

 Diagnostic Studies   Evidence Based Practice   Medications   Pediatric/Geriatric/Lifespan

11. National Institute of Mental Health (NIMH). (2018). Suicide in America: Frequently asked questions. *NIMH Brochure No. QF 18-6389.* Retrieved April 2018 from http://www.nimh.nih.gov/health/topics/suicide-prevention/issues-to-consider-in-intervention-research-with-persons-at-high-risk-for-suicidality.shtml.

12. Zai, C. C., Manchi, M., De Luca, V. (2011). The brain-derived neurotrophic factor gene in suicidal behaviour: A meta-analysis. *Int J Neuropsychopharmacol*, 15(8), 1037–1042.

13. Algreeshah, F. S., Benbadis, S. R. (Updated 2016). Psychiatric disorders associated with epilepsy (section on suicidal behaviors). Retrieved April 2018 from http://emedicine.medscape.com/article/1186336-overview#a1.

14. Sommers-Flannigan, J., Shaw, S. L. (2017). Suicide risk assessment: What psychologists should know. *Prof Psychol Res Pr*, 48(2), 98–106.

15. Centers for Disease Control and Prevention (CDC). (2015). Psychiatric disorders associated with epilepsy (section on suicidal behaviors). *CDC: National Center for Injury Control and Prevention; Division of Violence Prevention.* Retrieved April 2018 from https://www.cdc.gov/violenceprevention/pdf/suicide_factsheet-a.pdf.

16. Department of Veterans Affairs Department of Defense. (2013). VA/DoD clinical practice guideline for assessment and management of patients at risk for suicide. Retrieved April 2018 from https://www.healthquality.va.gov/guidelines/MH/srb/VADODCP_SuicideRisk_Full.pdf.

17. Tyrell, M., Elliot, R. (No date). Controlling depression with antidepressants. Retrieved April 2018 from http://www.clinical-depression.co.uk/dlp/treating-depression/controlling-depression-with-antidepressants/.

delayed Surgical Recovery

Taxonomy II: Safety/Protection—Class 2 Physical Injury (00100) **[Diagnostic Division:** Safety], Approved 1998; Revised 2006, 2013, 2017

DEFINITION: Extension of the number of postoperative days required to initiate and perform activities that maintain life, health, and well-being.

RELATED FACTORS
Malnutrition; obesity
Pain
Postoperative emotional response

DEFINING CHARACTERISTICS

Subjective
Discomfort
Loss of appetite
Postpones resumption of work

Objective
Evidence of interrupted healing of surgical area
Excessive time required for recuperation; inability to resume employment
Impaired mobility; requires assistance for self-care
At Risk Population: Extremes of age
History of delayed wound healing
Associated Condition: American Society of Anesthesiologists (ASA) Physical Status classification score ≥2
Diabetes mellitus
Edema or trauma at surgical site
Extensive or prolonged surgical procedure; surgical site contamination
History of delayed wound healing; perioperative surgical site infection
Impaired immobility
Persistent vomiting

 Acute Care
 Collaborative
 Community/Home Care
 Cultural

Pharmaceutical agent

Psychological disorder in perioperative period

Sample Clinical Applications: Major surgical procedures, traumatic injuries with surgical intervention, chronic conditions (e.g., diabetes mellitus, cancer, HIV/AIDS, chronic obstructive pulmonary disease [COPD])

DESIRED OUTCOMES/EVALUATION CRITERIA

Sample **NOC** linkages:

Self-Care: Activities of Daily Living (ADL): Personal actions to perform the most basic physical tasks and personal care activities independently with or without assistive device

Endurance: Capacity to sustain activity

Wound Healing: Primary Intention: Extent of regeneration of cells and tissues following intentional closure

Client Will (Include Specific Time Frame)

• Perform desired self-care activities.

• Report increased energy and be able to participate in usual (work or employment) activities in a timely manner.

• Display complete healing of surgical area.

ACTIONS/INTERVENTIONS

Sample **NIC** linkages:

Self-Care Assistance: Assisting another to perform activities of daily living

Energy Management: Regulating energy use to treat or prevent fatigue and optimize function

Wound Care: Prevention of wound complications and promotion of wound healing

NURSING PRIORITY NO. 1   To assess causative/contributing factors:

• Identify vulnerable client (e.g., low socioeconomic status or poverty; lack of insurance; inadequate transportation; lack of family or support system; severe trauma or prolonged hospitalization with multiple complicating factors; client with severe anxiety about diagnosis or outcome) *who is at higher risk for adverse outcomes.*[6]

• ∞ ▨ Determine age, developmental level, and general state of health *to help determine time that may be required for client to resume ADLs and other activities or expectation of time needed for healing. Note: The older adult undergoing surgical treatment is at greater risk for delayed recovery because of age-related changes in numerous systems and protective mechanisms that increase the potential for complications.*[1,7,16]

• ▨ Note underlying condition or pathology (e.g., cancer, burns, diabetes, hypothyroidism, obesity, steroid therapy, major trauma, infections, radiation therapy, cardiopulmonary disorders, debilitating illness) *that can adversely affect healing and prolong recuperation time. Note: One study found the incidence of surgical-site infection to be more than five times higher in obese patients and eight times higher in morbidly obese patients than in patients of normal weight. In this population, impaired pulmonary function, hyperglycemia, immobility, and nutritional deficits can compromise wound healing.*[3,8,12]

• ▨ Determine the length of operative procedure or time under anesthesia (e.g., typical or lengthy), type and severity of perioperative complications (e.g., trauma, other conditions requiring multiple surgeries; heavy bleeding during procedure), type of surgical wound (e.g., clean; clean-contaminated; grossly contaminated; acutely infected), and development of postoperative complications (e.g., surgical site infection, suture reactions, dehiscence, ventilator-associated pneumonia, deep vein thrombosis) *that can affect the pace of healing or prolong recovery.*[2,3,9]

 Diagnostic Studies   Evidence Based Practice   Medications   Pediatric/Geriatric/ Lifespan

- Evaluate circulation and sensation in surgical area, noting location of incision. *Lack of blood supply at the wound site can slow healing. Note: Some areas of the body, such as the face and neck, receive the most blood supply and heal the fastest, whereas other areas, such as extremities, take longer to heal. Poor circulation and impaired sensation in extremities, such as in the diabetic person, cause even longer healing times.*[14]

- Determine nutritional status and current intake *to ascertain if nutrition is adequate to support healing. Client may have preexisting nutritional concerns (e.g., elderly person, client with anorexia or morbid obesity) or may have been fasting perioperatively or experienced nausea, vomiting, and loss of appetite postoperatively, depending on the surgical procedure performed and client's reactions to medications (e.g., pain medications, antibiotics). Note: A lack of carbohydrates, proteins, zinc, and vitamins can cause a delay in healing.*[2,7,14]

- Review client's preoperative medications/other drug regimen *to ascertain that none could impede healing processes (e.g., aspirin and NSAIDs, chemotherapy agents) or increase bleeding time, (e.g., alcohol and some herbals such as garlic and ginkgo biloba can also be associated with bleeding complications).*[2]

- Perform pain assessment *to ascertain whether pain management is adequate to meet client's needs during recovery.*

- Evaluate client's cognitive and emotional state, noting presence of postoperative changes, including confusion, depression, apathy, and expressions of helplessness, *to determine need for further assessment of possible physical or psychological interferences.*

- Ascertain attitudes and cultural values of individual about condition. *Family beliefs and cultural values, stress and fear related to surgery (and the reason for it), possible stigma about relative condition or disease, or change in body image, as well as motivation to return to usual role and activities, all impact rate and expectations for sick role and recovery.*[5]

- Review results of laboratory tests (e.g., complete blood count, blood/wound cultures, serum glucose; hormones [e.g., cortisol, glucocorticoid and other hormones associated with inflammation and immune system dysfunction]) *to assess for presence and type of infections, immunosuppression, metabolic or endocrine dysfunction, or other conditions affecting body's ability to heal. Surgical site infections have been found to be tied to hyperglycemia that may impair phagocytosis, negatively affecting the body's normal defense mechanisms. Also, stress-impaired wound healing is mediated primarily through the hypothalamic-pituitary-adrenal hormones, and psychological response–induced unhealthy behaviors.*[11,16]

- Note allergies or history of skin reactions. Evaluate use of plastics (e.g., incontinence pads or moisture barriers), tape/adhesives, or latex materials. *Plastics retain heat and can enhance growth of pathogens in wound. Client sensitivity to adhesives and/or latex can cause skin or tissue reactions that delay primary wound healing and cause additional skin/tissue damage.*[15] Refer to NDs impaired Skin Integrity and Latex Allergy Response.

- Note lifestyle factors (e.g., obesity, cigarette smoking, alcohol abuse, lack of exercise/sedentary lifestyle) *that influence circulation and wound healing and can impede recovery.*[4,17]

NURSING PRIORITY NO. 2 To determine impact of delayed recovery:

- Note length of illness or hospitalization, time of discharge, and progress to date *to compare with general expectations for procedure and situation.*

- Determine client's/significant other's (SO's) expectations for recovery and specific stressors related to delay (e.g., return to work or school, home responsibilities, child care, financial difficulties, limited support system).

- Determine energy level and current participation in ADLs *to compare with usual level of function.*

- Ascertain whether client usually requires assistance in home setting and who provides it, as well as individual's current availability and capability.

- Note client/SO reports of helplessness or inability to cope with situation.

- Obtain psychological assessment of client's emotional status, noting potential problems arising from current situation.

 Acute Care   Collaborative   Community/Home Care   Cultural

NURSING PRIORITY NO. 3 To promote optimal recovery:

- 🟥🏠 Inspect incisions or wounds routinely, describing changes (e.g., deepening or healing, wound measurements, presence and type of drainage, development of necrosis).
- 📝 Practice and instruct client/caregiver(s) in proper hand hygiene and aseptic technique for incisional care *to reduce incidence of contamination and infection. Note: A recent study showed that while hand hygiene between patients remains a compliance issue in hospitals, healthcare workers have been found to be more motivated to perform hand hygiene to protect vulnerable patients than they are to protect their own health.*[4,13]
- 💊 Administer antibiotics as appropriate and medications to manage postoperative discomforts (e.g., pain, nausea, vomiting) and other concurrent or underlying conditions, such as diabetes, osteoporosis, heart failure, and COPD. *Several types of medications may be needed. For example, client may require antibiotics perioperatively, insulin to support tissue repair, and/or management of chronic pain to improve mobility and tissue recovery.*[10,11]
- 🏠 Instruct client/SO in necessary self-care of incisions and specific symptom management. *With short hospital stays, client/SO are usually expected to provide a great deal of postoperative care and monitoring at home.*[6]
- 🏠 Provide wound care expectations and instructions in verbal and written forms *to facilitate self-care and reduce likelihood of misinterpretation of information when client/SO is providing care at home.*[2]
- ♾️ Instruct client/SO in routine inspection of incision or wound and to report changes in wound indicative of failure to heal (e.g., deepening wound, local or systemic fever, exudates [noting color, amount, and odor], loss of approximation of wound edges) *to establish comparative baseline and allow for early intervention (e.g., antimicrobial therapy, wound irrigation or packing).*
- Avoid or limit use of plastics or latex materials in wound care, as appropriate. *Can delay healing and cause skin breakdown.*
- ♾️ Collaborate in treatment and assist with wound care, as indicated. *May require barrier dressings, skin-protective agents, wound vac for open or draining wounds, or surgical débridement.* Refer to/include wound care specialist or stomal therapist, as appropriate, *to address treatment interventions to deal with healing difficulties.*
- ♾️ Provide optimal nutrition with adequate protein *to provide a positive nitrogen balance, which aids in healing and contributes to general good health.*
- Encourage adequate fluid and electrolyte intake *to avoid dehydration of tissues and to promote optimal cellular and organ function.*
- Encourage early ambulation and regular exercise *to promote circulation, improve muscle strength and overall endurance, and reduce risks associated with immobility.*
- Recommend pacing (alternating activity with adequate rest periods) *to reduce fatigue and allow weakened muscles and tissues to recuperate.*
- Employ nonpharmacological healing measures as indicated (e.g., breathing exercises, listening to music, relaxation tapes, biofeedback, hot or cold applications) *to promote relaxation of muscles and tissue healing, as well as improve coping and outlook for positive healing experience.*
- ♾️ Refer for follow-up care, as indicated (e.g., telephone monitoring, home visit, wound care clinic, pain management program).

NURSING PRIORITY NO. 4 To promote wellness (Teaching/Discharge Considerations):

- 🏠 Discuss reality of recovery process and client's/SO's expectations. *Individuals are often unrealistic regarding energy and time required for healing and own abilities and responsibilities to facilitate process.*
- Involve client/SO(s) in setting incremental goals. *Enhances commitment to plan and reduces likelihood of frustration, thus blocking progress.*
- Demonstrate self-care skills and provide client/SO with health-related information and psychosocial support *to manage symptoms and pain, thus enhancing well-being.*
- ♾️ Refer to physical or occupational therapist and/or wound care specialist, as indicated *to address exercise program and home-care needs and identify assistive devices to facilitate independence in ADLs.*
- Identify suppliers for dressings and wound care items or assistive devices as needed.

 Diagnostic Studies   Evidence Based Practice   Medications   Pediatric/Geriatric/Lifespan

- Consult nutritionist for individual dietary plan *to meet increased nutritional needs that reflect personal situation and resources.*
- Evaluate home situation (e.g., lives alone, bedroom or bathroom on second floor, availability of assistance) where appropriate, *to evaluate for beneficial adjustments, such as moving bed to first floor, arranging for commode during recovery, and obtaining an in-home emergency call system.*
- Discuss alternative placement (e.g., convalescent or rehabilitation center, as appropriate). *Brief stay with concentrated support and therapy may speed recovery and return to home.*
- Identify community resources (e.g., visiting nurse, home healthcare agency, wound care, Meals on Wheels, respite care). *Facilitates adjustment to home setting.*
- Refer for counseling or support. *May need additional help to overcome feelings of discouragement, deal with changes in life, weight management, and/or smoking cessation.*

DOCUMENTATION FOCUS

Assessment/Reassessment
- Assessment findings, including status of wound healing, individual concerns, family involvement and support factors, availability of resources.
- Cultural expectations.
- Assistive device use or need.

Planning
- Plan of care and who is involved in planning.
- Teaching plan.

Implementation/Evaluation
- Responses of client/SO(s) to plan, interventions, teaching, and actions performed.
- Attainment or progress toward desired outcome(s).
- Modifications to plan of care.

Discharge Planning
- Long-term needs and who is responsible for actions to be taken.
- Specific referrals made.

References

1. Newfield, S. A., et al. (2007). ND: Surgical Recovery, delayed. *Cox's Clinical Applications of Nursing Diagnosis: Adult, Child, Women's, Psychiatric, Gerontic, and Home Health Considerations.* 5th ed. Philadelphia: F. A. Davis.
2. Semchyshyn, N. (2014, updated 2016). Dermatologic surgical complications. Retrieved April 2018 from http://emedicine.medscape.com/article/1128404-overview#a11.
3. Odom-Forren, J. (2006). Preventing surgical site infections. *Nursing,* 36(6), 59–63.
4. Stricker, L. J., Hocevar, B. J. (2017). Impediments to healing: Managing acute and chronic wounds. *Western Schools Continuing Education Course.* Bridgewater, MA: Specialty Catalog (S.C.) Publishing.
5. Purnell, L. D. (2011). *Guide to Culturally Competent Health Care.* 2nd ed. Philadelphia: F. A. Davis.
6. Pieper, B., et al. (2006). Discharge information needs of patients after surgery. *J Wound Ostomy Continence Nurs,* 33(3), 281–290.
7. Dunn, D. (2006). Age-smart care: Preventing perioperative complications in older adults. *Nursing Made Incredibly Easy!,* 4(3), 30–39.
8. Dunn, D. (2005). Preventing perioperative complications in special populations. *Nursing,* 35(1), 36–43.
9. Gray, M. (2005). Context for WOC practice: Synthesizing the evidence to guide facility wide policies for wound, ostomy and continence care. *J Wound Ostomy Continence Nurs,* 36(2), 123–125.
10. Sawyer, M., et al. (2012, updated 2014). Perioperative Protocol. *Institute for Clinical Systems Improvement.* Retrieved April 2018 from https://www.guideline.gov/summaries/summary/48408/perioperative-protocol-health-care-protocol.
11. Odom-Forren, J. (2005). Surgical-site infection: Still a reality. *Nurs Manage,* 36(11 Suppl, OR Insider), 16–20.
12. Gallagher, S., et al. (2004). Preplanning with protocols for skin and wound care in obese patients. *Adv Skin Wound Care,* 17(8), 442–443.
13. Association for Psychological Science. (2011). Patients' health motivates workers to wash their hands. Retrieved April 2018 from http://www.psychologicalscience.org/index.php/news/releases/patients-health-motivates-workers-to-wash-their-hands.html.

 Acute Care   Collaborative   Community/Home Care   Cultural

14. Satteson, E. S., Molnar, J. A. (2017). Materials for wound closure. Retrieved April 2018 from https://emedicine.medscape.com/article/1127693-overview#a2.

15. Glenn, Y. (2006). When your patient is sensitive to tape. *Nursing*, 36(1), 17.

16. Godbout, J. P., Glaser, R. (2006). Stress-induced immune dysregulation: implications for wound healing, infectious disease and cancer. *J Neuroimmune Pharmacol*, 1(4), 421–427.

17. Ahn, C., Mulligan, P., Salcido, R. S. (2008). Smoking—the bane of wound healing: Biomedical interventions and social influences. *Adv Skin Wound Care*, 21(5), 227–238.

risk for delayed **Surgical Recovery**

Taxonomy II: Safety/Protection—Class 2 Physical Injury (00246) **[Diagnostic Division:** Safety], Approved 2013, 2017

DEFINITION: Susceptible to an extension of the number of postoperative days required to initiate and perform activities that maintain life, health, and well-being, which may compromise health.

RISK FACTORS

Malnutrition; obesity

Pain

Postoperative emotional response

At Risk Population: Extremes of age

History of delayed wound healing

Associated Condition: American Society of Anesthesiologists (ASA) Physical Status classification score ≥2

Diabetes mellitus

Edema or trauma at surgical site

Extensive or prolonged surgical procedure; surgical site contamination

History of delayed wound healing; perioperative surgical site infection

Impaired immobility

Persistent vomiting

Pharmaceutical agent

Sample Clinical Applications: Major surgical procedures, traumatic injuries with surgical intervention, chronic conditions (e.g., diabetes mellitus, cancer, HIV/AIDS, chronic obstructive pulmonary disease [COPD])

DESIRED OUTCOMES/EVALUATION CRITERIA

Sample NOC linkages:

Self-Care: Activities of Daily Living (ADL): Ability to perform the most basic physical tasks and personal care activities independently with or without assistive device

Endurance: Capacity to sustain activity

Wound Healing: Primary Intention: Extent of regeneration of cells and tissues following intentional closure

Client Will (Include Specific Time Frame)

• Display complete healing of surgical area.

• Perform desired self-care activities.

• Report increased energy and be able to participate in usual (work or employment) activities in a timely manner.

(continues on page 868)

 Diagnostic Studies   Evidence Based Practice   Medications   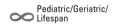 Pediatric/Geriatric/Lifespan

risk for delayed Surgical Recovery (continued)

ACTIONS/INTERVENTIONS

Sample **NIC** linkages:

Self-Care Assistance: Assisting another to perform activities of daily living

Energy Management: Regulating energy use to treat or prevent fatigue and optimize function

Wound Care: Prevention of wound complications and promotion of wound healing

NURSING PRIORITY NO. 1   To assess causative/contributing risk factors:

- Identify vulnerable client (e.g., low socioeconomic status or poverty, lack of insurance, inadequate transportation, lack of family or support system, severe trauma or prolonged hospitalization with multiple complicating factors, client with severe anxiety about diagnosis or outcome) *who is at higher risk for adverse outcomes.*[1]

- ∞ Determine age, developmental level, and general state of health *to help determine time that may be required for client to resume ADLs and other activities or expectation of time needed for healing. Note: The older adult undergoing surgical treatment is at greater risk for delayed recovery because of age-related changes in numerous body systems and protective mechanisms that increase the potential for complications.*[2-4]

- Note underlying condition or pathology (e.g., cancer, burns, diabetes, hypothyroidism, obesity, steroid therapy, major trauma, infections, radiation therapy, cardiopulmonary disorders, debilitating illness) *that can adversely affect healing and prolong recuperation time. Note: One study found the incidence of surgical-site infection to be more than five times higher in obese patients and eight times higher in morbidly obese patients than in patients of normal weight. In this population, impaired pulmonary function, hyperglycemia, immobility, and nutritional deficits can compromise wound healing.*[5-7,12]

- Determine the anticipated length of operative procedure or time under anesthesia (e.g., typical or lengthy), type and severity of perioperative complications (e.g., trauma or other conditions requiring multiple surgeries; heavy bleeding during procedure), and type of surgical wound (e.g., clean; clean-contaminated; grossly contaminated, acutely infected), *which can affect the pace of healing or prolong recovery.*[5,8,9]

- Determine nutritional status and current intake *to ascertain if nutrition is adequate to support healing. Client may have preexisting nutritional concerns (e.g., elderly person, client with anorexia or morbid obesity) or may have been fasting perioperatively or experienced nausea, vomiting, and loss of appetite postoperatively, depending on the surgical procedure performed and client's reactions to medications (e.g., pain medications, antibiotics). Note: A lack of carbohydrates, proteins, zinc, and vitamins can cause a delay in healing.*[3,7,8,12]

- Review client's preoperative medications/other drug regimen *to ascertain that none could impede healing processes (e.g., aspirin and NSAIDs, chemotherapy agents) or increase bleeding time (e.g., alcohol and some herbals such as garlic and ginkgo biloba can also be associated with bleeding complications).*[8]

- Ascertain attitudes and cultural values of individual about condition. *Family beliefs and cultural values, stress and fear related to surgery (and the reason for it), possible stigma about condition or disease, or change in body image all impact rate and expectations for sick role and recovery.*[10]

- Note allergies or history of skin reactions. Evaluate use of plastics (e.g., incontinence pads or moisture barriers), tape/adhesives, or latex materials. *Plastics retain heat and can enhance growth of pathogens in wound. Client sensitivity to adhesives and/or latex can cause skin or tissue reactions that delay primary wound healing and cause additional skin/tissue damage.*[11] Refer to NDs impaired Skin Integrity and Latex Allergy Response.

- Note lifestyle factors (e.g., obesity, poor dietary choices/malnutrition, cigarette smoking, alcohol abuse, lack of exercise/sedentary lifestyle) *that influence circulation and wound healing and can impede recovery.*[7,12]

 Acute Care   Collaborative   Community/ Home Care   Cultural

NURSING PRIORITY NO. 2 To promote optimal recovery:

- 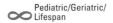 Inspect incisions or wounds routinely, describing changes (e.g., deepening or healing, wound measurements, presence and type of drainage, development of necrosis).
- Practice and instruct client/caregiver(s) in proper hand hygiene and aseptic technique for incisional care *to reduce incidence of contamination and infection. Note: A recent study showed that while hand hygiene between patients remains a compliance issue in hospitals, healthcare workers have been found to be more motivated to perform hand hygiene to protect vulnerable patients than they are to protect their own health.*[12,13]
- Instruct client/significant other (SO) in necessary self-care of incisions and specific symptom management. *With short hospital stays, client/SO are usually expected to provide a great deal of postoperative care and monitoring at home.*[1]
- Provide wound care expectations and instructions in verbal and written forms *to facilitate self-care and reduce likelihood of misinterpretation of information when client/SO is providing care at home.*[8]
- Instruct client/SO in routine inspection of incision or wound and to report changes in wound indicative of failure to heal (e.g., deepening wound, local or systemic fever, exudates [noting color, amount, odor], loss of approximation of wound edges) *to establish comparative baseline and allow for early intervention.*
- Avoid or limit use of plastics or latex materials in wound care, as appropriate. *Can delay healing and cause skin breakdown.*
- Provide optimal nutrition with adequate protein *to provide a positive nitrogen balance, which aids in healing and contributes to general good health.*
- Encourage adequate fluid and electrolyte intake *to avoid dehydration of tissues and to promote optimal cellular and organ function.*
- Encourage early ambulation and regular exercise *to promote circulation, improve muscle strength and overall endurance, and reduce risks associated with immobility.*
- Recommend pacing (alternating activity with adequate rest periods) *to reduce fatigue and allow weakened muscles and tissues to recuperate.*
- Refer for follow-up care, as indicated (e.g., telephone monitoring, home visit, pain management program).

NURSING PRIORITY NO. 3 To promote wellness (Teaching/Discharge Considerations):

- Discuss reality of recovery process and client's/SO's expectations. *Individuals are often unrealistic regarding energy and time required for healing and own abilities and responsibilities to facilitate process.*
- Demonstrate self-care skills and provide client/SO with health-related information and psychosocial support *to manage healing process.*
- Refer to physical or occupational therapist as indicated *to address recovery needs and identify assistive devices to facilitate independence.*
- Consult nutritionist for individual dietary plan *to meet increased nutritional needs that reflect personal situation and resources.*
- Discuss alternative placement (e.g., convalescent or rehabilitation center, as appropriate). *Brief stay with concentrated support and therapy may speed recovery and return to home.*
- Identify community resources (e.g., visiting nurse, home healthcare agency, wound care, Meals on Wheels, respite care). *Facilitates adjustment to home setting.*

DOCUMENTATION FOCUS

Assessment/Reassessment
- Assessment findings, including status of wound healing, individual concerns, family involvement and support factors, availability of resources.
- Cultural expectations.
- Assistive device use or need.

 Diagnostic Studies   Evidence Based Practice 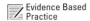 Medications ∞ Pediatric/Geriatric/Lifespan

Planning
- Plan of care and who is involved in planning.
- Teaching plan.

Implementation/Evaluation
- Responses of client/SO(s) to plan, interventions, teaching, and actions performed.
- Attainment or progress toward desired outcome(s).

Discharge Planning
- Long-term needs and who is responsible for actions to be taken.
- Specific referrals made.

References

1. Pieper, B., et al. (2006). Discharge information needs of patients after surgery. *J Wound Ostomy Continence Nurs*, 33(3), 281–290.
2. Newfield, S. A., et al. (2007). ND: Surgical Recovery, delayed. *Cox's Clinical Applications of Nursing Diagnosis: Adult, Child, Women's, Psychiatric, Gerontic, and Home Health Considerations*. 5th ed. Philadelphia: F. A. Davis.
3. Dunn, D. (2006). Age-smart care: Preventing perioperative complications in older adults. *Nursing Made Incredibly Easy!*, 4(3), 30–39.
4. Godbout, J. P., Glaser, R. (2006). Stress-induced immune dysregulation: Implications for wound healing, infectious disease and cancer. *J Neuroimmune Pharmacol*, 1(4), 421–427.
5. Odom-Forren, J. (2006). Preventing surgical site infections. *Nursing*, 36(6), 59–63.
6. Dunn, D. (2005). Preventing perioperative complications in special populations. *Nursing*, 35(1), 36–43.
7. Gallagher, S., et al. (2004). Preplanning with protocols for skin and wound care in obese patients. *Adv Skin Wound Care*, 17(8), 442–443.
8. Semchyshyn, N. (2016). Dermatologic surgical complications (various pages). Retrieved April 2018 from http://emedicine.medscape.com/article/1128404-overview#all.
9. Gray, M. (2005). Context for WOC practice: Synthesizing the evidence to guide facility wide policies for wound, ostomy and continence care. *J Wound Ostomy Continence Nurs*, 36(2), 123–125.
10. Purnell, L. D. (2011). *Guide to Culturally Competent Health Care*. 2nd ed. Philadelphia: F. A. Davis.
11. Glenn, Y. (2006). When your patient is sensitive to tape. *Nursing*, 36(1), 17.
12. Stricker, L. J., Hocevar, B. J. (2017). Impediments to healing: Managing acute and chronic wounds. *Western Schools Continuing Education Course*. Bridgewater, MA: Specialty Catalog (SC) Publishing.
13. Association for Psychological Science. (2011). Patients' health motivates workers to wash their hands. *Association for Psychological Science (APS)*. Retrieved April 2018 from http://www.psychologicalscience.org/index.php/news/releases/patients-health-motivates-workers-to-wash-their-hands.html.

risk for Surgical Site Infection

Taxonomy II: Safety/Protection—Class 1 Infection (002466) **[Diagnostic Division:** Safety**]**, Approved 2016

DEFINITION: Susceptible to invasion of pathogenic organisms at surgical site, which may compromise health.

RISK FACTORS
Alcoholism

Obesity

Smoking

At Risk Population: Cold temperature of operating room

Excessive number of personnel present during surgical procedure

Surgical wound contamination; increased environmental exposure to pathogens

Suboptimal American Society of Anesthesiologists (ASA) physical health status score

Associated Condition: Comorbidity; diabetes mellitus; hypertension; post-traumatic osteoarthritis; rheumatoid arthritis

Type of surgical procedure; duration of surgery; type of anesthesia

 Acute Care Collaborative Community/Home Care Cultural

Immunosuppression; infections at other surgical sites

Inadequate or ineffective antibiotic prophylaxis

Invasive procedure; use of implants and/or prostheses

Sample Clinical Applications: Surgical procedures, traumatic injuries with surgical intervention; fractures with surgical reduction

DESIRED OUTCOMES/EVALUATION CRITERIA

Sample NOC linkages:

Infection Severity: Severity of signs and symptoms of infection

Self-Management: Wound: Personal actions to manage a surgical incision, puncture, ulcer, or open wound following tissue injury

Client Will (Include Specific Time Frame)

- Be afebrile and free of signs/symptoms of infection, e.g., purulent drainage.
- Complete antibiotic therapy as directed.
- Engage in proper wound care techniques.
- Display complete healing of surgical incision.

ACTIONS/INTERVENTIONS

Sample NIC linkages:

Infection Control: Intraoperative: Preventing nosocomial infection in the operating room

Incision Site Care: Cleansing, monitoring, and promotion of healing in a wound that is closed with sutures, clips, or staples

Wound Care: Prevention of wound complications and promotion of wound healing

NURSING PRIORITY NO. 1   To assess causative/contributing factors:

- Determine reason for surgical intervention (e.g., trauma, elective joint replacement, traumatic amputation, colon resection) as well as comorbid conditions (e.g., obesity, current smoking, uncontrolled diabetes/hyperglycemia, advanced age, use of immunosuppressive drugs, poor nutritional status (especially low-protein and albumin levels), renal failure, client being carrier of *methicillin-resistant* Staphylococcus aureus *(MRSA)* or other antibiotic-resistant bacterium, *that could be a factor in development of postoperative site infections and identify needed interventions. Note: As recently as 2011, it was reported that in the United States approximately 157,500 surgical site infections (SSIs) occur after surgery each year.*[2,6]

NURSING PRIORITY NO. 2   To reduce risk of infection (**Perioperatively**):

- Prepare operative site according to specific procedure per agency protocol (e.g., scrubbing with liquid antibacterial soap, swabbing with betadine or other appropriate prep). *Minimizes bacterial count at operative site. Note: New Centers for Disease Control and Prevention (CDC) guidelines recommend skin prep in the OR should be performed using an alcohol-based agent unless contraindicated.*[2]
- Be aware of the type(s) of surgical wound(s). *Helps in predicting client's risk of surgical site infection (SSI). Note: The Centers of Disease Control and Prevention (CDC) has classified surgical wounds thus: "(1) Clean (Class I) not infected or inflamed at time of surgery; (2) clean-contaminated (Class II) involves entering the respiratory, gastrointestinal, genitourinary systems under controlled conditions; (3) contaminated (Class III) [including] open, fresh, accidental wounds, such as open fractures, or operations with . . . gross spillage from*

 Diagnostic Studies   Evidence Based Practice   Medications   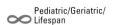 Pediatric/Geriatric/ Lifespan *the gastrointestinal tract, or incisions in which acute, non-purulent inflammation is encountered; (4) dirty-infected (Class IV) . . . is infected prior to surgical intervention, including old traumatic wounds with retained devitalized tissue or those that involve existing clinical infection or perforated viscera. . . ."[1–3]*

- Adhere to all surgical care policies and procedures *to prevent or reduce risks of infections. Note: The Surgical Care Improvement Project (SCIP) measures focus on reduction of surgically related infections through (1) use and timing of prophylactic antibiotics for selected procedures (e.g., cardiovascular, joint arthroplasty, colon resection); (2) appropriate hair removal and skin prep; (3) serum glucose management; (4) perioperative temperature management; and (5) timely removal of urinary catheters.[1,4,5]*

- Review laboratory studies for systemic infections or possible localized infections. *Increased white blood cell (WBC) count may indicate ongoing infection (e.g., appendicitis, abscess) or inflammation (e.g., recent trauma).*

- Maintain normal client temperature range as much as possible during surgery. *CDC recommends maintaining normothermia in all clients.[2] One study in 2011 found that patients who experienced mild hypothermia during surgery were three times more likely to have positive cultures from the surgical site.[5]*

- Identify breaks in aseptic technique and resolve immediately upon occurrence. *Contamination by environmental or personnel contact renders the operative field unsterile, thereby increasing the risk of infection.*

- Insert drain to evacuate wound bed, as necessary, via separate incision distant from the wound; remove the drain as soon as possible.

- Apply sterile dressings and maintain dressings according to facility protocol. *Prevents environmental contamination of fresh wound.*

- Administer appropriate antibiotics in timely manner, as indicated. *Antibiotics may be given prophylactically for (1) selected elective surgical procedures; (2) planned in client at high-risk for infection; or (3) when procedures need to be performed in the setting of known or suspected wound contamination. SCIP guidelines require the antibiotic to be administered within 1 hour of cut time (any time skin integrity is disrupted, such as in laparoscopic procedures)[2] with the belief that it provides opportunity for the medication to travel through the body and be available at the surgical site at the time of incision. Note: The CDC recommends that topical antimicrobial agents not be applied to the surgical incision.[2]*

NURSING PRIORITY NO. 3 To reduce risk of surgical site infections (**Postoperatively**):

- Obtain information from operating room staff regarding type of procedure performed (e.g., clean, contaminated, etc). *Different surgical types and sites may contribute to the development of infection. For example, elective procedures carry a lower risk of SSIs than do emergency procedures; cosmetic operations of the head and neck in otherwise healthy person pose a much lower risk of SSI than colon resection for cancer in elderly person with COPD and obesity.[4]*

- Determine presence and severity of comorbid conditions that may increase the incidence of surgical site infections (SSIs).

- Practice and promote hand washing before and after contact with any client. *Hand hygiene is the single most important factor in the reduction of SSIs. Skin contaminants on the client may be transferred to the caregiver and then passed on to another client if strict adherence to hand washing is not maintained.[7]*

- Perform ongoing assessments: (1) postoperative surgical dressing and surrounding areas immediately; (2) surgical incision when dressings are removed; (3) assessment of skin surrounding the incision *to evaluate any changes and/or to monitor trends in healing.*

- Protect primary closed incisions with a sterile dressing for 24 to 48 hr (or per surgeon instruction). Use sterile technique for wound dressing change.

- Monitor client's vital signs and skin color and warmth. *Provides information about systemic tissue perfusion, which impacts tissue healing.*

- Monitor lab values such as hematocrit, white blood cell count, serum glucose, serum albumin. *Provides information about fluid and circulatory status, immune and endocrine systems functioning, and nutrition needs.*

 Acute Care   Collaborative   Community/ Home Care   Cultural

- Administer blood products and fluids, as indicated *to reduce risk of tissue health problems associated with hypoxemia, hypovolemia, and dehydration.*
- Administer antibiotics as indicated. *Use of postoperative antibiotics is variable, and may be continued (1) if surgical wound was contaminated (either preoperatively or interpretively); (2) a high risk of infection is associated with the procedure (e.g., colon resection); or (3) consequences of infection are unusually severe (e.g., total joint replacement). Note: Postoperative administration of preventive systemic antibiotics beyond 24 hours has not been demonstrated to reduce the risk of SSIs.*[8]
- 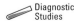 Maintain adequate control of serum blood glucose levels (usually less than 180 mg/dl) in all diabetic clients and avoid hyperglycemia perioperatively. *Hyperglycemia reduces the body's natural resistance to infection.*[8]
- 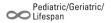 Provide nutrition by appropriate route (e.g., oral, enteral, parenteral) *to promote healing and general well-being.*
- Encourage early ambulation and resumption of activities *to reduce risks associated with immobility and stasis of body fluids.*

NURSING PRIORITY NO. 4 To promote wellness (Teaching/Discharge Considerations):

- Review client's specific surgical intervention and associated care needs *to promote client's informed self-care and reduce incidence of preventable complications.*
- Instruct client/care provider in incision care and receive return demonstration, as indicated.
- Review reportable symptoms (postdischarge) such as fever (especially if trending upward), increased pain in surgical site, hardness/redness/warmth of incision, development of drainage or change in character of drainage (e.g., from serosanguinous to blood-tinged pus). *Early intervention may prevent development of serious infectious complications.*
- Advise client to eat nutritious foods and snacks and have adequate fluid intake.
- Instruct client to get adequate rest and to increase activities gradually but steadily as tolerated.
- Ask client about home environment, support, and resources. *May reveal areas of concern (e.g., client unable to provide own incision care; has no access to nutritious food; cannot afford antibiotics).*

DOCUMENTATION FOCUS

Assessment/Reassessment
- Assessment findings, including vital signs, pain level, lab results/serum glucose levels,
- Character of wound and status of healing.
- Self-care ability, family support.
- Availability of resources.

Planning
- Plan of care and who is involved in planning.
- Teaching plan.

Implementation/Evaluation
- Responses of client/significant others to plan, interventions, teaching, and actions performed.
- Attainment or progress toward desired outcome(s).
- Modifications to plan of care.

Discharge Planning
- Long-term needs and who is responsible for actions to be taken.
- Specific referrals made.

Diagnostic Studies   Evidence Based Practice   Medications   Pediatric/Geriatric/Lifespan

References

1. Garner, J. S. (1985). Guideline for prevention of surgical wound infections, 1985 (archives). *Centers for Disease Control and Prevention (CDC)*. Retrieved May 2018 from https://wonder.cdc.gov/wonder/prevguid/p0000420/p0000420.aspl.
2. Berrios-Torres, S. I., et al. (2017). Centers for Disease Control and Prevention Guideline for the Prevention of Surgical Site Infection, 2017. *JAMA Surg*, 152(8), 784–791.
3. Smith, M. A., et al. (2013). Clinical practice guideline: Surgical site infection prevention. *Orthop Nurs*, 32(5), 242–248.
4. Fry, D. (2003). Surgical site infection: Pathogenesis and prevention CME/CE. Retrieved May 2018 from https://www.medscape.org/viewarticle/448981.
5. Drake, K. (2011). SCIP core measures: Deep impact. *Nurs Manage*, 42(5), 24–30.
6. Eislet, D. (2009). Presurgical skin preparation with a novel 2% chlorhexidine gluconate cloth reduces rates of surgical site infection in orthopedic surgical patients. *Orthop Nurs*, 28(3), 141–145.
7. Atkinson Smith, M., et al. (2017). Orthopaedic snafus: When adverse events happen in orthopaedics. *Orthop Nurs*, 36(2), 98–109.
8. Shanghai, H., Kaur, K. (2017). Wound infection (various pages). Retrieved May 2018 from https://emedicine.medscape.com/article/188988-overview.

---

impaired Swallowing

Taxonomy II: Nutrition—Class 1 Ingestion (00103) **[Diagnostic Division:** Food/Fluid**],** Approved 1986; Nursing Diagnosis Extension and Classification Revision 1998, 2017

DEFINITION: Abnormal functioning of the swallowing mechanism associated with deficits in oral, pharyngeal, or esophageal structure or function.

RELATED FACTORS
Behavioral feeding problem
Self-injurious behavior

DEFINING CHARACTERISTICS

Subjective
Third Stage: Esophageal
Reports "something stuck"; odynophagia [pain in esophagus on swallowing]
Food refusal; volume limiting
Heartburn; epigastric pain
Nighttime coughing or awakening

Objective
First Stage: Oral
Abnormal oral phase of swallow study
Prolonged bolus formation; tongue action ineffective in forming bolus; premature entry of bolus
Incomplete lip closure; insufficient chewing; piecemeal deglutition; food pushed out of or falls from mouth
Coughing, choking, or gagging prior to swallowing
Inability to clear oral cavity; pooling of bolus in lateral sulci; nasal reflux; drooling
Inefficient suck or nippling
Prolonged meal time with insufficient consumption
Second Stage: Pharyngeal
Abnormal pharyngeal phase of swallow study
Alteration in head position; inadequate laryngeal elevation
Choking; coughing; gagging sensation; nasal reflux; gurgly voice quality
Delayed or repetitive swallowing

 Acute Care   Collaborative   Community/Home Care   Cultural

Food refusal

Fevers of unknown etiology; recurrent pulmonary infection

Third Stage: Esophageal

Abnormal esophageal phase of swallow study

Difficulty swallowing

Hyperextension of head [e.g., arching during or after meals]

Repetitive swallowing; bruxism

Unexplained irritability surrounding mealtimes

Acidic-smelling breath; regurgitation; vomitus on pillow; vomiting; hematemesis

At Risk Population: Behavioral feeding problem; self-injurious behavior

Failure to thrive; developmental delay

History of enteral feeding

Prematurity

Associated Condition: Achalasia; laryngeal abnormality or defect; esophageal reflux disease

Acquired anatomic defect; oropharynx abnormality; nasopharyngeal cavity defect; tracheal or nasal defect; upper airway anomaly; congenital heart disease

Brain injury; cerebral palsy; cranial nerve involvement; conditions with significant hypotonia

Trauma; neurological problems; neuromuscular impairment

Mechanical obstruction

Sample Clinical Applications:

Brain injury/stroke, neuromuscular conditions (e.g., muscular dystrophy, cerebral palsy, Parkinson's disease, amyotrophic lateral sclerosis [ALS], Guillain-Barré syndrome), facial trauma, head/neck cancer, radical neck surgery/laryngectomy, cleft lip/palate, tracheoesophageal fistula, gastroesophageal reflux disease (GERD), dementia

DESIRED OUTCOMES/EVALUATION CRITERIA

Sample NOC linkages:

Swallowing Status: Safe passage of fluids and/or solids from the mouth to the stomach

Self-Care: Eating: Personal actions to prepare and ingest food and fluid independently with or without assistive device

Client Will (Include Specific Time Frame)

- Pass food and fluid from mouth to stomach safely.
- Maintain adequate hydration as evidenced by good skin turgor, moist mucous membranes, and individually appropriate urine output.
- Achieve or maintain desired body weight.

Sample NOC linkage:

Risk Control: Personal actions to understand, prevent, eliminate, or reduce modifiable health threats

Client/Caregiver Will (Include Specific Time Frame)

- Verbalize understanding of causative/contributing factors.
- Identify individually appropriate interventions/actions to promote intake and prevent aspiration.
- Demonstrate feeding methods appropriate to the individual situation.
- Demonstrate emergency measures in the event of choking.

(continues on page 876)

 Diagnostic Studies   Evidence Based Practice   Medications   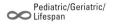 Pediatric/Geriatric/Lifespan

impaired Swallowing (continued)

ACTIONS/INTERVENTIONS

Sample NIC linkages:

Swallowing Therapy: Facilitating swallowing and preventing complications of impaired swallowing

Aspiration Precautions: Prevention or minimization of risk factors in the patient at risk for aspiration

Airway Suctioning: Removal of secretions by inserting a suction catheter into the patient's oral, nasopharyngeal, or tracheal airway

---

NURSING PRIORITY NO. 1 To assess causative/contributing factors and degree of impairment:

- ∞ Evaluate client's potential for swallowing problems, noting age and medical conditions (e.g., Parkinson's disease, multiple sclerosis, myasthenia gravis, other neuromuscular conditions). *Swallowing disorders are especially common in the elderly, possibly due to coexistence of variety of neurological, neuromuscular, and/or other conditions. Infants at risk include those born prematurely or born with tracheoesophageal fistula or lip and palate malformation. Persons with traumatic brain injuries often exhibit swallowing impairments regardless of gender or age.*[1,2,13]

- ▨ Determine current situation (e.g., intubation, surgery of head, neck, or jaw; cervical spine injury, vocal cord paralysis, problems with saliva production or management; pain with swallowing; mental or anxiety disorder) *that can affect swallowing. Note: Studies show that dysphagia has a significant impact on hospital stay and is a poor prognostic factor. Consequences include problems with nutrition, hydration, quality of life, and social issues.*[7,12]

- Assess client's cognitive and sensory-motor functional status. *Sensory awareness, orientation, concentration, and motor coordination affect desire and ability to swallow safely and effectively.*[4]

- Note voice quality and speech. *Abnormal voice (dysphonia) and abnormal speech patterns (dysarthria) are signs of motor dysfunction of structures involved in oral and pharyngeal swallowing.*[1]

- Note symmetry of facial structures and muscle tone. Assess strength and excursion of muscles involved in chewing and swallowing.

- Note hyperextension of head or arching of neck during or after meals or repetitive swallowing, *which suggests inability to complete swallowing process.*

- ∞ Determine infant's ability to initiate and sustain effective suck. *Weak suck results in inefficient nippling, suggesting ineffective movement of tongue and mouth muscles, impairing ability to swallow.*[2] Refer to ND ineffective infant Feeding Pattern.

- Ascertain presence and strength of cough and gag reflex. *Although absence of gag reflex is not necessarily predictive of client's eventual ability to swallow safely, it does increase client's potential for aspiration (overt or silent).*[1] *Coughing, drooling, double swallowing, decreased ability to move food in mouth, and throat clearing with or after swallowing is indicative of swallowing dysfunction and increases risk for aspiration.*[1]

- Auscultate breath sounds *to evaluate the presence of aspiration, especially if client is coughing with intake or has a "gurgly" or "gargly" voice.*

- Inspect oropharyngeal cavity for edema, inflammation, and altered integrity of oral mucosa or structures (e.g., lesions or tumors of the mouth or oral cavity and throat).[1,3]

- Evaluate state of dentition (e.g., poor or missing teeth, ill-fitting dentures) and adequacy of oral hygiene.

- 🥄 Review medications *that may affect (1) oropharyngeal function (e.g., benzodiazepines, neuroleptics, anticonvulsants, certain sedatives), (2) esophageal function (e.g., NSAIDs, iron preparations, tetracycline, calcium channel blockers), or (3) medications that can cause xerostomia (e.g., anticholinergics, opioids, antidepressants, antineoplastics, diuretics), thus impairing swallowing by means of sedation, pharyngeal weakness, inflammation, dry mouth, etc.*[1]

 Acute Care   Collaborative   Community/ Home Care   Cultural

- Review laboratory test results for underlying problems (e.g., complete blood count) *to screen for infectious or inflammatory conditions* or other metabolic and nutritional studies *that can affect swallowing.*[7]
- Prepare for or assist with diagnostic testing of swallowing activity (e.g., reflex cough test, swallowing electromyography, transnasal or esophageal endoscopy, videofluorographic swallow studies; fiber-optic endoscopic examination of swallowing) *to identify the pathophysiology of swallowing disorder.*[1,3,7]

NURSING PRIORITY NO. 2   To prevent aspiration and maintain airway patency:

- Withhold oral feedings until appropriate diagnostic workup is completed *to determine client's individual factors causing impaired swallowing and identify specific needs.*
- Consult with physician or dietitian regarding meeting current nutritional needs. *May need enteral (preferably by peripheral endoscopic gastrostomy tube) or parenteral feedings in order to obtain nutrition, while reducing risk of aspiration that could accompany nasogastric feedings.*[5]
- Move client to chair for meals, snacks, and drinks when possible; if client must be in bed, raise head of bed as upright as possible with head in anatomic alignment and slightly flexed forward during feeding. Keep client seated upright, or head of bed elevated for 30 to 45 min after feeding, if possible, *to reduce risk of regurgitation and aspiration.*[7,9]
- Instruct client to cough and expectorate *when secretion management is of concern.*
- Have suction equipment available during initial feeding attempts and as indicated. Suction oral cavity if client cannot clear secretions *to prevent aspiration.*
- Instruct client in self-suctioning techniques, when appropriate (e.g., for drooling, frequent choking, structural changes in mouth or throat). *Promotes independence and sense of control.*

NURSING PRIORITY NO. 3   To enhance swallowing ability to meet fluid and caloric body requirements:

- Consult with physician, speech pathologist, dysphagia specialist, gastroenterologist, or rehabilitation team, as indicated. *Therapies may consist of dietary modification, compensatory movements, medical or surgical procedures, etc. For example, medications may help with underlying condition (e.g., swallowing problem associated with Parkinson's disease), surgery (e.g., reconstructive facial surgery following trauma or to correct structural defect in infant), or esophageal dilatation when impaired sphincter function or esophageal strictures impede swallowing. Client/significant other (SO) may learn specific retraining or compensatory techniques (e.g., modifying head and neck posture, strengthening of swallowing muscles, techniques of food placement in mouth).*[1,3,8–10]
- Encourage a rest period before meals *if fatigue is interfering with efforts.*
- Provide analgesics (with caution) before feeding, as indicated, *to enhance comfort, but avoid decreasing awareness or sensory perception.*
- Implement dietary modifications as indicated:[1,3,8–11]
  Provide proper consistency of food and fluids. *Foods that can be formed into a bolus before swallowing, such as gelatin desserts prepared with less water than usual, pudding, and custard; thickened liquids (addition of thickening agent or yogurt, cream soups prepared with less water); thinned purees (hot cereal with water added) or thick drinks, such as nectars or fruit juices that have been frozen into "slush" consistency; and medium-soft boiled or scrambled eggs, canned fruit, and soft-cooked vegetables are most easily swallowed.*
  Feed one consistency or texture of food at a time. *Single-textured foods (e.g., pudding, hot cereal, pureed food) should be tolerated well before advancing to soft table foods.*[5]
  Avoid milk products and chocolate, *which may thicken oral secretions and impair swallowing,* and sticky foods (e.g., peanut butter, white bread) *that are difficult to swallow or need fluids to completely swallow.*[5]
  Ensure temperature (hot or cold versus tepid) of foods and fluids, *which will stimulate sensory receptors.*
  Avoid pouring liquid into the mouth or "washing food down" with liquid. *May cause client to lose control of food bolus, increasing risk of aspiration. Note: To avoid posterior head tilting while drinking, some people find drinking from a straw easier than sipping from a cup (if a straw is easier, consider using a flexible*

 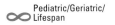

one-way straw); if a cup is easier, consider using a "nosey" cup that is double handled and made of durable plastic.

Feed smaller, more frequent meals *to limit fatigue associated with eating efforts and to promote adequate nutritional intake.*

Determine food preferences of client and present foods in an appealing, attractive manner. *Client may make effort to overcome swallowing problems when food is appealing and desired.*

- Provide or encourage use of proper food placement, chewing, and swallowing techniques:[1,3,8–10]

Provide cognitive cues and specific directions (e.g., remind client to open mouth, chew, or swallow), as indicated, *to enhance concentration and performance of swallowing sequence.*

Focus attention on feeding and swallowing activity by decreasing environmental stimuli, *which may be distracting during feeding. Also, if client is talking or laughing while eating, risk of aspiration is increased.*[6]

Position client on the unaffected side when appropriate, placing food in this side of mouth and having client use the tongue *to assist with managing the food when one side of the mouth is affected (e.g., hemiplegia).*

Manage size of bites—use a small spoon or cut all solid foods into small pieces (e.g., *small bites 1/2 tsp or less are usually easier to swallow*).

Place food midway in oral cavity *to adequately trigger the swallowing reflex.*

Massage the laryngopharyngeal musculature (sides of trachea and neck) gently (when prescribed) *to stimulate swallowing.*

Observe oral cavity after each bite and have client check around cheeks with tongue for remaining or unswallowed food *to prevent overloading mouth with food and reduce risk of aspiration.*

Allow ample time for eating (feeding). Incorporate client's eating style and pace when feeding *to avoid fatigue and frustration with process.*

Remain with client during meal *to reduce anxiety and provide assistance if needed.*

Provide positive feedback for client's efforts. *Encourages continuation of efforts and attainment of goals.*

Discontinue feeding and remove any food from mouth if client choking or unable to swallow *to reduce potential for aspiration.*

- Provide oral hygiene following each feeding *to clear mouth of retained food particles and reduce risk of infection and dental carries.*
- Monitor intake, output, and body weight *to evaluate adequacy of fluid and caloric intake and need for changes to therapeutic regimen.*
- Discuss use of tube feedings or parenteral solutions as indicated *for the client unable to achieve adequate nutritional intake.*
- Refer to lactation counselor or support group (e.g., La Leche League) *for breastfeeding guidance and problem-solving.* Refer to NDs ineffective Breastfeeding and ineffective infant Feeding Pattern for additional interventions for infants.

NURSING PRIORITY NO. 4   To promote safe swallowing (Teaching/Discharge Considerations):

- Consult with nutritionist *to establish optimum dietary plan considering specific pathology, nutritional needs, and available resources.* Refer to ND risk for imbalanced Nutrition: less than body requirements.
- Establish routine schedule for obtaining weight (same time of day and same clothes) and specific weight loss or gain to be reported to primary care provider. *Facilitates timely intervention to change regimen as needed.*
- Consult with pharmacist *to determine if pills may be crushed or if liquids or capsules are available.* Administer medication in gelatin, jelly, or puddings as appropriate.
- Instruct client and/or SO in specific feeding and swallowing techniques. *Enhances client safety and independence.*
- Instruct client/SO in emergency measures in event of choking *to prevent aspiration or more serious complications.*
- Encourage continuation of facial exercise program *to maintain or improve muscle strength.*

 Acute Care   Collaborative   Community/ Home Care   Cultural

- Recommend avoiding food intake within 3 hr of bedtime, eliminating alcohol and caffeine intake, reducing weight if needed, using stress-reduction techniques, and elevating head of bed during sleep *to limit potential for gastric reflux and aspiration.*

DOCUMENTATION FOCUS

Assessment/Reassessment
- Individual findings, including degree and characteristics of impairment, current weight and recent changes, and nutritional status.
- Effects on lifestyle and socialization.

Planning
- Plan of care and who is involved in planning.
- Teaching plan.

Implementation/Evaluation
- Response to interventions, teaching, and actions performed.
- Attainment or progress toward desired outcome(s).
- Modifications to plan of care.

Discharge Planning
- Long-term needs and who is responsible for actions to be taken.
- Available resources and specific referrals made.

References

1. Palmer, J. B., Drennen, J. C., Baba, M. (2000). Evaluation and treatment of swallowing impairments. *Am Fam Physician*, 61(8), 2453–2462.
2. Engel, J. (2002). *Pocket Guide to Pediatric Assessment*. 4th ed. St. Louis: Mosby.
3. Paik, N.-J., Dawodu, S. T. (2018). Dysphagia. Retrieved April 2018 from http://emedicine.medscape.com/article/2212409-overview.
4. Poertner, L. C., Coleman, R. F. (1998). Swallowing therapy in adults. *Otolaryngol Clin North Am*, 31(3), 56.
5. Fine, R., Ackley, B. J. (2002). ND: Impaired Swallowing. In Ackley, B. J., Ladwig, G. B. (eds). *Nursing Diagnosis Handbook: A Guide to Planning Care*. 5th ed. St. Louis: Mosby.
6. Galvan, T. J. (2001). Dysphagia: Going down and staying down. *Am J Nurs*, 101(1), 37–42.
7. Stoppler, M. C. (Reviewed 2017). Dysphagia (difficulty swallowing). Retrieved April 2018 from http://www.emedicinehealth.com/dysphagia_swallowing_problems/article_em.htm.
8. National Institute of Neurological Disorders and Stroke. (2018). Swallowing disorders information page. http://www.ninds.nih.gov/disorders/swallowing_disorders/swallowing_disorders.htm.
9. Searle, J. (No date). Eating and swallowing. Retrieved April 2018 from http://huntingtondisease.tripod.com/swallowing/id22.html.
10. McCarron, K. (2006). The shakedown on Parkinson's disease. *Nursing Made Incredibly Easy!*, 4(6), 40–49.
11. Garcia, J. M., Chambers, E. (2010). Managing dysphagia through diet modifications. *Am J Nurs*, 110(11), 26–33.
12. Altman, K. W., Yu, G. P., Schaefer, S. D. (2010). Consequence of dysphagia in the hospitalized patient. *Arch Otolaryngeal Head Neck Surg*, 136(8), 784–789.
13. Morgan, A., Ward, E., Murdoch, B. (2004). Clinical characteristics of acute dysphagia in pediatric patients following traumatic brain injury. *J Head Trauma Rehabil*, 19(3), 226–240.

 Diagnostic Studies
 Evidence Based Practice
 Medications
 Pediatric/Geriatric/Lifespan

risk for Thermal Injury

Taxonomy II: Safety/Protection—Class 5 Physical Injury (00220) [Diagnostic Division: Safety], Approved 2010; Revised 2013, 2017

DEFINITION: Susceptible to extreme temperature damage to skin and mucous membranes, which may compromise health.

RISK FACTORS
Inadequate supervision
Inadequate protective clothing [e.g., flame-retardant sleepwear, gloves, ear coverings]
Fatigue; inattentiveness
Insufficient knowledge of safety precautions; unsafe environment
Smoking
At Risk Population: Extremes of age
Extremes of environmental temperature
Associated Condition: Alcohol or drug intoxication
Alteration in cognitive functioning
Neuromuscular impairment; neuropathy
Treatment regimen
Sample Clinical Applications: Burns, face and head trauma, surgical procedure, radiation therapy, neonatal jaundice, frostbite, dementia/Alzheimer's, attempted suicide

DESIRED OUTCOMES/EVALUATION CRITERIA

Sample NOC linkages:
Tissue Integrity: Skin & Mucous Membrane: Structural intactness and normal physiological function of skin and mucous membranes
Risk Control: Personal actions to understand, prevent, eliminate, or reduce modifiable health threats

Client/Caregivers Will (Include Specific Time Frame)
• Be free of damage to skin or mucous membranes associated with extreme temperatures.
• Demonstrate behaviors and lifestyle changes to reduce risk factors and protect from injury.

ACTIONS/INTERVENTIONS

[This ND is a compilation of a number of situations that can result in injury. Refer to specific NDs, such as Hypothermia, risk for Injury; impaired Skin Integrity; impaired Tissue Integrity; and risk for physical Trauma, as appropriate, for more specific interventions.]
Sample NIC linkages:
Skin Surveillance: Collection and analysis of patient data to maintain skin and mucous membrane integrity
Risk Identification: Analysis of potential risk factors, determination of health risks, and prioritization of risk reduction strategies for an individual or group

NURSING PRIORITY NO. 1   To identify causative/precipitating factors related to risk:

• Identify client at risk (e.g., chronic illness conditions with weakness, prolonged immobility; acute or chronic confusion, mental illness, dementia, head injury; cultural, familial, and socioeconomic factors adversely affecting lifestyle and home; exposure to environmental chemicals).

 Acute Care   Collaborative   Community/ Home Care   Cultural

- ∞ Note chronological and developmental age of client. *Infants, young children, disabled, and debilitated aged or impaired individuals are not able to protect themselves and may not recognize and/or react appropriately in dangerous situations. Safe Kids Worldwide reported that in the United States in 2013, more than 126,000 children across the country (including more than 67,000 children age 4 and under) were injured due to a fire or burn.*[1,14]
- Evaluate client's/significant other's (SO's) level of cognition, competence, decision-making ability, and independence. *Determines ability to attend to safety issues.*
- Ascertain if client is using alcohol/other drugs or medications *that could impair ability to act in best interest of self or others.*
- Evaluate client's lifestyle practices, noting reports of risk-prone behavior (e.g., smoking in bed, failure to use safety equipment when working with chemicals, allowing child to play with matches, unprotected exposure to sun or cold environment) *that can place client or others at high risk for injury.*
- Ascertain knowledge of safety needs and injury prevention, as well as motivation to prevent injury. *Information may reveal areas of misinformation, lack of knowledge, and need for teaching.*

NURSING PRIORITY NO. 2   To assist client/caregiver to reduce or correct individual risk factors:

- Provide client/SO information regarding client's specific situation and consequences of continuing unsafe behaviors *to enhance decision making, clarify expectations and individual needs.*
- Review client's physical and psychological abilities or limitations *to determine adaptations that may be required by current situation.*
- Provide for client's safety while in facility care (e.g., apply hot and cold treatments judiciously, prevent/monitor smoking, supervise bath temperature in confused individuals, young children or elder adults, etc.) *to reduce risk of dermal injury.*
- Ensure client safety during **surgical procedures**:
    - Conduct a fire risk assessment at beginning of each surgical procedure, and continuously monitor for changes in risk during procedure. *The highest risks involve an ignition source (such as electrocautery device), delivery of supplemental oxygen, and the operation of the ignition source near the oxygen (e.g., head, neck, or upper chest surgery).*[2,4]
    - Provide supplemental oxygen safely, using the lowest concentration possible. Use a closed oxygen delivery system (e.g., endotracheal tube) when higher concentrations of oxygen are needed *to reduce amount of oxygen flowing into surgical field.*[2,4]
    - Verify electrical safety of equipment, including intact cords, grounds, and medical engineering verification labels. *Malfunction of equipment can occur during the operative procedure, causing burn injury or death. Note: Ignition sources include, but are not limited to, electrosurgery or electrocautery units and lasers.*[3,4]
    - Place dispersive electrode (electrocautery pad) over largest available muscle mass closest to surgical site, ensuring its contact. *Provides for shortest distance and maximum conductivity to ground to prevent electrical burns.*[4]
    - Ascertain that alcohol-containing skin prep solutions are not pooled under client or in surgical drapes and had sufficient drying time *to prevent sparking with electrocautery equipment activated.*[2,3]
    - Protect surrounding skin and anatomy appropriately when laser equipment is used in surgical procedures, utilizing wet towels, sponges, dams, and cottonoids *to prevent inadvertent skin integrity disruption, hair ignition, and adjacent anatomy injury. Surgical drapes should be configured to minimize the accumulation of oxidizers (oxygen and nitrous oxide) under the drapes and from flowing into the surgical site.*[4]
    - Apply eye protection before laser activation. *Eye protection for specific laser wavelength must be used to prevent injury.*[4]
- Implement skin care protocol for client receiving **radiation therapy**:
    - Assess skin frequently for side effects of therapy; note breakdown and delayed wound healing. Emphasize importance of reporting open areas to caregiver. *A reddening and/or tanning effect (radiation dermatitis) may develop within the field of radiation.*[5]

 Diagnostic Studies   Evidence Based Practice   Medications   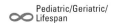 Pediatric/Geriatric/ Lifespan

Avoid rubbing the skin or use of soap, lotions, creams, ointments, powders, or deodorants on area; avoid applying heat or attempting to wash off marks/tattoos placed on skin to pinpoint location for radiation therapy. *These factors can potentiate or otherwise interfere with radiation delivery and may increase dermal reaction.*[5]

- Avoid application of lotion or oils to skin of infants receiving **phototherapy** for hyperbilirubinemia *to prevent dermal injury,* and cover male groin with small pad *to protect testes from heat-related injury.*[6]
- Provide or instruct in proper care of skin surfaces during exposure to very cold or hot weather. *Although everyone is at risk for frostbite or sunburn, individuals with impaired sensation or cognition and infants/young children require special attention to deal with extremes in weather (e.g., wearing gloves, boots, a face mask, and goggles when out in very cold weather to avoid frostbite; using sunscreen, limiting time in sun, and wearing light clothing to protect from dermal injury in summer).*[7]
- Discuss importance of self-monitoring of factors that can contribute to occurrence of injury (e.g., fatigue, anger). *Client/significant other (SO) may be able to modify risk through monitoring of actions or postponement of certain actions, especially during times when client is likely to be highly stressed.*
- Perform home assessment, if indicated *to address safety issues. Concerns vary widely and may include evaluation of fire alarms or extinguisher function, safe use of oxygen, checking hot water temperature, or obtaining medical alert device or home health services.*
- Review specific employment concerns or worksite issues and needs (e.g., properly fitting safety equipment, regular use of safety glasses or goggles, safe storage of hazardous substances).
- Discuss need for and refer to sources of supervision (e.g., before- and after-school programs for children, elder day programs, home-care assistance) *when client or care provider is unable or unwilling to attend to safety concerns.*

NURSING PRIORITY NO. 3. To promote wellness (Teaching/Discharge Criteria):

- Identify individual needs and resources for safety education.
- Prevent **burn injuries** (flame, scalding, chemical, electrical, sunburn):[8–12]
Install smoke alarms in kitchen, in every sleeping area, and on every floor of home.
Keep space heaters away from flammable materials and from at-risk persons.
Check all fuel-burning appliances, including fireplaces, for proper functioning.
Store combustibles away from all heat-producing appliances.
Prepare and practice an emergency escape plan.
Avoid smoking in bed. Get rid of used cigarettes carefully. *Fires caused by smoking materials are the leading cause of deaths in house fires.*[9]
Prevent small children from playing with matches or near open flame or stove.
Turn handles of pots and pans toward side of stove or use back burners.
Set the temperature on water heater to 120°F or use the "low-medium" setting.
Test water temperature before allowing child/impaired person into tub or shower.
Use cool-water humidifiers instead of hot-steam vaporizers.
Store cleaning supplies and other chemicals out of the reach of children *to prevent chemical burns.*
Avoid storing chemicals in food or drink containers; store in original containers with intact labels.
Wear gloves, safety glasses, and other protective clothing when handling chemicals.
Check electrical appliances for proper function and follow manufacturer's safety instructions. Discard frayed or damaged electrical cords *to reduce risk of electrical burn. Note: Most electrical injuries that occur in the home are low-voltage burns and almost exclusively involve either the hands or oral cavity.*[10]
Use child safety plugs in all outlets.
Avoid using electrical appliances while showering or when in other wet environmental conditions.
Stay out of midday sun. Avoid lengthy sun exposure/ultraviolet tanning, especially with specific disease conditions or treatments (e.g., systemic lupus, tetracycline or psychotropic drug use, radiation therapy) *to reduce risk of sunburn.*

 Acute Care   Collaborative   Community/ Home Care   Cultural

Start protecting child from the sun when he or she is a baby, dressing infants in lightweight long pants, long-sleeved shirts, and brimmed hats that shade the neck to prevent sunburn. Sunscreen is often not used in babies under the age of 6 months. *Because children spend a lot of time outdoors playing, they get most of their lifetime sun exposure in their first 18 years.*[11,13]

- Provide telephone numbers and other contact numbers as individually indicated (e.g., fire, police, physician).
- Refer to resources as indicated (e.g., substance recovery, anger management, or parenting classes) *to address conditions that could exacerbate risk of injury to self or others.*
- Recommend community education programs *to increase awareness of safety measures and available resources.*
- Identify emergency escape plans and routes for home and community *to be prepared in the event of natural or human-caused disaster (e.g., fire, toxic chemical release).*

DOCUMENTATION FOCUS

Assessment/Reassessment
- Individual risk factors identified.
- Client concerns or difficulty making and following through with plan.

Planning
- Plan of care and who is involved in planning.
- Teaching plan.

Implementation/Evaluation
- Response to interventions, teaching, and actions performed.
- Attainment or progress toward outcomes.

Discharge Planning
- Referrals to other resources.
- Long-term need and who is responsible for actions.

References

1. American Burn Association, National Burn Repository. (2016). Burn incidence and treatment in the United States. Retrieved May 2018 from http://ameriburn.org/who-we-are/media/burn-incidence-fact-sheet/.
2. Becker's ASC Review. (2011). 6 recommendations to prevent surgical fires. Ambulatory Surgical Center (ACS) News; for Food and Drug Administration (FDA) Retrieved May 2018 from https://www.beckersasc.com/asc-accreditation-and-patient-safety/6-recommendations-to-prevent-surgical-fires.html.
3. Grimes, B. (2007). Essentials of electrosurgical risks. *Perioperative Nursing Clinics*, 2(2), 119–125.
4. Caplan, R. A., et al. (2008). Practice advisory for the prevention and management of operating room fires. *Anesthesiology*, 108(5), 786–801.
5. Doenges, M. E., Moorhouse, M. F., Murr, A. C. (2010). Cancer. *Nursing Care Plans: Guidelines for Individualizing Client Care Across the Life Span*. 8th ed. Philadelphia: F. A. Davis.
6. No editors listed. (2008). Phototherapy. *Lippincott's Nursing Procedures*. 5th ed. Philadelphia: Williams & Wilkins, 895–897.
7. Geisbrecht, G. G., Wilkerson, J. A. (2006). *Hypothermia, Frostbite and Other Cold Injuries: Prevention, Survival, Rescue and Treatment*. 2nd ed. Seattle: The Mountaineers.
8. Safety for older consumers' home safety checklist. (No date). Consumer Product Safety Commission. Retrieved May 2018 from http://www.cpsc.gov//PageFiles/122038/701.pdf.
9. Familydoctor.org editorial staff. (2010, updated 2017). Burns: Preventing burns in your home. Retrieved May 2018 from http://familydoctor.org/familydoctor/en/prevention-wellness/staying-healthy/first-aid/burns-preventing-burns-in-your-home.html.
10. Edlich, R. F., et al. (2005). Modern concepts of treatment and prevention of electrical burns. *J Long Term Eff Med Implants*, 15(5), 511–532.
11. WebMD staff. (Updated 2013). Sunburn-prevention. Retrieved May 2018 from http://www.webmd.com/skin-problems-and-treatments/tc/sunburn-prevention.
12. Heller, J. L. (2011, updated 2015). Chemical burn or reaction. Retrieved May 2018 from https://uihc.org/adam/1/chemical-burn-or-reaction.
13. Gibson, L. (2016). When is it OK for a baby to wear sunscreen? *Mayo Clinic*. Retrieved May 2018 from http://www.mayoclinic.org/healthy-lifestyle/infant-and-toddler-health/expert-answers/baby-sunscreen/faq-20058159.
14. No author listed. (2013). Burns and scalds. *SafeKidsWorldwide*. Retrieved May 2108 from https://www.safekids.org/safetytips/field_risks/burns-and-scalds.

 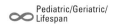

ineffective Thermoregulation

Taxonomy II: Safety/Protection—Class 6 Thermoregulation (00008) [**Diagnostic Division:** Safety], Approved 1986; Revised 2017

DEFINITION: Temperature fluctuation between hypothermia and hyperthermia.

RELATED FACTORS
Dehydration
Fluctuating environmental temperature; inappropriate clothing for environmental temperature
Inactivity or vigorous activity

DEFINING CHARACTERISTICS

Objective
Increase in body temperature above normal range; skin warm to touch; flushed skin; seizures
Reduction in body temperature below normal range; skin cool to touch; moderate pallor; mild shivering; piloerection; cyanotic nailbeds; slow capillary refill
Tachycardia; hypertension; increase in respiratory rate
At Risk Population: Extremes of age
Extremes of weight; increased body surface area-to-weight ratio; insufficient supply of subcutaneous fat
Extremes of environmental temperature
Associated Condition: Alteration in metabolic rate
Brain injury; sepsis; trauma
Condition affecting temperature regulation; decrease in sweat response; inefficient nonshivering thermogenesis
Pharmaceutical agent; sedation
Sample Clinical Applications: Prematurity, CNS trauma or diseases (e.g., stroke, brain or spinal cord injury, intracranial bleeding or surgery, Parkinson's disease, multiple sclerosis); lengthy anesthesia or sedation; prolonged cardiac arrest; infection or sepsis, major surgical procedures

DESIRED OUTCOMES/EVALUATION CRITERIA

Sample NOC linkages:
Thermoregulation: Balance among heat production, heat gain, and heat loss
Thermoregulation: Newborn: Balance among heat production, heat gain, and heat loss during the first 28 days of life

Client/Caregiver Will (Include Specific Time Frame)
• Verbalize understanding of individual factors and appropriate interventions.
• Demonstrate techniques or behaviors to correct underlying condition or situation.
• Maintain body temperature within normal limits.

ACTIONS/INTERVENTIONS

Sample NIC linkages:
Temperature Regulation: Attaining and/or maintaining body temperature within a normal range
Temperature Regulation: Perioperative: Attaining and maintaining desired body temperature throughout the surgical event
Fever Treatment: Management of symptoms and related conditions associated with an increase in body temperature mediated by endogenous pyrogens

 Acute Care Collaborative Community/Home Care Cultural

NURSING PRIORITY NO. 1 To identify causative/contributing factors:

- ∞ Note client's age (e.g., premature neonate, young child, aging individual), *as it can directly impact ability to maintain or regulate body temperature and respond to changes in environment.*[1,8]
- Obtain history concerning present symptoms and correlate with previous episodes or family history and diagnostic studies. *Thermoregulation is a controlled process that maintains the body's core temperature in the range at which most biochemical processes work best (97.7°F–99.5°F [36.5°C–37°C]).*[9]
- Determine specific factors involved in current temperature fluctuation (e.g., environmental factors [such as extreme heat or cold], surgery, infectious process, effects of drugs or toxins, brain or spinal cord injury; behaviors that can increase risk of exposure such alcoholism, illicit drug use; homelessness). *Thermoregulation is affected in two ways: (1) endogenous factors (via diseases or conditions of body/organ systems that affect temperature homeostasis) and (2) exogenous factors (via environmental exposures, medications, and nutrition).*[6,10] *Note: Understanding the current situation helps to determine the scope of interventions that may be needed (e.g., simple addition of warm blankets during or after surgery, hypothermia therapy following brain trauma).*
- ⟋ Review lab results (e.g., tests indicative of infection, thyroid or other endocrine tests, drug screens) *to identify potential internal causes of temperature imbalances.*

NURSING PRIORITY NO. 2 To assist with measures to correct/treat underlying cause:

- ∞ ▨ Monitor temperature by appropriate route (e.g., tympanic, rectal, oral), using the same site and device over time and noting variation from client's usual or normal temperature. *Oral temperature measurement has been shown to be more accurate than tympanic, axillary, or chemical dot thermometers. Rectal and tympanic temperatures most closely approximate core temperature; however, shell temperatures (oral, axillary, touch) are often measured at home and are predictive of fever or subnormal temperatures. Rectal temperature measurement may be the most accurate but is not always expedient (e.g., client declines, is agitated, has rectal lesions or surgery, parent is unskilled or uncomfortable with using rectal thermometer on child). Abdominal temperature monitoring may be done in the premature neonate.*[3,6,7]
- Ⓐ Collaborate in treatment of underlying conditions (e.g. sepsis, spinal cord injury, hormonal imbalances, severe malnourishment, dehydration) *that can cause or contribute to body temperature disturbances.*
- Ensure that cooling and warming equipment and supplies are readily available during childbirth and following procedures or surgery *to maintain or restore body temperature within normal range.*
- ✚ Ⓐ Initiate emergent or immediate interventions, such as cooling or warming measures, fluids, electrolytes, supplemental oral or enteral nutrition, medications (e.g., antipyretics, antibiotics), as indicated, *to restore body temperature within client's usual range, and to optimize organ function.*[1–4]
- ✚ ∞ Place newborn infant under radiant warmer, cover infant's head with cap, and use layers of lightweight blankets. *Newborns/infants have temperature instability, especially premature or very-low-birth-weight infants. Heat loss is greatest through the head and by evaporation and convection.*[5]
- Maintain and instruct care providers to environmental temperature in comfortable range *to prevent or compensate for client's heat production or heat loss (e.g., may need to add or remove clothing or blankets, avoid drafts, reduce or increase room temperature and humidity).*
- ∞ Ⓐ Ensure that elderly or fragile, high-risk, and debilitated client is evaluated for nutritional deficits, environmental safety, need for social or psychiatric interventions (e.g., need for home health assistance, referral for social services or substance abuse treatment). *Client needs may extend beyond what can be immediately met and require referral for long-term interventions and follow-up.*
- Refer to NDs risk for ineffective Thermoregulation, Hypothermia, or Hyperthermia for additional interventions.

NURSING PRIORITY NO. 3 To promote optimal body temperature (Teaching/Discharge Considerations):

- 🏠 Review causative or related factors with client/significant others (SOs). *Provides information about what, if any, measures can be implemented to protect client from harm or limit potential for problems associated with ineffective thermoregulation.*

 Diagnostic Studies   Evidence Based Practice   Medications   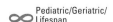 Pediatric/Geriatric/ Lifespan

- ∞ Review home management of temperature fluctuations in special population (e.g., newborn infant, person with spinal cord injury, frail elder). *Measures could include use of heating pads or ice bags, radiant heaters or fans, adding or removing clothing or blankets, cool or warm liquids and bath water, occlusive wrap in the delivery room, skin-to-skin contact in newborn, etc.*[2–4]
- Discuss with client/caregivers appropriate dressing for environment or weather conditions, as indicated, such as:

  Wearing layers of clothing that can be removed or added as needed;

  Donning hat and gloves in cold weather;

  Using water-resistant outer gear to protect from wet weather chill; and

  Dressing in light, loose protective clothing in hot weather.
- Provide oral and written information concerning client's disease processes, current therapies, and postdischarge precautions regarding hypothermia or hyperthermia, as appropriate to situation. *Allows for review of instructions for early intervention and implementation of preventive or corrective measures.*

DOCUMENTATION FOCUS

Assessment/Reassessment
- Individual findings, including nature of problem, degree of impairment, or fluctuations in temperature.

Planning
- Plan of care and who is involved in planning.
- Teaching plan.

Implementation/Evaluation
- Responses to interventions, teaching, and actions performed.
- Attainment or progress toward desired outcome(s).
- Modifications to plan of care.

Discharge Planning
- Long-term needs and who is responsible for actions to be taken.
- Specific referrals made.

References

1. Newfield, S. A., et al. (2007). *Cox's Clinical Applications of Nursing Diagnosis: Adult, Child, Women's, Psychiatric, Gerontic, and Home Health Considerations.* 5th ed. Philadelphia: F. A. Davis.
2. Helman, R. S., Habal, R. (Updated 2017). Heatstroke. Retrieved March 2018 from https://emedicine.medscape.com/article/166320-overview.
3. Galligan, M. (2006). Proposed guidelines for skin-to-skin treatment of neonatal hypothermia. *Amer J Matern Child Nurs,* 31(5), 298–304.
4. Jones, T. S. (2005). A bolt out of the blue: Dealing with the aftermath of spinal cord injury. *Nursing Made Incredibly Easy!,* 6(3), 14–28.
5. Bissinger, R. L., Annibale, D. J. (2010). Thermoregulation in very low-birth-weight infants during the gold hour results and implications. *Adv Neonatal Care,* 10(5), 230–238.
6. O'Grady, N. P., et al. (2008). Guidelines for evaluation of new fever in critically ill adult patients: 2008 update from the American College of Critical Care Medicine and the Infectious Disease Society of America. *Crit Care Med,* 36(4), 1330–1349.
7. Cunha, J. P. (Updated 2018). Fever. Retrieved March 2018 from http://www.medicinenet.com/aches_pain_fever/article.htm.
8. Smith, C. M., Cotter, V. (2008). Age-related changes in health. In Boltz, M., et al (eds). *Evidence-Based Geriatric Nursing Protocols for Best Practice.* New York: Springer.
9. Li, J., et al. (Updated 2017). Hypothermia. Retrieved March 2018 from https://emedicine.medscape.com/article/770542-overview#a5.
10. Harvard John, A. (No date). Thermoregulation. *Paulson School of Medicine.* Retrieved March 2018 from http://people.seas.harvard.edu/~jones/cscie129/pages/health/thermreg.htm.

 Acute Care   Collaborative   Community/ Home Care   Cultural

risk for ineffective Thermoregulation

Taxonomy II: Safety/Protection—Class 6 Physical Injury (00274) [**Diagnostic Division:** Safety], Approved 2016

DEFINITION: Susceptible to temperature fluctuation between hypothermia and hyperthermia, which may compromise health.

RISK FACTORS
Dehydration
Fluctuating environmental temperature; inappropriate clothing for environmental temperature
Inactivity or vigorous activity
Increase in oxygen demand
At Risk Population: Extremes of age
Extremes of weight; increased body surface area-to-weight ratio; insufficient supply of subcutaneous fat
Extremes of environmental temperature
Associated Condition: Alteration in metabolic rate
Brain injury; sepsis; trauma
Condition affecting temperature regulation; decrease is sweat response; inefficient nonshivering thermogenesis
Pharmaceutical agent; sedation
Sample Clinical Applications: Prematurity, brain injury, CVA, intracranial surgery (cerebral edema), infection or sepsis, major surgical procedures

DESIRED OUTCOMES/EVALUATION CRITERIA

Sample NOC linkages:
Thermoregulation: Balance among heat production, heat gain, and heat loss
Thermoregulation: Newborn: Balance among heat production, heat gain, and heat loss during the first 28 days of life

Client Will (Include Specific Time Frame)
• Maintain body temperature within normal limits.
• Verbalize understanding of risk factors and appropriate interventions.
• Demonstrate techniques or behaviors to correct underlying conditions or prevent hyperthermia or hypothermia.

ACTIONS/INTERVENTIONS

Sample NIC linkages:
Risk Identification: Analysis of potential risk factors, determination of health risks, and prioritization of risk reduction strategies for an individual or group
Temperature Regulation: Attaining or maintaining body temperature within a normal range

---

NURSING PRIORITY NO. 1   To identify causative/risk factors present:

• Note presence of condition that can affect body's heat production and heat dissipation (e.g., brain or spinal cord injury; burns or skin diseases; cardiac or endocrine disorders; neurological disorders, such as Parkinson's disease; kidney disease; being significantly overweight or underweight).[2,3]
• ∞ Note client's age (e.g., premature neonate, young child, aging individual), *as it can directly impact ability to maintain or regulate body temperature and respond to changes in environment.*[1,4,5]

 Diagnostic Studies   Evidence Based Practice   Medications   Pediatric/Geriatric/Lifespan

- Determine specific factors involved in current temperature fluctuation (e.g., environmental factors, surgery, infectious process, effects of drugs or toxins, brain or spinal cord injury). *Thermoregulation is affected in two ways: (1) endogenous factors (via diseases or conditions of body/organ systems that affect temperature homeostasis) and (2) exogenous factors (via environmental exposures, medications, and nutrition).*
- ✎ Review lab results (e.g., tests indicative of infection, thyroid, or other endocrine tests, drug screens) *to identify potential internal causes of temperature imbalances.*
- Assess nutritional status *to determine metabolism effect on body temperature and to identify foods or nutrient deficits that affect metabolism.*

NURSING PRIORITY NO. 2   To prevent occurrence of temperature alteration:

- ∞ ▨ Monitor temperature regularly, measuring core body temperature whenever needed to observe this vital sign. Exercise care in selecting appropriate thermometer for client's age and clinical condition, and observe for inconsistencies in readings obtained with various instruments. Observe temperature reading for trends, and avoid basing therapeutic decisions solely on thermometer readings. *Traditionally, temperature measurements have been taken orally (good in alert, oriented adults), rectally (accurate, but not always easy to obtain), or axillary (readings may be lower than core temperature), with each site offering advantages and disadvantages in terms of accuracy and safety. Newer technologies allow temperatures to be instantly measured. Tympanic temperature measurement is a noninvasive way to measure core temperature, as blood is supplied to the tympanic membrane by the carotid artery.*[3,5–8]
- Maintain comfortable ambient environment *to reduce effect on body temperature alterations:*
  Provide environmental heating or cooling measures, as needed, such as space heater or air conditioner or fans.
  ➕ Ascertain that cooling and warming equipment and supplies are available during or following procedures and surgery.
- Dress or discuss with client/caregivers appropriate dressing for client's condition:[2,6]
  Wear layers of clothing that can be removed or added as needed. Wear hat and gloves in cold weather; wear light, loose protective clothing in hot weather; and wear water-resistant outer gear *to protect from changes in weather or wet weather chill.*
  ∞ Cover infant's head with knit cap, use layers of lightweight blankets, and provide for skin-to-skin contact with mother. Place newborn infant under a radiant warmer. Teach parents to dress infant appropriately for weather and home environment. *Newborns/infants, especially very low-weight neonates, can have temperature instability, with heat loss greatest through head and by evaporation and convection.*[7]
  ∞ Limit clothing or remove blanket from premature infant placed in incubator *to prevent overheating in climate-controlled environment.*
- Maintain adequate fluid intake. Offer cool or warm liquids, as appropriate. *Hydration assists in maintaining normal body temperature. Note: Ambient temperature affects how much heat is lost through the skin and airways.*[2,3,4]
- 🌀 Maintain core temperature within client's normal range. (If temperature is below or above normal range, or parameters defined by physician, refer to NDs Hypothermia or Hyperthermia for additional interventions.)
- 🏠 Recommend lifestyle changes, such as cessation of substance use, normalization of body weight, nutritious meals, or regular exercise *to maximize metabolism and general health.*[4]
- 🌀 Refer at-risk persons to appropriate community resources (e.g., home care, social services, Foster Adult Care, housing agencies) *to provide assistance to meet individual needs.*[5]

NURSING PRIORITY NO. 3   To promote optimal body temperature (Teaching/Discharge Considerations):

- 🏠 Review potential problem or individual risk factors with client/significant others (SOs). *Provides information about what, if any, measures can be implemented to protect client from harm or limit potential for problems associated with ineffective thermoregulation.*
- ∞ Discuss effects of age and gender with client/caregiver, as appropriate. *Older or debilitated persons, infants, and young children typically feel more comfortable in higher ambient temperatures. Women notice*

 Acute Care   Collaborative   Community/ Home Care   Cultural

feeling cool quicker than men, which may be related to body size or to differences in metabolism and the rate that blood flows to extremities to regulate body temperature.[4,5]

- Instruct in measures to protect from identified risk factors. *Provides understanding for ways in managing lifestyle and environment (e.g., adding or removing clothing, adding or removing heat sources, evaluating home or shelter for ability to manage heat and cold, addressing nutritional and hydration status) and enhances self-care abilities.*

- Review client's medications for possible thermoregulatory side effects (e.g., diuretics, certain sedatives and antipsychotic agents, anticholinergics, anticonvulsants, some heart and blood pressure medications, anesthesia).[9]

- Review home management of temperature fluctuations in special population (e.g., newborn infant, person with spinal cord injury, frail elder). *Measures could include use of heating pads or ice bags, radiant heaters or fans, adding or removing clothing or blankets, cool or warm liquids and bath water, etc.*[1,6–8]

- Provide oral and written information concerning client's disease processes, current therapies, and postdischarge precautions regarding hypothermia or hyperthermia, as appropriate to situation. *Allows for review of instructions for early intervention and implementation of preventive or corrective measures.*

- Refer to teaching section in NDs ineffective Thermoregulation, Hypothermia, or Hyperthermia for related interventions as appropriate.

DOCUMENTATION FOCUS

Assessment/Reassessment
- Identified individual risk factors.
- Record of core temperature, initially and prn.

Planning
- Plan of care and who is involved in planning.
- Teaching plan, including best ambient temperature and ways to prevent hypothermia or hyperthermia.

Implementation/Evaluation
- Response to interventions, teaching, and actions performed.
- Attainment or progress toward desired outcome(s).
- Modifications to plan of care.

Discharge Planning
- Long-term needs and who is responsible for actions.
- Specific referrals made.

References

1. Galligan, M. (2006). Proposed guidelines for skin-to-skin treatment of neonatal hypothermia. *Amer J Matern Child Nurs*, 31(5), 298–304.
2. Jones, T. S. (2005). A bolt out of the blue: Dealing with the aftermath of spinal cord injury. *Nursing Made Incredibly Easy!*, 6(3), 14–28.
3. O'Grady, N. P., et al. (2008). Guidelines for evaluation of new fever in critically ill adult patients: 2008 update from the American College of Critical Care Medicine and the Infectious Disease Society of America. *Crit Care Med*, 36(4), 1330–1349.
4. Newfield, S. A., et al. (2007). *Cox's Clinical Applications of Nursing Diagnosis: Adult, Child, Women's, Psychiatric, Gerontic, and Home Health Considerations*. 5th ed. Philadelphia: F. A. Davis.
5. Smith, C. M., Cotter, V. (2008). Age-related changes in health. In Boltz, M., et al (eds). *Evidence-Based Geriatric Nursing Protocols for Best Practice*. New York: Springer.
6. Helman, R. S., Habal, R. (Updated 2017). Heatstroke. Retrieved March 2018 from https://emedicine.medscape.com/article/166320-overview.
7. Bissinger, R. L., Annibale, D. J. (2010). Thermoregulation in very low-birth-weight infants during the gold hour results and implications. *Adv Neonatal Care*, 10(5), 230–238.
8. Cunha, J. P. (Updated 2018). Fever. Retrieved March 2018 from http://www.medicinenet.com/aches_pain_fever/article.htm.
9. Westaway, K., Frank, O., Husband, A. (2015). Medicines can affect thermoregulation and accentuate the risk of dehydration and heat-related illness during hot weather. *J Clin Pharm Ther*, 40(4), 363–367.

 Diagnostic Studies   Evidence Based Practice   Medications   Pediatric/Geriatric/Lifespan

risk for venous Thromboembolism

Taxonomy II: Safety/Protection—Class 2 Physical Injury (00268) [Diagnostic Division: Safety], Approved 2016

DEFINITION: Susceptible to the development of a blood clot in a deep vein, commonly in the thigh, calf, or other extremity, which can break off and lodge in another vessel, which may compromise health.

RISK FACTORS
Dehydration
Impaired mobility
Obesity
At Risk Population: Age >60 years
Critical care admission
Current smoker
First-degree relative with history of venous thromboembolism; history of previous venous thromboembolism; history of cerebral vascular accident (CVA)
Less than 5 weeks postpartum
Associated Condition: Cerebral vascular accident (CVA); current cancer diagnosis; significant medical comorbidity; thrombophilia
Trauma below the waist or upper extremity; varicose veins
Postoperative for major or orthopedic surgery; surgery and total anesthesia time >90 minutes
Use of estrogen-containing contraceptive or hormone replacement therapy
Sample Clinical Applications: Cerebral vascular accident (CVA); current cancer diagnosis; pelvic trauma; upper or lower extremity crush injuries; orthopedic surgery; varicose veins.

DESIRED OUTCOMES/EVALUATION CRITERIA

Sample NOC linkages:
Knowledge: Thrombus Threat Reduction: Extent of understanding conveyed about causes, prevention, and early detection of blood clots within the circulatory system
Tissue Perfusion: Peripheral: Adequacy of blood flow through the small vessels of the extremities to maintain tissue function

Client Will (Include Specific Time Frame)
• Identify individual risk factors.
• Develop plan to reduce risk factors.
• Engage in activities/lifestyle changes to prevent thrombus/thromboembolism.
• Be free of signs/symptoms of thrombosis, e.g., extremity pulses/capillary refill equal bilaterally, free of erythema, edema, pain.

ACTIONS/INTERVENTIONS

Sample NIC linkages:
Embolus Precautions: Reduction of the risk of an embolus in a patient with thrombi or at risk for thrombus formation

NURSING PRIORITY NO. 1   To identify causative/risk factors

• Identify client at risk. *Conditions may include (1) past history of venous thromboembolism (VTE) or cessation of recent anticoagulant therapy or (2) predisposing factors (e.g., major surgery [especially orthopedic],*

 Acute Care   Collaborative   Community/Home Care   Cultural

trauma, extended travel; prolonged immobilization for any cause; spinal cord injury; pregnancy [especially when pregnant client has several conditions, including gestational hypertension, preeclampsia and eclampsia, cardiomyopathy, amniotic fluid embolism (not a complete listing)] use of oral contraceptives; valvular heart disease, heart failure, stroke; certain cancers or ongoing cancer treatments; clients requiring critical care for extended periods, indwelling central venous catheter use).[2,3]

- Evaluate client reports of calf pain or chest pain *symptoms that can be associated with VTE event.*
- Examine extremities in at-risk client *for signs potentially associated with development of deep vein thrombosis (DVT), such as asymmetry of calfs, edema, changes in skin color, obvious tissue injury, prominent veins.*
- Note client reports of shortness of breath.
- Review results of laboratory studies (such as hematocrit, coagulation profile, d-dimer assay). *Abnormalities in these tests (and others) point toward conditions associated with VTE, such as dehydration or clotting defects or other thrombotic processes,*[1]

NURSING PRIORITY NO. 2 To reduce risk/prevent VTE

- Initiate active or passive exercises while in bed or chair; for example, flex, extend, and rotate feet periodically.
- Promote early ambulation after any acute illness, surgery, or trauma
- Elevate legs when in bed or chair as indicated *to reduce edema*
- Caution client to avoid crossing legs or hyperflexing knee, such as when seated position with legs dangling, or lying in jackknife position.
- Increase fluid intake to at least 1500 to 2000 mL/day, within cardiac tolerance.
- Apply elastic support hose, compression stockings, or sequential compression devices, if indicated.
- Collaborate in treatment of underlying conditions *to manage/treat conditions that can cause or exacerbate risk of thromboembolism.*
- Provide DVT prophylaxis protocol, if indicated, and progressive mobility protocol where available. *While a prophylactic regimen of intermittent compression devices and chemical DVT prophylaxis is often standard practice in trauma intensive care units, studies suggest an additional benefit in VTE reduction with a focused progressive mobility protocol for this patient population.*[2]

NURSING PRIORITY NO. 3 To promote wellness (Teaching/Discharge Considerations):

- Instruct client/SO about client's particular condition and risk factors.
- Recommend continuation of prescribed treatments, exercises, and other measures to prevent immobility and stasis of body fluids.
- Review position recommendations, such as sitting with feet touching the floor, avoiding crossing of legs. *Prevents excess pressure on the popliteal space and enhances venous return.*
- Problem-solve solutions to predisposing factors that may be present, such as employment that requires prolonged standing or sitting, wearing restrictive clothing, use of oral contraceptives, obesity, prolonged immobility, smoking, and dehydration. *Actively involves client in identifying and initiating lifestyle and behavior changes to promote health and prevent recurrence of condition or development of complications.*

DOCUMENTATION FOCUS

Assessment/Reassessment
- Individual risk factors identified.
- Client concerns or difficulty making and following through with plan.

Planning
- Plan of care and who is involved in planning.
- Teaching plan.

 Diagnostic Studies   Evidence Based Practice   Medications 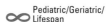 Pediatric/Geriatric/ Lifespan

Implementation/Evaluation
• Response to interventions, teaching, and actions performed.
• Attainment or progress toward outcomes.

Discharge Planning
• Referrals to other resources.
• Long-term need and who is responsible for actions.

References

1. Ouellette, D. R., Harrington, A., Kamangar, N. (2016). Pulmonary embolism. Retrieved May 2018 from http://emedicine.medscape.com/article/300901-overview.
2. Booth, K., et al. (2016). Progressive mobility protocol reduces venous thromboembolism rate in trauma intensive care patients: A quality improvement project. *J Trauma Nurs*, 23(5), 284–289.
3. Beal, C. C., Faucher, M. A. (2015). Stroke and pregnancy: An integrative review with implications for neuroscience nurses. *J Neurosci Nurs*, 47(2), 76–84.

impaired Tissue Integrity

Taxonomy II: Safety/Protection—Physical Injury 00044 [**Diagnostic Division:** Safety], Approved 1986; Revised 1998, 2013, 2017

DEFINITION: Damage to the mucous membrane, cornea, integumentary system, muscular fascia, muscle, tendon, bone cartilage, joint capsule, and/or ligament.

RELATED FACTORS
Imbalanced nutritional state [e.g., obesity, emaciation]
Chemical injury agent; high-voltage power supply; mechanical factor
Excessive or insufficient fluid volume; impaired circulation
Humidity
Insufficient knowledge about maintaining or protecting tissue integrity

DEFINING CHARACTERISTICS

Subjective
Acute pain

Objective
Bleeding; hematoma
Destroyed or damaged tissue
Localized area hot to touch; redness
At Risk Population: Extremes of age
Extremes of environmental temperature
Exposure to high-voltage power supply
Associated Condition: Alteration in metabolism
Alteration in sensation; peripheral neuropathy; impaired mobility
Arterial puncture; impaired circulation; vascular trauma
Radiation therapy; surgical procedure
Pharmaceutical agent

 Acute Care   Collaborative   Community/Home Care   Cultural

Sample Clinical Applications: Abscess, abuse (physical); traumatic injuries, amputation, anemias, burns, cataracts, deep vein thrombosis; diabetes; falls, frostbite; glaucoma, Parkinson's disease, poisoning; substance abuse, malnutrition; vascular occlusive disease

[Note: In reviewing this ND, it is apparent there is much overlap with other diagnoses. We have chosen to present generalized interventions. Although there are commonalities to injury situations, we suggest that the reader refer to other primary diagnoses as indicated, such as risk for Bleeding; risk for Contamination; risk for corneal Injury; risk for Dry Eye; risk for Falls; ineffective Health Maintenance; impaired Home Maintenance; risk for Infection; risk for Injury; impaired physical Mobility; risk for impaired oral Mucous Membrane Integrity; impaired/risk for impaired Parenting; ineffective Protection; risk for Poisoning; impaired/risk for impaired Skin/Tissue Integrity; risk for Surgical Site Infection; delayed/risk for delayed Surgical Recovery; risk for Perioperative Positioning Injury; risk for Pressure Ulcer; ineffective Tissue Perfusion; risk for Thermal Injury; risk for physical Trauma; risk for self- and other-directed Violence; risk for vascular Trauma for additional interventions.]

DESIRED OUTCOMES/EVALUATION CRITERIA

Sample NOC linkages:

Tissue Integrity: Skin & Mucous Membranes: Structural intactness and normal physiological function of skin and mucous membranes

Tissue Perfusion: Peripheral: Adequacy of blood flow through the small vessels of the extremities to maintain tissue function

Client/Caregiver Will (Include Specific Time Frame)
• Verbalize understanding of condition and causative factors.
• Identify interventions appropriate for specific condition.
• Demonstrate behaviors or lifestyle changes to promote healing and prevent complications.

ACTIONS/INTERVENTIONS

Sample NIC linkages:

Wound Care: Prevention of wound complications and promotion of wound healing

Incision Site Care: Cleansing, monitoring, and promotion of healing in a wound that is closed with sutures, clips, or staples

NURSING PRIORITY NO. 1 To identify causative/contributing factors:

• Identify underlying conditions or pathology. Assess for individual factors *that can result in tissue damage or can impede healing, such as (1) **trauma that causes internal tissue damage** (e.g., burns, high-velocity and penetrating trauma) and fractures (especially long-bone fractures) with hemorrhage, (2) **external pressures** (e.g., from tight dressings, splints or casting, burn eschar), (3) **immobility** (e.g., long-term bedrest, traction/cast), (4) presence of **conditions affecting peripheral circulation and sensation** (e.g., atherosclerosis, diabetes, venous insufficiency), (5) **lifestyle factors** (e.g., smoking, obesity, sedentary lifestyle), (6) **use of medications** (e.g., anticoagulants, corticosteroids, immunosuppressives, antineoplastics) that adversely affect healing, (7) **malnutrition** (deprives the body of protein and calories required for cell growth and repair), and (8) **dehydration** (impairs transport of oxygen and nutrients).*[1-4,11,13,26]

 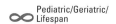

- ∞ ⧄ Note age, developmental stage, and gender. *Children, young adults, elderly persons, and men are at greater risk for injury, which may reflect client's ability or desire to protect self and influences choice of interventions or teaching.*[21,22]
- ⧄ Determine mechanism of traumatic injury where indicated (e.g., chemical burn affecting skin, mucous membranes; electrical/high-voltage injury, car crash, gunshot wound; environmental exposure to toxins or extreme temperatures). *Suggests initial treatment options and potential for tissue damage. Note: Information should include type of injuring agent (e.g., acid or base with route and length of exposure to offending agent; fire; penetration of contaminated object; possibility of coexisting injuries).*[26]
- Assess skin and mucous membranes for color, temperature, and sensation *for adequacy of blood supply and innervation.*
- Evaluate skin and mucous membranes for hydration status; note presence and degree of edema (1+ to 4+) and urine characteristics and output. *Determines presence of circulatory or metabolic imbalances resulting in fluid deficit or overload that can adversely affect cell or tissue health and organ function. Note: Edematous tissues are prone to breakdown.* Refer to NDs risk for imbalanced Fluid Volume, impaired Skin Integrity, and risk for Pressure Ulcer.
- Examine eyes for conjunctivitis, hemorrhage, burns, abrasions, or lacerations as indicated. Note reports of dry, scratchy eye, and vision impairment or pain. *May indicate injury to eye tissues, requiring more intensive evaluation and interventions.*[18] Refer to NDs risk for Dry Eye and risk for Corneal Injury for related interventions.
- ✎ ⧄ Evaluate pulses and calculate ankle-brachial index *to evaluate actual or potential for impairment of circulation to lower extremities. Result less than 0.9 indicates need for close monitoring or more aggressive intervention (e.g., tighter blood glucose and weight control in diabetic client).* Refer to NDs risk for peripheral Neurovascular Dysfunction and ineffective peripheral Tissue Perfusion.[6,11,13]
- 🌐 Determine race and ethnic background and family history for genetic factors *that may make individual vulnerable to particular conditions (e.g., sickle cell disease impairs circulation; systemic lupis erythematosis, Marfan syndrome)* and cultural or religious beliefs and practices regarding use of folk remedies or customs *that may damage tissues or impact choice of treatment options.*
- Determine nutritional status and impact of malnutrition on situation (e.g., pressure points on emaciated or elderly client, obesity, lack of activity, slow healing or failure to heal).
- Evaluate client's health and safety practices, noting lack of cleanliness, poor oral care, lack of foot and toenail care, unsafe sexual practices, failure to use safety equipment for occupational or sports-related activities, and unprotected exposure to sun or toxic substances, *that can place client at risk for injury to tissues or impaired function.*
- Note use of prosthetic, diagnostic, or external devices (e.g., artificial limbs, contacts, dentures, endotracheal airways, indwelling catheters, esophageal dilators), *which can cause pressure on/injure delicate tissues or provide entry point for infectious agents.*[10]

NURSING PRIORITY NO. 2 To assess degree of impairment:

- Obtain history of condition (e.g., pressure, venous, or diabetic wound; eye or oral lesions), including whether condition is acute or recurrent, original site and characteristics of wound, and duration of problem and changes that have occurred over time.
- Assess skin and tissues, bony prominences, and pressure areas, noting color, texture, and turgor. Assess areas of least pigmentation for color changes (e.g., sclera, conjunctiva, nailbeds, buccal mucosa, tongue, palms, and soles of feet).
- Assess wound/lesion, documenting (1) location; (2) dimensions and depth in centimeters; (3) exudates—color, odor, and amount; (4) margins—fixed or unfixed; (5) tunneling/tracts *(full extent of lesions of mucous membranes or subcutaneous tissue may not be visually discernible);* and (6) evidence of necrosis (e.g., color gray to black) or healing (e.g., pink or red granulation tissue) *in order to clarify treatment needs and establish a comparative baseline.*[3,4]

 Acute Care   Collaborative   Community/ Home Care   Cultural

- Classify/stage pressure ulcer(s) using an ulcer classification system, such as the Braden (or similar) scale. (See ND risk for Pressure Ulcer.) *Provides consistent terminology for risk assessment and documentation of pressure ulcers. Note: The National Pressure Ulcer Advisory Panel has updated the definition of a pressure ulcer and the stages of pressure ulcers based on current research and expert opinion. New definitions have been drafted to achieve accuracy, clarity, succinctness, clinical utility, and discrimination between and among the definitions of other pressure ulcer stages and other types of wounds. Deep tissue injury was also added as a distinct pressure ulcer in this updated system.*[5,16,19,20]
- Remeasure and photograph wound(s) periodically *to evaluate progress, development of complications, or delayed healing.*[17]
- Review diagnostic studies (e.g., x-rays, imaging scans, biopsies). *May be necessary to determine cause for and extent of impairment.*
- Obtain specimens of wound exudate or lesions for culture and sensitivity, when appropriate, *to identify effective antimicrobial therapies.*
- Monitor lab studies (e.g., complete blood count, electrolytes, glucose, cultures) *for systemic changes indicative of infection or other systemic complications.*
- Determine psychological effects of condition on the client and family. *Can be devastating for client's body or self-image and esteem—especially if condition is severe, disfiguring, or chronic—as well as costly and burdensome for SO/caregiver.*

NURSING PRIORITY NO. 3 To facilitate healing:

General[9–11,23–25]

- Modify or eliminate factors contributing to condition, if possible. Assist with treatment of underlying condition(s), as appropriate.
- Provide or encourage optimum nutrition (including protein, lipids, calories, trace minerals, and multivitamins) *to promote tissue health/healing. Nutrients should include adequate protein for tissue/organ maintenance, growth and repair, good immune function, and hormone production. High-quality fats improve energy production and reduction of inflammation. Good-quality carbohydrates provide immediate energy, stable blood sugar and insulin levels.*
- Provide/encourage adequate hydration *to reduce and replenish cellular water loss and enhance circulation. Note: Dehydration can reduce tissue perfusion at a wound site by reducing the blood volume, limiting the supply of oxygen and nutrients.*
- Provide or assist with oral care (e.g., teaching oral and dental hygiene, avoiding extremes of hot or cold, changing position of endotracheal and nasogastric tubes, lubricating lips) *to prevent damage to mucous membranes.* Refer to ND impaired oral Mucous Membranes for related interventions.
- Encourage adequate periods of rest and sleep *to promote healing and meet comfort needs.*
- Promote early and ongoing mobility. Assist with or encourage position changes and active or passive and assistive exercises *to promote circulation and prevent excessive tissue pressure.*

Incisions/wounds[9–12,20]

- Inspect lesions or wounds daily for changes (e.g., signs of infection, complications, or healing). *Promotes timely intervention and revision of plan of care.*
- Keep surgical area(s) clean and dry and change dressings or drainage appliances frequently, as indicated, *to prevent accumulation of secretions or excretions that can cause skin and tissue excoriation.*
- Practice aseptic technique for cleansing, dressing, and medicating wounds or lesions. *Reduces risk of infection and/or failure to heal.*
- Protect incision or wound approximation (e.g., use of Steri-Strips, splinting when coughing) and stimulate circulation to surrounding areas *to assist body's natural process of repair.*
- Collaborate with other healthcare providers (e.g., physician, burn specialist, ophthalmologist, infection or wound specialist, ostomy nurse), as indicated, *to assist with developing plan of care for problematic or potentially serious wounds. Note: A general surgeon or burn specialist/burn center may be needed for burns*

 Diagnostic Studies   Evidence Based Practice   Medications   Pediatric/Geriatric/Lifespan

(especially burns to hands, face, or perineum). Ophthalmological consultation is recommended for client with ocular burns from acids or bases if there is any significant degree of corneal or scleral injury. Caustic ingestions may require multiple specialties, including gastroenterology; gastrointestinal surgery; ear, nose, and throat; and surgery.[26]

- Apply appropriate barrier dressings or wound coverings (e.g., semipermeable, occlusive, wet-to-dry, hydrocolloid, hydrogel, polyacrylate moist wound dressing), drainage appliances, and skin-protective agents for open or draining wounds and stomas *to protect the wound and surrounding tissues from excoriating secretions or drainage and to enhance healing. Note: Recent studies are reporting that wet-to-dry dressings are beneficial only for mechanical débridement of wounds, can damage healthy granulation tissue, and can increase risk of infection.*[11,13–15]

- Assist with débridement or enzymatic therapy, as indicated (e.g., burns, severe pressure ulcer).

- Provide appropriate protective and healing devices (e.g., eye pads or goggles; heel protectors, padding, cushions, gel pads; therapeutic beds and mattresses; splints, chronic ulcer dressings, compression wrap).

- Refer to NDs dependent on individual situation (e.g., risk for Peripheral Neurovascular Dysfunction, risk for Perioperative Positioning Injury, risk for Pressure Ulcer, impaired physical/bed Mobility, impaired Skin Integrity, delayed Surgical Recovery; ineffective peripheral Tissue Perfusion, risk for Trauma, risk for Infection) *for related interventions.*

NURSING PRIORITY NO. 4   To correct hazards/minimize impairment:[3–5,7–10]

- Assess IV sites on regular basis for erythema, edema, tenderness, burning, etc., *which indicate infiltration or phlebitis, requiring immediate discontinuation of site use or interventions to heal the area.*

- Use appropriate catheter (e.g., peripheral or central venous) when infusing anticancer or other toxic drugs, and ascertain that IV is patent and infusing well *to prevent infiltration and extravasation with resulting tissue damage.*

- Inspect skin and tissues routinely around incisions and cast edges and traction devices *to ensure proper application and function; note possible development of pressure points.*

- Remove adhesive products with care, removing on horizontal plane and using mineral oil or Vaseline for softening, if needed, *to prevent abrasions or tearing of skin and damage to underlying tissues.*

- Monitor for correct placement of tubes, catheters, and other devices and assess skin tissues around these devices for effects of tape or fasteners or pressure from the devices *to prevent damage to skin and tissues as a result of pressure, friction, or shear forces.*

- Develop regularly timed repositioning schedule for client with mobility and sensation impairments, using adequate personnel and assistive devices as needed; encourage and assist with periodic weight shifts for client in chair *to reduce stress on pressure points and encourage circulation to tissues.*

- Use or demonstrate proper turning and transfer techniques *to avoid movements that cause friction or shearing (e.g., pulling client with parallel force, dragging movements).*

- Provide appropriate mattress (e.g., foam, flotation, alternating-pressure or air mattress) and appropriate padding devices (e.g., foam boots, heel protectors, ankle rolls), when indicated, *to reduce tissue pressure and enhance circulation to compromised tissues.*[13,20]

- Limit use of plastic material (e.g., rubber sheet, plastic-backed linen savers) and remove wet or wrinkled linens promptly. *Moisture potentiates skin and underlying tissues, increasing risk of breakdown and infection.*

- Avoid or restrict use of restraints; use adequate padding and evaluate circulation, movement, and sensation of extremity frequently when restraints are required. *Reduces risk of impaired circulation and tissue ischemia.*

- Elevate linens over affected extremity with bed cradle *to reduce pressure on and irritation of compromised tissues.*

- Encourage physical activity and exercise *to stimulate circulation, enhance organ function, and prevent/limit potential complications of immobility.*

- Provide or assist with oral care (e.g., oral and dental hygiene, avoiding extremes of hot or cold, change position of endotracheal/nasogastric tubes, lubricate lips) *to prevent damage to oral mucous membranes.* Refer to NDs impaired oral Mucous Membrane and risk for Pressure Ulcer for additional interventions.

 Acute Care   Collaborative   Community/ Home Care   Cultural

- Encourage use of adequate clothing or covers; protect from drafts and cold environment *to prevent vasoconstriction that can compromise circulation.*
- ∞ Provide or instruct in proper care of extremities during cold or hot weather. *Individuals with impaired sensation or young children/individuals unable to verbalize discomfort require special attention to deal with extremes in weather (e.g., dressing in layers and wearing gloves, clean dry socks, properly fitting shoes or boots, and a face mask in winter; using sunscreen and wearing light clothing to protect from dermal injury in summer).*
- Advise smoking cessation and refer for resources, if indicated. *Smoking causes vasoconstriction/interferes with healing.*

NURSING PRIORITY NO. 5   To promote wellness (Teaching/Discharge Considerations):

- Encourage verbalizations of feelings and expectations regarding condition and potential for recovery of structure and function.
- Help client and family to identify and implement successful coping skills *to reduce pain or discomforts and to improve quality of life.*
- Discuss importance of follow-up care (e.g., diabetic foot care clinic, wound care specialist, enterostomal therapist) as appropriate, self-monitoring, and reporting of changes in condition or pain characteristics. *Promotes early intervention and reduces potential for complications.*
- ∞ Educate the client/caregivers on proper safety precautions regarding hazardous materials, as indicated:[26] Inform client/caregivers of various substances in the home that are potentially dangerous.
  Counsel parents on how to keep chemicals out of the reach of children and cognitively impaired persons.
  Consult with local social services agency to evaluate child's home situation.
  Refer client to appropriate agencies for adequate training and protective equipment to protect against hazardous materials/agents in the community or employment setting.
- Review medical regimen (e.g., proper use of topical sprays, creams, ointments, soaks, or irrigations) with client/caregiver *to facilitate tissue healing and prevent complications associated with lack of knowledge about maintaining tissue integrity.*
- Identify required changes in lifestyle, occupation, or environment *necessitated by limitations imposed by condition or to avoid causative factors.*
- Refer to community or governmental resources as indicated (e.g., Public Health Department, Occupational Safety and Health Administration) *for information regarding specific conditions and to report hazards.*

DOCUMENTATION FOCUS

Assessment/Reassessment
- Individual findings, including history of condition, characteristics of wound or lesion, evidence of other organ or tissue involvement.
- Impact on functioning and lifestyle.
- Availability and use of resources.

Planning
- Plan of care and who is involved in planning.
- Teaching plan.

Implementation/Evaluation
- Responses to interventions, teaching, and actions performed.
- Attainment or progress toward desired outcome(s).
- Modifications to plan of care.

Discharge Planning
- Long-term needs and who is responsible for actions to be taken.
- Specific referrals made.

 Diagnostic Studies   Evidence Based Practice   Medications   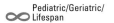 ∞ Pediatric/Geriatric/Lifespan

References

1. Fort, C. W. (2003). How to combat 3 deadly trauma complications. *Nursing*, 33(5), 58–63.
2. Rasul, A. T. (2014, updated 2018). Acute compartment syndrome. Retrieved May 2018 from http://emedicine.medscape.com/article/307668-overview.
3. Llewellyn, S. (2002). *Skin integrity and wound care (lecture materials)*. Chapel Hill, NC: Cape Fear Community College Nursing Program.
4. Colburn, L. (2001). Prevention for chronic wounds. In Krasner, D., Rodeheaver, G., Sibbald R. G. (eds). *Chronic Wound Care: A Clinical Source Book for Healthcare Professionals*. 2nd ed. Wayne, PA: Health Management.
5. Inouye, S. K., Studenski, S., Tinetti, M. E. (2007). Geriatric syndromes: Clinical, research and policy implications of a core geriatric concept. *J Am Geriatr Soc*, 55(5), 780–791.
6. Murabito, J. M., et al. (2003). The ankle-brachial index in the elderly and risk of stroke, coronary disease and death. *Arch Intern Med*, 163, 1939–1942.
7. Calianno, C. (2002). Patient hygiene, part 2—Skin care: Keeping the outside healthy. *Nursing*, 32(6). Suppl, June Clinical.
8. Wiersema, L. A., Stanley, M. (1999). The aging integumentary system. Stanley, M., Beare, P. G. (eds). *Gerontological Nursing: A Health Promotion/Protection Approach*. 2nd ed. Philadelphia: F. A. Davis, 102–111.
9. McGovern, C. (2014). Skin, hair and nail assessment. Unit 2 (lecture materials). Retrieved May 2018 from http://www10.homepage.villanova.edu/marycarol.mcgovern/2104/SkinHairNail2.htm.
10. Faller, N., Beitz, J. (2001). When a wound isn't a wound: Tubes, drains, fistulas and draining wounds. In Krasner, D., Rodeheaver, G., Sibbald, R. G. (eds). *Chronic Wound Care: A Clinical Source Book for Healthcare Professionals*. 2nd ed. Wayne, PA: Health Management.
11. Bonham, P. A., et al. (2009). What's new in lower-extremity arterial disease? WOCN's 2008 Clinical Practice Guideline. *J Wound Ostomy Continence Nurs*, 36(1), 37–44.
12. Okan, K., et al. (2007). The role of moisture balance in wound healing. *Adv Wound Care*, 20(1), 39–53.
13. Sieggreen, N. Y. (2006). Getting a leg up on managing venous ulcers. *Nursing Made Incredibly Easy!*, 4(6), 52–60.
14. Fleck, C. A. (2009). "Why wet to dry"? *J Am Coll Certified Wound Specialists*, 1(4), 109–113.
15. Cowan, L. G., Stechmiller, J. (2009). Prevalence of wet-to-dry dressings in wound care. *Adv Skin Wound Care*, 22(12), 567–573.
16. Black, J., Baharestani, M. M., Cudigan, J. (2007). From the NPUAP: National Pressure Ulcer Advisory Panel's Updated Pressure Ulcer Staging System. *Adv Skin Wound Care*, 20(5), 269–274.
17. Duncan, V., Lane, L., McKenzie, L. (2016). Skin & wound photographic recordings: Evidence informed practice tools. *Evidence Informed Practice Tools*. Retrieved May 2018 from http://www.wrha.mb.ca/extranet/eipt/files/EIPT-042.pdf.
18. Capão, F. J. A., et al. (2003). Modern sports eye injuries. *Br J Ophthalmol*, 87(11), 1336–1339.
19. Braden, B. J. (2003). The Braden Scale for predicting pressure sore risk: Reflections after 25 years. *Adv Skin Wound Care*, 25(2), 61.
20. National Pressure Ulcer Advisory Panel (NPUAP). (2014). Prevention and treatment of pressure ulcers: Clinical practice guideline (various pages). Retrieved May 2018 from http://www.npuap.org/resources/educational-and-clinical-resources/prevention-and-treatment-of-pressure-ulcers-clinical-practice-guideline/.
21. Schwebel, D. C., Barton, B. K. (2005). Contributions of multiple risk factors to child injury. *J Pediatr Psychol*, 25, 553–561.
22. Risolainen, L., et al. (2009). Gender differences in sport injury risk and types of injuries: A retrospective twelve-month study on cross-country skiers, long distance runners and soccer players. *J Sports Sci Med*, 8, 443–451.
23. Todorovic, V. (2003). Food and wounds: Nutritional factors in wound formation and healing. *Clin Nutr Update*, 8(2), 6–9.
24. Johnston, E. (2007). The role of nutrition in tissue viability. *Wound Essentials*, 2, 10–21.
25. Posthauer, M. (2007). Hydration: An essential nutrient. *Adv Skin Wound Care*, 18(1), 32–33.
26. Cox, R. D. (Update 2017). Chemical burns. Retrieved May 2018 from http://emedicine.medscape.com/article/769336-overview.

risk for impaired Tissue Integrity

Taxonomy II: Safety/Protection—Physical Injury 000248 [**Diagnostic Division:** Safety], Approved 2013; Revised 2017

DEFINITION: Susceptible to damage to the mucous membrane, cornea, integumentary system, muscular fascia, muscle, tendon, bone, cartilage, joint capsule, and/or ligament, which may compromise health.

RISK FACTORS
Imbalanced nutritional state [e.g., obesity, emaciation]
Chemical injury agent; high-voltage power supply; mechanical factor
Excessive or insufficient fluid volume; impaired circulation
Humidity

 Acute Care   Collaborative   Community/Home Care   Cultural

Insufficient knowledge about maintaining or protecting tissue integrity
At Risk Population: Extremes of age
Extremes of environmental temperature
Exposure to high-voltage power supply
Associated Condition: Alteration in metabolism
Alteration in sensation; peripheral neuropathy; impaired mobility
Arterial puncture; impaired circulation; vascular trauma
Radiation therapy; surgical procedure
Pharmaceutical agent
Sample Clinical Applications: Abscess, abuse (physical); traumatic injury, amputation, anemias, burns, cataracts, deep vein thrombosis; diabetes; falls, frostbite; glaucoma, Parkinson's disease, poisoning; substance abuse, malnutrition; vascular occlusive disease
[Note: In reviewing this ND, it is apparent there is much overlap with other diagnoses. We have chosen to present generalized interventions. Although there are commonalities to injury situations, we suggest that the reader refer to other primary diagnoses as indicated, such as risk for Bleeding; risk for Contamination; risk for corneal Injury; risk for Dry Eye; risk for Falls; ineffective Health Maintenance; impaired Home Maintenance; risk for Infection; risk for Injury; impaired physical Mobility; risk for impaired oral Mucous Membrane Integrity; impaired/risk for impaired Parenting; ineffective Protection; risk for Poisoning; impaired/risk for impaired Skin/Tissue Integrity; risk for Surgical Site Infection; delayed/risk for delayed Surgical Recovery; risk for Perioperative Positioning Injury; risk for Pressure Ulcer; ineffective Tissue Perfusion; risk for Thermal Injury; risk for physical Trauma; risk for self- and other-directed Violence; risk for Vascular Trauma for additional interventions.]

DESIRED OUTCOMES/EVALUATION CRITERIA

Sample NOC linkages:
Tissue Integrity: Skin & Mucous Membranes: Structural intactness and normal physiological function of skin and mucous membranes
Tissue Perfusion: Peripheral: Adequacy of blood flow through the small vessels of the extremities to maintain tissue function

Client/Caregiver Will (Include Specific Time Frame)
• Verbalize understanding of condition and causative factors.
• Identify interventions appropriate for specific condition.
• Demonstrate behaviors or lifestyle changes to promote healing and prevent complications or recurrence.

Sample NOC linkage:
Wound Healing: Secondary Intention: Extent of regeneration of cells and tissues in an open wound

ACTIONS/INTERVENTIONS

Sample NIC linkages:
Wound Care: Prevention of wound complications and promotion of wound healing
Incision Site Care: Cleansing, monitoring, and promotion of healing in a wound that is closed with sutures, clips, or staples

 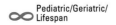

NURSING PRIORITY NO. 1   To identify risk factors:

- Identify underlying conditions or pathology. Assess for individual factors *that can result in tissue damage or can impede healing, such as (1)* **trauma that causes internal tissue damage** *(e.g., burns, high-velocity and penetrating trauma) and fractures (especially long-bone fractures) with hemorrhage, (2)* **external pressures** *(e.g., from tight dressings, splints or casting, burn eschar), (3)* **immobility** *(e.g., long-term bedrest, traction/cast), (4) presence of* **conditions affecting peripheral circulation and sensation** *(e.g., atherosclerosis, diabetes, venous insufficiency), (5)* **lifestyle factors** *(e.g., smoking, obesity, sedentary lifestyle), (6)* **use of medications** *(e.g., anticoagulants, corticosteroids, immunosuppressives, antineoplastics) that adversely affect healing, (7)* **malnutrition** *(deprives the body of protein and calories required for cell growth and repair); and (8)* **dehydration** *(impairs transport of oxygen and nutrients).*[1–7]
- Note age, developmental stage, and gender. *Children, young adults, elderly persons, and men are at greater risk for injury, which may reflect client's ability or desire to protect self, and influences choice of interventions or teaching.*[8,9]
- Assess skin and mucous membranes for color, temperature, and sensation *for adequacy of blood supply and innervation.*
- Evaluate skin and mucous membranes for hydration status; note presence and degree of edema (1+ to 4+) and urine characteristics and output. *Determines presence of circulatory or metabolic imbalances resulting in fluid deficit or overload that can adversely affect cell or tissue health and organ function. Note: Edematous tissues are prone to breakdown.* Refer to NDs risk for imbalanced Fluid Volume, impaired Skin Integrity, and risk for Pressure Ulcer.
- Assess skin over bony prominence and pressure areas, noting color, texture, and turgor. Assess areas of least pigmentation for color changes (e.g., nailbeds, buccal mucosa, tongue, palms, soles of feet).
- Evaluate pulses and calculate ankle-brachial index *to evaluate potential for impairment of circulation to lower extremities. Result less than 0.9 indicates need for close monitoring or more aggressive intervention (e.g., tighter blood glucose and weight control in diabetic client).*[5,6,10] Refer to NDs risk for Peripheral Neurovascular Dysfunction and ineffective peripheral Tissue Perfusion.
- Determine nutritional status and potential impact on situation (e.g., pressure points on emaciated or elderly client, obesity, lack of activity, history of slow healing or failure to heal).
- Evaluate client's health and safety practices, noting lack of cleanliness, poor oral care, lack of foot and toenail care, unsafe sexual practices, failure to use safety equipment for occupational or sports-related activities, and unprotected exposure to sun or toxic substances, *that can place client at risk for injury to tissues.*

NURSING PRIORITY NO. 2   To facilitate healing:

General[5,11–13]
- Assist with treatment of underlying condition(s), as appropriate.
- Provide or encourage optimum nutrition (including protein, lipids, calories, trace minerals, multivitamins) *to promote tissue health/healing* and adequate hydration *to reduce and replenish cellular water loss and enhance circulation.*
- Assess IV sites on regular basis for erythema, edema, tenderness, burning, etc., *which indicate infiltration or phlebitis, requiring immediate discontinuation of site use or interventions to heal the area.*
- Use appropriate catheter (e.g., peripheral or central venous) when infusing anticancer or other toxic drugs and ascertain that IV is patent and infusing well *to prevent infiltration and extravasation with resulting tissue damage.*
- Provide or assist with oral care (e.g., teaching oral and dental hygiene, avoiding extremes of hot or cold, changing position of endotracheal and nasogastric tubes, lubricating lips) *to prevent damage to mucous membranes.* Refer to ND impaired oral Mucous Membranes for related interventions.
- Inspect skin and tissues routinely around incisions and cast edges and traction devices *to ensure proper application and function; note possible development of pressure points.*

 Acute Care   Collaborative   Community/Home Care   Cultural

- Remove adhesive products with care, removing on horizontal plane and using mineral oil or Vaseline for softening, if needed, *to prevent abrasions or tearing of skin and damage to underlying tissues.*
- Monitor for correct placement of tubes, catheters, and other devices and assess skin tissues around these devices for effects of tape or fasteners or pressure from the devices *to prevent damage to skin and tissues as a result of pressure, friction, or shear forces.*
- Develop regularly timed repositioning schedule for client with mobility and sensation impairments, using adequate personnel and assistive devices as needed; encourage and assist with periodic weight shifts for client in chair *to reduce stress on pressure points and encourage circulation to tissues.*
- Use or demonstrate proper turning and transfer techniques *to avoid movements that cause friction or shearing (e.g., pulling client with parallel force, dragging movements).*
- Avoid or restrict use of restraints; use adequate padding and evaluate circulation, movement, and sensation of extremity frequently, when restraints are required. *Reduces risk of impaired circulation and tissue ischemia.*
- Encourage adequate periods of rest and sleep *to promote healing and meet comfort needs.*
- Promote early and ongoing mobility. Assist with or encourage position changes and active or passive and assistive exercises *to promote circulation and prevent excessive tissue pressure.*
  Incisions/Wounds[9–15]

  Inspect lesions or wounds daily for changes (e.g., signs of infection, complications, or healing). *Promotes timely intervention and revision of plan of care.*

  Keep surgical area(s) clean and dry and change dressings or drainage appliances frequently, as indicated, *to prevent accumulation of secretions or excretions that can cause skin and tissue excoriation.*

  Practice aseptic technique for cleansing, dressing, and medicating wounds or lesions. *Reduces risk of infection and/or failure to heal.*

  Protect incision or wound approximation (e.g., use of Steri-Strips, splinting when coughing) and stimulate circulation to surrounding areas *to assist body's natural process of repair.*

   Apply appropriate barrier dressings or wound coverings (e.g., semipermeable, occlusive, wet-to-dry, hydrocolloid, hydrogel, polyacrylate moist wound dressing), drainage appliances, and skin-protective agents for open or draining wounds and stomas *to protect the wound and surrounding tissues from excoriating secretions or drainage and to enhance healing.*

  Refer to NDs dependent on individual situation (e.g., risk for peripheral Neurovascular Dysfunction, risk for Perioperative Positioning Injury, risk for Pressure Ulcer, impaired physical/bed Mobility, impaired Skin Integrity, delayed Surgical Recovery, ineffective peripheral Tissue Perfusion, risk for physical Trauma, risk for Infection) *for related interventions.*

NURSING PRIORITY NO. 3 To promote wellness (Teaching/Discharge Considerations):

- 🏠 Review medical regimen (e.g., proper use of topical sprays, creams, ointments, soaks, or irrigations) with client/caregiver *to prevent complications associated with lack of knowledge about maintaining tissue integrity.*
- Discuss importance of follow-up care (e.g., diabetic foot care clinic, wound care specialist, enterostomal therapist) as appropriate, self-monitoring, and reporting of changes in condition or pain characteristics. *Reduces potential for complications.*
- Advise smoking cessation and refer for resources, if indicated. *Smoking causes vasoconstriction/interferes with healing.*
- Educate client/caregivers on proper safety precautions regarding hazardous materials, as indicated.

DOCUMENTATION FOCUS

Assessment/Reassessment
- Individual findings, characteristics of wound/incisions, etc.
- Impact on functioning and lifestyle.
- Availability and use of resources.

 Diagnostic Studies   Evidence Based Practice   Medications 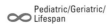 Pediatric/Geriatric/Lifespan

Planning
- Plan of care and who is involved in planning.
- Teaching plan.

Implementation/Evaluation
- Responses to interventions, teaching, and actions performed.
- Attainment or progress toward desired outcome(s).
- Modifications to plan of care.

Discharge Planning
- Long-term needs and who is responsible for actions to be taken.
- Specific referrals made.

References

1. Fort, C. W. (2003). How to combat 3 deadly trauma complications. *Nursing*, 33(5), 58–63.
2. Rasul, A. T. (2014, updated 2018). Acute compartment syndrome. Retrieved May 2018 from http://emedicine.medscape.com/article/307668-overview.
3. Llewellyn, S. (2002). *Skin integrity and wound care (lecture materials)*. Chapel Hill, NC: Cape Fear Community College Nursing Program.
4. Krasner, D. (ed.) (2007). Prevention for chronic wounds. *Chronic Wound Care: A Clinical Source Book for Health Care Professionals*. 4th ed. West Bloomfield, MI: HMP Communications, LLC.
5. Bonham, P. A., et al. (2009). What's new in lower-extremity arterial disease? WOCN's 2008 Clinical Practice Guideline. *J Wound Ostomy Continence Nurs*, 36(1), 37–44.
6. Sieggreen, N. Y. (2006). Getting a leg up on managing venous ulcers. *Nursing Made Incredibly Easy!*, 4(6), 52–60.
7. Cox, R. D. (2013, updated 2017). Chemical burns. Retrieved May 2018 from http://emedicine.medscape.com/article/769336-overview.
8. Schwebel, D. C., Barton, B. K. (2005). Contributions of multiple risk factors to child injury. *J Pediatr Psychol*, 25, 553–561.
9. Risolainen, L., et al. (2009). Gender differences in sport injury risk and types of injuries: A retrospective twelve-month study on cross-country skiers, long distance runners and soccer players. *J Sports Sci Med*, 8, 443–451.
10. Murabito, J. M., et al. (2003). The ankle-brachial index in the elderly and risk of stroke, coronary disease and death. *Arch Intern Med*, 163, 1939–1942.
11. McGovern, C. (2014). Skin, hair and nail assessment. Unit 2 (lecture materials). Retrieved May 2018 from http://www10.homepage.villanova.edu/marycarol.mcgovern/2104/SkinHairNail2.htm.
12. Faller, N., Beitz, J. (2001). When a wound isn't a wound: Tubes, drains, fistulas and draining wounds. In Krasner, D., Rodeheaver, G., Sibbald, R. G. (eds). *Chronic Wound Care: A Clinical Source Book for Healthcare Professionals*. 2nd ed. Wayne, PA: Health Management.
13. Posthauer, M. (2007). Hydration: An essential nutrient. *Adv Skin Wound Care*, 18(1), 32–33.
14. Okan, K., et al. (2007). The role of moisture balance in wound healing. *Adv Wound Care*, 20(1), 39–53.
15. National Pressure Ulcer Advisory Panel. (2014). Prevention and treatment of pressure ulcers: Clinical practice guideline (various pages). Retrieved May 2018 from http://www.npuap.org/resources/educational-and-clinical-resources/prevention-and-treatment-of-pressure-ulcers-clinical-practice-guideline/.

ineffective peripheral Tissue Perfusion

Taxonomy II: Activity/Rest—Class 4 Cardiovascular/Pulmonary Responses (00204) [**Diagnostic Division**: Circulation], Approved 2008; Revised 2010,2017

DEFINITION: Decrease in blood circulation to the periphery which may compromise health.

RELATED FACTORS
Excessive sodium intake
Insufficient knowledge of disease process or aggravating factors
Sedentary lifestyle; smoking

 Acute Care Collaborative Community/Home Care Cultural

DEFINING CHARACTERISTICS

Subjective
Extremity pain; intermittent claudication
Paresthesia

Objective
Decrease in or absence of peripheral pulses; ankle-brachial index <0.90; decrease in blood pressure in extremities; femoral bruit
Alteration in skin characteristics [e.g., color, elasticity, hair, moisture, nails, sensation, temperature]
Skin color pales with limb elevation; capillary refill time >3 sec; color does not return to lowered limb after 1 min leg elevation
Decrease in pain-free distances achieved in the 6-minute walk test; distance in the 6-minute walk test below normal range
Edema
Alteration in motor function
Delay in peripheral wound healing;
Associated Condition: Diabetes mellitus; hypertension
Endovascular procedure; trauma
Sample Clinical Applications: Atherosclerosis, anemias; arthritis; coronary artery disease; amputation; Buerger's disease, burns; CVA; COPD; CHF; diabetes mellitus, obesity; peripheral vascular disease, Raynaud's disease, thrombophlebitis

DESIRED OUTCOMES/EVALUATION CRITERIA

Sample NOC linkages:
Tissue Perfusion: Peripheral: Adequacy of blood flow through the small vessels of the extremities to maintain tissue function
Knowledge: Disease Process: Extent of understanding conveyed about a specific disease process and prevention of complications

Client Will (Include Specific Time Frame)
- Demonstrate increased perfusion as individually appropriate (e.g., skin warm and dry, peripheral pulses present and strong, absence of edema, free of pain or discomfort).
- Verbalize understanding of condition, therapy regimen, side effects of medications, and when to contact healthcare provider.
- Demonstrate behaviors or lifestyle changes to improve circulation (e.g., engage in regular exercise, cessation of smoking, weight reduction, disease management).

ACTIONS/INTERVENTIONS

Sample NIC linkages:
Circulatory Care: Arterial Insufficiency: Promotion of arterial circulation
Circulatory Care: Venous Insufficiency: Promotion of venous circulation

 Diagnostic Studies   Evidence Based Practice   Medications   Pediatric/Geriatric/Lifespan

NURSING PRIORITY NO. 1 To assess causative/contributing factors:

- Note current situation or presence of conditions that can affect perfusion to all body systems (e.g., congestive heart failure, lung disorders, major trauma, septic or hypovolemic shock, coagulopathies, sickle cell anemia) *affecting systemic circulation and perfusion.*
- Determine history of conditions associated with thrombus or emboli (e.g., problems with coronary or cerebral circulation, stroke; high-velocity trauma with fractures, abdominal or orthopedic surgery, long periods of immobility; inflammatory diseases; chronic lung disease; diabetes with coexisting peripheral vascular disease; estrogen therapy; cancer and cancer therapies; presence of central venous catheters) *to identify client at higher risk for venous stasis, vessel wall injury, and hypercoagulability.*[1,2,14,15]
- Identify presence of high-risk factors or conditions (e.g., smoking, uncontrolled hypertension, obesity, pregnancy, pelvic tumor, paralysis, hypercholesterolemia, varicose veins, arthritis, sepsis). *Places client at greater risk for developing peripheral vascular disease (PVD), including arterial blockage and chronic venous insufficiency, with associated complications.*[3,4,14]
- Note location of restrictive clothing, pressure dressings, circular wraps, and cast or traction device *that may restrict circulation to limb.*
- Ascertain impact on functioning and lifestyle. *For example, leg pain may restrict ambulation or person may develop skin ulceration and healing problems that seriously impact quality of life.*

NURSING PRIORITY NO. 2 To evaluate degree of impairment:

- Assess skin color, temperature, moisture, and whether changes are widespread or localized. *Helps in determining location and type of perfusion problem.*
- Compare skin temperature and color with other limb when assessing extremity circulation. *Helps differentiate type of problem (e.g., deep redness in both hands triggered by vibrating machinery is associated with functional PVD, such as Raynaud's disease; edema, redness, swelling in calf of one leg is associated with localized thrombophlebitis).*[1,5,14–16]
- Assess presence, location, and degree of swelling or edema formation. Measure circumference of extremities, noting differences in size. *Useful in identifying or quantifying edema in involved extremity.*
- Measure capillary refill *to determine adequacy of systemic circulation.*
- Note client's nutritional and fluid status. *Protein-energy malnutrition and weight loss make ischemic tissues more prone to breakdown. Dehydration reduces blood volume and compromises peripheral circulation.*[14]
- Inspect lower extremities for skin texture (e.g., atrophic; shiny appearance; lack of hair; dry, scaly, reddened skin) and skin breaks or ulcerations *that often accompany diminished peripheral circulation.*[2,3,6,14]
- Palpate arterial pulses (bilateral femoral, popliteal, dorsalis pedis, posterior tibial), using handheld Doppler if indicated *to determine level of circulatory problem (e.g., client with intermittent claudication may have palpable pulses that disappear after ambulation).*[2,5]
- Determine pulse equality as well as intensity (e.g., bounding, normal, diminished, absent) and compare with unaffected extremity *to evaluate distribution and quality of blood flow and success or failure of therapy.*[2]
- Evaluate extremity pain reports, noting associated symptoms (e.g., cramping or heaviness, discomfort with walking, progressive temperature or color changes, paresthesia). Determine time (day or night) that symptoms are worse, precipitating or aggravating events (e.g., walking), and relieving factors (e.g., rest, sitting down with legs in dependent position, oral analgesics) *to help isolate and differentiate problems such as intermittent chronic claudication versus loss of function and pain due to acute sustained ischemia related to loss of arterial blood flow.*[2,3]
- Assess motor and sensory function. *Problems with ambulation, hypersensitivity or loss of sensation, numbness and tingling are changes that can indicate neurovascular dysfunction or limb ischemia, requiring more evaluation for differentiation of problem.*[2,6]
- Check for calf tenderness or pain on dorsiflexion of foot (Homans' sign) and swelling and redness. *Indicators of deep vein thrombosis (DVT), although DVT is often present without a positive Homans' sign.*[1,15,18]
- Review lab studies (e.g., lipid profile, coagulation studies, hemoglobin/hematocrit, renal/cardiac function tests, inflammatory markers [e.g., D dimer, C-reactive protein]) and diagnostic studies (e.g., Doppler

 Acute Care   Collaborative   Community/ Home Care   Cultural

ultrasound, magnetic resonance angiography, venogram, contrast angiography, resting ankle-brachial index, leg segmental arterial pressure measurements) *to determine probability, location, and degree of impairment.*[1–3,6]

NURSING PRIORITY NO. 3   To maximize tissue perfusion:

- ✚ 🏠 Ⓐ Collaborate in treatment of underlying conditions, such as diabetes, hypertension, cardiopulmonary conditions, blood disorders, traumatic injury, hypovolemia, and hypoxemia *to maximize systemic circulation and organ perfusion.*
- 💊 📝 Administer medications such as antiplatelet agents, thrombolytics, and antibiotics *to improve tissue perfusion and organ function.*[1,2,4,6,15,16]
- Ⓐ Administer fluids, electrolytes, nutrients, and oxygen as indicated *to promote optimal blood flow, organ perfusion, and function.*
- Ⓐ Assist with or prepare for medical procedures such as endovascular stent placement, surgical revascularization procedures, thrombectomy, and sympathectomy *to improve peripheral circulation.*
- Ⓐ 📝 Assist with application of elasticized tubular support bandages, adhesive elastic or Velcro wraps (e.g., Circ-Aid), paste bandages (Unna's boot), multilayer bandage regimens, sequential pneumatic compression devices, and custom-fitted compression stockings as indicated *to provide graduated compression of lower extremity in presence of venous stasis ulcer.*[13,15]
- Ⓐ 📝 Collaborate with wound care specialist if arterial or venous ulcerations are present. *In-depth wound care may include débridement and various specialized dressings that provide optimal moisture for healing, prevention of infection and further injury.*[14,15]
- Provide interventions to promote peripheral circulation and limit complications:[1–3,7]

  📝 Encourage early ambulation when possible and recommend regular exercise. *Enhances venous return. Studies indicate exercise training may be an effective early treatment for intermittent claudication.*[8]

  Recommend or provide foot and ankle exercises when client unable to ambulate freely *to reduce venous pooling and increase venous return.*[15]

  Provide pressure-relieving devices for immobilized client (e.g., air mattress, foam or sheepskin padding, bed or foot cradle) *to reduce excessive tissue pressure that could lead to skin breakdown.*

  Ⓐ 📝 Apply intermittent compression devices or graduated compression stockings to lower extremities *to limit venous stasis, improve venous return, and reduce risk of DVT or tissue ulceration in client who is limited in activity or otherwise at risk.*[9,14–16]

  Assist with or cue client to change position at timed intervals rather than using presence of pain as signal to change positions *because sensation may be impaired.*[6]

  Elevate the legs when sitting, but avoid sharp angulation of the hips or knees *to enhance venous return and minimize edema formation.*

  Avoid massaging the leg in presence of thrombosis *to reduce risk for embolus.*

  Avoid, or carefully monitor, use of heat or cold, such as hot water bottle, heating pad, or ice pack. *Tissues may have decreased sensitivity due to ischemia, increasing risk of dermal injury.*
- Refer to NDs risk for peripheral Neurovascular Dysfunction, risk for impaired Skin Integrity, impaired Tissue Integrity, and [disturbed Sensory Perception] for additional interventions as appropriate.

NURSING PRIORITY NO. 4   To promote wellness (Teaching/Discharge Considerations):

- 🏠 Discuss relevant risk factors (e.g., family history, obesity, age, smoking, hypertension, diabetes, clotting disorders) and potential outcomes of atherosclerosis (e.g., systemic and peripheral vascular disease conditions). *Information necessary for client to make informed decisions concerning risk factors and to commit to lifestyle changes necessary to prevent onset of complications or manage symptoms when condition present.*[10,11]
- Identify necessary changes in lifestyle and assist client to incorporate disease management into activities of daily living. *Promotes independence and enhances self-concept regarding ability to deal with change and manage own needs.*

 Diagnostic Studies   Evidence Based Practice   Medications   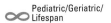 Pediatric/Geriatric/Lifespan

- Emphasize need for regular exercise program *to enhance circulation and promote general well-being.*[12]
- Refer to nutritionist for well-balanced, low-saturated-fat, low-cholesterol diet or other modifications as indicated *to promote weight loss and/or lower cholesterol levels.*
- Discuss care of dependent limbs and foot care as appropriate. *When circulation is impaired, changes in sensation place client at risk for development of lesions or ulcerations that are often slow to heal.*
- Discourage sitting or standing for long periods, wearing constrictive clothing, and crossing legs, *which can restrict circulation and lead to edema.*
- Provide education about relationship between smoking and peripheral vascular circulation, as indicated. *Smoking contributes to development and progression of PVD and is associated with higher rate of amputation in presence of Buerger's disease.*[10,17]
- Educate client/significant other (SO) in reportable symptoms, including any changes in pain level, difficulty walking, and nonhealing wounds, *to provide opportunity for timely evaluation and intervention.*
- Emphasize need for regular medical and laboratory follow-up *to evaluate disease progression and response to therapies, including medications for desired and untoward effects.*
- Review medication regimen with client/SO. *Client may be on various drugs (e.g., antiplatelet agents, blood viscosity–reducing agents, vasodilators, anticoagulants, cholesterol-lowering agents) for treatment of the particular vascular disorder. Any of these medications have harmful side effects and require client teaching and medical monitoring.*[5,14–16]
- Emphasize importance of avoiding use of aspirin, some over-the-counter drugs and supplements, and alcohol when taking anticoagulants.
- Refer to community resources such as smoking-cessation assistance, weight control program, and exercise group *to provide support for lifestyle changes.*

DOCUMENTATION FOCUS

Assessment/Reassessment
- Individual findings, noting nature, extent, and duration of problem, effect on independence and lifestyle.
- Characteristics of pain, precipitators, and what relieves pain.
- Pulses and blood pressure, including above and below suspected lesion as appropriate.

Planning
- Plan of care and who is involved in planning.
- Teaching plan.

Implementation/Evaluation
- Response to interventions/teaching, actions performed.
- Attainment or progress toward desired outcome(s).
- Modifications to plan of care.

Discharge Planning
- Long-term needs and who is responsible for actions to be taken.
- Available resources, specific referrals made.

References

1. Stockman, J. (2008). In too deep: Understanding deep vein thrombosis. *Nursing Made Incredibly Easy!*, 6(2), 29–38.
2. Sieggreen, M. (2008). Understanding critical limb ischemia. *Nursing*, 38(10), 50–55.
3. Stephens, E. (Updated 2017). Peripheral vascular disease. Retrieved May 2018 from http://emedicine.medscape.com/article/761556-overview.
4. Nieves, J., Capone-Swearer, D. (2006). The clot that changes lives. *Nurs 2006 Crit Care*, 1(3), 18–28.
5. American Heart Association. (Updated 2018). What is peripheral arterial disease? Retrieved Mary 2018 from http://www.heart.org/idc/groups/heart-public/@wcm/@hcm/documents/downloadable/ucm_300323.pdf.
6. Blach, D. A., Ignatavicius, D. D. (2006). Interventions for clients with vascular problems. In Ignatavicius, D. D., Workman, M. L. (eds). *Medical–Surgical Nursing: Critical Thinking for Collaborative Care.* 5th ed. St. Louis, MO: Elsevier Saunders.

 Acute Care   Collaborative   Community/Home Care   Cultural

7. Bartley, M. K. (2006). Keep venous thromboembolism at bay. *Nursing*, 36(10), 36–41.
8. Barclay, L. (2009). Hospital-supervised exercise may prevent need for surgery in patients with claudication. Retrieved May 2018 from hhttp://www.medscape.com/viewarticle/588053.
9. Sachdeva, A., Dalton, M., Amaragiri, S. V. (2010). Elastic compression stockings for prevention of deep vein thrombosis. *Cochrane Database Syst Rev*, 7.
10. Sieggreen, M. Y. (2006). Getting a leg up on managing venous ulcers. *Nursing Made Incredibly Easy!*, 4(6), 52–60.
11. Baldwin, K. M. (2006). Stroke: It's a knock-out punch. *Nursing Made Incredibly Easy!*, 4(2), 10–23.
12. Frost, K. L., Topp, R. (2006). A physical activity Rx for the hypertensive patient. *Nurse Pract*, 31(4), 29–37.
13. Moses, S. (Updated 2015). Unna's boot. Family practice notebook. Retrieved May 2018 from http://www.fpnotebook.com/surgery/Pharm/UnsBt.htm.
14. Calianno, C., Holton, S. J. (2007). Fighting the triple threat of lower extremity ulcers. *Nursing*, 37(3), 57–63.
15. Kehl-Pruett, W. (2006). Deep vein thrombosis in hospitalized patients: A review of evidence-based guidelines for prevention. *Dimens Crit Care Nurs*, 25(2), 53–59.
16. Wipke-Tevis, D. D., Sae-Sia, W. (2004). Caring for vascular leg ulcers. *Home Healthc Nurse*, 22(4), 237–247.
17. Johns Hopkins Vasculitis Center. (No date). Buerger's disease. Retrieved May 2018 from http://www.hopkinsvasculitis.org/types-vasculitis/buergers-disease/.
18. Patel, K., Chun, L. J. (Updated 2017). Deep venous thrombosis (DVT) clinical presentation. Retrieved May 2018 from https://emedicine.medscape.com/article/1911303-clinical.

risk for decreased cardiac Tissue Perfusion

Taxonomy II: Activity/Rest—Class 4 Cardiovascular/Pulmonary Responses (00200) [**Diagnostic Division:** Circulation], Approved 2008; Revised 2013, 2017

DEFINITION: Susceptible to a decrease in cardiac (coronary) circulation, which may compromise health.

RISK FACTORS
Insufficient knowledge of modifiable risk factors [e.g., smoking, sedentary lifestyle, obesity]
Substance misuse/abuse
At Risk Population: Family history of cardiovascular disease
Associated Condition: Coronary artery spasm; cardiovascular surgery; cardiac tamponade
Diabetes mellitus; hypertension
Hypovolemia; hypoxia/hypoxemia
Hyperlipidemia; increase in C-reactive protein
Pharmaceutical agent
Sample Clinical Applications: Angina, coronary artery disease, hypertension, congestive heart failure, diabetes, cardiac surgery, pericarditis, sepsis, anemia, hemorrhagic shock, cocaine use

DESIRED OUTCOMES/EVALUATION CRITERIA

Sample NOC linkages:
Tissue Perfusion: Cardiac: Adequacy of blood flow through the coronary vasculature to maintain heart function
Self-Management: Coronary Artery Disease: Personal actions to manage coronary artery disease, its treatment, and to prevent disease progression and complications

Client Will (Include Specific Time Frame)
• Demonstrate adequate coronary perfusion as individually appropriate (e.g., vital signs within client's normal range, free of chest pain or discomfort).
• Identify individual risk factors.
• Verbalize understanding of treatment regimen.
• Demonstrate behaviors or lifestyle changes to maintain or maximize circulation (e.g., cessation of smoking, relaxation techniques, exercise program, dietary plan).

(continues on page 908)

 Diagnostic Studies   Evidence Based Practice   Medications   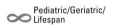 Pediatric/Geriatric/Lifespan

risk for decreased cardiac Tissue Perfusion (continued)

ACTIONS/INTERVENTIONS

Sample **NIC** linkages:

Cardiac Risk Management: Prevention of an acute episode of impaired cardiac function by minimizing contributing events and risk behaviors

Hemodynamic Regulation: Optimization of heart rate, preload, afterload, and contractility

NURSING PRIORITY NO. 1 To identify individual risk factors:

• Note presence of conditions such as heart failure, major trauma with blood loss, recent coronary artery bypass graft (CABG) surgery, use of intra-aortic balloon pump, chronic anemia, sepsis, etc. *Conditions such as these can affect systemic circulation, tissue oxygenation, and organ function.*[1,14]

• ∞ Note client's age and gender when assessing risk for coronary artery spasm or myocardial infarction. *Risk for heart disorders increases with age, and men are still considered at higher risk for myocardial infarction, and experience it earlier in life. Note: Although studies show that men have experienced a decline in coronary heart disease mortality in the last 2 decades, only 54% of women recognize that heart disease is their number one killer (based on 2010 data).*[3] *Studies continue to report the death rate from acute MI to be three times higher in men than in women until age 75.*[22] *And the American Heart Association (AHA) reported (2016) that "at older ages, women who have heart attacks are more likely than men are to die from them within a few weeks."*[2]

• Identify lifestyle issues such as obesity, smoking, high cholesterol, excessive alcohol intake, use of drugs such as cocaine, and physical inactivity *that can raise client's risk for coronary artery disease and impaired cardiac tissue perfusion.*[2]

• Determine presence of breathing problems, such as obstructive sleep apnea (OSA) with oxygen desaturation. *Can produce alveolar hypoventilation, respiratory acidosis, and hypoxia, which can result in cardiac dysrhythmias and cardiac dysfunction. Note: A recent study (2014) reported that "the strongest OSA-related predictor of cardiovascular events . . . was total sleep time spent with oxygen saturation below 90%, which increased the risk of a cardiovascular event or death by 50%."*[8]

• Determine if client is experiencing unusual long-term stress or may have underlying psychiatric disorder (e.g., anxiety or panic) *that may cause or exacerbate coronary artery disease and affect cardiac function.*[5]

• Review client's medications, noting current use of any vasoactive drugs such as amiodarone, dopamine, dobutamine, esmolol, lidocaine, nitroglycerin, and vasopressin. *These medications may be used in emergent situations or to manage blood pressure over time and can exert undesirable and potentially dangerous secondary effects in addition to their intended primary effects.*[9]

• Review diagnostic studies and lab tests (e.g., electrocardiogram; exercise tolerance tests, myocardial perfusion scan; echocardiogram, bubble echocardiogram; angiography, Doppler ultrasound, chest radiography; oxygen saturation, capnometry, or arterial blood gases; electrolytes, lipid profile; blood urea nitrogen/creatinine, cardiac enzymes) *to identify conditions requiring treatment, and response to therapies.*[7,10,11]

NURSING PRIORITY NO. 2 To determine changes in cardiac status:

• Investigate reports of chest pain, noting changes in characteristics of pain *to evaluate for potential myocardial ischemia or inadequate systemic oxygenation or perfusion of organs. Note: Chest pain is often difficult to diagnose due to variability in symptoms. Leading causes of chest pain (other than heart) include musculoskeletal, gastrointestinal, and pulmonary systems, as well as psychiatric disorders such as panic disorders.*[4–6]

 Acute Care   Collaborative   Community/ Home Care   Cultural

- Monitor vital signs, especially noting blood pressure changes, including hypertension or hypotension, *reflecting systemic vascular resistance problems that alter oxygen consumption and cardiac perfusion.*[1]
- Assess heart sounds and pulses for dysrhythmias. *Can be caused by inadequate myocardial or systemic tissue perfusion, electrolyte or acid-base imbalances.*[13]
- Assess for restlessness, fatigue, changes in level of consciousness; increased capillary refill time; diminished peripheral pulses; and pale, cool skin. *Signs and symptoms of inadequate systemic perfusion, which can cause or affect cardiac function.*[1]
- Inspect for pallor, mottling, cool and clammy skin, and diminished pulses. *Systemic vasoconstriction resulting from reduced cardiac output may be evidenced by poor skin or tissue perfusion and diminished pulses.*[13]
- Investigate reports of difficulty breathing; note respiratory rate outside of acceptable parameters, *which can be indicative of oxygen exchange problems with potential for cardiac dysfunction.*[7]

NURSING PRIORITY NO. 3   To maintain/maximize cardiac perfusion:

- Collaborate in treatment of underlying conditions such as hypovolemia, chronic obstructive pulmonary disease, diabetes, and chronic atrial fibrillation, *to correct or treat disorders that could influence cardiac perfusion or organ function.*
- Maintain hemodynamic stability when client is in postoperative phase of CABG surgery *to keep vital organs adequately perfused. Risk factors in this time frame include dysrhythmias, hypotension or hypertension, cardiac tamponade, and pulmonary dysfunction.*[12]
- Provide supplemental oxygen as indicated *to improve or maintain cardiac and systemic tissue perfusion.*
- Administer fluids and electrolytes as indicated *to maintain systemic circulation and optimal cardiac function.*
- Administer medications (e.g., antihypertensive agents, analgesics, antidysrhythmics, bronchodilators, fibrinolytic agents) *to treat underlying conditions, to prevent thromboembolic phenomena, and to maintain cardiac tissue perfusion and organ function.*[12,13,15]
- Collaborate with dietician or nutritionist to provide easily digestible diet sufficient in nutrients, low in cholesterol and fat, and high in complex carbohydrates *to provide energy and reduce substances harmful to coronary arteries.*[2,16]
- Provide periods of undisturbed rest and calming environment *to reduce myocardial workload.*

NURSING PRIORITY NO. 4   To promote heart health (Teaching/Discharge Considerations):

- Discuss the risk factors (e.g., family history, obesity, age, smoking, hypertension, diabetes, clotting disorders) and potential outcomes of atherosclerosis (e.g., systemic and cardiac disease conditions). *Information necessary for client to make informed decisions concerning risk factors and to commit to lifestyle changes necessary to prevent onset of complications or manage symptoms when condition present.*[2]
- Review difference between modifiable and nonmodifiable risk factors *to assist client/significant other (SO) in understanding those areas in which he/she can take action or make healthy choices*:
   Recommend maintenance of normal weight or weight loss if client is obese *to decrease risk associated with overweight and obesity.*[2]
  Review specific dietary concerns with client, such as reducing animal and dairy fats and increasing plant foods—fruits, vegetables, olive oil, and nuts.[16]
  Encourage smoking cessation, when indicated, offering information about stop-smoking aids and programs. *Smoking cessation is important in the medical management of many contributors to heart attack (e.g., vasoconstriction [which can reduce coronary perfusion], atherosclerosis, thrombosis, coronary artery spasm, and cardiac dysrhythmias).*[17]
  Encourage client to engage in regular exercise *to enhance circulation and promote general well-being.*[18]
   Review medications on regular basis *to manage those that affect cardiac function or those given to prevent blood pressure or thromboembolic problems.*

 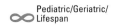

Discuss drug use where indicated (including cocaine, methamphetamines, alcohol) *to educate client regarding effect of drug on the heart. Note: Studies have found a substantial association between self-reported cocaine use and physician-diagnosed myocardial infarction. Another study indicates that when methamphetamine is used with alcohol, increased psychological and cardiac effects are observed.*[19–21]

Discuss coping and stress tolerance. Demonstrate and encourage use of relaxation or stress management techniques *to decrease tension level, thereby improving heart health.*

Encourage client in high-risk categories (e.g., strong family history, diabetic, prior history of cardiac event) to have regular medical examinations *to provide timely intervention, when needed.*

- Refer to educational or community resources, as indicated. *Client/SO may benefit from instruction and support provided by agencies to engage in healthier heart activities (e.g., weight loss, smoking cessation, exercise).*
- Instruct in blood pressure monitoring at home if indicated; advise purchase of home monitoring equipment; refer to community resources as indicated. *Facilitates management of hypertension, which is a major risk factor for damage to blood vessels or organ function.*[13]

DOCUMENTATION FOCUS

Assessment/Reassessment
- Individual findings, noting specific risk factors.
- Vital signs, cardiac rhythm, presence of dysrhythmias.

Planning
- Plan of care and who is involved in planning.
- Teaching plan.

Implementation/Evaluation
- Response to interventions, teaching, and actions performed.
- Attainment or progress toward desired outcome(s).
- Modifications to plan of care.

Discharge Planning
- Long-term needs and who is responsible for actions to be taken.
- Available resources, specific referrals made.

References

1. Breitenbach, J. E. (2007). Putting an end to perfusion confusion. *Nursing Made Incredibly Easy!*, 5(3), 50–60.
2. American Heart Association. (2016). Understand your risks to prevent a heart attack. Retrieved May 2018 from http://www.heart.org/HEARTORG/Conditions/HeartAttack/UnderstandYourRiskstoPreventaHeartAttack/Understand-Your-Risks-to-Prevent-a-Heart-Attack_UCM_002040_Article.jsp#.WurqWkxFzIU.
3. Centers for Disease Control and Prevention (CDC). (2017). Women and heart disease fact sheet. *CDC: Division for Heart Disease and Stroke Prevention.* Retrieved May 2018 from https://www.cdc.gov/dhdsp/data_statistics/fact_sheets/fs_women_heart.htm.
4. Fagring, A. J., et al. (2005). Description of unexplained chest pain and its influence on daily life in men and women. *Eur J Cardiovasc Nurs*, (4), 337–344.
5. Katerndahl, D. (2004). Panic and plaques: Panic disorder and coronary artery disease in patients with chest pain. *J Am Board Fam Pract*, 17(2), 114–126.
6. Cayley, W. E. (2005). Diagnosing the cause of chest pain. *J Am Fam Physician*, 72(10), 2012–2021.
7. Schulman, C. (2002). End points of resuscitation: Choosing the right parameters to monitor. *Dimens Crit Care Nurs*, 21(1), 2–10.
8. Kendzesrka, T., et al. (2014). Obstructive sleep apnea and risk of cardiovascular events and all-cause mortality: A decade-long historical cohort study. *PLoS Med*, 11(2), e1001599.
9. Miller, J. (2007). Keeping your patient hemodynamically stable. *Nursing*, 37(5), 36–41.
10. Morici, B. (2014). Diagnosis and management of acute pulmonary embolism. *JAAPA*, 27(4), 18–22.
11. Goldrich, G. (2006). Understanding the 12-lead ECG, part I. *Nursing*, 36(11), 36–41.
12. Mullen-Fortino, M., O'Brien, N. (2008). Caring for the patient after coronary artery bypass graft. *Nursing*, 38(3), 46–52.
13. Bartley, M. K. (2006). Keep venous thromboembolism at bay. *Nursing*, 10(3), 36–41.
14. Eberhardt, R. T., Raffetto, J. D. (2005). Chronic venous insufficiency. *Circulation*, 111(18), 2398–2409.
15. Baldwin, K. M. (2006). Stroke: It's a knock-out punch. *Nursing Made Incredibly Easy!*, 4(2), 10–23.

 Acute Care   Collaborative   Community/Home Care   Cultural

16. Sacks, F. M., Katan, M. (2002). Randomized clinical trials on the effects of dietary fat and carbohydrate on plasma proteins and cardiovascular disease. *Am J Med*, Suppl 9B, 13–24.
17. Centers for Disease Control and Prevention (CDC). (Updated 2018). Smoking and tobacco use: Heart disease and stroke. Retrieved May 2018 from http://www.cdc.gov/tobacco/basic_information/health_effects/heart_disease/.
18. Frost, K. L., Topp, R. (2006). A physical activity Rx for the hypertensive patient. *Nurs Pract*, 31(4), 29–37.
19. Aslibekyan, S., Levitan, E. B., Mittleman, M. A. (2008). Prevalent cocaine use and myocardial infarction. *Am J Cardiol*, 102(8), 966–969.
20. Wright, M. N. J., et al. (2007). Cocaine and thrombosis: A narrative systematic review of clinical and in-vivo studies. *Subst Abuse Treat Prevent Policy*, 2:27.
21. Richards, J. R., Derlet, R. W., Albertson, T. E. (Updated 2017). Methamphetamine toxicity. Retrieved May 2018 from http://emedicine.medscape.com/article/820918-overview.
22. Lloyd-Jones, D., et al. (2010). Executive summary: heart disease and stroke statistics–2010 update: A report from the American Heart Association. *Circulation*, 121(7), 948–954.

risk for ineffective cerebral Tissue Perfusion

Taxonomy II: Activity/Rest—Class 4 Cardiovascular/Pulmonary Responses (00201) [**Diagnostic Division:** Circulation], Approved 2008; Revised 2013, 2018

DEFINITION: Susceptible to a decrease in cerebral tissue circulation, which may compromise health.

RISK FACTORS

Substance misuse [abuse]

At Risk Population: Recent myocardial infarction; [cerebral vascular accident (CVA)/stroke]

Associated Conditions: Abnormal partial thromboplastin time (PTT); abnormal prothrombin time (PT); coagulopathy; disseminated intravascular coagulopathy; hypercholesterolemia

Akinetic left ventricular wall segment; dilated cardiomyopathy; atrial myxoma; infective endocarditis; aortic atherosclerosis

Arterial dissection; carotid stenosis; cerebral aneurysm; brain injury, brain neoplasm; embolism

Hypertension

Pharmaceutical agent; treatment regimen

Sample Clinical Applications: Traumatic brain injury, stroke; atherosclerosis, hypertension, atrial fibrillation, mitral valve stenosis or replacement, transient ischemic attack, cerebral vascular accident (CVA)/stroke; sickle cell anemia, cocaine use

DESIRED OUTCOMES/EVALUATION CRITERIA

Sample NOC linkages:

Tissue Perfusion: Cerebral: Adequacy of blood flow through the cerebral vasculature to maintain brain function

Risk Control: Personal actions to understand, prevent, eliminate, or reduce modifiable health threats

Client Will (Include Specific Time Frame)

- Display neurological signs within client's normal range.
- Verbalize understanding of condition, therapy regimen, side effects of medications, and when to contact healthcare provider.
- Demonstrate behaviors or lifestyle changes to improve circulation (e.g., cessation of smoking, relaxation techniques, exercise program, dietary plan).

(continues on page 912)

 Diagnostic Studies   Evidence Based Practice   Medications 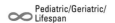 Pediatric/Geriatric/Lifespan

risk for ineffective cerebral Tissue Perfusion (continued)

ACTIONS/INTERVENTIONS

Sample **NIC** linkages:

Cerebral Perfusion Promotion: Promotion of adequate perfusion and limitation of complications for a patient experiencing or at risk for inadequate cerebral perfusion

Surveillance: Purposeful and ongoing acquisition, interpretation, and synthesis of patient data for clinical decision making

Cerebral Edema Management: Limitation of secondary cerebral injury resulting from swelling of brain tissue

NURSING PRIORITY NO. 1   To assess causative/contributing factors:

- Determine history of conditions associated with thrombus or emboli such as stroke, complicated pregnancy, sickle cell disease, fractures (especially long bones or pelvis) *to identify client at higher risk for decreased cerebral perfusion related to bleeding and/or coagulation problems.*
- Note current situation or presence of conditions (e.g., congestive heart failure, major trauma, sepsis, hypertension) *that can affect all body systems and systemic circulation and perfusion.*
- Ascertain potential for presence of acute neurological conditions, such as traumatic brain injury, tumors, hemorrhage, anoxic brain injury associated with cardiac arrest, and toxic or viral encephalopathies. *These conditions alter the relationship between intracranial volume and pressure, potentially increasing intracranial pressure and decreasing cerebral perfusion.*[1]
- Investigate client reports of headache, particularly when accompanied by loss of coordination, confusion, visual disturbances, difficulty understanding or using language, or a range of progressive neurological deficits. *These symptoms may accompany cerebral perfusion deficits associated with conditions such as stroke, transient ischemic attack, brain trauma, or cerebral arteriovenous malformations.*[2,5]
- Ascertain if client has history of cardiac problems (e.g., recent myocardial infarction, heart failure, heart valve dysfunction or replacement, chronic atrial fibrillation), *which can impair systemic and cerebral blood flow or cause thromboembolic events to brain.*[3]
- Determine presence of cardiac dysrhythmias (e.g., chronic atrial fibrillation, bradycardia). *Can be caused by inadequate myocardial perfusion, electrolyte imbalances, or be associated with brain injury (e.g., bradycardia can accompany traumatic injury; stroke can be precipitated by dysrhythmias).*[3]
- Assess level of consciousness, mental status, speech, and behavior. *Clinical symptoms of decreased cerebral perfusion include fluctuations in consciousness and cognitive functions.*[11]
- Evaluate blood pressure. *Chronic or severe acute hypertension can precipitate cerebrovascular spasm and stroke. Low blood pressure or severe hypotension causes inadequate perfusion of brain, with adverse changes in consciousness/mentation.*[4]
- Verify proper use of antihypertensive medications. *Individuals may stop medication because of lack of symptoms, presence of undesired side effects, and/or cost of drug, potentiating risk of stroke.*
- Review medication regimen noting use of anticoagulants or antiplatelet agents and other drugs *that could cause intracranial bleeding.*
- Review pulse oximetry or arterial blood gases, noting oxygenation level and saturation. *Hypoxia (PaO_2 level less than 60 mg Hg, or O_2 saturation level less than 90%) is associated with reduced cerebral perfusion and increased morbidity and mortality from severe brain injury.*[3,4]
- Review lab studies (e.g., coagulation profiles, complete blood count, electrolytes, lipids, B-type natriuretic peptide) *to identify disorders that increase risk of clotting or bleeding or other conditions contributing to causing decreased cerebral perfusion.*

 Acute Care   Collaborative   Community/ Home Care   Cultural

- Review results of diagnostic studies (e.g., ultrasound or other imaging scans such as echocardiography, computed tomography [CT], or magnetic resonance angiography [MRA]; diffusion and perfusion magnetic resonance imaging) *to determine location and severity of disorder that can cause or exacerbate cerebral perfusion problems.*[10]

NURSING PRIORITY NO. 2   To maximize tissue perfusion:

- Collaborate in treatment of underlying conditions (e.g., carotid stent placement, medical or surgical reperfusion procedures, treatment of infections) as indicated *to improve systemic perfusion and organ function.*[1,16]
- Restore or maintain fluid balance *to maximize cardiac output and prevent decreased cerebral perfusion associated with hypovolemia.*[1,2]
- Assist with treatment/management of cardiac dysrhythmias (such as with medication administration, pacemaker insertion). *Reduces risk of diminished cerebral perfusion due to blood clots or low cardiac output.*[1,2]
- Restrict fluids and administer diuretics as indicated *to prevent diminished cerebral perfusion associated with hypertension, and cerebral edema.*[1,2]
- Keep head in midline position, when indicated, *to promote venous drainage, preventing or reducing risk of elevated intracranial pressure.*[1,2]
- Maintain optimal head of bed (HOB) placement (e.g., 0, 15, 30 degrees). *Various studies demonstrate different perfusion responses to HOB placement but indicate that cerebral perfusion is reduced when HOB elevated greater than 30 degrees. Note: A recent study showed that routine nursing of patients with severe head injury at 30 degrees of head elevation within 24 hr after trauma leads to a consistent reduction of intracranial pressure (statistically significant) and an improvement in cerebral perfusion (although not statistically significant) without concomitant deleterious changes in cerebral oxygenation.*[6,12]
- Control fever, monitor hypothermia therapy, and provide supplemental oxygen, as indicated, *to decrease cerebral metabolism and cerebral edema.*[1,2]
- Administer vasoactive medications, as indicated, *to increase cardiac output and/or adequate mean arterial pressure to maintain cerebral perfusion.*[1,2]
- Administer other medications as indicated. *Cortiocosteroids may be used to reduce cerebral edema, antihypertensives may be used to manage high blood pressure, and anticoagulants may be used to prevent cerebral embolus.*[1,2]
- Prepare client for surgery as indicated (e.g., carotid endarterectomy, evacuation of hematoma or space-occupying lesion; thrombectomy following stroke) *to improve cerebral perfusion.*[1,16]
- Refer to NDs decreased Cardiac Output and decreased Intracranial Adaptive Capacity for additional interventions.

NURSING PRIORITY NO. 3   To promote optimal perfusion (Teaching/Discharge Considerations):

- Review modifiable risk factors, as indicated: *Information can help client make informed choices about remedial actions to reduce risk factors and to commit to lifestyle changes as appropriate.*[2,7]

  Uncontrolled hypertension: *Incidence of stroke increases with systolic blood pressure greater than 140/90 mmHg. Client at risk can learn to self-monitor blood pressure, take prescribed antihypertensive agents consistently, and identify symptoms to report to physician.*

  Smoking: *Smoking causes vasoconstriction and increased arterial wall stiffness, increasing fibrinogen levels and platelet aggregation, and abnormal blood lipids. Numerous recent studies have confirmed a relationship between active and passive smoking, with the maximum risk period being middle life. Smoking cessation immediately lowers risk of stroke.*[8] *Note: A report of a clinical trial (2012) reported that "50% of stroke patients in this trial who claimed to be motivated to quit at the time of discharge [after stroke] relapsed in three weeks. If a patient resumed smoking within 10 days of discharge, their risk of death in the following year was five times greater than those who managed to abstain."*[15]

  Obesity and unhealthy diet: *Abdominal obesity has been associated with increased risk for ischemic stroke.*[8] *Diet high in cholesterol contributes to development of cerebral atherosclerosis. High intake of sodium can contribute to hypertension.*

 Diagnostic Studies   Evidence Based Practice   Medications   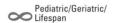 Pediatric/Geriatric/Lifespan

Physical inactivity: *Contributes to obesity and hypertension.*

Excessive alcohol intake: *Linked to higher risk of stroke because it can cause hypertension, which is a major risk factor. Note: Alcohol intake consumption at higher amounts is associated with increased risk of atrial fibrillation, ventricular fibrillation, dilated cardiomyopathy, hypertension, dyslipidemia, and a systemic anticoagulant effect, all of which increase the risk of stroke.*[7,14]

Illicit drug use: *Can significantly boost the risk of a deadly or debilitating stroke. Note: Many illicit drugs have been linked to increased stroke risk (i.e., cocaine, amphetamines, opiates, phencyclidine, marijuana).*[9]

- Discuss impact of unmodifiable risk factors such as family history, age, and race. *Understanding effects and interrelationship of all risk factors may encourage client to address what can be changed to improve general well-being and reduce individual risk.*
- Assist client to incorporate disease management into activities of daily living, including regular exercise. *Promotes independence and enhances self-concept regarding ability to deal with change and manage own needs.*
- Emphasize necessity of routine follow-up and laboratory monitoring as indicated. *Important for effective disease management and possible changes in therapeutic regimen.*
- Refer to educational or community resources as indicated. *Client/SO may benefit from instruction and support provided by agencies to engage in healthy activities (e.g., weight loss, smoking cessation, exercise).*

DOCUMENTATION FOCUS

Assessment/Reassessment
- Individual findings, noting specific risk factors.
- Vital signs, blood pressure, cardiac rhythm.
- Medication regimen.
- Diagnostic studies, laboratory results.

Planning
- Plan of care and who is involved in planning.
- Teaching plan.

Implementation/Evaluation
- Response to interventions, teaching, and actions performed.
- Attainment or progress toward desired outcome(s).
- Modifications to plan of care.

Discharge Planning
- Long-term needs and who is responsible for actions to be taken.
- Available resources, specific referrals made.

References

1. Editorial Staff. (2007). Patho puzzler: Don't let your head explode over increased ICP. *Nursing Made Incredibly Easy!*, 5(2), 21–25.
2. Nieves, J., Capone-Swearer, D. (2006). The clot that changes lives. *Nurs 2006 Crit Care*, 1(3), 18–28.
3. Dumitru, I., Baker, M. M. (2018). Heart Failure (various pages). Retrieved May 2018 from https://emedicine.medscape.com/article/163062-overview.
4. Hemphill, J. C., et al. (2015). Guidelines for the management of spontaneous intracerebral hemorrhage: A guideline for healthcare professionals from the American Heart Association/American Stroke Association (online version). Retrieved May 2018 from http://stroke.ahajournals.org/content/early/2015/05/28/STR.0000000000000069.
5. Vacca, V. M., Violett, S. (2008). Teamwork integral to treating cerebral arteriovenous malformation. *Nursing*, 3(3), 20–27.
6. McIlvoy, L. H., Meyer, K. (2008). Cerebral perfusion promotion. In Ackley, B. J., et al. (eds) *Evidence-Based Nursing Care Guidelines: Medical-Surgical Interventions*. St. Louis, MO: Mosby Elsevier.
7. National Stroke Association. (Updated 2018). Lifestyle risk factors (various monographs regarding controllable risk factors). Retrieved May 2018 from http://www.stroke.org/understand-stroke/preventing-stroke/lifestyle-risk-factors.
8. Roger, V. L., Go, A. S., Lloyd-Jones, D. M. (2011). Heart disease and stroke statistics—2011 update: A report from the American Heart Association. *Circulation*, 123, e18–e209.

 Acute Care   Collaborative   Community/Home Care   Cultural

9. de los Rios, F., et al. (2014). Trends in substance abuse preceding stroke among young adults: A population-based study. Retrieved May 2018 from http://stroke.ahajournals.org/content/43/12/3179.long.

10. Kochan, J. P., Kanamalla, U. S. (Updated 2016). Cerebral revascularization imaging. Retrieved May 2018 from http://emedicine.medscape.com/article/420186-overview.

11. Sakowitz, O., Unterberg, A. (2006). Detecting and treating microvascular ischemia after subarachnoid hemorrhage. *Curr Opin Crit Car*, 12(2), 103–111.

12. Ng, I. F., Lim, J. B., Wong, H. B. (2004). Effects of head posture on cerebral hemodynamics: Its influences on intracranial pressure, cerebral perfusion pressure, and cerebral oxygenation. *Neurosurgery*, 54(3), 593–599.

13. Girot, M. (2009). Smoking and stroke. *Presse Med*, 38(7–8), 1120–1125.

14. Di Minno, M. N., et al. (2011). Alcohol dosing and the heart: Updating clinical evidence. *Semin Thromb Hemost*, 37(8), 875–884.

15. Walton-Shirley, M. (2012). Smoking: Worse than bad after stroke. Retrieved May 2018 from https://www.medscape.com/viewarticle/801900.

16. Powers, W. J., et al. (2018). 2018 Guidelines for the early management of patients with acute ischemic stroke: A guideline for healthcare professionals. *The American Heart Association/American Stroke Association*. Retrieved May 2018 from http://www.acc.org/latest-in-cardiology/ten-points-to-remember/2018/01/29/12/45/2018-guidelines-for-the-early-management-of-stroke.

risk for ineffective peripheral Tissue Perfusion

Taxonomy II: Activity/Rest—Class 4 Cardiovascular/Pulmonary Responses (00228) [**Diagnostic Division:** Circulation], Approved 2010; Revised 2013, 2017

DEFINITION: Susceptible to a decrease in blood circulation to the periphery, which may compromise health.

RISK FACTORS
Sedentary lifestyle; smoking
Endovascular procedure; trauma
Excessive sodium intake
Insufficient knowledge of disease process, risk factors, or aggravating factors (e.g., smoking, sedentary lifestyle, trauma, obesity, salt intake, immobility)
Associated Condition: Diabetes mellitus; hypertension
Endovascular procedure; trauma
Sample Clinical Applications: Atherosclerosis, coronary artery disease, Raynaud's disease, peripheral vascular disease, Buerger's disease, thrombophlebitis, diabetes mellitus, sickle cell anemia

DESIRED OUTCOMES/EVALUATION CRITERIA

Sample NOC linkages:
Tissue Perfusion; Peripheral: Adequacy of blood flow through the small vessels of the extremities to maintain tissue perfusion
Knowledge: Disease Process: Extent of understanding conveyed about a specific disease process and prevention of complications

Client Will (Include Specific Time Frame)
• Demonstrate adequate perfusion as individually appropriate (e.g., peripheral pulses present and strong, absence of edema, free of pain or discomfort).
• Verbalize understanding of risk factors and when to contact healthcare provider.
• Demonstrate behaviors or lifestyle changes to improve circulation (e.g., engage in regular exercise, cessation of smoking, weight reduction, disease management).

(continues on page 916)

 Diagnostic Studies   Evidence Based Practice   Medications   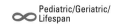 Pediatric/Geriatric/Lifespan

risk for ineffective peripheral Tissue Perfusion (continued)

Sample NIC linkages:

Circulatory Care: Arterial Insufficiency: Promotion of arterial circulation

Circulatory Care: Venous Insufficiency: Promotion of venous circulation

Teaching: Disease Process: Assisting the patient to understand information related to a specific disease process

NURSING PRIORITY NO. 1   To identify causative/precipitating factors related to risk:

- Note current situation or presence of conditions that can affect perfusion to all body systems (e.g., client admitted for endovascular procedure such as angiography or placement of stent, history or presence of congestive heart failure, lung disorders, major trauma, septic or hypovolemic shock, coagulopathies, sickle cell anemia) *affecting systemic circulation and perfusion.*
- Determine history of conditions associated with thrombus or emboli (e.g., problems with coronary or cerebral circulation, stroke; high-velocity trauma with fractures, abdominal or orthopedic surgery, long periods of immobility; inflammatory diseases; chronic lung disease; diabetes with coexisting peripheral vascular disease (PVD); estrogen therapy; cancer and cancer therapies; presence of central venous catheters) *to identify client at higher risk for venous stasis, vessel wall injury, and hypercoagulability.*[1-4]
- Identify presence of high-risk factors or conditions (e.g., smoking, uncontrolled hypertension, obesity, pregnancy, pelvic tumor, paralysis, hypercholesterolemia, varicose veins, arthritis, sepsis). *Places client at greater risk for developing PVD (including arterial blockage and chronic venous insufficiency) with associated complications.*[3,5,6]

NURSING PRIORITY NO. 2   To assess for and reduce risk of perfusion complications:

- Evaluate reports of extremity pain promptly, noting any associated symptoms (e.g., cramping or heaviness, discomfort with walking, progressive temperature or color changes, paresthesia) *to help isolate and differentiate problems.*
- Note presence and location of restrictive pressure dressings, circular wraps, cast or traction device *that may impede circulation to limb.*
- Assess skin color and temperature in all extremities *for changes that might indicate circulation problem.*
- Compare skin temperature and color with other limb *if developing problem is suspected (e.g., edema, redness, swelling in calf of one leg is associated with localized thrombophlebitis).*[1,3,7]
- Palpate arterial pulses—bilateral radial, femoral, popliteal, dorsalis pedis, and posterior tibial—comparing equality as well as intensity (e.g., bounding, normal, diminished, absent). *Assesses distribution and quality of blood flow.*[2]
- Inspect lower extremities for skin texture (e.g., atrophic; shiny appearance; lack of hair; dry, scaly, reddened skin) and skin breaks or ulcerations *that often accompany diminished peripheral circulation.*[3,5,8]
- Note client's nutritional and fluid status. *Protein-energy malnutrition and weight loss make ischemic tissues more prone to breakdown. Dehydration reduces blood volume and compromises peripheral circulation.*[3,5,8]
- Review lab studies such as lipid profile, coagulation studies, hemoglobin/hematocrit, renal/cardiac function tests, inflammatory markers (e.g., D dimer, C-reactive protein) *to determine potential for circulatory impairment.*

NURSING PRIORITY NO. 3   To maximize tissue perfusion or reduce risk of perfusion complications:

- Collaborate in treatment of underlying conditions, such as diabetes, hypertension, cardiopulmonary conditions, blood disorders, traumatic injury, hypovolemia, and hypoxemia *to maximize systemic circulation and organ perfusion.*

 Acute Care   Collaborative   Community/ Home Care   Cultural

- Administer fluids, electrolytes, nutrients, and oxygen as indicated *to promote optimal blood flow and organ and peripheral tissue perfusion and function.*
- Provide interventions to promote peripheral circulation and limit complications:[1,2,4,5,9]

  Encourage early ambulation when possible. *Enhances venous return.*

  Recommend or provide foot and ankle exercises when client unable to ambulate freely *to reduce venous pooling and increase venous return.*

  Provide pressure-relieving/reducing devices for immobilized client (e.g., air mattress, gel or foam padding, bed or foot cradle) *to reduce excessive tissue pressure that could lead to skin breakdown.*

  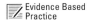 Apply intermittent compression devices or graduated compression stockings to lower extremities *to limit venous stasis, improve venous return, and reduce risk of deep vein thrombosis or tissue ulceration in client who is limited in activity or otherwise at risk.*[4,10,11]

  Assist with or cue client to change position at timed intervals rather than using presence of pain as signal to change positions, *if sensation is/could be impaired.*

  Elevate the legs when sitting, but avoid sharp angulation of the hips or knees *to enhance venous return and minimize edema formation.*

  Discuss/monitor use of heat or cold, such as hot water bottle, heating pad, or ice pack. *Reduces risk of dermal injury if client has condition associated with decreased sensation or neuropathy.*
- 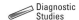 Refer to dietitian or nutritionist to discuss dietary needs such as a well-balanced, low-saturated-fat, low-cholesterol diet or other modifications as indicated *to promote weight loss and/or lower cholesterol levels to improve tissue perfusion.*
- Refer to NDs ineffective peripheral Tissue Perfusion, risk for peripheral Neurovascular Dysfunction, risk for impaired Skin Integrity, impaired Tissue Integrity, and [disturbed Sensory Perception] for additional interventions as appropriate.

NURSING PRIORITY NO. 4 To promote and maintain optimal perfusion (Teaching/discharge Considerations):

- Discuss relevant risk factors (e.g., family history, obesity, age, smoking, hypertension, diabetes, clotting disorders) and potential outcomes of atherosclerosis (e.g., systemic and peripheral vascular disease conditions). *Information necessary for client to make informed choices about risk factors and commit to lifestyle changes as appropriate to prevent onset of complications or manage symptoms when condition is present.*[2,12]
- Identify necessary changes in lifestyle and assist client to incorporate disease management into activities of daily living. *Promotes independence and enhances self-concept regarding ability to deal with change and manage own needs.*
- Emphasize need for regular exercise program *to enhance circulation and promote general well-being.*[13]
- Discourage sitting or standing for long periods, wearing constrictive clothing and crossing legs, *which can restrict circulation and lead to edema.*
- Provide education about relationship between smoking and peripheral vascular circulation, as indicated. *Smoking contributes to development and progression of PVD.*[2,14]
- Educate client/significant other in reportable symptoms, including any changes in pain level, difficulty walking, and nonhealing wounds *to provide opportunity for timely evaluation and intervention.*
- Refer to community resources such as smoking-cessation assistance, weight control program, diabetic educator, and/or exercise group *to provide support for lifestyle changes.*

DOCUMENTATION FOCUS

Assessment/Reassessment
- Individual risk factors identified.
- Client concerns or difficulty making and following through with plan.

Planning
- Plan of care and who is involved in planning.
- Teaching plan.

Implementation/Evaluation
- Response to interventions, teaching, and actions performed.
- Attainment or progress toward outcomes.

Discharge Planning
- Referrals to other resources.
- Long term need and who is responsible for actions.

References

1. Stockman, J. (2008). In too deep: Understanding deep vein thrombosis. *Nursing Made Incredibly Easy!*, 6(2), 29–38.
2. Sieggreen, M. (2008). Understanding critical limb ischemia. *Nursing*, 38(10), 50–55.
3. Calianno, C., Holton, S. J. (2007). Fighting the triple threat of lower extremity ulcers. *Nursing*, 37(3), 57–63.
4. Kehl-Pruett, W. (2006). Deep vein thrombosis in hospitalized patients: A review of evidence-based guidelines for prevention. *Dimens Crit Care Nurs*, 25(2), 53–59.
5. StephensE.Peripheral vascular disease. (Updated 2017). Retrieved May 2018 from http://emedicine.medscape.com/article/761556-overview.
6. Nieves, J., Capone-Swearer, D. (2006). The clot that changes lives. *Nurs 2006 Crit Care*, 1(3), 18–28.
7. American Heart Association. (Updated 2018). What is peripheral arterial disease? Retrieved Mary 2018 from http://www.heart.org/idc/groups/heart-public/@wcm/@hcm/documents/downloadable/ucm_300323.pdf.
8. Sieggreen, M. Y. (2006). Getting a leg up on managing venous ulcers. *Nursing Made Incredibly Easy!*, 4(6), 52–60.
9. Barclay, L. (2009). Hospital-supervised exercise may prevent need for surgery in patients with claudication. Retrieved May 2018 from http://www.medscape.com/viewarticle/588053.
10. Sachdeva, A., et al. (2010). Elastic compression stockings for prevention of deep vein thrombosis. *Cochrane Database Syst Rev*, 7(7), CDOO1484.
11. Wipke-Tevis, D. D., Sae-Sia, W. (2004). Caring for vascular leg ulcers. *Home Healthc Nurse*, 22(4), 237–247.
12. Baldwin, K. M. (2006). Stroke: It's a knock-out punch. *Nursing Made Incredibly Easy!*, 4(2), 10–23.
13. Frost, K. L., Topp, R. (2006). A physical activity Rx for the hypertensive patient. *Nurse Pract*, 31(4), 29–37.
14. Johns Hopkins Vasculitis Center. (No date). Buerger's disease. Retrieved May 2018 from http://www.hopkinsvasculitis.org/types-vasculitis/buergers-disease/.

impaired Transfer Ability

Taxonomy II: Activity/Rest—Class 2 Activity/Exercise (00090) [**Diagnostic Division:** Activity/Rest], Approved 1998; Revised 2006, 2017

DEFINITION: Limitation of independent movement between two nearby surfaces.

RELATED FACTORS
Insufficient muscle strength; physical deconditioning
Pain
Obesity
Insufficient knowledge of transfer techniques
Environmental barrier [e.g., bed height, inadequate space, wheelchair type, treatment equipment, restraints]

DEFINING CHARACTERISTICS

Subjective or Objective
Impaired ability to transfer between bed and chair, bed and standing position; between chair and car, chair and floor, or chair and standing; on or off a toilet or commode; in or out of bathtub or shower; between uneven levels

 Acute Care Collaborative Community/Home Care Cultural

Associated Condition: Alteration in cognitive function
Impaired vision
Musculoskeletal, neuromuscular impairment
Note: Specify level of independence using a standardized functional scale—[refer to ND impaired physical Mobility for suggested functional level classification]
Sample Clinical Applications: Arthritis, fractures, amputation, neuromuscular diseases (e.g., multiple sclerosis [MS], amyotrophic lateral sclerosis [ALS], Guillain-Barré syndrome), paralysis, glaucoma, macular degeneration, dementias

DESIRED OUTCOMES/EVALUATION CRITERIA

Sample NOC linkages:
Transfer Performance: Ability to change body location independently with or without assistive device
Balance: Ability to maintain body equilibrium
Body Positioning: Self-Initiated: Personal actions to change own body position independently with or without assistive device

Client/Caregiver Will (Include Specific Time Frame)
• Verbalize understanding of situation and appropriate safety measures.
• Master techniques of transfer successfully.
• Make desired transfer safely.

ACTIONS/INTERVENTIONS

Sample NIC linkages:
Self-Care Assistance: Transfer: Assisting a patient with limitation of independent movement to learn to change body location
Body Mechanics Promotion: Facilitating the use of posture and movement in daily activities to prevent fatigue and musculoskeletal strain or injury
Exercise Promotion: Strength Training: Facilitating regular resistive muscle training to maintain or increase muscle strength

NURSING PRIORITY NO. 1 To assess causative/contributing factors:

• Determine presence of conditions that contribute to transfer problems. *Neuromuscular and musculoskeletal problems (such as MS, fractures with splints or casts, back injuries, knee/hip replacement surgery, amputation, quadriplegia or paraplegia, contractures or spastic muscles); agedness (diminished faculties; multiple medications; painful conditions; decreased balance, muscle mass, tone, or strength), and effects of dementias, brain injury, etc., can seriously impact balance and physical and psychological well-being.*[3]
• Evaluate perceptual and cognitive impairments and ability to follow directions. *Plan of care and choice of interventions is dependent upon nature of condition—acute, chronic, or progressive; for example, client with severe brain injury may have permanent limitations because of impaired cognition affecting memory, judgment, problem-solving, and motor coordination, requiring more intensive inpatient and long-term care.*
• Note factors complicating current situation. *Recent surgery or traction apparatus, debilitating illness or weakness, and mechanical ventilation or multiple IV/indwelling tubings can restrict movement.*
• Review medication regimen and schedule *to determine possible side effects or drug interactions impairing balance and/or muscle tone.*

Diagnostic Studies   Evidence Based Practice   Medications   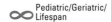Pediatric/Geriatric/ Lifespan

NURSING PRIORITY NO. 2   To assess functional ability:

- Perform the "Timed Up and Go" (TUG) test, as indicated, *to assess client's basic ability to transfer and ambulate safely, and risks of falling. In this test, the client is asked to get up from a seated position in a chair, stand still momentarily, walk forward 10 feet, turn around, walk back to the chair, turn, and sit down. Factors assessed include sitting balance, ability to transfer from sitting to standing and back to sitting, the pace and stability of ambulation, and the ability to turn without staggering. If the client is not safe with ambulation, assistance may also be required with transfers.*[1,7] *Note: Client may perform this test adequately and still have difficulty with some transfers, such as in or out of a car or bathtub or from floor to chair.*
- Determine degree of impairment using a 0–4 scale, noting muscle strength and tone, joint mobility, cardiovascular status, balance, and endurance. *Identifies strengths and deficits (e.g., ability to ambulate with assistive devices or problems with balance, failure to attend to one side, inability to bear weight [client is non-weight-bearing or partial weight-bearing]) and may provide information regarding potential for recovery.*[3,8]
- Observe movement when client is unaware of observations *to note any incongruence with reported abilities.*
- Note emotional and behavioral responses of client/significant other to problems of immobility. *Restrictions or limitations imposed by immobility can cause physical, social, emotional, and financial difficulties for everyone.*

NURSING PRIORITY NO. 3   To promote optimal level of movement:

- Assist with treatment of underlying condition causing dysfunction. *Treatment of condition (e.g., surgery for hip replacement, therapy for unilateral neglect following stroke) can alleviate or improve difficulties with transfer activity.*
- Consult with physical and occupational therapists or rehabilitation team *to develop general and specific muscle strengthening and range-of-motion exercises and transfer training and techniques, as well as recommendations and provision of balance, gait, and mobility aids or adjunctive devices.*[1]
- Position devices (e.g., call light, bed-positioning switch) in easy reach on the bed or chair. *Facilitates transfer and allows client to obtain assistance for transfer as needed.*
- Use appropriate number of people to assist with transfers and correct equipment (e.g., mechanical lift/sling, gait belt, sitting or standing disk pivot) *to safely transfer the client in a particular situation (e.g., chair to bed, chair to car, in or out of shower or tub).*[4–6,8]
- Demonstrate and assist with use of side rails or stand pole, overhead trapeze, and transfer or sit-to-stand hoist; specialty slings; and/or cane, walker, wheelchair, or crutches, as necessary, *to protect client or care providers from injury during transfers and movements.*[4,5,8]
- Provide instruction and reinforce information for client and caregivers regarding body and equipment positioning *to improve or maintain balance during transfers.*
- Monitor body alignment, posture, and balance and encourage wide base of support *when standing to transfer.*
- Use full-length mirror, as needed, *to facilitate client's view of own postural alignment.*

NURSING PRIORITY NO. 4   To maintain safety (Teaching/Discharge Considerations):

- Instruct client/caregiver in appropriate safety measures. *Actions (e.g., proper use of transfer board; locking wheels on bed or chair; correct placement of equipment for optimal body mechanics of client and caregivers(s); use of gait belt, supportive nonslip footwear; good lighting; clearing floor of clutter) are important to facilitating transfers and reducing the possibility of fall and subsequent injury to client and caregiver.*[2]
- Discuss need for and sources of care or supervision. *Home-care agency, before- and after-school programs, senior day care, personal companions, etc., may be required to assist with or monitor activity.*
- Refer to appropriate community resources *for evaluation and modification of environment (e.g., roll-in-shower or tub, correction of uneven floor surfaces and steps, installation of ramps, use of standing tables or lifts).*
- Refer also to NDs impaired bed/physical/wheelchair Mobility, Unilateral Neglect, risk for Falls, impaired Sitting; impaired Standing; impaired Walking for additional interventions.

 Acute Care   Collaborative   Community/ Home Care   Cultural

DOCUMENTATION FOCUS

Assessment/Reassessment
- Individual findings, including level of function and ability to participate in desired transfers.
- Mobility aides and transfer devices used.

Planning
- Plan of care and who is involved in the planning.
- Teaching plan.

Implementation/Evaluation
- Responses to interventions, teaching, and actions performed.
- Attainment or progress toward desired outcome(s).
- Modifications to plan of care.

Discharge Planning
- Discharge and long-term needs, noting who is responsible for each action to be taken.
- Specific referrals made.
- Sources of and maintenance for assistive devices.

References

1. Cruise, C. M., Koval, K. J. (1998). Rehabilitation of the elderly. *Arch Am Acad Orthop Surg*, 2(1), 103–107.
2. Patient safety during transfers. (2000). *Policy/Operations Manual*. Galveston, TX: UTMB Department of Rehabilitation Services.
3. Kourouche, S., et al. (2011). Identifying risk and raising awareness in older person trauma: A trauma center initiative. *J Trauma Nurs*, 18(3), 163–170.
4. Parsons, K. S., Galinsky, T. L., Waters, T. (2006). Suggestions for preventing musculoskeletal disorders in home healthcare workers, Part 1: Lift and transfer assistance for partially weight-bearing home care patients. *Home Healthc Nurse*, 24(3), 158–164.
5. Parsons, K. S., Galinsky, T. L., Waters, T. (2006). Suggestions for preventing musculoskeletal disorders in home healthcare workers, Part 2: Lift and transfer assistance for non-weight-bearing home care patients. *Home Healthc Nurse*, 24(4), 227–233.
6. Patterson, M., et al. (2006). Safe vertical transfer of patient with extremity cast or splint. *Orthop Nurs*, 28(2 Suppl), S18–S23.
7. Zasadazska, E., et al. (2015). Assessment of the risk of falling with the use of timed up and go test in the elderly with lower extremity osteoarthritis. *Clin Interv Aging*, 10, 1289–1298.
8. Venema, D. M., Hassel, J., Jones, K. J. (2013). Best practices in safe transfers and mobility to decrease fall risk. Retrieved May 2018 from https://www.unmc.edu/patient-safety/_documents/safe-transfers-mobility-handout.pdf.

---

risk for physical Trauma

Taxonomy II: Safety/Protection—Class 2 Physical Injury (00038) **[Diagnostic Division:** Safety**]**, Submitted 1980; Revised 2013, 2017

DEFINITION: Susceptible to physical injury of sudden onset and severity, which requires immediate attention.

RISK FACTORS
Internal
Emotional disturbance
Impaired balance; weakness; insufficient vision
Insufficient knowledge of safety precautions

(continues on page 922)

 Diagnostic Studies   Evidence Based Practice   Medications 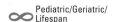 Pediatric/Geriatric/Lifespan

risk for Physical Trauma (continued)

External:

Absent or dysfunctional call-for-aid device; bed in high position; struggling with restraints

Absence of stairway gate or window guard; inadequate stair rails; slippery floor; insufficient anti-slip material in bathroom; use or throw rugs; obstructed passageway; insufficient lighting; unstable chair or ladder

Access to weapon; high crime neighborhood

Insufficient protection from heat source; bathing in very hot water; pot handle facing front of stove; use of cracked dishware; flammable object; wearing loose clothing around open flame; inadequately stored combustible

Children riding in front seat of car; nonuse or misuse of seat restraint; misuse of headgear [e.g., hard hat, motorcycle helmet]

Defective appliance; delay in ignition of gas appliance; grease on stove; electrical hazard;

Exposure to corrosive product or toxic chemical; inadequately stored corrosive; exposure to radiation

Icicles hanging from roof

Playing with dangerous object or explosive

Proximity to vehicle pathway [e.g., driveway, railroad track]; unsafe road or walkway; unsafe operation of heavy equipment

Smoking in bed or near oxygen

At Risk Population: Economically disadvantaged

Extremes of environmental temperature

Gas leak

High crime neighborhood

History of trauma

Associated Condition: Alteration in cognitive function; alteration in sensation

Decrease in eye-hand coordination; decrease in muscle coordination

Sample Clinical Applications: Substance intoxication or abuse, peripheral neuropathy, cataracts, glaucoma, macular degeneration, Parkinson's disease, seizure disorder, dementia, major depression, developmental delay

DESIRED OUTCOMES/EVALUATION CRITERIA

Sample NOC linkages:

Physical Injury Severity: Severity of signs and symptoms of injuries to the body

Personal Safety Behavior: Personal actions to prevent unintentional physical injury to self

Knowledge: Personal Safety: Extent of understanding conveyed about risk reduction and prevention of unintentional injuries to self

Client/Caregiver Will (Include Specific Time Frame)

• Identify and correct potential risk factors in the environment.
• Demonstrate appropriate lifestyle changes to reduce risk of injury.
• Identify resources to assist in promoting a safe environment.
• Recognize need for and seek assistance to prevent accidents/injuries.

ACTIONS/INTERVENTIONS

[This ND is a compilation of a number of situations that can result in injury. Refer to specific NDs, such as risk for imbalanced Body Temperature; risk for Contamination; risk for Falls; impaired Home Maintenance; Hyperthermia; Hypothermia; risk for Injury; impaired physical Mobility; risk for impaired Parenting; risk for Poisoning; risk for Thermal Injury, [disturbed Sensory Perception]; impaired Skin Integrity;

 Acute Care Collaborative Community/ Home Care Cultural

risk for Suffocation; impaired Tissue Integrity; risk for self-/other-directed Violence; impaired Walking, as appropriate, for more specific interventions.]

Sample NIC linkages:

Environmental Management: Safety: Monitoring and manipulation of the physical environment to promote safety

Environmental Management: Worker Safety: Monitoring and manipulation of the worksite environment to promote safety and health of workers

Teaching: Infant [or] Toddler Safety [specify age]: Instruction on safety during first or second and third years of life

NURSING PRIORITY NO. 1 To assess causative/contributing factors:

- Determine factors related to individual situation and extent of risk for trauma. *Influences scope and intensity of interventions to manage threats to safety, which are dynamic and constants in every life and situation. Clients interfacing with the healthcare system are at higher risk for trauma for any number of reasons (e.g., illness state, cognitive function, family structure, information and training) and require protection in numerous ways.*[1]
- ∞ ▨ Note client's age, gender, developmental stage, decision-making ability, level of cognition and competence *to determine client's ability to recognize danger and to protect self. Note: Children, young adults, older persons, and men are at greater risk for injury, which may reflect client's ability or desire to protect self, and influences choice of interventions or teaching.*[12,13]
- Ascertain client's/significant other's (SO's) knowledge of safety needs, injury prevention, and ways of looking at and improving own environment. *Lack of appreciation of significance of individual hazards increases risk of traumatic injury.*[1]
- Assess influence of stressors (e.g., physical, mental, peer related, work related, financial) *that can impair judgment and greatly increase client's potential for injury.*
- ▨ Assess mood, coping abilities, and personality styles (i.e., temperament, aggression, impulsive behavior, level of self-esteem). *May result in carelessness or increased risk-taking without consideration of consequences.*[10,11]
- Evaluate individual's emotional and behavioral response to violence in surroundings (e.g., neighborhood, television, peer group). *May affect client's view of and regard for own/others' safety.*[10–12]
- 🏠 Evaluate environment (home, neighborhood, work, transportation) *for obvious safety hazards, as well as situations that can exacerbate injury or adversely affect client's well-being. Unsafe factors include a vast array of possibilities (e.g., unsafe heating appliances, smoking and unattended smoking materials, toxic substances and chemicals, open flames, knives, improperly stored weapons, overloaded electrical outlets, dangerous neighborhoods, unsupervised children).*[1]
- 🏠 Review potential occupational risk factors (e.g., works with dangerous tools and machinery, electricity, explosives; police, fire, emergency medical service officers; working with hazardous chemicals, various inhalants, or radiation).
- Note history of accidents during specific period of time, noting circumstances of the accident (e.g., time of day that falls occur, activities going on, who was present). *Investigation of such events can provide clues for client's risk for subsequent events and potential for enhanced safety by a change in the people or environment involved (e.g., client may need assistance when getting up at night, increased playground supervision may be required).*
- ∞ Determine potential for abusive behavior by family members/SO(s)/peers. Be prepared for assessment of persons in abusive/violent situations and reporting and referral to appropriate social and law enforcement services. *Anyone, but especially child/frail elder, may require placement if incurring repeated injuries in family/ community setting.*

 Diagnostic Studies   Evidence Based Practice   Medications 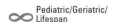 Pediatric/Geriatric/ Lifespan

- Note socioeconomic status and availability and use of resources. *Lack of resources, including financial, may limit ability to meet safety needs (e.g., proper child safety seat, appliance repairs, window grates).*
- ✎ Review diagnostic studies and laboratory results, noting impairments or imbalances *that may result in or exacerbate conditions, such as confusion, tetany, pathological fractures, etc.*

NURSING PRIORITY NO. 2   To enhance safety in healthcare environment:

- 🟥🏠∞📝 Screen client for safety concerns (e.g., risk for falls, cognitive, developmental, vision/other sensory impairments upon admission and during stay in healthcare facility). Assess for and report changes in client's functional status. Perform thorough assessments regarding safety issues when planning for client discharge. *Failure to accurately assess and intervene or refer regarding these issues can place the client at needless risk and creates negligence issues for the healthcare practitioner.*[8,9,14]
- 🟥 Monitor client's therapeutic regimen on a continual basis when under direct care (e.g., client's vital signs, medications, treatment modalities, infusions, nutrition, physical environment) *to prevent healthcare-related complications:*[9,14]
- 🐾 Collaborate in treatment of underlying medical, surgical, or psychiatric conditions *to improve cognition and thinking processes, musculoskeletal function, awareness of own safety needs, and general well-being.*
- 🐾 Refer to physical or occupational therapist as appropriate *to identify high-risk tasks, conduct site visits, select, create, or modify equipment; and provide education about body mechanics and musculoskeletal injuries, as well as provide needed therapies.*[2]
- Emphasize with client importance of obtaining assistance when weak or sedated and when problems of balance, coordination, or postural hypotension are present *to reduce risk of syncope and falls.*
- Provide quiet environment and reduced stimulation as indicated. *Helps limit confusion or overstimulation for clients at risk for such conditions as seizures, tetany, and autonomic hyperreflexia.*
- Demonstrate and encourage use of techniques to reduce or manage stress and vent emotions such as anger and hostility *to reduce risk of violence to self/others.*
- Provide for routine safety needs:[2–7]

  Provide adequate supervision and frequent observation.

  ∞ Place young children and confused client/person with dementia near nurses' station.

  Provide for appropriate communication tools (e.g., call light, cell phone; writing implements and paper; computer/tablet, alphabet picture board).

  Demonstrate use and place call bell/light or phone within client's reach.

  Orient or reorient client to environment as needed.

  Encourage client's use of corrective vision and hearing aids.

  Keep bed in low position or place mattress on floor as appropriate.

  Maintain correct body alignment and mechanics.

  Provide positioning as required by situation (e.g., immobilization of fractures).

  Implement appropriate measures to maintain skin and tissue health.

  Protect client (with sensory impairments) from injury due to heat and cold.

  Provide seizure precautions when indicated.

  Lock wheels on bed, wheelchair, and movable furniture.

  Assist with activities and transfers as needed.

  Provide well-fitting, nonskid footwear.

  Demonstrate and monitor use of assistive devices, such as cane, walker, crutches, wheelchair, and safety bars.

  Clear travel paths, pick up small items from floor; keep furniture in one place and door in one position (completely open or closed).

  Provide adequate area lighting.

  Follow facility protocol and closely monitor use of restraints when required (e.g., vest, limb, belt, mitten).
- Administer treatments, medications, and therapies in a therapeutic manner.
- Dispose of sharp implements in appropriate container.

 Acute Care   Collaborative   Community/ Home Care   Cultural

NURSING PRIORITY NO. 3   To enhance safety for client in community care setting:

- Provide information to caregivers regarding client's specific disease or condition(s) and associated risks. *For example, postural hypotension, muscle weakness (e.g., multiple sclerosis), dementia, osteoporosis, and head injury can impair function or cognition, impacting client's ability to protect self.*
- Identify interventions and safety devices to promote safe physical environment and individual safety:[5,6,8–11]
  Recommend wearing visual or hearing aids *to maximize sensory input.*
  Ensure availability of communication devices (e.g., telephone, computer, alarm system, or medical emergency alert device).
  Install and maintain electrical and fire safety devices, extinguishers, and alarms. Participate in fire drills and planning for fire evacuation routes.
  Review smoking safety rules, as indicated, especially as relates to unsafe places to smoke, including while in bed or when oxygen is in use.
  Identify environmental needs (e.g., decals on glass doors *to show when they are closed;* adequate lighting of stairways, handrails, ramps, bathtub safety tapes *to reduce risk of falls;* lowering temperature on hot water heater *to prevent accidental burns;* creation of ergonomic workstation).
  Obtain seat raisers for chairs; ergonomic beds or chairs.
  Encourage participation in back-safety classes, injury-prevention exercises, and/or mobility or transfer device training.
  Install locked cabinets for medications and toxic household substances and use tamper-proof medication containers.
  Review proper storage and disposal of volatile liquids, installation of proper ventilation for use when mixing or using toxic substances, and use of safety glasses or goggles.
  Emphasize importance of appropriate use of car restraints and bicycle, skating, or skiing helmets.
  Discuss swimming pool fencing and supervision; attending first-aid and cardiopulmonary resuscitation classes.
  Obtain trigger locks or gun safes for firearms.
- Initiate appropriate teaching and referrals, *if reckless behavior is occurring or likely to occur (e.g., smoking in bed, driving without safety belts, working with chemicals without safety goggles).*
- Encourage participation in self-help programs *to address individual risks (e.g., assertiveness training, positive self-image to enhance self-esteem, smoking cessation, weight management).*
- Refer to counseling or psychotherapy, as needed, *especially when individual is "accident-prone" or violent or self-destructive behavior is noted.* Refer to NDs risk for self-directed/other-directed Violence.

NURSING PRIORITY NO. 4   To promote optimal safety (Teaching/Discharge Considerations):

- Discuss importance of self-monitoring of conditions or emotions that can contribute to occurrence of injury to self/others (e.g., fatigue, anger, irritability). *Client/SO may be able to modify risk through monitoring of actions or postponement of certain actions, especially during times when client is likely to be highly stressed.*
- ∞ Review expectations caregivers have of children, cognitively impaired, or older family members *to identify needed information, required assistance with care, and follow-up that may be needed to provide safe environment for client.*
- ∞ Problem-solve with client/parent *to provide adequate child supervision after school, during working hours, and on school holidays.*
- ∞ Discuss need for and sources of adult supervision (e.g., senior day care, home health aide, or companion).
- Encourage client's family to identify neighbors or friends willing *to assist elderly/individuals with disabilities in providing such things as checking on client who lives alone, removing snow and ice from walks and steps, assisting with structural maintenance, etc.*

 Diagnostic Studies   Evidence Based Practice   Medications   Pediatric/Geriatric/Lifespan

- Explore behaviors related to use of alcohol, tobacco, and recreational drugs and other substances. *Provides opportunity to review consequences of previously determined risk factors (e.g., increase in oral cancer among teenagers using smokeless tobacco, potential consequences of illegal activities, effects of smoking on health of family members as well as fire danger; occurrence of spontaneous abortion, fetal alcohol syndrome or neonatal addiction in prenatal women using tobacco, alcohol, and other drugs).*[10–12]
- Encourage development of fire safety program. *Participation in family fire drills, use of smoke detectors, yearly chimney cleaning, purchase of fire-retardant clothing (especially children's nightwear), fireworks safety, safe use of in-home oxygen or propane sources, etc., enhances home safety.*
- Recommend use of seat belts and approved infant seat in appropriate position in vehicle; fitted helmets for cyclists, motorcyclists, and skateboarders; wearing necessary visual aids; driver training course for new and mature drivers; avoidance of hitchhiking; and substance-abuse program as indicated *to promote transportation safety.*
- Identify community resources (e.g., financial, volunteer) *to assist with necessary home improvements or equipment purchases.*
- Refer to other resources as indicated (e.g., counseling/psychotherapy, parenting classes, budget counseling).
- Provide client/caregiver with emergency contact numbers as individually indicated (e.g., doctor, 911, poison control, police).
- Provide client/caregiver with bibliotherapy and written resources *for later review and self-paced learning.*
- Encourage involvement in community awareness programs and problem-solving of identified community needs:

    Participate in self-help programs (e.g., Neighborhood Watch, Helping Hand, after-school activities). *Programs based on identified needs enhance support of community members and potential funding sources.*

    Promote educational opportunities *geared toward increasing awareness of safety measures (e.g., firearms safety) and resources available to the individual.*

    Seek out and involve businesses in volunteer outreach activities such as building safe playgrounds, community or street cleanup, home repair or improvement for frail elders, etc.

    Advocate for and promote solutions for problems of design of buildings, equipment, transportation, and workplace practices *that contribute to accidents.*

DOCUMENTATION FOCUS

Assessment/Reassessment
- Individual risk factors, past and recent history of injuries, awareness of safety needs.

Planning
- Plan of care and who is involved in the planning.
- Teaching plan.

Implementation/Evaluation
- Responses to interventions, teaching, and actions performed.
- Attainment or progress toward desired outcome(s).
- Modifications to plan of care.

Discharge Planning
- Long-term needs and who is responsible for actions to be taken.
- Available resources, specific referrals made.

References

1. Ebright, P. R., Patterson, E. S., Render, M. L. (2002). The "New Look" approach to patient safety: A guide for clinical specialist leadership. *Clin Nurs Spec*, 16(5), 247–253.

2. Nelson, A., (ed.). (2006). *Safe Patient Handling and Movement: A Practical Guide for Health Care Professionals.* New York: Springer.

 Acute Care   Collaborative   Community/Home Care   Cultural

3. Walton, J. (2001). Helping high-risk surgical patients beat the odds. *Nursing*, 31(3), 54–59.
4. Wright, A. (1998). Nursing interventions with advanced osteoporosis. *Home Healthc Nurse*, 16(3), 144–151.
5. Munche, J. A., McCarty, S. M. (2015, updated 2017). Geriatric Rehabilitation. Retrieved April 2018 from http://emedicine .medscape.com/article/318521-overview.
6. Consumer Product Safety Commission. (No date). Safety for older consumers' home safety checklist. Retrieved April 2018 from http://www.cpsc.gov//PageFiles/122038/701.pdf.
7. Daus, C. (1999). Maintaining mobility: Assistive equipment helps the geriatric population stay active and independent. *Rehabil Manage*, 12(5), 58–61.
8. Horn, L. B. (2000). Reducing the risk of falls in the elderly. *Rehabil Manage*, 13(3), 36–38.
9. Kizer, K. W., Blum, L. N. (2005). Safe practices for better health care. Abstract for a portion of the Consensus Report. *Agency for Healthcare Research and Quality*. Retrieved April 2018 from http://www.ncbi.nlm.nih.gov/books/ NBK20613/.
10. Gorman-Smith, D., Henry, D. B., Tolan, P. H. (2004). Exposure to community violence and violence perpetration: The protective effects of family functioning. *J Clin Child Psychol*, 33(3), 439–449.
11. Centers for Disease Control and Prevention (CDC). (2015, updated 2017). School violence: Risk and protective factors. Injury Center: Violence prevention. Retrieved April 2018 from http://www.cdc.gov/violenceprevention/youthviolence/ riskprotectivefactors.html#RiskFactors.
12. Schwebel, D. C., Barton, B. K. (2005). Contributions of multiple risk factors to child injury. *J Pediatr Psychol*, 30(7), 553–561.
13. Ristolainen, L., et al. (2009). Gender differences in sport injury risk and types of injuries: A retrospective twelve-month study on cross-country skiers, long distance runners and soccer players. *J Sports Sci Med*, 8, 443–451.
14. Austin, S. (2008). Seven legal tips for safe nursing practice. *Nursing*, 38(3), 34–39.

risk for vascular Trauma

Taxonomy II: Safety/Protection—Class 2 Physical Injury [**Diagnostic Division:** Safety], Approved 2008; Revised 2013, 2017

DEFINITION: Susceptible to damage to vein and its surrounding tissues related to the presence of a catheter and/or infused solutions, which may compromise health.

RISK FACTORS
Inadequate available insertion site
Prolonged period of time catheter is in place
Irritating solution
Rapid infusion rate
Sample Clinical Applications: Surgery, trauma, cancer/chemotherapy, pneumonia, sepsis, dehydration, heat stroke

DESIRED OUTCOMES/EVALUATION CRITERIA

Sample **NOC** linkages:
Risk Control: Personal actions to understand, prevent, eliminate, or reduce modifiable health threats
Knowledge: Treatment Procedure: Extent of understanding conveyed about a procedure required as part of a treatment regimen
Self-Care: Parenteral Medication: Personal actions to administer parenteral medications to meet therapeutic goals independently with or without assistive device

Client Will (Include Specific Time Frame)
• Identify sign/symptoms to report to healthcare provider.
• Be free of signs/symptoms associated with venipuncture, infusion solution, or local infection.
• Develop plan for home therapy where indicated and demonstrate appropriate procedures.

(continues on page 928)

 Diagnostic Studies   Evidence Based Practice   Medications   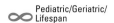 Pediatric/Geriatric/ Lifespan

risk for vascular Trauma (continued)

ACTIONS/INTERVENTIONS

Sample **NIC** linkages:

Intravenous (IV) Insertion: Insertion of a cannulated needle into a peripheral vein for the purpose of administering fluids, blood, or medications

Intravenous (IV) Therapy: Administration and monitoring of intravenous fluids and medications

Medication Administration: Intravenous: Preparing and giving medications via the intravenous route

NURSING PRIORITY NO. 1 To assess risk factors:

- Determine presence of medical condition(s) requiring IV therapy, such as dehydration, trauma, and surgery; long-term antibiotic treatment of severe infections; cancer therapies; and pain management when oral drugs not effective or practical.
- ∞ Note client's age, body size, and weight. *Very young and elderly clients are at risk because of lack of subcutaneous tissue surrounding veins, and veins may be fragile or ropy, causing difficulties with insertion. Forearm veins may be difficult to see in obese, edematous, or dark-skinned individuals.*[3,4]
- Identify particular issues, such as client's emotional state (including fear of needles) and mental or developmental status, *that might interfere with client's ability to cooperate with procedures,* and IV site choices that interfere with client's mobility *to prevent or limit potential for vascular damage.*[3]
- Determine type(s) of solutions being used or planned. *Certain infusates are associated with greater risk of vein irritation and pain (e.g., potassium, contrast media); others are associated with tissue injury, especially upon infiltration into surrounding tissues, including certain antibiotics (e.g., nafcillin, cloxacillin, vancomycin). Hyperosmolar solutions such as total parenteral nutrition can cause tissue damage by altering osmotic pressure. Most cancer chemotherapeutic agents cause direct cellular toxicity after extravasation, and some have potential for causing substantial tissue necrosis (e.g., doxorubicin, vincristine).*[5] *Note: Therapies not appropriate for peripheral short catheters include continuous vesicant therapy, parenteral nutrition, infusates with a pH less than 5 or greater than 9, and solutions with an osmolarity greater than 600 mOsm/L.*[6,7]
- Assess peripheral IV site when one is already in place to determine potential for complications. *Reddened, blanched, tight, translucent, or cool skin; swelling; pain; numbness; streak formation; and a palpable venous cord or purulent drainage are indicative of problem with IV requiring immediate intervention.*[1]
- Assess central venous access device (CVAD), if present, to determine potential for complications. *Inability to aspirate; slowed or absent solution flow; site pain; and engorged veins or swelling in upper arm, chest wall, neck, or jaw on side of catheter insertion may indicate vein or catheter-related thrombus, requiring immediate intervention.*[1,2]

NURSING PRIORITY NO. 2 To reduce potential complications:

- Determine appropriate site choice:
  - Identify extremities and sites that have impaired circulation or injury, such as lymphedema, postoperative swelling, recent trauma, hematoma, axillary lymph node dissection, open wounds, etc.[4] *Leg veins should be avoided in adults due to potential for thrombophlebitis. Antecubital veins should be avoided for peripheral catheters where possible because they limit client's movement and are easily dislodged.*[6]
  - Inspect and palpate chosen veins to determine size and condition. *Vein that is scarred, lumpy, or small and fragile can not only cause problems upon cannulation but also can impede effectiveness of infusion.*[1,6]
  - Avoid inserting needle in vein valve site. *Damage to this area can cause blood pooling and increase risk of thrombosis.*[3]

 Acute Care   Collaborative   Community/Home Care   Cultural

- Use a best-practice approach to IV insertion and therapies:

  📝 Determine best type of access when IV therapy is to be initiated. *Peripheral catheter in forearm is recommended for short-duration, nonirritating solutions of less than 7 days. CVAD placed so that tip is in or near the superior vena cava is appropriate for infusing many kinds of solutions over long periods of time.*[4,8,9]

  📝 Choose appropriate needle or catheter for situation considering planned length and type of therapy, avoiding steel butterfly needles when possible *to reduce risk of vein injury and infiltration.*[1,2,4] *Over-the-needle catheter for hand or forearm may be ideal for most solutions over a short length of time, while midline catheter may be chosen for chemotherapy or when antibiotic therapy is planned for 1 to 4 weeks; a central venous catheter is used for infusates and other substances that are too irritating to peripheral veins, when client has suffered multiple peripheral sticks, or when one extremity is not available (e.g., amputation, dialysis shunt in one arm).*[4,8]

  📝 Use appropriate needle gauge. *Size should be smallest diameter possible for chosen vein and solution to be infused to deliver solution at appropriate rate, to promote hemodilution of fluid(s) at the catheter tip, and to reduce mechanical and chemical irritation to vein wall.*[1,3,4]

  📝 Make use of equipment (e.g., ultrasound, near-infrared technology, transillumination), as indicated/available, when venous access is difficult and/or after failed venous access attempts *to reduce client's trauma (both physical and emotional), and potential for excess vein damage affiliated with multiple attempts (2016 Infusion Nurses Society [INS] Standards of Practice, Standard 22).*[6]

  ♾📝 Clean site and follow agency policy for the use of a local anesthetic (e.g., buffered 1% lidocaine) before venipuncture *to reduce risk of infection and pain with needle or cannula insertion. Note: Nursing research is being conducted on the use of lidocaine or normal saline injection for the reduction of the discomfort of venipuncture. One recent small study found intradermal lidocaine superior to bacteriostatic normal saline as an anesthetic pretreatment; however, this study demonstrated that normal saline can provide reasonable pain relief and is thus a practical alternative when intradermal lidocaine is not available or the patient has an allergy to lidocaine.*[10]

  Stretch and immobilize skin and tissues *to stabilize vein and prevent rolling, requiring multiple sticks.*

  Insert needle bevel up and hold at a 3- to 10-degree angle *to prevent "blowing" the vein by piercing the back wall.*[2]

  Release tourniquet immediately when insertion is complete *to prevent intravascular pressure from causing bleeding into surrounding tissues.*[1]

  Observe for hematoma development and/or reports of pain and discomfort during insertion, *indicating vein damage with bleeding into tissues.*[4]

  Secure needle or cannula with tape or other securement device *to prevent dislodging and extend catheter dwell time.*[6]

  Avoid placing tape entirely around arm to anchor catheter. *This may impede venous return and cause venous stasis, pooling of fluid, and infiltration or extravasation into surrounding tissues.*[4]

  Utilize transparent dressing over insertion site *to protect from external contaminants and to easily observe for potential complications.*

  💊📝 Adhere to recommended infusions, dilutions, and administration rates for medications or irritating substances such as potassium *to reduce incidence of tissue irritation and sloughing.*[2,4,6]

- ♾ Consult with IV nurse or other medical provider *to problem-solve issues that arise with IVs and/or when different access should be considered (e.g., midline catheter for continuous infusion of irritating solutions, peripheral intravenous central catheter [PICC] for parenteral nutrition) or for evaluation and interventions for complications such as thrombus development in central catheter tip or in the vein around the catheter.*[4,9]

NURSING PRIORITY NO. 3   To promote optimum therapeutic effect:

- ➕ Observe IV site on a regular basis and instruct client/caregiver to report any discomfort, bruising, redness, swelling, bleeding, or other fluid leaking from site *to allow for prompt intervention and limit serious complications.*

 Diagnostic Studies   Evidence Based Practice   Medications   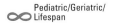 Pediatric/Geriatric/Lifespan

- Replace peripheral catheters every 72 to 96 hr (or per agency policy) *to prevent thrombophlebitis and catheter-related infections.*[4]
- Apply pressure to site when IV is discontinued for sufficient time *to prevent bleeding, especially in client with coagulopathies or on anticoagulants.*[4]
- Adhere to specific protocols related to infection control *to promote safe infusion of solutions or medications and prevent complications.* Refer to ND risk for Infection.
- Identify community resources and suppliers *to support home therapy regimen.*

DOCUMENTATION FOCUS

Assessment/Reassessment
- Assessment findings pre/postinsertion, site choice, use of local anesthetic, type and gauge of needle or cannula inserted, number of sticks required, dressing applied.
- Type, amount, and rate of solution administered, presence of additives.
- Client's response to procedure.

Planning
- Plan of care, specific interventions, and who is involved in the planning.
- Teaching plan as appropriate.

Implementation/Evaluation
- Attainment or progress toward desired outcome(s).
- Modifications to plan of care.

Discharge Planning
- Long-range needs, identifying who is responsible for actions to be taken.
- Community resources for equipment and supplies for home therapy.
- Specific referrals made.

References

1. Hadaway, L. C. (2005). Reopen the pipeline for I.V. therapy. *Nursing*, 35(8), 54–61.
2. Hadaway, L. C., Millam, D. A. (2007). On the road to successful I.V. starts. *Nursing*, 37(8 Suppl), 1–14.
3. Rosenthal, K. (2005). Tailor your I.V. insertion techniques for special populations. *Nursing*, 35(5), 36–41.
4. Horattas, M., Hale, K. L (2012; reviewed 2017). Venous access devices. Retrieved May 2018 from https://www.emedicinehealth.com/venous_access_devices/article_em.htm#venous_access_device_chart.
5. Dychter, S. S., Gold, D. A., Carson, D. (2012). Intravenous therapy: A review of complications and economic considerations of peripheral access. *J Infus Nurs*, 35(2), 84–91.
6. Infusion Nurses Society (INS). (2016). Overview of the New 2016 INS Standards of Practice (in brief). *Infusion Knowledge Inc.* Retrieved May 2018 from https://www.uwcne.org/sites/uwcne.org/files/users/9/new-standards.pdf.
7. Gorski, L. A. (2008). Intravenous therapy. In Ackley, B. J., et al. (eds). *Evidence-Based Nursing Care Guidelines: Medical-Surgical Interventions.* St. Louis, MO: Mosby Elsevier.
8. Cook, L. S. (2007). Choosing the right intravenous catheter. *Home Healthc Nurse*, 25(8), 523–531.
9. Hadaway, L. C. (2008). Targeting therapy with central venous access devices. *Nursing*, 38(6), 34–40.
10. Burke, S. D., et al. (2011). Original research: Local anesthesia before IV catheterization. *Am J Nurs*, 111(2), 40–45.

 Acute Care Collaborative Community/Home Care Cultural

Unilateral Neglect

Taxonomy II: Perception/Cognition—Class 1 Attention (00123) **[Diagnostic Division:** Neurosensory**]**, Submitted 1986; Revised 2006

DEFINITION: Impairment in sensory and motor response, mental representation, and spatial attention to the body and the corresponding environment, characterized by inattention to one side and overattention to the opposite side. Left-side neglect is more severe and persistent than right-side neglect.

RELATED FACTORS
To Be Developed

DEFINING CHARACTERISTICS

Objective
Left hemiplegia from cerebrovascular accident; unilateral visuospatial neglect
Hemianopsia; marked deviation of the eyes or trunk to stimuli on the non-neglected side
Failure to move eyes, head, limbs, or trunk in the neglected hemisphere; failure to notice people approaching from the neglected side
Disturbance of sound lateralization
Unaware of positioning of neglected limb
Alteration in safety behavior on neglected side
Failure to: eat food from portion of plate on neglected side; dress or groom neglected side
Use of vertical half of page only when writing; impaired performance on line cancellation, line bisection, and target cancellation tests; substitution of letters to form alternative words when reading
Omission of drawing on the neglected side; representational neglect [e.g., distortion of drawing on the neglected side]
Perseveration
Transfer of pain sensation to the non-neglected side
Associated Condition: Brain injury
Sample Clinical Applications: Traumatic brain injury, CVA/ruptured cerebral aneurysm, brain tumor, glaucoma

DESIRED OUTCOMES/EVALUATION CRITERIA

Sample NOC linkages:
Heedfulness of Affected Side: Personal actions to acknowledge, protect, and cognitively integrate affected body part(s) into self
Self-Care: Activities of Daily Living (ADL): Personal actions to perform the most basic physical tasks and personal care activities independently with or without assistive device

Client/Caregiver Will (Include Specific Time Frame)
• Acknowledge presence of sensory-perceptual impairment.
• Identify adaptive and protective measures for individual situation.
• Demonstrate behaviors and lifestyle changes necessary to promote physical safety.

Client Will (Include Specific Time Frame)
• Verbalize positive realistic perception of self, incorporating the current dysfunction.
• Perform self-care within level of ability.

(continues on page 932)

 Diagnostic Studies   Evidence Based Practice   Medications 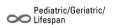 Pediatric/Geriatric/Lifespan

Unilateral Neglect (continued)

ACTIONS/INTERVENTIONS

Sample NIC linkages:

Unilateral Neglect Management: Protecting and safely reintegrating the affected part of the body while helping the patient adapt to disturbed perceptual abilities

Positioning: Deliberative placement of the patient or a body part to promote physiological and/or psychological well-being

Environmental Management: Safety: Monitoring and manipulation of the physical environment to promote safety

NURSING PRIORITY NO. 1   To assess the extent of altered perception and the related degree of disability:

- Identify underlying condition or reason for alterations in sensory/motor/behavioral perceptions as noted in Related Factors. *The client with injury to either side of the brain may experience spatial neglect, but more commonly, it occurs when brain injury affects the right cortical hemisphere, causing left hemiparesis.*[10]
- Observe client's behaviors (as noted in Defining Characteristics) *to determine the extent of impairment (e.g., failure to respond to stimuli, objects, or people on the contralesional side).*
- Ascertain client's/significant other's (SO's) perception of problem and changes and impact on life and future, noting differences in perceptions. *Client is often not aware of, or able to express, spatial perception problems or understand potential effect on future expectations.*
- Assist with/review results of early screening tests. *Tests (often performed at the bedside) may include (and are not limited to) observation to determine if client shows evidence of body neglect such as asymmetric shaving/grooming. Reading test might reveal that client begins reading in the middle of the page. Client may not be able to count fingers on both hands or perceive finger snapping at both ears. Paper and pencil testing may reveal hemispatial neglect through line dissection.*[1,9]
- Assess ability to distinguish between right and left. *Unilateral spatial neglect is observed in stroke, brain tumor, or accident victims with damage to the right parietal or parietal-occipital lobe, resulting in misperceptions of space opposite to brain damage. The individual with this condition has information from the left hemispace but no conscious awareness of the information; thus, he/she will pay no attention to the left space.*[1–4]
- Assess sensory awareness (e.g., response to stimulus of hot and cold, dull or sharp); note problems with awareness of motion and proprioception. *Disturbances in these areas may be result of spinal cord injury (where loss of sensation affects body awareness) or brain lesion (where sensation may be intact but awareness is impaired).*
- Note physical signs of neglect (e.g., inability to maintain normal posture; disregard for position of affected limb[s], bumping into objects or walls on the left when ambulating, skin irritation/damage on the left side, indicating lack of awareness of injury).
- Observe ability to function within limits of impairment. Compare with client's perception of own abilities. *Client may or may not be able to learn from mistakes or from observing others depending on the location and severity of the brain lesion.*[5]
- Explore and encourage verbalization of feelings *to identify meaning of loss, dysfunction, or change to the client and impact it may have on assuming ADLs. Note: Expression of loss may be difficult for the client for a variety of reasons. For example, some emotional disturbances and personality changes are caused by the physical effects of brain damage, or the client may be hyperemotional or depressed or be unable to express feelings in the same manner as prior to brain injury.*[5]

 Acute Care   Collaborative   Community/ Home Care   Cultural

- 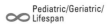 Review results of testing (e.g., computed tomography or magnetic resonance imaging scanning, complete neuropsychological tests) *done to determine cause or type of neglect syndrome (e.g., sensory, motor, representational, personal, spatial, behavioral inattention).*[6–9]

NURSING PRIORITY NO. 2 To promote optimal comfort and safety for the client in the environment:

- Engage in treatment strategies *focused on training of attention to the neglected hemispace:*[1–5,8,9]
Encourage use of vision and hearing aids if condition requires or client usually wears them *to improve sensory input and interpretation.*
Remove excess stimuli from the environment *to decrease confusion and reactive stress.*
Orient or reorient to physical environment and persons interacting with client. *Client with unilateral neglect can also have numerous other cognitive defects affecting ability to think, remember, speak or understand language, and/or interpret environment.*[5]
Approach client and instruct others to approach client from the unaffected side (e.g., right side, side where vision is not impaired) *to enhance client's awareness and potential for communication.*
Encourage client to turn head and eyes in full rotation and "scan" the environment *to compensate for visual field loss or when neglect therapies include scanning.*
Position bedside table and objects (e.g., telephone, call bell, tissues) *within functional field of vision or awareness to facilitate self-care. Note: Therapies may include orienting the client's environment leftward in attempt to help client perceive the neglected space.*
Place nonessential items (e.g., television, pictures, hairbrush) on affected side during postacute phase once client begins to cross midline *to encourage continuation of retraining behaviors.*
Discuss affected side while touching, manipulating, and stroking affected side *to focus client's attention on area* and provide objects of various weight, texture, and size for the client to handle *to provide tactile stimuli.*
Describe where affected areas of body are *when moving or repositioning client.*
Use descriptive terms to identify body parts rather than "left" and "right"; for example, "Lift this leg" (point to leg) or "Lift your affected leg."
Encourage client to accept affected limb or side as part of self even when it no longer feels like it belongs. Have client look at and handle affected side *to stimulate awareness* and bring the affected limb across the midline *for client to visualize during care.*
Provide visual cues and assist client to position the affected extremity carefully and teach to routinely visualize placement of the extremity.
Use a mirror to help client adjust position *by visualizing both sides of the body.*
- Provide assistance with ADLs (e.g., feeding, bathing, dressing, grooming, toileting), *which helps client tend to affected side or compensate for client's impairments. Note: Studies show that unilateral neglect is a major factor limiting ADLs and in client being at increased risk for falls.*[11]
- Monitor neglected body part(s) for positioning and anatomic alignment, pressure points, skin irritation or injury, and dependent edema. *Increased risk of injury and pressure ulcer formation necessitates close observation and timely intervention.* (Refer to NDs risk for Peripheral Neurovascular Dysfunction and impaired Tissue Integrity.)
- Assist with ambulation or movement, using appropriate mobility and assistive devices *to promote safety of client and caregiver.*
- Protect from falls and/or collision with objects:
Position furniture and equipment *so travel path is unobstructed.*
Remove articles that may create a safety hazard (e.g., footstool, throw rug).
Ensure adequate lighting in the environment.
Keep doors wide open or completely closed.
- Refer to NDs impaired Environmental Interpretation Syndrome, risk for Falls/Injury, and Self-Care Deficit (specify) for additional interventions regarding comfort and safety.
- Collaborate with rehabilitation team in strategies (e.g., sensory stimulation techniques such as tapping or stroking, patching one half of each eye, auditory stimulation, wedge prism adaptation techniques, virtual reality technology) *to assist client to overcome or compensate for deficits.*[5,12,13]

 Diagnostic Studies   Evidence Based Practice   Medications   Pediatric/Geriatric/ Lifespan

NURSING PRIORITY NO. 3   To promote optimal functioning (Teaching/Discharge Considerations):

- 🏠 Acknowledge and accept feelings of despondency, grief, and anger. *When feelings are openly expressed, client can deal with them and move forward.* (Refer to ND Grieving as appropriate.)
- Encourage family members/SO(s) to treat client normally, to urge client to perform own care as able, and to include client in family activities and outings. *Promotes sense of self-worth and encourages participation in life activities to limit withdrawal and depression.*
- Reinforce to client the reality of the dysfunction and need to compensate. Avoid participating in the client's use of denial. *Delays dealing with reality of situation and limits progress toward goals.*
- 🅐📝 Encourage client to continue rehabilitative services *to maximize recovery and enhance independence. Note: Research indicates that most clients with neglect show early recovery, particularly within the first month, and marked improvement within 3 months. In approximately 5% of clients, classic (more severe) symptoms of spatial neglect persist after 6 months or longer. In these individuals, the deficit may be regarded as chronic neglect.*[9]
- Discuss and prepare for ongoing safety issues. *Client may continue to have some functional problems after apparent recovery of spatial neglect, including difficulty with navigating in familiar and unfamiliar environments or safe driving.*[9]
- 🅐 Identify additional resources to meet individual needs (e.g., Meals on Wheels, home-care rehabilitation services) *to maximize independence and allow client to return to and succeed in community setting.*

DOCUMENTATION FOCUS

Assessment/Reassessment
- Individual findings, including extent of altered perception, degree of disability, effect on independence and participation in ADLs.

Planning
- Plan of care and who is involved in the planning.
- Teaching plan.

Implementation/Evaluation
- Responses to intervention, teaching, and actions performed.
- Attainment or progress toward desired outcome(s).
- Modifications to plan of care.

Discharge Planning
- Long-term needs and who is responsible for actions to be taken.
- Available resources, specific referrals made.

References

1. Walker, R. (1994). Unilateral neglect: Clinical and experimental studies. *Review for Psyche: An Interdisciplinary Journal of Research on Consciousness.* Retrieved July 2018 from https://www.routledge.com/Unilateral-Neglect-Clinical-And-Experimental-Studies/Marshall-Robertson/p/book/9780863772184.
2. Mansoori, L. (2010). *Hemispatial neglect syndrome. Student lecture for Brain, Thought and Action (MCDB 3650).* Boulder: University of Colorado.
3. Ricci, R., Calhoun, J., Chatterjee, A. (2000). Orientation bias in unilateral neglect: Representational contributions. *Cortex,* 36(5), 671–677.
4. Sinclair, C. (2001). *Brain organization as seen in unilateral spatial neglect.* Retrieved July 2018 from http://serendip.brynmawr.edu/bb/neuro/neuro01/web2/Sinclair.html.
5. National Institute for Neurological Disorders and Stroke (NINDS). (2014). *Post-stroke rehabilitation fact sheet.*
Retrieved July 2018 from http://stroke.nih.gov/materials/rehabilitation.htm.
6. Bates, B., Choi, J. Y., Duncan, P. W. (2005). Veterans Affairs/Department of Defense clinical practice guidelines for the management of adult stroke rehabilitation care: An executive summary. *Stroke,* 36(9), 2049–2056.
7. Plummer, P., Morris, M. E., Dunai, J. (2003). Assessment of unilateral neglect. *Phys Ther,* 83(8), 732–740.
8. Swan, L. (2001). Unilateral spatial neglect. *Phys Ther,* 81(9), 1572–1580.
9. Barrett, A. M. (2007, updated 2018). *Spatial neglect.* Retrieved July 2018 from http://emedicine.medscape.com/article/1136474-overview.
10. Vocat, R., et al. (2010). Anosognosia for hemiplegia: A clinical-anatomical prospective study. *Brain,* 133, 3578–3597.

 Acute Care   Collaborative   Community/Home Care   Cultural

11. Czernuszenko, A. (2007). Risk factors for falls in post-stroke patients treated in a neurorehabilitation ward. *Neurol Neurochir Pol*, 41(1), 28–35.

12. Tsirlin, I., et al. (2009). Uses of virtual reality for diagnosis, rehabilitation and study of unilateral spacial neglect: Review and analysis. *Cyberpsychol Behav*, 12(2), 175–181.

13. Mizuno, K., et al. (2011). Prism adaptation therapy enhances rehabilitation of stroke patients with unilateral spatial neglect: A randomized controlled trial. *Neurorehabil Neural Repair*, 25(8), 711–720.

impaired spontaneous Ventilation

Taxonomy II: Activity/Rest—Class 2 Cardiovascular/Pulmonary Response (00033) [**Diagnostic Division:** Respiration], Approved 1992; Revised 2017

DEFINITION: Inability to initiate and/or maintain independent breathing that is adequate to support life.

RELATED FACTORS
Respiratory muscle fatigue

DEFINING CHARACTERISTICS

Subjective
Dyspnea
Apprehensiveness

Objective
Alteration in metabolic rate
Increase in heart rate
Restlessness
Increase in accessory muscle use
Decrease in tidal volume
Decrease in partial pressure of oxygen (PO_2), arterial oxygen saturation (SaO_2); increase in partial pressure of carbon dioxide (PCO_2)
Associated Condition: Alteration in metabolism
Sample Clinical Applications: Chronic obstructive pulmonary disease (COPD), asthma, pulmonary embolus, acute respiratory distress syndrome, brain injury, chest trauma or surgery, Guillain-Barré syndrome, amyotrophic lateral sclerosis (ALS)

DESIRED OUTCOMES/EVALUATION CRITERIA

Sample NOC linkages:
Mechanical Ventilation Response: Adult: Alveolar exchange and tissue perfusion are effectively supported by mechanical ventilation
Respiratory Status: Ventilation: Movement of air in and out of the lungs
Endurance: Capacity to sustain activity

Client Will (Include Specific Time Frame)
• Reestablish and maintain effective respiratory pattern via ventilator, with absence of retractions or use of accessory muscles, cyanosis, or other signs of hypoxia, and with arterial blood gases (ABGs)/SaO_2 within acceptable range.
• Participate in efforts to wean (as appropriate) within individual's ability.

(continues on page 936)

 Diagnostic Studies   Evidence Based Practice   Medications   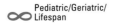 Pediatric/Geriatric/Lifespan

impaired spontaneous Ventilation (continued)

Energy Conservation: Personal actions to manage energy for initiating and sustaining activity

Caregiver Will (Include Specific Time Frame)
• Demonstrate behaviors necessary to maintain client's respiratory function.

ACTIONS/INTERVENTIONS

Ventilation Assistance: Promotion of an optimal spontaneous breathing pattern that maximizes oxygen and carbon dioxide exchange in the lungs

Mechanical Ventilation Management: Invasive: Assisting the patient receiving artificial breathing support through a device inserted into the trachea

Respiratory Monitoring: Collection and analysis of patient data to ensure airway patency and adequate gas exchange

NURSING PRIORITY NO. 1 To determine degree of impairment:

• Identify client with impending respiratory failure (e.g., developing apnea or slow, shallow breathing; declining mentation or obtunded with need for airway protection).[5]

• Determine presence of conditions that could be associated with hypoventilation. *Causes include (1) central alveolar hypoventilation as a result of congenital defects, drugs, and central nervous system disorders (e.g., stroke, trauma, neoplasms); (2) obesity hypoventilation syndrome is another well-known cause of hypoventilation; (3) chest wall deformities (e.g., kyphoscoliosis, changes after thoracic surgery) can be associated with alveolar hypoventilation, leading to respiratory insufficiency and failure; and (4) neuromuscular diseases that can cause alveolar hypoventilation include myasthenia gravis, ALS, Guillain-Barré, and muscular dystrophy.*[5]

• Assess spontaneous respiratory pattern, noting rate, depth, rhythm, symmetry of chest movement, and use of accessory muscles. *Tachypnea, shallow breathing, and demonstrated or reports of dyspnea (using a numeric or similar scale); increased heart rate and dysrhythmias; pallor or cyanosis; and intercostal retractions and use of accessory muscles indicate increased work of breathing or impaired gas exchange. Note: Studies to date show that no one specific scale has been developed to cover all aspects of breathlessness, but asking the client to rate it some way may be helpful in differentiating this episode from others.*[5,8]

• Auscultate breath sounds, noting presence or absence and equality of breath sounds and adventitious breath sounds (e.g., wheezing) *to evaluate presence and degree of ventilatory impairment.*

• Evaluate ABGs or pulse oximetry and capnography *to determine presence and degree of arterial hypoxemia (PaO$_2$ less than 55%) and hypercapnia (PaCO$_2$ greater than 45%), resulting in impaired ventilation requiring support.*[6,7]

• Obtain or review results of pulmonary function studies (e.g., lung volumes, inspiratory and expiratory pressures, forced vital capacity), as appropriate, *to assess presence and degree of respiratory insufficiency. Note: Pulmonary function tests revealing (1) PaO$_2$<55 mmHg; (2) vital capacity less than 10 mL/kg; (3) negative inspiratory force <25 cm H$_2$O; and (4) FEV$_1$ less than 10 mL/kg are standard indicators for intubation and ventilatory management.*[7]

• Investigate etiology of current respiratory failure (e.g., exacerbation of COPD, pneumonia, pulmonary embolus, heart failure, trauma) *to determine client's ventilation needs and most appropriate type of ventilatory support.*

 Acute Care   Collaborative   Community/Home Care   Cultural

- Review serial chest x-rays and imaging scans (e.g., magnetic resonance imaging, computed tomography) that may be performed *to diagnose underlying disorder and monitor response to treatment.*
- Note response to current measures and respiratory therapy (e.g., bronchodilators, supplemental oxygen, intermittent positive pressure breathing treatments). *Client may already be receiving treatments to maintain airway patency and enhance gas exchange or may have respiratory failure associated with sudden event (e.g., severe trauma, sudden onset respiratory illness, surgery with complications).*
- Ascertain desires of client/significant others (SOs) regarding plan for treatment of respiratory failure, as indicated. *Client may have advance directives and/or prior stated decisions about the level of therapy aggressiveness that he or she desires if situation is chronic or long term. Family members may help in decision-making processes if client is a minor or is incapacitated.*

NURSING PRIORITY NO. 2 To provide/maintain ventilatory support:

- Collaborate with physician and respiratory care practitioners regarding effective mode of ventilation (e.g., noninvasive oxygenation via continuous positive airway pressure [CPAP] and biphasic positive airway pressure [BIPAP]) or intubation and mechanical ventilation (e.g., continuous mandatory, assist control, intermittent mandatory [IMV], pressure support). *Specific mode is determined by client's respiratory requirements, presence of underlying disease process, and the extent to which client can participate in ventilatory efforts. Goals of therapy depend on the reason for mechanical ventilation (e.g., to improve oxygenation, permit sedation, reverse respiratory muscle fatigue).*[9]
- Ensure effective ventilation:[1,7,9]

  Ensure that ventilator settings and parameters are correct as ordered by client situation, including respiratory rate and fraction of inspired oxygen (FIO_2, expressed as a percentage; tidal volume); peak inspiratory pressure.

  Observe overall breathing pattern, distinguishing between spontaneous respirations and ventilator breaths. *Client may be completely dependent on the ventilator or able to take breaths but have poor oxygen saturation without the ventilator. The client on assist-control ventilation mode can still experience hyper/hypoventilation or "air hunger" and attempt to correct deficiency by overbreathing.*[7]

  Verify that client's respirations are in phase with the ventilator. *Decreases work of breathing, maximizes O_2 delivery when client is not fighting the ventilator.*

  Inflate tracheal or endotracheal tube cuff properly using minimal leak or occlusive technique *to ensure adequate ventilation and delivery of desired tidal volume.*

  Check cuff inflation periodically per facility protocol, and whenever cuff is deflated then reinflated *to prevent risks associated with under/overinflation.*

  Check tubings for obstruction (e.g., kinking or accumulation of water) *that can impede flow of oxygen.* Drain tubing, as indicated; refrain from draining toward the client or back into the reservoir, *which can result in contamination and provide medium for growth of bacteria.*

  Check ventilator alarms for proper functioning. Do not turn off alarms, even for suctioning. Verify that alarms can be heard in the nurses' station by care providers *to ensure care provider is alerted to emergent situation or ventilator disconnect.*

  Suction only as needed, using lowest pressure possible, *to clear secretions if client is coughing excessively, has visible secretions, or is tripping high-pressure alarm on ventilator.*

  Remove from ventilator and ventilate manually *if source of ventilator alarm cannot be quickly identified and rectified.*

  Verify that oxygen line is in proper outlet or tank; monitor in-line oxygen analyzer or perform periodic oxygen analysis *to deliver an acceptable oxygen percentage and saturation for client's specific needs.*

  Assess ventilator settings routinely and readjust, as indicated, *according to client's primary disease and results of diagnostic testing.*

  Verify tidal volume set to volume needed for individual situation and proper functioning of spirometer, bellows, or computer readout of delivered volume *to reduce risk of complications associated with alteration in lung compliance or leakage through machine or around tube cuff.*

 Diagnostic Studies   Evidence Based Practice   Medications   Pediatric/Geriatric/ Lifespan

> Monitor airway pressure for developing complications or equipment problems (e.g., increased airway resistance, retained secretions, decreased lung compliance, client out of phase or off ventilator).
>
> Promote periodic maximal ventilation of alveoli; check sigh rate intervals (usually 1 1/2 to 2 times tidal volume). *Reduces risk of atelectasis and helps mobilize secretions.*
>
> Note inspired humidity and temperature; maintain hydration *to prevent excessive drying of mucosa and secretions.*

- Auscultate breath sounds periodically. Note frequent crackles or rhonchi that do not clear with coughing or suctioning. *May indicate developing complications (e.g., atelectasis, pneumonia, acute bronchospasm, pulmonary edema).*
- Note changes in chest symmetry. *May indicate improper placement of endotracheal tube or development of barotrauma.*
- Keep resuscitation bag at bedside *to allow for manual ventilation whenever indicated (e.g., if client is removed from ventilator or troubleshooting equipment problems).*
- Administer and monitor response to medications that promote airway patency and gas exchange *to determine efficacy and need for change.*
- Administer sedation, as required, *to synchronize respirations and reduce work of breathing and energy expenditure.*
- Refer to NDs ineffective Airway Clearance, ineffective Breathing Pattern, and impaired Gas Exchange for related interventions.

NURSING PRIORITY NO. 3   To prepare for/assist with weaning process if appropriate:

- Determine client's physical and psychological readiness to wean soon after intubation, whenever possible, *to limit complications associated with long-term mechanical ventilation. Successful weaning is based on parameters such as (1) evidence for some reversal of the underlying cause of respiratory failure, (2) adequate oxygenation and normal pH, (3) hemodynamic stability, (4) capability and willingness to initiate inspiratory effort, (5) absence of excessive secretions, and (6) nutritional status sufficient to maintain work of breathing.*[1–4,5,7,9]
- Determine mode for weaning. *Recent studies indicate that pressure support mode or multiple daily T-piece trials may be superior to IMV, low-level pressure support may be beneficial for spontaneous breathing trials, and early extubation and institution of noninvasive positive pressure ventilation may have substantial benefits in alert, cooperative client.*[2,4,5]
- Explain to client/SO weaning activities and techniques, individual plan, and expectations. *Reduces fear of unknown, provides opportunities to deal with concerns, clarifies reality of fears, and helps reduce anxiety to a more manageable level.*[3,7]
- Engage client in specialized exercise program *to enhance respiratory muscle strength and general endurance.*
- Maximize weaning effort:

> Elevate head of bed/place in orthopedic chair, if possible, or position *to alleviate dyspnea and to facilitate oxygenation.*
>
> Coach client in "taking control" of breathing during weaning periods (e.g., to take slower, deeper breaths; practice abdominal or pursed-lip breathing; assume position of comfort) *to maximize respiratory function and reduce anxiety.*
>
> Instruct in or assist client to perform effective coughing techniques. *Necessary for secretion management after extubation.*
>
> Provide quiet environment, calm approach, and undivided attention of nurse. *Promotes relaxation, decreasing energy and oxygen requirements.*
>
> Involve family/SO(s) as appropriate. Provide diversionary activity. *Helps client focus on something other than breathing.*
>
> Instruct client in use of energy-saving techniques during care activities *to limit oxygen consumption and fatigue associated with work of breathing.*

 Acute Care   Collaborative   Community/Home Care   Cultural

- Acknowledge and provide ongoing encouragement for client's efforts. Communicate hope for successful weaning response (even partial). *Emotional support can enhance client's commitment to continue weaning activity, maximizing outcomes.*

NURSING PRIORITY NO. 4 To prepare for discharge on ventilator when indicated:

- Ascertain plan for discharge placement (e.g., return home, short-term admission to subacute or rehabilitation center, permanent placement in extended-care facility). *Helps to determine care needs and fiscal impact of home care versus extended-care facility.*
- Review layout of home, noting size of rooms, doorways, placement of furniture, and number and type of electrical outlets *to identify necessary modifications and safety needs.*
- Determine specific equipment needs and resources for equipment and maintenance. Arrange for delivery before client discharge *to allow SO/caregivers to prepare for transfer.*
- Allow sufficient opportunity for SO(s)/family to practice new skills. Role-play potential crisis situations *to enhance confidence in ability to handle client's needs.*
- Demonstrate airway management techniques and proper equipment cleaning practices *to reduce risk of infection.*
- Instruct SO(s)/caregivers in pulmonary physiotherapy measures, as indicated. Refer for home respiratory therapy support, as needed.
- Provide positive feedback and encouragement for efforts of SO(s)/caregivers. *Promotes continuation of desired behaviors.*
- List names and phone numbers for identified contact persons and resources. *Can reduce sense of isolation and enhance likelihood of obtaining assistance and support when needed.*
- Review and provide written or audiovisual materials regarding proper ventilator management, maintenance, and safety for reference in home setting. *Provides information to enhance client's/SO's level of comfort with challenging tasks.*
- Identify signs/symptoms requiring prompt medical evaluation or intervention. *Timely treatment may prevent progression of problem or untoward complications.*
- Obtain no-smoking signs to be posted in home, and remind family members to refrain from smoking *to reduce risk of fire.*
- Have family/SO(s) notify utility company and fire department of presence of ventilator in home. *Client will be placed in high-risk list for follow-up in case of power outage or fire.*

NURSING PRIORITY NO. 5 To promote wellness (Teaching/Discharge Considerations):

- Discuss impact of specific activities on respiratory status and problem-solve solutions *to maximize weaning effort or to reduce incidence of respiratory distress or failure.*
- Monitor health of visitors and persons involved in care *to protect client from sources of infection.*
- Encourage time-out or respite for caregivers *so they may attend to personal needs, wellness, and growth.* Refer to ND risk for caregiver Role Strain.
- Provide opportunities for client/SO(s) to discuss advance directives. *Clarifies parameters for termination of therapy or other end-of-life decisions, as desired.*
- Recommend involvement in support group; introduce to other ventilator-dependent individuals who are successfully managing home ventilation, if desired, *to answer questions, provide role model, assist with problem-solving, and offer encouragement and hope for the future.*

DOCUMENTATION FOCUS

Assessment/Reassessment
- Baseline findings, subsequent alterations in respiratory function.
- Results of diagnostic testing.
- Individual risk factors and concerns.

 Diagnostic Studies   Evidence Based Practice   Medications   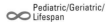 Pediatric/Geriatric/Lifespan

Planning
- Plan of care and who is involved in planning.
- Teaching plan.

Implementation/Evaluation
- Client's/other's responses to interventions, teaching, and actions performed.
- Skill level and assistance needs of SO(s)/family.
- Attainment or progress toward desired outcome(s).
- Modifications to plan of care.

Discharge Planning
- Discharge plan, including appropriate referrals, action taken, and who is responsible for each action.
- Equipment needs and source.
- Resources for support persons or home-care providers.

References

1. Epstein, S. K. (2002). Weaning from mechanical ventilation. *Respir Care*, 47(4), 454–466.
2. MacIntyre, N. R. (2001). Evidence-based guidelines for weaning and discontinuation of ventilatory support. *Chest*, 120(6 Suppl), S385–S484.
3. Tasota, F. J., Dobbin, D. (2000). Weaning your patient from mechanical ventilation. *Nursing*, 30(10), 41–46.
4. Stawicki, S. P. (2007). Mechanical ventilation: Weaning and extubation. *OPUS 12 Scientist*, 1(2), 13–16.
5. Fayyaz, J., Lessnau, K.-D. (Updated 2017). Hypoventilation syndromes. Retrieved May 2018 from http://emedicine .medscape.com/article/304381-overview.
6. D'Arcy, Y. (2007). Eye on capnography. *Men Nurs*, 2(2), 25–29.
7. Amitai, A., et al. (Updated 2017). Ventilator management. Retrieved May 2018 from http://emedicine.medscape.com/ article/810126-overview.
8. Bausewein, C., et al. (2007). Measurement of breathlessness in advanced disease: A systematic review. *Resp Med*, 101(3), 399–410.
9. Parker, L. C. (2012). Top 10 care essentials for ventilator patients: Evidence-based interventions and teamwork are crucial when caring for patients on mechanical ventilation. Retrieved May 2018 from http://www.medscape.com/viewarticle/761358_2.

dysfunctional Ventilatory Weaning Response

Taxonomy II: Activity/Rest—Class 4 Cardiovascular/Pulmonary Responses (00034) [**Diagnostic Division:** Respiration], Approved 1992; Revised 2017

DEFINITION: Inability to adjust to lowered levels of mechanical ventilator support that interrupts and prolongs the weaning process.

RELATED FACTORS
Physiological
Ineffective airway clearance
Alteration in sleep pattern; [fatigue]
Inadequate nutrition
Pain
Psychological
Insufficient knowledge of the weaning process
Uncertainty about ability to wean; [unprepared for weaning attempt]
Decrease in motivation; low self-esteem
Anxiety; fear; insufficient trust in healthcare professionals
Hopelessness; powerlessness
Situational
Uncontrolled episodic energy demands

 Acute Care   Collaborative 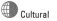 Community/Home Care Cultural

Inappropriate pace of weaning process
Insufficient social support
Environmental barrier [e.g., distractions, low nurse to patient ratio, unfamiliar healthcare staff]

DEFINING CHARACTERISTICS

Mild
Subjective
Perceived need for increase in oxygen; breathing discomfort; fatigue, warmth
Fear of machine malfunction
Objective
Restlessness
Mild increase of respiratory rate from baseline
Increase in focus on breathing

Moderate
Subjective
Apprehensiveness
Objective
Increase in blood pressure (<20 mmHg)/heart rate (<20 beats/min) from baseline
Moderate increase in respiratory rate over baseline; minimal use of respiratory accessory muscles; decrease in air entry on auscultation
Hyperfocused on activities; facial expression of fear
Impaired ability to cooperate or respond to coaching
Diaphoresis
Abnormal skin color

Severe
Objective
Agitation; decrease in level of consciousness
Deterioration in arterial blood gases from baseline
Increase in blood pressure (≥20 mmHg)/heart rate (≥20 beats/min) from baseline
Significant increase in respiratory rate above baseline; use of significant respiratory accessory muscles; shallow breathing; gasping breaths; paradoxical abdominal breathing
Adventitious breath sounds
Asynchronized breathing with the ventilator
Profuse diaphoresis
Abnormal skin color
Associated Condition: History of unsuccessful weaning attempt
History of ventilator dependence >4 days
Sample Clinical Applications: Traumatic brain injury, stroke, substance overdose, chronic obstructive pulmonary disease (COPD), crushing chest trauma, respiratory or cardiac arrest

DESIRED OUTCOMES/EVALUATION CRITERIA

Sample **NOC** linkages:
Mechanical Ventilation Weaning Response: Adult: Respiratory and psychological adjustment to progressive removal of mechanical ventilation
Respiratory Status: Ventilation: Movement of air in and out of the lungs

(continues on page 942)

 Diagnostic Studies   Evidence Based Practice   Medications   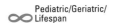 Pediatric/Geriatric/Lifespan

dysfunctional Ventilatory Weaning Response (continued)

Respiratory Status: Gas Exchange: Alveolar exchange of carbon dioxide and oxygen to maintain arterial blood gas concentrations

Client Will (Include Specific Time Frame)
- Actively participate in the weaning process.
- Reestablish independent respiration with arterial blood gases (ABGs) within client's normal range and be free of signs of respiratory failure.
- Demonstrate increased tolerance for activity and participate in self-care within level of ability.

ACTIONS/INTERVENTIONS

Sample NIC linkages:

Mechanical Ventilation Management: Invasive: Assisting the patient receiving artificial breathing support through a device inserted into the trachea

Mechanical Ventilatory Weaning: Assisting the patient to breathe without the aid of a mechanical ventilator

Energy Management: Regulating energy use to treat or prevent fatigue and optimize function

---

NURSING PRIORITY NO. 1   To identify contributing factors/degree of dysfunction:

- Determine extent and nature of underlying disorders or factors (e.g., respiratory pump insufficiency [control of breathing, respiratory muscles, lung/chest wall mechanics or, rarely, gas exchange], cardiovascular dysfunction, neuromuscular disorders, psychological factors [such as depressive disorders or delirium] as well as metabolic/endocrine diseases, alone or combined) *that contribute to client's reliance on mechanical support, thus affecting weaning efforts.*[7] *Note: Recent studies have reported on various predictors of weaning outcome, which included maximal inspiratory pressure, rapid shallow breathing index, fluid balance, comorbidity burden, severity of illness, emphysematous changes, and low serum albumin. Age, in and of itself, was not a predictor of weaning from mechanical ventilation in six studies.*[4]
- Note length of time client has been on ventilator. Review previous episodes of extubation and reintubation. *Previous unsuccessful weaning attempts (e.g., due to inability to protect airway or clear secretions; oxygen saturation less than 50% on room air) can influence weaning interventions. Although most individuals remain on the ventilator for 7 days or less, some require support for several weeks or more. Note studies have shown that if client fails to wean from ventilator dependence within 60 days, he/she will probably not do so later.*[1,8,15]
- Complete Burns Weaning Assessment Program (BWAP) or similar checklist (e.g., stability of vital signs, factors that increase metabolic rate [e.g., sepsis, fever]; hydration status; need for or recent use of analgesia or sedation; nutritional state, muscle strength, and activity level) *to assess systemic parameters that may affect readiness for weaning. Note: A recent study of the use of BWAP score in five adult critical care units found that a score of 50 or higher was linked to successful weaning outcomes.*[1,2,9–11,13]
- Ascertain client's awareness and understanding of weaning process, expectations, and concerns. *Client/significant other (SO) may need specific and repeated instructions during process to allay fears and enhance cooperation. Unrealistic expectations or unvoiced concerns can impair weaning process or willingness to participate.*
- Determine psychological readiness and presence/degree of anxiety. *Weaning provokes anxiety regarding ability to breathe on own and likelihood of ventilator dependence. The client must be highly motivated, be able to actively participate in the weaning process, and be physically comfortable enough to work at weaning.*[3]
- Review lab studies, such as complete blood count, *to determine number and integrity of red blood cells for oxygen transport;* electrolytes; and nutritional markers, such as serum protein and albumin, *to determine if client has sufficient nutritional stores to meet demands of spontaneous breathing and weaning.*[13,10]

 Acute Care   Collaborative   Community/ Home Care   Cultural

• ✏️▤ Review chest radiograph, pulse oximetry or ABGs, and/or capnometry. *Before weaning attempts, chest radiograph should show clear lungs or marked improvement in pulmonary congestion. ABGs should document satisfactory oxygenation on an FIO_2 of 40% or less. Capnometry measures end-tidal carbon dioxide values and can be used to confirm correct placement of endotracheal tube and monitor integrity of ventilation equipment.*[3,8]

NURSING PRIORITY NO. 2 To support weaning process:

• Discuss with client/SO individual plan and expectations. *May reduce client's anxiety about process and ultimate outcome and support willingness to work at spontaneous breathing trials.*

• ⊘▤ Consult with dietitian and nutritional support team for adjustments in composition of diet prior to weaning *to support respiratory muscle strength and work of breathing and to prevent excessive production of CO_2, which could alter respiratory drive. Individuals on long-term ventilation may require enteral feedings with high intake of carbohydrates, protein, and calories to improve respiratory muscle function.*[3,8]

• ⊘▤ Collaborate in implementing weaning protocols and mode (e.g., spontaneous breathing trials, automatic tube compensation, partial client support by means of synchronized intermittent mandatory ventilation, pressure support ventilation during client's spontaneous breathing) *to optimize the work of breathing and to provide support for spontaneous ventilation.*[4,7,10–12]

• Note response to activity or client care during weaning and limit, as indicated. Provide undisturbed rest or sleep periods. Avoid stressful procedures or situations and nonessential activities *to prevent excessive oxygen consumption or demand with increased possibility of weaning failure.*

• Discuss impact of specific activities on respiratory status, and problem-solve solutions to maximize weaning effort.

• 💊 Time medications during weaning efforts *to minimize sedative effects.*

• Provide quiet room, calm approach, and undivided attention. *Enhances relaxation, thereby conserving energy.*

• Involve SO(s)/family, as appropriate (e.g., sit at bedside, provide encouragement, help monitor client status).

• Provide diversionary activity (e.g., watching TV, listening to audiobooks, music) *to focus attention away from breathing when not actively working at breathing exercises.*

• Acknowledge and provide ongoing encouragement for client's efforts.

• Minimize setbacks and focus client attention on gains and progress to date *to reduce frustration that may further impair progress.*

NURSING PRIORITY NO. 3 To prepare for discharge on ventilator when indicated:

• 🏠⊘▤ Prepare client/SO for alternative actions when client is unable to resume spontaneous ventilation (e.g., tracheostomy with long-term ventilation support in alternate care setting or home, palliative care or end-of-life procedures). *Numerous studies report that despite meeting all weaning criteria and succeeding in a weaning trial, failure of planned extubation occurs in about 10% to 20% of cases.*[15] *Therefore long-term strategies may be required. Client discharged from intensive care unit may sent to specialized units (so-called long-term acute care), extended care facilities, or home. Customized discharge planning for people new to home ventilation is essential. This must include assessment of the environment, assessment of resources, assessment of caregivers, education and training, and a plan of care.*[5,7,14]

• Ascertain that all needed equipment is in place, caregivers are trained, and safety concerns have been addressed (e.g., alternative power source, backup equipment, client call or alarm system, established means of client/caregiver communication) *to ease the transfer when client is going home on ventilator.*

• Evaluate caregiver capabilities and burden when client requires long-term ventilator in the home *to determine potential or presence of skill-related problems or emotional issues (e.g., caregiver overload, burnout, or depression). Note: All home caregivers (professionals, family, friends) should receive a comprehensive orientation before caring for someone using a home ventilator. This includes familiarization with the ventilator; alarms and the subsequent actions that must be taken; tracheostomy care; safe transfer of the ventilator user; suctioning techniques; and bag-valve-mask ventilation (use of an Ambu bag) in the case of an emergency, such as accidental disconnection of the ventilator circuit.*[6,14]

• Refer to ND impaired spontaneous Ventilation for additional interventions.

 Diagnostic Studies   Evidence Based Practice   Medications   Pediatric/Geriatric/ Lifespan

NURSING PRIORITY NO. 4 To promote optimal ventilation (Teaching/Discharge Considerations):

- Encourage client/SO(s) to evaluate impact of ventilatory dependence on their lifestyle and what changes they are willing or unwilling to make when client is discharged on ventilator. *Quality-of-life issues must be examined, including issues of privacy and intimacy, and resolved by the ventilator-dependent client and SO(s). All parties need to understand that ventilatory support is a 24-hr job that ultimately affects everyone.*[14]
  A recent study of 160 caregivers (age, 50–53 years) of clients receiving home mechanical ventilation reported insufficient sleep, physical exhaustion, back pain, and significantly higher physical burden levels than respiratory care ward caregivers. Findings may dictate alternative placement is desirable or needed.[16]
- Discuss importance of time for self and identify appropriate sources for respite care. *Initially, caregivers have limited understanding of the magnitude of the demands on their time and energy. Knowing support is available enhances coping abilities.* Refer to ND risk for caregiver Role Strain.
- Emphasize to client/SO(s) importance of monitoring health of visitors and persons involved in care, avoiding crowds during flu season, obtaining immunizations, etc., *to protect client from sources of infection.*
- Engage in rehabilitation program *to enhance respiratory muscle strength and general endurance or to compensate for deficits.*
- Encourage client/SO(s) to discuss advance directives and ascertain that all care providers are aware of the plan of care. *Clarifies parameters for emergency situations, termination of therapy, or other end-of-life decisions, as desired.*
- Recommend involvement in support group (may be online) and introduce to other ventilator-dependent individuals who are successfully managing home ventilation, if desired, *to answer questions, provide role models, assist with problem-solving, and offer encouragement and hope for the future.*
- Identify conditions requiring immediate medical intervention *to treat developing complications and potentially prevent respiratory failure.*

DOCUMENTATION FOCUS

Assessment/Reassessment
- Baseline findings and subsequent alterations.
- Results of diagnostic testing and procedures.
- Individual risk factors.

Planning
- Plan of care, specific interventions, and who is involved in the planning.
- Teaching plan.

Implementation/Evaluation
- Client response to interventions.
- Attainment or progress toward desired outcome(s).
- Modifications to plan of care.

Discharge Planning
- Status at discharge, long-term needs and referrals, indicating who is to be responsible for each action.
- Equipment needs and supplier.

References

1. Ambrosino, N., Gabbrielli, L. (2010). The difficult-to-wean patient. Retrieved May 2018 from https://www.medscape.com/viewarticle/730317_7.
2. MacIntyre, N. R., et al. (2001). Evidence-based guidelines for weaning and discontinuation of ventilatory support. *Chest*, 120(6 Suppl), S375–S395.
3. Frakes, M. A. (2001). Measuring end-tidal carbon dioxide: Clinical applications and usefulness. *Crit Care Nurse*, 21(5), 23–35.
4. Stieff, K.V., Lim, F., Chen, L. (2017). Factors influencing weaning older adults from mechanical ventilation: An integrative review. *Crit Care Nurs Q*, 40(2), 165–177.

 Acute Care   Collaborative   Community/Home Care   Cultural

5. Iregui, M., et al. (2002). Determinants of outcome for patients admitted to a long-term ventilator unit. *South Med J*, 95(3), 310–317.

6. Douglas, S. L., Daly, B. J. (2003). Caregivers of long-term ventilator patients: Physical and psychological outcomes. *Chest*, 123, 1073–1081.

7. Perren, A., Brochard, L. (2013). Managing the apparent and hidden difficulties of weaning from mechanical ventilation. *Intensive Care Med*, 39, 1885–1895.

8. McLean, S. E., et al. (2006). Improving adherence to a mechanical ventilation weaning protocol for critically ill adults: Outcomes after an implementation program. *Am J Crit Care*, 15(3), 299–309.

9. Burns, S. M. (2005). Mechanical ventilation of clients with acute respiratory distress syndrome and patents requiring weaning: The evidence guiding practice. *Crit Care Nurse*, 25(4), 14–24.

10. Epstein, C. D., Peerless, J. R. (2006). Weaning readiness and fluid balance in older critically ill surgical clients. *Am J Crit Care*, 15(1), 54–64.

11. Stawicki, S. P. (2007). Mechanical ventilation: Weaning and extubation. *OPUS 12 Scientist*, 1(2), 13–16.

12. Unoki, T., Serita, A., Grap, M. J. (2008). Automatic tube compensation during weaning from mechanical ventilation: Evidence and clinical implications. *Crit Care Nurs*, 28(4), 34–42.

13. Burns, S. M., Fisher, C., Tribble, S. S. E. (2010). Multifactor clinical score and outcome of mechanical ventilation weaning trials: Burns Wean Assessment Program. *Am J Crit Care*, 19(431), 439.

14. Stuban, S. L. (2010). Home mechanical ventilation. *Am J Nurs*, 110(5), 63–67.

15. Thille, A. W., Cortes-Puch, I., Estaban, A. (2017). Weaning from the ventilator and extubation in ICU. *Curr Opin Crit Care*, 19(1), 57–64.

16. Liu, J. F., et al. (2017). Burden on caregivers of ventilator-dependent patients: A cross-sectional study. *Medicine*, 96(27), e7396.

risk for other-directed Violence

Taxonomy II: Safety/Protection—Class 3 Violence (00138) [**Diagnostic Division:** Safety], Approved 1980; Revised 1996, 2013, 2017

DEFINITION: Susceptible to behaviors in which an individual demonstrates that he or she can be physically, emotionally, or sexually harmful to others.

RISK FACTORS
Suicidal behavior; impulsiveness; access to weapon

Negative body language [e.g., rigid posture, clenching of fists/jaw, pacing, threatening stances]; suicidal behavior

Pattern of violent anti-social behavior

Pattern of indirect violence [e.g., tearing objects off walls, urinating/defecating on floor, temper tantrum] or other-directed violence [e.g., hitting/kicking/spitting/scratching others, throwing objects, sexual molestation]; threatening violence [e.g., verbal threats against property/people, threatening notes/gestures]

At Risk Population: History of childhood abuse; witnessing family violence

History of cruelty to animals; fire-setting; motor vehicle offense

History of substance misuse [abuse]

Associated Condition: Alteration in cognitive functioning; neurological impairment; psychotic disorder [panic states; rage reactions; manic excitement]

Pathological intoxication [toxic reaction to pharmaceutical agent]

Prenatal or perinatal complications

Sample Clinical Applications: Psychotic conditions (e.g., schizophrenia, paranoia), antisocial personality disorder, dementia, substance abuse (e.g., phencyclidine [PCP], delirium tremens), postpartum psychosis, premenstrual syndrome [PMS], brain injured

[****Note: NANDA has separated the diagnosis of Violence with its two elements—other-directed and self-directed. However, the interventions in general address both situations and have been left in one block following the Desired Outcomes section of risk for self-directed Violence.]

 Diagnostic Studies   Evidence Based Practice   Medications   Pediatric/Geriatric/Lifespan

risk for self-directed Violence

Taxonomy II: Safety/Protection—Class 3 Violence (00140) [**Diagnostic Division:** Safety], Approved 1994; Revised 2013, 2017

DEFINITION: Susceptible to behaviors in which an individual demonstrates that he or she can be physically, emotionally, or sexually harmful to self.

RISK FACTORS

Behavioral clues [e.g., writing forlorn love notes, giving away personal items, taking out a large life insurance policy]

Conflict about sexual orientation; engagement in autoerotic sexual acts

Conflict in interpersonal relationship(s); employment concern

Insufficient personal resources [e.g., achievement, insight, affect unavailable and poorly controlled]; social isolation

Suicidal ideation; verbal cues of suicidal intent [e.g., talking about death, "better off without me," asking about lethal dosages of medication]; suicidal plan

At Risk Population: Age 15 to 19, ≥45

Marital status; pattern of difficulties in family background; occupation [e.g., executive, professional, semi-skilled worker]

History of multiple suicide attempts

Associated Condition: Mental health issue [e.g., substance abuse]; psychological disorder [e.g., depression, psychosis, severe personality disorder]; physical disorder

Sample Clinical Applications: Major depression, postpartum depression/psychosis, Munchausen syndrome, psychosis, substance abuse (e.g., phencyclidine [PCP]), abuse or neglect

DESIRED OUTCOMES/EVALUATION CRITERIA (FOR OTHER-/SELF-DIRECTED VIOLENCE)

Sample NOC linkages:

Aggression Self-Restraint: Personal actions to refrain from assaultive, combative, or destructive behaviors toward others

Abusive Behavior Self-Restraint: Personal actions to refrain from abusive and neglectful behaviors toward others

Impulse Self-Control: Self-restraint of compulsive or impulsive behaviors

Depression Self-Control: Personal actions to minimize melancholy and maintain interest in life events

Client Will (Include Specific Time Frame)
- Acknowledge realities of the situation.
- Verbalize understanding of why behavior occurs.
- Identify precipitating factors in individual situation.
- Express realistic self-evaluation and increased sense of self-esteem.
- Participate in care and meet own needs in an assertive manner.
- Demonstrate self-control as evidenced by relaxed posture, nonviolent behavior or verbalizations.
- Use resources and support systems in an effective manner.

 Acute Care
 Collaborative
 Community/Home Care
 Cultural

ACTIONS/INTERVENTIONS (ADDRESSES BOTH OTHER- AND SELF-DIRECTED)

Sample **NIC** linkages:

Anger Control Assistance: Facilitation of the expression of anger in an adaptive, nonviolent manner

Environmental Management: Violence Prevention: Monitoring and manipulation of the physical environment to decrease the potential for violent behavior directed toward self, others, or environment

Behavior Management: Self-Harm: Assisting the patient to decrease or eliminate self-mutilating or self-abusive behaviors

NURSING PRIORITY NO. 1   To assess causative/contributing factors:

- Determine underlying dynamics as listed in Risk Factors.
- Identify conditions, such as acute or chronic brain syndrome, panic state, hormonal imbalance, premenstrual syndrome, postpartum psychosis, drug-induced psychotic states, and postanesthesia or postseizure confusion, *that may interfere with ability to control own behavior and lead to violent episodes.*[1,12]
- Review lab findings (e.g., blood alcohol, drug/tox screen, blood glucose, arterial blood gases, electrolytes, renal function tests). *Provides information about possible treatable sources of behavior.*[2,6]
- Ascertain client's perception of self and situation. Note use of defense mechanisms. *Individuals who are prone to violent behavior may see themselves as victims (denial), may blame others (projection), may not follow social norms, and may be impulsive.*[1]
- Observe and listen for early cues of distress or increasing anxiety. *Behaviors, such as irritability, lack of cooperation, and demanding behavior, and body posture or expression may signal escalating potential for violent behavior and need for immediate intervention.*[1,6]
- Observe for signs of suicidal or homicidal intent. *Perceived morbid or anxious feelings while with the client; warning from the client, "It doesn't matter," "I'd/They'd be better off dead"; mood swings; "accident-prone" or self-destructive behavior; and possession of alcohol or other drug(s) by known substance abuser needs to be noted, taken seriously, and treated appropriately.*[1,6] Refer to ND risk for Suicide.
- Note family history of suicidal or homicidal behavior. *Dynamics in family of origin and current family and parental deprivation or abuse in the early years of an individual's life may contribute to violent behavior in current situation as individual uses violence as a means of solving problems.*[1,10]
- Ask directly if the person is thinking of acting on thoughts or feelings. *Can determine reality and urgency of violent intent and importance of immediate intervention.*[6]
- Determine availability of suicidal means. *Identifies urgency of situation and need to intervene by removing lethal means, possibly hospitalizing client, or instituting other measures to ensure safety of client and others.*[1,6,8]
- Assess client coping behaviors. *Client believes there are no alternatives other than violence and has been dealing with frustration and anger in unacceptable ways (yelling, hitting, other violent behaviors) and needs to learn alternative coping skills.*[1,9]
- Identify risk factors and assess for indicators of child abuse or neglect (e.g., unexplained or frequent injuries, failure to thrive). *Visible evidence of physical abuse or neglect makes it more easily recognized; however, behaviors of withdrawal and acting out may also signal the presence of abuse.*[6,9,12]
- Determine presence, extent, and acceptance of violence in the client's culture. *Youth violence has become a national concern with widely publicized school shootings and an increase in arrests of both boys and girls for violent crimes and weapons violations. Young people who are at risk for violence need to be identified, and positive programs aimed at promoting emotional wellness need to be instituted in schools, parent education meetings, churches, and community centers.*[3,7,11]

 Diagnostic Studies   Evidence Based Practice   Medications   Pediatric/Geriatric/ Lifespan

NURSING PRIORITY NO. 2 To assist client to accept responsibility for impulsive behavior and potential for violence:

• Develop therapeutic nurse-client relationship. Provide consistent caregiver when possible. *Promotes sense of trust, allowing client to discuss feelings openly and to begin to identify sources of anger and more acceptable ways of dealing with it.*[1,6]

• Maintain straightforward communication. *Avoids reinforcing manipulative behavior. Manipulation is used for management of powerlessness because of distrust of others, fear of loss of power or control, fear of intimacy, and search for approval.*[4,6]

• Discuss motivation for change (e.g., failing relationships, job loss, involvement with judicial system). *Crisis situation can provide impetus for change but requires timely therapeutic intervention to sustain efforts.*[7,8]

• Make time to listen to expressions of feelings. Acknowledge reality of client's feelings and that feelings are okay. (Refer to ND Self-Esteem, specify.) *Promotes understanding of how feelings lead to actions and that individual is responsible for controlling behavior in acceptable ways.*[6]

• Help client recognize that client's actions may be in response to his/her fear (may be afraid of own behavior, loss of control), dependency, and feeling of powerlessness. *Promotes understanding of self and ability to deal with feelings in acceptable ways.*[6,13]

• Confront client's tendency to minimize situation or behavior. *Individuals often want to say that things "are not as bad" as portrayed. By confronting this minimization, the reality of the situation can be brought out and discussed, leading to better understanding of the situation and changes in behavior.*[1,6]

• Identify feelings or events (e.g., individual's view of self, hallucinations, individual/family or peer conflict, aggressive behavior) involved in precipitating violent behavior. *By identifying the factors involved in current situation, an appropriate plan can be made to change actions to prevent future violent behavior.*[1,7]

• Discuss impact of behavior on others and consequences of actions. *Discussing these issues openly can help client to develop empathy and understand other person's reactions and begin to change behaviors that can lead to violence.*[5,8]

• Acknowledge reality of suicide or homicide as an option. Discuss consequences of actions if they were to follow through on intent. Ask how it will help client to resolve problems. *Acknowledging the reality of individual's thoughts provides opportunity to look at how actions would affect others, ability to control own behavior, and make choices to live and make a better life for self.*[6,11]

• Accept client's anger without reacting on emotional basis. Give permission to express angry feelings in acceptable ways and let client know that staff will be available to assist in maintaining control. *Promotes acceptance and sense of safety. Client's anger is usually directed at the situation and not at the caregiver, and by remaining separate, the therapist can be more helpful for resolution of the anger.*[6,9]

• Help client identify more appropriate solutions/behaviors. *Motor activities or exercise can lessen sense of anxiety and associated physical manifestations, thus diminishing feelings of anger.*[8]

• Provide directions for actions client can take, avoiding negatives, such as "do nots." *Discussing positive ideas to help client begin to look toward a better future can provide hope that violent behaviors can be changed, promoting feelings of self-worth and belief in control of own self.*[5,13]

NURSING PRIORITY NO. 3 To assist client in controlling behavior:

• Contract with client regarding safety of self/others. *Making a contract in which the individual agrees to refrain from any violent behavior for a specified period of time, from Day 1 through the entire course of treatment, and that is written and signed by each party may help the client to follow through with therapy to find more effective ways of resolving conflict. Although there is little research on the effectiveness of these contracts, they are frequently used.*[6,7]

• Give client as much control as possible within constraints of individual situation. *Because control issues are a factor in violent behavior, giving client control in appropriate ways can enhance self-esteem and promote confidence in ability to change behavior.*[7]

 Acute Care   Collaborative   Community/ Home Care   Cultural

- Be truthful when giving information and dealing with individual. *Builds trust, enhancing therapeutic relationship, and prevents manipulative behavior.*[5]
- Identify current and past successes and strengths. Discuss effectiveness of coping techniques used and possible changes. Refer to ND ineffective Coping. *Client is often not aware of positive aspects of life, and once recognized, they can be used as a basis for change.*[8]
- Give positive reinforcement for client's efforts. *Encourages continuation of desired behaviors.*[1]
- Assist client to distinguish between reality and hallucinations or delusions. *Violent behavior in clients with major mental disorders (schizophrenia, mania) may be in response to command hallucinations and may require more aggressive treatment or hospitalization until behavior is under control.*[1,6]
- Approach in positive manner, acting as if the client has control and is responsible for own behavior. Be aware, though, that the client may not have control, especially if under the influence of drugs (including alcohol). *Individuals will often respond to a positive expectation, reducing threatening actions. Staff needs to be trained in management of this behavior and be prepared to take control of the situation if client is out of control.*[1,6]
- Maintain distance and do not touch client when situation indicates client does not tolerate such closeness. *Individuals who have experienced traumatic events, such as rape, or suffer from posttrauma response may fear close contact even with trusted persons.*[1,6]
- Remain calm and state limits on inappropriate behavior (including consequences) in a firm manner. *Calm manner enables client to de-escalate anger, and knowing what the consequences will be gives an opportunity to choose to change behavior and deal appropriately with situation. Consequences need to be decided beforehand and agreed to by client or they may sound like punishment and be counterproductive.*[1,6,12]
- Direct client to stay in view of staff, when indicated. *Intervention may be needed to maintain safety of client and others.*[1,6] Refer to ND risk for Suicide.
- [Z]Administer prescribed medications (e.g., anti-anxiety or antipsychotic), taking care not to oversedate client. *May be least restrictive way to help client control violent behaviors while learning new coping skills to handle anger and impulsive behavior. The chemistry of the brain is changed by early violence and has been shown to respond to serotonin as well as related neurotransmitter systems, which play a role in restraining aggressive impulses.*[1,6,9]
- Monitor for possible drug interactions and cumulative effects of drug regimen (e.g., anticonvulsants, antidepressants). *May be contributing factor in violent behavior.*[1,6]

NURSING PRIORITY NO. 4   To assist client/SO(s) to correct/deal with existing situation:

- Gear interventions to individual(s) involved based on age, relationship, etc. *Conflict-resolution skills can be learned by all age groups when age-appropriate materials are used.*[5,8]
- Maintain calm, matter-of-fact, nonjudgmental attitude. *Decreases defensive response, allowing individual to think about own responsibility in the conflict and choose positive behaviors instead of usual angry reaction.*[4,5,8]
- [Z] Notify potential victims in the presence of serious homicidal threat in accordance with legal and ethical guidelines. *Various Tarasoff statutes exist in many states requiring therapists/healthcare providers to report specific threats to both the individual named and law enforcement when client expresses homicidal intent overtly or covertly in addition to helping the client realize that the proposed action is not wise or in his or her own best interest.*[1]
- Discuss situation with abused or battered person, providing accurate information about choices and effective actions that can be taken. *Promotes understanding of options, giving hope and support for planning for a violence-free future.*[2]
- Assist individual to understand that angry, vengeful feelings are appropriate in the situation and need to be expressed but not acted on. (Refer to ND Post-Trauma Syndrome, as psychological responses may be very similar.) *Helps client accept feelings as natural and begin to learn effective coping skills, and promotes sense of control over situation.*[2]
- Identify resources available for assistance (e.g., battered women's shelter, social services, financial). *Helps client to manage immediate needs such as food, shelter, and safety with a long-range goal of attaining or maintaining independence and violence-free life.*[2]

NURSING PRIORITY NO. 5 To promote safety in event of violent behavior:

- Provide a safe, quiet environment and remove items from the client's environment that could be used to inflict harm to self/others. *Reducing stimuli can help client to calm down, and removing articles provides for safety of client and staff.*[1,6]
- Maintain distance from client who is striking out or hitting and take evasive or controlling actions, as indicated. *Staff safety is of prime importance, and avoiding physical confrontation until client regains control or take-down team is assembled can prevent injury.*[6]
- Call for additional staff/security personnel. *Having sufficient people available to handle the situation may defuse client's anger, allowing situation to calm down without further action. All personnel need to be trained in take-down techniques.*[6]
- Approach aggressive or attacking client from the front, just out of reach, in a commanding posture with palms down. *Safety is a prime concern, and these actions may defuse the situation.*[6]
- Tell client *"Stop"* in a firm voice. *This may be sufficient to help client control own actions.*[6]
- Maintain direct and constant eye contact when appropriate. *Assists in identifying client's intentions and conveys sense of caring. Eye contact may be perceived as threatening, so it needs to be used cautiously.*[2,6]
- Speak in a low, commanding voice. *Tone of voice conveys message of control and concern and can help to calm the client's anger.*[6]
- Provide client with a sense that caregiver is in control of the situation. *Client is feeling out of control, and seeing that staff are in control provides a feeling of safety.*[6]
- Maintain clear route for staff and client and be prepared to move quickly. *Safety for all is of prime importance, and staff may need to leave the room to regroup while continuing to protect the client. Take-down needs to be done quickly to gain control of the individual.*[6]
- Hold client, using restraints or seclusion when necessary until client regains self-control. *Brief period of physical restraint may be required until client regains control or other therapeutic interventions take effect.*[6]
- Administer medication, as indicated. *Client may require chemical restraint until control is regained.*[1,6]
- Discuss event with client after situation is calmed down and control is regained. *Helping client to understand how feelings of anger had gotten out of control and what can be done to prevent a recurrence can provide a learning opportunity for the individual.*[2,6]

NURSING PRIORITY NO. 6 To promote wellness (Teaching/Discharge Considerations):

- Promote client involvement in planning care within limits of situation, allowing for meeting own needs for enjoyment. *Individuals often believe they are not entitled to pleasure and good things in their lives and need to learn how to meet these needs in acceptable ways.*[6,13]
- Assist client to learn assertive behaviors. *Manipulative, nonassertive, or aggressive behaviors lead to anger, which can result in violence. Learning assertiveness skills can facilitate change, increase self-esteem, and promote interpersonal relationships.*[1,13]
- Provide information about conflict-resolution skills and help client learn how to use them effectively. *Conflict is always present in human relationships, and learning how to manage conflict is one of the most important tools we can use to solve disagreements and improve relationships.*[4,5,8]
- Discuss reasons for client's behavior with SO(s). Determine desire and commitment of involved parties to sustain current relationships. *Family members may believe individual is purposefully behaving in angry ways, and understanding underlying reasons for behavior can defuse feelings of anger on their part, leading to willingness to resolve problems.*[1,4]
- Develop strategies to help parents learn more effective parenting skills. *Participating in parenting classes and learning appropriate ways of dealing with frustrations can improve family relationships and prevent angry interactions and the possibility of violent behavior.*[4,5]
- Identify support systems. *Presence of family/friends and clergy who can serve as mentors and listen to individual nonjudgmentally can help client defuse angry feelings and learn appropriate ways of dealing with them.*[1]

 Acute Care   Collaborative   Community/ Home Care   Cultural

Note: Not just the client needs help; those around them also need to learn how to provide positive role models and display a broader array of skills for resolving problems.

- 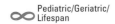 Refer to formal resources, as indicated. *May need individual or group psychotherapy, substance-abuse treatment program, anger-management class, social services, and/or safe house to facilitate change.*[1]
- Promote violence prevention and emotional literacy programs in the schools and community. *These programs are based on the premise that intelligent management of emotions is critical to successful living. Aggressive youth lack skills in arousal management and nonviolent problem-solving, which can be learned in programs and reinforced by the adults in their lives.*[7,11,13]
- Refer to NDs impaired Parenting, family Coping [specify], and Post-Trauma Syndrome.

DOCUMENTATION FOCUS

Assessment/Reassessment
- Individual findings, including nature of concern (e.g., suicidal, homicidal), behavioral risk factors, and level of impulse control, plan of action, and means to carry out plan.
- Client's perception of situation, motivation for change.
- Family history of violence.
- Availability and use of resources.

Planning
- Plan of care and who is involved in the planning.
- Details of contract regarding violence to self/others.
- Teaching plan.

Implementation/Evaluation
- Actions taken to promote safety, including notification of parties at risk.
- Response to interventions, teaching, and actions performed.
- Attainment or progress toward desired outcome(s).
- Modifications to plan of care.

Discharge Planning
- Long-term needs and who is responsible for actions to be taken.
- Available resources, specific referrals made.

References

1. Townsend, M. C. (2003). *Psychiatric Mental Health Nursing Concepts of Care*. 4th ed. Philadelphia: F. A. Davis.
2. Newfield, S. A., et al. (2007). *Cox's Clinical Applications of Nursing Diagnosis: Adult, Child, Women's, Psychiatric, Geron- tic, and Home Health Considerations*. 5th ed. Philadelphia: F. A. Davis.
3. Zoucha, R. (2006). Considering culture in understanding per- sonal violence. *J Forensic Nurs*, 4(2), 195–196.
4. Doll, L. S., et al. (ed). (2007). *Handbook of Injury and Vio- lence Prevention*. New York: Springer.
5. Stinnet, W. D. (2011). Turning conflict into cooperation. *Gor- don Training Books: Leadership Effectiveness Training*. Solano Beach, CA: Gordon Training International.
6. Doenges, M. E., Townsend, M. C., Moorhouse, M. F. (1998). *Psychiatric Care Plans: Guidelines for Individualizing Care*. 3rd ed. Philadelphia: F. A. Davis.
7. Thomas, S. P. (2003). Identifying and intervening with girls at risk for violence. *J School Nurs*, 19(3), 130–139.
8. Heathfield, S. (2011, updated 2018). Resolutions: Avoid these actions to create effective conflict resolution. Retrieved May 2018 from http://humanresources.about.com/od/ managementtips/a/conflict_solue.htm.
9. Goleman, D. (1995). Early violence leaves its mark on the brain. *New York Times*. Retrieved May 2018 from archives http://www.nytimes.com/1995/10/03/science/early-violence- leaves-its-mark-on-the-brain.html?pagewanted=1.
10. No author listed. (2014). What is neuroscience? *Psychology Career Center*. Retrieved May 2018 from https://www .psychologycareercenter.org/what-is-neuroscience.html.
11. Croft, H. (Updated 2014). Thinking about violence in our schools. *National Institute of Mental Health (NIMH)*. Retrieved May 2018 from https://www.healthyplace.com/parenting/nimh/ thinking-about-violence-in-our-schools/.
12. Roberts, A. R., Kim, J. H. (2006). Exploring the effects of head injuries among battered women. *J Soc Serv Res*, 32(1), 33–47.
13. Goleman, D. (2006). *Emotional Intelligence: Why It Matters More Than IQ*. 10th Anniversary ed. New York: Bantam.

 Diagnostic Studies   Evidence Based Practice   Medications Pediatric/Geriatric/Lifespan

impaired Walking

Taxonomy II: Activity/Rest—Class 2 Activity/Exercise (00088) [Diagnostic Division: Activity/Rest], Approved 1998; Revised 2006, 2017

DEFINITION: Limitation of independent movement within the environment on foot.
[*** Specify level of independence using a standardized functional scale.]

RELATED FACTORS

Insufficient muscle strength
Decrease in endurance; physical deconditioning
Fear of falling
Pain
Obesity
Alteration in mood
Insufficient knowledge of mobility strategies
Environmental barrier

DEFINING CHARACTERISTICS

Subjective or Objective
Impaired ability to walk required distance, walk on incline or decline, walk on uneven surface, navigate curbs, climb stairs
Associated Condition: Alteration in cognitive functioning
Musculoskeletal, neuromuscular functioning
Impaired balance, vision
Sample Clinical Applications: Arthritis, obesity, amputation, brain injury, stroke, traumatic injury, fractures, chronic pain, peripheral vascular disease (PVD), spinal nerve compression, multiple sclerosis (MS), cerebral palsy, Parkinson's disease, macular degeneration, dementia

DESIRED OUTCOMES/EVALUATION CRITERIA

Sample NOC linkages:
Ambulation: Personal actions to walk from place to place independently with or without assistive device
Mobility: Ability to move purposefully in own environment independently with or without assistive device
Balance: Ability to maintain body equilibrium

Client Will (Include Specific Time Frame)
• Be able to move about within environment as needed or desired within limits of ability or with appropriate adjuncts.
• Verbalize understanding of situation, risk factors, and safety measures.

ACTIONS/INTERVENTIONS

Sample NIC linkages:
Exercise Therapy: Ambulation: Promotion and assistance with walking to maintain or restore autonomic and voluntary body functions during treatment and recovery from illness or injury
Body Mechanics Promotion: Facilitating the use of posture and movement in daily activities to prevent fatigue and musculoskeletal strain or injury
Exercise Therapy: Balance: Use of specific activities, postures, and movements to maintain, enhance, or restore balance

 Acute Care
 Collaborative
 Community/Home Care
 Cultural

NURSING PRIORITY NO. 1   To assess causative/contributing factors:

- Identify conditions or diagnoses (e.g., advanced age, sensory impairments, pain, obesity, chronic fatigue, cognitive dysfunction, acute illness with weakness, chronic illness [e.g., cardiopulmonary disorders, cancer], musculoskeletal injuries or surgery [e.g., sprains, fractures, tendon or ligament injury; total joint replacement, surgical repair of fractured bone; amputation], balance problems [e.g., inner ear infection, brain injury, stroke], nerve disorders [e.g., MS, Parkinson's disease, cerebral palsy], spinal abnormalities [disease, trauma, degeneration], impaired circulation or neuropathies [e.g., peripheral, diabetic, alcoholic], degenerative bone or muscle disorders [e.g., osteoporosis, muscular dystrophy, myositis], foot conditions [e.g., plantar warts, bunions, ingrown toenails, pressure ulcers]) *that contribute to walking impairment and identify specific needs and appropriate interventions.*[1–6]
- Determine ability to follow directions and presence of emotional or behavioral responses *that may be affecting client's ability or desire to engage in activity.*
- Note client's particular symptoms (e.g., unable to bear weight, can't walk usual distance, limping, staggering, stiff leg, leg pain, shuffling, asymmetric or unsteady gait; can walk on certain surfaces, but not on others). *Influences choice of interventions.*[4–6,8]

NURSING PRIORITY NO. 2   To assess functional ability:

- Perform "Timed Up and Go" (TUG) test, as indicated, to assess client's basic ability to ambulate safely. *Factors assessed include sitting balance, ability to transfer from sitting to standing and back to sitting, the pace and stability of ambulation, and the ability to turn without staggering. Additional testing is indicated for individuals requiring more than 20 sec to complete the test.*[7]
- Evaluate components of walking (e.g., gait, distance covered over time). Determine muscle strength and tone, joint mobility, cardiovascular status, balance, endurance, and use of assistive device. *Identifies strengths and deficits (e.g., ability to ambulate with/without assistive devices) and may provide information regarding potential for recovery (e.g., client with severe brain injury may have permanent limitations because of impaired cognition affecting memory, judgment, problem-solving, and motor planning, requiring more intensive inpatient and long-term care).*[6]
- Note whether impairment is temporary or permanent. *Condition may be caused by reversible condition (e.g., weakness associated with acute illness or fractures/surgery with weight-bearing restrictions), or walking impairment can be permanent (e.g., congenital anomalies, amputation, severe rheumatoid arthritis).*[6]
- Assist with or review results of mobility testing (e.g., timing of walking over fixed distance, distance walked over set period of time [endurance], limb movement analysis, leg strength and speed of walking, ambulatory activity monitoring with pedometer) *for differential diagnosis and to guide treatment interventions.*[6,7]
- Note emotional or behavioral responses of client/significant other (SO) to problems of mobility. *Walking impairments can negatively affect self-concept and self-esteem, autonomy, and independence. Social, occupational, and relationship roles can change, leading to isolation, depression, and economic consequences.*

NURSING PRIORITY NO. 3   To promote safe, optimal level of independence in walking:

- Assist with treatment of underlying condition as needed or indicated by individual situation. *Treatment can often reverse or limit dysfunction.*
- Consult with physical therapist, occupational therapist, or rehabilitation team *to develop individual program (e.g., to improve general conditioning, coordination and balance, range-of-motion exercises, specific muscle strengthening), to instruct in specific tasks (e.g., stair climbing or gait training), and to identify and develop appropriate adjunctive devices (e.g., shoe insert, leg brace for proper foot alignment; customized cane, crutches, or walker).*[1]
- Monitor client's cardiopulmonary tolerance for walking. *Increased pulse rate, chest pain, breathlessness, and irregular heartbeat is indicative of need to reduce level of activity.* Refer to ND Activity Intolerance and decreased Cardiac Output for related interventions.

 Diagnostic Studies   Evidence Based Practice   Medications   Pediatric/Geriatric/Lifespan

- Encourage adequate rest and gradual increase in walking distance *to reduce fatigue or leg pain associated with walking, and to improve stamina.*[3,4] Refer to NDs Fatigue and risk for peripheral neurovascular Dysfunction.
- Administer medication, as indicated, *to manage pain and maximize level of functioning.* Refer to NDs acute/chronic Pain; chronic Pain Syndrome.
- Implement fall precautions for high-risk clients (e.g., frail or ill elderly, visually or cognitively impaired, person on multiple medications, presence of balance disorders) *to reduce risk of accidental injury.*[3] Refer to NDs risk for Falls and risk for Disuse Syndrome for related interventions.
- Instruct in proper application of prostheses, immobilizers (e.g., walking cast or boot), and braces before walking *to maintain joint stability or immobilization or to maintain alignment during movement.*[2]
- Demonstrate and remind client to properly use assistive devices (e.g., cane, crutches, walker) *individually prescribed and fitted to improve balance, reduce limb pain and dysfunction, and provide support during ambulation.*[1]
- Use adequate personnel and safety devices (e.g., gait belt, properly fitted nonslip shoes, handrail) when ambulating *to prevent injury to client or caregivers.*[1,3,8]
- Limit distractions and provide safe environment. *Allows client to concentrate on walking activities or learning use of assistive devices.*[1]
- Provide cueing as indicated. *Client may need reminders (e.g., lift foot higher, look where going, walk tall) to concentrate on/perform tasks of walking, especially when balance or cognition is impaired.*
- Provide ample time to perform mobility-related tasks *to reduce risk of falling and manage fatigue or pain.*
- Provide positive, constructive feedback *to encourage continuation of efforts and enhance client's self-sufficiency.*[3]
- Assist client to obtain needed information, such as handicap placard for close-in parking, sources for mobility scooter, or special public transportation options, when indicated, *to deal with temporary or permanent disability access.*

NURSING PRIORITY NO. 4 To promote wellness (Teaching/Discharge Considerations):

- Evaluate client's home (or work) environment for barriers to walking (e.g., uneven surfaces, many steps, no ramps, long distances between places client needs to walk) *to determine needed changes and make recommendations for client safety.*
- Involve client/SO in problem solving, assisting them to learn ways of managing deficits, *to enhance safety for client with long-term or permanent impairments.*
- Encourage participation in regular active and passive exercise program. Advance levels of exercise, as able, *to improve muscle tone and strength and increase stamina and endurance.*
- Discuss appropriate use of electric scooter, if indicated. *Enhances mobility, especially over distances, to maintain independence and socialization.*
- Identify appropriate resources for obtaining and maintaining appliances, equipment, and environmental modifications *to promote safe mobility.*
- Instruct client/SO in safety measures in home, as individually indicated (e.g., maintaining safe travel pathway, proper lighting, wearing glasses, handrails on stairs, grab bars in bathroom, using walker instead of cane when tired or walking on uneven surface) *to reduce risk of falls.*
- Discuss need for emergency call/support system (e.g., Lifeline, HealthWatch) *to provide immediate assistance for falls and other home emergencies when client lives alone.*

DOCUMENTATION FOCUS

Assessment/Reassessment
- Individual findings, including level of function and ability to participate in specific or desired activities.
- Equipment and assistive device needs.

 Acute Care   Collaborative   Community/Home Care   Cultural

Planning

- Plan of care and who is involved in the planning.
- Teaching plan.

Implementation/Evaluation

- Responses to interventions, teaching, and actions performed.
- Attainment or progress toward desired outcome(s).
- Modifications to plan of care.

Discharge Planning

- Discharge and long-term needs, noting who is responsible for each action to be taken.
- Specific referrals made.
- Sources of and maintenance for assistive devices.

References

1. Bradley, S. M., Hernandez, C. R. (2011). Geriatric assistive devices. *Am Fam Physician*, 84(4), 405–411.
2. Teplicky, R., Law, M., Russell, D. (2002). The effectiveness of casts, orthotics, and splints for children with neurological disorders. *Infants Young Child*, 15(1), 42–50.
3. Jitramontree, N. (2001). *Evidence-Based Protocol. Exercise Promotion: Walking in Elders [Research Dissemination Core, 53].* Iowa City, IA: University of Iowa Gerontological Nursing Interventions Research Center.
4. Eberhardt, R. T. (2002). Exercise for intermittent claudication: Walking for life? [Editorial]. *J Cardiopulm Rehabil*, 22(3), 199–200.
5. No author listed. (No date). Walking disorders (various pages). Retrieved May 2018 from http://www.rightdiagnosis.com/sym/walking_disorders.htm.
6. Pearsen, O. R., Busse, M. E., van Deuresn, R. W. M. (2004). Quantification of walking mobility in neurological disorders. *Q J Med*, 97, 463–475.
7. Baer, H. R., Wolf, S. L. (2001). Modified Emory Functional Ambulation Profile: An outcome measure for the rehabilitation of poststroke gait dysfunction. *Stroke*, 32, 973–979.
8. McGuire, J. (2010). Transitional off-loading: An evidence-based approach to pressure redistribution in the diabetic foot. *Adv Skin Wound Care*, 23(4), 175–188.

Wandering [Specify Level]

Taxonomy II: Activity/Rest—Class 3 Energy Balance (00154) [**Diagnostic Division:** Safety], [Approved 2000; Revised 2017]

DEFINITION: Meandering, aimless, or repetitive locomotion that exposes the individual to harm; frequently incongruent with boundaries, limits, or obstacles.

RELATED FACTORS

Alteration in sleep-wake cycle; physiological state [e.g., hunger/thirst, cold, pain, need to urinate]
Desire to go home; separation from familiar environment
Overstimulating environment

DEFINING CHARACTERISTICS

Objective

Frequent or continuous movement from place to place; pacing
Persistent locomotion in search of something; scanning or searching behavior
Haphazard or fretful locomotion; long periods of locomotion without an apparent destination
Locomotion into unauthorized spaces; trespassing
Locomotion resulting in getting lost; eloping behavior
Impaired ability to locate landmarks in a familiar setting
Locomotion that cannot be easily dissuaded; shadowing a caregiver's locomotion

(continues on page 556)

 Diagnostic Studies   Evidence Based Practice   Medications   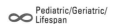 Pediatric/Geriatric/Lifespan

Wandering [Specify Level] (continued)

Hyperactivity

Periods of locomotion interspersed with periods of nonlocomotion (e.g., sitting, standing, sleeping)

At Risk Population: Premorbid behavior

Associated Condition: Alteration in cognitive functioning; cortical atrophy; psychological disorder

Sedation

Sample Clinical Applications: Brain injury, dementias, developmental delays, major depression, substance abuse, amnesia, fugue

DESIRED OUTCOMES/EVALUATION CRITERIA

Sample NOC linkage:

Physical Injury Severity: Severity of injuries from accidents and trauma

Client Will (Include Specific Time Frame)

• Be free of injury, or unplanned exits.

Sample NOC linkages:

Safe Home Environment: Physical arrangements to minimize environmental factors that might cause physical injury in the home

Safe Wandering: Safe, socially acceptable moving about without apparent purpose in an individual with cognitive impairment

Caregiver(s) Will (Include Specific Time Frame)

• Modify environment, as indicated, to enhance safety.

• Provide for maximal independence of client.

ACTIONS/INTERVENTIONS

Sample NIC linkages:

Elopement Precautions: Minimizing the risk of a patient leaving a treatment setting without authorization when departure presents a threat to the safety of patient or others

Area Restriction: Use of least restrictive limitation of patient mobility to a specified area for purposes of safety or behavior management

Environmental Management: Safety: Monitoring and manipulation of the physical environment to promote safety

---

NURSING PRIORITY NO. 1   To assess degree of impairment/stage of disease process:

• Ascertain history of client's memory loss and cognitive changes.

• ✐ 📝 Review responses of collaborative diagnostic examinations (e.g., cognition, functional capacity, behavior, memory impairments, reality orientation, general physical health, and quality of life). *A combination of tests is often needed to complete an evaluation of client's overall condition relating to chronic or irreversible condition. These tests include (but are not limited to) Mini-Mental State Examination, Alzheimer's Disease Assessment Scale cognitive subsection, Functional Assessment Questionnaire, Clinical Global Impression of Change, and Neuropsychiatric Inventory.*[1,2]

• 📝 Evaluate client's past history (e.g., individual was very active physically and socially or reacted to stress with physical activity rather than emotional reactions) *to help identify likelihood of wandering. Note: One*

 Acute Care   Collaborative   Community/Home Care   Cultural

study showed that a history of prior wandering incidents is a high predictor (72%) for further wandering incidents.[2,5]

- ∞ Note client's age. *Results of a study in selected nursing homes revealed that subjects' age was found to have significant negative correlations with the Revised Algase Wandering Scale—Nursing Home Version overall, suggesting that younger persons with dementia were likely to show more wandering behavior than older ones.*[2,6,7]
- Determine presence of depression. *Research supports the idea that wandering develops more often in depressed client with Alzheimer's disease.*[2]
- Evaluate client's mental status during both daytime and nighttime, noting when client's confusion is most pronounced and when and how long client sleeps. *Information about cognition and behavioral habits can reveal circumstances under which client is likely to wander.*[7]
- Identify client's reason for wandering, if possible. *Client may demonstrate searching behavior (e.g., looking for lost item, pursuing certain unattainable activity), inexhaustible drive to do things and remain busy, or be experiencing sensations (e.g., hunger, thirst, discomfort) without ability to express the actual need.*[2]
- Determine bowel and bladder elimination pattern, timing of incontinence, and presence of constipation *for possible correlation to wandering behavior.*
- Note timing and pattern of wandering behavior. *Client attempting to leave at 5:00 p.m. every day may believe he is going home from work; client may be goal directed (e.g., searching for person or object, escaping from something) or nongoal directed (wandering aimlessly). Knowledge of patterns can prompt caregivers to anticipate need for personal attention.*[2,5]
- Ascertain if client has delusions due to shadows, lights, and noises *to determine necessary changes to environment.*
- Evaluate usual travel patterns. *Activity may be (1) direct (from one location to another without diversion), (2) random (random direction with no obvious stopping point), (3) pacing (back and forth within limited area), or (4) lapping (circling large areas).*[2,5,6]
- Assist with or review results of specific testing (e.g., Revised Algase Wandering Scale, Need-Driven Dementia-Compromised Behavior, similar tool), as indicated. *Researchers are using adjunct tools for clinical assessment that quantify wandering in several domains (as reported by caregivers) to determine individual risks and safety needs.*[2,6]
- Monitor client's need for and use of assistive devices, such as glasses, hearing aids, cane, safe walking shoes, comfortable clothing, etc. *Wandering client is at high risk for falls due to cognitive impairments and the fatigue related to functional decline or forgetting necessary assistive devices or how to properly use them.*

NURSING PRIORITY NO. 2 To assist client/caregiver to deal with wandering:

- Provide a structured daily routine:
  Encourage participation in family activities and familiar routines, such as folding laundry, listening to music, or shared-walking time outdoors. *Activities and exercises may reduce anxiety, depression, and restlessness. Note: Repetitive activity (e.g., rocking, folding laundry, paperwork) may help client with "lapping"—wandering to reduce energy expenditure and fatigue. In addition, studies reveal that wandering may be an adaptive behavior that reflects continuity of premorbid personality traits and lifelong patterns of coping with stress.*[3,7]

  Offer food, fluids, and toileting on a regular schedule when client is unable to verbalize, *as agitation, pacing, or wandering may be associated with these basic needs.*[3]

  Sit with client and talk *when client is socially gregarious, enjoys conversation, or reminiscence is calming.*

  Provide television, radio, or music, *which may be more effective than talking or reading to decrease wandering.*[1]

  Monitor activities, loud conversations, and number of visitors at one time *to prevent overstimulation or increased agitation.*

  Remove items from immediate environment (e.g., coat, hat, keys) *to reduce stimulus for leaving the site.*

 Diagnostic Studies   Evidence Based Practice   Medications   Pediatric/Geriatric/Lifespan

- Provide safe place for client to wander:

Remove environmental safety hazards such as hot water faucets and knobs on kitchen stove, gate or block open stairways, etc.[1,2]

Keep area free of clutter and place comfortable furniture and other items against the wall or out of travel path *to accommodate safe walking and promote rest periods during times of continual lapping.*[1]

Install safety locks or latches on doors and windows (*door latches are complex and less accessible*); equip exits with alarms (always turned on; pressure-sensitive doormats that sound an alarm).[1-3]

Provide for 24-hr supervision, as indicated. *Client can be awake at any time and fail to recognize day or night routines.*

Consider use of GPS device. Register client with community and national resources such as SafeReturn Program administered by the Alzheimer's Association. *Program registers persons with dementia and operates a 24-hr helpline to facilitate the return of lost persons (800-272-3900).*[2,4,5]

- Ascertain client history of wandering when admitted to facility:

Place in room near monitoring station; check client location on frequent basis.

Assign consistent staff as much as possible.

Create a "wanderer's lounge" or large safe walking area with inaccessible exits or outside gated area.

Avoid overstimulation from activities or new partner/roommate during rest periods. *Client who is used to wandering in usual living setting may react with increased agitation and emotional outbreaks when admitted to an unfamiliar setting and restricted from wandering. This places both the client and caregivers at risk for injury.*[1-3]

- Use technology to promote safety:

Provide pressure-sensitive bed or chair alarms *to alert caregivers of movement, especially when client frequently gets up at night or when no one is present.*

Provide client ID bracelet or necklace with updated photograph, client name, and emergency contact *to assist with identification efforts, particularly when progressive dementia produces marked changes in client's appearance.*[4]

Obtain electronic locator devices *to find client when there is the potential for client to get lost or go missing.*[4]

Install verbal door alarm system. *Voice command is more effective at redirecting client and less likely to increase agitation than loud sound.*[1]

- Use universal symbols, large-print signs, portrait-like photographs, pictures, and signs *to assist client in finding way, especially when client has diminished ability or has lost ability to read*

- Avoid using physical or chemical restraints (sedatives) to control wandering behavior. *May increase agitation, sensory deprivation, and falls, and can aggravate wandering behavior.*

NURSING PRIORITY NO. 3   To enhance safety (Teaching/Discharge Considerations):

- Identify problems that are remediable and assist client/significant other (SO) to seek appropriate assistance and access resources. *Encourages problem-solving to improve condition rather than accept the status quo.*

- Notify neighbors about client's condition and request that they contact client's family or local police if they see client outside alone. *Community awareness can prevent or reduce risk of client being lost or hurt.*

- Help client/SO and family members develop plan of care when problem is progressive. *Client may initially need part-time assistance at home, progressing to enrollment in day-care program, and then full-time home care or placement in care facility.*

- Refer to community resources, such as day-care programs, support groups, respite care, etc. *Caregiver(s) will require access to multiple kinds of assistance and opportunities to promote problem-solving, enhance coping, and obtain necessary respite.*

- Refer to NDs acute/chronic Confusion, risk for Falls, risk for Injury, and [disturbed Sensory Perception (specify)].

 Acute Care   Collaborative   Community/ Home Care   Cultural

DOCUMENTATION FOCUS

Assessment/Reassessment
- Assessment findings, including individual concerns, family involvement, and support factors.
- Availability and use of resources.

Planning
- Plan of care and who is involved in planning.
- Teaching plan.

Implementation/Evaluation
- Responses of client/SO(s) to plan interventions and actions performed.
- Attainment or progress toward desired outcome(s).
- Modifications to plan of care.

Discharge Planning
- Long-term needs and who is responsible for actions to be taken.
- Specific referrals made.

References

1. alz.org. (2018). Health care professionals and Alzheimer's (various pages). Retrieved May 2018 from http://www.alz.org/health-care-professionals/health-care-clinical-medical-resources.asp.
2. Mayo Clinic Staff. (2015). Alzheimer's: Understand wandering and how to address it. Retrieved May 2018 from http://www.mayoclinic.org/healthy-lifestyle/caregivers/in-depth/alzheimers/art-20046222.
3. Cox, H. C., et al. (2002). ND: Wandering. *Clinical Applications of Nursing Diagnosis: Adult, Child, Women's, Psychiatric, Gerontic, and Home Health Considerations*. 4th ed. Philadelphia: F. A. Davis.
4. Rowe, M. A. (2003). People with dementia who become lost. *Am J Nurs*, 103(7), 32–39.
5. Alzheimer's Disease and Related Disorders SAR Research. (No date). Wandering. Retrieved May 2018 from http://www.dbs-sar.com/SAR_Research/wandering.htm.
6. Algase, D. L., Beel-Bates, C., Beattie, E. (2003). Wandering in long term care. *Ann Long Term Care*, 11(1), 33–39.
7. Song, J. A., Algase, D. (2008). Premorbid characteristics and wandering behavior in persons with dementia. *Arch Psychiatr Nurs*, 22(6), 318–327.

 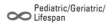

CHAPTER 6

Health Conditions and Client Concerns With Associated Nursing Diagnoses

This chapter presents 850 disorders/health conditions and life situations reflecting all specialty areas, with associated nursing diagnoses written as client problem/need statements that include the "related to" and "evidenced by" components.

This section facilitates and helps validate the assessment and diagnosis steps of the nursing process. Because the nursing process is perpetual and ongoing, other nursing diagnoses may be appropriate based on changing individual situations. Therefore, the nurse must continually assess, identify, and validate new client needs and evaluate subsequent care.

To facilitate access to the health conditions/concerns and nursing diagnoses, the conditions are listed alphabetically and coded to identify nursing specialty areas.

MS: Medical-Surgical
PED: Pediatric
OB/GYN: Obstetric/Gynecological
CH: Community/Home
PSY: Psychiatric/Behavioral

There is no separate category for geriatrics because concerns and conditions in this population are subsumed under the other specialty areas and because elderly persons are susceptible to the majority of these problems.

Abdominal hysterectomy   MS
Refer to Hysterectomy

Abdominal perineal resection   MS
Also refer to Surgery, general
disturbed Body Image may be related to alteration in self-perception, cultural or spiritual incongruence, possibly evidenced by verbalizations of feelings or perceptions, fear of reaction by others, preoccupation with change.

risk for Constipation possibly evidenced by risk factors of decreased physical activity and gastric motility, abdominal muscle weakness (associated with surgery), insufficient fluid intake, change in usual foods or eating pattern.

risk for Sexual dysfunction possibly evidenced by associated conditions of altered body structure or function (e.g., radical resection or treatment procedures), vulnerability, psychological concern about response of significant other(s), and disruption of sexual response pattern (e.g., erection difficulty).

Abortion, elective termination   OB
risk for Decisional Conflict possibly evidenced by unclear personal values/beliefs, lack of experience or interference with decision making, information from divergent sources, deficient support system.

deficient Knowledge regarding reproduction, contraception, self-care, and Rh factor may be related to lack of exposure or recall, misinterpretation of information, possibly evidenced by request for information, statement reflecting misconception, inaccurate follow-through of instructions, development of preventable complications.

risk for Moral Distress possibly evidenced by conflicting information available for ethical decision making, difficulty reaching treatment decision, [perception of moral or ethical implications of therapeutic procedure], time constraints for decision making.

Anxiety [specify level] may be related to threat to personal status, fear of unspecific consequences, value conflicts or beliefs possibly evidenced by increased tension, apprehension, sympathetic stimulation, focus on self.

impaired Comfort may be related to aftereffects of procedure, drug effect, possibly evidenced by verbal report, distraction behaviors, changes in muscle tone, changes in vital signs.

risk for [maternal] Injury possibly evidenced by surgical procedure, effects of anesthesia or medications.

Abortion, spontaneous termination   OB
risk for Bleeding possibly evidenced by pregnancy complication.

risk for Spiritual distress possibly evidenced by stressors [e.g., challenged beliefs/values, blame directed at self or higher power]; loss.

deficient Knowledge regarding cause of abortion, self-care, contraception, and future pregnancy may be related to lack of familiarity with new self-healthcare needs, sources for support, possibly evidenced by requests for information and statement of concern or misconceptions, development of preventable complications.

Grieving may be related to loss of significant other [e.g., perinatal loss], possibly evidenced by anger, crying, disorganization, expressions of sorrow/distress, or alteration in sleep patterns.

risk for Sexual dysfunction possibly evidenced by vulnerability [increasing fear of pregnancy or repeat loss, impaired relationship with SO(s), self-doubt regarding own femininity].

Abruptio placentae   OB
Also refer to Hemorrhage, prenatal
risk for Bleeding possibly evidenced by pregnancy complication—abruptio placentae.

Fear related to [threat of death to fetus/self], possibly evidenced by apprehensiveness, feeling of alarm or dread, avoidance behaviors.

acute Pain may be related to biological injury: collection of blood between uterine wall and placenta, possibly evidenced by verbal reports, abdominal guarding, muscle tension, or alterations in vital signs.

risk for disturbed Maternal-Fetal Dyad possibly evidenced by pregnancy complications, compromised fetal oxygen transport.

Abscess, brain (acute)   MS
acute Pain may be related to physical injury agent: inflammation, edema of tissues, possibly evidenced by reports of headache, restlessness, irritability, and moaning.

risk for Hyperthermia possibly evidenced by increase in metabolic rate and dehydration.

acute Confusion may be related to (delirium [cerebral edema, altered perfusion, fever]), possibly evidenced by fluctuation in cognition or level of consciousness, increased agitation, restlessness, hallucinations.

risk for Trauma possibly evidenced by (alteration in cognitive functioning, [disease process, seizure activity]).

Abscess, gingival   CH
impaired Dentition may be related to inadequate oral hygiene, insufficient knowledge of dental health, inadequate dietary habits barrier to self-care or [professional care] possibly evidenced by toothache, dental or root caries, halitosis.

risk for imbalanced Nutrition: less than body requirements possibly evidenced by insufficient dietary intake.

Abscess, skin/tissue   CH/MS
impaired Skin/Tissue Integrity may be related to [infection], alteration in fluid volume, inadequate nutrition (impaired circulation or vascular trauma, immunodeficiency); possibly evidenced by acute pain, alteration in skin integrity, hematoma/bleeding, redness, localized area hot to touch.

risk for Infection [spread] possibly evidenced by exposure to toxins, alteration in skin integrity, malnutrition, insufficient knowledge to avoid exposure to pathogens.

Abuse, physical   CH/PSY
Also refer to Battered child syndrome
risk for physical Trauma possibly evidenced by [vulnerable client, recipient of verbal threats], history of physical abuse.

Powerlessness may be related to insufficient interpersonal interactions, ineffective coping strategies, insufficient knowledge to manage a situation, low self-esteem social marginalization, [lifestyle of helplessness] as evidenced by verbal expressions of insufficient control, alienation, dependency, shame, [reluctance to express true feelings, apathy, passivity].

chronic low Self-Esteem may be related to inadequate belonging or affection received, inadequate respect from others [continual negative evaluation of self or capabilities, personal vulnerability, willingness to tolerate possible life-threatening domestic violence] as evidenced by nonassertive behavior, overly conforming, passivity, underestimating ability to deal with situation; [self-negative verbalization, evaluation of self as unable to deal with events, rejects positive feedback about self].

ineffective Coping may be related to high degree of threat or inadequate threat appraisal, insufficient sense of control, inadequate resources or social support possibly evidenced by change in communication pattern, risk-taking or destructive behaviors toward self/others, inability to ask for help or deal with the situation.

Sexual dysfunction may be related to ineffectual or absent role model, vulnerability, physical abuse possibly evidenced by verbalizations, change in sexual behaviors or activities, inability to achieve desired satisfaction.

Abuse, psychological   CH/PSY
ineffective Coping may be related to high degree of threat or inadequate threat appraisal, insufficient sense of control, inadequate resources or social support possibly evidenced by change in communication pattern, frequent illness, risk-taking or destructive behaviors toward self/others, inability to ask for help or deal with the situation.

Powerlessness may be related to insufficient interpersonal interactions, ineffective coping strategies, insufficient knowledge to manage a situation, low self-esteem social marginalization, [lifestyle of helplessness] as evidenced by verbal expressions of insufficient control, alienation, dependency, shame, [reluctance to express true feelings, apathy, passivity].

Sexual dysfunction may be related to ineffectual or absent role model, vulnerability, [psychological abuse (harmful relationship)], possibly evidenced by alteration in sexual function or satisfaction, seeking confirmation of desirability.

[esophageal] Achalasia (cardiospasm)   MS
impaired Swallowing may be related to (neuromuscular impairment, trauma, oropharynx abnormality), possibly evidenced by observed difficulty in swallowing, heartburn/regurgitation.

imbalanced Nutrition: less than body requirements may be related to insufficient dietary intake; inability/reluctance to ingest food, possibly evidenced by perceived inability to ingest food, food aversion, weight loss, and pale conjunctiva and mucous membranes.

acute Pain may be related to spasm of the lower esophageal sphincter, possibly evidenced by reports of substernal pressure, recurrent heartburn, or gastric fullness (gas pains).

Anxiety [specify level]/Fear may be related to stressors [e.g., recurrent pain, choking sensation, threat to health status], possibly evidenced by verbalizations of distress, apprehension, restlessness, or insomnia.

risk for Aspiration possibly evidenced by incompetent lower esophageal sphincter, [regurgitation or spillover of esophageal contents].

deficient Knowledge regarding condition, prognosis, self-care, and treatment needs may be related to lack of familiarity with pathology and treatment of condition, possibly evidenced by requests for information, statement of concern, or development of preventable complications.

Acidosis, metabolic   MS
Refer to underlying cause/condition, e.g., Diabetic ketoacidosis; Renal failure, Dialysis

Acidosis, respiratory   MS
(Also refer to underlying cause/condition)
impaired Gas Exchange may be related to (ventilation-perfusion imbalance, alveolar-capillary membrane changes), [decreased oxygen-carrying capacity of blood, altered oxygen supply], possibly evidenced by dyspnea, irritability, tachycardia, hypoxia, hypercapnia.

Acne   CH/PED
impaired Skin Integrity may be related to secretions, [infectious process] as evidenced by alteration in skin integrity.

disturbed Body Image may be related to alteration in self-perception, possibly evidenced by verbalizations of feelings or perceptions, fear of reaction by others, preoccupation with change in visual appearance as evidenced by fear of rejection of others, focus on past appearance, negative feelings about body, change in social involvement.

situational low Self-Esteem may be related to adolescence, negative perception of appearance as evidenced by self-negating verbalizations, expressions of helplessness.

Acoustic neuroma   MS
Also refer to Surgery, general
[disturbed auditory Sensory Perception] may be related to altered sensory reception (compression of eighth cranial nerve), possibly evidenced by unilateral sensorineural hearing loss, tinnitus.

risk for Falls possibly evidenced by hearing difficulties, dizziness, sense of unsteadiness.

Acquired immune deficiency syndrome   CH
Refer to AIDS

Acromegaly   CH
chronic Pain may be related to soft tissue swelling, joint degeneration, peripheral nerve compression, possibly evidenced by verbal reports, altered ability to continue previous activities, changes in sleep pattern, fatigue.

　　disturbed Body Image may be related to alteration in self-perception, cultural or spiritual incongruence possibly evidenced by verbalizations of feelings or perceptions, fear of rejection or reaction by others.

　　risk for Sexual dysfunction possibly evidenced by altered body structure, perceived sexual limitation, changes in libido.

Acute respiratory distress syndrome   MS
Refer to Respiratory distress syndrome, acute

Adams-Stokes syndrome   CH
Refer to Dysrhythmia, cardiac

ADD   PED
Refer to Attention deficit disorder

Addiction   CH/PSY
Refer to specific substance used; Substance dependence/abuse rehabilitation

Addison's disease   MS
deficient Fluid Volume [hypertonic] may be related to vomiting, diarrhea, increased renal losses, possibly evidenced by delayed capillary refill, poor skin turgor, dry mucous membranes, report of thirst.

　　risk for Electrolyte Imbalance possibly evidenced by vomiting, diarrhea, endocrine dysfunction.

　　decreased Cardiac Output may be related to hypovolemia and altered electrical conduction (dysrhythmias) or diminished cardiac muscle mass, possibly evidenced by alterations in vital signs, changes in mentation, and irregular pulse or pulse deficit.

CH

　　Fatigue may be related to decreased metabolic energy production, altered body chemistry (fluid, electrolyte, and glucose imbalance), possibly evidenced by unremitting overwhelming lack of energy, inability to maintain usual routines, decreased performance, impaired ability to concentrate, lethargy, and disinterest in surroundings.

　　disturbed Body Image may be related to alteration in self-perception, cultural or spiritual incongruence, possibly evidenced by verbalizations of feelings or perceptions, fear of reaction by others, preoccupation with changes (i.e., in skin pigmentation, mucous membranes, loss of axillary and pubic hair), and impaired social involvement.

　　risk for impaired physical Mobility possibly evidenced by neuromuscular impairment (muscle wasting, weakness) and dizziness, syncope.

　　imbalanced Nutrition: less than body requirements may be related to inadequate dietary intake, (inability to absorb nutrients [glucocorticoid deficiency; abnormal fat, protein, and carbohydrate metabolism]); possibly evidenced by weight loss, muscle wasting, abdominal cramping, diarrhea, and [hypoglycemia].

　　risk for impaired Home Maintenance possibly evidenced by effects of disease process, impaired cognitive functioning, and inadequate support systems.

Adenoidectomy   PED/MS
Anxiety [specify level]/Fear may be related to threat to current status/unmet needs [e.g., separation from supportive others, unfamiliar surroundings, and perceived threat of injury or abandonment], possibly evidenced by crying, apprehension, trembling, and sympathetic stimulation (pupil dilation, increased heart rate).

　　risk for ineffective Airway Clearance possibly evidenced by sedation, collection of secretions and blood in oropharynx, and vomiting.

　　risk for deficient Fluid Volume possibly evidenced by operative trauma to highly vascular site, hemorrhage.

　　acute Pain may be related to physical trauma to oronasopharynx, presence of packing, possibly evidenced by restlessness, crying, and facial mask of pain.

Adjustment disorder   PED/PSY
Refer to Anxiety disorders

Adoption/loss of child custody   PSY
risk for complicated Grieving possibly evidenced by emotional disturbance, depression, self-blame, separation distress [due to actual loss of child, expectations for future of child/self, thwarted grieving response to loss].

　　risk for Powerlessness possibly evidenced by [perceived lack of options, no input into decision process, no control over outcome].

Adrenal crisis, acute   MS
Also refer to Addison's disease; Shock
deficient Fluid Volume [hypertonic] may be related to
failure of regulatory mechanism (damage to or suppression of adrenal gland), inability to concentrate
urine, possibly evidenced by decreased venous filling,
pulse volume and pressure; hypotension, dry mucous
membranes, changes in mentation, decreased serum
sodium.

    acute Pain may be related to effects of disease
process and metabolic imbalances, decreased tissue
perfusion, possibly evidenced by reports of severe pain
in abdomen, lower back, or legs.

    impaired physical Mobility may be related
to neuromuscular impairment, decreased muscle
strength and control, possibly evidenced by generalized weakness, inability to perform desired activities
or movements.

    risk for Hyperthermia possibly evidenced by
increase in metabolic rate [illness or infectious pro-
cess], dehydration.

    risk for ineffective Protection possibly evidenced
by hormone deficiency, drug therapy, nutritional or
metabolic deficiencies.

Adrenalectomy   MS
ineffective Tissue Perfusion (specify) may be related
to hypovolemia and vascular pooling of blood [vaso-
dilation], possibly evidenced by diminished pulse,
pallor or cyanosis, hypotension, and changes in
mentation.

    risk for Infection possibly evidenced by altera-
tion in skin integrity, invasive procedure (incision,
traumatized tissues).

    *deficient Knowledge regarding condition, prog-
nosis, self-care, and treatment needs* may be related
to unfamiliarity with long-term therapy requirements,
possibly evidenced by request for information and
statement of concern or misconceptions.

Adrenal insufficiency   CH
Refer to Addison's disease

Affective disorder   PSY
Refer to Bipolar disorder; Depression, major

Affective disorder, seasonal   PSY
Also refer to Depression, major
[intermittent] ineffective Coping may be related to ineffective pattern of tension release strategies, inadequate
resources, possibly evidenced by alteration in sleep
pattern (too little or too much), fatigue, insufficient
problem resolution, [behavioral changes-irritability,
discouragement].

Agoraphobia   PSY
Also refer to Phobia
Anxiety [panic] may be related to threat to current
status (i.e., contact with feared situation [public place,
crowds]), possibly evidenced by tachycardia, chest
pain, dyspnea, gastrointestinal distress, faintness, sense
of impending doom.

Agranulocytosis   MS
risk for Infection possibly evidenced by (suppressed
inflammatory response).

    *risk for impaired oral Mucous Membrane
Integrity* possibly evidenced by (immunodeficiency),
[infection].

AIDS (acquired immunodeficiency   MS
syndrome)
Also refer to HIV infection
*risk for Infection [onset of new opportunistic infec-
tion]* possibly evidenced by chronic illness, suppressed
inflammatory response, malnutrition, insufficient
knowledge to avoid exposure to pathogens, use of
antimicrobial agents.

    risk for deficient Fluid Volume possibly evi-
denced by risk factors of excessive losses—copious
diarrhea, profuse sweating, vomiting, hypermetabolic
state or fever; and restricted intake—nausea, anorexia,
lethargy.

    acute/chronic Pain may be related to tissue
inflammation or destruction: infections, internal or
external cutaneous lesions, rectal excoriation, malignancies, necrosis, peripheral neuropathies, myalgias
and arthralgias, possibly evidenced by verbal reports,
narrowed focus, alteration in muscle tone, paresthesias,
paralysis, guarding behaviors, changes in vital signs
(acute), autonomic responses, and restlessness.

    risk for ineffective Breathing Pattern possibly
evidenced by (neuromuscular impairment [wasting of
respiratory musculature]); fatigue, respiratory muscle
fatigue, pain.

                               CH

    *imbalanced Nutrition: less than body require-
ments* may be related to insufficient dietary intake,
(altered ability to ingest, digest, or absorb nutrients);
[increased metabolic rate and nutritional needs (fever,
infection)], possibly evidenced by perceived inability

to ingest food/food aversion, body weight 20% or more below ideal weight range, altered taste sensation; abdominal cramping, hyperactive bowel sounds, diarrhea, sore buccal cavity, [abnormal laboratory results—vitamin, mineral, and protein deficiencies; electrolyte imbalances].

Fatigue may be related to decreased metabolic energy production, increased energy requirements (hypermetabolic state), overwhelming psychological or emotional demands, altered body chemistry (side effects of medication, chemotherapy), sleep deprivation, possibly evidenced by unremitting or overwhelming lack of energy, inability to maintain usual routines, decreased performance, impaired ability to concentrate, lethargy, listlessness, and disinterest in surroundings.

ineffective Protection may be related to chronic disease affecting immune and neurological systems, inadequate nutrition, drug therapies, possibly evidenced by deficient immunity, impaired healing, neurosensory alterations, maladaptive stress response, fatigue, anorexia, disorientation.

PSY

Social Isolation may be related to alterations in physical appearance, mental status, state of wellness; perceptions of unacceptable social behavior or values [phobic fear of others (transmission of disease)], possibly evidenced by expressed feelings of aloneness or rejection, absence of supportive SO(s), and withdrawal from usual activities.

chronic Confusion may be related to physiological changes (hypoxemia, central nervous system infection by HIV, brain malignancies, or disseminated systemic opportunistic infection); altered drug metabolism and excretion, accumulation of toxic elements (renal failure, severe electrolyte imbalance, hepatic insufficiency), possibly evidenced by clinical evidence of organic impairment, altered response to stimuli, memory deficit, and altered personality.

AIDS dementia   CH
Also refer to Dementia, HIV
chronic Confusion/impaired Memory related to physiological changes (neuronal degeneration), possibly evidenced by inaccurate interpretation of or response to stimuli, progressive or long-standing cognitive impairment, short-term memory deficit, impaired socialization, altered personality, and clinical evidence of organic impairment.

ineffective Protection may be related to immune disorder, inadequate nutrition, drug therapies, possibly evidenced by deficient immunity, impaired healing, neurosensory alterations, maladaptive stress response, fatigue, anorexia, disorientation.

Alcohol abuse/withdrawal   CH/MS/PSY
Refer to Alcohol intoxication, acute; Delirium tremens; Substance dependence/abuse rehabilitation

Alcohol intoxication, acute   MS
Also refer to Delirium tremens
acute Confusion may be related to alteration in sleep-wake cycle, sensory deprivation, impaired mobility, dehydration, malnutrition, substance misuse/[abuse], inappropriate use of restraints, possibly evidenced by hallucinations, exaggerated emotional response, fluctuation in cognition or level of consciousness, increased agitation.

risk for ineffective Breathing Pattern possibly evidenced by (hypoventilation syndrome, neuromuscular impairment), fatigue.

risk for Aspiration possibly evidenced by ineffective cough (decrease in level of consciousness, depressed gag reflexes, delayed gastric emptying).

Alcoholism   CH
Refer to Substance dependence/abuse rehabilitation

Aldosteronism, primary   MS
deficient Fluid Volume may be related to increased urinary losses, possibly evidenced by dry mucous membranes, poor skin turgor, dilute urine, excessive thirst, weight loss.

impaired physical Mobility may be related to neuromuscular impairment, decreased muscle strength, and pain, possibly evidenced by limited range of motion, slowed movement, limited ability to perform gross/fine motor skills.

risk for decreased Cardiac Output possibly evidenced by risk factors of altered preload and altered heart rhythm.

Alkalosis, metabolic   MS
Refer to underlying cause/condition, e.g., Renal failure, Dialysis

Alkalosis, respiratory   MS
(Also refer to underlying cause/condition.)
impaired Gas Exchange may be related to (ventilation-perfusion imbalance, alveolar-capillary membrane

changes [decreased oxygen-carrying capacity of blood, altered oxygen supply]), possibly evidenced by low respiratory rate, tachypnea, changes in mentation.

Allergies, seasonal   CH
Refer to Hay fever

Alopecia   CH
disturbed Body Image may be related to alteration in self-perception, possibly evidenced by verbalizations of feelings or concerns, fear of reaction by others, preoccupation with change in appearance [e.g., effects of illness, therapy, or aging process]; focus on past appearance, preoccupation with change, feelings of helplessness.

ALS   CH
Refer to Amyotrophic lateral sclerosis

Alzheimer's disease   CH
Also refer to Dementia, presenile/senile
risk for Injury/Trauma possibly evidenced by insufficient knowledge of modifiable factors [inability to recognize or identify danger in environment, disorientation, confusion, impaired judgment, weakness, muscular incoordination, balancing difficulties, altered perception].

chronic Confusion related to physiological changes [neuronal degeneration], possibly evidenced by inaccurate interpretation of or response to stimuli, progressive or long-standing cognitive impairment, short-term memory deficit, impaired socialization, altered personality, and clinical evidence of organic impairment.

[disturbed Sensory Perception (specify)] may be related to altered sensory reception, transmission, or integration (neurological disease, deficit), socially restricted environment (homebound or institutionalized), sleep deprivation, possibly evidenced by changes in usual response to stimuli, change in problem-solving abilities, exaggerated emotional responses (anxiety, paranoia, hallucinations), inability to tell position of body parts, diminished or altered sense of taste.

Sleep deprivation may be related to sensory impairment, changes in activity patterns, psychological stress [neurological impairment], possibly evidenced by wakefulness, disorientation [day/night reversal], increased aimless wandering, inability to identify need or time for sleeping, changes in behavior, lethargy, dark circles under eyes, and frequent yawning.

ineffective Health Maintenance may be related to deterioration affecting ability in all areas, including coordination, communication, and cognition; ineffective individual or family coping, possibly evidenced by reported or observed inability to take responsibility for meeting basic health practices, lack of equipment/ financial or other resources, and impairment of personal support system.

    PSY

risk for Stress overload possibly evidenced by inadequate resources, chronic illness, physical demands, threats of violence.

compromised family Coping/caregiver Role Strain may be related to disruptive behavior of client, family grief about their helplessness watching loved one deteriorate, prolonged disease or disability progression that exhausts the supportive capacity of SO or family, highly ambivalent family relationships, possibly evidenced by verbalizations of frustrations in dealing with day-to-day care, reports of conflict, feelings of depression, expressed anger/guilt directed toward client, and withdrawal from interaction with client or social contacts.

risk for Relocation Stress Syndrome possibly evidenced by little or no preparation for transfer to a new setting, changes in daily routine, sensory impairment, physical deterioration, separation from support systems.

Amenorrhea (secondary or pathological)   GYN
Also refer to Anorexia nervosa
imbalanced Nutrition: less than body requirements may be related to (inability to ingest food or absorb nutrients), possibly evidenced by body weight 20% or more below ideal weight range, aversion to eating, lack of interest in food, [excessive hair growth or lanugo], pale conjunctiva and mucous membranes, [abnormal lab studies].

risk for Sexual dysfunction possibly evidenced by alteration in body function.

Amphetamine abuse   PSY
Refer to Stimulant abuse

Amputation   MS
risk for ineffective peripheral Tissue Perfusion possibly evidenced by reduced arterial or venous blood flow, tissue edema, hematoma formation, hypovolemia.

acute Pain may be related to physical injury agent (tissue and nerve trauma), [psychological impact of loss of body part], possibly evidenced by reports of incisional or phantom pain, guarding or protective behavior, narrowed or self-focus, and autonomic responses.

impaired physical Mobility may be related to loss of limb, altered sense of balance, pain or discomfort, possibly evidenced by reluctance to attempt movement, impaired coordination; decreased muscle strength, control, and mass.

disturbed Body Image may be related to alteration in self-perception, (alteration in body function, injury/trauma), possibly evidenced by preoccupation with loss; negative feeling about body; focus on past strength, function, or appearance; fear of reaction by others; avoids looking at or touching one's body.

Amyotrophic lateral sclerosis (ALS)   MS

impaired physical Mobility may be related to muscle wasting, weakness, possibly evidenced by impaired coordination, limited range of motion, and impaired purposeful movement.

ineffective Breathing Pattern/impaired spontaneous Ventilation may be related to neuromuscular impairment, decreased energy, fatigue, tracheobronchial obstruction, possibly evidenced by shortness of breath, fremitus, respiratory depth changes, and reduced vital capacity.

impaired Swallowing may be related to (neurological problem), possibly evidenced by delayed/repetitive swallowing, coughing, choking, and recurrent pulmonary infection.

PSY

Powerlessness may be related to anxiety, insufficient knowledge to manage a situation, ineffective coping skills, insufficient social support, pain, [chronic and debilitating nature of illness, lack of control over outcome], possibly evidenced by expressions of frustration about inability to perform previous activities, inadequate participation in care, dependency, and depression.

Grieving may be related to anticipatory loss of significant object [self and physiopsychosocial well-being], possibly evidenced by distress, despair, anger, detachment.

CH

impaired verbal Communication may be related to physical barrier (neuromuscular impairment), possibly evidenced by impaired articulation, inability to speak in sentences, and use of nonverbal cues (changes in facial expression).

risk for caregiver Role Strain possibly evidenced by illness severity of care receiver, complexity and amount of home-care needs, duration of caregiving required, caregiver is spouse, family/caregiver isolation, lack of respite or recreation for caregiver.

Anaphylaxis   CH
Also refer to Shock

ineffective Airway Clearance may be related to airway spasm (bronchial), laryngeal edema, possibly evidenced by diminished or adventitious breath sounds, cough ineffective or absent, difficulty vocalizing, wide-eyed.

decreased Cardiac Output may be related to decreased preload—increased capillary permeability (third spacing) and vasodilation, possibly evidenced by tachycardia/palpitations, changes in blood pressure, anxiety, restlessness.

Anemia   CH

Activity Intolerance may be related to imbalance between oxygen supply and demand, possibly evidenced by reports of fatigue and weakness, abnormal heart rate or blood pressure response to activity, [decreased exercise or activity level, and exertional discomfort] or dyspnea.

imbalanced Nutrition: less than body requirements may be related to inadequate dietary intake, (inability to digest food or absorb nutrients), possibly evidenced by [weight loss or weight below normal for age]; pale oral mucous membranes, sore buccal cavity; insufficient muscle tone, [fatigue].

deficient Knowledge regarding condition, prognosis, self-care, and treatment needs may be related to inadequate understanding or misinterpretation of dietary or physiological needs, possibly evidenced by inadequate dietary intake, request for information, and development of preventable complications.

Anemia, iron-deficiency   CH
Also refer to Anemia

Fatigue may be related to anemia, malnutrition, possibly evidenced by feeling tired, inability to maintain usual routines or level of physical activity.

risk for deficient Fluid Volume possibly evidenced by active or chronic blood loss.

risk for impaired oral Mucous Membrane Integrity possibly evidenced by dehydration, malnutrition, [vitamin deficiency].

Anemia, pernicious CH

Also refer to Anemia

[disturbed kinesthetic/visual Sensory Perception] may be related to changes in reception or perception, possibly evidenced by paresthesia, inability to tell position of extremities (proprioception), loss of vibratory sensation, changes in sensory acuity (yellow-blue color blindness).

risk for Constipation/Diarrhea possibly evidenced by muscular weakness, changes in gastrointestinal motility, neurological impairment.

risk for Injury/Falls possibly evidenced by malnutrition [with generalized weakness, paresthesia of extremities, loss of proprioception, ataxia].

Anemia, sickle cell MS

impaired Gas Exchange may be related to ventilation-perfusion imbalance, possibly evidenced by dyspnea, abnormal breathing pattern, signs of hypoxia—abnormal skin color, tachycardia, confusion, and restlessness.

ineffective Tissue Perfusion (specify) may be related to stasis, vaso-occlusive nature of sickling, inflammatory response, atrioventricular shunts in pulmonary and peripheral circulation, myocardial damage (small infarcts, iron deposits, fibrosis), possibly evidenced by signs and symptoms dependent on system involved; for example, renal—decreased specific gravity and pale urine in face of dehydration; cerebral—paralysis and visual disturbances; peripheral—distal ischemia, tissue infarctions, ulcerations, bone pain; cardiac—angina, palpitations.

CH

acute/chronic Pain may be related to physical injury agent [intravascular sickling with localized vascular stasis, occlusion, infarction or necrosis and deprivation of oxygen and nutrients, accumulation of noxious metabolites], possibly evidenced by reports of localized, generalized, or migratory joint or abdominal/back pain; guarding and distraction behaviors (moaning, crying, restlessness); facial grimacing; narrowed focus; and autonomic responses.

deficient Knowledge regarding disease process, genetic factors, prognosis, self-care, and treatment needs may be related to lack of exposure or recall, misinterpretation of information, unfamiliarity with resources, possibly evidenced by questions, statements of concern or misconceptions, exacerbation of condition, inadequate follow-through of therapy instructions, and development of preventable complications.

risk for sedentary Lifestyle possibly evidenced by lack of interest or motivation, resources; lack of training or knowledge of specific exercise needs, safety concerns, fear of injury.

PED

risk for delayed Development possibly evidenced by inadequate nutrition, chronic illness.

compromised family Coping may be related to chronic nature of disease and disability, family disorganization, presence of other crises or situations impacting significant person or parent, lifestyle restrictions, possibly evidenced by SO expressing preoccupation with own reaction and displaying protective behavior disproportionate to client's ability or need for autonomy.

Anencephaly OB

Also refer to Fetal demise

Anxiety [specify level] may be related to situational crisis, threat of fetal death, interpersonal transmission or contagion, possibly evidenced by increased tension, apprehension, feelings of inadequacy, somatic complaints, difficulty sleeping.

risk for Decisional Conflict possibly evidenced by threat to value/belief system, multiple or divergent sources of information, support system deficit, feelings of guilt (particularly regarding moral/ethical issues such as termination of pregnancy, organ donation).

Aneurysm, abdominal aortic MS

Refer to Aortic aneurysm, abdominal

Aneurysm, cerebral MS

Refer to Cerebrovascular accident

Aneurysm, ventricular MS

decreased Cardiac Output may be related to altered stroke volume (decreased contractility, increased systemic vascular resistance), changes in heart rate or rhythm, possibly evidenced by dyspnea, adventitious breath sounds, S_3/S_4 heart sounds, changes in hemodynamic measurements, dysrhythmias.

ineffective Tissue Perfusion (specify) may be related to decreased arterial blood flow, possibly evidenced by blood pressure changes, diminished pulses, edema, dyspnea, dysrhythmias, altered mental status, decreased renal function.

Activity Intolerance may be related to imbalance between oxygen supply and demand, possibly evidenced by weakness, fatigue, abnormal heart rate/

blood pressure response to activity, electrocardiogram changes (dysrhythmias, ischemia).

Angina pectoris   MS

acute Pain may be related to physical injury agent [decreased myocardial blood flow, increased cardiac workload and oxygen consumption], possibly evidenced by verbal reports, narrowed focus, distraction behavior (restlessness, moaning), and autonomic responses (diaphoresis, changes in vital signs).

risk for decreased Cardiac Output possibly evidenced by transient or prolonged myocardial ischemia and effects of medications, alterations in rate, rhythm, and electrical conduction.

Anxiety [specify level] may be related to stressors, change in health status or threat of death; possibly evidenced by apprehensiveness, expressed concerns, facial tension, extraneous movements, and self-focused.

                                                          CH

Activity Intolerance may be related to imbalance between oxygen supply and demand, possibly evidenced by exertional dyspnea, abnormal pulse/blood pressure response to activity, and electrocardiogram changes.

deficient Knowledge regarding condition, prognosis, self-care, and treatment needs may be related to lack of exposure, inaccurate/misinterpretation of information, possibly evidenced by questions, request for information, statement of concern, and inaccurate follow-through of instructions.

risk for sedentary Lifestyle possibly evidenced by lack of training or knowledge of specific exercise needs, safety concerns, fear of myocardial injury.

risk for risk-prone Health Behavior possibly evidenced by condition requiring long-term therapy/change in lifestyle, multiple stressors, assault to self-concept, and altered locus of control.

Anorexia nervosa   MS

imbalanced Nutrition: less than body requirements may be related to (physiological disorder), possibly evidenced by weight loss, insufficient muscle tone, food aversion/intake less than recommended daily allowance, [amenorrhea, electrolyte imbalance, cardiac irregularities, hypotension].

risk for deficient Fluid Volume possibly evidenced by inadequate intake of food and liquids, chronic laxative or diuretic use.

disturbed Body Image may be related to alteration in self-perception, cultural or spiritual incongruence possibly evidenced by verbalizations of feelings or perceptions (e.g., rejection by others, perceptual developmental changes), perceptions reflecting altered view of body appearance, refusal to verify actual change.

chronic low Self-Esteem may be related to inadequate affection received, inadequate respect from others, receiving insufficient approval from others, possibly evidenced by reports of exaggerated negative feedback about self, overly conforming, passivity, shame.

impaired Parenting may be related to issues of control in family, situational or maturational crises, history of inadequate coping methods, possibly evidenced by enmeshed family; dissonance among family members; focus on "identified patient"; family developmental tasks not being met; family members acting as enablers; ill-defined family rules, functions, and roles.

Anthrax, cutaneous   MS/CH

impaired Skin/Tissue Integrity may be related to [chemical injury agent], possibly evidenced by acute pain, alteration in skin integrity, alteration in sensation, [damage to tissues].

impaired Comfort may be related to local edema, effects of circulating toxins, possibly evidenced by reports of headache, muscle aches, nausea, malaise.

risk for Infection [spread/sepsis] possibly evidenced by alteration in skin integrity, suppression, lack of immunity, [presence of infective agent].

Anthrax, gastrointestinal   MS

Anxiety [moderate to severe]/Fear may be related to threat of death, interpersonal transmission or contagion, possibly evidenced by expressed concerns, apprehension, uncertainty, fear, increased tension, restlessness.

risk for deficient Fluid Volume possibly evidenced by decreased intake (nausea), excessive loss—bloody vomit or diarrhea, hypermetabolic state.

imbalanced Nutrition: less than body requirements may be related to inadequate dietary intake, [inability to ingest food or absorb nutrients], possibly evidenced by [loss of appetite, nausea, vomiting], abdominal pain, diarrhea.

impaired oral Mucous Membrane Integrity may be related to effects of infection, dehydration, possibly evidenced by oropharyngeal ulcerations, oral pain, difficulty swallowing.

Health Conditions and Client Concerns With Associated Nursing Diagnoses

Anthrax, inhalation (pulmonary)   MS

Also refer to Ventilator assist/dependence

impaired Comfort may be related to effects of inflammatory response, possibly evidenced by fever, malaise, weakness, fatigue, mild chest pain.

Anxiety [moderate to severe]/Fear may be related to threat of death, interpersonal transmission or contagion, possibly evidenced by expressed concerns, apprehension, uncertainty, fear, increased tension, restlessness, blocking of thought.

impaired Gas Exchange may be related to (alveolar-capillary membrane changes [fluid collection or shifts into interstitial space or alveoli]), possibly evidenced by dyspnea, restlessness, irritability, abnormal breathing and skin color, hypoxia, lethargy, confusion.

risk for impaired spontaneous Ventilation possibly evidenced by decrease in arterial oxygen saturation, respiratory muscle fatigue, decrease in tidal volume [widening of mediastinum].

Antisocial personality disorder   PSY

risk for other-directed Violence possibly evidenced by contempt for authority or rights of others, inability to tolerate frustration, need for immediate gratification, easy agitation, vulnerable self-concept, inability to verbalize feelings, use of maladjusted coping mechanisms, history of substance abuse.

ineffective Coping may be related to ineffective tension release strategies, insufficient sense of control, (situational crisis), possibly evidenced by ineffective coping strategies, insufficient problem-solving skills, risk-taking behavior, destructive behaviors toward self/others.

chronic low Self-Esteem may be related to [lack of positive or repeated negative feedback, unmet dependency needs, retarded ego development, dysfunctional family system], possibly evidenced by acting-out behaviors (e.g., substance abuse, sexual promiscuity, feelings of inadequacy, nonparticipation in therapy)].

compromised/disabled family Coping may be related to family disorganization or role changes, highly ambivalent family relationships, client providing little support in turn for the primary person(s), history of abuse or neglect in the home, possibly evidenced by expressions of concern or complaints, preoccupation of primary person with own reactions to situation, display of protective behaviors disproportionate to client's abilities or need for autonomy.

impaired Social Interaction may be related to inadequate personal resources (shallow feelings), immature interests, underdeveloped conscience, unaccepted social values, possibly evidenced by difficulty meeting expectations of others, lack of belief that rules pertain to self, sense of emptiness or inadequacy covered by expressions of self-conceit, arrogance, contempt; behavior unaccepted by dominant cultural group.

Anxiety disorder, generalized   PSY

Anxiety [specify level]/Powerlessness may be related to real or perceived threat to physical integrity or self-concept, values or beliefs conflicts; possibly evidenced by sympathetic stimulation, extraneous movements, persistent expression of apprehension and uneasiness, poor eye contact, focus on self, impaired functioning, and nonparticipation in decision making.

ineffective Coping may be related to inaccurate threat appraisal, inadequate resources or social support systems, possibly evidenced by inability to ask for help, attend to information or deal with a situation, ineffective coping strategies, risk-taking behavior, substance misuse.

Insomnia may be related to stress, repetitive thoughts, possibly evidenced by reports of difficulty in falling/staying asleep, dissatisfaction with sleep, nonrestorative sleep, lack of energy.

risk for compromised family Coping possibly evidenced by inadequate or incorrect information or understanding by a support person, temporary family disorganization and role changes, exhaustion of support person.

impaired Social Interaction/Social Isolation may be related to low self-concept, inadequate personal resources, misinterpretation of internal or external stimuli, hypervigilance, possibly evidenced by discomfort in social situations, withdrawal from or reported change in pattern of interactions, dysfunctional interactions; expressed feelings of difference from others; sad, dull affect.

Anxiety disorders   PED/PSY

Anxiety [severe/panic] may be related to [situational or maturational crisis], interpersonal transmission or contagion, threat to current status, unmet needs, possibly evidenced by increase in tension, awareness of physiological symptoms, extraneous movement, diminished ability to learn, apprehensiveness, distress, fear.

ineffective Coping may be related to [maturational crisis], inadequate confidence in ability to deal with situation, insufficient sense of control, possibly evidenced by inability to deal with a situation, inability to meet role expectation, insufficient access of social support, [panic attacks].

impaired Social Interaction may be related to disturbance in self-concept, disturbance in thought processes possibly evidenced by discomfort in social situations, dissatisfaction with social engagement; impaired social functioning.

risk for Self-Mutilation/self-directed Violence possibly evidenced by panic states, dysfunctional family, history of self-destructive behaviors, emotional disturbance, increasing motor activity.

compromised/disabled family Coping may be related to [situational or developmental crisis], family disorganization, differing coping styles, [high-risk family situations–neglect or abuse, substance abuse], possibly evidenced by protective behavior by support person incongruent with client's abilities/ need for autonomy, family behaviors detrimental to well-being.

Anxiolytic abuse   PSY
Refer to Depressant abuse

Aortic aneurysm, abdominal (AAA)   MS
risk for ineffective Tissue Perfusion (Specify: cardiovascular, cerebral, peripheral) possibly evidenced by hypertension, hypovolemia, hypoxia.

risk for Bleeding possibly evidenced by abnormal blood profile; treatment regimen [e.g., surgery, medications, administration of platelet-deficient blood products]

acute Pain may be related to physical injury agent (vascular enlargement-dissection or rupture), possibly evidenced by verbal coded reports, guarding behavior, facial mask, change in vital signs.

Aortic aneurysm repair, abdominal   MS
Also refer to Surgery, general
Anxiety may be related to threat to change in status, threat of death, possibly evidenced by expressed concerns, apprehensiveness, increase in tension, changes in vital signs.

risk for Bleeding possibly evidenced by (aneurysm, treatment regimen [e.g., surgery, failure of vascular repair]).

risk for ineffective Tissue Perfusion (Specify) possibly evidenced by (hypertension, treatment regimen—surgery, hypovolemia, hypoxia).

Aortic insufficiency   MS/CH
Refer to Valvular heart disease

Aortic stenosis   MS
Also refer to Valvular heart disease
decreased Cardiac Output may be related to altered contractility, altered preload or afterload possibly evidenced by fatigue, dyspnea, changes in vital signs, jugular vein distension, increased CVP/PAWP, and syncope.

risk for impaired Gas Exchange possibly evidenced by (alveolar-capillary membrane changes).

CH
risk for acute Pain possibly evidenced by physical injury agent (episodic myocardial ischemia, stretching of left atrium).

Activity Intolerance may be related to imbalance between oxygen supply and demand [decreased or fixed cardiac output], possibly evidenced by exertional dyspnea, fatigue, weakness, and abnormal blood pressure or electrocardiogram changes, dysrhythmias in response to activity.

Aplastic anemia   CH
Also refer to Anemia
risk for ineffective Protection possibly evidenced by (abnormal blood profile, pharmaceutical agent [antineoplastics, antibiotics, NSAIDs, anticonvulsants].

Fatigue may be related to anemia, disease states, malnutrition, possibly evidenced by verbalization of overwhelming lack of energy, inability to maintain usual routines or level of physical activity, tired, compromised libido, lethargy, increase in physical complaints.

Appendectomy   MS
Also refer to Surgery, general
risk for Infection possibly evidenced by alteration in skin/tissue integrity, [release of pathogenic organisms into peritoneal cavity].

Appendicitis   MS
acute Pain may be related to physical injury agent [distention of intestinal tissues/inflammation], possibly evidenced by verbal reports, guarding behavior, narrowed focus, and autonomic responses (diaphoresis, changes in vital signs).

risk for deficient Fluid Volume possibly evidenced by excessive losses through normal routes (vomiting), deviations affecting intake of fluids (nausea, anorexia), and factors influencing fluid needs [hypermetabolic state].

risk for Infection possibly evidenced by alteration in tissue integrity, (invasive procedure, suppressed inflammatory response and exposure to pathogens [release of pathogenic organisms into peritoneal cavity]).

ARDS   MS
Refer to Respiratory distress syndrome, acute

Arrhythmia, cardiac   MS/CH
Refer to Dysrhythmia, cardiac

Arterial occlusive disease, peripheral   CH
ineffective peripheral Tissue Perfusion may be related to deficient knowledge of disease process [PAD], hypertension, smoking, sedentary lifestyle, possibly evidenced by skin characteristics, diminished pulses, claudication, delayed peripheral wound healing.

risk for impaired Walking possibly evidenced by decrease in endurance, pain.

risk for impaired Skin/Tissue Integrity possibly evidenced by (impaired circulation, and alteration of sensation).

Arthritis, gouty   CH
Refer to Gout

Arthritis, juvenile rheumatoid   PED/CH
Also refer to Arthritis, rheumatoid
risk for delayed Development possibly evidenced by chronic illness, effects of required therapy.

risk for Social Isolation possibly evidenced by delay in accomplishing developmental task, altered state of wellness, and alterations in physical appearance.

Arthritis, rheumatoid   CH
acute/chronic Pain may be related to accumulation of fluid, inflammatory process, degeneration of joint, and deformity, possibly evidenced by verbal reports, narrowed focus, guarding or protective behavior, and physical and social withdrawal.

impaired physical Mobility may be related to musculoskeletal deformity, pain or discomfort, decreased muscle strength, possibly evidenced by limited range of motion, impaired coordination, reluctance to attempt movement, and decreased muscle strength, control, and mass.

Self-Care deficit [specify] may be related to musculoskeletal impairment, decreased strength and endurance, limited range of motion, pain on movement, possibly evidenced by inability to manage activities of daily living.

disturbed Body Image/ineffective Role Performance may be related to change in body structure and function, impaired mobility or ability to perform usual tasks, focus on past strength, function, or appearance, possibly evidenced by negative self-talk, feelings of helplessness, change in lifestyle and physical abilities, dependence on others for assistance, decreased social involvement.

Arthritis, septic   CH
acute Pain may be related to physical injury agent (joint inflammation), possibly evidenced by verbal or coded reports, guarding behavior, restlessness, narrowed focus.

impaired physical Mobility may be related to joint stiffness, pain or discomfort, reluctance to initiate movement, possibly evidenced by limited range of motion, slowed movement.

Self-Care deficit [specify] may be related to musculoskeletal impairment, pain or discomfort, decreased strength, impaired coordination, possibly evidenced by inability to perform desired activities of daily living.

risk for Infection, spread possibly evidenced by presence of chronic disease state, suppressed inflammatory response.

Arthroplasty   MS
risk for Surgical Site Infection possibly evidenced by comorbidity (e.g., arthritis), duration/type of surgical procedure, use of implants/prosthesis, [stasis of body fluids at operative site, and altered inflammatory response].

risk for Bleeding possibly evidenced by (surgical procedure, trauma to vascular area).

impaired physical Mobility may be related to decreased strength, pain, musculoskeletal changes, possibly evidenced by impaired coordination and reluctance to attempt movement.

acute Pain may be related to physical injury agent (tissue trauma, local edema), possibly evidenced by verbal reports, narrowed focus, guarded movement, and autonomic responses (diaphoresis, changes in vital signs).

Arthroscopy, knee   MS
deficient Knowledge regarding procedure, outcomes, and self-care needs may be related to unfamiliarity with information or resources, misinterpretations, possibly evidenced by questions and requests for information, misconceptions.

risk for impaired Walking possibly evidenced by (musculoskeletal impairment), pain, physical deconditioning, fear of falling.

Asbestosis   CH

impaired Gas Exchange may be related to (alveolar-capillary membrane changes, ventilation-perfusion imbalance, possibly evidenced by dyspnea, tachypnea, restlessness, abnormal arterial blood gases [clubbing of fingers].

Activity Intolerance may be related to imbalance between oxygen supply and demand, possibly evidenced by exertional dyspnea, generalized weakness, abnormal vital sign response to activity.

ineffective Airway Clearance may be related to inflammatory response to inhaled foreign body, smoking or secondhand smoke, infection, possibly evidenced by dyspnea, adventitious breath sounds, increased sputum.

risk for Infection possibly evidenced by stasis of body fluids, (decrease in ciliary action, chronic illness), malnutrition, insufficient knowledge to avoid exposure to pathogen.

acute Pain may be related to physical injury agent (inflammation or irritation of the parietal pleura), possibly evidenced by verbal reports, guarding or distraction behavior, self-focused, and autonomic responses (changes in vital signs).

Asperger's disorder   PED/PSY
(now Autism spectrum disorder)

impaired Social Interaction may be related to insufficient skills to enhance mutuality, communication barriers, social dissonance, possibly evidenced by discomfort in social situations, dysfunctional interaction with others, impaired social functioning.

risk for delayed Development possibly evidenced by behavior disorder.

risk for Injury possibly evidenced by insufficient knowledge of modifiable factors [rituals, repetitive motor mannerisms, clumsiness, poor coordination, vulnerability to manipulation or peer pressure], (alteration in cognitive functioning).

Aspiration, foreign body   CH

ineffective Airway Clearance may be related to presence of foreign body, possibly evidenced by dyspnea, ineffective cough, diminished or adventitious breath sounds.

Anxiety [specify] may be related to threat of death, possibly evidenced by apprehensiveness, fearfulness, pupil dilation, increase in tension.

risk for Suffocation possibly evidenced by lack of safety education or precautions, eating large mouthfuls or pieces of food.

Asthma   MS
Also refer to Emphysema

ineffective Airway Clearance may be related to (airway spasm, allergic airway/asthma), excessive mucus, retained secretions, possibly evidenced by dyspnea, ineffective cough, difficulty verbalizing, diminished/adventitious breath sounds, alteration in respiratory pattern.

impaired Gas Exchange may be related to (ventilation-perfusion imbalance [e.g., altered delivery of inspired oxygen, air trapping]), possibly evidenced by dyspnea, restlessness, abnormal skin color, [reduced tolerance for activity], abnormal arterial blood gases, changes in vital signs.

Anxiety [specify level] may be related to threat to current status, threat of death, possibly evidenced by apprehensiveness, distress, fear, self-focused, extraneous movement, restlessness.

                                       CH

Activity Intolerance may be related to imbalance between oxygen supply and demand, possibly evidenced by fatigue and exertional dyspnea.

risk for Contamination possibly evidenced by (exposure to atmospheric pollutants), environmental contaminants in the home (e.g., smoking or secondhand smoke).

Atelectasis   MS

impaired Gas Exchange may be related to (alveolar-capillary membrane changes [e.g., inflammatory process, stasis of secretions, hypoventilation], possibly evidenced by restlessness, dyspnea, tachycardia, abnormal skin color (pallor, cyanosis), abnormal arterial blood gases, hypoxia.

Atherosclerosis   CH/MS
Refer to Coronary artery disease: Peripheral vascular disease

Athlete's foot   CH

impaired Skin Integrity may be related to [fungal invasion], humidity, secretions, possibly evidenced by alteration in skin integrity, [painful itching].

risk for Infection [spread] possibly evidenced by alteration in skin integrity [exposure to moist, warm environment].

Atrial fibrillation   CH
Also refer to Dysrhythmia, cardiac

risk for Activity Intolerance may be related to imbalance between oxygen supply and demand, exertional dyspnea, (circulatory problem).

---

risk for ineffective cerebral Tissue Perfusion possibly evidenced by arterial fibrillation, embolism, thrombolytic therapy.

Atrial flutter CH

Also refer to Dysrhythmia, cardiac

Anxiety [specify] may be related to threat to change in status, possibly evidenced by expressed concerns, apprehensiveness, awareness of physiological symptoms (palpitations, dizziness, presyncope or syncopal episodes), self-focused.

Atrial tachycardia CH

Refer to Dysrhythmia, cardiac

Attention deficit disorder PED/PSY

ineffective Coping may be related to (situational or maturational crisis), ineffective tension release strategies, inadequate confidence in ability to deal with situation, possibly evidenced by alteration in concentration, inability to attend to information, insufficient goal directed behavior.

chronic low Self-Esteem may be related to (psychiatric disorder, repeated negative reinforcement), possibly evidenced by poor eye contact, exaggerates negative feedback about self, rejection of positive feedback, hesitant to try new experiences, indecisive or nonassertive behavior.

deficient Knowledge regarding condition, prognosis, and therapy may be related to misinformation or misinterpretations, unfamiliarity with resources, possibly evidenced by verbalization of problems or misconceptions, poor school performance, unrealistic expectations of medication regimen.

Autism spectrum disorder PED/PSY

impaired Social Interaction may be related to communication barrier, insufficient skills to enhance mutuality, disturbance in thought processes, disturbance in self-concept, absence of significant other, possibly evidenced by dysfunctional interactions with others, discomfort in social situations.

impaired verbal Communication may be related to alteration in self-concept, low self-esteem, emotional disturbance, absence of significant others, possibly evidenced by difficulty speaking, forming words/sentences, difficulty in use of facial/body expressions, inappropriate verbalizations, stuttering.

risk for Self-Mutilation possibly evidenced by inability to express tension verbally, ineffective coping strategies, requires rapid stress reduction, impaired

self-esteem, perfectionism, (individuals with autism, borderline personality disorder, character disorder, developmental delay).

disturbed Personal Identity may be related to low self-esteem, dysfunctional family processes, cultural incongruence, (developmental transition, organic brain disorder), possibly evidenced by fluctuating feelings about self, delusional description of self, unable to distinguish between internal and external stimuli, ineffective relationships.

compromised family Coping may be related to exhaustion of supportive person's capacity, family disorganization, insufficient understanding of information by a support person, coexisting situations affecting the significant other, possibly evidenced by support person reports insufficient knowledge, or inadequate understanding, that interferes with effective behaviors, support person reports preoccupation with personal reactions to client's needs; protective behavior by support person incongruent with client's abilities.

Bacteremia MS

Refer to Sepsis

Barbiturate abuse CH/PSY

Refer to Depressant abuse

Battered child syndrome PED/CH

Also refer to Abuse, physical

risk for other-directed Violence possibly evidenced by pattern of indirect violence or threatening violence, [vulnerability (e.g., congenital problems/chronic illness)], (history of childhood abuse or neglect).

[risk for disproportionate Growth] and/or delayed Development possibly evidenced by presence of abuse, exposure to violence, inadequate nutrition/malnutrition; caregiver mental health issue, substance abuse, unplanned/unwanted pregnancy.

interrupted Family Processes/impaired Parenting may be related to poor role model, unrealistic expectations, presence of stressors, and lack of support, possibly evidenced by verbalization of negative feelings, inappropriate caretaking behaviors, and evidence of physical or psychological trauma to child.

PSY

chronic low Self-Esteem may be related to inadequate affection received, (repeated negative reinforcement, exposure to traumatic situation), possibly evidenced by poor eye contact, exaggerates negative feedback about self, guilt/shame, nonassertive, indecisive, or overly conforming behavior.

Post-Trauma Syndrome may be related to sustained or recurrent physical or emotional abuse; possibly evidenced by acting-out behavior, development of phobias, poor impulse control, and emotional numbness.

Bedsores CH/MS
Refer to Ulcer, pressure

Bed-wetting PED
Refer to Enuresis

Benign prostatic hyperplasia CH/MS
[acute/chronic] urinary Retention/overflow urinary Incontinence may be related to blockage in urinary tract [enlarged prostate], decompensation of detrusor musculature, inability of bladder to contract adequately, possibly evidenced by frequent voiding, hesitancy, inability to empty bladder completely, incontinence or dribbling, nocturia, bladder distention, residual urine.

acute Pain may be related to physical injury agent [mucosal irritation, bladder distention, colic, urinary infection, radiation therapy], possibly evidenced by verbal reports, narrowed focus, altered muscle tone, grimacing, distraction behavior, restlessness, and autonomic responses.

risk for deficient Fluid Volume/Electrolyte Imbalance possibly evidenced by active fluid volume loss—postobstructive diuresis, endocrine or renal dysfunction.

Fear/Anxiety [specify level] may be related to threat to current status; embarrassment, concern about sexual ability, and fear of unspecific consequences, possibly evidenced by increase in tension, apprehensiveness, worry, expressed concerns regarding perceived changes.

Besnier-Boeck disease CH
Refer to Sarcoidosis

Biliary calculus CH/MS
Refer to Cholelithiasis

Biliary cancer MS
Also refer to Cancer
imbalanced Nutrition: less than body requirements may be related to insufficient dietary intake, (inability to ingest or absorb nutrients), abdominal discomfort, possibly evidenced by food aversion, food intake less than recommended, insufficient muscle tone, weight loss with adequate food intake, and [imbalances in nutritional studies].

risk for impaired Skin Integrity possibly evidenced by chemical injury agent (accumulation of bile salts in skin), alteration in fluid volume (poor skin turgor), pressure over bony prominence.

Death Anxiety may be related to lack of successful treatment options, poor prognosis, possibly evidenced by fear of the process of dying, leaving SO/family alone after death, negative death images, concern of overworking caregiver, deep sadness.

Binge-eating disorder PSY
Refer to Bulimia nervosa

Bipolar disorder PSY
ineffective Impulse Control may be related to mood disorder, (alteration in cognitive functioning, development; personality disorder), possibly evidenced by acting without thinking, temper outbursts, violent behavior.

imbalanced Nutrition: less than body requirements may be related to insufficient dietary intake, (psychological disorder), possibly evidenced by insufficient information, misinformation/misperceptions, insufficient interest in food, food intake less than recommended daily allowance, body weight 20% or more below ideal weight range, [laboratory evidence of nutritional deficits or imbalances].

risk for Poisoning [lithium toxicity] possibly evidenced by [narrow therapeutic range of drug], emotional disturbance, insufficient knowledge of pharmaceutical agent.

Sleep Deprivation may be related to overstimulating environment, sustained circadian asynchrony, sustained inadequate sleep hygiene, possibly evidenced by agitation, irritability, restlessness, decrease in functional ability, alteration in concentration.

[disturbed Sensory Perception (specify)]/Stress overload may be related to psychological stress, [sleep deprivation], biochemical imbalances [e.g., increased norepinephrine levels in the brain], insufficient environmental stimulation, possibly evidenced by restlessness, poor concentration, disorientation, change in usual response to stimuli, sensory distortions, hallucination, change in behavior pattern, motor incoordination.

interrupted Family Processes may be related to shift in family roles, (situational crises, shift in health status of family member, change in family finances), possibly evidenced by change in communication pattern, changes in relationship pattern, decrease in mutual support, assigned tasks change, changes in participation for problem-solving/decision making.

Bladder cancer   MS
Also refer to Cancer; Urinary diversion

impaired urinary Elimination may be related to presence of tumor, possibly evidenced by frequent,voiding burning, dysuria.

acute/chronic urinary Retention may be related to blockage of urethra, possibly evidenced by sensation of fullness, bladder distention, residual urine, dysuria.

Body dysmorphic disorder   PSY
Refer to Hypochondriasis

Bone cancer   MS/CH
Also refer to Myeloma, multiple; Amputation

acute Pain may be related to physical injury agent [bone, tissue, and nerve destruction], possibly evidenced by verbal or coded report, protective behavior, autonomic responses.

impaired Walking may be related to (musculoskeletal impairment [amputation], impaired balance), possibly evidenced by impaired ability to climb stairs, navigate curbs, walk on incline or decline, or uneven surface.

Bone marrow transplantation   MS/CH
Also refer to Transplantation, recipient

risk for Injury possibly evidenced by (immune dysfunction or suppression, abnormal blood profile, [action of donor T cells]).

decreased Diversional Activity Engagement may be related to hospitalization or length of treatment, restriction of visitors, limitation of activities, possibly evidenced by expressions of boredom, restlessness, withdrawal, and requests for something to do.

risk for imbalanced Nutrition: less than body requirements possibly evidenced by (inability to ingest food or absorb nutrients), [increased metabolic needs for healing], nausea, vomiting, insufficient interest in food, alteration in taste sensations, sore buccal cavity.

Borderline personality disorder   PSY
risk for ineffective Impulse Control possibly evidenced by acting without thinking, sexual promiscuity, gambling, irritability, temper outbursts, violent behavior, (alteration in cognitive functioning).

Anxiety [severe to panic] may be related to threat to current status, value conflict, unmet needs, substance misuse, possibly evidenced by self-focused,

poor eye contact, hypervigilance, diminished ability to problem-solve, tendency to blame others, alteration in concentration, increase in tension, cardiac excitation.

chronic low Self-Esteem may be related to receiving insufficient approval from others, (repeated negative reinforcement, psychiatric disorder), possibly evidenced by rejection of positive feedback, excessive seeking of reassurance, underestimates ability to deal with situation, repeatedly unsuccessful in life events.

Social Isolation may be related to developmentally inappropriate interests, social behavior incongruent with norms, insufficient personal resources, and inability to engage in satisfying personal relationships, possibly evidenced by inability to meet expectations of others, feeling difference from others, aloneness imposed by others.

Botulism (foodborne)   MS
deficient Fluid Volume may be related to active losses (vomiting, diarrhea, decreased intake), nausea, dysphagia, possibly evidenced by reports of thirst; dry skin or mucous membranes, decreased blood pressure and urine output, change in mental state, increased hematocrit.

impaired physical Mobility may be related to neuromuscular impairment, possibly evidenced by limited ability to perform gross or fine motor skills.

Anxiety [specify level]/Fear may be related to threat of death, possibly evidenced by expressed concerns, apprehensiveness, awareness of physiological symptoms, self-focused.

risk for impaired spontaneous Ventilation possibly evidenced by [neuromuscular impairment, presence of infectious process].

CH

Contamination may be related to lack of proper precautions in food storage or preparation as evidenced by gastrointestinal and neurological effects of exposure to biological agent.

Bowel obstruction   MS
Refer to Ileus

Bowel resection   CH
Refer to Intestinal surgery (without diversion)

BPH   CH/MS
Refer to Benign prostatic hyperplasia

Brachytherapy (radioactive implants;   **MS**
also called internal radiation therapy)

risk for Injury [to others] possibly evidenced by risk factors of [radiation emitted by client (depending on type of procedure)].

risk for impaired physical Mobility possibly evidenced by prescribed restrictions [48 hours for low-dose implants], reluctance to move [fear of dislodging implants], decreased strength or endurance, depressed mood.

Bradycardia   **CH**
Refer to Dysrhythmia, cardiac

Brain attack   **MS**
Refer to Cerebrovascular accident

Brain tumor   **MS**
Also refer to Cancer

acute Pain may be related to physical injury agent [pressure on brain tissues], possibly evidenced by verbal/coded reports, facial mask, narrowed focus, and autonomic responses [changes in vital signs].

impaired Memory may be related to (neurological impairment, brain injury), possibly evidenced by persistent forgetfulness, persistent inability to recall events/factual information.

[disturbed Sensory Perception (specify)] may be related to altered sensory reception/integration, possibly evidenced by changes in sensory acuity, change in behavior pattern, poor concentration/problem-solving abilities, disorientation.

risk for deficient Fluid Volume, possibly evidenced by insufficient fluid intake, (active fluid volume loss [recurrent vomiting]).

Self-Care deficit [specify] may be related to pain, weakness, (neuromuscular impairment, alteration in cognitive functioning), possibly evidenced by inability to perform necessary steps for activities of daily living.

Breast cancer   **MS/CH**
Also refer to Cancer

Anxiety [specify level] may be related to change in status, threat of death, stressors, interpersonal transmission, possibly evidenced by expressed concerns, apprehensiveness, uncertainty, self-focused, diminished productivity.

deficient Knowledge regarding diagnosis, prognosis, and treatment options may be related to lack of

exposure or unfamiliarity with information resources, information misinterpretation, cognitive limitation, anxiety, possibly evidenced by verbalizations, statements of misconceptions, inappropriate behaviors.

risk for disturbed Body Image possibly evidenced by surgical or other treatment/procedure, alteration in self-perception or role perception.

risk for Sexual dysfunction possibly evidenced by health-related changes, medical treatments, perceived sexual limitation; change in sexual role, activity, or satisfaction; concern about relationship with SO.

Bronchitis   **CH**
ineffective Airway Clearance may be related to excessive, thickened mucous secretions, possibly evidenced by presence of rhonchi, tachypnea, and ineffective cough.

Activity Intolerance [specify level] may be related to imbalance between oxygen supply/demand, physical deconditioning, possibly evidenced by fatigue, exertional dyspnea, generalized weakness, and abnormal vital sign response to activity.

Bronchogenic carcinoma   **· MS/CH**
Also refer to Cancer

impaired Gas Exchange may be related to (ventilation-perfusion imbalance), possibly evidenced by abnormal breathing pattern, [diminished or adventitious breath sounds, decreased chest expansion], abnormal arterial blood gases.

risk for ineffective Airway Clearance possibly evidenced by retained secretions, inflammatory exudate, bronchial narrowing, pain, smoking or second-hand smoke, infection.

risk for Infection [spread] possibly evidenced by stasis of body fluids, malnutrition and (chronic illness), decrease in ciliary action, immunosuppression.

Bronchopneumonia   **MS/CH**
Also refer to Bronchitis

ineffective Airway Clearance may be related to tracheal bronchial inflammation, edema formation, increased sputum production, pleuritic pain, decreased energy, fatigue, possibly evidenced by changes in rate and depth of respirations, abnormal breath sounds, use of accessory muscles, dyspnea, cyanosis, cough with or without sputum production.

impaired Gas Exchange may be related to (alveolar-capillary membrane changes, ventilation-perfusion imbalance), possibly evidenced by restlessness, confusion, abnormal breathing pattern (dyspnea), and skin color, (pallor, cyanosis), and arterial blood gas or hypoxia.

risk for Infection [spread] possibly evidenced by stasis of body fluids, malnutrition and associated condition of chronic illness, decrease in ciliary action, immunosuppression.

Brown-Sequard syndrome   MS/CH
Also refer to Paraplegia; Quadriplegia

impaired physical Mobility may be related to (neuromuscular and sensoriperceptual impairment), possibly evidenced by limited motion, weakness, or paralysis (hemiparaplegia).

[disturbed kinesthetic/tactile Sensory Perception] may be related to altered sensory transmission [e.g., neurological trauma, ischemia, inflammation, infection], possibly evidenced by reported change in sensory acuity—loss of touch, vibration, and position on one side of the body, loss of pain and temperature sensation on opposite side of body (hemianesthesia).

Buck's traction   MS
Refer to Traction

Buerger's disease   CH
Refer to Peripheral vascular disease

Bulimia nervosa   PSY/MS
Also refer to Anorexia nervosa

impaired Dentition may be related to inadequate dietary habits/malnutrition; barrier to self-care, inadequate oral hygiene; and associated condition of chronic vomiting, possibly evidenced by erosion of tooth enamel, multiple caries, abraded teeth.

impaired oral Mucous Membrane Integrity may be related to malnutrition or vitamin deficiency, poor oral hygiene, chronic vomiting, possibly evidenced by sore, inflamed buccal mucosa; swollen salivary glands; ulcerations of mucosa; reports of constant sore mouth or throat.

risk for deficient Fluid Volume possibly evidenced by (fluid loss through abnormal route [consistent self-induced vomiting], pharmaceutical agent [laxative or diuretic use], active fluid volume loss [esophageal erosion or tear]).

deficient Knowledge regarding condition, prognosis, complications, and treatment may be related to lack of exposure or recall, unfamiliarity with information about condition, learned maladaptive coping skills, possibly evidenced by verbalization of misconception of relationship of current situation and bingeing and purging behaviors, distortion of body image, verbalization of the problem.

Bunion   CH
impaired Walking may be related to inflammation and degeneration of joint, inappropriate footwear, possibly evidenced by inability to walk required distances.

Bunionectomy   MS
Also refer to Surgery, general; Postoperative recovery period

impaired Walking may be related to pain, possibly evidenced by inability to walk required distances, navigate curbs, climb stairs.

Burns (dependent on type, degree,   MS/CH
and severity of the injury)
risk for deficient Fluid Volume/Bleeding possibly evidenced by loss of fluids through wounds, capillary damage and evaporation, hypermetabolic state, insufficient intake, hemorrhagic losses.

risk for ineffective Airway Clearance possibly evidenced by tracheobronchial obstruction—mucosal edema and loss of ciliary action with smoke inhalation; circumferential full-thickness burns of the neck, thorax, and chest, with compression of the airway or limited chest excursion, trauma—direct upper airway injury by flame, steam, chemicals or gases; fluid shifts, pulmonary edema, decreased lung compliance.

risk for Infection possibly evidenced by alteration in skin integrity, (decreased hemoglobin, suppressed inflammatory response, invasive procedures).

acute/chronic Pain may be related to destruction of skin, tissue, and nerves; edema formation; and manipulation of injured tissues, possibly evidenced by verbal/coded reports, narrowed focus, distraction and guarding behavior, facial mask, and changes in vital signs.

risk for imbalanced Nutrition: less than body requirements possibly evidenced by (inability to ingest or digest food), [hypermetabolic state as much as 50% to 60% higher than normal proportional to the severity of injury, protein catabolism, anorexia], restricted oral intake.

Post-Trauma Syndrome may be related to life-threatening event, possibly evidenced by reexperiencing the event, repetitive dreams or nightmares, psychic or emotional numbness, and sleep disturbance.

ineffective Protection may be related to extremes of age, inadequate nutrition, anemia, impaired immune system, possibly evidenced by impaired healing, deficient immunity, fatigue, anorexia.

PED

decreased Diversional Activity Engagement may be related to (prolonged hospitalization, therapeutic isolation), impaired mobility, physical discomfort, insufficient energy, possibly evidenced by boredom, discontent with situation.

risk for delayed Development possibly evidenced by [effects of physical disability, separation from SO(s), and environmental deficiencies].

Bursitis   CH

acute/chronic Pain may be related to inflammation of affected joint, possibly evidenced by verbal/coded reports, guarding behavior, and narrowed focus.

impaired physical Mobility may be related to inflammation and swelling of joint and pain, possibly evidenced by diminished range of motion, reluctance to attempt movement, and imposed restriction of movement by medical treatment.

CABG   MS

Refer to Coronary artery bypass surgery

CAD   CH/MS

Refer to Coronary artery disease

Calculi, urinary   CH/MS

acute Pain may be related to physical injury agent [increased frequency or force of ureteral contractions, tissue trauma, edema formation, cellular ischemia], possibly evidenced by verbal/coded reports of pain; guarding and distraction behavior; self-focused; and autonomic responses.

impaired urinary Elimination may be related to multiple causality, (anatomic obstruction), possibly evidenced by urgency and frequent voiding, urinary retention, [hematuria].

risk for deficient Fluid Volume possibly evidenced by stimulation of renal-intestinal reflexes causing nausea, vomiting, and diarrhea; changes in urinary output, postobstructive diuresis.

deficient Knowledge regarding condition, prognosis, self-care, and treatment needs may be related to lack of exposure or recall and information misinterpretation, possibly evidenced by requests for information, statements of concern, and recurrence or development of preventable complications.

Cancer   MS

Also refer to Chemotherapy; Radiation therapy

Fear/Death Anxiety may be related to learned response to threat, uncertainty of prognosis, possibly evidenced by apprehensiveness, feeling of fear/dread, anorexia, increase in tension, fear of pain/suffering related to dying, increase in blood pressure.

Grieving may be related to psychological distress with potential loss of physiological well-being, change in lifestyle, perceived potential death, possibly evidenced by anger, sadness, withdrawal, choked feelings, changes in eating or sleep patterns, activity level, libido, and communication patterns.

acute/chronic Pain may be related to the disease process [compression of nerve tissue, infiltration of nerves or their vascular supply, obstruction of a nerve pathway, inflammation], or side effects of therapeutic agents, possibly evidenced by verbal/coded reports, self-focused or narrowed focus, alteration in muscle tone, facial expression of pain, distraction or guarding behavior, autonomic responses, and restlessness.

Fatigue may be related to decreased metabolic energy production, increased energy requirements—hypermetabolic state; overwhelming psychological or emotional demands, and altered body chemistry—side effects of medications, chemotherapy, radiation therapy, biotherapy, possibly evidenced by unremitting or overwhelming lack of energy, inability to maintain usual routines, decreased performance, impaired ability to concentrate, lethargy, listlessness, and disinterest in surroundings.

impaired Home Maintenance may be related to debilitation, lack of resources, or inadequate support systems, possibly evidenced by verbalization of problem, request for assistance, and lack of necessary equipment or aids.

PED

risk for interrupted Family Processes possibly evidenced by (situational or transitional crises—long-term illness, change in roles or economic status; developmental—anticipated loss of a family member).

readiness for enhanced family Coping possibly evidenced by expresses desire to acknowledge growth impact of crisis.

Candidiasis   CH

Also refer to Thrush

impaired Skin/Tissue Integrity may be related to [infectious lesions], possibly evidenced by alteration in

---

Health Conditions and Client Concerns With Associated Nursing Diagnoses skin and mucous membrane integrity [rashes, patchy lesions, blisters, pustules].

acute Pain/impaired Comfort may be related to exposure of irritated skin and mucous membranes to excretions (urine, feces), possibly evidenced by verbal or coded reports, restlessness, guarding behaviors.

risk for Sexual dysfunction possibly evidenced by alteration in body function [e.g., presence of infectious process, vaginal discomfort].

Cannabis abuse   CH
Refer to Depressant abuse

Carbon monoxide poisoning   MS
impaired Gas Exchange may be related to [altered oxygen-carrying capacity of blood], possibly evidenced by headache, confusion, somnolence, [elevated carbon monoxide levels].

Activity Intolerance may be related to imbalance between oxygen supply and demand, possibly evidenced by fatigue, exertional dyspnea.

risk for Trauma/Suffocation possibly evidenced by insufficient knowledge of safety precautions.

Cardiac catheterization   MS
Anxiety [specify] may be related to threat to change in status, stressors, possibly evidenced by expressed concerns, apprehensiveness, uncertainty, self-focused.

risk for decreased Cardiac Output possibly evidenced by altered heart rate or rhythm [vasovagal response, ventricular dysrhythmias], decreased myocardial contractility [ischemia].

risk for decreased cardiac Tissue Perfusion (specify) may be related to coronary artery spasm, hypovolemia, hypoxia [thrombosis, emboli].

risk for Adverse Reaction to Iodinated Contrast Media possibly evidenced by heart disease, concurrent use of pharmaceutical agents [e.g., beta blockers, metformin], history of allergies.

Cardiac conditions, prenatal   OB
Also refer to Pregnancy, high-risk
risk for Cardiac Output [decompensation] possibly evidenced by increased circulating volume, dysrhythmias, altered myocardial contractility, inotropic changes in the heart.

risk for excess Fluid Volume possibly evidenced by increasing circulating volume, changes in renal function, dietary indiscretion.

risk for ineffective [uteroplacental] Tissue Perfusion possibly evidenced by changes in circulating volume, right-to-left shunt.

risk for Activity Intolerance possibly evidenced by (circulatory problem), physical deconditioning, previous episodes of intolerance.

Cardiac inflammatory disease   MS
Refer to Endocarditis; Myocarditis; Pericarditis

Cardiac surgery   MS/PED
risk for decreased Cardiac Output possibly evidenced by altered myocardial contractility [ventricular wall surgery, recent myocardial infarction, response to certain medications or drug interactions]; altered preload—hypovolemia, and afterload—systemic vascular resistance; altered heart rate or rhythm—dysrhythmias.

risk for Bleeding/deficient Fluid Volume possibly evidenced by [intraoperative bleeding with inadequate blood replacement; bleeding related to insufficient heparin reversal, fibrinolysis, or platelet destruction]; or volume depletion [effects of intraoperative or postoperative diuretic therapy].

risk for impaired Gas Exchange possibly evidenced by (alveolar-capillary membrane changes [atelectasis, interstitial edema]), abnormal breathing pattern [inadequate function or premature discontinuation of chest tubes], [anemia], hypoxemia.

acute Pain/impaired Comfort may be related to [tissue inflammation or trauma, edema formation, intraoperative nerve trauma, and myocardial ischemia], possibly evidenced by reports of incisional discomfort or pain in chest and donor site; paresthesia or pain in hand, arm, shoulder, anxiety, restlessness, irritability; distraction behaviors, and changes in heart rate and blood pressure.

impaired Skin/Tissue Integrity may be related to [mechanical trauma (surgical incisions, puncture wounds) and edema] possibly evidenced by acute pain, alteration in skin/tissue integrity, hematoma.

Cardiogenic shock   MS
Refer to Shock, cardiogenic

Cardiomyopathy   CH/MS
decreased Cardiac Output may be related to altered contractility, possibly evidenced by dyspnea, fatigue, chest pain, dizziness, syncope.

Activity Intolerance may be related to imbalance between oxygen supply and demand, possibly evidenced by generalized weakness, fatigue, exertional dyspnea, abnormal heart rate or blood pressure response to activity, electrocardiogram changes.

ineffective Role Performance may be related to changes in physical health, stress, demands of job and life, possibly evidenced by change in usual patterns of responsibility, role strain, change in capacity to resume role.

Carotid endarterectomy MS
Also refer to Surgery, general
risk for ineffective cerebral Tissue Perfusion possibly evidenced by (carotid stenosis, embolism, treatment regimen [thrombolytic therapy]).

Carpal tunnel syndrome CH/MS
acute/chronic Pain may be related to pressure on median nerve, possibly evidenced by verbal/coded reports, reluctance to use affected extremity, guarding behavior, expressed fear of reinjury, altered ability to continue previous activities.

impaired physical Mobility may be related to (neuromuscular impairment) and pain, possibly evidenced by decreased hand strength, weakness, limited range of motion, and reluctance to attempt movement.

risk for peripheral Neurovascular Dysfunction possibly evidenced by (mechanical compression [e.g., brace, repetitive tasks or motions], immobilization).

deficient Knowledge regarding condition, prognosis, and treatment and safety needs may be related to lack of exposure or recall, information misinterpretation, possibly evidenced by questions, statements of concern, request for information, inaccurate follow-through of instructions, development of preventable complications.

Casts CH/MS
Also refer to Fractures
risk for peripheral Neurovascular Dysfunction possibly evidenced by (fracture, mechanical compression [cast], tissue trauma, immobilization, vascular obstruction).

risk for impaired Skin Integrity possibly evidenced by [pressure of cast], humidity, [debris under cast, objects inserted under cast to relieve itching], (altered sensation or circulation, vascular trauma).

Self-Care deficit [specify] may be related to impaired ability to perform self-care tasks, possibly evidenced by statements of need for assistance and difficulty in performing activities of daily living.

Cataract CH
[disturbed visual Sensory Perception] may be related to altered sensory reception or status of sense organs, possibly evidenced by diminished acuity, visual distortions, and change in usual response to stimuli.

risk for physical Trauma possibly evidenced by insufficient knowledge of safety precautions, insufficient vision.

Anxiety [specify level]/Fear may be related to alteration in visual acuity, threat of loss of vision and independence, possibly evidenced by expressed concerns, apprehension, and feelings of uncertainty.

deficient Knowledge regarding ways of coping with altered abilities, therapy choices, and lifestyle changes may be related to lack of exposure or recall, misinterpretation, or cognitive limitations, possibly evidenced by requests for information, statement of concern, inaccurate follow-through of instructions, development of preventable complications.

Cataract extraction (postoperative care) MS
risk for Injury possibly evidenced by [increased intraocular pressure, intraocular hemorrhage, vitreous loss].

risk for Infection possibly evidenced by alteration in skin/tissue integrity, invasive procedure.

[disturbed visual Sensory Perception] may be related to altered sensory reception (use of eyedrops, cataract glasses), therapeutically restricted environment (surgical procedure, patching), possibly evidenced by visual distortions or blurring, visual confusion, change in depth perception.

Cat scratch disease CH
acute Pain may be related to physical injury agent: effects of circulating toxins [fever, headache, and lymphadenitis], possibly evidenced by verbal/coded reports, guarding behavior, and autonomic response (changes in vital signs).

Hyperthermia may be related to inflammatory process, possibly evidenced by increased body temperature, flushed warm skin, tachypnea, and tachycardia.

Celiac disease CH
imbalanced Nutrition: less than body requirements may be related to insufficient dietary intake, (inability to absorb nutrients, mucosal damage, loss of villi, proliferation of crypt cells, shortened transit time through gastrointestinal tract, possibly evidenced by weight loss, [abdominal distention, steatorrhea, anemia, vitamin deficiencies]).

Diarrhea may be related to irritation, malabsorption, possibly evidenced by abdominal pain, hyperactive bowel sounds, at least three loose stools per day.

risk for deficient Fluid Volume possibly evidenced by mild to massive steatorrhea, diarrhea.

Cellulitis   **CH/MS**

risk for *Infection [abscess, bacteremia]* possibly evidenced by alteration in skin integrity, (chronic illness), insufficient knowledge to avoid exposure to pathogens.

acute Pain/impaired Comfort may be related to physical injury agent (inflammatory process, circulating toxins), possibly evidenced by verbal/coded reports of pain, headache, guarding behavior, restlessness, autonomic responses.

impaired Tissue Integrity may be related to [trauma, inflammation, or invasion of tissues by infectious bacterial agent], or (impaired circulation), possibly evidenced by redness, localized area hot to touch, tenderness, or pain.

Cerebral embolism   **MS/CH**
Refer to Cerebrovascular accident

Cerebral palsy   **PED/CH**
Refer to Palsy, cerebral

Cerebrovascular accident   **MS**
ineffective cerebral Tissue Perfusion may be related to (embolism, cerebral aneurysm, brain injury[edema]), possibly evidenced by altered level of consciousness, changes in vital signs, changes in motor or sensory responses, restlessness, memory loss; sensory, language, intellectual, and emotional deficits.

impaired physical Mobility may be related to (neuromuscular impairment, sensory-perceptual impairment, alteration in cognitive functioning), possibly evidenced by decrease in fine/gross motor skills, decrease in range of motion; uncoordinated movement.

impaired verbal [and/or written] Communication may be related to (central nervous system impairment, physical barrier [loss of facial or oral muscle tone and control; generalized weakness]), possibly evidenced by difficulty forming words, difficulty speaking (dysarthria); inappropriate verbalization, difficulty comprehending written/spoken language; [inability to produce written communication].

Self-Care deficit [specify] may be related to (neuromuscular impairment, perceptual disorders, alteration in cognitive functioning), weakness, impaired mobility/ability to transfer, pain, possibly evidenced by inability to perform activities of daily living.

risk for *impaired Swallowing* possibly evidenced by (neuromuscular impairment).

risk for *Unilateral Neglect* possibly evidenced by visual field impairment.

                                       CH

situational low Self-Esteem/disturbed Body Image may be related to functional impairment, loss, focus on past function/strength, and (cognitive or perceptual impairment), possibly evidenced by actual change in function, self-negating verbalizations, report of perceptions reflecting altered view of body function.

Grieving may be related to alteration in neuroendocrine functioning, loss of processes of body, [neuromuscular impairments], and psychological distress, loss of job, role function, status, or independence, possibly evidenced by despair, anger, disorganization.

impaired Home Maintenance may be related to condition of individual family member, insufficient finances, family organization or planning; unfamiliarity with resources, and inadequate support systems, possibly evidenced by members expressing difficulty in managing home in a comfortable manner, requesting assistance with home maintenance, disorderly surroundings, and overtaxed family members.

Cervix, dysfunctional   **OB**
Refer to Dilation of Cervix, premature

Cesarean birth   **OB**
Also refer to Cesarean birth, unplanned/postpartal
deficient Knowledge regarding surgical procedure, expectation, postoperative routines and therapy, and self-care needs may be related to insufficient information, insufficient knowledge of resources, misinformation presented by others, possibly evidenced by insufficient knowledge, inappropriate behavior.

risk for *deficient Fluid Volume/Bleeding* possibly evidenced by restriction of oral intake, blood loss.

risk for *impaired Attachment* possibly evidenced by parent-child separation, insufficient privacy, (premature infant).

Cesarean birth, postpartal   **OB**
Also refer to Postpartum periods
risk for *impaired Attachment* possibly evidenced by anxiety, parent-child separation, [situational crisis (e.g., surgical intervention)].

acute Pain/impaired Comfort may be related to physical agent [e.g., surgical trauma, bladder or abdominal distention], chemical agent [e.g., effects of anesthesia], biological agent [hormonal effects], possibly evidenced by verbal/coded reports of pain, guarding or distraction behavior, irritability, facial expression of pain.

risk for situational low Self-Esteem possibly evidenced by, unrealistic self-expectations; physical condition; decrease in control over current situation.

risk for Injury possibly evidenced by (biochemical dysfunction [e.g., orthostatic hypotension, development of preeclampsia or eclampsia]), tissue hypoxia [e.g., effects of anesthesia, thromboembolism], abnormal blood profile [anemia, excessive blood loss, rubella sensitivity, Rh incompatibility], tissue trauma.

risk for Infection possibly evidenced by [tissue trauma], malnutrition, and associated conditions of decreased hemoglobin, invasive procedures or [increased environmental exposure, prolonged rupture of amniotic membranes], malnutrition.

Self-Care deficit (specify) may be related to effects of anesthesia, decreased strength and endurance, physical discomfort, possibly evidenced by inability to perform desired activities of daily living.

Cesarean birth, unplanned   OB
Also refer to Cesarean birth, postpartal
deficient Knowledge regarding underlying procedure, pathophysiology, and self-care needs may be related to incomplete or inadequate information, possibly evidenced by request for information, verbalization of concerns or misconceptions, and inappropriate or exaggerated behavior.

Anxiety [specify level] may be related to threat to current status—mother/fetus, emotional threat to self-esteem, unmet needs, interpersonal transmission, possibly evidenced by sympathetic stimulation, increase in tension, apprehensiveness, expressions of inadequacy, and restlessness.

Powerlessness may be related to anxiety, insufficient knowledge to manage a situation, insufficient interpersonal interactions, possibly evidenced by verbalization of sufficient sense of control, inadequate participation in care [or decision making].

risk for disturbed Maternal-Fetal Dyad possibly evidenced by (compromised fetal oxygen transport, pregnancy complication).

risk for labor Pain possibly evidenced by risk factors of increased or prolonged contractions, psychological reaction.

risk for Infection possibly evidenced by [tissue trauma], malnutrition, (decreased hemoglobin, invasive procedures or prolonged rupture of amniotic membranes), malnutrition.

Chemical dependence   PSY/CH
Refer to specific agents; Substance dependence/abuse rehabilitation

Chemotherapy   MS/CH
Also refer to Cancer
risk for deficient Fluid Volume possibly evidenced by gastrointestinal losses (vomiting), interference with adequate intake (stomatitis, anorexia), losses through abnormal routes (indwelling tubes, wounds, fistulas), hypermetabolic state.

imbalanced Nutrition: less than body requirements may be related to insufficient dietary intake, (inability to ingest food), [hypermetabolic state], possibly evidenced by weight loss (wasting), food aversion, alteration in taste sensation, sore buccal cavity; diarrhea or constipation.

impaired oral Mucous Membrane Integrity may be related to side effects of therapeutic agents or radiation, dehydration, and malnutrition, possibly evidenced by ulcerations, leukoplakia, decreased salivation, and reports of pain.

disturbed Body Image may be related to alteration in self-perception, cultural or spiritual incongruence possibly evidenced by verbalizations of feelings or perceptions, fear of reaction by others, preoccupation with change (e.g., anatomical or structural changes; loss of hair and weight), negative feelings about body, feelings of helplessness, hopelessness, and change in social environment.

ineffective Protection may be related to inadequate nutrition, drug therapy, radiation, abnormal blood profile, disease state (cancer), possibly evidenced by impaired healing, deficient immunity, anorexia, fatigue.

readiness for enhanced Hope possibly evidenced by expressed desire to enhance belief in possibilities or sense of meaning to life.

Chickenpox   CH/PED
Refer to Measles

Chlamydia trachomatis infection   CH
Refer to Sexually transmitted infection

Cholecystectomy   MS
acute Pain may be related to physical injury agent (interruption in skin and tissue layers with mechanical closure [sutures, staples] and invasive procedures including T-tube/nasogastric tube), possibly evidenced

by verbal reports, guarding or distraction behaviors, and autonomic responses—changes in vital signs.

ineffective Breathing Pattern may be related to pain, muscular impairment, decreased energy, fatigue, ineffective cough, possibly evidenced by fremitus, tachypnea, decreased respiratory depth and vital capacity, holding breath, reluctance to cough.

risk for deficient Fluid Volume/Bleeding possibly evidenced by losses from vomiting or nasogastric aspiration, medically restricted intake, altered coagulation.

Cholelithiasis   CH

acute Pain may be related to [obstruction or ductal spasm, inflammatory process, tissue ischemia, necrosis] possibly evidenced by verbal reports, guarding or distraction behavior, narrowed focus, and changes in vital signs.

risk for imbalanced Nutrition: less than body requirements possibly evidenced by [self-imposed or prescribed dietary restrictions, nausea and vomiting], food aversion, indigestion, abdominal pain.

deficient Knowledge regarding pathophysiology, therapy choices, and self-care needs may be related to lack of information or recall, misinterpretation, possibly evidenced by verbalization of concerns, questions, and recurrence of condition.

Cholera   CH/MS

deficient Fluid Volume may be related to active volume loss—profuse watery diarrhea, vomiting, possibly evidenced by intense thirst, marked loss of tissue turgor, decreased urine output (oliguria, anuria), change in mental state, hemoconcentration.

risk for Shock possibly evidenced by hypotension, hypovolemia, sepsis.

Christmas disease   CH

Refer to Hemophilia

Chronic obstructive lung disease   CH/MS

ineffective Airway Clearance may be related to bronchospasm, increased production of tenacious secretions, retained secretions, and decreased energy, fatigue, possibly evidenced by presence of wheezes, crackles, tachypnea, dyspnea, changes in depth of respirations, use of accessory muscles, persistent cough, and chest radiograph findings.

impaired Gas Exchange may be related to (alveolar-capillary membrane changes, altered oxygen delivery–[retained secretions/bronchospasm, air

trapping] and alveoli destruction), possibly evidenced by abnormal breathing pattern, restlessness, confusion, hypoxia, hypercapnia.

Activity Intolerance may be related to imbalance between oxygen supply and demand, and physical deconditioning, possibly evidenced by generalized weakness, fatigue, exertional dyspnea, and abnormal vital sign response.

imbalanced Nutrition: less than body requirements may be related to insufficient dietary intake, (inability to ingest food/adequate nutrients), possibly evidenced by weight loss, alteration in taste sensation, food aversion/insufficient interest in food, [decreased muscle mass and subcutaneous fat, poor muscle tone].

risk for Infection possibly evidenced by stasis of body fluid and malnutrition, (chronic illness), and decreased ciliary action.

Circumcision   PED

deficient Knowledge regarding surgical procedure, prognosis, and treatment may be related to lack of exposure, misinterpretation, unfamiliarity with information resources, possibly evidenced by request for information, verbalization of concern or misconceptions, inaccurate follow-through of instructions.

acute Pain may be related to physical injury agent (trauma to and edema of tender tissues), possibly evidenced by crying, changes in sleep pattern, refusal to eat.

impaired urinary Elimination may be related to tissue injury, inflammation, development of urethral fistula, possibly evidenced by edema, difficulty voiding.

risk for Bleeding possibly evidenced by insufficient knowledge of bleeding precautions [related to circumcision, decreased clotting factors immediately after birth, previously undiagnosed problems with bleeding or clotting].

risk for Infection possibly evidenced by [immature immune system], (invasive procedure/tissue trauma).

Cirrhosis   MS

Also refer to Substance dependence/abuse rehabilitation; Hepatitis, acute viral

risk for impaired Liver Function possibly evidenced by (viral infection), substance misuse.

                                                        CH

imbalanced Nutrition: less than body requirements may be related to insufficient dietary intake, (inability to ingest food or absorb nutrients), possibly evidenced by food aversion, food intake less than recommended daily allowance, satiety immediately upon ingesting food, [muscle wasting, weight loss, and imbalances in nutritional studies].

excess Fluid Volume may be related to compromised regulatory mechanism [syndrome of inappropriate antidiuretic hormone, decreased plasma proteins, malnutrition] and excess sodium or fluid intake, possibly evidenced by generalized or abdominal edema, weight gain, dyspnea, blood pressure changes, positive hepatojugular reflex, change in mentation, altered electrolytes, changes in urine specific gravity, and pleural effusion.

risk for impaired Skin Integrity possibly evidenced by impaired circulation, alteration in metabolism, alteration in skin turgor, pressure over bony prominence, and [presence of edema, ascites, accumulation of bile salts in skin].

risk for Bleeding possibly evidenced by impaired liver function. inherent coagulopathy, [portal hypertension, development of esophageal varices].

risk for acute Confusion possibly evidenced by substance misuse, malnutrition, impaired metabolic functioning.

Self-Esteem (specify)/disturbed Body Image may be related to alteration in self-perception, cultural or spiritual incongruence possibly evidenced by verbalizations of feelings or perceptions (e.g., fear of rejection or reaction by others), preoccupation with biophysical changes, altered physical appearance, uncertainty of prognosis, changes in role function, personal vulnerability, self-destructive behavior, changes in lifestyle.

Cleft lip/palate   PED/MS
Also refer to Newborn, special needs
ineffective infant Feeding Pattern may be related to anatomic abnormality, possibly evidenced by inability to sustain an effective suck, inability to coordinate sucking, swallowing, and breathing.

risk for Aspiration possibly evidenced by (impaired ability to swallow).

risk for impaired verbal Communication possibly evidenced by (oropharyngeal defect), difficulty forming words.

risk for disturbed Body Image/Social Isolation possibly evidenced by altered appearance, anatomic deficit, significance of body part (face).

Cocaine hydrochloride poisoning, acute   MS
Also refer to Stimulant abuse; Substance dependence/abuse rehabilitation

ineffective Breathing Pattern may be related to pharmacological effects on respiratory center of the brain, possibly evidenced by tachypnea, altered depth of respiration, shortness of breath, and abnormal arterial blood gases.

risk for decreased Cardiac Output possibly evidenced by drug effect on myocardium (degree dependent on drug purity/quality used); alterations in electrical rate, rhythm, or conduction; preexisting myocardiopathy.

CH

risk for impaired Liver Function possibly evidenced by cocaine abuse, effect of drug on liver.

Coccidioidomycosis   CH
(San Joaquin Valley/Valley Fever)
acute Pain may be related to physical injury agent (inflammation), possibly evidenced by verbal/coded reports of pain, distraction behavior, and narrowed focus.

Fatigue may be related to (illness), stressors, possibly evidenced by insufficient energy, impaired ability to maintain usual routines, lethargy, alteration in concentration, alteration in libido.

deficient Knowledge regarding nature and course of disease, therapy, and self-care needs may be related to lack of information, possibly evidenced by statements of concern and questions.

Colectomy   MS
Refer to Intestinal surgery (without diversion)

Colitis, ulcerative   MS
Diarrhea may be related to inflammation or malabsorption of the bowel, presence of toxins or segmental narrowing of the lumen, possibly evidenced by increased bowel sounds and peristalsis; frequent, watery stools (acute phase); abdominal pain; urgency; cramping.

acute/chronic Pain may be related to physical agent—inflammation of the intestines, hyperperistalsis, prolonged diarrhea, and anal or rectal irritation, fissures, fistulas, possibly evidenced by verbal/coded reports of pain, guarding or distraction behavior, restlessness, self-focused.

risk for deficient Fluid Volume possibly evidenced by continued gastrointestinal losses—severe diarrhea, vomiting; capillary plasma loss, restricted intake—nausea, anorexia, hypermetabolic state (inflammation, fever).

CH

imbalanced Nutrition: less than body requirements may be related to insufficient dietary intake, (inability to ingest food or absorb nutrients), and [hypermetabolic state], possibly evidenced by [weight loss, decreased subcutaneous fat or muscle mass], insufficient muscle tone, hyperactive bowel sounds, pale mucous membranes, and food aversion.

ineffective Coping may be related to [chronic nature and indefinite outcome of disease, multiple stressors (repeated over time), personal vulnerability, severe pain, inadequate sleep], lack of or ineffective support systems, possibly evidenced by verbalization of inability to cope with the situation, frequent illness, insufficient coping strategies, [depression and recurrent exacerbation of symptoms].

risk for Powerlessness possibly evidenced by (progressive illness, unpredictably of illness trajectory, complex treatment regimen).

Collagen disorders   CH
Refer to Arthritis, rheumatoid/juvenile rheumatoid; Lupus erythematosus, systemic; Polyarteritis nodosa; Temporal arteritis

Colorectal cancer   MS
Refer to Cancer; Colostomy

Colostomy   MS
risk for impaired Skin Integrity possibly evidenced by risk factors of chemical injury agent (absence of sphincter at stoma, character and flow of effluent and flatus from stoma, reaction to product or removal of adhesive, and improperly fitting appliance).

risk for Diarrhea/Constipation possibly evidenced by interruption or alteration of normal bowel function (placement of ostomy), changes in dietary or fluid intake, and effects of medication.

                                                          CH

deficient Knowledge regarding changes in physiological function and self-care/treatment needs may be related to lack of exposure or recall, information misinterpretation, possibly evidenced by questions, statement of concern, inaccurate follow-through of instruction or performance of ostomy care, development of preventable complications.

disturbed Body Image may be related to alteration in self-perception possibly evidenced by verbalizations of feelings or perceptions, preoccupation with biophysical changes (presence of stoma, loss of control of bowel elimination) and psychosocial factors negative feelings about body, fear of rejection or reaction of others, not touching or looking at stoma, and refusal to participate in care.

impaired Social Interaction may be related to fear of embarrassing situation secondary to altered bowel control with loss of contents, odor, possibly evidenced by reduced participation and verbalized or observed discomfort in social situations.

risk for Sexual dysfunction possibly evidenced by (alteration in body structure and function), vulnerability, [concern about response of SO, and disruption of sexual response pattern (e.g., erection difficulty)].

Coma   MS
risk for Suffocation possibly evidenced by cognitive impairment, loss of protective reflexes and purposeful movement.

risk for deficient Fluid Volume/imbalanced Nutrition: less than body requirements possibly evidenced by inability to ingest food or fluids, increased needs—hypermetabolic state.

[total] Self-Care deficit may be related to cognitive impairment and absence of purposeful activity, evidenced by inability to perform activities of daily living.

risk for ineffective cerebral Tissue Perfusion possibly evidenced by brain injury, substance abuse, embolism, cerebral aneurysm, brain tumor/neoplasm.

risk for Infection possibly evidenced by stasis of body fluids (oral, pulmonary, urinary), malnutrition, and associated condition of invasive procedures.

Coma, diabetic   MS
Refer to Diabetic ketoacidosis

Compartment syndrome, abdominal   MS
acute Pain may be related to physical agent [increasing abdominal distention and edema formation, inflammation], possibly evidenced by reports of pain, guarding behavior, restlessness, narrowed focus.

risk for dysfunctional Gastrointestinal Motility possibly evidenced by (decrease in gastrointestinal circulation).

ineffective Breathing Pattern may be related to abdominal distention, pain possibly evidenced by dyspnea, tachypnea, altered chest excursion.

risk for Shock possibly evidenced by hypotension, hypovolemia.

Compartment syndrome, extremity   MS
acute Pain may be related to physical injury agent (increasing pressure within muscle) possibly evidenced by reports of progressing pain [distal to injury unrelieved by routine analgesics].

ineffective peripheral Tissue Perfusion may be related to interruption of arterial blood flow, elevated tissue pressures, possibly evidenced by absent or diminished distal pulses, erythema, pain.

risk for peripheral Neurovascular Dysfunction possibly evidenced by reduction or interruption of blood flow (direct vascular injury, tissue trauma, excessive edema, elevated tissue pressures, hypovolemia).

Complex regional pain syndrome   CH

acute/chronic Pain may be related to physical agent (continued nerve stimulation), possibly evidenced by verbal reports, distraction or guarding behavior, narrowed focus, changes in sleep pattern, and altered ability to continue previous activities.

ineffective peripheral Tissue Perfusion may be related to reduction of arterial blood flow (arteriole vasoconstriction), possibly evidenced by extremity pain, altered skin characteristics, diminished pulses, and edema.

[disturbed tactile Sensory Perception] may be related to altered sensory reception (neurological deficit, pain), possibly evidenced by change in usual response to stimuli—abnormal sensitivity of touch, physiological anxiety, and irritability.

risk for ineffective Role Performance possibly evidenced by risk factors of situational crisis, chronic disability, debilitating pain.

risk for compromised family Coping possibly evidenced by family disorganization, (family role change, and prolonged disability that exhausts capacity of support person).

Concussion, brain   CH

Also refer to Postconcussion syndrome

acute Pain may be related to trauma to/edema of cerebral tissue, possibly evidenced by reports of headache, guarding or distraction behaviors, and narrowed focus.

risk for deficient Fluid Volume possibly evidenced by vomiting, decreased intake, and hypermetabolic state (fever).

risk for impaired Memory possibly evidenced by (brain injury, neurological impairment).

deficient Knowledge regarding condition, treatment, safety needs, and potential complications may be related to lack of recall, misinterpretation, cognitive limitation, possibly evidenced by questions, statement of concerns, development of preventable complications.

Conduct disorder (childhood,   PSY/PED
adolescence)

risk for self-/other-directed Violence: possibly evidenced by conflict in interpersonal relationships, pattern of indirect violence, impulsivity, suicide behavior, (pattern of difficulties in family background, mental health issues, psychological disorder).

defensive Coping may be related to inadequate coping strategies, maturational crisis, multiple life changes/losses, lack of control of impulsive actions, and personal vulnerability, possibly evidenced by inappropriate use of defense mechanisms; inability to meet role expectations; poor self-esteem; failure to assume responsibility for own actions; hypersensitivity to slight or criticism; and excessive smoking, drinking, or drug use.

ineffective Impulse Control may be related to chronic low self-esteem, anger, disorder of development, mood, personality possibly evidenced by acting without thinking, irritability, temper outbursts.

chronic low Self-Esteem may be related to cultural incongruence, inadequate belonging or affection, receiving insufficient approval of others, possibly evidenced by exaggerated negative feedback about self, excessive seeking of reassurance, rejection of positive feedback, underestimates ability to deal with situations.

CH

compromised/disabled family Coping may be related to excessive guilt, anger, or blaming among family members; parental inconsistencies; disagreements regarding discipline, limit setting, and approaches; and exhaustion of parental resources [prolonged coping with disruptive child], possibly evidenced by unrealistic parental expectations; rejection or overprotection of child; and exaggerated expressions of anger, disappointment, or despair regarding child's behavior or ability to improve or change.

impaired Social Interaction may be related to retarded ego development, developmental state (adolescence), lack of social skills, low self-concept, dysfunctional family system, and neurological impairment, possibly evidenced by dysfunctional interaction with others, difficulty playing quietly and maintaining attention to task or play activity, and interrupting or intruding on others.

Congestive heart failure   MS

Refer to Heart failure, chronic

Conjunctivitis, bacterial   CH

acute Pain/impaired Comfort may be related to inflammation, ocular irritation, edema, possibly evidenced by verbal reports, irritability, guarding behavior.

risk for Infection [spread] possibly evidenced by insufficient knowledge to avoid spread.

risk for ineffective Health Management possibly evidenced by length of therapy, perceived benefit.

Connective tissue disease   CH

Refer to Arthritis, rheumatoid/juvenile rheumatoid; Lupus erythematosus, systemic; Polyarteritis nodosa; Temporal arteritis

Conn's syndrome   MS/CH

Refer to Aldosteronism, primary

Constipation   CH

Constipation may be related to weak abdominal musculature, gastrointestinal obstructive lesions, pain on defecation, medications, diagnostic procedures, pregnancy, possibly evidenced by change in character and frequency of stools, feeling of abdominal or rectal fullness or pressure, changes in bowel sounds, abdominal distention.

acute Pain may be related to physical agent (abdominal fullness or pressure, straining to defecate, and trauma to delicate tissues), possibly evidenced by verbal reports, reluctance to defecate, and distraction behavior.

deficient Knowledge regarding dietary needs, bowel function, and medication effect may be related to lack of information, misconceptions, possibly evidenced by development of problem and verbalization of concerns, questions.

Conversion disorder   PSY

Refer to Somatoform disorders

Convulsions   CH

Refer to Seizure disorder

COPD   CH

Refer to Chronic obstructive lung disease

Corneal transplantation   MS

risk for Injury possibly evidenced by intraocular hemorrhage, edema/swelling, changes in visual acuity, increased intraocular pressure, glaucoma.

risk for Infection possibly evidenced by (type of surgical procedure, and use of implants; inadequate or ineffective antibiotic prophylaxis).

[disturbed visual Sensory Perception] may be related to altered sensory reception (use of eyedrops, edema, swelling), therapeutically restricted environment (patching), possibly evidenced by visual distortions, blurring, change in acuity.

Coronary artery bypass surgery   MS

risk for decreased Cardiac Output possibly evidenced by decreased myocardial contractility, diminished circulating volume (preload), alterations in electrical conduction, and increased systemic vascular resistance (afterload).

acute Pain may be related to physical injury agent [direct chest tissue and bone trauma, invasive tubes and lines, donor site incision, tissue inflammation, edema formation, intraoperative nerve trauma], possibly evidenced by verbal reports, changes in vital signs, distraction behaviors, restlessness, irritability.

[disturbed Sensory Perception (specify)] may be related to restricted environment (postoperative), sleep deprivation, effects of medications, continuous environmental sounds and activities, and psychological stress of procedure, possibly evidenced by disorientation, alterations in behavior, exaggerated emotional responses, and visual or auditory distortions.

    CH

ineffective Role Performance may be related to situational crises (dependent role), recuperative process, uncertainty about future, possibly evidenced by delay or alteration in physical capacity to resume role, change in usual role or responsibility, change in self-/others' perception of role.

Coronary artery disease   CH

Activity Intolerance may be related to imbalance between oxygen supply and demand, sedentary lifestyle, possibly evidenced by exertional discomfort, pain, fatigue, abnormal heart rate response, electrocardiogram changes—dysrhythmias, ischemia.

risk for decreased Cardiac Output possibly evidenced by altered heart rate or rhythm, altered contractility, increased peripheral vascular resistance.

Cor pulmonale   CH/MS

Also refer to Heart failure, chronic; Chronic obstructive lung disease

Activity Intolerance may be related to imbalance between oxygen supply and demand, generalized weakness, [chest pain], possibly evidenced by exertional discomfort and dyspnea, fatigue.

excess Fluid Volume may be related to compromised regulatory mechanism, possibly evidenced by shortness of breath, dependent edema, jugular vein distention, positive hepatojugular reflux, abnormal breath sounds, change in mental status.

impaired Gas Exchange may be related to (ventilation perfusion imbalance [heart failure]), possibly evidenced by abnormal breathing (dyspnea) and skin color (cyanosis), restlessness, somnolence, abnormal arterial blood gas values (hypoxemia, hypercapnia, acidosis), polycythemia.

Cradle cap   CH
Refer to Dermatitis, seborrheic

Craniotomy   MS
Also refer to Surgery, general
risk for decreased intracranial Adaptive Capacity possibly evidenced by brain injuries, systemic hypotension with intracranial hypertension.

[disturbed Sensory Perception (specify)] may be related to altered sensory reception, transmission or integration (neurological deficit), possibly evidenced by disorientation to time, place, person; motor incoordination, altered communication patterns, restlessness, irritability, change in behavior pattern.

risk for Infection possibly evidenced by [traumatized tissues], alteration in skin integrity and (invasive procedures), and [altered integrity of closed system (cerebrospinal fluid leak)].

Creutzfeldt-Jakob disease   CH
impaired Memory may be related to neurological deficits, possibly evidenced by observed experiences of forgetting, inability to perform previously learned skills, inability to recall factual information or recent or past events.

Fear may be related to [diminished functional abilities, progressive deterioration, lack of treatment options], possibly evidenced by apprehension, irritability, defensiveness, suspiciousness, aggressive behavior, social isolation.

impaired Walking may be related to changes in muscle coordination and balance, visual changes, impaired judgment, myoclonic seizures, possibly evidenced by inability to walk desired distances, climb stairs, navigate uneven surfaces.

[disturbed visual Sensory Perception] may be related to altered sensory reception or integration (neurological disease), possibly evidenced by change in sensory acuity (visual field defects, diplopia, dimness, blurring, visual agnosia), change in usual response to stimuli.

[total] Self-Care deficit may be related to cognitive decline, physical limitations, frustration over loss of independence, depression, possibly evidenced by impaired ability to perform activities of daily living, unkempt appearance, poor hygiene, apathy.

risk for caregiver Role Strain possibly evidenced by illness severity of care receiver, duration of caregiving required, care receiver exhibiting deviant or bizarre behavior; family/caregiver isolation, lack of respite or recreation, spouse is caregiver.

Crohn's disease   MS/CH
Also refer to Colitis, ulcerative
imbalanced Nutrition: less than body requirements may be related to insufficient dietary intake due to [intestinal pain after eating, decreased transit time through bowel, fear that eating may cause diarrhea], possibly evidenced by [weight loss, decreased subcutaneous fat and muscle mass], insufficient muscle tone, food aversion.

Diarrhea may be related to inflammation of small intestines, presence of toxins, irritation—particular dietary intake, malabsorption of the bowel, segmental narrowing of the lumen, possibly evidenced by hyperactive bowel sounds, increased peristalsis, cramping, and frequent loose liquid stools.

deficient Knowledge regarding condition, nutritional needs, and prevention of recurrence may be related to misinterpretation of information, lack of recall, unfamiliarity with resources, possibly evidenced by statements of concern, questions, inaccurate follow-through of instructions, and development of preventable complications or exacerbation of condition.

Croup   PED/CH
ineffective Airway Clearance may be related to presence of thick, tenacious mucus and swelling or spasms of the epiglottis, possibly evidenced by harsh, brassy cough; tachypnea; use of accessory breathing muscles; and presence of wheezes.

deficient Fluid Volume may be related to decreased ability or aversion to swallowing, presence of fever, and increased respiratory losses, possibly evidenced by dry mucous membranes; poor skin turgor; and scanty, concentrated urine.

Croup, membranous   PED/CH
Also refer to Croup

risk for Suffocation possibly evidenced by inflammation of larynx with formation of false membrane.

Anxiety [specify level]/Fear may be related to perceived threat [to self (difficulty breathing), and transmission of anxiety of adults], possibly evidenced by restlessness, facial tension, crying, and sympathetic stimulation.

C-section   **OB**
Refer to Cesarean birth, unplanned

Cubital tunnel syndrome   **CH**
acute/chronic Pain may be related to physical agent (pressure on ulnar nerve at elbow), possibly evidenced by verbal reports, reluctance to use affected extremity, guarding behaviors, expressed fear of reinjury, altered ability to continue previous activities.

impaired physical Mobility may be related to (neuromuscular impairment), and pain, possibly evidenced by decreased pinch or grasp strength, hand fatigue, and reluctance to attempt movement.

risk for peripheral Neurovascular Dysfunction possibly evidenced by mechanical compression (e.g., brace, repetitive tasks or motions), immobilization.

Cushing's syndrome   **CH/MS**
risk for excess Fluid Volume possibly evidenced by compromised regulatory mechanism (fluid and sodium retention).

risk for Infection possibly evidenced by (suppressed inflammatory response), [skin and capillary fragility, and negative nitrogen balance].

imbalanced Nutrition: less than body requirements may be related to insufficient dietary intake, (biological factors [disturbance of carbohydrate metabolism]), possibly evidenced by [decreased muscle mass and laboratory evidence of increased resistance to insulin].

Self-Care deficit [specify] may be related to muscle wasting, generalized weakness, fatigue, and demineralization of bones, possibly evidenced by statements of or observed inability to complete or perform activities of daily living.

disturbed Body Image may be related to alteration in self-perception (e.g., change in structure or appearance [effects of disease process, drug therapy], possibly evidenced by negative feelings about body, feelings of helplessness, and changes in social involvement).

Sexual dysfunction may be related to (altered body function [loss of libido, impotence, and cessation of menses]), possibly evidenced by verbalization of undesired change in sexual function or desire [alteration in relationship with SO].

risk for physical Trauma [fractures] possibly evidenced by impaired balance and associated conditions of decrease in muscle coordination and [increased protein breakdown and demineralization of bones].

CVA   **MS/CH**
Refer to Cerebrovascular accident

Cyclothymic disorder   **PSY**
Refer to Bipolar disorder

Cystic fibrosis   **CH/PED**
ineffective Airway Clearance may be related to excessive production of thick mucus and decreased ciliary action, possibly evidenced by abnormal breath sounds, ineffective cough, cyanosis, and altered respiratory rate and depth.

risk for Infection possibly evidenced by stasis of body fluids (respiratory secretions), insufficient knowledge to avoid exposure to pathogens.

imbalanced Nutrition: less than body requirements may be related to insufficient dietary intake, (inability to digest food/absorb nutrients) possibly evidenced by [failure to gain weight, muscle wasting, and retarded physical growth].

deficient Knowledge regarding pathophysiology of condition, medical management, and available community resources may be related to insufficient information, misconceptions, possibly evidenced by statements of concern, questions; inaccurate follow-through of instructions, development of preventable complications.

compromised family Coping may be related to chronic nature of disease and disability, inadequate or incorrect information or understanding by a primary person, and possibly evidenced by SO attempting assistive or supportive behaviors with less than satisfactory results, protective behavior disproportionate to client's abilities or need for autonomy.

Cystitis   **CH**
acute Pain may be related to physical injury agent [inflammation and bladder spasms], possibly evidenced by verbal reports, distraction behaviors, and narrowed focus.

impaired urinary Elimination may be related to inflammation or irritation of bladder, possibly evidenced by frequency, nocturia, and dysuria.

deficient Knowledge regarding condition, treatment, and prevention of recurrence may be related to inadequate information, misconceptions, possibly evidenced by statements of concern and questions; recurrent infections.

Cytomegalic inclusion disease   CH
Refer to Cytomegalovirus infection

Cytomegalovirus (CMV) infection   CH
[risk for disturbed visual Sensory Perception] possibly evidenced by inflammation of the retina.

risk for fetal Infection possibly evidenced by risk factors of transplacental exposure, contact with blood or body fluids.

D&C   OB/GYN
Refer to Dilation and curettage

Deep vein thrombosis   CH/MS
Refer to Thrombophlebitis

Degenerative disc disease   CH/MS
Refer to Herniated nucleus pulposus

Degenerative joint disease   CH
Refer to Arthritis, rheumatoid
(Although this is a degenerative process versus the inflammatory process of rheumatoid arthritis, nursing concerns are the same.)

Dehiscence, abdominal wound   MS
impaired Skin Integrity may be related to alteration in fluid volume (circulation), inadequate nutrition (obesity, malnutrition), and [physical stress on incision], possibly evidenced by [poor or delayed wound healing and disruption of skin surface or wound closure].

risk for Infection possibly evidenced by risk factors of alteration in skin/tissue integrity (separation of incision) and associated conditions of invasive procedure [traumatized intestines, environmental exposure].

Fear/Anxiety [severe] may be related to learned response to threat [health crisis, potential threat of death], possibly evidenced by apprehensiveness, feeling of dread, restless behaviors, and sympathetic stimulation.

deficient Knowledge regarding condition, prognosis, and treatment needs may be related to lack of information or recall and misinterpretation of information, possibly evidenced by development of preventable complications, requests for information, and statement of concern.

Dehydration   PED/CH
deficient Fluid Volume [specify] may be related to etiology as defined by specific situation, possibly evidenced by dry mucous membranes, poor skin turgor, decreased pulse volume and pressure, and thirst.

risk for impaired oral Mucous Membrane Integrity possibly evidenced by risk factors of dehydration and decreased salivation.

deficient Knowledge regarding fluid needs may be related to lack of information/misinterpretation, possibly evidenced by questions, statement of concern, and inadequate follow-through of instructions, development of preventable complications.

Delirium tremens   MS/PSY
Also refer to Alcohol intoxication, acute
Anxiety [severe/panic]/Fear may be related to cessation of alcohol intake, physiological withdrawal, threat to self-concept, perceived threat of death, possibly evidenced by increased tension; apprehension; expressions of shame, self-disgust, or remorse; fear of unspecified consequences.

[disturbed Sensory Perception (specify)] may be related to exogenous (alcohol consumption and sudden cessation) or endogenous factors (electrolyte imbalance, elevated ammonia and blood urea nitrogen), chemical alterations, sleep deprivation, and psychological stress, possibly evidenced by disorientation, restlessness, irritability, exaggerated emotional responses, bizarre thinking, and visual and auditory distortions or hallucinations.

risk for decreased Cardiac Output possibly evidenced by direct effect of alcohol on heart muscle, altered systemic vascular resistance, presence of dysrhythmias.

risk for Falls possibly evidenced by risk factors of history of falls, (alteration in cognitive functioning, impaired balance, anemia).

imbalanced Nutrition: less than body requirements may be related to insufficient dietary intake (inability to digest food, absorb nutrients) possibly evidenced by inadequate food intake, alteration in taste sensation, food aversion, [debilitated state, decreased subcutaneous fat or muscle mass, signs of mineral or electrolyte deficiency].

Delivery, precipitous/out of hospital   OB
Also refer to Labor, precipitous; Labor stages I–IV
risk for deficient Fluid Volume/Bleeding possibly evidenced by nausea/vomiting, lack of intake, excessive vascular loss (pregnancy complication [e.g., abruptio placenta], postpartum complication [e.g., lacerations]).

risk for Infection possibly evidenced by alteration in skin integrity, increased environmental exposure, (rupture of amniotic membranes).

risk for fetal Injury possibly evidenced by physical factors (e.g., rapid descent, pressure changes), (tissue hypoxia).

Delusional disorder   PSY
risk for self-/other-directed Violence possibly evidenced by perceived threats of danger, increased feelings of anxiety, acting out in an irrational manner.

[severe] Anxiety may be related to stressors, unmet needs, value conflict, threat to current status, (maturational/situational crisis), possibly evidenced by feeling of inadequacy, facial tension, poor eye contact, preoccupation, rumination, blocking of thoughts.

Powerlessness may be related to insufficient interpersonal interaction, anxiety, (complex treatment regimen), possibly evidenced by insufficient sense of control, alienation.

impaired Social Interaction may be related to disturbance in thought processes, insufficient skills to enhance mutuality, possibly evidenced by discomfort in social situations, dysfunctional interaction with others, dissatisfaction with social engagement.

Dementia, HIV   CH/PSY
Also refer to Dementia, presenile/senile
acute/chronic Confusion may be related to alteration in sleep-wake cycle, dehydration, malnutrition, (infection, cerebrovascular accident, impaired metabolic functioning), possibly evidenced by misperception, alteration/progressive impairment in cognitive functioning, agitation, restlessness, alteration in behavior/personality.

[mild to severe] Anxiety may be related to unmet needs, threat to change in current status, threat of death, interpersonal transmission/contagion, possibly evidenced by increase in tension, apprehensiveness, distress, increase in wariness, restlessness, extraneous movement, cardiovascular excitation.

compromised family Coping/caregiver Role Strain may be related to increase in care needs/ around-the-clock responsibilities, exhaustion of support person's capacity, family disorganization, isolation/alienation, possibly evidenced by family conflict, emotional vacillation, support person withdraws from client.

Dementia, presenile/senile   CH/PSY
Also refer to Alzheimer's disease
impaired Memory may be related to (mild cognitive impairment, neurological impairment), possibly evidenced by persistent forgetfulness, persistent inability to recall if a behavior was performed, persistent inability to perform a previously learned skill, persistent inability to recall factual information or events.

Fear may be related to [diminished functional abilities, public disclosure of disabilities, further mental or physical deterioration], possibly evidenced by social isolation, apprehension, irritability, defensiveness, suspiciousness, aggressive behavior.

Self-Care deficit [specify] may be related to decrease in motivation, anxiety, (alteration in cognitive functioning, fatigue, perceptual disorders), possibly evidenced by impaired ability to perform activities of daily living.

risk for Injury/physical Trauma possibly evidenced by emotional disturbance, impaired balance, weakness, malnutrition, (alteration in cognitive functioning).

risk for caregiver Role Strain possibly evidenced by (care receiver illness severity, cognitive disorder), complexity or of care activities, family/caregiver isolation, insufficient respite or recreation.

Grieving may be related to anticipatory loss (e.g., decline in memory, loss of job/status, and independence; family perception of potential loss of loved one, possibly evidenced by psychological distress, anger, despair, and alteration in sleep patterns).

Dementia, vascular   CH/PSY
Refer to Alzheimer's disease

Depersonalization disorder   PSY
Refer to Dissociative disorders

Depressant abuse   CH/PSY
Also refer to Drug overdose, acute (depressants)
ineffective Denial may be related to threat of unpleasant reality, insufficient sense of control, ineffective coping strategies, possibly evidenced by does not admit impact of condition on life, minimizes symptoms, refusal of healthcare.

ineffective Coping may be related to inaccurate threat appraisal, ineffective tension release strategies, possibly evidenced by substance misuse, insufficient goal-directed behavior, insufficient problem-solving skills, destructive behavior toward self.

imbalanced Nutrition: less than body requirements may be related to insufficient dietary intake [use of substance in place of nutritional food] possibly evidenced by loss of weight, pale mucous membranes, [laboratory evidence of electrolyte imbalances, anemias].

risk for Injury possibly evidenced by exposure to toxic chemical [CNS depressant, CNS agitation], (alteration in cognitive functioning).

Depression, major   PSY
risk for Suicide possibly evidenced by marked changes in attitude/behavior, hopelessness, grieving, sudden euphoric recovery from depression.

[moderate to severe] Anxiety may be related to stressors, conflict about life goals, value conflict, unmet needs, threat to current status, interpersonal transmission/contagion, possibly evidenced by feeling of inadequacy, fear, increase in tension, hypervigilance, alteration in concentration, decrease in productivity, diminished ability to problem-solve, rumination.

Insomnia may be related to stressors, depression, physical discomfort, average daily physical activity is less than recommended for gender/age, alcohol consumption, possibly evidenced by difficulty initiating/maintaining sleep state, early awakening, nonrestorative sleep pattern, insufficient energy, alteration in concentration, increase in accidents/absenteeism.

Social Isolation/impaired Social Interaction may be related to disturbance in self-concept, disturbance in thought processes [depressed mood], communication barrier, insufficient skills to enhance mutuality, possibly evidenced by discomfort in social situations, dissatisfaction with social engagement, impaired social functioning, and dysfunctional interaction with others.

interrupted Family Processes may be related to (situational/developmental crises, change in family social status), shift in family roles, power shift among family members, shift in health status of a family member, possibly evidenced by decrease in available emotional support, change in communication pattern, changes in participation for decision making, alteration in family satisfaction.

Depression, postpartum   OB/PSY
Also refer to Depressive disorders
risk for impaired Attachment possibly evidenced by anxiety [associated with the parent role], inability to meet personal needs, perceived guilt regarding relationship with infant.

Fatigue may be related to stressors, sleep deprivation, depression as evidenced by insufficient energy, impaired inability to maintain usual routines, increase in physical symptoms.

situational low Self-Esteem may be related to (developmental transition), alteration in body image, possibly evidenced by underestimates ability to deal with situation, self-negating verbalizations, helplessness.

risk for other-directed Violence possibly evidenced by hopelessness, increased anxiety, mood swings, despondency, severe depression, (psychotic disorder).

Depressive disorders   PSY
Refer to Depression, major; Bipolar disorder; Premenstrual dysphoric disorder

de Quervain's syndrome   CH
acute/chronic Pain may be related to physical agent (inflammation of tendon sheath, swelling), possibly evidenced by verbal reports of pain, reluctance to use affected hand, guarding behavior, expressed fear of reinjury, altered ability to continue previous activities.

impaired physical Mobility may be related to (musculoskeletal impairment), swelling, pain, numbness of thumb and index finger, possibly evidenced by decreased grasp or pinch strength, weakness, limited range of motion, and reluctance to attempt movement.

Dermatitis, contact   CH
acute Pain/impaired Comfort may be related to [cutaneous inflammation and irritation] possibly evidenced by verbal reports, irritability, and scratching.

impaired Skin Integrity may be related to chemical injury agent (exposure to chemicals or environmental allergens) possibly evidenced by [inflammation, epidermal edema, development of vesicles or bullae].

risk for Infection possibly evidenced by alteration in skin/tissue and suppressed inflammatory response.

Social Isolation may be related to alterations in physical appearance, possibly evidenced by expressed feelings of rejection and decreased interaction with peers.

Dermatitis, seborrheic   CH

impaired Skin Integrity may be related to chronic inflammatory condition of the skin, possibly evidenced by disruption of skin surface with dry or moist scales, yellowish crusts, erythema, and fissures.

Developmental disorders, pervasive PED/PSY

Refer to Autism spectrum disorder; Rett's syndrome; Asperger's disorder

Diabetes, gestational   OB

Also refer to Diabetes mellitus

risk for unstable Blood Glucose Level possibly evidenced by (pregnancy), insufficient knowledge of diabetes management, inadequate blood glucose monitoring.

risk for disturbed Maternal-Fetal Dyad possibly evidenced by (alteration in glucose metabolism, compromised fetal oxygen transport; treatment regimen).

readiness for enhanced Knowledge regarding diabetic condition, prognosis, and self-care treatment needs possibly evidenced by expresses desire to enhance learning.

Diabetes insipidus   MS/CH

deficient Fluid Volume [hypertonic] may be related to failure of regulatory mechanisms and hormone imbalance (e.g., brain injury, medication, sickle cell anemia, hypothyroidism), possibly evidenced by urinary frequency, thirst, polydipsia, dilute urine, dry skin and mucous membranes, decreased skin turgor, nocturia, increased serum sodium.

risk for ineffective Health Management possibly evidenced by complexity of medication regimen, presence of side effects, economic difficulties, inadequate knowledge, perceived seriousness and benefits.

Diabetes, juvenile   PED

Also refer to Diabetes mellitus

risk-prone Health Behavior may be related to inadequate comprehension, negative attitude toward healthcare, multiple stressors and life changes, possibly evidenced by failure to take action that prevents health problems, minimizes health status change, failure to achieve optimal sense of control.

risk for Injury possibly evidenced by ineffective control or swings in serum glucose level, changes in mentation, developmental age, risk-taking behaviors.

ineffective Coping may be related to (maturational crisis), inadequate level of perception of control, gender differences in coping strategies, possibly evidenced by ineffective coping strategies, insufficient problem-solving skills, risk-taking/destructive behavior toward self [inadequate diabetic control].

compromised family Coping may be related to insufficient information or understanding by support person, (situational or developmental crises faced by support person), possibly evidenced by assistive behaviors by support person produce unsatisfactory results; support person reports inadequate understanding that interferes with effective behaviors; support person reports preoccupation with own reaction to client's need, protective behavior by support person incongruent with client's abilities or need for autonomy.

Diabetes mellitus   CH/PED

deficient Knowledge regarding disease process/treatment and individual care needs may be related to unfamiliarity with information, lack of recall, misinterpretation, possibly evidenced by requests for information, statements of concern, misconceptions, inadequate follow-through of instructions, and development of preventable complications.

risk for unstable Blood Glucose Level possibly evidenced by nonadherence to diabetes management plan, ineffective medication management, inadequate blood glucose monitoring, average daily physical activity is less than recommended for gender/age, health status, stress, rapid growth periods.

risk for ineffective Health Management possibly evidenced by complexity and duration of treatment, perceived excessive demands made on individual, powerlessness, perceived susceptibility to complications.

risk for Infection possibly evidenced by associated conditions of (chronic illness, leukopenia, impaired circulation), and [delayed healing].

[risk for disturbed Sensory Perception (specify)] possibly evidenced by endogenous chemical alteration (glucose, insulin, or electrolyte imbalance).

Diabetes mellitus, intrapartum   OB

Also refer to Diabetes mellitus

risk for physical Trauma/impaired fetal Gas Exchange possibly evidenced by inadequate maternal diabetic control, presence of macrosomia, or intrauterine growth retardation.

risk for maternal Injury possibly evidenced by inadequate diabetic control (hypertension, severe edema, ketoacidosis, uterine atony or overdistention, dystocia).

[mild to moderate] Anxiety may be related to (situational "crisis"), threat to health status (maternal/fetus), possibly evidenced by increase in tension, apprehensiveness, fear of unspecific consequences, sympathetic stimulation.

Diabetes mellitus, postpartum   OB
risk for unstable Blood Glucose Level possibly evidenced by insufficient knowledge of disease management, ineffective medication management, [increased metabolic demands (recuperation, lactation)].

risk for Injury possibly evidenced by (biochemical or regulatory dysfunction—uterine atony/hemorrhage, gestational hypertension, hyperglycemia).

risk for impaired Attachment possibly evidenced by interruption in bonding process, physical illness, changes in physical abilities.

Diabetic ketoacidosis   CH/MS
deficient Fluid Volume [specify] may be related to hyperosmolar urinary losses, gastric losses, and inadequate intake, possibly evidenced by increased urinary output, dilute urine; reports of weakness, thirst; sudden weight loss; hypotension; tachycardia; delayed capillary refill; dry mucous membranes; poor skin turgor.

unstable Blood Glucose Level may be related to ineffective medication management, insufficient diabetes management, inadequate blood glucose monitoring, possibly evidenced by elevated serum glucose level, ketones in urine, nausea, weight loss, blurred vision, irritability.

Fatigue may be related to (illness), stressors, possibly evidenced by insufficient energy, impaired ability to maintain usual routines, ineffective role performance, alteration in concentration, lethargy.

risk for Infection possibly evidenced by stasis of body fluids, [high glucose levels], leukopenia, invasive procedures.

Dialysis, general   CH
Also refer to Dialysis, peritoneal; Hemodialysis
imbalanced Nutrition: less than body requirements may be related to insufficient dietary intake, (inability to ingest food or absorb nutrients), possibly evidenced by food intake less than recommended daily allowance, satiety immediately upon ingesting food, food aversion, alteration in taste sensation, insufficient muscle tone, weakness, sore buccal cavity, pale mucous membranes.

Grieving may be related to (loss of significant object—chronic disease; anticipatory loss—potentially fatal illness, possibly evidenced by distress, despair, alteration in sleep/dream pattern, alteration in activity level, and anger.

disturbed Body Image/situational low Self-Esteem may be related to alteration in self-perception, cultural or spiritual incongruence possibly evidenced by verbalizations of feelings or perceptions [or actions], (e.g., fear of reaction by others), preoccupation with changes in usual roles and body image, negative feelings about body, feelings of helplessness, powerlessness, extension of body boundary to incorporate environmental objects (e.g., dialysis setup), change in social involvement, overdependence on others for care, not taking responsibility for self-care, lack of follow-through, and self-destructive behavior).

Self-Care deficit [specify] may be related to (perceptual disorders, alteration in cognitive functioning [accumulated toxins]); fatigue, pain, discomfort, decrease in motivation, possibly evidenced by reported inability to perform activities of daily living.

ineffective Health Management may be related to difficulty managing complex treatment regimen or navigating complex healthcare systems, excessive demands, powerlessness; perceived seriousness of condition, perceived benefit [of treatment], possibly evidenced by difficulty with prescribed regiment, failure to include treatment regimen in daily living, ineffective choices for meeting health goal.

compromised/disabled family Coping may be related to insufficient or incorrect information or understanding by support person, family disorganization, (family role change), insufficient reciprocal, exhaustion of support person's capacity, possibly evidenced by client concern about support person's response to health problem, neglect of treatment regimen, intolerance or rejection, and protective behavior by support person incongruent with client's abilities or need for autonomy.

Dialysis, peritoneal   MS/CH
Also refer to Dialysis, general
risk for excess Fluid Volume possibly evidenced by inadequate osmotic gradient of dialysate, fluid retention—malpositioned, kinked, or clotted catheter; bowel distention, peritonitis, scarring of peritoneum; excessive PO/IV intake.

risk for physical Trauma possibly evidenced by risk factors of improper placement during insertion or manipulation of catheter.

acute Pain/impaired Comfort may be related to physical injury agent (catheter irritation, improper catheter placement, presence of edema, abdominal distention, inflammation, or infection; rapid infusion or infusion of cold or acidic dialysate) possibly evidenced by verbal reports, guarding or distraction behaviors, and self-focus.

risk for Infection [peritonitis] possibly evidenced by [contamination of catheter or infusion system, skin contaminants].

risk for ineffective Breathing Pattern possibly evidenced by increased abdominal pressure restricting diaphragmatic excursion, rapid infusion of dialysate, pain or discomfort, inflammatory process (e.g., atelectasis/pneumonia).

Diaper rash   PED
Refer to Candidiasis

Diaphragmatic hernia   CH/MS
Refer to Hernia, hiatal

Diarrhea   PED/CH
deficient Knowledge regarding causative or contributing factors and therapeutic needs may be related to lack of information, misconceptions, possibly evidenced by statements of concern, questions, and development of preventable complications.

risk for deficient Fluid Volume possibly evidenced by excessive losses through gastrointestinal tract, altered intake.

impaired Skin Integrity may be related to effects of excretions on delicate tissues, possibly evidenced by reports of acute pain and/or bleeding, and alteration in skin integrity.

DIC   MS
Refer to Disseminated intravascular coagulation

Diffuse axonal (brain) injury   MS
Refer to Traumatic brain injury; Cerebrovascular accident

Digitalis toxicity   MS/CH
decreased Cardiac Output may be related to altered myocardial contractility and electrical conduction, possibly evidenced by changes in rate, rhythm, and conduction (development or worsening of dysrhythmias), changes in mentation, [elevated serum drug levels].

risk for imbalanced Fluid Volume possibly evidenced by excessive losses from vomiting or diarrhea, decreased intake, nausea, decreased plasma proteins, malnutrition, continued use of diuretics; excess sodium and fluid retention.

risk for Poisoning [drug toxicity] possibly evidenced by access to pharmaceutical agent; insufficient knowledge of pharmacological agent or poisoning prevention.

deficient Knowledge regarding condition, therapy, and self-care needs may be related to information misinterpretation and lack of recall, possibly evidenced by inaccurate follow-through of instructions and development of preventable complications.

Dilation and curettage   OB/GYN
Also refer to Abortion, elective or spontaneous termination
deficient Knowledge regarding surgical procedure, possible postprocedural complications, and therapeutic needs may be related to lack of exposure or unfamiliarity with information, possibly evidenced by requests for information and statements of concern, misconceptions.

Dilation of cervix, premature   OB
Also refer to Preterm labor
Anxiety [specify level] may be related to (situational crisis), threat of death or fetal loss, possibly evidenced by increase in tension, apprehensiveness, feeling of inadequacy, sympathetic stimulation, and repetitive questioning.

risk for disturbed Maternal-Fetal Dyad possibly evidenced by (treatment regimen—surgical intervention, use of tocolytic drugs).

Grieving may be related to (anticipatory potential fetal loss), possibly evidenced by expression of distress, anger, blaming.

Dislocation/subluxation of joint   CH
acute Pain may be related to [lack of continuity of bone/joint, muscle spasms, edema], possibly evidenced by verbal or coded reports, guarded or protective behavior, narrowed focus, autonomic responses.

risk for Injury possibly evidenced by nerve impingement, improper fitting of splint device.

impaired physical Mobility may be related to immobilization device, activity restrictions, pain, edema, decreased muscle strength, possibly evidenced by limited range of motion, limited ability to perform motor skills, gait changes.

Disruptive behavior disorder   PED/PSY
Refer to Oppositional defiant disorder

Disseminated intravascular coagulation   **MS**

risk for Shock possibly evidenced by failure of regulatory mechanism (coagulation process) and active loss, hemorrhage.

ineffective Tissue Perfusion (specify) may be related to alteration of arterial or venous flow (microemboli throughout circulatory system, and hypovolemia), possibly evidenced by changes in respiratory rate and depth, changes in mentation, decreased urinary output, and development of acral cyanosis and focal gangrene.

Anxiety [specify level]/Fear may be related to learned response to threat [sudden change in health status/threat of death], possibly evidenced by sympathetic stimulation, restlessness, focus on self, and apprehension.

risk for impaired Gas Exchange possibly evidenced by [reduced oxygen-carrying capacity, development of acidosis, fibrin deposition in microcirculation, and ischemic damage of lung parenchyma].

acute Pain may be related to physical injury agent (bleeding into joints/muscles, with hematoma formation, and ischemic tissues with areas of acral cyanosis and focal gangrene), possibly evidenced by verbal reports, narrowed focus, alteration in muscle tone, guarding or distraction behaviors, restlessness, autonomic responses.

Dissociative disorders   **PSY**

[severe/panic] Anxiety/Fear may be related to a threat to current status, value conflict(s), unmet needs, (learned response to threat or phobic stimulus), possibly evidenced by maladaptive response to stress [e.g., dissociating self, fragmentation of the personality].

risk for self-directed Violence possibly evidenced by suicidal ideation/behavior, (mental health issues [e.g., dissociative state/conflicting personalities, depression, substance misuse]), panic states, and suicidal or homicidal behaviors.

disturbed Personal Identity may be related to low self-esteem, dysfunctional family processes, (dissociative identity disorder), possibly evidenced by fluctuating feelings about self, confusion about goals, inability to distinguish between internal and external stimuli, ineffective relationships, inconsistent behavior.

disabled family Coping may be related to ambivalent family relationships, differing coping styles between support persons, chronically unexpressed feelings, possibly evidenced by abandonment, rejection, aggression, hostility; disregard for client's needs, neglect of relationship with family member.

Diverticulitis   **CH**

acute Pain may be related to physical injury agent (inflammation of intestinal mucosa), possibly evidenced by verbal reports, guarding or distraction behavior, autonomic responses, and narrowed focus.

Diarrhea/Constipation may be related to altered structure and function, and presence of inflammation, possibly evidenced by signs and symptoms dependent on specific problem (e.g., increase or decrease in frequency of stools and change in consistency).

deficient Knowledge regarding disease process, potential complications, therapy, and self-care needs may be related to lack of information, misconceptions, possibly evidenced by statements of concern, request for information, and development of preventable complications.

risk for ineffective Health Management possibly evidenced by difficulty with prescribed regimen, ineffective choices in daily living for meeting health goal; insufficient knowledge of therapeutic regimen; perceived seriousness of condition [chronic nature of disease process and recurrent episodes despite cooperation with medical regimen].

Down syndrome   **PED/CH**

Also refer to Mental delay (formerly retardation)

risk for disproportionate Growth and/or delayed Development possibly evidenced by (genetic disorder).

risk for physical Trauma possibly evidenced by cognitive difficulties and poor muscle tone or coordination, weakness.

risk for imbalanced Nutrition: less than body requirements possibly evidenced by inability to ingest food, insufficient muscle tone and protruding tongue, [weak or ineffective sucking/swallowing].

interrupted Family Processes may be related to (situational or developmental crises, shift in health status of a family member), shift in family roles, possibly evidenced by decrease in mutual support, ineffective task completion, change in family satisfaction/relationship pattern.

risk for complicated Grieving [parent/caregiver] possibly evidenced by emotional disturbance [loss of "the perfect child," chronic condition requiring long-term care, and unresolved feelings].

risk for impaired Attachment possibly evidenced by ill infant/child who is unable to effectively initiate parental contact, disorganized infant behavioral, inability of parents to meet personal needs.

---

risk for Social Isolation possibly evidenced by withdrawal from usual social interactions and activities, assumption of total child care, and becoming overindulgent or overprotective.

Dressler's syndrome   CH

acute Pain may be related to physical injury (tissue inflammation) possibly evidenced by verbal reports of chest pain, guarding or distraction behavior, self-focused, and changes in vital signs.

Anxiety [specify level] may be related to threat to current status, possibly evidenced by increase in tension, apprehensiveness, restlessness, distress, and uncertainty.

risk for ineffective Breathing Pattern possibly evidenced by pain on inspiration.

risk for impaired Gas Exchange possibly evidenced by (ventilation perfusion imbalance—pleural effusion, pulmonary infiltrates).

Drug overdose, acute (depressants)   MS/PSY

Also refer to Substance dependence/abuse rehabilitation

ineffective Breathing Pattern/impaired Gas Exchange may be related to (ventilation-perfusion imbalance [neuromuscular impairment, central nervous system depression, decreased lung expansion]), possibly evidenced by changes in respirations, cyanosis, and abnormal arterial blood gases.

risk for physical Trauma/Suffocation/Poisoning possibly evidenced by central nervous system depression, agitation, hypersensitivity to the drug(s), psychological stress.

risk for self-/other-directed Violence possibly evidenced by suicidal behaviors, toxic reactions to drug(s).

risk for Infection possibly evidenced by [drug injection techniques, impurities in injected drugs, localized trauma]; malnutrition, immunosuppression.

Drug withdrawal   CH/MS

[disturbed Sensory Perception (specify)] may be related to biochemical imbalance, altered sensory integration possibly evidenced by sensory distortions, poor concentration, irritability, hallucinations.

risk for Injury possibly evidenced by central nervous system agitation (depressants).

risk for Suicide possibly evidenced by alcohol or substance abuse, legal or disciplinary problems, depressed mood (stimulants).

acute Pain/impaired Comfort may be related to biochemical changes [cessation of drug use], possibly evidenced by reports of muscle aches, malaise.

Self-Care deficit (specify) may be related to perceptual or cognitive impairment, therapeutic management (restraints), possibly evidenced by inability to meet own physical needs.

Insomnia may be related to cessation of substance use, fatigue, possibly evidenced by reports of insomnia or hypersomnia, decreased ability to function, increased irritability.

Fatigue may be related to altered body chemistry (drug withdrawal), sleep deprivation, malnutrition, poor physical condition, possibly evidenced by verbal reports of overwhelming lack of energy, inability to maintain usual level of physical activity, inability to restore energy after sleep, compromised concentration.

DTs   MS/PSY

Refer to Delirium tremens

Duchenne's muscular dystrophy   PED/CH

Refer to Muscular dystrophy (Duchenne's)

Duodenal ulcer   MS/CH

Refer to Ulcer, peptic

DVT   CH/MS

Refer to Thrombophlebitis

Dysmenorrhea   GYN

acute Pain may be related to physical/biological agent—exaggerated uterine contractions, muscular contractions, possibly evidenced by verbal reports, guarding or distraction behavior, narrowed focus, and changes in vital signs.

ineffective Coping may be related to ineffective tension release strategies, insufficient sense of control, (situational "crisis," possibly evidenced by ineffective coping strategies, inability to deal with a situation, insufficient problem resolution).

Dyspareunia   GYN/PSY

Sexual dysfunction may be related to (alteration in body function), vulnerability, psychosocial abuse, possibly evidenced by alteration in sexual satisfaction, decrease in sexual desire, alteration in sexual activity.

Anxiety [specify] may be related to threat to current status, unmet needs, possibly evidenced by expressed concerns, distress, expressions of inadequacy.

Dysrhythmia, cardiac   CH/MS

risk for decreased Cardiac Output possibly evidenced by altered electrical conduction and reduced myocardial contractility.

deficient Knowledge regarding medical condition and therapy needs may be related to lack of information, misinterpretation, and unfamiliarity with information resources, possibly evidenced by questions, statement of misconception, failure to improve on previous regimen, and development of preventable complications.

risk for Activity Intolerance possibly evidenced by imbalance between oxygen supply and demand, and [cardiac depressant effects of certain drugs (beta blockers, antidysrhythmics)].

risk for Poisoning [digitalis toxicity] possibly evidenced by limited range of therapeutic effectiveness, lack of education or proper precautions, reduced vision, cognitive limitations.

Dysthymic disorder PSY/CH
Refer to Depression, major

Dystocia OB
Also refer to Labor, stage I [latent/active phases]
risk for maternal Injury possibly evidenced by alteration of muscle tone/contractile pattern, mechanical obstruction to fetal descent, maternal fatigue.

risk for fetal Injury possibly evidenced by prolonged labor, fetal malpresentations, tissue hypoxia and acidosis, abnormalities of the maternal pelvis, cephalopelvic disproportion.

risk for deficient Fluid Volume possibly evidenced by hypermetabolic state, vomiting, profuse diaphoresis, restricted oral intake, mild diuresis associated with oxytocin administration.

Eating disorders CH/PSY
Refer to Anorexia nervosa; Bulimia nervosa

Ebola MS
Also refer to Disseminated intravascular coagulation; Multiple organ dysfunction syndrome
acute Pain/impaired Comfort may be related to (illness-related symptoms), possibly evidenced by reports of distressing symptoms, anxiety, report of pain, facial expression of pain, self-focused.

Hyperthermia may be related to inflammatory process, possibly evidenced by increased body temperature, warm skin, headache.

risk for deficient Fluid Volume possibly evidenced by inadequate intake (nausea, painful swallowing, abdominal pain), increased losses (vomiting, diarrhea, hemorrhage/disseminated intravascular coagulation), hypermetabolic state (fever).

risk for Infection [spread of or secondary] possibly evidenced by (exposure to disease outbreak), insufficient knowledge [or resources] to avoid exposure to pathogens, malnutrition, (invasive procedure).

acute Confusion may be related to dehydration, malnutrition, (delirium or impaired metabolic functioning, infection), possibly evidenced by alterations in level of consciousness or cognition, restlessness/agitation, hallucinations.

Eclampsia OB
Also refer to Hypertension, gestational
Anxiety [specify]/Fear may be related to (situational crisis), threat of change in current status or death (self/fetus)], separation from support system, possibly evidenced by expressed concerns, apprehensiveness, increase in tension, decreased self-assurance, difficulty concentrating.

risk for maternal Injury possibly evidenced by tissue edema, hypoxia–tonic-clonic convulsions; abnormal blood profile–altered clotting factors.

impaired physical Mobility may be related to prescribed physical restrictions, discomfort, anxiety, possibly evidenced by difficulty turning, postural instability.

risk for Self-Care deficit (specify) possibly evidenced by weakness, discomfort, physical restrictions.

ECT PSY
Refer to Electroconvulsive therapy

Ectopic pregnancy (tubal) OB
Also refer to Abortion, spontaneous termination
acute Pain may be related to physical injury agent (distention/rupture of fallopian tube) possibly evidenced by verbal reports, guarding or distraction behavior, facial expression of pain, diaphoresis, and changes in vital signs.

risk for Bleeding/deficient Fluid Volume possibly evidenced by (pregnancy complication), hemorrhagic losses, and decreased or restricted intake.

Anxiety [specify level]/Fear may be related to threat of death and possible threat to current status (e.g., loss of ability to conceive), possibly evidenced by increase in tension, apprehensiveness, sympathetic stimulation, restlessness, and self-focused.

Eczema CH
Refer to Dermatitis, contact/seborrheic
impaired Comfort may be related to [cutaneous inflammation and irritation] possibly evidenced by verbal reports, irritability, and scratching.

---

risk for Infection possibly evidenced by alteration in skin integrity.

Social Isolation may be related to alterations in physical appearance, possibly evidenced by expressed feelings of rejection and decreased interaction with peers.

Edema, pulmonary   MS

excess Fluid Volume may be related to decreased cardiac functioning, excessive fluid and sodium intake, possibly evidenced by dyspnea, presence of crackles (rales), pulmonary congestion on radiograph, restlessness, anxiety, and increased central venous pressure and pulmonary pressures.

impaired Gas Exchange may be related to (alveolar-capillary changes and ventilation-perfusion imbalance–fluid collection or shifts into interstitial space and alveoli), possibly evidenced by hypoxia, restlessness, and confusion.

Anxiety [specify level]/Fear may be related to stressors perceived threat of death [inability to breathe], possibly evidenced by responses ranging from apprehension to panic state, restlessness, and focus on self.

Elder abuse   CH/PSY

Refer to Abuse, physical/psychological

Electrical injury   MS

Also refer to Burns

risk for decreased Cardiac Output possibly evidenced by altered heart rate and rhythm (ventricular fibrillation, asystole).

impaired [internal] Tissue Integrity may be related to thermal injury (along path of current), altered circulation (massive edema), possibly evidenced by damaged or destroyed tissue, necrosis.

risk for ineffective peripheral Tissue Perfusion possibly evidenced by reduction of venous or arterial blood flow (vein coagulation, muscle edema), increased tissue pressure (compartment syndrome).

risk for physical Trauma/Suffocation possibly evidenced by muscle paralysis (central nervous system damage), loss of large- or small-muscle coordination (seizures).

Electroconvulsive therapy   PSY

Decisional Conflict may be related to lack of relevant or multiple and divergent sources of information, mistrust of regimen or healthcare personnel, sense of powerlessness, support system deficit.

acute Confusion may be related to [direct effects of electric shock on the central nervous system, medications, and anesthesia], possibly evidenced by fluctuation in cognition, agitation.

impaired Memory may be related to neurological disturbance (electrical shock), possibly evidenced by reported or observed experiences of forgetting, difficulty recalling recent events or factual information.

Emphysema   CH/MS

impaired Gas Exchange may be related to (alveolar capillary membrane changes [or destruction]), possibly evidenced by abnormal breathing pattern (dyspnea), restlessness, [changes in mentation], abnormal arterial blood gas values.

ineffective Airway Clearance may be related to increased production and retained tenacious secretions, decreased energy level, and muscle wasting, possibly evidenced by abnormal breath sounds (rhonchi), ineffective cough, changes in rate and depth of respirations, and dyspnea.

Activity Intolerance may be related to imbalance between oxygen supply and demand and physical deconditioning, possibly evidenced by reports of fatigue or generalized weakness, exertional dyspnea, and abnormal vital sign response to activity.

imbalanced Nutrition: less than body requirements may be related to insufficient dietary intake, inability to ingest food, possibly evidenced by insufficient interest in food, alteration in taste sensation, insufficient muscle tone, [fatigue, and weight loss].

risk for Infection possibly evidenced by stasis of body fluids, malnutrition (decrease in ciliary action, and chronic illness).

ineffective Health Management may be related to difficulty managing complex treatment regimen or navigating complex healthcare systems, excessive demands, powerlessness; perceived seriousness of condition, perceived benefit [of treatment], possibly evidenced by difficulty with prescribed regiment, failure to include treatment regimen in daily living, ineffective choices for meeting health goal.

Encephalitis   MS

risk for ineffective cerebral Tissue Perfusion possibly evidenced by cerebral edema altering or interrupting cerebral arterial or venous blood flow, hypovolemia, exchange problems at cellular level (acidosis).

Hyperthermia may be related to increased metabolic rate, illness, and dehydration, possibly evidenced by increased body temperature; flushed, warm skin; and increased pulse and respiratory rates.

acute Pain may be related to physical injury agent (inflammation or irritation of the brain and cerebral edema) possibly evidenced by verbal reports of pain, photophobia, distraction behavior, restlessness, and changes in vital signs.

risk for physical Trauma/Suffocation possibly evidenced by restlessness, clonic-tonic activity, altered sensorium, cognitive impairment, generalized weakness, ataxia, vertigo.

Encopresis   PSY/PED

bowel Incontinence may be related to [situational or maturational crisis], stressors (predisposing vulnerability, threat to physical integrity—child/sexual abuse), possibly evidenced by involuntary passage of stool at least once monthly, strong odor of feces on client, hiding soiled clothing in inappropriate places.

disturbed Body Image/chronic low Self-Esteem may be related to negative view of self, maturational expectations, social factors, stigma attached to loss of body function in public, family's belief that condition is volitional, shame related to body odor, possibly evidenced by angry outbursts or oppositional behavior, verbalization of powerlessness, reluctance to engage in social activities.

compromised family Coping may be related to inadequate or incorrect information or understanding of condition, belief that behavior is volitional, disagreement regarding treatment or coping strategies, possibly evidenced by increasingly ineffective attempts to intervene with child, significant person describes preoccupation with personal reaction (excessive guilt, anger, blame regarding child's condition or behavior), overprotective behavior.

Endocarditis   MS

risk for decreased Cardiac Output possibly evidenced by inflammation of lining of heart and structural change in valve leaflets.

Anxiety [specify level] may be related to change in current status and threat of death, possibly evidenced by apprehensiveness, expressed concerns, and self-focused.

acute Pain may be related to physical injury agent (inflammatory process and effects of embolic phenomena), possibly evidenced by verbal reports, narrowed focus, distraction behavior, and autonomic responses (changes in vital signs).

risk for Activity Intolerance possibly evidenced by risk factors of imbalance between oxygen supply and demand, [debilitating condition].

risk for ineffective Tissue Perfusion (specify) possibly evidenced by embolic interruption of arterial flow (embolization of thrombi or valvular vegetations).

End-of-life care   CH

Refer to Hospice care

Endometriosis   GYN

acute/chronic Pain may be related to pressure of concealed bleeding, formation of adhesions, possibly evidenced by verbal reports (pain between and with menstruation), guarding or distraction behaviors, and narrowed focus.

Sexual dysfunction may be related to (alteration in body function, presence of adhesions, painful menses), possibly evidenced by undesired change in sexual function, decrease in sexual desire, change in interest toward others.

deficient Knowledge regarding pathophysiology of condition and therapy needs may be related to lack of information, misinterpretations, possibly evidenced by statements of concern and misconceptions.

Enteral feeding   MS/CH

imbalanced Nutrition: less than body requirements may be related to insufficient dietary intake, possibly evidenced by body weight 10% or more under ideal, [decreased subcutaneous fat or muscle mass, changes in gastric motility and stool characteristics].

risk for Infection possibly evidenced by malnutrition, chronic illness, and associated conditions of invasive procedure, [surgical placement of feeding tube].

risk for Aspiration possibly evidenced by (presence of feeding tube, enteral feedings, increase in intragastric pressure, delayed gastric emptying, treatment regimen).

risk for imbalanced Fluid Volume possibly evidenced by active loss or failure of regulatory mechanisms (specific to underlying disease process or trauma), inability to obtain or ingest fluids.

Fatigue may be related to decreased metabolic energy production, increased energy requirements (hypermetabolic state, healing process), altered body chemistry (medications, chemotherapy), possibly evidenced by overwhelming lack of energy, inability to maintain usual routines or accomplish routine tasks, lethargy, impaired ability to concentrate.

Enteritis　　　　　　　　　　　　　**MS/CH**
Refer to Colitis, ulcerative; Crohn's disease

Enuresis　　　　　　　　　　　　**PSY/PED**
impaired urinary Elimination may be related to multiple causality—situational or maturational crisis, psychogenic factors (predisposing vulnerability, threat to physical integrity—abuse), possibly evidenced by nocturnal or diurnal enuresis, strong odor of urine on client, hiding soiled clothing in inappropriate places.

　　disturbed Body Image/chronic low Self-Esteem may be related to negative view of self, maturational expectations, social factors, stigma attached to loss of body function in public, family's belief condition is volitional, shame related to body odor, possibly evidenced by angry outbursts or oppositional behavior, verbalization of powerlessness, reluctance to engage in social activities.

　　compromised family Coping may be related to inadequate or incorrect information or understanding of condition, belief that behavior is volitional, disagreement regarding treatment or coping strategies, possibly evidenced by increasingly ineffective attempts to intervene with child, SO describes preoccupation with personal reaction (excessive guilt, anger, blame regarding child's condition or behavior), overprotective behavior.

Epididymitis　　　　　　　　　　　　　　**MS**
acute Pain may be related to [inflammation, edema formation, and tension on the spermatic cord] possibly evidenced by verbal reports, guarding or distraction behaviors (restlessness), and changes in vital signs.

　　risk for Infection [spread] possibly evidenced by insufficient knowledge to avoid spread of infection.

　　deficient Knowledge regarding pathophysiology, outcome, and self-care needs may be related to lack of information, misinterpretations, possibly evidenced by statements of concern, misconceptions, and questions.

Epilepsy　　　　　　　　　　　　　　**CH**
Refer to Seizure disorder

Episiotomy　　　　　　　　　　　　　　**OB**
acute Pain may be related to physical injury agent (tissue trauma, edema, surgical incision) possibly evidenced by self-report of pain, guarding behavior, self-focused.

　　risk for Infection possibly evidenced by alteration in skin/traumatized tissue, [body excretions, inadequate hygiene].

risk for Sexual dysfunction possibly evidenced by associated condition of alteration in body structure (recent childbirth, presence of incision).

Epistaxis　　　　　　　　　　　　　　**CH**
[mild to moderate] Anxiety may be related to (situational crisis), threat to current status, interpersonal transmission, possibly evidenced by expressed concerns, apprehension, anxiety.

　　risk for Aspiration possibly evidenced by (uncontrolled nasal bleeding).

Epstein-Barr virus　　　　　　　　　　**CH**
Refer to Mononucleosis, infectious

Erectile dysfunction　　　　　　　　**CH/PSY**
Sexual dysfunction may be related to (altered body function), [side effects of medication], possibly evidenced by reports of disruption of sexual response pattern, inability to achieve desired satisfaction.

　　situational low Self-Esteem may be related to functional impairment, perceived failure to perform satisfactorily, rejection of other(s), possibly evidenced by self-negating verbalizations, expressions of helplessness, powerlessness.

Esophageal reflux disease　　　　　　　**CH**
Refer to Gastroesophageal reflux disease

Esophageal varices　　　　　　　　**CH/MS**
Refer to Varices, esophageal

Esophagitis　　　　　　　　　　　　　**CH**
Refer to Gastroesophageal reflux disease; Achalasia

ETOH withdrawal　　　　　　　　　　**MS/CH**
Refer to Alcohol intoxication, acute; Substance dependence/abuse rehabilitation

Evisceration　　　　　　　　　　　　　**MS**
Refer to Dehiscence, abdominal wound

Facial reconstructive surgery　　　　**MS/CH**
Also refer to Surgery, general; Intermaxillary fixation
risk for ineffective Airway Clearance possibly evidenced by soft tissue edema, airway trauma, retained secretions.

　　impaired Skin Integrity may be related to [traumatic injury, surgical procedure (incisions/grafts), edema, altered circulation, possibly evidenced by disruption or destruction of skin layers].

　　Fear/Anxiety may be related to (situational crisis), memory of traumatic event, threat to self-concept [disfigurement], possibly evidenced by expressed concerns, apprehension, uncertainty, decreased self-assurance, restlessness.

disturbed Body Image may be related to alteration in self-perception, cultural or spiritual incongruence, (trauma), possibly evidenced by negative feelings about body, fear of reaction by others, preoccupation with change, change in social involvement.

risk for Social Isolation possibly evidenced by feeling different from others, alteration in physical appearance.

Failure to thrive, adult　　　　　　　CH/MS
Frail Elderly Syndrome may be related to depression, apathy, aging process, fatigue, degenerative condition, possibly evidenced by expressed lack of appetite, difficulty performing self-care tasks, altered mood state, inadequate intake, weight loss, physical decline.

ineffective Protection may be related to inadequate nutrition, anemia, extremes of age, possibly evidenced by fatigue, weakness, deficient immunity, impaired healing, pressure sores.

Failure to thrive, infant/child　　　　　PED
imbalanced Nutrition: less than body requirements may be related to insufficient dietary intake, (inability to ingest/digest food, or absorb nutrients); [physical deprivation; psychosocial factors], possibly evidenced by [lack of appropriate weight gain or weight loss], insufficient muscle tone, pale conjunctiva or mucous membranes, and [laboratory tests reflecting nutritional deficiency].

[risk for disproportionate Growth] and/or delayed Development possibly evidenced by maladaptive feeding behavior, economically disadvantaged, caregiver mental health issue, presence of abuse (physical, psychological, sexual).

risk for impaired Parenting possibly evidenced by lack of knowledge, inadequate bonding, unrealistic expectations for self/infant, and lack of appropriate response of child to relationship.

deficient Knowledge regarding pathophysiology of condition, nutritional needs, growth/development expectations, and parenting skills may be related to lack of information, misinformation, or misinterpretation, possibly evidenced by verbalization of concerns, questions, misconceptions; or development of preventable complications.

Fat embolism syndrome　　　　　　　MS
Refer to Pulmonary embolus; Respiratory distress syndrome, acute

Fatigue syndrome, chronic　　　　　　CH
Fatigue may be related to disease state, inadequate sleep, possibly evidenced by verbalization of unremitting or overwhelming lack of energy, inability to maintain usual routines, listlessness, compromised concentration.

chronic Pain may be related to chronic physical disability, possibly evidenced by verbal reports of headache, sore throat, arthralgias, abdominal pain, muscle aches, altered ability to continue previous activities, changes in sleep pattern.

Self-Care deficit [specify] may be related to tiredness, pain, discomfort, possibly evidenced by reports of inability to perform desired activities of daily living.

risk for ineffective Role Performance possibly evidenced by health alterations, stress.

Febrile seizure　　　　　　　　　　PED
Hyperthermia may be related to illness, dehydration, decreased ability to perspire, possibly evidenced by increase in body temperature; flushed, warm skin; seizures.

Fecal diversion　　　　　　　　　　MS/CH
Refer to Colostomy

Fecal impaction　　　　　　　　　　CH
Constipation may be related to irregular defecation habits, decreased activity, dehydration, abdominal muscle weakness, neurological impairment, possibly evidenced by inability to pass stool, abdominal distention, tenderness or pain, nausea, vomiting, anorexia.

Femoral popliteal bypass　　　　　　MS
Also refer to Surgery, general
risk for ineffective peripheral Tissue Perfusion possibly evidenced by interruption of arterial blood flow, hypovolemia.

risk for peripheral Neurovascular Dysfunction possibly evidenced by vascular obstruction, immobilization, mechanical compression, dressings.

impaired Walking may be related to surgical incisions, dressings, possibly evidenced by inability to walk desired distance, climb stairs, negotiate inclines.

Fetal alcohol syndrome　　　　　　　PED
risk for Injury [central nervous system damage] possibly evidenced by external chemical factors (alcohol intake by mother), placental insufficiency, fetal drug withdrawal in utero or postpartum, and prematurity.

---

disorganized infant Behavior may be related to prematurity, environmental overstimulation, lack of containment or boundaries, possibly evidenced by change from baseline physiological measures, tremors, startles, twitches, hyperextension of arms and legs, deficient self-regulatory behaviors, deficient response to visual or auditory stimuli.

risk for impaired Parenting possibly evidenced by mental or physical illness, inability of mother to assume the overwhelming task of unselfish giving and nurturing, presence of stressors (financial or legal problems), lack of available or ineffective role model, interruption of bonding process, lack of appropriate response of child to relationship.

PSY

ineffective [maternal] Coping may be related to personal vulnerability, low self-esteem, inadequate coping skills, and multiple stressors (repeated over period of time), possibly evidenced by inability to meet basic needs, fulfill role expectations, or problem-solve; and excessive use of drug(s).

dysfunctional Family Processes may be related to lack of or insufficient support from others, mother's drug problem and treatment status, together with poor coping skills, lack of family stability, overinvolvement of parents with children and multigenerational addictive behaviors, possibly evidenced by abandonment, rejection, neglectful relationships with family members, and decisions and actions by family that are detrimental.

Fetal demise   OB
Refer to Perinatal loss/death of child

Fetal transfusion syndrome   OB
Refer to Twin-twin transfusion syndrome

Fibrocystic breast disease   CH
[mild to moderate] Anxiety may be related to situational crisis, threat to health status, family heredity, interpersonal transmission, possibly evidenced by expressed concerns, apprehension, uncertainty, fearfulness, focus on self, increased tension.

acute/chronic Pain may be related to physical agents (edema formation, nerve irritation), possibly evidenced by verbal reports, guarded or protective behavior, expressive behavior, self-focusing.

Fibroids, uterine   GYN
Refer to Uterine myomas

Fibromyalgia syndrome, primary   CH
acute/chronic Pain may be related to idiopathic diffuse condition, possibly evidenced by reports of achy pain in fibrous tissues (muscles, tendons, ligaments), muscle stiffness or spasm, disturbed sleep, guarding behaviors, fear of reinjury or exacerbation, restlessness, irritability, self-focusing, reduced interaction with others.

Fatigue may be related to disease state, stress, anxiety, depression, sleep deprivation, possibly evidenced by verbalization of overwhelming lack of energy, inability to maintain usual routines or level of physical activity, tired, feelings of guilt for not keeping up with responsibilities, increase in physical complaints, listlessness.

risk for Hopelessness possibly evidenced by chronic debilitating physical condition, prolonged activity restriction (possibly self-induced), creating isolation, lack of specific therapeutic cure, prolonged stress.

Flail chest   MS
Refer to Hemothorax; Pneumothorax

Food poisoning   CH/MS
Refer to Gastroenteritis

Fractures   MS/CH
Also refer to Casts; Traction
risk for physical Trauma [additional injury] possibly evidenced by insufficient knowledge of safety precautions, weakness, [loss of skeletal integrity, movement of skeletal fragments, use of traction apparatus].

acute Pain may be related to physical injury agent (muscle spasms, movement of bone fragments, tissue trauma, edema, traction or immobility device, stress, and anxiety), possibly evidenced by verbal reports, distraction behavior, self-focused or narrowed focus, facial expression of pain, guarding or protective behavior, alteration in muscle tone, and changes in vital signs.

risk for peripheral Neurovascular Dysfunction possibly evidenced by reduction or interruption of blood flow (direct vascular injury, tissue trauma, excessive edema, thrombus formation, hypovolemia).

impaired physical Mobility may be related to neuromuscular or skeletal impairment, pain, discomfort, restrictive therapies (bedrest, extremity immobilization), and psychological immobility, possibly evidenced by inability to purposefully move within the physical environment, imposed restrictions, reluctance to attempt movement, limited range of motion, and decreased muscle strength or control.

risk for impaired Gas Exchange possibly evidenced by (alveolar-capillary membrane changes [interstitial or pulmonary edema, congestion]) or possibly (ventilation-perfusion imbalance [altered blood flow, blood or fat emboli]).

deficient Knowledge regarding healing process, therapy requirements, potential complications, and self-care needs may be related to lack of exposure or recall, misinterpretation of information, possibly evidenced by statements of concern, questions, and misconceptions.

Frostbite   MS/CH

impaired Tissue Integrity may be related to altered circulation and thermal injury, possibly evidenced by damaged or destroyed tissue.

acute Pain may be related to physical injury agent (tissue ischemia or necrosis and edema formation) possibly evidenced by verbal reports, guarding or distraction behaviors, narrowed focus, and changes in vital signs.

risk for Infection possibly evidenced by alteration in skin/tissue integrity and associated conditions of impaired circulation, and [compromised immune response in affected area].

Fusion, cervical   MS
Refer to Laminectomy, cervical

Fusion, lumbar   MS
Refer to Laminectomy, lumbar

Gallstones   CH
Refer to Cholelithiasis

Gangrene, dry   MS

ineffective peripheral Tissue Perfusion may be related to interruption in arterial flow, possibly evidenced by cool skin temperature, change in color (black), atrophy of affected part, and presence of pain.

acute Pain may be related to physical injury agent (tissue hypoxia and necrotic process), possibly evidenced by verbal reports, guarding or distraction behaviors, narrowed focus, and changes in vital signs.

Gangrene, gas   MS

impaired Tissue Integrity may be related to trauma, surgery, infection, altered circulation, possibly evidenced by edema, brown or serous exudate, bronze or blackish green skin color, gas bubbles or crepitation, pain.

[severe] Anxiety/Fear may be related to learned response to threat (situational crisis), threat of death, possibly evidenced by expressed concerns, distress, apprehension, fearfulness, restlessness, irritability, focus on self.

risk for Injury possibly evidenced by [therapeutic intervention (hyperbaric oxygen therapy)].

Gas, lung irritant   MS/CH

ineffective Airway Clearance may be related to irritation or inflammation of airway, possibly evidenced by marked cough, abnormal breath sounds (wheezes), dyspnea, and tachypnea.

risk for impaired Gas Exchange possibly evidenced by (alveolar-capillary membrane changes [irritation or inflammation dependent on type of agent and length of exposure]).

Anxiety [specify level] may be related to threat to change in current status and threat of death, possibly evidenced by verbalizations, increased tension, apprehension, and sympathetic stimulation.

Gastrectomy, subtotal   MS
Also refer to Surgery, general

risk for imbalanced Nutrition: less than body requirements possibly evidenced by (inability to ingest food or absorb nutrients), restricted oral intake, early satiety, change in digestive process.

risk for Fatigue possibly evidenced by malnutrition, anemia.

risk for Diarrhea possibly evidenced by malabsorption.

Gastric partitioning   MS
Refer to Gastroplasty

Gastric resection   MS
Refer to Gastrectomy, subtotal

Gastric ulcer   MS/CH
Refer to Ulcer, peptic

Gastrinoma   MS/CH
Refer to Zollinger-Ellison syndrome

Gastritis, acute   MS

acute Pain may be related to physical injury agent (inflammation of gastric mucosa), possibly evidenced by verbal reports, guarding or distraction behaviors, and changes in vital signs.

risk for deficient Fluid Volume/Bleeding possibly evidenced by excessive losses through vomiting and

---

diarrhea, continued bleeding, reluctance to ingest or restrictions of oral intake.

Gastritis, chronic CH
risk for imbalanced Nutrition: less than body requirements possibly evidenced by (inability to ingest food or absorb nutrients), prolonged nausea, vomiting, anorexia, epigastric pain.

deficient Knowledge regarding pathophysiology, psychological factors, therapy needs, and potential complications may be related to lack of information or recall, unfamiliarity with information resources, information misinterpretation, possibly evidenced by verbalization of concerns, questions, and continuation of problem or development of preventable complications.

Gastroenteritis CH/MS
Diarrhea may be related to toxins, contaminants, travel, infectious process, parasites, possibly evidenced by at least three loose liquid stools per day, hyperactive bowel sounds, abdominal pain.

risk for deficient Fluid Volume possibly evidenced by excessive losses (diarrhea, vomiting), hypermetabolic state (infection), decreased intake (nausea, anorexia), extremes of age or weight.

risk for Infection [transmission] possibly evidenced by alteration in peristalsis, inadequate vaccination, insufficient knowledge to prevent contamination (inappropriate hand hygiene and food handling).

Gastroesophageal reflux disease (GERD) CH
acute/chronic Pain may be related to acidic irritation of mucosa, muscle spasm, recurrent vomiting, possibly evidenced by reports of heartburn, distraction behaviors.

impaired Swallowing may be related to (esophageal reflux disease [GERD], achalasia) possibly evidenced by reports of heartburn or epigastric pain, "something stuck" when swallowing, food refusal or volume limiting, nighttime coughing or awakening.

risk for imbalanced Nutrition: less than body requirements possibly evidenced by insufficient dietary intake, food aversion, [recurrent vomiting].

risk for Insomnia possibly evidenced by physical discomfort [nighttime heartburn, regurgitation of stomach contents].

risk for Aspiration possibly evidenced by (incompetent lower esophageal sphincter, increase in gastric residual).

Gastrointestinal hemorrhage MS
Refer to Gastritis, acute or chronic; Ulcer, peptic; Colitis, ulcerative; Crohn's disease; Varices, esophageal

Gastroplasty MS
Also refer to Surgery, general
ineffective Breathing Pattern may be related to decreased lung expansion, pain, anxiety, decreased energy, fatigue, tracheobronchial obstruction, possibly evidenced by dyspnea, tachypnea, changes in respiratory depth, reduced vital capacity, wheezes, rhonchi, abnormal arterial blood gases.

risk for ineffective peripheral Tissue Perfusion possibly evidenced by diminished blood flow, hypovolemia, immobility or bedrest, interruption of venous blood flow (thrombus).

risk for deficient Fluid Volume possibly evidenced by excessive gastric losses, nasogastric suction, diarrhea, reduced intake.

risk for imbalanced Nutrition: less than body requirements possibly evidenced by inability to ingest food or absorb nutrients [restricted oral intake, early satiety, change in digestive process].

Diarrhea may be related to treatment regimen [changes in dietary fiber and bulk], malabsorption, possibly evidenced by loose liquid stools >3 in 24 hours, bowel urgency, hyperactive bowel sounds.

Gender dysphoria PSY
(For individuals experiencing persistent and marked distress regarding uncertainty about issues relating to personal identity, e.g., sexual orientation and behavior.)
Anxiety [specify level] may be related to value conflict, threat to current status, unmet needs, possibly evidenced by increase in tension, helplessness, feeling of inadequacy, uncertainty, insomnia, self-focused.

ineffective Role Performance/disturbed Personal Identity may be related to (developmental crisis), conflict, inadequate role preparation, possibly evidenced by role confusion, uncertainty, insufficient knowledge of role requirements, insufficient external support for role enactment, ineffective adaptation to change.

ineffective Sexuality Pattern may be related to inadequate model, conflict about sexual orientation or variant preference, impaired relationship with a significant other, possibly evidenced by value conflict, change in sexual role, difficulty with sexual behavior.

risk for compromised/disabled family Coping possibly evidenced by insufficient information available or misunderstanding of information by support person, family disorganization and role changes, and insufficient reciprocal support.

readiness for enhanced family Coping possibly evidenced by expresses desire to acknowledge growth impact of crisis/situation, to enhance connection with others who have experienced a similar situation.

Genetic disorder   CH/OB

Anxiety may be related to presence of specific risk factors (e.g., exposure to teratogens), situational crisis, threat to self-concept, conscious or unconscious conflict about essential values and life goals, possibly evidenced by increased tension, apprehension, uncertainty, feelings of inadequacy, expressed concerns.

deficient Knowledge regarding purpose and process of genetic counseling may be related to lack of awareness of ramifications of diagnosis, process necessary for analyzing available options, and information misinterpretation, possibly evidenced by verbalization of concerns, statement of misconceptions, request for information.

risk for interrupted Family Processes possibly evidenced by (situational crisis), individual/family vulnerability, difficulty reaching agreement regarding options.

Grieving may be related to anticipatory or actual loss [e.g., childbearing or reproductive issues], possibly evidenced by suffering, blame, despair, change in usual routines and activities of daily living.

Spiritual distress may be related to intense inner conflict about the outcome, normal grieving for the loss of the perfect child, anger that is often directed at God/greater power, religious beliefs or moral convictions, possibly evidenced by verbalization of inner conflict about beliefs, questioning of the moral and ethical implications of therapeutic choices, viewing situation as punishment, anger, hostility, and crying.

Genital herpes   CH
Refer to Herpes simplex; Sexually transmitted infection

Genital warts (human papillomavirus)   CH
Refer to Sexually transmitted infection

GERD   CH
Refer to Gastroesophageal reflux disease

GI bleeding   MS
Refer to Gastritis, acute or chronic; Ulcer, peptic

Gigantism   CH
Refer to Acromegaly

Gingivitis   CH
impaired oral Mucous Membrane Integrity may be related to ineffective oral hygiene, ill-fitting dentures, decreased salivation, hormonal changes, possibly evidenced by edema, gingival bleeding, hyperplasia, oral pain.

Glaucoma   CH
[disturbed visual Sensory Perception] may be related to altered sensory reception and altered status of sense organ (increased intraocular pressure, atrophy of optic nerve head), possibly evidenced by progressive loss of visual field.

Anxiety [specify level] may be related to change in current status, pain, unmet needs, possibly evidenced by apprehensiveness, uncertainty, and expressed concern regarding changes in life event.

Glomerulonephritis   PED
excess Fluid Volume may be related to failure of regulatory mechanism (inflammation of glomerular membrane inhibiting filtration), possibly evidenced by weight gain, edema, anasarca, intake greater than output, and blood pressure changes.

acute Pain may be related to physical injury agent (circulating toxins and edema), possibly evidenced by verbal reports, guarding or distraction behaviors, and changes in vital signs.

imbalanced Nutrition: less than body requirements may be related to (inability to ingest food or absorb nutrients [anorexia and dietary restrictions]) possibly evidenced by food aversion, alteration in taste sensation, and weight loss.

decreased Diversional Activity Engagement may be related to treatment modality and restrictions, fatigue, and malaise, possibly evidenced by statements of boredom, restlessness, and irritability.

Gluten sensitive enteropathy   CH
Refer to Celiac disease

Goiter   CH
disturbed Body Image may be related to alteration in self-perception possibly evidenced by verbalizations of feelings or perceptions, fear of reaction by others, preoccupation with change (e.g., visible swelling in neck, possibly actual change in structure).

Anxiety may be related to change in current status, progressive growth of mass, perceived threat of death.

risk for ineffective Airway Clearance possibly evidenced by tracheal compression or obstruction.

Gonorrhea   CH
Also refer to Sexually transmitted infection

risk for Infection [dissemination/bacteremia] possibly evidenced by [presence of infectious process in highly vascular area] and lack of knowledge to avoid exposure to pathogens.

acute Pain may be related to physical injury agent (inflammation of mucosa, effects of circulating toxins), possibly evidenced by verbal reports of genital or pharyngeal irritation, perineal or pelvic pain, guarding or distraction behaviors.

deficient Knowledge regarding disease cause, transmission, therapy, and self-care needs may be related to lack of information, misinterpretation, denial of exposure, possibly evidenced by statements of concern, questions, misconceptions, and inaccurate follow-through of instructions, development of preventable complications.

Gout   CH
acute Pain may be related to physical injury agent (inflammation of joint[s]) possibly evidenced by verbal reports, guarding or distraction behaviors, and changes in vital signs.

impaired physical Mobility may be related to joint pain, edema, possibly evidenced by reluctance to attempt movement, limited range of motion, and therapeutic restriction of movement.

deficient Knowledge regarding cause, treatment, and prevention of condition may be related to lack of information, misinterpretation, possibly evidenced by statements of concern, questions, misconceptions, and inaccurate follow-through of instructions.

Grand mal seizures   CH/PED
Refer to Seizure disorder

Grave's disease   CH
Refer to Hyperthyroidism

Guillain-Barré syndrome   MS
(acute polyneuritis)
risk for ineffective Breathing Pattern/Airway Clearance possibly evidenced by weakness or paralysis of respiratory muscles, impaired gag or swallow reflexes, decreased energy, fatigue.

[disturbed Sensory Perception (specify)] may be related to altered sensory reception, transmission, or integration (altered status of sense organs, sleep deprivation); therapeutically restricted environment; endogenous chemical alterations (electrolyte imbalance, hypoxia); and psychological stress, possibly evidenced by reported or observed change in usual response to stimuli, altered communication patterns, and measured change in sensory acuity and motor coordination.

impaired physical Mobility may be related to neuromuscular impairment, pain, discomfort, possibly evidenced by impaired coordination, partial or complete paralysis, decreased muscle strength or control.

Anxiety [specify level]/Fear may be related to change in current status, threat of death, possibly evidenced by increased tension, restlessness, helplessness, apprehension, uncertainty, fearfulness, focus on self, and sympathetic stimulation.

risk for Disuse Syndrome possibly evidenced by paralysis and pain.

Gulf War syndrome   CH/MS
[chronic] Fatigue may be related to unknown environmental exposure, stress, anxiety, disease state, possibly evidenced by overwhelming lack of energy, inability to maintain usual routines or level of physical activity, lethargic, compromised concentration.

Anxiety [specify] may be related to exposure to toxins, change in current status, threat of death, change in role function or economic status, unmet needs, possibly evidenced by expressed concerns, apprehension, uncertainty, fear of unspecific consequences, sleep disturbance, irritability, preoccupation.

impaired Memory may be related to neurological disturbances, possibly evidenced by reported or observed experiences of forgetting, inability to recall recent events.

chronic Pain may be related to chronic physical condition, possibly evidenced by verbal reports of muscle or joint pain, headaches, altered ability to continue previous activities, fatigue, reduced interaction with others.

Diarrhea may be related to environmental exposure to toxins, high stress levels/anxiety, possibly evidenced by liquid stools, abdominal pain.

[disturbed visual Sensory Perception] may be related to altered sensory reception, possibly evidenced by blurred vision, photosensitivity.

Hallucinogen abuse   CH/PSY

Also refer to Substance dependence/abuse rehabilitation
Anxiety/Fear may be related to substance misuse, stressors, sensory deficit, response to phobic stimulus, threat to change in current status, threat of death, possibly evidenced by apprehensiveness, restlessness, feeling of alarm, terror, attack behavior, sympathetic stimulation.

Self-Neglect may be related to substance misuse, deficient executive function, possibly evidenced by inadequate personal/environmental hygiene, nonadherence to health activity.

Self-Care deficit (specify) may be related to (perceptual disorders, alteration in cognitive functioning), environmental barrier (restraints), possibly evidenced by inability to meet own physical needs.

Hand-foot-mouth disease   PED/CH

Also refer to Meningitis, acute meningococcal
impaired oral Mucous Membrane Integrity may be related to infection, dehydration, possibly evidenced by oral lesions, ulcers, pain, difficulty eating.

risk for Infection [transmission] possibly evidenced by insufficient knowledge to avoid exposure to pathogens, [inadequate acquired immunity].

risk for deficient Fluid Volume possibly evidenced by deviations affecting intake (oral ulcers and pain), increased fluid needs (hypermetabolic state, fever).

Hansen's disease   CH

impaired Skin/Tissue integrity may be related to immunodeficiency, impaired circulation, alteration in sensation and pigmentation; and [invasion of tissues by bacterial infection], possibly evidenced by alteration in skin integrity, destroyed tissue.

risk for Infection [spread/transmission] possibly evidenced by insufficient knowledge to avoid exposure to/early treatment of infectious bacterial [*Mycobacterium leprae*] agent.

impaired physical Mobility may be related to neuromuscular and sensoriperceptual impairments, possibly evidenced by muscular weakness, or numbness or absence of sensation in hands, arms, legs, feet.

disturbed Body Image may be related to alteration in self-perception (e.g., due to biophysical illness, trauma, actual change in structure, missing body part) possibly evidenced by verbalizations fear of reaction or rejection by others, preoccupation with change.

Hantavirus   MS

Refer to Hantavirus pulmonary syndrome

Hantavirus pulmonary syndrome   MS

Also refer to Disseminated intravascular coagulation
acute Pain/impaired Comfort may be related to physical injury agent (inflammatory process, circulating toxins), possibly evidenced by reports of headache, myalgia, gastrointestinal distress, fever.

impaired Gas Exchange may be related to associated condition of alveolar-capillary membrane changes (fluid collection or shifts into interstitial space or alveoli), possibly evidenced by abnormal breathing pattern (dyspnea, abnormal rate or depth of respirations), restlessness, irritability, somnolence, confusion.

[moderate to severe] Anxiety may be related to threat to current status, threat of death, interpersonal transmission, possibly evidenced by expressed concerns, distressed, apprehensiveness, extraneous movement.

risk for impaired spontaneous Ventilation possibly evidenced by respiratory muscle fatigue, problems with secretion management.

Hashimoto's thyroiditis   CH

Refer to Hypothyroidism; Goiter

Hay fever   CH

impaired Comfort may be related to noxious environmental stimuli irritation or inflammation of upper airway mucous membranes and conjunctiva, possibly evidenced by distressing symptoms, irritability, itching, and restlessness.

deficient Knowledge regarding underlying cause, appropriate therapy, and required lifestyle changes may be related to lack of information, possibly evidenced by statements of concern, questions, and misconceptions.

Headache   CH/MS

Also refer to Temporal arteritis
acute/chronic Pain may be related to biological/physical injuring agents [tension, nerve irritation or pressure, vasospasm, increased intracranial pressure], possibly evidenced by verbal or coded reports, pallor, facial expression of pain, guarding or distraction behavior, restlessness, self-focused, changes in sleep pattern or appetite, preoccupation with pain.

risk for ineffective Coping possibly evidenced by (situational crisis), personal vulnerability, inadequate resources, insufficient sense of control, ineffective tension release, overwhelming threat to self.

deficient Knowledge regarding condition, prognosis, and treatment needs may be related to lack of exposure or recall, unfamiliarity with information or resources, cognitive limitations, possibly evidenced by request for information, statement of misconceptions, inaccurate follow-through of instructions, development of preventable complications.

Head injury   MS/CH
Refer to Traumatic brain injury

Heart attack   MS
Refer to Myocardial infarction

Heart failure, chronic   MS
decreased Cardiac Output may be related to altered myocardial contractility, inotropic changes; alterations in rate, rhythm, and electrical conduction; and structural changes (valvular defects, ventricular aneurysm), possibly evidenced by tachycardia, dysrhythmias, changes in blood pressure, extra heart sounds, decreased urine output, diminished peripheral pulses, cool and ashen skin, orthopnea, crackles; dependent or generalized edema and chest pain.

excess Fluid Volume may be related to reduced glomerular filtration rate, increased antidiuretic hormone production, and sodium/water retention, possibly evidenced by orthopnea and abnormal breath sounds, S_3 heart sound, jugular vein distention, positive hepatojugular reflex, weight gain, hypertension, oliguria, generalized edema.

risk for impaired Gas Exchange possibly evidenced by (alveolar-capillary membrane changes [fluid collection or shifts into interstitial space and alveoli]).

CH

Activity Intolerance may be related to imbalance between oxygen supply and demand, physical deconditioning, sedentary lifestyle, possibly evidenced by weakness, fatigue; changes in vital signs in response to activity (dysrhythmias; exertional dyspnea, pallor, diaphoresis).

risk for impaired Skin Integrity possibly evidenced by alteration in fluid volume, inadequate nutrition, pressure over bony prominences, [prolonged chair or bedrest] and (impaired circulation).

deficient Knowledge regarding cardiac function, disease process, therapy, and self-care needs may be related to lack of information, misinterpretation, possibly evidenced by questions, statements of concern or

misconceptions; development of preventable complications or exacerbations of condition.

Heart transplantation   MS/CH
Refer to Cardiac surgery; Transplantation, recipient

Heat exhaustion   CH/MS
deficient Fluid Volume may be related to excessive losses (profuse sweating), hypermetabolic state (core temperature 101°F to 105°F [38.3°C to 40.6°C]), lack of intake, extremes of age, possibly evidenced by weakness, fatigue, slow pulse, decreased blood pressure, changes in mentation.

Heatstroke   MS
Hyperthermia may be related to prolonged exposure to hot environment, vigorous activity with failure of regulating mechanism of the body, possibly evidenced by high body temperature (greater than 105°F [40.6°C]), flushed/hot skin, tachycardia, and seizure activity.

decreased Cardiac Output may be related to functional stress of hypermetabolic state, altered circulating volume and venous return, and direct myocardial damage secondary to hyperthermia, possibly evidenced by decreased peripheral pulses, dysrhythmias, tachycardia, and changes in mentation.

Hematoma, epidural   MS
acute Confusion may be related to (alteration in cognitive functioning), possibly evidenced by alteration in level of consciousness, agitation, restlessness, misperception.

risk for decreased intracranial Adaptive Capacity possibly evidenced by brain injury, decreased cerebral perfusion pressure, systemic hypotension with intracranial hypertension).

risk for ineffective Breathing Pattern possibly evidenced by (neuromuscular impairment [injury to respiratory center of brain]), abnormal breathing pattern.

risk for deficient Fluid Volume possibly evidenced by restricted oral intake, hypermetabolic state, loss of fluid through normal or abnormal routes.

Hematoma, subdural-acute   MS
Refer to Traumatic brain injury

Hematoma, subdural-chronic   CH
acute/chronic Pain may be related to physical agent (space-occupying clot), possibly evidenced by reports of increasing daily headache.

acute/chronic Confusion may be related to head injury, alcohol abuse, possibly evidenced by fluctuations in cognition, increased agitation, restlessness, misperceptions, inappropriate responses.

impaired physical Mobility may be related to neuromuscular impairment (hemiparesis), decreased muscle strength, cognitive impairment, possibly evidenced by limited ability to perform gross or fine motor skills, gait changes, postural instability.

Hemiplegia, spastic PED/CH
Refer to Palsy, cerebral

Hemodialysis MS/CH
Also refer to Dialysis, general

risk for Injury [loss of vascular access] possibly evidenced by clotting or thrombosis, infection, disconnection, hemorrhage.

risk for deficient Fluid Volume possibly evidenced by excessive fluid losses or shifts via ultrafiltration, fluid restrictions, altered coagulation, disconnection of shunt.

risk for excess Fluid Volume possibly evidenced by rapid or excessive fluid intake—IV, blood, plasma expanders, or saline given to support blood pressure during procedure.

ineffective Protection may be related to chronic disease state, drug therapy, abnormal blood profile, inadequate nutrition, possibly evidenced by altered clotting, impaired healing, deficient immunity, fatigue, anorexia.

Hemophilia PED
risk for Bleeding/deficient Fluid Volume possibly evidenced by (inherent coagulopathy, trauma/[hemorrhagic losses]).

risk for acute/chronic Pain possibly evidenced by nerve compression from hematomas, nerve damage, or hemorrhage into joint space.

risk for impaired physical Mobility possibly evidenced by joint hemorrhage, swelling, degenerative changes, and muscle atrophy.

ineffective Protection may be related to abnormal blood profile, possibly evidenced by altered clotting.

compromised family Coping may be related to prolonged nature of condition that exhausts the supportive capacity of significant person(s), possibly evidenced by protective behaviors disproportionate to client's abilities or need for autonomy.

Hemorrhage, postpartum OB
risk for Shock possibly evidenced by (hypovolemia, hypotension).

[moderate] Anxiety may be related to (situational crisis), threat to current status or of death, interpersonal transmission or contagion, possibly evidenced by increased in tension, apprehensiveness, feeling of inadequacy, helplessness, sympathetic stimulation, self-focused.

risk for Infection possibly evidenced by alteration in skin integrity/traumatized tissue, stasis of body fluids (lochia), and (decreased hemoglobin, invasive procedure).

risk for impaired Attachment possibly evidenced by interruption in bonding process, physical condition, perceived threat to own survival.

Hemorrhage, prenatal OB
risk for Shock possibly evidenced by (hypovolemia, hypotension—ectopic or molar pregnancy, abruptio placentae).

risk for disturbed Maternal-Fetal Dyad possibly evidenced by (pregnancy complication, compromised fetal oxygen transport—hypovolemia).

Anxiety may be related to threat of death [self/fetus], possibly evidenced by apprehensiveness, fear, increase in tension, sympathetic stimulation.

acute Pain may be related to physical agent (muscle contractions/cervical dilation, tissue trauma] possibly evidenced by self report, distraction behavior, and change in blood pressure/pulse.

risk for imbalanced Fluid Volume possibly evidenced by (treatment regimen—excessive or rapid replacement of fluid losses).

Hemorrhagic fever, viral MS
Refer to Ebola; Hantavirus pulmonary syndrome

Hemorrhoidectomy MS/CH
acute Pain may be related to physical injury agent (edema, surgical tissue trauma), possibly evidenced by verbal reports, guarding or distraction behaviors, self-focused, and changes in vital signs.

risk for urinary Retention possibly evidenced by perineal trauma, edema or swelling, and pain.

deficient Knowledge regarding therapeutic treatment and potential complications may be related to lack of information, misconceptions, possibly evidenced by statements of concern and questions.

Hemorrhoids CH/OB
acute Pain may be related to [inflammation and edema of prolapsed varices], possibly evidenced by verbal reports and guarding or distraction behaviors.

Constipation may be related to pain on defecation and reluctance to defecate, possibly evidenced by frequency, less than usual pattern, and hard, formed stools.

Hemothorax   MS
Also refer to Pneumothorax
risk for physical Trauma/Suffocation possibly evidenced by concurrent disease or injury process, dependence on external device (chest drainage system), and lack of safety education or precautions.

Anxiety [specify level] may be related to threat to current status and threat of death, possibly evidenced by increase in tension, restlessness, expressed concern, sympathetic stimulation, and self-focused.

Hepatitis, acute viral   MS/CH
impaired Liver Function related to (viral infection) as evidenced by jaundice, hepatic enlargement, abdominal pain, marked elevations in serum liver function tests.

Fatigue may be related to decreased metabolic energy production, discomfort, altered body chemistry—changes in liver function, effect on target organs, possibly evidenced by reports of lack of energy, inability to maintain usual routines, decreased performance, and increased physical complaints.

imbalanced Nutrition: less than body requirements may be related to inability to (ingest food or absorb nutrients); [hypermetabolic state], possibly evidenced by food aversion or insufficient interest in food, alteration in taste sensation, [observed lack of intake, and weight loss].

acute Pain/impaired Comfort may be related to biological agent—inflammation and swelling of the liver, arthralgias, urticarial eruptions, and pruritus, possibly evidenced by verbal reports, guarding or distraction behaviors, focus on self, and changes in vital signs.

risk for Infection possibly evidenced by immunosuppression, malnutrition, insufficient knowledge to avoid exposure to pathogens or spread to others.

risk for impaired Tissue Integrity possibly evidenced by [bile salt accumulation in the tissues].

deficient Knowledge regarding disease process and transmission, treatment needs, and future expectations may be related to lack of information or recall, misinterpretation, unfamiliarity with resources, possibly evidenced by questions, statement of concerns, misconceptions, inaccurate follow-through of instructions, and development of preventable complications.

Hepatorenal syndrome   MS
Refer to Cirrhosis; Renal failure, acute

Hernia, hiatal   CH
chronic Pain may be related to injury agent [regurgitation of acidic gastric contents], possibly evidenced by self-reports, alteration in sleep pattern, facial expression of pain, and self-focused.

deficient Knowledge regarding pathophysiology, prevention of complications, and self-care needs may be related to lack of information, misconceptions, possibly evidenced by statements of concern, questions, and recurrence of condition.

Hernia, inguinal   MS
Refer to Herniorrhaphy

Herniated nucleus pulposus   CH/MS
(ruptured intervertebral disc)
acute/chronic Pain may be related to injury agent [nerve compression/irritation and muscle spasms], possibly evidenced by self-reports, guarding or distraction behavior, preoccupation with pain, self-focused, narrowed focus, changes in vital signs [when pain is acute], altered muscle tone or function, changes in eating or sleeping patterns and libido, and physical or social withdrawal.

impaired physical Mobility may be related to pain (muscle spasms), therapeutic restrictions (e.g., rest, braces, or traction), muscular impairment, and depressive mood state, possibly evidenced by reports of pain on movement, reluctance to attempt or difficulty with purposeful movement, decreased muscle strength, impaired coordination, and limited range of motion.

decreased Diversional Activity Engagement may be related to length of recuperation period and therapy restrictions, physical limitations, pain and depression, possibly evidenced by statements of boredom, disinterest, "nothing to do," and restlessness, irritability, withdrawal.

Herniorrhaphy   MS/PED
acute Pain may be related to physical injury agent (surgical disruption of skin, tissue, and muscle integrity), possibly evidenced by verbal or coded reports, alteration in muscle tone, distraction or guarding behaviors, narrowed focus, and autonomic responses.

risk for Injury possibly evidenced by surgical repair, insertion of graft, increased intra-abdominal pressure (straining at stool, heavy lifting, strenuous activity).

Heroin abuse   **CH**

risk for Infection possibly evidenced by malnutrition, altered immune state, insufficient knowledge or motivation to avoid pathogens, and environmental exposure [injection, reuse, or sharing of needles].

imbalanced Nutrition: less than body requirements may be related to insufficient dietary intake, (economically disadvantaged, psychological disorder), possibly evidenced by [substituting drug for food], insufficient interest in food, weight loss, insufficient muscle tone.

risk for physical Trauma possibly evidenced by personal vulnerability, cigarette smoking, lack of safety precautions, driving impaired or under the influence, high-crime neighborhood.

risk for ineffective Protection possibly evidenced by effects of substance use, malnutrition, chronic disease, lifestyle choices, unhealthy environment.

Heroin withdrawal   **CH/MS**

acute Pain/impaired Comfort may be related to [cessation of drug, drug cravings] possibly evidenced by self-reports, tremors, twitching; hot and cold flashes, diaphoresis, lacrimation, rhinorrhea.

[severe] Anxiety may be related to central nervous system hyperactivity, possibly evidenced by apprehensiveness, pervasive anxious feelings, jittery, restlessness, weakness, insomnia, anorexia.

risk for ineffective Health Management possibly evidenced by protracted withdrawal, economic difficulties, family or social support deficits, perceived barriers or benefits.

Herpes simplex   **CH**

acute Pain may be related to physical injury agent (localized inflammation and open lesions), possibly evidenced by verbal reports, distraction behaviors, and restlessness.

risk for [secondary] Infection possibly evidenced by broken or traumatized tissue, altered immune response, and untreated infection or treatment failure.

risk for Sexual dysfunction possibly evidenced by vulnerability (e.g., lack of knowledge, values conflict, or fear of transmitting the disease).

Herpes zoster (shingles)   **CH**

acute Pain may be related to inflammation, local lesions along sensory nerve(s), possibly evidenced by verbal reports, guarding or distraction behaviors, narrowed focus, and changes in vital signs.

deficient Knowledge regarding pathophysiology, therapeutic needs, and potential complications may be related to lack of information, misinterpretation, possibly evidenced by statements of concern, questions, and misconceptions.

High altitude pulmonary edema (HAPE)   **MS**

Also refer to Mountain sickness, acute

impaired Gas Exchange may be related to (ventilation-perfusion imbalance and alveolar-capillary membrane changes), possibly evidenced by abnormal breathing (dyspnea) and skin color (cyanosis), confusion, tachycardia, abnormal arterial blood gases.

excess Fluid Volume may be related to compromised regulatory mechanism, possibly evidenced by shortness of breath, anxiety, edema, abnormal breath sounds, pulmonary congestion.

High altitude sickness   **MS**

Refer to Mountain sickness, acute; High altitude pulmonary edema

High-risk pregnancy   **OB**

Refer to Pregnancy, high-risk

Hip replacement   **MS**

Refer to Total joint replacement

HIV infection   **CH**

Also refer to AIDS

risk-prone Health Behavior may be related to stressors, low self-efficacy, social anxiety, insufficient social support; negative perception of recommended healthcare strategy, possibly evidenced by nonacceptance of or minimizes health status change, failure to take action that prevents health problem.

deficient Knowledge regarding disease, prognosis, and treatment needs may be related to lack of exposure or recall, information misinterpretation, unfamiliarity with information resources, or cognitive limitation, possibly evidenced by statement of misconception, request for information, inappropriate or exaggerated behaviors (hostile, agitated, hysterical, apathetic), inaccurate follow-through of instructions, development of preventable complications.

risk for ineffective Health Management possibly evidenced by difficulty navigating complex healthcare systems, economically disadvantaged; difficulty managing complex treatment regimen, perceived seriousness of condition, perceived benefit/barrier, decisional conflict.

risk for complicated Grieving possibly evidenced by emotional disturbance and insufficient social support.

Hodgkin's disease   CH/MS
Also refer to Cancer; Chemotherapy

Anxiety [specify level]/Fear may be related to threat to self-concept and threat of death, possibly evidenced by apprehensiveness, insomnia, self-focused, and increase in tension.

deficient Knowledge regarding diagnosis, pathophysiology, treatment, and prognosis may be related to lack of information, misinterpretation, possibly evidenced by statements of concern, questions, and misconceptions.

acute Pain/impaired Comfort may be related to physical injury agents (inflammatory response [fever, chills, night sweats] and pruritus), possibly evidenced by self-reports, distraction behavior, and self-focused.

risk for ineffective Breathing Pattern/Airway Clearance possibly evidenced by tracheobronchial obstruction (enlarged mediastinal nodes or airway edema).

Hospice/End-of-life care   CH
acute/chronic Pain may be related to biological, physical, psychological agent; chronic physical disability, possibly evidenced by verbal or coded report, preoccupation with pain, changes in appetite, sleep pattern, altered ability to continue desired activities, guarded or protective behavior, restlessness, irritability, narrowed focus—altered time perception, impaired thought processes.

Activity Intolerance/Fatigue may be related to, [bedrest or immobility, pain, progressive disease state or debilitating condition, depressive state], imbalance between oxygen supply and demand, possibly evidenced by generalized weakness/inability to maintain usual routine, verbalized [lack of desire or interest in activity, decreased performance, lethargy].

Grieving/Death Anxiety may be related to (terminal illness, anticipated loss) perceived imminence of death, anticipation of pain/suffering, possibly evidenced by anger, blaming, despair, alteration in sleep pattern, fear of pain/suffering related to dying; powerlessness, worried about the impact of one's death on significant other.

compromised/disabled family Coping/caregiver Role Strain may be related to prolonged disease or disability progression, family disorganization, ineffective family adaptation, increase in care needs, possibly evidenced by difficulty performing/completing required tasks, protective behavior by support person incongruent with client's abilities/need for autonomy, family conflict.

risk for Spiritual distress possibly evidenced by stressors ineffective relationships, loneliness, perception of having unfinished business; separation from support system, social isolation, inability to forgive.

risk for Moral Distress possibly evidenced by conflicting information available for moral decision making; difficulty reaching end-of-life decisions; conflict among decision-makers, cultural incongruence.

Huntington's disease   CH
Hopelessness may be related to chronic progressive debilitating condition, possibly evidenced by despondent verbalizations, withdrawal from environs, angry outbursts.

impaired Walking may be related to movement disorder (altered gait, ataxia, dystonia), possibly evidenced by inability to walk required distances, navigate curbs or uneven surfaces, climb stairs.

chronic Confusion may be related to dementia, possibly evidenced by altered interpretation, progressive cognitive impairment, altered personality, impaired memory, impaired socialization.

imbalanced Nutrition: less than body requirements may be related to insufficient dietary intake, (inability to ingest food [difficulty swallowing, cognitive decline]), possibly evidenced by food aversion, food intake less than recommended daily allowance, [weight loss, decreased subcutaneous fat or muscle mass].

[total] Self-Care deficit may be related to neuromuscular impairment, cognitive decline, possibly evidenced by inability to perform desired activities of daily living.

risk for caregiver Role Strain possibly evidenced by (chronic illness), unpredictably of illness trajectory, extended duration of caregiving activities, complexity care activities, caregiver's competing role commitments, family isolation, lack of respite or recreation for caregiver, bizarre behavior of care receiver.

Hydrocephalus   PED/MS
ineffective cerebral Tissue Perfusion may be related to decreased arterial or venous blood flow (compression of brain tissue), possibly evidenced by changes in mentation, restlessness, irritability, reports of headache, pupillary changes, and changes in vital signs.

[disturbed visual Sensory Perception] may be related to pressure on sensory or motor nerves, possibly evidenced by reports of double vision, development of strabismus, nystagmus, pupillary changes, and optic atrophy.

risk for impaired physical Mobility possibly evidenced by neuromuscular impairment, decreased muscle strength, and impaired coordination.

risk for decreased intracranial Adaptive Capacity possibly evidenced by brain injury, changes in perfusion pressure and intracranial pressure.

CH

risk for Infection possibly evidenced by (invasive procedure—presence of shunt).

deficient Knowledge regarding condition, prognosis, long-term therapy needs, and medical follow-up may be related to lack of information, misperceptions, possibly evidenced by questions, statement of concern, request for information, and inaccurate follow-through of instructions, development of preventable complications.

Hydrophobia   CH/MS
Refer to Rabies

Hyperactivity disorder   PED/PSY
ineffective Impulse Control may be related to compunction, possibly evidenced by acting without thinking, temper outbursts.

defensive Coping may be related to mild neurological deficits, dysfunctional family system, abuse or neglect, possibly evidenced by denial of obvious problems, projection of blame or responsibility, grandiosity, difficulty in reality testing perceptions.

impaired Social Interaction may be related to disturbance in thought processes, sociocultural dissonance, possibly evidenced by discomfort in social situations, dysfunctional interaction with others.

compromised family Coping may be related to insufficient understanding of information by support person, exhaustion of support person's capacity, family disorganization, possibly evidenced by assistive behaviors by support person produce unsatisfactory results, support person reports inadequate understanding that interferes with effective behaviors, limitation between support person and client.

Hyperbilirubinemia   PED
neonatal Hyperbilirubinemia may be related to (premature infant, age ≤ 7 days, populations living at high altitude, blood type incompatibility between mother and infant), deficient feeding pattern, delay in meconium passage, possibly evidenced by abnormal blood profile (elevated blood urea nitrogen), yellow-orange skin color, and yellow mucous membranes/sclera.

risk for Injury [effects of treatment] possibly evidenced by physical properties of phototherapy and effects on body regulatory mechanisms, invasive procedure (exchange transfusion), abnormal blood profile, chemical imbalances.

deficient Knowledge regarding condition prognosis, treatment, and safety needs may be related to lack of exposure or recall and information misinterpretation, possibly evidenced by questions, statement of concern, and inaccurate follow-through of instructions, development of preventable complications.

Hyperemesis gravidarum   OB
deficient Fluid Volume may be related to excessive gastric losses and reduced intake, possibly evidenced by dry mucous membranes, decreased and concentrated urine, decreased pulse volume and pressure, thirst, and hemoconcentration.

risk for Electrolyte Imbalance possibly evidenced by vomiting, dehydration.

imbalanced Nutrition: less than body requirements may be related to insufficient dietary intake, (inability to ingest or digest food, or absorb nutrients), possibly evidenced by food intake less than recommended daily allowance, insufficient interest in food or food aversion, and [weight loss].

risk for ineffective Coping possibly evidenced by (situational or maturational crisis [pregnancy, change in health status, projected role changes, concern about outcome]).

Hyperparathyroidism, primary   MS
risk for deficient Fluid Volume possibly evidenced by excessive losses through normal routes (vomiting, diarrhea, gastric bleed).

risk for Electrolyte Imbalance possibly evidenced by impaired regulatory mechanism, vomiting.

impaired urinary Elimination may be related to anatomic obstruction (renal calculi), possibly evidenced by decreased renal function.

risk for physical Trauma possibly evidenced by decreased calcium levels, bone fragility.

Hypertension   CH
deficient Knowledge regarding condition, therapeutic regimen, and potential complications may be related

to lack of information or recall, misinterpretation, cognitive limitations, or denial of diagnosis, possibly evidenced by statements of concern, questions, and misconceptions, inaccurate follow-through of instructions, and lack of blood pressure control.

risk-prone Health Behavior may be related to inadequate comprehension, low self-efficacy, negative perception of recommended healthcare strategy, (economically disadvantaged), possibly evidenced by minimizes/nonacceptance of health status change, failure to take action that prevents health problem.

risk for Activity Intolerance possibly evidenced by imbalance between oxygen supply and demand and physical deconditioning.

risk for Sexual dysfunction possibly evidenced by vulnerability (side effects of medications).

MS

risk for decreased Cardiac Output possibly evidenced by increased afterload (vasoconstriction), fluid shifts, hypovolemia, myocardial ischemia, ventricular hypertrophy and rigidity.

Hypertension, gestational   OB/CH
Also refer to Eclampsia

deficient Fluid Volume may be related to (compromised regulatory mechanisms [e.g., plasma protein loss, decreasing osmotic pressure]), possibly evidenced by increase in hematocrit, decrease in urine output, increase in urine concentration, sudden weight gain [edema, third spacing].

decreased Cardiac Output may be related to alteration in preload, afterload, possibly evidenced by preload—increase in hemodynamic readings, weight gain/edema, afterload—alteration in blood pressure, dyspnea.

risk for disturbed Maternal-Fetal Dyad possibly evidenced by pregnancy complication [e.g., compromised oxygen transport—vasospasm of spiral arteries, and maternal hypovolemia, hypertension].

deficient Knowledge regarding pathophysiology of condition, therapy, self-care, nutritional needs, and potential complications may be related to lack of information or recall, misinterpretation, possibly evidenced by statements of concern, questions, misconceptions, inaccurate follow-through of instructions, development of preventable complications.

Hypertension, intrapartum   OB
risk for imbalanced Fluid Volume possibly evidenced by compromised regulatory mechanism, fluid shifts, excessive fluid intake, effects of drug therapy (oxytocin infusion).

risk for impaired fetal Gas Exchange possibly evidenced by altered blood flow, vasospasms, prolonged uterine contractions.

impaired urinary Elimination may be related to fluid shifts, hormonal changes, effects of medication, possibly evidenced by changes in amount and frequency of voiding, bladder distention, changes in urine specific gravity, presence of albumin.

risk for maternal Injury possibly evidenced by tonic-clonic convulsions, altered clotting factors (release of thromboplastin from placenta).

Hypertension, prenatal   OB
Refer to Hypertension, gestational

Hypertension, pulmonary   CH/MS
Refer to Pulmonary hypertension

Hyperthyroidism   CH
Also refer to Thyrotoxicosis

Fatigue may be related to hypermetabolic imbalance with increased energy requirements, irritability of central nervous system, and altered body chemistry, possibly evidenced by verbalization of overwhelming lack of energy to maintain usual routine, decreased performance, emotional lability and irritability, and impaired ability to concentrate.

Anxiety [specify level] may be related to stressors (e.g., hypermetabolic state, pseudocatecholamine effect of thyroid hormones), possibly evidenced by increased feelings of apprehension, overexcitement, or distress; irritability; emotional lability; restless movements; tremors.

risk for imbalanced Nutrition: less than body requirements possibly evidenced by inability to ingest adequate food for [hypermetabolic rate, constant activity level, impaired absorption of nutrients (vomiting, diarrhea), hyperglycemia, relative insulin insufficiency].

risk for Dry Eye possibly evidenced by autoimmune diseases (thyroid disease), lack of spontaneous blink reflex, ocular surface damage.

Hypervolemia   CH/MS
excess Fluid Volume may be related to excess fluid and sodium intake, compromised regulatory mechanisms (renal failure, increased antidiuretic hormone), decreased plasma proteins, rapid or excessive administration of isotonic parenteral fluids, possibly evidenced by edema,

abnormal breath sounds, S$_3$ heart sound, shortness of breath, positive hepatojugular reflex—elevated central venous pressure, change in mental status.

Hypochondriasis   PSY
Refer to Somatoform disorders

Hypoglycemia   CH
acute Confusion may be related to (impaired metabolic functioning), possibly evidenced by restlessness, misperception, alteration in cognitive functioning/level of consciousness.

risk for unstable Blood Glucose Level possibly evidenced by insufficient diabetes management, inadequate blood glucose monitoring, ineffective medication management.

deficient Knowledge regarding pathophysiology of condition, therapy, and self-care needs may be related to lack of information or recall, misinterpretations, possibly evidenced by development of hypoglycemia and statements of questions, misconceptions.

Hypoparathyroidism (acute)   MS
risk for Electrolyte Imbalance possibly evidenced by impaired regulatory mechanism.

risk for Injury possibly evidenced by neuromuscular excitability—tetany and formation of renal stones.

acute Pain may be related to physical agent [recurrent muscle spasms], possibly evidenced by verbal reports, distraction behaviors, and narrowed focus.

risk for ineffective Airway Clearance possibly evidenced by spasm of the laryngeal muscles.

Anxiety [specify level] may be related to threat to current status, physiological responses.

Hypophysectomy   MS
Also refer to Surgery, general; Cancer
Fear/Anxiety may be related learned response to threat [situational crisis (nature of diagnosis and procedure), change in health status, perceived threat of death, separation from support system], possibly evidenced by expressed concerns, apprehension, being scared, increased tension, extraneous movement, difficulty concentrating.

risk for deficient Fluid Volume possibly evidenced by failure of regulatory mechanism (decreased antidiuretic hormone).

risk for Infection possibly evidenced by (invasive procedure, immunosuppression, chronic illness).

Sexual dysfunction may be related to altered body function (loss of anterior pituitary), possibly evidenced by [sterility, decreased libido, impotence (male), infertility, atrophy of vaginal mucosa (female)].

Hypothermia (systemic)   CH
Also refer to Frostbite
Hypothermia may be related to exposure to cold environment, inadequate clothing, age extremes (very young or elderly), damage to hypothalamus, consumption of alcohol or medications causing vasodilation, possibly evidenced by reduction in body temperature below normal range, shivering, cool skin, pallor.

deficient Knowledge regarding risk factors, treatment needs, and prognosis may be related to lack of information or recall, misinterpretation, possibly evidenced by statement of concerns, misconceptions, occurrence of problem, and development of complications.

Hypothyroidism   CH
Also refer to Myxedema
Fatigue may be related to decreased metabolic energy production, possibly evidenced by verbalization of unremitting or overwhelming lack of energy, inability to maintain usual routines, impaired ability to concentrate, decreased libido, irritability, listlessness, decreased performance, increase in physical complaints.

Constipation may be related to decreased peristalsis, lack of physical activity, possibly evidenced by frequency less than usual pattern, decreased bowel sounds, hard dry stools, and development of fecal impaction.

impaired physical Mobility may be related to weakness, fatigue, muscle aches, altered reflexes, and mucin deposits in joints and interstitial spaces, possibly evidenced by decreased muscle strength or control and impaired coordination.

[disturbed Sensory Perception (specify)] may be related to mucin deposits and nerve compression, possibly evidenced by paresthesias of hands and feet or decreased hearing.

Hypovolemia   CH/MS
deficient Fluid Volume may be related to active fluid loss (hemorrhage, vomiting, gastric intubation, diarrhea, burns, wounds, fistulas), regulatory failure (adrenal disease, recovery phase of acute renal failure, diabetic ketoacidosis, hyperosmolar nonketotic coma,

diabetes insipidus, sepsis), possibly evidenced by thirst, weight loss, poor skin turgor, dry mucous membranes, tachycardia, tachypnea, fatigue, decreased central venous pressure.

Hysterectomy GYN/MS
Also refer to Surgery, general
acute Pain may be related to physical injury agent (tissue trauma, abdominal incision), possibly evidenced by verbal reports, guarding or distraction behaviors, and changes in vital signs.

risk for perioperative positioning Injury possibly evidenced by immobilization, lithotomy position.

impaired urinary Elimination/risk for [acute] urinary Retention possibly evidenced by mechanical trauma, surgical manipulation, presence of localized edema or hematoma, or nerve trauma with temporary bladder atony.

risk for Sexual dysfunction possibly evidenced by (altered body function and structure), vulnerability [perceived changes in femininity], decrease in sexual desire, and alteration in sexual excitation/satisfaction.

Ileal conduit MS/CH
Refer to Urinary diversion

Ileocolitis MS/CH
Refer to Crohn's disease

Ileostomy MS/CH
Refer to Colostomy

Ileus MS
acute Pain may be related to physical injury agent: (ischemia of intestinal tissue), possibly evidenced by verbal reports, guarding/distraction behaviors, narrowed focus, and changes in vital signs.

Diarrhea/Constipation may be related to presence of obstruction, changes in peristalsis, possibly evidenced by changes in frequency and consistency or absence of stool, alterations in bowel sounds, presence of pain, and cramping.

risk for deficient Fluid Volume possibly evidenced by risk factors of increased intestinal losses (vomiting, diarrhea) and decreased intake.

Immersion foot MS
impaired Skin/Tissue Integrity may be related to hypothermia and moisture (cold and wet environment [above freezing], possibly evidenced by acute pain, [tissue maceration, soggy edema]).

[disturbed peripheral Sensory Perception] may be related to altered sensory reception, possibly evidenced by paresthesia, numbness.

risk for ineffective Health Maintenance possibly evidenced by lack of material resources, poor coping skills, inadequate knowledge of safety needs.

Impetigo PED/CH
impaired Skin Integrity may be related to presence of [infectious process and pruritus], possibly evidenced by open, crusted lesions.

acute Pain may be related to physical agent (inflammation), possibly evidenced by verbal reports, distraction behavior, and self-focused.

risk for [secondary] Infection possibly evidenced by broken skin, traumatized tissue, altered immune response, and virulence or contagious nature of causative organism.

risk for Infection [transmission] possibly evidenced by insufficient knowledge to prevent infection of others.

Impotence CH
Refer to Erectile dysfunction

Infant (at 4 weeks) PED
readiness for enhanced Knowledge regarding infant care, developmental expectations, safety, and well-being possibly evidenced by expresses desire to enhance learning.

risk for imbalanced Nutrition (specify) possibly evidenced by inability to ingest, digest, or absorb adequate calories—insufficient intake, malabsorption, congenital problem, neglect or emotional abuse, or failure to thrive; obesity in one or both parents, rapid transition across growth percentiles.

risk for acute Pain possibly evidenced by [accumulation of gas in confined space with cramping of intestinal musculature].

risk for Infection possibly evidenced by [immature immunological response, increased environmental exposure].

risk for Sudden Infant Death possibly evidenced by sleeping position, secondhand smoke exposure, type of bedding used.

risk for disorganized infant Behavior possibly evidenced by immature development of sensory organs, inappropriate or inadequate environmental stimuli, effects of prenatal or intrapartal complications, drugs.

Infant of addicted mother   **OB/PED**

Neonatal Abstinence Syndrome may be related to (in-utero substance exposure secondary to maternal substance use), possibly evidenced by disorganized infant behavior, ineffective infant feeding pattern, impaired skin integrity, risk for impaired attachment.

ineffective Airway Clearance/impaired Gas Exchange may be related to [excess mucus production, depression of cough reflex and respiratory center, intrauterine asphyxia], possibly evidenced by abnormal breathing pattern (tachypnea, grunting respirations) and skin color (cyanosis), nasal flaring, hypoxia, acidosis.

impaired Parenting may be related to lack of available or ineffective role model, unmet emotional maturation needs of parent, lack of support between or from SO, interruption in bonding process, lack of appropriate response of infant, possibly evidenced by reports of role inadequacy or inability to care for infant, inattention to infant needs, inappropriate caretaking behaviors, lack of parental attachment behaviors.

disabled family Coping may be related to SO with chronically unexpressed feelings of guilt, anxiety, hostility, despair; dissonant discrepancy of coping styles; high-risk family situations, possibly evidenced by intolerance, rejection, abandonment, or desertion, neglectful relationships between family members, neglectful care of infant, distortion of reality of parent's health problem or substance use.

Infant of HIV-positive mother   **OB/PED**

Also refer to AIDS

risk for Infection possibly evidenced by [immature immune system, inadequate acquired immunity], (suppressed inflammatory response, invasive procedures), malnutrition.

risk for imbalanced Nutrition: risk for less than body requirements possibly evidenced by (inability to ingest, digest, or absorb nutrients [e.g., impaired suck or swallow, gastrointestinal infection, malabsorption, diarrhea]).

risk for delayed Development possibly evidenced by separation from SO, inadequate caretaking, inconsistent responsiveness, multiple caretakers, environmental and stimulation deficiencies, effects of chronic condition or disabilities.

deficient Knowledge regarding condition, prognosis, and treatment needs may be related to lack of exposure, misinterpretation, unfamiliarity with resources, lack of recall or interest in learning, possibly evidenced by questions, statements of misconceptions, inaccurate follow-through of instructions, development of preventable complications.

Infection, ear   **PED**

Refer to Otitis media

Infection, prenatal   **OB**

Also refer to AIDS

risk for disturbed Maternal-Fetal Dyad possibly evidenced by inadequate prenatal care, (pregnancy complication-rupture of amniotic membranes, treatment-related side effects).

deficient Knowledge regarding treatment, prevention, and prognosis of condition may be related to lack of exposure to information or unfamiliarity with resources, misinterpretation, possibly evidenced by verbalization of problem, inaccurate follow-through of instructions, development of preventable complications, continuation of infectious process.

impaired Comfort may be related to body response to infective agent, properties of infection (e.g., skin or tissue irritation, development of lesions), possibly evidenced by verbal reports, illness-related symptoms, restlessness, withdrawal from social contacts.

Infection, puerperal   **OB/CH**

risk for Infection [spread/sepsis] possibly evidenced by alteration in skin integrity/traumatized tissues, (invasive procedures/increased environmental exposure, anemia, chronic disease).

acute Pain may be related to physical injury agent (infective agent and toxins), possibly evidenced by verbalizations, restlessness, guarding behavior, self-focusing, and changes in vital signs.

imbalanced Nutrition: less than body requirements may be related to insufficient dietary intake, possibly evidenced by food aversion, insufficient or lack of oral intake, [unanticipated weight loss].

risk for impaired Attachment possibly evidenced by interruption in bonding process, separation, physical barriers, maternal fatigue or apathy.

Infection, wound   **MS/CH**

risk for Surgical Site Infection/Infection [sepsis] possibly evidenced by presence of infection, broken skin, or traumatized tissues, stasis of body fluids, invasive procedures, increased environmental exposure, chronic disease (e.g., diabetes, anemia, malnutrition), altered immune response, and untoward effect of medications (e.g., opportunistic or secondary infection).

impaired Skin/Tissue Integrity may be related to alteration in fluid volume (circulation) inadequate nutrition; and [presence of systemic or local infection, wound drainage], possibly evidenced by [delayed healing, damaged tissues, invasion of body structures].

risk for delayed Surgical Recovery possibly evidenced by presence of infection, activity restrictions or limitations, nutritional deficiency.

Infertility   CH
situational low Self-Esteem may be related to functional impairment (inability to conceive), unrealistic self-expectations, sense of failure, possibly evidenced by self-negating verbalizations, expressions of helplessness, perceived inability to deal with situation.

chronic Sorrow may be related to perceived physical disability (inability to conceive), possibly evidenced by expressions of anger, disappointment, emptiness, self-blame, helplessness, sadness, feelings interfering with client's ability to achieve maximum well-being.

risk for Spiritual distress possibly evidenced by anxiety, ineffective relationships, pain, separation from support system, social isolation, anxiety, low self-esteem, [deteriorating relationship with SO, viewing situation as deserved or punishment for past behaviors].

Inflammatory bowel disease   CH
Refer to Colitis, ulcerative; Crohn's disease

Influenza   CH
acute Pain/impaired Comfort may be related to physical injury agent (inflammation, circulating toxins), possibly evidenced by verbal reports, distraction behaviors, and narrowed focus.

risk for deficient Fluid Volume possibly evidenced by excessive gastric losses, hypermetabolic state, and altered intake.

Hyperthermia may be related to effects of circulating toxins and dehydration, possibly evidenced by increased body temperature; warm, flushed skin; and tachycardia.

risk for ineffective Breathing Pattern possibly evidenced by response to infectious process, decreased energy, fatigue.

Inhalant intoxication/abuse   CH/PSY
Refer to Stimulant abuse

Insomnia, acute   CH
Insomnia may be related to daytime activity pattern, social or work schedule inconsistent with chronotype, travel across time zones, fatigue, life change, physical conditions (dyspnea, gastroesophageal reflux, night sweats), possibly evidenced by verbal reports of difficulties, not feeling well-rested, less than age-normed total sleep time, changes in behavior and performance, physical signs (dark circles under eyes, frequent yawning).

Insomnia, chronic   CH
Sleep deprivation may be related to sustained environmental stimulation, sustained circadian asynchrony, prolonged use of pharmacological or dietary antisoporifics, prolonged pain, sleep apnea, dementia, narcolepsy, possibly evidenced by daytime drowsiness, decreased ability to perform, lethargy, slowed reaction, apathy.

Insulin resistance syndrome   CH
Refer to Metabolic syndrome

Insulin shock   MS/CH
Refer to Hypoglycemia

Intermaxillary fixation   MS/CH
Also refer to Surgery, general
risk for ineffective Airway Clearance possibly evidenced by soft tissue trauma, retained secretions.

risk for Aspiration possibly evidenced by (facial trauma or oral surgery, wired jaw), ineffective cough.

impaired Tissue Integrity may be related to tissue trauma or damage, intraoperative manipulation, mechanical fixation device, altered circulation, nutritional deficit, possibly evidenced by edema, hematoma, ecchymosis, erythema, inflammation, delayed healing.

impaired verbal Communication may be related to wiring of jaws, edema of mouth and surrounding structures, pain, possibly evidenced by inability or reluctance to talk.

risk for imbalanced Nutrition: less than body requirements possibly evidenced by inability to ingest food, weakness of muscles required for mastication/swallowing, insufficient interest in food.

Intervertebral disc excision   MS
Refer to Laminectomy, cervical or lumbar

Intestinal obstruction   MS
Refer to Ileus

Intestinal surgery (without diversion)   MS
Also refer to Surgery, general
risk for deficient Fluid Volume possibly evidenced by excessive losses through normal routes (vomiting,

diarrhea), excessive losses through abnormal routes (indwelling drains, nasogastric/intestinal suctioning, hemorrhage), insufficient replacement, fever.

risk for Infection possibly evidenced by (chronic disease), malnutrition, stasis of body fluids, altered peristalsis, and [opening of abdominal cavity and bowel].

Constipation/Diarrhea may be related to effects of anesthesia, surgical manipulation, decreased dietary intake or bulk, physical inactivity, irritation, malabsorption, pain, effects of medication, possibly evidenced by change in bowel habits, change in stool characteristics, hyper-/hypoactive bowel sounds, abdominal pain.

Intracranial infections   MS
Refer to Abscess, brain [acute]; Encephalitis; Meningitis, acute meningococcal

Irritable bowel syndrome   CH
acute Pain may be related to physical injury agent (increased sensitivity of intestine to distention, hypersensitivity to hormones gastrin and cholecystokinin, skin or tissue irritation, perirectal excoriation), possibly evidenced by verbal reports, guarding behavior, expressive behavior (restlessness, moaning, irritability).

Constipation may be related to motor abnormalities of longitudinal muscles, changes in frequency and amplitude of contractions, dietary restrictions, stress, possibly evidenced by change in bowel pattern—decreased frequency, sensation of incomplete evacuation, abdominal pain and distention.

Diarrhea may be related to motor abnormalities of longitudinal muscles, changes in frequency and amplitude of contractions, stress, possibly evidenced by precipitous passing of liquid stool on rising or immediately after eating, rectal urgency, incontinence, bloating.

Kanner's syndrome   PED/PSY
Refer to Autistic spectrum disorder

Kaposi's sarcoma, AIDS-related   CH/MS
Also refer to Chemotherapy
disturbed Body Image may be related to actual change in structure, (e.g., widely disseminated lesions of varied color in skin and mucous membranes), possibly evidenced by verbalizations, fear of rejection or reaction of others, negative feelings about body, hiding body parts, change in social involvement.

risk for deficient Fluid Volume possibly evidenced by extensive bleeding of visceral lesions.

Kawasaki disease   PED
Hyperthermia may be related to increased metabolic rate and dehydration, possibly evidenced by increased body temperature greater than normal range, flushed skin, increased respiratory rate, and tachycardia.

acute Pain may be related to physical injury agent (inflammation of blood vessels, and swelling of tissues) possibly evidenced by verbal reports, restlessness, guarding behaviors, and narrowed focus.

impaired Skin Integrity may be related to [inflammatory process], and alteration in fluid volume [edema formation], (impaired circulation), possibly evidenced by alteration in skin integrity (macular rash and desquamation).

impaired oral Mucous Membrane Integrity may be related to inflammatory process, dehydration, and mouth breathing, possibly evidenced by pain, hyperemia, and fissures of lips.

risk for decreased Cardiac Output possibly evidenced by structural changes and inflammation of coronary arteries, and alterations in rate and rhythm or conduction.

Ketoacidosis   CH
Refer to Diabetic ketoacidosis

Kidney disease, polycystic   CH
risk for [urinary tract] Infection possibly evidenced by inadequate primary defenses (traumatized tissue, stasis of body fluids), inadequate secondary defenses (suppressed inflammatory response), chronic disease.

acute/chronic Pain may be related to injuring agents—presence of cysts in kidneys or other organs, possibly evidenced by verbal report of back or lower side pain, headaches beyond tolerance, guarded or protective behavior, narrowed focus, sleep disturbance, distraction behaviors.

risk for excess Fluid Volume possibly evidenced by oliguria, edema, abnormal breath sounds, jugular vein distention, hypertension.

Kidney failure, acute   MS
Refer to Renal failure, acute

Kidney failure, chronic   CH/MS
Refer to Renal failure, chronic

Kidney stone(s)   CH
Refer to Calculi, urinary

Knee replacement   MS
Refer to Total joint replacement

Kwashiorkor   **PED**

imbalanced Nutrition: less than body requirements may be related to insufficient dietary intake (economically disadvantaged), possibly evidenced by food intake less than recommended daily allowances, body weight 20% or more below ideal weight range, insufficient muscle tone, [decreased subcutaneous fat or muscle mass, abnormal laboratory studies].

risk for Infection possibly evidenced by malnutrition.

risk for disproportionate Growth possibly evidenced by malnutrition, caregiver maladaptive feeding behaviors, deprivation, poverty, impaired insulin response, infection.

Labor, breech presentation   **OB**

Anxiety [specify level] may be related to situational crisis, threat to self/fetus, interpersonal transmission, possibly evidenced by increased tension, apprehension, fearfulness, restlessness, sympathetic stimulation.

risk for fetal Injury possibly evidenced by risk factors of entrapment of head, stretching of brachial plexus or spinal cord (nerve damage), hypoxia (brain damage).

Labor, dysfunctional   **OB**

Refer to Dystocia

Labor, induced/augmented   **OB**

deficient Knowledge regarding procedure, treatment needs, and possible outcomes may be related to lack of exposure or recall, information misinterpretation, and unfamiliarity with information resources, possibly evidenced by questions, statement of concern, misconception, and exaggerated behaviors.

risk for maternal Injury possibly evidenced by physical factor [e.g., adverse effects or response to therapeutic interventions].

risk for disturbed Maternal-Fetal Dyad possibly evidenced by (compromised fetal oxygen transport [e.g., altered placental perfusion, cord prolapse]).

labor Pain may be related to physical agent [e.g., characteristics of chemically stimulated contractions], cervical dilation, possibly evidenced by verbal reports, alteration in muscle tension, distraction or expressive behavior, and narrowed focus.

Labor, precipitous   **OB**

Anxiety [specify level] may be related to (situational crisis), threat to current status [self/fetus], interpersonal transmission, possibly evidenced by increase in

tension; apprehensiveness, uncertainty, fear, restless, sympathetic stimulation.

risk for impaired Skin/Tissue Integrity possibly evidenced by [mechanical factors (e.g., pressure, shearing forces)].

labor Pain may be related to physical agent [e.g., rapid, strong uterine contractions], cervical dilation, fetal expulsion; psychological factors (anxiety), possibly evidenced by pain, sympathetic stimulation, expressive behavior (e.g., moaning, restlessness), self-focused.

Labor, preterm   **OB/CH**

risk for disturbed Maternal-Fetal Dyad possibly evidenced by (compromised fetal oxygen transport, treatment regimen [side effects of tocolytics]).

risk for Poisoning possibly evidenced by dose-related toxic or side effects of tocolytics.

risk for fetal Injury possibly evidenced by (tissue hypoxia; chemical [e.g., pharmaceutical agents]).

Anxiety [specify level] may be related to (situational crisis), threat to change in current status [self/fetus], and interpersonal transmission, possibly evidenced by increase in tension, apprehensiveness, distress, uncertainty, restlessness, and changes in vital signs.

readiness for enhanced Knowledge regarding preterm labor treatment needs and prognosis possibly evidenced by expresses desire to enhance learning.

Labor, stage I (active phase)   **OB**

labor Pain may be related to physical agent [e.g., tissue dilation, muscle hypoxia, and pressure on adjacent structures and nerve endings], possibly evidenced by uterine contraction, expressive behavior (restlessness), and narrowed focus, positioning to ease pain, alteration in vital signs.

impaired urinary Elimination may be related to multiple causality [e.g., altered intake, fluid shifts, hormonal changes, mechanical compression of bladder, and effects of regional anesthesia], possibly evidenced by frequent voiding, urinary urgency, urinary retention.

risk for ineffective [individual/couple] Coping possibly evidenced by (situational crises), uncertainty, inadequate confidence in ability to deal with situation, inability to conserve adaptive energies.

Labor, stage I (latent phase)   **OB**

readiness for enhanced Childbearing Process possibly evidenced by expresses desire to enhance proactivity during labor and delivery.

risk for [mild] Anxiety possibly evidenced by (situational crisis), unmet needs, stressors, interpersonal transmission.

risk for ineffective Coping possibly evidenced by (situational crisis), insufficient sense of control, inadequate confidence in ability to deal with situation.

Labor, stage I (transition phase)   OB
labor Pain may be related to physical agent (e.g., mechanical pressure of presenting part, tissue dilation/stretching and tissue hypoxia, possibly evidenced by uterine contraction pain, expressive behavior, narrowed focus, changes in vital signs).

Fatigue may be related to (pregnancy), stressors, anxiety, increased physical exertion, possibly evidenced by lack of energy, compromised concentration, lethargy, increase in physical complaints.

risk for imbalanced Fluid Volume possibly evidenced by [reduced intake, excess fluid loss/hemorrhage, excess fluid retention], (treatment regimen—rapid fluid administration).

risk for decreased Cardiac Output possibly evidenced by (alteration in preload [e.g., decreased venous return, hypovolemia, changes in systemic vascular resistance]).

Labor, stage II (expulsion)   OB
labor Pain may be related to physical agents [e.g., pressure of presenting part, tissue stretching/dilation, and muscle hypoxia], possibly evidenced by uterine contraction, perineal pressure, facial expression of pain, expressive behavior (e.g., restlessness), narrowed focus, changes in vital signs, and autonomic responses (diaphoresis).

risk for decreased Cardiac Output possibly evidenced by (altered preload [e.g., fluctuations in venous return], altered afterload, altered heart rate).

risk for disturbed Maternal-Fetal Dyad possibly evidenced by (compromised fetal oxygen transport [e.g., mechanical compression of head or cord, prolonged labor, reduced placental perfusion, and maternal hyperventilation]).

risk for impaired Skin/Tissue Integrity possibly evidenced by mechanical factors–pressure, precipitous labor, large fetus, and application of forceps.

Fatigue may be related to stressors, sleep deprivation, increase in physical exertion, possibly evidenced by insufficient energy, tiredness.

Labor, stage III (placental expulsion)   OB
labor Pain may be related to physical agent [e.g., tissue trauma, physiological response following delivery], possibly evidenced by pain, expressive behavior, uterine contraction.

risk for deficient Fluid Volume/Bleeding possibly evidenced by insufficient fluid intake, (excessive losses through normal routes [e.g., vomiting, diaphoresis, increased insensible water loss], pregnancy complication [e.g., uterine atony, lacerations of the birth canal, retained placental fragments]).

risk for maternal Injury possibly evidenced by physical factors [e.g., positioning during delivery and transfers], abnormal blood profile, exposure to pathogens.

readiness for enhanced Childbearing Process possibly evidenced by expresses desire to enhance: proactivity during labor and delivery, attachment behavior.

Labor, stage IV (first 4 hr following delivery of placenta)   OB
Fatigue may be related to increased physical exertion, sleep deprivation, stressors, environmental stimuli, [hormonal changes], possibly evidenced by insufficient energy, alteration in concentration, lethargy/tiredness.

acute Pain may be related to chemical agent [e.g., effects of hormones and medications], physical factor [e.g., mechanical trauma, tissue edema, exhaustion, edema], psychological factor [anxiety], possibly evidenced by reports of self-report of pain, cramping (afterpains), expressive behavior, facial expression of pain.

risk for deficient Fluid Volume possibly evidenced by insufficient fluid intake, insufficient knowledge about fluid needs, (active fluid volume loss [e.g., myometrial fatigue, continued uteroplacental circulation, incomplete vasoconstriction], failure of regulatory mechanism [e.g., effects of pregnancy-induced hypertension]).

readiness for enhanced Childbearing Process possibly evidenced by expresses desire to enhance: attachment behavior, baby feeding techniques.

Laceration   CH
impaired Skin/Tissue Integrity may be related to [trauma], possibly evidenced by alteration in skin integrity, [invasion of body structures].

risk for Infection possibly evidenced by [trauma, tissue destruction, increased environmental exposure].

Laminectomy, cervical   MS
Also refer to Laminectomy, lumbar
risk for perioperative Positioning Injury possibly evidenced by immobilization, muscle weakness, obesity, advanced age.

risk for ineffective Airway Clearance possibly evidenced by retained secretions, pain, muscular weakness.

risk for impaired Swallowing possibly evidenced by (trauma [operative edema, pain], neuromuscular impairment).

Laminectomy, lumbar   MS
Also refer to Surgery, general
risk for ineffective Tissue Perfusion (specify) possibly evidenced by diminished or interrupted blood flow—pressure dressing, edema of operative site, hematoma formation; hypovolemia.

risk for [spinal] Trauma possibly evidenced by temporary weakness of spinal column, balancing difficulties, changes in muscle tone and coordination.

acute Pain may be related to physical injury agent (surgical manipulation, harvesting bone graft; localized inflammation, edema), possibly evidenced by altered muscle tone, verbal reports, distraction or guarding behaviors, autonomic changes—changes in vital signs, diaphoresis, pallor.

impaired physical Mobility may be related to imposed therapeutic restrictions, neuromuscular impairment, and pain, possibly evidenced by limited range of motion, decreased muscle strength and control, impaired coordination, and reluctance to attempt movement.

risk for [acute] urinary Retention possibly evidenced by reduced mobility, restrictions of position.

Laryngectomy   MS
Also refer to Cancer; Chemotherapy
ineffective Airway Clearance may be related to excessive mucus, retained secretions; (foreign body in airway—tracheotomy), possibly evidenced by dyspnea; alteration in respiratory rate and pattern; ineffective cough; diminished breath sounds; and cyanosis.

impaired Skin/Tissue Integrity may be related to [surgical removal of tissues and grafting, effects of radiation or chemotherapeutic agents], inadequate nutrition, and associated conditions of impaired circulation, [edema formation, and pooling or continuous drainage of secretions], possibly evidenced by disruption and destruction of skin and tissue layers.

impaired oral Mucous Membrane Integrity/risk for Dry Mouth may be related to dehydration, decrease in salivation, inadequate oral hygiene, surgical procedure, nil per os (NPO), and malnutritional, possibly evidenced by xerostomia (dry mouth), oral discomfort/ pain, mucosal denudation, impaired ability to swallow, and halitosis.

CH

impaired verbal Communication may be related to anatomic deficit (removal of vocal cords), physical barrier (tracheostomy tube), and required voice rest, possibly evidenced by inability to speak, change in vocal characteristics, and impaired articulation.

risk for Aspiration possibly evidenced by ineffective cough, (neck/oral surgery, impaired ability to swallow, enteral feedings), [tracheostomy].

Laryngitis   CH/PED
Refer to Croup

Latex allergy   CH
Latex Allergy Reaction may be related to hypersensitivity to latex rubber protein, possibly evidenced by contact dermatitis—erythema, blisters; type IV reaction—eczema, irritation; hypersensitivity—generalized edema, wheezing, bronchospasm, hypotension, cardiac arrest.

risk for risk-prone Health Behavior possibly evidenced by health status requiring change in occupation.

Laxative abuse   CH
perceived Constipation may be related to health beliefs, faulty appraisal, impaired cognition/thought processes, possibly evidenced by expectation of daily bowel movement, expected passage of stool at same time every day.

Lead poisoning, acute   PED/CH
Also refer to Lead poisoning, chronic
Contamination may be related to flaking or peeling paint (young children), improperly lead-glazed ceramic pottery, unprotected contact with lead (e.g., battery manufacture or recycling, bronzing, soldering or welding), imported herbal products or medicinals, possibly evidenced by abdominal cramping, headache, irritability, decreased attentiveness, constipation, tremors.

risk for physical Trauma possibly evidenced by loss of coordination, altered level of consciousness, clonic or tonic muscle activity, neurological damage.

risk for deficient Fluid Volume possibly evidenced by excessive vomiting, diarrhea, or decreased intake.

deficient Knowledge regarding sources of lead and prevention of poisoning may be related to lack of information, misinterpretation, possibly evidenced by statements of concern, questions, and misconceptions.

Lead poisoning, chronic   CH
Also refer to Lead poisoning, acute
Contamination may be related to flaking or peeling paint (young children), improperly lead-glazed ceramic pottery, unprotected contact with lead (e.g., battery manufacture or recycling, bronzing, soldering or welding), imported herbal products or medicinals, possibly evidenced by chronic abdominal cramping, headache, personality changes, cognitive deficits, seizures, neuropathy.

imbalanced Nutrition: less than body requirements may be related to insufficient dietary intake, (inability to absorb nutrients—chemically induced changes in the gastrointestinal tract), possibly evidenced by food intake less than recommended daily allowance, abdominal discomfort, alteration in taste sensation, and [weight loss].

chronic Pain may be related to deposition of lead in soft tissues and bone, possibly evidenced by verbal reports, distraction behaviors, and focus on self.

risk for delayed Development/[disproportionate Growth] possibly evidenced by (lead poisoning, chronic illness).

Legionnaires' disease   CH/MS
Hyperthermia may be related to illness and inflammatory process, possibly evidenced by increased body temperature; flushed, warm skin; chills.

acute Pain/impaired Comfort may be related to [infectious agent and inflammatory response, effects of circulating toxins] possibly evidenced by reports of headache, myalgia, high fever, diaphoresis.

ineffective Airway Clearance may be related to excessive mucus, retained secretions, (infection—inflammation, edema formation), possibly evidenced by alteration in respiratory rate/pattern, abnormal breath sounds, dyspnea, cyanosis, ineffective cough.

impaired Gas Exchange may be related to (alveolar-capillary membrane changes–inflammatory process), and [hypoventilation], possibly evidenced by restlessness, [changes in mentation], dyspnea, tachycardia, abnormal skin color (pallor, cyanosis), and hypoxia.

Diarrhea may be related to infectious process, possibly evidenced by liquid stools, abdominal cramping.

risk for Infection [spread] possibly evidenced by stasis of body fluids/(decreased ciliary action, [secretions]), [presence of existing infection].

Leprosy   CH
Refer to Hansen's disease

Leukemia, acute   MS
Also refer to Chemotherapy
risk for Infection possibly evidenced by associated conditions of [alterations in mature white blood cells, increased number of immature lymphocytes, immunosuppression and bone marrow suppression, invasive procedures, and malnutrition].

Anxiety [specify level]/Fear may be related to change in current status, threat of death, and (situational crisis), possibly evidenced by sympathetic stimulation, apprehensiveness, helplessness, self-focused, and insomnia.

Activity Intolerance may be related to reduced energy stores, increased metabolic rate], imbalance between oxygen supply and demand (anemia, hypoxia); sedentary lifestyle due to therapeutic restrictions (isolation, bedrest), [effect of drug therapy], possibly evidenced by generalized weakness, reports of fatigue and exertional dyspnea, abnormal heart rate or blood pressure response.

acute Pain may be related to physical injury agents—infiltration of tissues, organs, central nervous system, or expanding bone marrow; chemical agents (antileukemic treatments)]; psychological manifestations—anxiety, fear, possibly evidenced by verbal reports of abdominal discomfort, arthralgia, bone pain, headache; distraction behaviors, narrowed focus, and autonomic responses—changes in vital signs.

risk for deficient Fluid Volume/Bleeding possibly evidenced by xcessive losses (vomiting, hemorrhage, diarrhea, coagulopathy), decreased intake (nausea, anorexia), increased fluid need (hypermetabolic state/fever), predisposition for kidney stone formation and tumor lysis syndrome.

Leukemia, chronic   CH
ineffective Protection may be related to abnormal blood profiles, drug therapy (cytotoxic agents, steroids), radiation treatments, possibly evidenced by deficient immunity, impaired healing, altered clotting, weakness.

Fatigue may be related to disease state, anemia, possibly evidenced by verbalizations, inability to maintain usual routines, listlessness.

imbalanced Nutrition: less than body require-ments may be related to insufficient dietary intake, possibly evidenced by insufficient interest in food, [anorexia, weight loss, abdominal fullness, pain].

Lice, head   PED/CH
Refer to Pediculosis capitis

Lice, pubic   CH
Refer to Pediculosis capitis

Lightning injury   MS
Also refer to Electrical injury
acute Confusion may be related to [alteration in neuropsychological functioning—central nervous system involvement], possibly evidenced by alteration in consciousness and cognitive functioning, agitation, inability to initiate or sustain goal-directed behavior, misperceptions.
   impaired Memory may be related to acute hypoxia, decreased cardiac output, electrolyte imbalance, neurological disturbance, possibly evidenced by inability to recall recent events, amnesia.

Liver failure   MS/CH
Refer to Cirrhosis; Hepatitis, acute viral

Liver transplantation   MS/CH
Refer to Transplantation, recipient

Lockjaw   MS
Refer to Tetanus

Long-term care   CH
(Also refer to condition requiring/contributing to need for facility placement.)
Anxiety [specify level]/Fear may be related to threat to current status, (situational crisis, major change—role functioning, socioeconomic status); unmet needs; possibly evidenced by apprehensiveness, restlessness, insomnia, repetitive questioning, pacing, purposeless activity, and self-focused.
   Grieving may be related to [perceived, actual, or potential loss of physiopsychosocial well-being, personal possessions, and SO(s)], possibly evidenced by denial of feelings, depression, sorrow, guilt; alterations in activity level, sleep patterns, eating habits, and libido.
   risk for Poisoning [drug toxicity] possibly evidenced by effects of aging (reduced metabolism, impaired circulation, precarious physiological balance, presence of multiple diseases and organ involvement)

and use of multiple prescribed and over-the-counter drugs.
   impaired Memory may be related to neurological disturbances, hypoxia, fluid imbalance, possibly evidenced by inability to recall events/factual information, reports experience of forgetting.
   Insomnia may be related to internal factors (illness, psychological stress, inactivity) and external factors (environmental changes, facility routines), possibly evidenced by reports of difficulty in falling asleep, not feeling rested, interrupted sleep, awakening earlier than desired, change in behavior or performance, increasing irritability, and listlessness.
   risk for Relocation Stress Syndrome possibly evidenced by temporary or permanent move that may be voluntary or involuntary, lack of predeparture counseling, multiple losses, feeling of powerlessness, lack of or inappropriate use of support system, decreased psychosocial or physical health status.
   risk for impaired Religiosity possibly evidenced by life transition, ineffective support or coping, lack of social interaction, depression.

LSD (lysergic acid diethylamide)   MS/PSY
intoxication
Also refer to Hallucinogen abuse
risk for physical Trauma possibly evidenced by perceptual distortion, impaired judgment, dangerous decision making, changes in mood.
   Anxiety [panic attack] may be related to substance use/stressors (e.g., drug side effects), possibly evidenced by severe apprehensiveness, fear of unspecific consequences, central nervous system excitation, central autonomic hyperactivity.

Lung cancer   MS/CH
Refer to Bronchogenic carcinoma

Lung transplantation   MS/CH
Also refer to Transplantation, recipient
risk for impaired Gas Exchange possibly evidenced by (ventilation-perfusion imbalance, [stenosis of bronchial or tracheal anastomosis]).
   risk for Infection possibly evidenced by [immunosuppression, suppressed inflammatory response, antibiotic therapy, invasive procedures, chronic illness].

Lupus erythematosus, systemic (SLE)   CH
Fatigue may be related to inadequate energy production, increased energy requirements (chronic inflammation), overwhelming psychological or emotional

demands, states of discomfort, and altered body chemistry (including effects of drug therapy), possibly evidenced by reports of unremitting and overwhelming lack of energy, inability to maintain usual routines, decreased performance, lethargy, and decreased libido.

acute Pain may be related to physical injury agent (widespread inflammatory process affecting connective tissues, blood vessels, serosal surfaces and mucous membranes) possibly evidenced by verbal reports, guarding or distraction behaviors, self-focusing, and changes in vital signs.

impaired Skin/Tissue Integrity may be related to (immunodeficiency, and impaired circulation), possibly evidenced by presence of skin rash or lesions, ulcerations of mucous membranes, and photosensitivity.

disturbed Body Image may be related to (illness), possibly evidenced by alteration in body structure [e.g., presence of rash, lesions, ulcers, purpura, mottled erythema of hands, alopecia], hiding of body parts, negative feeling about body, fear of reaction by others, and change in social involvement.

Lyme disease   CH/MS

acute/chronic Pain may be related to systemic effects of toxins, presence of rash, urticaria, and joint swelling and inflammation, possibly evidenced by verbal reports, guarding behaviors, autonomic responses, and narrowed focus.

Fatigue may be related to increased energy requirements, altered body chemistry, and states of discomfort evidenced by reports of overwhelming lack of energy, inability to maintain usual routines, decreased performance, lethargy, and malaise.

risk for decreased Cardiac Output possibly evidenced by alteration in cardiac rate, rhythm, or conduction.

Lymphedema   CH

disturbed Body Image may be related to alteration in self-perception, and [physical changes—chronic swelling of extremity], possibly evidenced by fear of reaction by others, negative feeling about body, hiding body part, change in social involvement.

impaired Walking may be related to chronic or progressive swelling of lower extremity, possibly evidenced by difficulty walking required distances, climbing stairs, navigating uneven surfaces and declines.

risk for impaired Skin Integrity possibly evidenced by alteration in fluid volume (significant edema) and associated conditions of altered circulation, alteration in sensation.

Macular degeneration   CH

[disturbed visual Sensory Perception] may be related to altered sensory reception, possibly evidenced by reported or measured change in sensory acuity, change in usual response to stimuli.

Anxiety [specify level] may be related to (situational crisis), threat to current status, possibly evidenced by expressed concerns, apprehensiveness, feelings of inadequacy, diminished productivity, alteration in attention.

risk for impaired Social Interaction possibly evidenced by limited physical mobility, environmental barriers.

Malaria   MS/CH

Hyperthermia may be related to inflammatory process, possibly evidenced by increased body temperature (106°F [41.1°C]); flushed, warm skin; tachycardia; headache; altered consciousness.

acute Pain/impaired Comfort may be related to physical injury agent (infection, inflammatory response), possibly evidenced by reports of headache, backache, myalgia, malaise, high fever, shaking chills, abdominal discomfort.

risk for deficient Fluid Volume possibly evidenced by decreased intake (nausea, abdominal pain, prostration), excessive losses (vomiting, diarrhea), hypermetabolic state.

Fatigue may be related to disease state, anemia, lack of restful sleep, possibly evidenced by verbalization of unremitting or overwhelming lack of energy, inability to restore energy even after sleep, lethargy.

Mallory-Weiss syndrome   MS

Also refer to Achalasia (cardiospasm)

risk for deficient Fluid Volume possibly evidenced by excessive vascular losses, presence of vomiting, and reduced intake.

deficient Knowledge regarding causes, treatment, and prevention of condition may be related to lack of information, misinterpretation, possibly evidenced by statements of concern, questions, and recurrence of problem.

Malnutrition   CH

Also refer to Anorexia nervosa

Frail Elderly Syndrome may be related to depression, apathy, aging process, fatigue, degenerative condition, possibly evidenced by expressed lack of appetite, difficulty performing self-care tasks, altered mood state, inadequate intake, weight loss, physical decline.

---

ineffective Protection may be related to inadequate nutrition, anemia, extremes of age, possibly evidenced by fatigue, weakness, deficient immunity, impaired healing, pressure sores.

Marburg disease   MS
Refer to Ebola

Mastectomy   MS
impaired Skin/Tissue Integrity may be related to surgical procedure—removal of skin and tissue), impaired circulation, alteration in skin turgor and alteration in sensation possibly evidenced by alteration in skin and tissue integrity, tissue damage.

impaired physical Mobility may be related to neuromuscular impairment, pain, and edema formation, possibly evidenced by reluctance to attempt movement, limited range of motion, and decreased muscle mass and strength.

bathing/dressing Self-Care deficit may be related to temporary decreased range of motion of one or both arms, possibly evidenced by statements of inability to perform or complete self-care tasks.

disturbed Body Image/situational low Self-Esteem may be related to alteration in self-perception (e.g., loss of body part denoting femininity), behaviors inconsistent with self-value system possibly evidenced by not looking at or touching area, self-negating verbalizations, preoccupation with loss, and change in social involvement or relationship.

Mastitis   OB/GYN
acute Pain may be related to physical agent—inflammation and edema of breast tissues, possibly evidenced by self-report of pain, guarding or expressive behavior, self-focused, and changes in vital signs.

risk for Infection [spread/abscess formation] possibly evidenced by [traumatized tissues], stasis of body fluid, and insufficient knowledge to prevent complications.

deficient Knowledge regarding pathophysiology, treatment, and prevention may be related to lack of information, misinterpretation, possibly evidenced by statements of concern, questions, and misconceptions.

risk for ineffective Breastfeeding possibly evidenced by inability to feed on affected side, interruption in breastfeeding.

Mastoidectomy   PED/MS
Also refer to Surgery, general
risk for Infection [spread] possibly evidenced by [preexisting infection, surgical trauma], and stasis of body fluids.

acute Pain may be related to physical injury agent (infection and edema formation), possibly evidenced by self-report of pain, distraction behavior, restlessness, self-focused, and changes in vital signs.

[disturbed auditory Sensory Perception] may be related to presence of surgical packing, edema, and surgical disturbance of middle ear structures, possibly evidenced by reported or tested hearing loss in affected ear.

Measles   CH/PED
acute Pain/impaired Comfort may be related to physical injury agent (viral infection) causing inflammation of mucous membranes, conjunctiva, and presence of extensive skin rash with pruritus, possibly evidenced by verbal/coded reports, distraction behaviors, self-focusing, and changes in vital signs.

Hyperthermia may be related to presence of viral toxins and inflammatory response, possibly evidenced by increased body temperature; flushed, warm skin; and tachycardia.

risk for [secondary] Infection possibly evidenced by altered immune response and traumatized dermal tissues.

deficient Knowledge regarding condition, transmission, and possible complications may be related to lack of information, misinterpretation, possibly evidenced by statements of concern, questions, misconceptions, and development of preventable complications.

Measles, German   PED/CH
Refer to Rubella

Melanoma, malignant   MS/CH
Refer to Cancer; Chemotherapy

Ménière's disease   CH
Also refer to Vertigo
[disturbed auditory Sensory Perception] may be related to altered state of sensory organ or sensory reception, possibly evidenced by change in sensory acuity, tinnitus, vertigo.

Nausea may be related to inner ear disturbance, possibly evidenced by verbal reports, vomiting.

risk for [total] Self-Care deficit possibly evidenced by perceptual impairment, recurrent nausea, general weakness.

Meningitis, acute meningococcal   MS
risk for Infection [spread] possibly evidenced by [hematogenous dissemination of pathogen], stasis of body fluids, (suppressed inflammatory response), and [exposure of others to pathogens].

risk for ineffective cerebral Tissue Perfusion possibly evidenced by cerebral edema altering or interrupting cerebral arterial or venous blood flow, hypovolemia, exchange problems at cellular level (acidosis).

Hyperthermia may be related to infectious process (increased metabolic rate) and dehydration, possibly evidenced by increased body temperature; warm, flushed skin; and tachycardia.

acute Pain may be related to physical injury agent bacterial or viral infection with inflammation and irritation of the meninges, with headache and spasm of extensor muscles (neck, shoulders, and back), possibly evidenced by verbal reports, guarding or distraction behaviors, narrowed focus, photophobia, and changes in vital signs.

risk for physical Trauma/Suffocation possibly evidenced by alterations in level of consciousness, possible development of clonic-tonic muscle activity (seizures), generalized weakness, prostration, ataxia, vertigo.

Meniscectomy   MS/CH

impaired Walking may be related to pain, joint instability, and imposed medical restrictions of movement, possibly evidenced by impaired ability to move about environment as needed or desired.

deficient Knowledge regarding postoperative expectations, prevention of complications, and self-care needs may be related to lack of information, possibly evidenced by statements of concern, questions, and misconceptions.

Menopause   GYN

ineffective Thermoregulation may be related to fluctuation of hormonal levels, possibly evidenced by skin flushed/warm to touch, diaphoresis, night sweats, cold hands and feet.

Fatigue may be related to change in body chemistry, lack of sleep, depression, possibly evidenced by reports of lack of energy, tiredness, inability to maintain usual routines, decreased performance.

risk for Sexual dysfunction possibly evidenced by lack of/misinformation about sexual function, perceived altered body function, changes in physical/sexual response, impaired/absent relationship with SO.

risk for stress urinary Incontinence possibly evidenced by changes in pelvic muscles and loss of structural support.

readiness for enhanced Health Management possibly evidenced by expresses desire to enhance management of symptoms.

Mental delay (formerly retardation)   CH
Also refer to Down syndrome

impaired verbal Communication may be related to developmental delay or impairment of cognitive and motor abilities, possibly evidenced by impaired articulation, difficulty with phonation, and inability to modulate speech or find appropriate words (dependent on degree of retardation).

risk for Self-Care deficit [specify] possibly evidenced by impaired cognitive ability and motor skills.

risk for Overweight or Obesity possibly evidenced by decreased metabolic rate coupled with impaired cognitive development, dysfunctional eating patterns, and sedentary activity level.

risk for sedentary Lifestyle possibly evidenced by lack of interest or motivation, resources; lack of training or knowledge of specific exercise needs, safety concerns, fear of injury.

impaired Social Interaction may be related to impaired thought processes, communication barriers, and knowledge or skill deficit about ways to enhance mutuality, possibly evidenced by dysfunctional interactions with peers, family, and/or SO(s), and verbalized or observed discomfort in social situation.

compromised family Coping may be related to chronic nature of condition and degree of disability that exhausts supportive capacity of SO(s), other situational or developmental crises or situations SO(s) may be facing, unrealistic expectations of SO(s), possibly evidenced by preoccupation of SO with personal reaction, SO(s) withdraw(s) or enter(s) into limited interaction with individual, protective behavior disproportionate (too much or too little) to client's abilities or need for autonomy.

impaired Home Maintenance may be related to impaired cognitive functioning, insufficient finances/family organization or planning, lack of knowledge, and inadequate support systems, possibly evidenced by requests for assistance, expression of difficulty in maintaining home, disorderly surroundings, and over-taxed family members.

risk for Sexual dysfunction possibly evidenced by risk factors of [biopsychosocial alteration of sexuality], inadequate or absent role models, misinformation/

lack of knowledge about sexual function, [absence of SO(s) and lack of appropriate behavior control].

Mesothelioma CH/MS
Also refer to Asbestosis; Cancer

acute Pain may be related to physical injury agent (cancer of mesothelium of chest and abdominal cavity or around heart), possibly evidenced by reports of chest pain (initially nonpleuritic), irritability, self-focusing, autonomic responses.

Activity Intolerance may be related to imbalance between oxygen supply and demand, possibly evidenced by exertional dyspnea, fatigue.

Metabolic syndrome CH
risk for unstable Blood Glucose Level possibly evidenced by ineffective medication management, excessive weight gain, average daily physical activity is less than recommended for gender/age.

sedentary Lifestyle may be related to deficient knowledge of health benefits of physical exercise, lack of interest, motivation, or resources, possibly evidenced by verbalized preference for activities low in physical activity, choosing a daily routine lacking physical exercise.

risk for ineffective Tissue Perfusion (specify) possibly evidenced by arterial plaque formation (elevated triglycerides, low levels of high-density lipoprotein), prothrombotic state, proinflammatory state.

Migraine CH/MS
Refer to Headache

Miscarriage OB
Refer to Abortion, spontaneous termination

Mitral insufficiency MS/CH
Refer to Valvular heart disease

Mitral stenosis MS/CH
Activity Intolerance may be related to imbalance between oxygen supply and demand, possibly evidenced by reports of fatigue, generalized weakness, exertional dyspnea, and abnormal heart rate response to activity.

impaired Gas Exchange may be related to [altered blood flow], possibly evidenced by abnormal breathing patterns (orthopnea, paroxysmal nocturnal dyspnea), restlessness, and hypoxia.

decreased Cardiac Output may be related to impeded blood flow as evidenced by jugular vein distention, peripheral or dependent edema, orthopnea, paroxysmal nocturnal dyspnea.

deficient Knowledge regarding pathophysiology, therapeutic needs, and potential complications may be related to lack of information or recall, misinterpretation, possibly evidenced by statements of concern, questions, inaccurate follow-through of instructions, and development of preventable complications.

Mitral valve prolapse (MVP) CH
Refer to Valvular heart disease

Mononucleosis, infectious CH
Fatigue may be related to decreased energy production, states of discomfort, and increased energy requirements (inflammatory process), possibly evidenced by reports of overwhelming lack of energy, inability to maintain usual routines, lethargy, and malaise.

acute Pain/impaired Comfort may be related to physical injury agent (viral infection) causing inflammation of lymphoid and organ tissues, irritation of oropharyngeal mucous membranes, possibly evidenced by verbal reports, distraction behaviors, and self-focusing.

Hyperthermia may be related to inflammatory process, possibly evidenced by increased body temperature; warm, flushed skin; and tachycardia.

deficient Knowledge regarding disease transmission, self-care needs, medical therapy, and potential complications may be related to lack of information, misinterpretation, possibly evidenced by statements of concern, misconceptions, and inaccurate follow-through of instructions.

Mood disorders PSY
Refer to Depression, major; Bipolar disorder; Premenstrual dysphoric disorder

Mountain sickness, acute (AMS) CH/MS
acute Pain may be related to physical injury agent (effect of lower levels of oxygen and reduced air pressure at high altitude), possibly evidenced by reports of headache, dizziness [and other discomforts, such as shortness of breath, nausea, swelling of extremities].

Fatigue may be related to stressors, increase in physical exertion, sleep deprivation, possibly evidenced by insufficient energy, nonrestorative sleep pattern, alteration in concentration, decreased performance.

risk for deficient Fluid Volume possibly evidenced by increased water loss (e.g., overbreathing dry air), exertion, inadequate fluid intake (nausea).

Multiple organ dysfunction syndrome　　**MS**
Also refer to specific organs involved; Sepsis; Ventilator assist/dependence

ineffective peripheral Tissue Perfusion may be related to hypovolemia, selective vasoconstriction, microvascular embolization, possibly evidenced by cool skin, diminished pulses.

impaired Gas Exchange may be related to (ventilation-perfusion imbalance), possibly evidenced by dyspnea, irritability, confusion, abnormal arterial blood gases.

Activity Intolerance may be related to imbalance between oxygen supply and demand, [bedrest], pain, possibly evidenced by abnormal heart rate and blood pressure response to activity, pallor, exertional discomfort, electrocardiogram changes (dysrhythmias, ischemia).

[severe] Anxiety/Fear may be related to (situational crisis), threat to current status, threat of death, unfamiliar setting, separation from support system, possibly evidenced by expressed concerns, apprehensiveness, increase in tension, fearfulness, restlessness, decreased perceptual field.

imbalanced Nutrition: less than body requirements may be related to insufficient dietary intake, (inability to digest food or absorb nutrients) and [increased metabolic demands], possibly evidenced by [weight loss, decreased subcutaneous fat and muscle mass, abnormal laboratory studies].

risk for Infection possibly evidenced by malnutrition and stasis of body fluids; (immunosuppression, invasive devices/[procedures, environmental exposure]).

Multiple personality　　**PSY**
Refer to Dissociative disorders

Multiple sclerosis　　**CH**
Fatigue may be related to decreased energy production, increased energy requirements to perform activities, psychological and emotional demands, pain or discomfort, medication side effects, possibly evidenced by verbalization of overwhelming lack of energy, inability to maintain usual routine, decreased performance, impaired ability to concentrate, increase in physical complaints.

[disturbed visual/kinesthetic/tactile Sensory Perception] may be related to delayed or interrupted neuronal transmission, possibly evidenced by impaired vision, diplopia, disturbance of vibratory or position sense, paresthesias, numbness, and blunting of sensation.

impaired physical Mobility may be related to neuromuscular impairment, discomfort or pain, sensoriperceptual impairments, decreased muscle strength, control, or mass, deconditioning, as evidenced by limited ability to perform motor skills, limited range of motion, gait changes, postural instability.

Powerlessness/Hopelessness may be related to chronic stress, prolonged activity restriction, social isolation, and associated condition of deterioration in physiological condition, possibly evidenced by dependency, depression, frustration about ability to perform previous activities, insufficient sense of control, inadequate participation in care.

impaired Home Maintenance may be related to effects of debilitating disease, impaired cognitive or emotional functioning, insufficient finances, and inadequate support systems, possibly evidenced by reported difficulty, observed disorderly surroundings, and poor hygienic conditions.

compromised/disabled family Coping may be related to situational crises, temporary family disorganization, and role changes, client providing little support in turn for SO(s), prolonged disease and disability progression that exhausts the supportive capacity of SO(s), feelings of guilt, anxiety, hostility, despair, and highly ambivalent family relationships, possibly evidenced by client who expresses or confirms concern about SOs' response to client's illness, SO(s) preoccupied with own personal reactions, intolerance, abandonment, neglectful care of the client, and distortion of reality regarding client's illness.

Mumps　　**PED/CH**
acute Pain may be related to physical injury agent (viral infection) with [inflammation, and enlargement of salivary glands], possibly evidenced by self-reports of pain, guarding or distraction behavior, self-focused, and autonomic responses (changes in vital signs).

Hyperthermia may be related to inflammatory process (increased metabolic rate) and dehydration, possibly evidenced by increased body temperature; warm, flushed skin; and tachycardia.

risk for deficient Fluid Volume possibly evidenced by factors influencing fluid needs—hypermetabolic state, and insufficient fluid intake.

Muscular dystrophy (Duchenne's)　　**PED/CH**
impaired physical Mobility may be related to musculoskeletal impairment and weakness, possibly evidenced by decreased muscle strength, control, and mass; limited range of motion; and impaired coordination.

---

risk for delayed Development possibly evidenced by genetic disorder/chronic illness, learning disability, altered ability to perform self-care or self-control activities appropriate to age.

risk for Overweight or Obesity possibly evidenced by sedentary lifestyle and dysfunctional eating patterns.

compromised family Coping may be related to [emotional conflicts–hereditary nature of condition], family disorganization, exhaustion of support person's capacity, possibly evidenced by support person reports preoccupation with own reaction to client's need, protective behavior by support person incongruent with client's abilities/need for autonomy.

Myasthenia gravis   MS

ineffective Breathing Pattern/Airway Clearance may be related to neuromuscular weakness and decreased energy, fatigue, possibly evidenced by dyspnea, changes in rate and depth of respiration, ineffective cough, and adventitious breath sounds.

impaired verbal Communication may be related to neuromuscular weakness, fatigue, and physical barrier (intubation), possibly evidenced by facial weakness, impaired articulation, hoarseness, and inability to speak.

impaired Swallowing may be related to (neuromuscular impairment—laryngeal and pharyngeal muscle abnormalities/fatigue), possibly evidenced by difficulty swallowing, coughing, choking, and recurrent pulmonary infection.

Anxiety [specify level]/Fear may be related to stressors, (major change), threat to current status, separation from support systems, and [inability to communicate], possibly evidenced by expressed concerns, increase in tension, restlessness, apprehensiveness, sympathetic stimulation, crying, self-focused, uncooperative behavior, withdrawal, anger.

CH

deficient Knowledge regarding drug therapy, potential for crisis (myasthenic or cholinergic), and self-care management may be related to inadequate information, misinterpretation, possibly evidenced by statements of concern, questions, and misconceptions; development of preventable complications.

impaired physical Mobility may be related to neuromuscular impairment, possibly evidenced by reports of progressive fatigue with repetitive or prolonged muscle use, impaired coordination, and decreased muscle strength and control.

[disturbed visual Sensory Perception] may be related to neuromuscular impairment, possibly evidenced by visual distortions (diplopia) and motor incoordination.

Myelitis, transverse   MS/CH

Refer to Paraplegia

Myeloma, multiple   MS/CH

Also refer to Cancer

acute/chronic Pain may be related to physical agent—destruction of tissues and bone, side effects of therapy, possibly evidenced by verbal or coded reports, guarding or protective behavior, changes in appetite, weight, sleep; reduced interaction with others.

impaired physical Mobility may be related to loss of integrity of bone structure, pain, deconditioning, depressed mood, possibly evidenced by verbalizations, limited range of motion, slowed movement, gait changes.

risk for ineffective Protection possibly evidenced by cancer, drug therapies, radiation treatments, inadequate nutrition.

Myocardial infarction   MS

Also refer to Myocarditis

acute Pain may be related to physical injury agent (ischemia of myocardial tissue), possibly evidenced by verbal reports, guarding or distraction behaviors (restlessness), facial mask of pain, self-focusing, and autonomic responses (diaphoresis, changes in vital signs).

Anxiety [specify level]/Fear may be related to threat of death, threat to current status; possibly evidenced by increase in tension, fearful attitude, apprehensiveness, expressed concerns or uncertainty, restlessness, sympathetic stimulation, and somatic complaints.

risk for decreased Cardiac Output possibly evidenced by changes in rate and electrical conduction, reduced preload, increased systemic vascular resistance, altered muscle contractility, depressant effects of some medications, infarcted or dyskinetic muscle, structural defects.

CH

risk for sedentary Lifestyle possibly evidenced by lack of resources; lack of training or knowledge of specific exercise needs, safety concerns, fear of injury

Myocarditis   MS

Also refer to Myocardial infarction

Activity Intolerance may be related to imbalance in oxygen supply and demand (myocardial inflammation or damage, cardiac depressant effects of certain drugs), and sedentary lifestyle (enforced bedrest), possibly evidenced by reports of fatigue, exertional dyspnea, abnormal heart rate and ECG response to activity (tachycardia, dysrhythmias, and palpitations) and generalized weakness.

risk for decreased Cardiac Output possibly evidenced by altered contractility, altered stroke volume.

deficient Knowledge regarding pathophysiology of condition, prognosis, treatment, self-care needs, and lifestyle changes may be related to lack of information, misinterpretation, possibly evidenced by statements of concern, misconceptions, inaccurate follow-through of instructions, and development of preventable complications.

Myoclonus, nocturnal   CH

Sleep deprivation may be related to nonrestorative sleep pattern, (condition with periodic limb movement), possibly evidenced by irritability, drowsiness, decrease in functional ability, alteration in concentrate.

Myofascial pain syndrome   CH

Also refer to Fibromyalgia
acute/chronic Pain may be related to physical agent—nocturnal bruxism, possibly evidenced by self-reports of pain (temporomandibular region), headache, muscular tenderness to palpation, limitation in opening mouth.

risk for impaired Dentition possibly evidenced by (bruxism), inadequate oral hygiene (limitations in opening mouth).

Myringotomy   PED/MS

Refer to Mastoidectomy

Myxedema   CH

Also refer to Hypothyroidism
disturbed Body Image may be related to (alteration in body structure or function [loss of hair, thickening of skin, masklike facial expression, enlarged tongue, menstrual and reproductive disturbances]), possibly evidenced by negative feeling about body, fear of reaction by others, and change in social involvement.

Overweight may be related to decreased metabolic rate and activity level, possibly evidenced by weight gain greater than ideal for height and frame.

risk for decreased Cardiac Output possibly evidenced by alteration in heart rhythm, altered contractility.

Narcolepsy   CH

Sleep deprivation may be related to (narcolepsy, nightmares), norestorative sleep pattern, possibly evidenced by drowsiness[/hypersomnia], decrease in functional ability, hallucinations.

risk for physical Trauma possibly evidenced by sudden loss of muscle tone, momentary paralysis (cataplexy), sudden inappropriate sleep episodes.

Near drowning   MS

impaired Gas Exchange may be related to (ventilation perfusion imbalance, and alveolar-capillary membrane changes), possibly evidenced by severe hypoxia, abnormal skin color (pale or dusky skin), change in mentation (confusion to coma).

risk for Hypothermia possibly evidenced by submersion in very cold water.

NEC   PED

Refer to Necrotizing enterocolitis

Necrotizing cellulitis/fasciitis   MS

Also refer to Cellulitis; Sepsis
Hyperthermia may be related to inflammatory process, response to circulating toxins, possibly evidenced by body temperature above normal range; flushed, warm skin; tachycardia; altered mental status.

impaired Tissue Integrity may be related to inflammation and edema (infection), ischemia, possibly evidenced by damaged or destroyed tissue, dermal gangrene.

Necrotizing enterocolitis   PED

Also refer to Sepsis
imbalanced Nutrition: less than body requirements may be related to insufficient dietary intake, (inability to digest food or absorb nutrients), possibly evidenced by abdominal pain, [gastric residuals after feedings, failure to gain weight].

risk for deficient Fluid Volume possibly evidenced by vomiting, third-space fluid losses (bowel inflammation, peritonitis), lack of oral intake.

Neglect/abuse   CH/PSY

Refer to Abuse, Battered child syndrome

Nephrectomy   MS

acute Pain may be related to physical injury agent (surgical tissue trauma), possibly evidenced by verbal reports, guarding or distraction behavior, self-focused, and changes in vital signs.

risk for deficient *Fluid Volume* possibly evidenced by excessive vascular losses and restricted intake.

ineffective Breathing Pattern may be related to incisional pain with decreased lung expansion, possibly evidenced by tachypnea, fremitus, changes in respiratory depth and chest expansion, and changes in arterial blood gases.

Constipation may be related to reduced dietary intake, decreased mobility, gastrointestinal obstruction (paralytic ileus), and incisional pain with defecation, possibly evidenced by decreased bowel sounds; reduced frequency/amount of stool; and hard, formed stool.

Nephrolithiasis   MS/CH
Refer to Calculi, urinary

Nephrotic syndrome   MS/CH
Also refer to Renal failure, acute/chronic
excess Fluid Volume may be related to compromised regulatory mechanism with changes in hydrostatic or oncotic vascular pressure and increased activation of the renin-angiotensin-aldosterone system, possibly evidenced by edema, anasarca, effusions, ascites, weight gain, intake greater than output, and blood pressure changes.

imbalanced Nutrition: less than body requirements may be related to insufficient dietary intake, (inability to ingest food or absorb adequate nutrients), possibly evidenced by [weight loss, muscle wasting (may be difficult to assess due to edema)], insufficient interest in food, alteration in taste sensation, and food intake less than recommended daily allowance.

risk for Infection possibly evidenced by (chronic illness and suppressed inflammatory responses).

risk for impaired Skin Integrity possibly evidenced by alteration in fluid volume, inadequate nutrition and associated conditions of immunodeficiency, and alteration in skin turgor.

Neuralgia, trigeminal   CH
acute Pain may be related to physical agent—sudden violent muscle spasm, possibly evidenced by verbal reports, guarding or distraction behavior, self-focused, and changes in vital signs.

deficient Knowledge regarding control of recurrent episodes, medical therapies, and self-care needs may be related to lack of information or recall and misinterpretation, possibly evidenced by statements of concern, questions, and exacerbation of condition.

Neural tube defect   PED
Refer to Spina bifida

Neuritis   CH
acute/chronic Pain may be related to (damage to the nervous system), possibly evidenced by verbal reports, guarding or distraction behavior, self-focused, and changes in vital signs.

deficient Knowledge regarding underlying causative factors, treatment, and prevention may be related to lack of information, misinterpretation, possibly evidenced by statements of concern, questions, and misconceptions.

Newborn, growth deviations   PED
Also refer to Newborn, premature
[disproportionate Growth] may be related to maternal nutrition, substance use or abuse, multiple gestation, prematurity, maternal conditions (e.g., pregnancy-induced hypertension, diabetes), possibly evidenced by birth weight at or below 10th percentile or at or above 90th percentile (considering gestational age, ethnicity, etc.).

imbalanced Nutrition: less than body requirements may be related to [decreased nutritional stores, hyperplasia of pancreatic beta cells, and increased insulin production], possibly evidenced by [weight deviation from expected, decreased muscle mass/fat stores, electrolyte imbalance].

risk for ineffective Tissue Perfusion (specify) possibly evidenced by interruption of arterial or venous blood flow (hyperviscosity associated with polycythemia).

risk for physical Injury possibly evidenced by altered growth, delayed central nervous system or neurological development, abnormal blood profile.

risk for disorganized infant Behavior possibly evidenced by functional limitations related to growth deviations (restricting neonate's opportunity to seek out, recognize, and interpret stimuli), electrolyte imbalance, psychological stress, low energy reserves, poor organizational ability, limited ability to control environment.

Newborn, normal   PED
risk for impaired Gas Exchange possibly evidenced by [prenatal or intrapartal stressors, excess production of mucus, or cold stress].

risk for Hypothermia possibly evidenced by large body surface in relation to mass, limited amounts of insulating subcutaneous fat, nonrenewable sources of brown fat and few white fat stores, thin epidermis with close proximity of blood vessels to the skin, inability to shiver, and movement from a warm uterine environment to a much cooler environment.

risk for impaired Attachment possibly evidenced by developmental transition or gain of a family member, anxiety associated with the parent role, lack of privacy (healthcare interventions, intrusive family/visitors).

readiness for enhanced Childbearing Process-possibly evidenced by expresses desire to enhance baby feeding/care techniques and environmental safety for the baby.

Newborn at 1 week   PED
Also refer to Newborn, normal
risk for Injury possibly evidenced by physical (hyperbilirubinemia), environmental (inadequate safety precautions), chemical (drugs in breast milk), psychological (inappropriate parental stimulation or interaction).

risk for Constipation/Diarrhea possibly evidenced by type and amount of oral intake, medications or dietary intake of lactating mother, presence of allergies, infection.

risk for impaired Skin Integrity possibly evidenced by excretions (ammonia formation from urea), moisture, chemical injury agent (laundry detergent or diapering material), [mechanical factors (e.g., long fingernails)].

Newborn, postmature   PED
risk for impaired Gas Exchange possibly evidenced by (ventilation perfusion imbalances [meconium aspiration, pneumonitis]).

Hypothermia may be related to decreased subcutaneous fat stores, poor metabolic reserves, exposure to cool environment, decreased ability to shiver, possibly evidenced by reduction in body temperature, cool skin, pallor.

risk for imbalanced Nutrition: less than body requirements possibly evidenced by [placental insufficiency, decreased subcutaneous fat stores, decreased glycogen stores at birth (neonatal hypoglycemia)].

risk for impaired Skin Integrity possibly evidenced by alteration in skin turgor (dry, peeling skin); [long fingernails, absence of vernix caseous].

Newborn, premature   PED
impaired Gas Exchange may be related to (alveolar-capillary membrane changes [inadequate surfactant levels]), (ventilation-perfusion imbalance [immaturity

of pulmonary arteriole musculature]), possibly evidenced by [respiratory difficulties, inadequate oxygenation of tissues, and acidemia].

ineffective Breathing Pattern may be related to immaturity of the respiratory center, poor positioning, drug-related depression and metabolic imbalances, decreased energy, fatigue, possibly evidenced by dyspnea, tachypnea, periods of apnea, nasal flaring, use of accessory muscles, cyanosis, abnormal arterial blood gases, and tachycardia.

risk for ineffective Thermoregulation possibly evidenced by immature central nervous system development (temperature regulation center), decreased ratio of body mass to surface area, decreased subcutaneous fat, limited brown fat stores, inability to shiver or sweat, poor metabolic reserves, muted response to hypothermia, and frequent medical/nursing manipulations and interventions.

risk for deficient Fluid Volume possibly evidenced by extremes of age and weight, excessive fluid losses (thin skin, lack of insulating fat, increased environmental temperature, immature kidney/failure to concentrate urine).

risk for ineffective infant Feeding Pattern possibly evidenced by decreased energy, fatigue; poor positioning; drug-related depression; inability to coordinate sucking, swallowing, and breathing.

risk for disorganized infant Behavior possibly evidenced by prematurity (immaturity of central nervous system, hypoxia), lack of containment or boundaries, pain, overstimulation, separation from parents.

risk for Injury [central nervous system damage] possibly evidenced by tissue hypoxia, altered clotting factors, metabolic imbalances (hypoglycemia, electrolyte shifts, elevated bilirubin).

Newborn, small for gestational age   PED
Refer to Newborn, growth deviations

Newborn, special needs   PED
(Also refer to specific condition.)
[family] Grieving may be related to [perceived loss of the perfect child, alterations of future expectations], possibly evidenced by expression of distress at loss, sorrow, guilt, anger, choked feelings; interference with life activities, crying.

deficient parental Knowledge regarding condition and infant care may be related to lack of or unfamiliarity with information resources, misinterpretation, possibly evidenced by questions, concerns, misconceptions, hesitancy, or inadequate performance of activities.

risk for impaired Attachment possibly evidenced by delay or interruption in bonding process (separation, physical barriers), perceived threat to infant's survival, stressors (financial, family needs), lack of appropriate response of newborn, lack of support between or from SOs.

risk for ineffective family Coping possibly evidenced by situational crises, temporary preoccupation of SO trying to manage emotional conflicts and personal suffering, being unable to perceive or act effectively in regard to infant's needs, temporary family disorganization.

risk for (parental) Social Isolation possibly evidenced by perceived situational crisis, assuming sole or full-time responsibility for infant's care, lack of or inappropriate use of resources.

Nicotine abuse   CH
risk-prone Health Behavior may be related to lack of motivation to change behavior, low state of optimism, absence of social/SO support for change, failure to intend to change behavior, possibly evidenced by denial of health problem, failure to take action, failure to achieve optimal sense of control.

risk for Injury possibly evidenced by smoking habits (e.g., in bed, while driving, near combustible chemicals or oxygen), children playing with cigarettes or matches.

risk for impaired Gas Exchange possibly evidenced by [progressive airflow obstruction, decreased oxygen supply (carbon monoxide)].

risk for ineffective peripheral Tissue Perfusion possibly evidenced by reduction of arterial or venous blood flow.

Nicotine withdrawal   CH
readiness for enhanced Health Management (smoking cessation) possibly evidenced by expresses desire to enhance choices of daily living for meeting goals.

risk for Overweight possibly evidenced by eating in response to internal cues (substitution of food for activity of smoking).

risk for ineffective Health Management possibly evidenced by economic difficulties, lack of support from SO/friends, continued environmental exposure to secondhand smoke or smoking activity.

Nonketotic hyperosmolar syndrome   MS
deficient Fluid Volume may be related to excessive renal losses, inadequate oral intake, extremes of age,

presence of infection, possibly evidenced by sudden weight loss, dry skin and mucous membranes, poor skin turgor, hypotension, increased pulse, fever, change in mental status (confusion to coma).

decreased Cardiac Output may be related to decreased preload (hypovolemia), altered heart rhythm (hyper-/hypokalemia), possibly evidenced by decreased hemodynamic pressures (e.g., central venous pressure), electrocardiogram changes, dysrhythmias.

imbalanced Nutrition: less than body requirements may be related to insufficient dietary intake, [inadequate utilization of nutrients (insulin deficiency)], possibly evidenced by [recent weight loss, imbalance between glucose and insulin levels].

risk for physical Trauma possibly evidenced by weakness, cognitive limitations, altered consciousness, loss of large- or small-muscle coordination (risk for seizure activity).

Obesity   CH
Obesity may be related to excessive intake in relation to metabolic needs, possibly evidenced by weight 20% greater than ideal for height and frame, sedentary activity level, reported or observed dysfunctional eating patterns, and excess body fat by triceps skinfold or other measurements.

sedentary Lifestyle may be related to lack of interest or motivation, resources; lack of training or knowledge of specific exercise needs, safety concerns or fear of injury, possibly evidenced by demonstration of physical deconditioning, choice of a daily routine lacking physical exercise.

Activity Intolerance may be related to imbalance between oxygen supply and demand, and sedentary lifestyle, possibly evidenced by fatigue or weakness, exertional discomfort, and abnormal heart rate and blood pressure response to activity.

risk for Sleep deprivation possibly evidenced by nonrestorative sleep pattern, (sleep apnea).

                                                     PSY
disturbed Body Image may be related to alteration in self-perception [view of self in contrast to societal values], possibly evidenced by negative feeling about body, fear of reaction of others [lack of follow through with treatment plan].

impaired Social Interaction may be related to disturbance in self-concept, (absence of significant other), impaired mobility, possibly evidenced by dissatisfaction with social engagement, discomfort in social situations, dysfunctional interactions with others.

Obesity-hypoventilation syndrome   CH
Refer to Pickwickian syndrome

Obsessive-compulsive disorder   PSY
[severe] Anxiety may be related to earlier life conflicts, possibly evidenced by repetitive actions, recurring thoughts, decreased social and role functioning.

    risk for impaired Skin/Tissue Integrity possibly evidenced by risk factors of psychogenic factors (repetitive behaviors related to cleansing [e.g., hand washing, brushing teeth, showering]).

    risk for ineffective Role Performance possibly evidenced by stressors, anxiety, ineffective coping strategies.

Opioid abuse   CH/PSY
Refer to Depressant abuse; Heroin abuse/withdrawal

Oppositional defiant disorder   PED/PSY
ineffective Coping may be related to (situational or maturational crisis), ineffective tension release strategies, insufficient sense of control, insufficient social support, possibly evidenced by inability to meet role expectations, ineffective coping strategies, insufficient problem-solving skills, risk-taking behavior.

    impaired Social Interaction may be related to disturbance in self-concept, sociocultural dissonance, insufficient skills to enhance mutuality, disturbance in thought processes, possibly evidenced by discomfort in social situations, impaired social functioning, dysfunctional interactions with others.

    chronic low Self-Esteem may be related to inadequate respect from others, receiving insufficient approval from others, (repeated negative reinforcement, psychiatric disorder), possibly evidenced by exaggerates negative feedback about self [or brags about self, grandiosity], poor eye contact, repeatedly unsuccessful in life events [projection of blame/responsibility for problems].

    disabled family Coping may be related to chronically unexpressed feelings by support person, ambivalent family relationships, differing coping styles between support persons, possibly evidenced by intolerance, rejection, hostility, aggression, depression, disregard for client's needs, family behaviors detrimental to well-being.

Organic brain syndrome   CH
Refer to Alzheimer's disease

Osgood-Schlatter disease   PED
acute Pain may be related to physical agent inflammation and swelling [region of patellar tendon], possibly evidenced by verbal reports, protective behavior, change in muscle tone.

    impaired Walking may be related to inflammatory process (knee), possibly evidenced by impaired ability to walk desired distances, climb or descend stairs.

    risk for ineffective Health Management possibly evidenced by age (adolescence), perceived seriousness or benefit, failure to include treatment regimen in daily living.

Osteitis deformans   CH
Refer to Paget's disease, bone

Osteoarthritis (degenerative joint disease) CH
Refer to Arthritis, rheumatoid

    (Although this is a degenerative process versus the inflammatory process of rheumatoid arthritis, nursing concerns are the same.)

Osteomalacia   CH
Refer to Rickets

Osteomyelitis   MS/CH
acute Pain may be related to physical injury agent (typically bacterial infection), possibly evidenced by verbal reports, guarding or distraction behavior, self-focused, and autonomic responses (changes in vital signs).

    Hyperthermia may be related to increased metabolic rate and infectious process, possibly evidenced by increased body temperature and warm, flushed skin.

    ineffective bone Tissue Perfusion may be related to inflammatory reaction with thrombosis of vessels, destruction of tissue, edema, and abscess formation, possibly evidenced by bone necrosis, continuation of infectious process, and delayed healing.

    risk for impaired Walking possibly evidenced by inflammation and tissue necrosis, pain, joint instability.

    deficient Knowledge regarding pathophysiology of condition, long-term therapy needs, activity restriction, and prevention of complications may be related to lack of information, misinterpretation, possibly evidenced by statements of concern, questions, and misconceptions, and inaccurate follow-through of instructions.

Osteoporosis   CH
risk for Trauma possibly evidenced by loss of bone density and integrity increasing risk of fracture with minimal or no stress.

acute/chronic Pain may be related to physical agent—vertebral compression on spinal nerve, muscles, or ligaments; spontaneous fractures, possibly evidenced by verbal reports, guarding or distraction behaviors, self-focus, and changes in sleep pattern.

impaired physical Mobility may be related to pain and musculoskeletal impairment, possibly evidenced by limited range of motion, reluctance to attempt movement, expressed fear of reinjury, and imposed restrictions or limitations.

Otitis media   PED

acute Pain may be related to physical injury agent (infection, allergy or blockage) possibly evidenced by verbal or coded report, guarding behavior, restlessness, crying.

[disturbed auditory Sensory Perception] may be related to decreased sensory reception, possibly evidenced by reported change in sensory acuity, auditory distortions, change in usual response to stimuli.

risk for delayed Development possibly evidenced by auditory impairment, frequent ear infections.

Ovarian cancer   MS

Also refer to Cancer

disturbed Body Image may be related to alteration in self-perception, possibly evidenced by alteration in body function, negative feeling about body, preoccupation with change/loss, and change in social involvement.

Sexual dysfunction may be related to (alteration in body function), vulnerability, insufficient knowledge/misinformation about sexual function, possibly evidenced by verbalizations of problem, alteration in sexual satisfaction, perceived sexual limitation, undesired change in sexual function.

Paget's disease, bone   CH

acute Pain may be related to physical agent—compression/entrapment of nerves, joint deformities, possibly evidenced by reports of headache, back or joint pain.

Fatigue may be related to disease state and hypermetabolic condition, possibly evidenced by overwhelming lack of energy, inability to maintain usual routines, tired.

disturbed Body Image may be related to alteration in self-perception, cultural incongruence, possibly evidenced by alteration in structure—enlarged skull, bowing of long bones, alteration in view of one's body, negative feeling about body, fear of reaction of others, change in social involvement.

[disturbed auditory Sensory Perception] may be related to altered sensory reception or transmission (nerve compression), possibly evidenced by decreased auditory acuity.

risk for impaired Walking possibly evidenced by bowing of long bones, hobbling gait, joint stiffness and pain, paresis or paralysis.

risk for Injury/Falls possibly evidenced by bone deformity or fragility, joint stiffness and pain, altered gait.

risk for decreased Cardiac Output possibly evidenced by excessive circulatory demands (metabolically active and highly vascular nature of lesions).

Palliative care   CH

Refer to Hospice care

Palsy, cerebral   PED/CH

impaired physical Mobility may be related to muscular weakness or hypertonicity, increased deep tendon reflexes, tendency to contractures, and underdevelopment of affected limbs, possibly evidenced by decreased muscle strength, control, mass; limited range of motion, and impaired coordination.

compromised family Coping may be related to permanent nature of condition, situational crisis, emotional conflicts, temporary family disorganization, and incomplete information or understanding of client's needs, possibly evidenced by verbalized anxiety or guilt regarding client's disability, inadequate understanding and knowledge base, and displaying protective behaviors disproportionate (too little or too much) to client's abilities or need for autonomy.

risk for delayed Development possibly evidenced by congenital disorder/brain injury, seizure disorder, visual/hearing impairment.

Pancreas transplantation   MS/CH

Refer to Transplantation, recipient

Pancreatic cancer   MS

Also refer to Cancer

acute Pain/impaired Comfort may be related to physical injury agent (tumor involving or invading nerves or organs that lie near the pancreas) possibly evidenced by verbal reports, guarding or distraction behavior, self-focused, and autonomic responses (changes in vital signs).

imbalanced Nutrition: less than body requirements may be related to insufficient dietary intake, (inability to ingest or digest food, or absorb nutrients), possibly evidenced by food intake less than recommended daily allowance, [anorexia, abdominal pain after eating, weight loss, cachexia].

risk for Infection possibly evidenced by stasis of body fluids (biliary obstruction), malnutrition.

risk for impaired Tissue Integrity possibly evidenced by poor skin turgor, skeletal prominence, presence of edema, ascites, bile salt accumulation in the tissues.

Pancreatitis   MS

acute Pain may be related to physical agent—obstruction of pancreatic and biliary ducts, chemical agent—contamination of peritoneal surfaces by pancreatic exudate, autodigestion of pancreas, extension of inflammation to the retroperitoneal nerve plexus, possibly evidenced by verbal reports, guarding or distraction behaviors, self-focused, grimacing, changes in vital signs, and alteration in muscle tone.

risk for deficient Fluid Volume/Bleeding possibly evidenced by excessive gastric losses (vomiting, nasogastric suctioning), increase in size of vascular bed (vasodilation, effects of kinins), third-space fluid transudation, ascites formation, alteration of clotting process, hemorrhage.

risk for unstable Blood Glucose Level possibly evidenced by (compromised physical health status), excessive stress, ineffective medication management.

imbalanced Nutrition: less than body requirements may be related to insufficient dietary intake, (inability to ingest or digest food, or absorb nutrients), possibly evidenced by food aversion, food intake less than recommended daily allowance, [anorexia, abdominal pain after eating, weight loss, cachexia].

risk for Infection possibly evidenced by stasis of body fluids, altered peristalsis, malnutrition, (alteration in pH of secretions, immunosuppression, and chronic illness).

Panic disorder   PSY

Fear may be related to response to phobic stimulus (unfounded morbid dread of a seemingly harmless object or situation, possibly evidenced by physiological symptoms, mental or cognitive behaviors indicative of panic, withdrawal from or total avoidance of situations that place client in contact with feared object).

[severe to panic] Anxiety may be related to stressors, contact with feared object or situation, limitations placed on ritualistic behavior, possibly evidenced by attacks of immobilizing apprehension,

physical, mental, or cognitive behaviors indicative of panic; expressed feelings of terror or inability to cope.

Paralysis, infantile   PED
Refer to Poliomyelitis

Paranoid personality disorder   PSY

risk for other-/self-directed Violence possibly evidenced by perceived threats of danger, paranoid delusions, and increased feelings of anxiety.

[severe] Anxiety may be related to unmet needs—has not mastered tasks of trust versus mistrust, possibly evidenced by [rigid delusional system (serves to provide relief from stress that justifies the delusion)], apprehensiveness, fear, uncertainty.

Powerlessness may be related to insufficient interpersonal interactions, anxiety, social marginalization, (comples treatment regimen), possibly evidenced by alienation, insufficient sense of control.

[disturbed Sensory Perception (specify)] may be related to psychological stress, possibly evidenced by change in behavior pattern/usual response to stimuli.

compromised family Coping may be related to family disorganization/role changes, prolonged progression of condition that exhausts the supportive capacity of SO(s), possibly evidenced by family system not meeting physical, emotional, or spiritual needs of its members; inability to express or to accept wide range of feelings; inappropriate boundary maintenance; SO(s) describe(s) preoccupation with personal reactions.

Paranoid schizophrenia   PSY
Refer to Schizophrenia (schizophrenic disorders)

Paraphilias   PSY

ineffective Sexuality Pattern may be related to conflict with sexual orientation or variant preferences, possibly evidenced by alterations in achieving sexual satisfaction, difficulty achieving desired satisfaction in socially acceptable ways.

situational low Self-Esteem may be related to behavior inconsistent with values, (history of rejection, pattern of failure), possibly evidenced by situational challenge to self-worth, self-negating verbalizations, helplessness.

interrupted Family Processes may be related to (situational crisis [e.g., revelation of sexual deviance or dysfunction]), shift in family roles, (change in family social status), possibly evidenced by change in communication pattern, change in family conflict resolution, change in family satisfaction, change in intimacy.

Paraplegia   MS/CH
Also refer to Quadriplegia

impaired Transfer Ability may be related to loss of muscle function and control, injury to upper extremity joints (overuse).

[disturbed kinesthetic/tactile Sensory Perception] may be related to neurological deficit with loss of sensory reception and transmission, psychological stress, possibly evidenced by reported or measured change in sensory acuity, change in usual response to stimuli, anxiety, disorientation, bizarre thinking, exaggerated emotional responses.

reflex urinary Incontinence/impaired urinary Elimination may be related to disruption of bladder innervation, bladder atony, fecal impaction, possibly evidenced by lack of awareness of bladder distention, retention, incontinence, or overflow, urinary tract infections—kidney stone formation, renal dysfunction.

situational low Self-Esteem may be related to alteration in body function, (functional impairment), possibly evidenced by self-negating verbalizations, situational challenge to self-worth, helplessness.

Sexual dysfunction may be related to (alteration in function), and vulnerability, possibly evidenced by seeking confirmation of desirability, perceived sexual limitation, and change in interest in self/others.

Parathyroidectomy   MS
acute Pain may be related to physical agent—surgical incision and effects of calcium imbalance [bone pain, tetany], possibly evidenced by verbal reports, guarding or distraction behavior, self-focused, and changes in vital signs.

risk for excess Fluid Volume possibly evidenced by preoperative renal involvement, stress-induced release of antidiuretic hormone, and changing calcium or other electrolyte levels.

risk for ineffective Airway Clearance possibly evidenced by edema formation and laryngeal nerve damage.

deficient Knowledge regarding postoperative care, complications, and long-term needs may be related to lack of information or recall, misinterpretation, possibly evidenced by statements of concern, questions, and misconceptions.

Parent-child relational problem   PED/PSY
impaired Parenting may be related to lack of or ineffective role model, lack of support between or from SO, interruption in bonding process, unrealistic expectations for self/child/partner, presence of stressors, lack of appropriate response of child to parent, possibly evidenced by frequent verbalization of disappointment in child, inability to care for or discipline child, lack of parental attachment behaviors, child abuse or abandonment.

ineffective Role Performance may be related to conflict, inadequate role model, domestic violence, insufficient role preparation, resources or rewards, low self-esteem [psychiatric or physical illness of the child], possibly evidenced by change in usual pattern of responsibility, role ambivalence/strain, uncertainty, inappropriate developmental expectations, ineffective adaptation to change.

interrupted Family Process may be related to situational crisis of child/adolescent, maturational crisis (e.g., adolescence, midlife), possibly evidenced by expressions of confusion and difficulty coping with situation; family system not meeting physical, emotional, or security needs of members; difficulty accepting help; parents not respecting each other's parenting practices.

compromised/disabled family Coping may be related to individual preoccupation with own emotional conflicts and personal suffering or anxiety about the crisis, temporary family disorganization, exhausted supportive capacity of members, highly ambivalent family relationships, possibly evidenced by detrimental decisions or actions, neglected relationships, intolerance, agitation, depression, hostility, aggression.

readiness for enhanced family Coping possibly evidenced by expresses desire to enhance contact with others who have experienced a similar situation.

Parenteral feeding   MS/CH
imbalanced Nutrition: less than body requirements may be related to insufficient dietary intake, (inability to ingest/digest food, or absorb nutrients), possibly evidenced by [body weight 10% or more under ideal, decreased subcutaneous fat or muscle mass].

risk for Infection possibly evidenced by malnutrition, (invasive procedure), and (chronic illness).

risk for Injury [multifactor] possibly evidenced by catheter-related complications (air emboli, septic thrombophlebitis).

risk for imbalanced *Fluid Volume* possibly evidenced by active loss or failure of regulatory mechanisms (specific to underlying disease process or trauma), complications of therapy—high glucose solutions or hyperglycemia (hyperosmolar nonketotic syndrome and severe dehydration), inability to obtain or ingest fluids.

Fatigue may be related to decreased metabolic energy production, increased energy requirements (hypermetabolic state, healing process), altered body chemistry (medications, chemotherapy), possibly evidenced by overwhelming lack of energy, inability to maintain usual routines or accomplish routine tasks, lethargy, impaired ability to concentrate.

Parkinson's disease   CH

impaired Walking may be related to neuromuscular impairment (muscle weakness, tremors, bradykinesia) and musculoskeletal impairment (joint rigidity), possibly evidenced by inability to move about the environment as desired, increased occurrence of falls.

impaired Swallowing may be related to neuromuscular impairment, muscle weakness, possibly evidenced by reported or observed difficulty in swallowing, drooling, evidence of aspiration (choking, coughing).

impaired verbal Communication may be related to muscle weakness and incoordination, possibly evidenced by impaired articulation, difficulty with phonation, and changes in rhythm and intonation.

risk for Stress overload possibly evidenced by inadequate resources, chronic illness, physical demands.

caregiver Role Strain may be related to illness, severity of care receiver, psychological/cognitive problems in care receiver, caregiver is spouse, duration of caregiving required, lack of respite or recreation for caregiver, possibly evidenced by feeling stressed, depressed, worried; lack of resources or support, family conflict.

Passive-aggressive personality disorder   PSY

[moderate to severe] Anxiety may be related to conflict about life goals, unmet needs, threat to current status, stressors, possibly evidenced by worried about change in life event, blocking of thoughts, feeling of inadequacy, extraneous movements, irritability, tendency to blame others.

ineffective Coping may be related to insufficient sense of control, ineffective tension release strategies,

possibly evidenced by ineffective coping strategies; insufficient problem-solving skills.

chronic low Self-Esteem may be related to inadequate affection received; receiving insufficient approval from others, (psychiatric disorder), possibly evidenced by rejective of positive feedback, underestimates ability to deal with situation, passivity, non-assertive/indecisive behavior, dependent on others' opinions, (repeated negative reinforcement).

Powerlessness may be related to insufficient interpersonal interactions, possibly evidenced by alienation, insufficient sense of control, depression, inadequate participation in care, dependency.

PCP (phencyclidine) intoxication   MS/PSY
Also refer to Hallucinogen abuse
risk for self-/other-directed Violence possibly evidenced by negative body language, impulsiveness, (history of substance misuse, alteration in cognitive functioning, mental health issue.

risk for physical Trauma/Suffocation/Poisoning possibly evidenced by risk factors of impaired balance, alteration in cognitive functioning, alteration in sensation [decrease in pain perception], [increase in muscle strength, myoclonic jerks or convulsions].

risk for ineffective cerebral Tissue Perfusion possibly evidenced by substance abuse, (hypertensive crisis).

Pediculosis capitis   PED/CH

impaired Skin Integrity related to [presence of nits, intense itching, and scratching]; possibly evidenced by redness, [excoriation, disruption of skin surface].

risk for Infection [spread] possibly evidenced by insufficient knowledge to avoid exposure or transmission of parasite.

Pediculosis pubis   CH
Refer to Pediculosis capitis

Pelvic inflammatory disease   OB/GYN/CH
risk for Infection [spread] possibly evidenced by [presence of infectious process in highly vascular pelvic structures, delay in seeking treatment].

acute Pain may be related to inflammation, edema, and congestion of reproductive and pelvic tissues, possibly evidenced by verbal reports, guarding or distraction behaviors, self-focus, and changes in vital signs.

Hyperthermia may be related to inflammatory process and hypermetabolic state, possibly evidenced by increased body temperature; warm, flushed skin; and tachycardia.

risk for situational low Self-Esteem possibly evidenced by perceived stigma of physical condition (infection of reproductive system).

deficient Knowledge regarding cause/complications of condition, therapy needs, and transmission of disease to others may be related to lack of information, misinterpretation, possibly evidenced by statements of concern, questions, misconceptions, and development of preventable complications.

Periarteritis nodosa   MS/CH
Refer to Polyarteritis nodosa

Pericarditis   MS
acute Pain may be related to physical agent—tissue inflammation and presence of effusion, possibly evidenced by verbal reports of pain, guarding or distraction behavior, self-focused, and changes in vital signs.

Activity Intolerance may be related to imbalance between oxygen supply and demand (restriction of cardiac filling and ventricular contraction, reduced cardiac output), possibly evidenced by reports of weakness, fatigue, exertional dyspnea, abnormal heart rate or blood pressure response (signs of heart failure).

risk for decreased Cardiac Output possibly evidenced by accumulation of fluid (effusion), restricted cardiac filling, and contractility.

Anxiety [specify level] may be related to threat to current status, threat of death, possibly evidenced by increased tension, apprehension, restlessness, and expressed concerns.

Perinatal loss/death of child   OB/CH
Grieving may be related to death of significant other—fetus/infant, possibly evidenced by distress, anger, blaming, alteration in sleep pattern.

situational low Self-Esteem may be related to unrealistic self-expectation, (developmental transition), possibly evidenced by self-negating verbalizations, helplessness, indecisive behavior, situational challenge to self-worth.

risk for ineffective Role Performance possibly evidenced by stressors, ineffective coping strategies, insufficient support system.

risk for interrupted Family Processes possibly evidenced by (situational crisis, developmental transition [loss of child]), shift in family roles.

risk for Spiritual distress possibly evidenced by stressors, depression, (loss of child, unexpected life event), separation from support system.

Peripheral arterial occlusive disease   CH
Refer to Arterial occlusive disease, peripheral

Peripheral vascular disease   CH
(atherosclerosis)
ineffective peripheral Tissue Perfusion may be related to reduction or interruption of arterial or venous blood flow, possibly evidenced by changes in skin temperature and color, lack of hair growth, blood pressure and pulse changes in extremity, presence of bruits, and reports of claudication.

Activity Intolerance may be related to imbalance between oxygen supply and demand, possibly evidenced by reports of fatigue, weakness and exertional discomfort (claudication).

risk for impaired Skin/Tissue Integrity possibly evidenced by impaired circulation and alteration insensation.

Peritonitis   MS
risk for Infection [spread/sepsis/septic shock] possibly evidenced by alteration in skin integrity or traumatized tissue, altered peristalsis, and associated condition of immunosuppression and invasive procedures.

deficient Fluid Volume [mixed] may be related to fluid shifts from extracellular, intravascular, and interstitial compartments into intestines or peritoneal space, excessive gastric losses (vomiting, diarrhea, nasogastric suction), fever, hypermetabolic state, and restricted intake, possibly evidenced by dry mucous membranes, poor skin turgor, delayed capillary refill, weak peripheral pulses, diminished urinary output, dark, concentrated urine; hypotension, and tachycardia.

acute Pain may be related to chemical irritation of parietal peritoneum, trauma to tissues, abdominal distention—accumulation of fluid in abdominal or peritoneal cavity, possibly evidenced by verbal reports, muscle guarding or rebound tenderness, distraction behaviors, facial mask of pain, self-focus, and changes in vital signs.

risk for imbalanced Nutrition: less than body requirements possibly evidenced by (inability to ingest/digest food), abdominal pain, insufficient interest in food/food aversion.

Persian Gulf syndrome   CH/MS
Refer to Gulf War syndrome

Personality disorders; or   **PSY**

Refer to Antisocial; Borderline; Obsessive-compulsive; Passive-aggressive; or Paranoid personality disorders

Pertussis   **PED**

ineffective Airway Clearance may be related to retained secretions, excessive thick tenacious mucus, infection, possibly evidenced by dyspnea, adventitious breath sounds, hacking/paroxysmal cough.

deficient Fluid Volume may be related to decreased intake, anorexia, vomiting, increased insensible losses (fever, diaphoresis), possibly evidenced by decreased urine output and increased specific gravity, decreased blood pressure, increased pulse rate, decreased skin and tongue turgor, dry skin and mucous membranes.

risk for Infection [transmission/secondary] possibly evidenced by stasis of body fluids, malnutrition, insufficient knowledge to avoid exposure to pathogens.

risk for imbalanced Nutrition: less than body requirements possibly evidenced by inability to ingest food or absorb nutrients (anorexia, vomiting), and [increased metabolic demands].

risk for impaired Gas Exchange possibly evidenced by (ventilation perfusion imbalance–atelectasis).

Pervasive developmental disorders   **PED/PSY**

Refer to Autism spectrum disorder; Rett's syndrome; Asperger's disorder

Pheochromocytoma   **MS**

Anxiety [specify level] may be related to excessive physiological (hormonal) stimulation of the sympathetic nervous system, situational crises, threat to or change in health status, possibly evidenced by apprehension, shakiness, restlessness, focus on self, fearfulness, diaphoresis, and sense of impending doom.

deficient Fluid Volume [mixed] may be related to excessive gastric losses (vomiting, diarrhea), hypermetabolic state, diaphoresis, and hyperosmolar diuresis, possibly evidenced by hemoconcentration, dry mucous membranes, poor skin turgor, thirst, and weight loss.

decreased Cardiac Output/ineffective Tissue Perfusion (specify) may be related to altered preload—decreased blood volume, altered systemic vascular resistance, and increased sympathetic activity (excessive secretion of catecholamines), possibly evidenced by cool, clammy skin, change in blood pressure (hypertension, postural hypotension), visual disturbances, severe headache, and angina.

deficient Knowledge regarding pathophysiology of condition, outcome, and preoperative and postoperative care needs may be related to lack of information or recall, possibly evidenced by statements of concern, questions, and misconceptions.

Phlebitis   **CH**

Refer to Thrombophlebitis

Phobia   **PSY**

Also refer to Anxiety disorder, generalized

Fear may be related to learned response to phobic stimulus, unfounded morbid dread of a seemingly harmless object or situation, possibly evidenced by sympathetic stimulation and reactions ranging from apprehension to panic, withdrawal from or total avoidance of situations that place individual in contact with feared object.

impaired Social Interaction may be related to intense fear of encountering feared object, activity or situation; and anticipated loss of control, possibly evidenced by reported change of style or pattern of interaction, discomfort in social situations, and avoidance of phobic stimulus.

Physical abuse   **CH/PSY**

Refer to Abuse, physical; Battered child syndrome

Pickwickian syndrome   **CH**

ineffective Breathing Pattern may be related to obesity, hypoventilation, possibly evidenced by decreased pulmonary function, hypercapnia, hypoxia, reduced effect of carbon dioxide in stimulating respirations.

PID   **GYN/OB/CH**

Refer to Pelvic inflammatory disease

Pinkeye   **CH**

Refer to Conjunctivitis, bacterial

Placenta previa   **OB**

risk for Bleeding/Shock possibly evidenced by (pregnancy complication), hypotension, hypovolemia.

risk for disturbed Maternal-Fetal Dyad may be related to (pregnancy complication, alteration in fetal oxygen transport).

[severe] Anxiety may be related to threat of death, threat to current status, interpersonal contagion, stressors, possibly evidenced by distress, increase in tension, hypervigilance, sympathetic stimulation.

Plague, bubonic   **MS**

Hyperthermia may be related to illness, dehydration, possibly evidenced by increased body temperature, tachycardia, chills, confusion.

    acute Pain may be related to inflammatory process, enlarged lymph nodes, possibly evidenced by verbal or coded reports, expressive behavior, autonomic responses.

    risk for deficient Fluid Volume possibly evidenced by fever, decreased oral intake.

    risk for impaired Skin Integrity possibly evidenced by (impaired circulation and immunodeficiency—infectious process).

Plague, pneumonic   **MS**

risk for Infection [spread] possibly evidenced by [contagious nature of disease, close contact with others].

    Hyperthermia may be related to illness, dehydration, possibly evidenced by increased body temperature, tachycardia, chills, severe headache, confusion.

    impaired Gas Exchange may be related to (alveolar-capillary membrane changes), possibly evidenced by abnormal breathing patterns (tachypnea, dyspnea, stridor), abnormal skin color (cyanosis), [hemoptysis].

    deficient Fluid Volume may be related to fever, hypermetabolic state, decreased intake, bleeding diathesis (disseminated intravascular coagulation), possibly evidenced by weakness, decreased venous filling, decreased blood pressure, decreased skin turgor, dry mucous membranes, change in mental state.

Plantar fasciitis   **CH**

acute/chronic Pain may be related to inflammation, possibly evidenced by report of stabbing, burning pain, guarding or protective behavior, change in posture and gait, altered ability to continue previous activities.

    impaired Walking may be related to musculoskeletal impairment, impaired balance, pain, possibly evidenced by impaired ability to walk required distances or climb stairs.

Pleural effusion   **CH/MS**

Also refer to Hemothorax

acute Pain may be related to inflammation/irritation of the parietal pleura, possibly evidenced by verbal reports, guarding or distraction behaviors, self-focus, and changes in vital signs.

    ineffective Breathing Pattern may be related to pain on inspiration, possibly evidenced by decreased respiratory depth, tachypnea, and dyspnea.

    risk for impaired Gas Exchange possibly evidenced by (ventilation perfusion imbalance).

Pleurisy   **CH**

acute Pain may be related to inflammation and irritation of the parietal pleura, possibly evidenced by verbal reports, guarding or distraction behaviors, self-focus, and changes in vital signs.

    ineffective Breathing Pattern may be related to pain on inspiration, possibly evidenced by decreased respiratory depth, tachypnea, and dyspnea.

    risk for Infection [pneumonia] possibly evidenced by stasis of pulmonary secretions, decreased lung expansion, and ineffective cough.

PMDD   **GYN/PSY**

Refer to Premenstrual dysphoric disorder

PMS   **GYN/PSY**

Refer to Premenstrual dysphoric disorder

Pneumoconiosis (black lung)   **CH**

Refer to Pulmonary fibrosis

Pneumonia   **CH/MS**

Refer to Bronchitis; Bronchopneumonia

Pneumonia, ventilator associated   **CH**

Refer to Bronchopneumonia

Pneumothorax   **MS**

Also refer to Hemothorax

ineffective Breathing Pattern may be related to decreased lung expansion (air accumulation), musculoskeletal impairment, pain, inflammatory process, possibly evidenced by dyspnea, tachypnea, altered chest excursion, respiratory depth changes, use of accessory muscles, nasal flaring, cough, cyanosis, and abnormal arterial blood gases.

    risk for decreased Cardiac Output possibly evidenced by compression or displacement of cardiac structures.

    acute Pain may be related to irritation of nerve endings within pleural space by foreign object (chest tube), possibly evidenced by verbal reports, guarding or distraction behaviors, self-focus, and changes in vital signs.

Poliomyelitis   **CH**

Also refer to Postpolio syndrome

ineffective Breathing Pattern may be related to neuromuscular dysfunction and intercostal muscle impairment, hypoventilation syndrome, possibly evidenced by dyspnea, decreased depth of breathing, altered chest excursion, respiratory failure.

impaired physical Mobility related to neuromuscular dysfunction and musculoskeletal impairment, decreased muscle strength, control or mass; contracture, decreased endurance, pain, prescribed movement restriction or bracing, possibly evidenced by limited ability to move, uncoordinated or jerky movements, gait changes, exaggerated lateral postural sway, postural instability.

Self-Care deficit [specify] may be related to neuromuscular impairment, weakness, pain, fatigue, possibly evidenced by reported or observed inability to perform specified activities.

Polyarteritis nodosa   MS/CH
ineffective Tissue Perfusion (specify) may be related to reduction or interruption of blood flow, possibly evidenced by organ tissue infarctions, changes in organ function, and development of organic psychosis.

Hyperthermia may be related to widespread inflammatory process, possibly evidenced by increased body temperature and warm, flushed skin.

acute Pain may be related to inflammation, tissue ischemia, and necrosis of affected area, possibly evidenced by verbal reports, guarding or distraction behaviors, self-focus, and changes in vital signs.

Polycythemia vera   CH
Activity Intolerance may be related to imbalance between oxygen supply and demand, possibly evidenced by reports of fatigue, weakness.

ineffective Tissue Perfusion (specify) may be related to reduction or interruption of arterial or venous blood flow (insufficiency, thrombosis, or hemorrhage), possibly evidenced by pain in affected area, impaired mental ability, visual disturbances, and color changes of skin and mucous membranes.

Polyradiculitis, acute inflammatory   MS
Refer to Guillain-Barré syndrome

Postconcussion syndrome   CH
acute/chronic Pain may be related to neuronal damage, possibly evidenced by reports of headache.

Anxiety [specify level] may be related to stressors (e.g., situational crisis, change in health status, ongoing nature of disability, unmet needs), possibly evidenced by expressed concerns, apprehensiveness, uncertainty, feeling of inadequacy, self-focused, difficulty concentrating.

impaired Memory may be related to neurological disturbances possibly evidenced by inability to recall events/factual information, reports experience of forgetting.

Postmaturity syndrome   PED
Refer to Newborn, postmature

Postmyocardial syndrome   CH
Refer to Dressler's syndrome

Postoperative recovery period   MS
ineffective Breathing Pattern may be related to neuromuscular and perceptual or cognitive impairment, decreased lung expansion and energy, and tracheobronchial obstruction, possibly evidenced by changes in respiratory rate and depth, reduced vital capacity, apnea, cyanosis, and noisy respirations.

risk for imbalanced Body Temperature possibly evidenced by exposure to cool environment, effect of medications and anesthetic agents, extremes of age or weight, and dehydration.

risk for acute Confusion possibly evidenced by (pharmaceutical agents—anesthesia), pain.

risk for deficit Fluid Volume possibly evidenced by restriction of oral intake, loss of fluid through abnormal routes (indwelling tubes, drains) and normal routes (vomiting, loss of vascular integrity, changes in clotting ability), extremes of age and weight.

acute Pain may be related to disruption of skin, tissue, and muscle integrity; musculoskeletal or bone trauma; and presence of tubes and drains, possibly evidenced by verbal reports, alteration in muscle tone, facial mask of pain, distraction or guarding behaviors, narrowed focus, and autonomic responses.

impaired Skin/Tissue Integrity may be related to [mechanical interruption of skin or tissues (surgical incision)], (impaired circulation, pharmaceutical agent, alteration in metabolism) possibly evidenced by alteration in skin and tissue integrity, acute pain.

risk for Surgical Site Infection possibly evidenced by increased environmental exposure to pathogens, surgical wound contamination, and associated conditions of type and duration of surgery, type of anesthesia and comorbidities, immunosuppression.

Postpartum blues   OB/PSY
Refer to Depression, postpartum

Postpartum period, 4 to 48 hours   OB/CH
acute Pain/impaired Comfort may be related to tissue trauma, edema, muscle contractions, bladder fullness,

and physical or psychological exhaustion, possibly evidenced by reports of cramping (afterpains), self-focusing, alteration in muscle tone, distraction behaviors, and changes in vital signs.

Breastfeeding (specify) may be related to level of knowledge, previous experiences, infant gestational age, level of support, physical structure or characteristics of the maternal breasts, possibly evidenced by maternal verbalization regarding level of satisfaction, observations of breastfeeding process, infant response and weight gain.

risk for impaired Attachment possibly evidenced by lack of support between or from SO(s), ineffective or no role model, anxiety associated with the parental role, unrealistic expectations, unmet social or emotional maturation needs of client/partner, presence of stressors (e.g., financial, housing, employment).

risk for deficient Fluid Volume/Bleeding possibly evidenced by excessive blood loss during delivery, reduced intake or inadequate replacement, nausea, vomiting, increased urine output, and insensible losses.

impaired urinary Elimination may be related to hormonal effects (fluid shifts, continued elevation in renal plasma flow), mechanical trauma, tissue edema, and effects of medication or anesthesia, possibly evidenced by frequency, dysuria, urgency, incontinence, or retention.

Constipation may be related to decreased muscle tone associated with diastasis recti, prenatal effects of progesterone, dehydration, excess analgesia or anesthesia, pain (hemorrhoids, episiotomy, or perineal tenderness), prelabor diarrhea and lack of intake, possibly evidenced by frequency less than usual pattern, hard-formed stool, straining at stool, decreased bowel sounds, and abdominal distention.

Insomnia may be related to pain, discomfort, intense exhilaration or excitement, anxiety, exhausting process of labor and delivery, and needs or demands of family members, possibly evidenced by verbal reports of difficulty in falling asleep or staying asleep, not feeling well-rested, interrupted sleep, lack of energy.

Postpartum period, 4 to 6 weeks OB/CH
readiness for enhanced family Coping possibly evidenced by family member(s) moving in direction of health-promoting and enriching lifestyle.

disturbed Body Image may be related to unrealistic expectations, permanency of some changes, possibly evidenced by negative feeling about body, feeling of helplessness, preoccupation with change, focus on past appearance, fear of reaction of others.

risk for Sexual dysfunction possibly evidenced by [health-related transition (changes in body function including lactation)], lack of privacy, fear of pregnancy.

readiness for enhanced Parenting possibly evidenced by expressed desire to enhance parenting.

Postpartum period, postdischarge OB/CH to 4 weeks
risk for Fatigue possibly evidenced by physical and emotional demands of infant and other family members, psychological stressors, continued discomfort.

Breastfeeding (specify) may be related to level of knowledge and support, previous experiences, infant gestational age, physical structure or characteristics of maternal breast, demands of home life and employment, possibly evidenced by maternal verbalizations regarding level of satisfaction, observations of feeding process, infant response, and weight gain.

risk for imbalanced Nutrition: less than body requirements possibly evidenced by [intake insufficient to meet metabolic demands or correct existing deficiencies (e.g., lactation, anemia, excessive blood loss, infection, excessive tissue trauma, desire to regain prenatal weight)].

risk for Infection possibly evidenced by malnutrition, alteration in skin integrity/tissue trauma, and associated conditions of premature or prolonged rupture of amniotic membranes, decreased Hb, invasive procedures, increased environmental exposure.

risk for compromised family Coping possibly evidenced by (situational or developmental changes), family disorganization/role change, insufficient reciprocal support.

risk for impaired Parenting possibly evidenced by situational crisis—addition and demands of new family member, changes in responsibilities of family members; sleep disruption, lack of support from SO/family members, young parental age, life stressors—financial, employment, home environment, lack of resources.

Postpartum psychosis OB/PSY
Also refer to Depression, postpartum
ineffective Coping may be related to inadequate level of confidence in ability to cope with situation, inadequate sense of control, possibly evidenced by inability to meet basic needs, insufficient problem-solving skills, alteration in sleep pattern and/or concentration.

risk for other-directed Violence possibly evidenced by mood swings, increased anxiety, despondency, hopelessness, psychotic symptomatology.

Postpolio syndrome   CH

Fatigue may be related to disease state, stress, anxiety, sleep deprivation, depression, possibly evidenced by overwhelming lack of energy, inability to maintain usual routines or level of physical activity, difficulty concentrating.

chronic Pain may be related to chronic physical disability, joint degeneration, possibly evidenced by reports of deep aching pain, altered ability to continue previous activities, change in sleep patterns, reduced interaction with others.

impaired Walking/physical Mobility may be related to neuromuscular impairment, decreased muscle strength and atrophy, decreased endurance, pain, inability to stand erect (flat back syndrome), possibly evidenced by gait disturbances, joint or postural instability, decreased ability to perform gross motor skills.

Sleep deprivation may be related to sleep apnea (central and obstructive), chronic pain, possibly evidenced by daytime drowsiness, decreased ability to function, inability to concentrate.

impaired Swallowing may be related to neuromuscular impairment, pharyngeal muscle weakness, possibly evidenced by coughing, choking, recurrent pulmonary infections.

ineffective Airway Clearance may be related to neuromuscular dysfunction (muscle weakness and atrophy), retained secretions, possibly evidenced by diminished or adventitious breath sounds (chronic microatelectasis), poor cough (decreased pulmonary compliance, increased chest wall tightness).

Post-traumatic stress disorder   PSY

Post-Trauma Syndrome may be related to perceives event as traumatic, serious injury to loved one/self, survivor role, (history of abuse, witnessing violent death, exposure to war), possibly evidenced by anxiety, irritability, aggression, anger, avoidance behavior, denial, depression, repression, exaggerated startle response, flashbacks, intrusive dreams/thoughts, substance misuse.

risk for self-/other-directed Violence possibly evidenced by impulsiveness, access to weapon, conflict in interpersonal relation(s), insufficient personal resources, pattern of threatening violence, suicidal ideation.

ineffective Coping may be related to high-degree of threat, inaccurate threat appraisal, inadequate confidence in ability to cope with situation, insufficient sense of control, possibly evidenced by inability to meet basic needs, insufficient problem-solving skills, alteration in sleep pattern and/or concentration, substance misuse.

complicated Grieving may be related to insufficient social support, emotional disturbance, possibly evidenced by depression, anxiety, anger, mistrust, self-blame, traumatic distress, feeling of detachment from others, decrease in functioning in life roles, insufficient sense of well-being.

interrupted Family Processes may be related to shift in family roles, power shift among family members, (situational crisis, shift in health status of a family member), possibly evidenced by change in communication pattern, change in family satisfaction, changes in participation for decision making, decrease in emotional support, change in stress-reduction behavior.

Preeclampsia   OB

Refer to Hypertension, gestational; Abruptio placentae

Pregnancy, 1st trimester   OB/CH

risk for imbalanced Nutrition: less than body requirements possibly evidenced by insufficient intake (nausea, vomiting, inadequate financial resources and nutritional knowledge).

impaired Comfort may be related to hormonal influences, physical changes, possibly evidenced by verbal reports (nausea, breast changes, leg cramps, hemorrhoids, nasal stuffiness), alteration in muscle tone, inability to relax.

risk for disturbed Maternal-Fetal Dyad possibly evidenced by environmental or hereditary factors, problems of maternal well-being (e.g., malnutrition, substance use).

[maximally compensated] Cardiac Output may be related to increased fluid volume, maximal cardiac effort and hormonal effects of progesterone and relaxin (places the client at risk for hypertension and/or circulatory failure), and changes in peripheral resistance (afterload), possibly evidenced by variations in blood pressure and pulse, syncopal episodes, presence of pathological edema.

readiness for enhanced family Coping possibly evidenced by expresses desire to enhance health promotion, and choose experiences that optimize wellness.

risk for Constipation possibly evidenced by changes in dietary or fluid intake, smooth muscle relaxation, decreased peristalsis, and effects of medications (e.g., iron).

Fatigue/Insomnia may be related to increased carbohydrate metabolism, altered body chemistry, increased energy requirements to perform activities of daily living, discomfort, anxiety, inactivity, possibly evidenced by reports of overwhelming lack of energy, inability to maintain usual routines, difficulty falling asleep, dissatisfaction with sleep, decreased quality of life.

risk for ineffective Role Performance possibly evidenced by maturational crisis, developmental level, history of maladaptive coping, absence of support systems.

readiness for enhanced Childbearing process possibly evidenced by expresses desire to enhance: knowledge of childbearing process, management of unpleasant pregnancy symptoms.

Pregnancy, 2nd trimester OB/CH
Also refer to Pregnancy, 1st trimester
ineffective Breathing Pattern may be related to impingement of the diaphragm by enlarging uterus, possibly evidenced by reports of shortness of breath, dyspnea, and changes in respiratory depth.

risk for [decompensated] Cardiac Output possibly evidenced by increased circulatory demand, changes in preload (decreased venous return) and afterload (increased peripheral vascular resistance), and ventricular hypertrophy.

risk for excess Fluid Volume possibly evidenced by changes in regulatory mechanisms, sodium and water retention.

Sexual dysfunction may be related to conflict regarding changes in sexual desire and expectations, fear of physical injury to woman/fetus, possibly evidenced by reported difficulties, limitations or changes in sexual behaviors or activities.

Pregnancy, 3rd trimester OB/CH
Also refer to Pregnancy, 1st and 2nd trimesters
readiness for enhanced Childbearing Process possibly evidenced by expresses desire to enhance preparation for labor/delivery, newborn.

impaired urinary Elimination may be related to uterine enlargement, increased abdominal pressure, fluctuation of renal blood flow, and glomerular filtration rate, possibly evidenced by urinary frequency, urgency, dependent edema.

risk for ineffective Coping/compromised family Coping possibly evidenced by (situational or maturational crisis), vulnerability, insufficient sense of control, insufficient social support.

risk for disturbed Maternal-Fetal Dyad possibly evidenced by risk factors of (pregnancy complication—hypertension, infection, abnormal blood profile), substance misuse.

Pregnancy, adolescent OB/CH
Also refer to Pregnancy, 1st, 2nd, and 3rd trimesters
interrupted Family Processes may be related to (situational or developmental transition, shift in health status of a family member); shift in family roles, possibly evidenced by change in expression of conflict within family, change in communication pattern, changes in participation for problem-solving or decision making, decrease in available emotional support.

Social Isolation may be related to (alterations in physical appearance), perceived incongruent social behavior with norms, insufficient personal resources, possibly evidenced by aloneness imposed by others, inability to meet expectations of others; withdrawn; desires to be alone; and absence of support system.

situational low Self-Esteem may be related to (developmental transition), alteration in body image, social role; behavior inconsistent with values, unrealistic self-expectations possibly evidenced by self-negating verbalizations, underestimates ability to deal with situation, situational challenge to self-worth, and [lack of follow-through or nonparticipation in prenatal care].

ineffective Childbearing Process may be related to insufficient knowledge of childbearing process, (unplanned/unwanted pregnancy), inadequate maternal nutrition, low maternal confidence, insufficient cognitive readiness for parenting, insufficient support system, possibly evidenced by inadequate prenatal care/lifestyle, unrealistic birth plan, inadequate preparation of home environment/newborn care items.

risk for impaired Parenting possibly evidenced by (young parental age, insufficient cognitive readiness for parenting; low educational level, unplanned pregnancy), insufficient knowledge about parenting skills, father of child uninvolved.

Pregnancy, high-risk OB/CH
Also refer to Pregnancy, 1st, 2nd, and 3rd trimesters
Anxiety [specify level] may be related to (situational crisis), threat to current status, interpersonal transmission or contagion, possibly evidenced by increase

in tension, apprehensiveness, feeling of inadequacy, alteration in sleep pattern.

readiness for enhanced Knowledge regarding high-risk situation and preterm labor possibly evidenced by expresses desire to enhance learning.

risk for disturbed Maternal-Fetal Dyad possibly evidenced by (pregnancy complication—alteration in glucose metabolism, compromised fetal oxygen transport), substance misuse, physical abuse.

risk for maternal Injury possibly evidenced by physical—preexisting medical conditions, complications of pregnancy; insufficient knowledge of modifiable factors.

risk for Activity Intolerance possibly evidenced by imbalance between oxygen supply and demand; (circulatory or respiratory problems).

risk for compromised family Coping possibly evidenced by (situational crisis), family disorganization, insufficient support given by client to support person, family role change.

risk for ineffective Health Management possibly evidenced by difficulty managing complex treatment regimen, decisional conflicts, insufficient social support, economically disadvantaged, perceived seriousness of condition/susceptibility.

Pregnancy-induced hypertension   OB/CH
Refer to Hypertension, gestational

Pregnancy, postmaturity   OB
Anxiety [specify level] may be related to (situational crisis), threat to current status, interpersonal transmission or contagion, possibly evidenced by increase in tension, apprehensiveness, irritability, feeling of inadequacy, somatic complaints.

ineffective [uteroplacental] Tissue Perfusion may be related to placental involution, multiple infarcts, and villous degeneration, possibly evidenced by decrease in fetal motion, meconium staining of amniotic fluid, intrauterine growth restriction, late decelerations on fetal monitor.

risk for maternal Injury possibly evidenced by dysfunctional or prolonged labor.

risk for fetal Injury possibly evidenced by prolonged labor (tissue hypoxia, acidosis), meconium aspiration.

Premature ejaculation   CH
Sexual dysfunction may be related to altered body function, partner-related issues, possibly evidenced by

reports of disruption of sexual response pattern, inability to achieve desired satisfaction.

situational low Self-Esteem may be related to functional impairment, perceived failure to perform satisfactorily, rejection of other(s), possibly evidenced by self-negating verbalizations, expressions of helplessness, powerlessness.

Premature infant   OB/PED
Refer to Newborn, premature

Premenstrual dysphoric disorder   GYN/PSY
chronic Pain may be related to cyclic changes in female hormones affecting other systems (e.g., vascular congestion, spasms), vitamin deficiency, fluid retention, possibly evidenced by increased tension, apprehension, jitteriness, verbal reports, distraction behaviors, somatic complaints, self-focusing, physical and social withdrawal.

[moderate to panic] Anxiety may be related to cyclic changes in female hormones affecting other systems, possibly evidenced by feelings of inability to cope or loss of control, depersonalization, increased tension, apprehension, jitteriness, somatic complaints, and impaired functioning.

ineffective Coping may be related to inaccurate threat appraisal, ineffective tension release strategies, [threat to self-concept, multiple stressors], possibly evidenced by reports of inability to cope, inadequate problem-solving skills, alteration in sleep pattern.

excess Fluid Volume may be related to abnormal alterations of hormonal levels, possibly evidenced by edema formation, weight gain, and periodic changes in emotional status/irritability.

deficient Knowledge regarding pathophysiology of condition and self-care and treatment needs may be related to lack of information, misinterpretation, possibly evidenced by statements of concern, questions, misconceptions, and continuation of condition, exacerbating symptoms.

Premenstrual tension syndrome   GYN/PSY
Refer to Premenstrual dysphoric disorder

Prenatal substance abuse   OB
Refer to Substance dependence/abuse, prenatal

Pressure ulcer or sore   CH
Also refer to Ulcer, decubitus
ineffective peripheral Tissue Perfusion may be related to reduced or interrupted blood flow, possibly evidenced by presence of inflamed, necrotic lesion.

deficient Knowledge regarding cause, prevention of condition, and potential complications may be related to lack of information or misinterpretation, possibly evidenced by statements of concern, questions, misconceptions, and inaccurate follow-through of instructions.

Preterm labor OB/CH
Refer to Labor, preterm

Prostate cancer MS
Also refer to Cancer; Prostatectomy
[acute/chronic] urinary Retention may be related to blockage of urethra, possibly evidenced by sensation of bladder fullness, dysuria, small and frequent voiding, residual urine, bladder distention.

acute Pain may be related to physical agent—destruction of tissues, pressure on surrounding structures, bladder distention, possibly evidenced by verbal reports of pain, restlessness, irritability, autonomic responses.

Prostatectomy MS
Also refer to Surgery, general
impaired urinary Elimination may be related to mechanical obstruction (blood clots, edema, trauma, surgical procedure, pressure or irritation of catheter and balloon) and loss of bladder tone, possibly evidenced by dysuria, frequency, dribbling, incontinence, retention, bladder fullness, suprapubic discomfort.

risk for Bleeding/deficient Fluid Volume possibly evidenced by trauma [to highly vascular area], restricted intake, postobstructive diuresis].

acute Pain may be related to irritation of bladder mucosa and tissue trauma/edema, possibly evidenced by verbal reports (bladder spasms), distraction behaviors, self-focus, and autonomic responses (changes in vital signs).

disturbed Body Image may be related to alteration in self-perception (e.g., perceived threat of altered body and sexual function) expression of negative feelings about body, and statements of concern regarding functioning.

CH
risk for Sexual dysfunction possibly evidenced by alteration in body function (e.g., incontinence, leakage of urine after catheter removal, involvement of genital area) and threat to self-concept, change in health status.

Prostatitis, acute CH
Also refer to Cystitis
acute Pain/impaired Comfort may be related to inflammatory response, possibly evidenced by reports of low back and pelvic pain, arthralgia, myalgia.

impaired urinary Elimination may be related to localized swelling, urinary tract infection, possibly evidenced by dysuria or burning on urination, frequency, urgency, nocturia, obstructed voiding.

Hyperthermia may be related to illness, possibly evidenced by high fever; chills; flushed, warm skin.

risk for ineffective Health Management possibly evidenced by length of therapy, perceived seriousness or benefits.

Prostatitis, chronic CH
Also refer to Cystitis
impaired Comfort/acute Pain may be related to inflammatory response, possibly evidenced by reports of back, pelvic, or scrotal discomfort; low-grade fever.

impaired urinary Elimination may be related to localized swelling, urinary tract infection, possibly evidenced by dysuria, frequency, urgency.

Pruritus CH
acute Pain may be related to cutaneous hyperesthesia and inflammation, possibly evidenced by verbal reports, distraction behaviors, and self-focus.

risk for impaired Skin Integrity possibly evidenced by [mechanical trauma (scratching) and development/rupture of vesicles or bullae].

Psoriasis CH
impaired Skin Integrity may be related to [increased epidermal cell proliferation and absence of normal protective skin layers], possibly evidenced by alteration in skin integrity, redness [scaling papules and plaques].

disturbed Body Image may be related to cosmetically unsightly skin lesions, possibly evidenced by hiding affected body part, negative feelings about body, feelings of helplessness, and change in social involvement.

Psychological abuse CH/PSY
Refer to Abuse, psychological

PTSD PSY
Refer to Post-traumatic stress disorder

Pulmonary edema MS
impaired Gas Exchange may be related to (alveolar-capillary membrane changes), possibly evidenced by

abnormal breathing pattern (changes in rate and depth of respirations, dyspnea), restlessness, irritability, confusion.

[moderate to severe] Anxiety may be related to threat to current status, threat of death, interpersonal transmission, possibly evidenced by expressed concerns, distress, apprehensiveness, extraneous movement.

risk for impaired spontaneous Ventilation possibly evidenced by respiratory muscle fatigue, problems with secretion management.

Pulmonary edema, high altitude   MS
Refer to High altitude pulmonary edema

Pulmonary embolus   MS
ineffective Breathing Pattern may be related to tracheobronchial obstruction (inflammation, copious secretions or active bleeding), decreased lung expansion, inflammatory process, possibly evidenced by changes in depth or rate of respiration, dyspnea, use of accessory muscles, altered chest excursion, abnormal breath sounds (crackles, wheezes), and cough (with or without sputum production).

impaired Gas Exchange may be related to (ventilation-perfusion imbalance and alveolar-capillary membrane changes), possibly evidenced by abnormal breathing patterns (profound dyspnea), restlessness, somnolence, cyanosis, hypoxemia, and hypercapnia.

Fear/Anxiety [specify level] may be related to dyspnea, inability to breathe normally, threat of death, threat to current status, physiological response to hypoxemia, acidosis, and concern regarding unknown outcome of situation, possibly evidenced by restlessness, irritability, sympathetic stimulation (cardiovascular excitation, pupil dilation, sweating), crying impending sense of doom.

Pulmonary fibrosis   CH
impaired Gas Exchange may be related to (alveolar-capillary membrane changes, ventilation-perfusion imbalance), possibly evidenced by abnormal breathing pattern (dyspnea), [nonproductive cough], abnormal skin color (cyanosis).

Anxiety [specify]/Fear may be related to threat to current status, threat of death, possibly evidenced by expressed concerns, apprehension, uncertainty, increased tension.

Activity Intolerance may be related to imbalance between oxygen supply and demand, possibly evidenced by, generalized weakness, exertional dyspnea,

abnormal heart rate and blood pressure response to activity, [cyanosis].

risk for Infection possibly evidenced by stasis of body fluids (secretions), (chronic illness), [drug therapies—corticosteroids, cytotoxins].

Pulmonary hypertension   CH/MS
impaired Gas Exchange may be related to (alveolar-capillary changes), and [increased pulmonary vascular resistance], possibly evidenced by abnormal breathing pattern (dyspnea), irritability, somnolence, abnormal arterial blood gases.

decreased Cardiac Output may be related to increased pulmonary vascular resistance, decreased blood return to left side of heart, possibly evidenced by increased heart rate, dyspnea, fatigue.

Activity Intolerance may be related to imbalance between oxygen supply and demand, possibly evidenced by reports of weakness, fatigue, abnormal vital signs with activity.

[mild to moderate] Anxiety may be related to threat to current status, stress, threat to self-concept, possibly evidenced by expressed concerns, uncertainty, anxiety, awareness of physiological symptoms, diminished productivity and ability to problem-solve.

Pulmonic insufficiency   MS/CH
Refer to Valvular heart disease

Pulmonic stenosis   MS/CH
Refer to Valvular heart disease

Purpura, idiopathic thrombocytopenic   CH
ineffective Protection may be related to abnormal blood profile, drug therapy (corticosteroids or immunosuppressive agents), possibly evidenced by altered clotting, fatigue, deficient immunity.

Activity Intolerance may be related to imbalance between oxygen supply and demand, possibly evidenced by weakness, fatigue, abnormal vital signs with activity.

deficient Knowledge regarding therapy choices, outcomes, and self-care needs may be related to lack of information, misinterpretation, possibly evidenced by statements of concern, questions, and misconceptions.

Pyelonephritis   MS
acute Pain may be related to acute inflammation of renal tissues, possibly evidenced by verbal reports, guarding or distraction behaviors, self-focus, and changes in vital signs.

Hyperthermia may be related to inflammatory process and increased metabolic rate, possibly evidenced by increase in body temperature; warm, flushed skin; tachycardia; and chills.

impaired urinary Elimination may be related to inflammation and irritation of bladder mucosa, possibly evidenced by dysuria, urgency, and frequency.

deficient Knowledge regarding therapy needs and prevention may be related to lack of information, misinterpretation, possibly evidenced by statements of concern, questions, misconceptions, and recurrence of condition.

Pyloric stenosis   PED

deficient Fluid Volume may be related to excessive projectile vomiting, possibly evidenced by decreased, concentrated urine; poor skin turgor, dry skin and mucous membranes, lethargy.

imbalanced Nutrition: less than body requirements may be related to insufficient dietary intake, (inability to digest food or absorb nutrients), possibly evidenced by [weight loss], insufficient muscle tone, pale mucous membranes.

Quadriplegia   MS/CH

Also refer to Paraplegia

ineffective Breathing Pattern may be related to (spinal cord injury, neurological impairment), respiratory muscle fatigue[/weakness], possibly evidenced by abnormal breathing pattern, altered chest excursion, decreased in vital capacity, dyspnea, and [abnormal arterial blood gases].

risk for physical Trauma [additional spinal injury] possibly evidenced by weakness, [instability of spinal column].

Grieving may be related to [perceived loss of self, anticipated alterations in lifestyle and expectations, and limitation of future options and choices], possibly evidenced by expressions of distress, anger, sorrow; choked feelings; and changes in eating habits, sleep, communication patterns.

[total] Self-Care deficit related to (neuromuscular impairment) weakness, evidenced by inability to perform self-care tasks.

bowel Incontinence/Constipation may be related to disruption of nerve innervation, perceptual impairment, changes in dietary and fluid intake, change in activity level, possibly evidenced by inability to evacuate bowel voluntarily; increased abdominal pressure and distention; dry, hard formed stool; change in bowel sounds.

impaired bed/wheelchair Mobility may be related to loss of muscle function and control.

risk for Autonomic Dysreflexia possibly evidenced by risk factors of altered nerve function (spinal cord injury at T6 or above); bladder, bowel, or skin stimulation (tactile, pain, thermal).

impaired Home Maintenance may be related to permanent effects of injury, inadequate or absent support systems and finances, and lack of familiarity with resources, possibly evidenced by expressions of difficulties, requests for information and assistance, outstanding debts or financial crisis, and lack of necessary aids and equipment.

Rabies   CH/MS

Hyperthermia may be related to infection, possibly evidenced by fever, malaise.

risk for ineffective Airway Clearance possibly evidenced by excessive salivation, muscle spasms (laryngeal, pharyngeal).

deficient Fluid Volume related to inability to drink (severe painful pharyngeal muscle spasms), excessive salivation, possibly evidenced by extreme thirst, decreased skin turgor, decreased output/concentrated urine.

risk for physical Trauma possibly evidenced by progressive restlessness, uncontrollable excitement, inability to utilize physical restraints for safety.

Radiation syndrome/poisoning   MS

(Dependent on dose and duration of exposure)

[severe] Anxiety/Fear may be related to (situational crisis), threat of death, interpersonal transmission and contagion, unmet needs, possibly evidenced by expressed concerns, fearfulness, hopelessness, restlessness, agitation, anguish, increased tension, awareness of physiological symptoms.

deficient Fluid Volume may be related to intractable nausea, vomiting, diarrhea (gastrointestinal tissue necrosis and atrophy), interference with adequate intake (stomatitis, anorexia), hemorrhagic losses (thrombocytopenia), possibly evidenced by dry skin and mucous membranes, poor skin turgor, decreased venous filling, reduced pulse volume and pressure, hypotension, weakness, change in mentation.

acute Confusion may be related to (alteration in cognitive functioning, impaired metabolic functioning), possibly evidenced by alteration in level of consciousness, agitation, misperception.

ineffective Protection may be related to effects of radiation, abnormal blood profile (leukopenia, thrombocytopenia, anemia), inadequate nutrition, possibly evidenced by neurosensory alterations, anorexia, deficient immunity, impaired healing, altered clotting, disorientation.

risk for Infection possibly evidenced by stasis of body fluids, altered peristalsis, and associated conditions decreased hemoglobin/anemia, leukopenia.

Sexual dysfunction may be related to altered body function, possibly evidenced by amenorrhea, decreased libido, infertility.

Radiation therapy   CH
Also refer to Brachytherapy; Cancer

Nausea may be related to therapeutic procedure, irritation to gastrointestinal system, possibly evidenced by verbal reports, vomiting, gastric stasis.

imbalanced Nutrition: less than body requirements may be related to insufficient dietary intake, (inability to ingest food or absorb nutrients), possibly evidenced by [weight loss], food aversion, reported altered taste sensation, sore buccal cavity, diarrhea.

impaired oral Mucous Membrane Integrity may be related to side effects of radiation, dehydration, and malnutrition, possibly evidenced by ulcerations, leukoplakia, decreased salivation, and reports of pain.

ineffective Protection may be related to inadequate nutrition, radiation, abnormal blood profile, disease state (cancer), possibly evidenced by impaired healing, deficient immunity, anorexia, fatigue.

Radical neck surgery   MS
Refer to Laryngectomy

Rape   CH
deficient Knowledge regarding required medical/legal procedures, prophylactic treatment for individual concerns (sexually transmitted infection, pregnancy), and community resources and supports may be related to lack of information, possibly evidenced by statements of concern, questions, misconceptions, and exacerbation of symptoms.

Rape-Trauma Syndrome related to actual or attempted sexual penetration without consent, possibly evidenced by wide range of emotional reactions, including anxiety, fear, anger, embarrassment, and multisystem physical complaints.

risk for impaired Tissue Integrity possibly evidenced by forceful sexual penetration and trauma to fragile tissues.

ineffective Coping may be related to high degree of threat, [personal vulnerability, unmet expectations, unrealistic perceptions, inadequate social support systems or coping methods, multiple stressors repeated over time], possibly evidenced by verbalizations of inability to cope or difficulty asking for help, inability to deal with a situation or meet role expectations, destructive behaviors toward self/others.

Sexual dysfunction may be related to biopsychosocial alteration of sexuality (stress of posttrauma response), vulnerability, loss of sexual desire, impaired relationship with SO, possibly evidenced by alteration in achieving sexual satisfaction, change in interest in self/others, preoccupation with self.

Raynaud's disease   CH
acute/chronic Pain may be related to vasospasm and altered perfusion of affected tissues, and ischemia or destruction of tissues, possibly evidenced by verbal reports, guarding of affected parts, self-focusing, and restlessness.

ineffective peripheral Tissue Perfusion may be related to periodic reduction of arterial blood flow to affected areas, possibly evidenced by pallor, cyanosis, coolness, numbness, paresthesia, slow healing of lesions.

deficient Knowledge regarding pathophysiology of condition, potential for complications, treatment, and self-care needs may be related to lack of information, misinterpretation, possibly evidenced by statements of concern, questions, and misconceptions; development of preventable complications.

Raynaud's phenomenon   CH
Refer to Raynaud's disease

Reactive attachment disorder   PED/PSY
Refer to Anxiety disorders—PED

Reflex sympathetic dystrophy   CH
Refer to Complex regional pain syndrome

acute/chronic Pain may be related to continued nerve stimulation, possibly evidenced by verbal reports, distraction or guarding behaviors, narrowed focus, changes in sleep patterns, and altered ability to continue previous activities.

ineffective peripheral Tissue Perfusion may be related to reduction of arterial blood flow (arteriole vasoconstriction), possibly evidenced by reports of pain, decreased skin temperature and pallor, diminished arterial pulsations, and tissue swelling.

[disturbed tactile Sensory Perception] may be related to altered sensory reception (neurological deficit, pain), possibly evidenced by change in usual response to stimuli, abnormal sensitivity of touch, physiological anxiety, and irritability.

risk for ineffective Role Performance possibly evidenced by situational crisis, chronic disability, debilitating pain.

risk for compromised family Coping possibly evidenced by temporary family disorganization and role changes and prolonged disability that exhausts the supportive capacity of SO(s).

Regional enteritis   CH
Refer to Crohn's disease

Renal disease, end-stage   CH/MS
Also refer to Renal failure, chronic
Death Anxiety may be related to progressive debilitating disease, unmet needs, inadequate support system, personal vulnerability, past negative experiences, possibly evidenced by fear of the process of dying or loss of abilities, concerns of unfinished business, powerlessness, loss of control, denial of impending death.

Renal failure, acute (Kidney injury, acute) MS
excess Fluid Volume may be related to compromised regulatory mechanisms (decreased kidney function), possibly evidenced by weight gain, edema, anasarca, intake greater than output, venous congestion, changes in blood pressure and central venous pressure, altered electrolyte levels, decreased hemoglobin and hematocrit, pulmonary congestion on x-ray.

risk for imbalanced Nutrition: less than body requirements possibly evidenced by (inability to ingest or digest foods or absorb nutrients), food aversion, sore buccal cavity, [therapeutic dietary restrictions].

risk for Infection possibly evidenced by malnutrition, immunosuppression, (invasive procedures or devices).

risk for acute Confusion possibly evidenced by (impaired metabolic functioning), malnutrition (electrolyte imbalance, increased blood urea nitrogen/creatinine, azotemia).

Renal failure, chronic   CH/MS
Also refer to Dialysis, general
risk for decreased Cardiac Output possibly evidenced by fluid imbalances affecting circulating volume, myocardial workload, and systemic vascular resistance; alterations in rate, rhythm, and cardiac conduction (electrolyte imbalances, hypoxia); accumulation of toxins (urea); soft calcification.

risk for Bleeding possibly evidenced by inherent coagulopathy.

risk for chronic Confusion possibly evidenced by [long-term or progressive impairment in cognitive functioning associated with electrolyte imbalance, increased blood urea nitrogen/creatinine, azotemia, malnutrition, decreased hemoglobin].

risk for impaired Skin Integrity possibly evidenced by alteration in metabolism, immunodeficiency, impaired circulation and sensation, alteration in skin turgor, [reduced activity, immobility, accumulation of toxins in the skin].

risk for impaired oral Mucous Membrane Integrity possibly evidenced by decreased or lack of salivation, fluid restrictions, chemical irritation (conversion of urea in saliva to ammonia).

Renal transplantation   MS
Also refer to Transplantation, recipient
risk for excess Fluid Volume possibly evidenced by compromised regulatory mechanism (implantation of new kidney requiring adjustment period for optimal functioning).

disturbed Body Image may be related to alteration in self-perception (e.g., failure and subsequent replacement of body part and medication-induced changes in appearance), possibly evidenced by preoccupation with loss or change, negative feelings about body, and focus on past strength and function.

Fear may be related to [threat to health status—potential for transplant rejection or failure; and threat of death], possibly evidenced by increased tension, apprehension, concentration on source, and verbalizations of concern.

risk for Infection possibly evidenced by alteration in skin/tissue integrity, stasis of body fluids, malnutrition and associated conditions of immunosuppression, invasive procedures and chronic illness.

                                                            CH
risk for ineffective Coping/compromised family Coping possibly evidenced by (situational crises), family disorganization and role changes, prolonged disease exhausting supportive capacity of SO/family, therapeutic restrictions/long-term therapy needs.

Repetitive motion injury   CH
Refer to Carpal tunnel syndrome

Respiratory distress syndrome, acute   MS

ineffective Airway Clearance may be related to loss of ciliary action, increased amount and viscosity of secretions, and increased airway resistance, possibly evidenced by presence of dyspnea, changes in depth and rate of respiration, use of accessory muscles for breathing, wheezes, crackles, cough with or without sputum production.

impaired Gas Exchange may be related to changes in (ventilation—perfusion imbalance), possibly evidenced by abnormal breathing patterns (tachypnea, use of accessory muscles), and abnormal skin color (cyanosis, hypoxia per arterial blood gases or oximetry), [anxiety and changes in mentation].

risk for deficient Fluid Volume possibly evidenced by active loss from diuretic use and restricted intake.

risk for decreased Cardiac Output possibly evidenced by alteration in preload (hypovolemia, vascular pooling, diuretic therapy, and increased intrathoracic pressure, use of ventilator, and positive end-expiratory pressure [PEEP]).

Anxiety [specify level]/Fear may be related to physiological factors (effects of hypoxemia), situational crisis, change in health status/threat of death, possibly evidenced by increased tension, apprehension, restlessness, focus on self, and sympathetic stimulation.

risk for [pulmonary] Injury possibly evidenced by increased airway pressure associated with mechanical ventilation (PEEP).

Respiratory distress syndrome (premature infant)   PED

Also refer to Newborn, premature
impaired Gas Exchange may be related to (alveolar-capillary membrane changes, ventilation-perfusion imbalance), possibly evidenced by abnormal breathing patterns (tachypnea, use of accessory muscles and retractions, expiratory grunting), abnormal skin color (pallor or cyanosis), abnormal arterial blood gases, and tachycardia.

impaired Spontaneous Ventilation may be related to respiratory muscle fatigue and metabolic factors, possibly evidenced by dyspnea, increased metabolic rate, restlessness, use of accessory muscles, and abnormal arterial blood gases.

risk for Infection possibly evidenced by stasis of body fluids, malnutrition (absence of nutrient stores, increased metabolic demands), and invasive procedures.

risk for dysfunctional Gastrointestinal Mobility possibly evidenced by (decrease in gastrointestinal circulation).

risk for impaired Attachment possibly evidenced by premature/ill infant who is unable to effectively initiate parental contact (altered behavioral organization), separation, physical barriers, anxiety associated with the parental role and demands of infant.

Respiratory syncytial virus   PED

impaired Gas Exchange may be related to (ventilation-perfusion imbalance), possibly evidenced by abnormal breathing patterns (dyspnea, apnea) abnormal arterial blood gases/hypoxia.

ineffective Airway Clearance may be related to infection, retained secretions, exudate in alveoli, inflammation of airways, possibly evidenced by dyspnea, adventitious breath sounds, cough.

risk for deficient Fluid Volume possibly evidenced by increased insensible losses (fever, diaphoresis), decreased oral intake.

Restless leg syndrome   CH

Refer to Myoclonus, nocturnal

Retinal detachment   CH

[disturbed visual Sensory Perception] related to decreased sensory reception, possibly evidenced by visual distortions, decreased visual field, and changes in visual acuity.

[mild to moderate] Anxiety may be related to (situational crisis), threat to current status and role function, possibly evidenced by expressed concerns, apprehensiveness, uncertainty, self-focused.

deficient Knowledge regarding therapy, prognosis, and self-care needs may be related to lack of information, misconceptions, possibly evidenced by statements of concern and questions.

risk for impaired Home Maintenance possibly evidenced by visual limitations, activity restrictions.

Rett's syndrome   PED/PSY

Also refer to Autism spectrum disorder
delayed Development may be related to effects of physical and mental disability, possibly evidenced by delay or inability in performing skills and self-care or self-control activities appropriate for age.

impaired Walking/physical Mobility may be related to neuromuscular impairment, joint stiffness, contractures, disuse, possibly evidenced by limited range of motion, inability to perform gross motor skills, walk, or reposition self.

risk for physical Trauma possibly evidenced by cognitive deficits, lack of muscle tone and coordination, seizure activity.

ineffective infant Feeding Pattern/imbalanced Nutrition: less than body requirements may be related to (neurological impairment), insufficient dietary intake, possibly evidenced by inability to coordinate sucking, swallowing, and breathing; weakness of muscles required for mastication/swallowing, food intake less than recommended daily allowance, [weight loss or failure to gain].

risk for complicated Grieving possibly evidenced by emotional disturbance [loss of "the perfect child," chronic condition requiring long-term care].

Reye's syndrome   PED

deficient Fluid Volume may be related to failure of regulatory mechanism (diabetes insipidus), excessive gastric losses (pernicious vomiting), and altered intake, possibly evidenced by increased and dilute urine output, sudden weight loss, decreased venous filling, dry mucous membranes, decreased skin turgor, hypotension, and tachycardia.

ineffective cerebral Tissue Perfusion may be related to diminished arterial or venous blood flow and hypovolemia, possibly evidenced by memory loss, altered consciousness, and restlessness, agitation.

risk for physical Trauma possibly evidenced by generalized weakness, reduced coordination, and cognitive deficits.

ineffective Breathing Pattern may be related to decreased energy and fatigue, cognitive impairment, tracheobronchial obstruction, and inflammatory process (aspiration pneumonia), possibly evidenced by tachypnea, abnormal arterial blood gases, cough, and use of accessory muscles.

Rheumatic fever   PED

acute Pain may be related to migratory inflammation of joints, possibly evidenced by verbal reports, guarding or distraction behaviors, self-focus, and changes in vital signs.

Hyperthermia may be related to inflammatory process, hypermetabolic state, possibly evidenced by increased body temperature; warm, flushed skin; and tachycardia.

Activity Intolerance may be related to physical deconditioning (generalized weakness, joint pain, and

medical restrictions or bedrest), possibly evidenced by reports of fatigue, exertional discomfort, and abnormal heart rate in response to activity.

risk for decreased Cardiac Output possibly evidenced by altered contractility.

Rheumatic heart disease   PED/MS

Also refer to Valvular heart disease

Activity Intolerance may be related to imbalance between oxygen supply and demand, physical deconditioning (generalized weakness), or sedentary lifestyle (prolonged bedrest), possibly evidenced by reported or observed weakness, fatigue, abnormal vital signs in response to activity (dysrhythmias, dyspnea, pallor).

risk-prone Health Behavior may be related to health status requiring change in lifestyle or restriction of desired activities, unrealistic expectations, negative attitudes, possibly evidenced by denial of situation, demonstration of nonacceptance of health status, failure to achieve optimal sense of control.

risk for ineffective Health Management possibly evidenced by complexity and duration of therapeutic regimen, imposed restrictions or limitations, economic difficulties, family patterns of healthcare, perceived seriousness or benefits.

risk for impaired Gas Exchange possibly evidenced by (alveolar-capillary membrane changes).

Rhinitis, allergic   CH

Refer to Hay fever

Rickets   PED

risk for [disproportionate Growth]/delayed Development possibly evidenced by inadequate nutrition, economically disadvantaged, chronic illness, prematurity.

deficient Knowledge regarding cause, pathophysiology, therapy needs and prevention may be related to lack of information, possibly evidenced by statements of concern, questions, misconceptions, and inaccurate follow-through of instructions.

Ringworm, tinea   CH

Also refer to Athlete's foot

impaired Skin Integrity may be related to [fungal infection of the dermis], possibly evidenced by alteration in skin integrity (presence of lesions).

deficient Knowledge regarding infectious nature, therapy, and self-care needs may be related to lack of information, misinformation, possibly evidenced by statements of concern, questions, and recurrence and spread.

Rocky Mountain spotted fever   CH/MS
Refer to Typhus

RSD   CH
Refer to Reflex sympathetic dystrophy

RSV   PED
Refer to Respiratory syncytial virus

Rubella   PED/CH
acute Pain/impaired Comfort may be related to inflammatory effects of viral infection and presence of desquamating rash, possibly evidenced by verbal reports, distraction behaviors, restlessness.

deficient Knowledge regarding contagious nature, possible complications, and self-care needs may be related to lack of information, misinterpretations, possibly evidenced by statements of concern, questions, and inaccurate follow-through of instructions.

Rubeola   PED/CH
Refer to Measles

Ruptured intervertebral disc   CH/MS
Refer to Herniated nucleus pulposus

Sarcoidosis   CH
Also refer to Pulmonary fibrosis
Fatigue may be related to disease state, anemia, possibly evidenced by lack of energy, lethargy, decreased performance, inability to maintain usual routines.

risk for Injury possibly evidenced by autoimmune dysfunction, abnormal blood profile—thrombocytopenia, leukopenia, anemia; sensory dysfunction.

SARS (sudden acute respiratory syndrome)   MS
Hyperthermia may be related to inflammatory process, possibly evidenced by high fever, chills, rigors, headache.

acute Pain/impaired Comfort may be related to inflammation and circulating toxins, possibly evidenced by reports of myalgia, headache, malaise.

impaired Gas Exchange may be related to (ventilation-perfusion imbalance), possibly evidenced by dyspnea, confusion, restlessness, hypoxemia.

risk for impaired spontaneous Ventilation possibly evidenced by hypermetabolic state, infection, depletion of energy stores, respiratory muscle fatigue.

Death Anxiety may be related to uncertainty of prognosis, possibly evidenced by report of apprehension; increased pulse and respiratory rate, muscle tension, pupil dilation.

risk for ineffective Protection possibly evidenced by inadequate nutrition, abnormal blood profile (leukopenia, thrombocytopenia).

Scabies   CH
impaired Skin Integrity may be related to [presence of invasive parasite and development of pruritus], possibly evidenced by alteration in skin integrity, redness.

deficient Knowledge regarding communicable nature, possible complications, therapy, and self-care needs may be related to lack of information, misinterpretation, possibly evidenced by questions and statements of concern about spread to others.

Scarlet fever   PED
Hyperthermia may be related to effects of circulating toxins, possibly evidenced by increased body temperature; warm, flushed skin; and tachycardia.

acute Pain/impaired Comfort may be related to inflammation of mucous membranes and effects of circulating toxins (malaise, fever), possibly evidenced by verbal reports, distraction behaviors, guarding (decreased swallowing), and self-focus.

risk for deficient Fluid Volume possibly evidenced by hypermetabolic state (hyperthermia) and reduced intake.

Schizoaffective disorder   PSY
risk for other-/self-directed Violence possibly evidenced by depressed mood, feelings of worthlessness, hopelessness, unsatisfactory parent-child relationship, feelings of abandonment by SOs, anger turned inward or directed at the environment, punitive superego, irrational feelings of guilt, numerous failures, misinterpretation of reality.

Social Isolation may be related to developmental regression, depressed mood, feelings of worthlessness, egocentric behaviors (offending others and discouraging relationships), delusional thinking, fear of failure, unresolved grief, possibly evidenced by sad, dull affect; absence of support systems; uncommunicative, withdrawn, or catatonic behavior; absence of eye contact; preoccupation with own thoughts; repetitive or meaningless actions.

imbalanced Nutrition: less than body requirements may be related to insufficient dietary intake, (psychological disorder [e.g., lack of attention to or recognition of hunger cues], possibly evidenced by insufficient interest in food, weight loss, pale mucous membranes, insufficient muscle tone [amenorrhea, abnormal laboratory studies].

Schizophrenia (schizophrenic disorders)   PSY

ineffective Impulse Control may be related to mood disorder, (alteration in cognitive functioning, personality disorder), possibly evidenced by acting without thinking, irritability, temper outbursts, violent behavior, sexual promiscuity.

[disturbed Sensory Perception (specify)] may be related to biochemical/electrolyte imbalance, psychological stress, possibly evidenced by disorientation to space/time, hallucinations, change in behavior pattern.

impaired verbal Communication may be related to low self-esteem, vulnerability, (alteration in perception, psychotic disorder), possibly evidenced by inappropriate verbalizations, difficulty comprehending communication, difficulty in use of facial/body expressions.

Social Isolation may be related to (alterations in mental status), social behavior incongruent with norms, values incongruent with cultural norms, insufficient personal resources, and inability to engage in satisfying personal relationships, possibly evidenced by sad or flat affect, poor eye contact, withdrawn, desire to be alone, hostility, cultural incongruence, member of subculture, and history of rejection.

risk for self-/other-directed Violence possibly evidenced by insufficient personal resources, lack of social resources, social isolation, pattern of threatening violence, (psychological disorder, psychotic disorder, alteration in cognitive functioning).

ineffective Coping may be related to inaccurate threat appraisal, inadequate resources, insufficient social support, inadequate confidence in ability to deal with situation, possibly evidenced by difficulty organizing/inability to attend to information, insufficient problem-solving skills, inability to meet basic needs or role expectations, insufficient assess of social support, risk-taking behavior, destructive behavior toward others/self.

CH

disabled family Coping may be related to ambivalent family relationships, differing coping styles between support persons, or between support person and client, chronically unexpressed feelings, possibly evidenced by family behaviors detrimental to well-being, client dependence, prolonged hyperfocus on client, depression, rejection, abandonment.

ineffective Health Management may be related to difficulty managing complex treatment regimen, perceived barrier/benefit, family conflict, insufficient social support, possibly evidenced by failure to include treatment regimen in daily living, ineffective choices in daily living for meeting health goals, failure to take action to reduce risk factors.

Self-Neglect may be related to stressors, deficient executive function, inability to maintain control, (alteration in cognitive functioning), possibly evidenced by insufficient personal hygiene, nonadherence to health activity, insufficient environmental hygiene.

Sciatica   CH

acute/chronic Pain may be related to peripheral nerve root compression, possibly evidenced by verbal reports of pain, guarding or distraction behavior, and self-focused.

impaired physical Mobility may be related to neurological pain and muscular involvement, possibly evidenced by reluctance to attempt movement and decreased muscle strength and mass.

Scleroderma   CH

Also refer to Lupus erythematosus, systemic (SLE)

impaired physical Mobility may be related to musculoskeletal impairment and associated pain, possibly evidenced by decreased strength, decreased range of motion, and reluctance to attempt movement.

ineffective Tissue Perfusion (specify) may be related to reduced arterial blood flow (arteriolar vasoconstriction), possibly evidenced by changes in skin temperature and color, ulcer formation, and changes in organ function (cardiopulmonary, gastrointestinal, renal).

imbalanced Nutrition: less than body requirements may be related to insufficient dietary intake, (inability to ingest or digest food, or absorb nutrients), possibly evidenced by difficulty swallowing, food intake less than recommended daily allowance and [weight loss].

risk-prone Health Behavior may be related to stressors, inadequate comprehension, insufficient social support, possibly evidenced by nonacceptance of/minimizes health status change, failure to achieve optimal sense of control, failure to take action to prevent/[manage] health problem.

disturbed Body Image may be related to alteration in self-perception (e.g., skin changes, loss of hair; skin/muscle contractures), possibly evidenced by negative feeling about body; focus on past strength, function, or appearance; expressions of fear of reaction by others; hiding body part; and change in social involvement.

Scoliosis   PED
disturbed Body Image may be related to alteration in self-perception (e.g., altered body structure), treatment regimen, possibly evidenced by negative feeling about body, change in social involvement, and preoccupation with situation or refusal to acknowledge problem.

deficient Knowledge regarding pathophysiology of condition, therapy needs, and possible outcomes may be related to lack of information, misinterpretation, possibly evidenced by statements of concern, questions, misconceptions, and inaccurate follow-through of instructions.

risk-prone Health Behavior may be related to inadequate comprehension, negative perception of recommended healthcare strategy, possibly evidenced by minimizing health status change, failure to take action that manages health problem.

Seasonal affective disorder   PSY
Refer to Affective disorder, seasonal

Sedative intoxication/abuse   CH/PSY
Refer to Depressant abuse

Seizure disorder   CH
deficient Knowledge regarding condition and medication control may be related to lack of information, misinterpretations, scarce financial resources, possibly evidenced by questions, statements of concern, misconceptions, incorrect use of anticonvulsant medication, recurrent episodes, or uncontrolled seizures.

disturbed Personal Identity may be related to perceived prejudice (stigma associated with condition, perception of being out of control or helpless), possibly evidenced by ineffective coping strategies, verbalization about feeling of strangeness (changed lifestyle, fear of rejection), [denial of problem resulting in lack of follow-through or nonparticipation in therapy].

impaired Social Interaction may be related to unpredictable nature of condition and self-concept disturbance, possibly evidenced by decreased self-assurance, verbalization of concern, discomfort in social situations, inability to receive or communicate a satisfying sense of belonging and caring, and withdrawal from social contacts and activities.

risk for Trauma/Suffocation possibly evidenced by weakness, balancing difficulties, cognitive limitations, altered consciousness, loss of large- or small-muscle coordination (during seizure).

Separation anxiety disorder   PED/PSY
Refer to Anxiety disorders—PED

Sepsis   MS
Also refer to Sepsis, puerperal
risk for deficient Fluid Volume possibly evidenced by marked increase in vascular compartment—massive vasodilation, vascular shifts to interstitial space, and reduced intake.

risk for decreased Cardiac Output possibly evidenced by decreased preload (venous return and circulating volume), altered afterload (increased systemic vascular resistance), negative inotropic effects of hypoxia, complement activation, and lysosomal hydrolase.

risk for Shock possibly evidenced by infection/ sepsis, hypovolemia—fluid shifts or third spacing; hypotension, hypoxemia.

Sepsis, puerperal   OB
risk for Infection [spread] possibly evidenced by [presence of infection], alteration in skin integrity, (premature/prolonged rupture of amniotic membranes), stasis of body fluids, (invasive procedures, chronic illness [e.g., diabetes mellitus]).

Hyperthermia may be related to inflammatory process, hypermetabolic state, dehydration, effect of circulating endotoxins on the hypothalamus, possibly evidenced by increase in body temperature, warm, flushed skin; increased respiratory rate and tachycardia.

risk for impaired Attachment possibly evidenced by interruption in bonding process, physical illness, perceived threat to own survival.

risk for ineffective peripheral Tissue Perfusion possibly evidenced by interruption or reduction of blood flow—presence of infectious thrombi.

risk for Shock possibly evidenced by infection, hypovolemia, hypotension, hypoxemia.

Septicemia   MS
Refer to Sepsis

Serum sickness   CH
acute Pain may be related to physical agent—inflammation of the joints and skin eruptions, possibly evidenced by verbal reports of pain, guarding or distraction behavior, and self-focused.

---

deficient Knowledge regarding nature of condition, treatment needs, potential complications, and prevention of recurrence may be related to lack of information, misinterpretation, possibly evidenced by statements of concern, questions, misconceptions, and inaccurate follow-through of instructions.

Severe acute respiratory syndrome   **MS**
Refer to SARS

Sexual desire disorder   **PSY**
Sexual dysfunction may be related to insufficient knowledge/misinformation about sexual function, inadequate role model, (absence of significant other), vulnerability, presence of abuse, value conflict, possibly evidenced by alterations in sexual activity/sexual satisfaction, perceived sexual limitation.

Anxiety [moderate to severe] may be related to threat to current status, value conflict, unmet needs, (major change), possibly evidenced by increase in [sexual] tension, feeling of inadequacy, self-focused, extraneous movement, poor eye contact, glancing about, hypervigilance, cardiovascular excitation.

situational low Self-Esteem may be related to behavior inconsistent with values, (history of rejection, pattern of failure), possibly evidenced by situational challenge to self worth, helplessness, self-negating verbalizations.

Sexual dysfunctions   **PSY**
Refer to Dyspareunia; Erectile dysfunction; Sexual desire disorder; Vaginismus

Sexually transmitted infection   **GYN/CH**
risk for Infection [transmission] possibly evidenced by [contagious nature of infecting agent] and insufficient knowledge to avoid exposure to or transmission of pathogens.

impaired Skin/Tissue Integrity may be related to invasion of and irritation by pathogenic organism(s), possibly evidenced by [inflammation (e.g., in gonorrhea or chlamydial infection) or ulceration (e.g., in herpes simplex, syphilis)].

deficient Knowledge regarding condition, prognosis, potential complications, therapy needs, and transmission may be related to lack of information, misinterpretation, lack of interest in learning, possibly evidenced by statements of concern, questions, misconceptions, inaccurate follow-through of instructions, and development of preventable complications.

Shingles   **CH**
Refer to Herpes zoster

Shock   **MS**
Also refer to Shock, cardiogenic; Shock, hypovolemic/hemorrhagic; Sepsis
risk for Infection [progression] may be related to alteration in peristalsis or skin integrity; stasis of body fluids, malnutrition, possibly associated with immunosuppression.

ineffective Tissue Perfusion (specify) may be related to changes in circulating volume or vascular tone, possibly evidenced by changes in skin color and temperature and pulse pressure, reduced blood pressure, changes in mentation, and decreased urinary output.

risk for Shock may be related to alteration in peristalsis or skin integrity; stasis of body fluids, malnutrition, possibly associated with immunosuppression.

Shock, cardiogenic   **MS**
Also refer to Shock
decreased Cardiac Output may be related to structural damage, decreased myocardial contractility, and presence of dysrhythmias, possibly evidenced by electrocardiogram changes, variations in hemodynamic readings, jugular vein distention, cold and clammy skin, diminished peripheral pulses, and decreased urinary output.

risk for impaired Gas Exchange possibly evidenced by (ventilation-perfusion imbalance, alveolar-capillary membrane changes).

Shock, hypovolemic/hemorrhagic   **MS**
Also refer to Shock
deficient Fluid Volume may be related to excessive vascular loss, inadequate intake or replacement, possibly evidenced by hypotension, tachycardia, decreased pulse volume and pressure, change in mentation, and decreased, concentrated urine.

Shock, septic   **MS**
Refer to Sepsis

Sicca syndrome   **CH**
Refer to Sjögren syndrome

Sick building syndrome   **CH**
Contamination may be related to presence of atmospheric or environmental contaminants (e.g., volatile organic compounds, carbon monoxide, asbestos, dust, fungi, molds, pollens, tobacco smoke), carpeted

flooring, inadequate ventilation, possibly evidenced by dermatological/gastrointestinal/pulmonary/neurological effects of contaminating agent(s).

Fatigue may be related to stressors [place of employment/residence], possibly evidenced by tiredness, lethargy, insufficient energy; impaired ability to maintain usual physical activity/routines.

Sick sinus syndrome   MS
Also refer to Dysrhythmia, cardiac

decreased Cardiac Output may be related to alterations in rate, rhythm, and electrical conduction, possibly evidenced by electrocardiogram indication of dysrhythmias, reports of palpitations, weakness, changes in mentation or consciousness, and syncope.

risk for Trauma possibly evidenced by changes in cerebral perfusion with altered consciousness, loss of balance.

SIDS   PED
Refer to Sudden infant death

Sinusitis, chronic   CH
acute/chronic Pain may be related to physical agent—inflammatory process, possibly evidenced by reports of [headache and facial] pain, irritability, alteration in sleep pattern, fatigue.

risk for Infection [spread] possibly evidenced by stasis of body fluids, [low-level chronic infection; improper handling of infectious material].

Sjögren syndrome   CH
*impaired oral Mucous Membrane Integrity/Dry Mouth*may be related to decreased salivation, possibly evidenced by xerostomia (dry mouth), oral pain or discomfort, self-report of bad or diminished taste, difficulty eating and swallowing.

risk for impaired Tissue Integrity/Dry Eye (cornea, mucous membranes) possibly evidenced by impaired production of tears, mucus.

risk for Infection possibly evidenced by [decreased secretions, tissue dryness and damage].

[risk for disturbed visual Sensory Perception] possibly evidenced by risk factors of altered sensory reception (light sensitivity, blurred vision, corneal ulcers).

Skin cancer   CH
impaired Skin Integrity may be related to [invasive growth, surgical excision], possibly evidenced by alteration of skin integrity [destruction of dermis].

risk for acute Pain possibly evidenced by ulceration of skin, surgical incision.

risk for disturbed Body Image possibly evidenced by skin lesion, surgical intervention.

deficient Knowledge regarding condition, prognosis, treatment, and prevention may be related to lack of information, misinterpretation, possibly evidenced by statements of concern, questions, misconceptions, inaccurate follow-through of instructions, development of preventable complications, or recurrence.

SLE   CH
Refer to Lupus erythematosus, systemic

Sleep apnea   CH
Sleep deprivation may be related to nonrestorative sleep pattern, (sleep apnea), possibly evidenced by drowsiness, fatigue, decrease in functional ability, alteration in concentration.

impaired Gas Exchange may be related to [altered oxygen supply—recurrent apneic episodes lasting 10 seconds to 2 minutes], possibly evidenced by abnormal breathing pattern, headache upon awakening, confusion, hypoxemia, hypercapnia, [dysrhythmias (e.g., extreme bradycardia, ventricular tachycardia)].

risk for ineffective Health Management possibly evidenced by difficulty managing treatment regimen, perceived seriousness or benefit.

Smallpox   MS
risk of Infection [spread] possibly evidenced by [contagious nature of organism], inadequate vaccination, (chronic illness, immunosuppression).

deficient Fluid Volume may be related to hypermetabolic state, decreased intake (pharyngeal lesions, nausea), increased losses (vomiting), fluid shifts from vascular bed, possibly evidenced by reports of thirst; decreased blood pressure, venous filling, and urinary output; dry mucous membranes; decreased skin turgor; change in mental state; elevated hematocrit.

impaired Tissue Integrity may be related to immunological deficit, possibly evidenced by disruption of skin surface, cornea, mucous membranes.

                                           CH
interrupted Family Processes may be related to changes in interaction with community, shift in family roles, (situational crisis, shift in health status of family member), possibly evidenced by change in participation for problem-solving, change in family satisfaction, change in stress-reduction behavior, decrease in mutual support.

ineffective community Coping may be related to (exposure to disaster [bioterrorism]), inadequate resources for problem-solving, possibly evidenced by deficient community participation, elevated community illness rate, excessive community conflict, perceived community vulnerability or powerlessness.

Snake bite, venomous   MS
[severe] Anxiety/Fear may be related to (situational crisis), threat of death, possibly evidenced by uncertainty, apprehensiveness, irritability, jitteriness, increase in tension, tremors.

acute Pain/impaired Comfort may be related to effects of toxins [e.g., edema, erythema, nausea, fever, diaphoresis, muscle fasciculations], possibly evidenced by reports of pain and paresthesias, guarded behavior, restlessness, autonomic responses.

impaired Skin Integrity may be related to [snake bite] possibly evidenced by alteration in skin integrity, acute pain, redness.

risk for deficient Fluid Volume possibly evidenced by excessive losses (vomiting, edema formation, hemorrhage from mucous membranes).

Snow blindness   CH
[disturbed visual Sensory Perception] may be related to altered status of sense organ (irritation of the conjunctiva, hyperemia), possibly evidenced by intolerance to light (photophobia) and decreased or loss of visual acuity.

acute Pain may be related to irritation and vascular congestion [conjunctiva], possibly evidenced by verbal reports of pain, guarding or distraction behavior, and self-focused.

Somatoform disorders   PSY
ineffective Coping may be related to inadequate confidence to deal with situation, ineffective tension release strategies, possibly evidenced by inability to deal with situation, insufficient problem resolution/problem-solving skills, insufficient goal directed behavior, frequent illness, destructive behavior toward self, substance misuse.

chronic Pain may be related to alteration in sleep pattern, fatigue, emotional distress [severe level of repressed anxiety], social isolation, possibly evidenced by verbal reports of pain; facial expression of pain, self-focusing, alteration in ability to continue previous activities.

[disturbed Sensory Perception (specify)] may be related to psychological stress (narrowed perceptual fields, expression of stress as physical problems or deficits), poor quality of sleep, presence of chronic pain, possibly evidenced by reported change in voluntary motor or sensory function (paralysis, anosmia, aphonia, deafness, blindness, loss of touch or pain sensation), la belle indifférence (lack of concern over functional loss).

impaired Social Interaction may be related to insufficient knowledge about ways, or skills, to enhance mutuality, communication barriers, sociocultural dissonance, disturbance in thought processes, possibly evidenced by dysfunctional interactions with others, dissatisfaction with social engagement, impaired social functioning, family reports change in interaction.

Spina bifida   PED
Also refer to Paraplegia; Newborn, special needs
bowel Incontinence/Constipation may be related to disruption of nerve innervation, perceptual impairment, reduced activity level, possibly evidenced by inability to evacuate bowel voluntarily, increased abdominal pressure or distention, dry and hard formed stool, change in bowel sounds.

risk for impaired Walking/physical Mobility possibly evidenced by neuromuscular impairment, developmental delay, musculoskeletal impairments—clubfoot, hip dislocation, joint deformities, kyphosis.

risk for decreased intracranial Adaptive Capacity possibly evidenced by structural changes (aqueductal stricture, malformation of brainstem).

risk for Infection possibly evidenced by (increased environmental exposure, invasive procedures, [cerebrospinal fluid leak]).

Spinal cord injury (SCI)   MS/CH
Refer to Paraplegia; Quadriplegia

Splenectomy   MS/CH
Refer to Surgery, general
risk for Infection possibly evidenced by insufficient knowledge to avoid exposure to pathogens and (invasive procedure/surgery, type of anesthesia, immunosuppression).

risk for ineffective Health Management possibly evidenced by length of therapy, economically disadvantaged, perceived benefits.

Spongiform encephalopathy   CH
Refer to Creutzfeldt-Jakob disease

Sprain of ankle or foot   **CH**

acute Pain may be related to physical injury agent—trauma, possibly evidenced by verbal reports of pain, guarding or distraction behavior, self-focused, and changes in vital signs.

impaired Walking may be related to (musculoskeletal injury), pain, and [therapeutic restrictions], possibly evidenced by impaired ability to walk required distance, on uneven surface, or climb stairs.

Sprue, nontropical   **CH**

Refer to Celiac disease

Stapedectomy   **MS**

risk for Trauma possibly evidenced by increased middle-ear pressure with displacement of prosthesis and balancing difficulties, dizziness.

risk for Infection possibly evidenced by (invasive procedure), and environmental exposure to pathogens.

acute Pain may be related to surgical trauma, edema, and [presence of packing], possibly evidenced by verbal reports of pain, guarding or distraction behavior, and self-focused.

Stasis dermatitis   **CH**

Also refer to Venous insufficiency

impaired Skin Integrity may be related to alteration in fluid volume, and (impaired circulation), possibly evidenced by alteration in skin integrity, redness, alteration in pigmentation and sensation.

risk for Infection possibly evidenced by [circulatory stasis, edema formation (small-vessel vasoconstrictive reflexes) in lower extremities, persistent inflammation, tissue destruction].

STI   **CH**

Refer to Sexually transmitted infection

Stillbirth   **OB**

Refer to Perinatal loss/death of child

Stimulant abuse   **CH**

Also refer to Cocaine hydrochloride poisoning, acute; Substance dependence/abuse rehabilitation

imbalanced Nutrition: less than body requirements may be related to insufficient dietary intake, possibly evidenced by [substituting drug for food], food intake less than recommended daily allowance, (economically disadvantaged), [weight loss], insufficient muscle tone, (psychological disorder).

risk for Infection possibly evidenced by altered immune state; malnutrition; (exposure to disease

[e.g., injection techniques, impurities of drugs; tissue trauma].

Insomnia may be related to substance consumption, anxiety/fear, stressors, physical discomfort, possibly evidenced by difficulty initiating sleep, dissatisfaction with sleep, insufficient energy, alteration in concentration, alteration in affect, [denial of need to sleep, racing thoughts].

                             PSY

Fear/Anxiety [specify] may be related to substance misuse; stressors; unmet needs; threat to change in current status, threat of death, (exposure to toxins, situational crisis), possibly evidenced by awareness of physiological symptoms; fear; cardiovascular excitation; increased respiration, restlessness, apprehensiveness, increase in wariness, alteration in sleep pattern.

ineffective Coping may be related to inaccurate threat appraisal/high degree of threat; ineffective tension release strategies; insufficient social support, possibly evidenced by substance misuse; ineffective coping skills; inability to meet basic needs; insufficient access of social support; risk-taking behavior/destructive behavior toward self.

[disturbed Sensory Perception (specify)] may be related to exogenous chemical, altered sensory reception, transmission, or integration (hallucination), altered status of sense organs, possibly evidenced by responding to internal stimuli from hallucinatory experiences, bizarre thinking, anxiety, panic changes in sensory acuity (sense of smell, taste).

Stomatitis   **CH**

impaired oral Mucous Membrane Integrity may be related to [infection], inadequate nutrition [vitamin deficiency], alcohol consumption, smoking, barrier to dental care, mouth breathing, possibly evidenced by oral pain; difficulty eating; oral lesions, ulcers; white patches or plaques in mouth, coated tongue.

risk for deficient Fluid Volume possibly evidenced by oral pain, difficulty swallowing.

Strep throat   **CH**

Hyperthermia may be related to illness and effects of toxins, inability to ingest sufficient fluids, possibly evidenced by body temperature above normal range, flushed dry skin, decreased urine output.

acute Pain may be related to injuring biological agent, possibly evidenced by self-report of pain, change in ability to eat, crying.

risk for Infection [transmission] possibly evidenced by insufficient knowledge to avoid exposure to or transmission of pathogen.

Stress disorder, acute   PSY
Refer to Post-traumatic stress disorder

Substance dependence/abuse, prenatal   OB
imbalanced Nutrition: less than body requirements may be related to insufficient dietary intake, possibly evidenced by [substituting drug for food], anorexia, economically disadvantaged, [low weight gain or weight loss, protein/vitamin deficiencies].

risk for disturbed Maternal-Fetal Dyad possibly evidenced by substance misuse, (treatment regimen).

ineffective Denial/Coping may be related to insufficient sense of control, threat of unpleasant reality, excessive stress, ineffective tension release strategies, possibly evidenced by delay in seeking healthcare, does not admit impact of disease on life, ineffective coping strategies, substance misuse, risk-taking behavior, insufficient access of social support.

Powerlessness may be related to illness [substance addiction], ineffective coping strategies, low self-esteem, social marginalization/stigmatization, possibly evidenced by dependency, inadequate participation in care, insufficient sense of control.

chronic low Self-Esteem may be related to [social stigma attached to substance abuse, social expectation that one controls own behavior, continual negative evaluation of self, personal vulnerabilities], possibly evidenced by [not taking responsibility for self, lack of follow-through, self-destructive behavior, denial that substance use is a problem].

disabled Family Coping may be related to ambivalent family relationships, differing coping styles between support person(s)/client, family disorganization, possibly evidenced by client dependence, distortion of reality about client's health problem, family behaviors detrimental to well-being, neglect of treatment regimen.

Substance dependence/   PSY/CH
abuse rehabilitation
(Following acute detoxification)
ineffective Denial may be related to threat of unpleasant reality, insufficient emotional support, excessive stress, possibly evidenced by does not admit impact of disease on life, delay in seeking healthcare.

Powerlessness may be related to ineffective coping strategies, low self-esteem, social marginalization, stigmatization, possibly evidenced by dependency, insufficient sense of control, doubt about role performance, shame.

imbalanced Nutrition: less than body requirements may be related to insufficient dietary intake, possibly evidenced by food intake less than recommended daily allowance [substituting drug for food], economically disadvantaged, alteration in taste sensation, weight loss, insufficient muscle tone.

Sexual dysfunction may be related to altered body function (neurological damage and debilitating effects of drug use), vulnerability, value conflict, possibly evidenced by alteration in sexual activity/satisfaction, decrease in sexual desire, undesired change in sexual function.

dysfunctional Family Processes may be related to substance misuse, addictive personality, (family history of substance misuse), ineffective coping strategies, insufficient problem-solving skills, possibly evidenced by anger, frustration, self-blame, shame, embarrassment, repressed emotions, guilt, vulnerability, rationalization, controlling communication pattern, manipulation, blaming, enabling substance use pattern, inability to accept or receive help appropriately.

                               OB
risk for fetal Injury possibly evidenced by drug or alcohol use, exposure to teratogens.

deficient Knowledge regarding condition, effects on pregnancy, prognosis, and treatment needs may be related to lack or misinterpretation of information, lack of recall, cognitive limitations, interference with learning, possibly evidenced by statements of concern, questions, misconceptions, inaccurate follow-through of instructions, development of preventable complications, continued use in spite of complications.

Sudden infant death   PED
complicated Grieving may be related to emotional disturbance [unexpected loss of child], possibly evidenced by distress about the deceased person, feeling of emptiness, anger; self-blame, rumination.

risk for impaired Parenting possibly evidenced by recent crisis, change in family unit, maladaptive coping strategies, sleep disruption, depression.

risk for interrupted Family Processes possibly evidenced by situational crisis, loss of a family member.

risk for chronic Sorrow possibly evidenced by death of a loved one, anniversary dates (birth, death, etc.), trigger events (e.g., infants on TV, at play).

Suicide attempt   **MS**

Also refer to specific means, e.g., Drug overdose, acute; Wound, gunshot

PSY

Hopelessness may be related to long-term stress, abandonment, deteriorating physical or mental condition, challenged value or belief system, possibly evidenced by verbal cues, passivity, lack of involvement or withdrawal, angry outbursts.

risk for Suicide possibly evidenced by prior or current attempt, marked changes in behavior, attitude, or performance, impulsiveness, sudden euphoric recovery from major depression, living alone, loss of independence, economic instability, substance abuse, has a plan and available means.

chronic/situational low Self-Esteem may be related to losses, functional impairment, developmental changes, failures or rejection, possibly evidenced by evaluating self as unable to deal with events, expressions of helplessness, uselessness, shame, or guilt; self-negating verbalizations.

compromised family Coping may be related to family disorganization, role changes, prolonged disease or disability, (situational or developmental crises), possibly evidenced by client expressing concern about SO's response to problems, SO confirms ineffective supportive behaviors, SO withdraws from client.

Sunstroke   **MS**

Refer to Heatstroke

Surgery, general   **MS**

Also refer to Postoperative recovery period
deficient Knowledge regarding surgical procedure and expectation, postoperative routines, therapy, and self-care needs may be related to lack of information, misinterpretation, possibly evidenced by statements of concern, questions, and misconceptions.

Anxiety [specify level]/Fear may be related to (situational crisis), unfamiliarity with environment, threat to current status or threat of death and separation from support system, possibly evidenced by increase in tension, apprehensiveness, decreased self-assurance, fear, self-focused, sympathetic stimulation, and restlessness.

risk for perioperative Positioning Injury possibly evidenced by disorientation, immobilization, muscle weakness, obesity, edema.

risk for Injury possibly evidenced by physical factor—wrong client, procedure, site, implants, equipment or materials; interactive conditions between individual and environment; external environment—physical design, structure of environment, exposure to equipment, instrumentation, positioning, use of pharmaceutical agents; internal environment—tissue hypoxia, abnormal blood profile or altered clotting factors, broken skin.

risk for imbalanced Fluid Volume possibly evidenced by preoperative fluid deprivation, blood loss, and excessive gastrointestinal losses—vomiting or gastric suction; inappropriate or rapid replacement.

Syndrome X   **CH**

Refer to Metabolic syndrome

Synovitis (knee)   **CH**

acute Pain may be related to physical agent—inflammation, effusion, possibly evidenced by verbal reports of pain, guarding or distraction behavior, self-focused, and changes in vital signs.

impaired Walking may be related to pain and insufficient [joint] strength, possibly evidenced by impaired ability to walk required distance.

Syphilis, congenital   **PED**

Also refer to Sexually transmitted infection
acute Pain may be related to physical agent—inflammation, edema, and development of skin lesions, possibly evidenced by self-report of pain, expressive/guarding behavior, facial expression of pain, and autonomic responses (changes in vital signs).

impaired Skin/Tissue Integrity may be related to [exposure to pathogens during vaginal delivery] possibly evidenced by alteration in skin integrity/tissue damage.

risk for [disproportionate Growth]/delayed Development] possibly evidenced by congenital disorder, malnutrition, seizure disorder.

deficient Knowledge regarding pathophysiology of condition, transmissibility, therapy needs, expected outcomes, and potential complications may be related to caretaker/parental lack of information, misinterpretation, possibly evidenced by statements of concern, questions, and misconceptions.

Syringomyelia   **MS**

[disturbed Sensory Perception (specify)] may be related to altered sensory perception (neurological lesion), possibly evidenced by change in usual response to stimuli and motor incoordination.

---

impaired physical Mobility may be related to neuromuscular and sensory impairment, possibly evidenced by decreased muscle strength, control, and mass; and impaired coordination.

Self-Care deficit [specify] may be related to neuromuscular and sensory impairments, possibly evidenced by statement of inability to perform care tasks.

Tarsal tunnel syndrome CH

acute/chronic Pain may be related to physical agent—pressure on nerve, possibly evidenced by verbal reports of pain, guarding behavior, alteration in ability to continue previous activities.

impaired Walking may be related to (neuromuscular impairment) and pain, possibly evidenced by impaired ability to walk desired distances, climb stairs, navigate curbs or uneven surfaces.

Tay-Sachs disease PED

risk for delayed Development possibly evidenced by risk factors of genetic disorder, seizure disorder, visual/hearing impairment.

[disturbed visual Sensory Perception] may be related to neurological deterioration of optic nerve, possibly evidenced by loss of visual acuity.

CH

family Grieving may be related to anticipatory loss of significant other [infant/child], possibly evidenced by distress, anger, despair, blaming; alteration in sleep pattern, disorganization.

[family] Powerlessness may be related to (progressive illness, unpredictably of illness trajectory), [absence of therapeutic interventions], possibly evidenced by insufficient sense of control, and depression.

risk for Spiritual distress possibly evidenced by stressors [challenged belief and value system], illness, [anticipated] death.

compromised family Coping may be related to (situational crisis faced by support person), exhaustion of support person's capacity; family disorganization; possibly evidenced by support person reports preoccupations with reaction to client's need, and altered communication patterns.

TBI MS/CH

Refer to Traumatic brain injury

Temporal arteritis CH

acute Pain may be related to physical agent—arterial inflammation, possibly evidenced by reports of pain. facial expression of pain.

[risk for disturbed visual Sensory Perception]: possibly evidenced by altered reception (arterial inflammation, ischemic optic neuropathy).

risk for ineffective Health Management risk factors may include medication side effects, economic difficulties, perceived seriousness or benefits.

Temporomandibular joint syndrome CH

chronic Pain may be related to (chronic musculoskeletal condition), possibly evidenced by reports of pain, self-focused.

risk for imbalanced Nutrition: less than body requirements possibly evidenced by risk factors of inability to ingest food, food intake less than recommended daily allowance, weakness of muscles required for mastication.

[risk for disturbed auditory Sensory Perception] possibly evidenced by altered sensory reception (tinnitus, occasional deafness).

Tendonitis CH

acute/chronic Pain may be related to physical agent—inflammation, swelling of tendon, possibly evidenced by verbal reports of pain, guarding or protective behavior, alteration in ability to continue previous activities.

impaired physical Mobility may be related to pain, joint stiffness, musculoskeletal impairment, prescribed movement restrictions, possibly evidenced by limited range of motion, limited ability to perform fine or gross motor skills.

risk for ineffective Role Performance possibly evidenced by health alterations, fatigue, pain.

Testicular cancer MS

Also refer to Cancer

disturbed Body Image may be related to (surgical procedure), alteration in self-perception, possibly evidenced by negative feeling about body, preoccupation with change, fear of reaction of others, and change in social environment.

Sexual dysfunction may be related to alteration in body structure/function, vulnerability, possibly evidenced by alteration in sexual satisfaction/activity.

Tetanus MS

acute Pain may be related to biological injury agent—neurotoxic bacterium, possibly evidenced by self-report of pain, narrowed focus, facial expression of pain.

bowel/urinary Incontinence may be related to abnormally high abdominal/intestinal pressure possibly evidenced by urgency, inability to delay elimination.

risk for impaired Swallowing possibly evidenced by (neuromuscular impairment).

risk for impaired spontaneous Ventilation possibly evidenced by respiratory muscle fatigue/muscle spasms.

Tetraplegia   MS/CH
Refer to Quadriplegia

Thoracotomy   MS
Refer to Surgery, general; Hemothorax

Thrombophlebitis   CH/MS/OB
ineffective peripheral Tissue Perfusion may be related to interruption of venous blood flow, venous stasis, possibly evidenced by changes in skin color and temperature over affected area, development of edema, pain, diminished peripheral pulses, slow capillary refill.

acute Pain/impaired Comfort may be related to physical agent—vascular inflammation, edema formation, possibly evidenced by self-report, of pain, guarding or distraction behavior, restlessness, and self-focused.

risk for impaired physical Mobility possibly evidenced by pain and discomfort, restrictive therapies, and safety precautions.

deficient Knowledge regarding pathophysiology of condition, therapy, self-care needs, and risk of embolization may be related to lack of information or misinterpretation, possibly evidenced by statements of concern, questions, inaccurate follow-through of instructions, and development of preventable complications.

Thrombosis, venous   MS
Refer to Thrombophlebitis

Thrush   CH
impaired oral Mucous Membrane Integrity may be related to (infection) as evidenced by white patches or plaques, oral discomfort, mucosal irritation, bleeding.

risk for imbalanced Nutrition: less than body requirements possibly evidenced by inability to ingest food, food aversion.

Thyroidectomy   MS
Also refer to Hyperthyroidism; Hypoparathyroidism (acute), Hypothyroidism
risk for ineffective Airway Clearance possibly evidenced by tracheal obstruction—edema, hematoma formation, laryngeal spasms.

impaired verbal Communication may be related to (physiological condition—tissue edema, pain, vocal cord injury or laryngeal nerve damage), possibly evidenced by difficulty/inability to speak.

risk for Injury [tetany] possibly evidenced by chemical imbalance—hypocalcemia, increased release of thyroid hormones; excessive central nervous system stimulation.

risk for head/neck physical Trauma possibly evidenced by loss of muscle control and support, and position of suture line.

acute Pain may be related to physical injury agent—manipulation of tissues and muscles, postoperative edema; (surgical procedure), possibly evidenced by verbal reports of pain, guarding or distraction behavior, narrowed focus, and autonomic responses—changes in vital signs.

Thyrotoxicosis   MS
Also refer to Hyperthyroidism
risk for decreased Cardiac Output possibly evidenced by uncontrolled hypermetabolic state increasing cardiac workload; changes in venous return and systemic vascular resistance; and alterations in rate, rhythm, and electrical conduction.

Anxiety [specific level] may be related to threat to current status, physiological factors and central nervous system stimulation (hypermetabolic state and pseudocatecholamine effect of thyroid hormones), possibly evidenced by apprehensiveness, uncertainty, alteration in concentration, extraneous movements, restlessness, and tremors.

deficient Knowledge regarding condition, treatment needs, and potential for complications or crisis situation may be related to lack of information or recall, misinterpretation, possibly evidenced by statements of concern, questions, misconceptions, and inaccurate follow-through of instructions.

TIA   CH
Refer to Transient ischemic attack

Tic douloureux   CH
Refer to Neuralgia, trigeminal

TMJ syndrome   CH
Refer to Temporomandibular joint syndrome

Tonsillectomy   PED/MS
Refer to Adenoidectomy

Tonsillitis   PED
acute Pain may be related to biological injury agent [bacteria or virus causing inflammation], possibly

evidenced by verbal reports of pain, guarding or distraction behavior, self-focused, and changes in vital signs.

Hyperthermia may be related to presence of inflammatory process, hypermetabolic state and dehydration, possibly evidenced by increased body temperature; warm, flushed skin; and tachycardia.

deficient Knowledge regarding cause/transmission, treatment needs, and potential complications may be related to lack of information, misinterpretation, possibly evidenced by statements of concern, questions, inaccurate follow-through of instructions, and recurrence of condition.

Total joint replacement   MS
risk for Infection possibly evidenced by alteration in skin integrity, immunosuppression (long-term corticosteroid use), invasive procedures and surgical manipulation, implantation of foreign body, and [decreased mobility].

impaired physical Mobility may be related to pain and discomfort, musculoskeletal impairment, and surgery and restrictive therapies, possibly evidenced by reluctance to attempt movement, difficulty with purposefully moving within the physical environment, reports of pain or discomfort on movement, limited range of motion, and decreased muscle strength and control.

risk for ineffective peripheral Tissue Perfusion possibly evidenced by reduced arterial or venous blood flow, direct trauma to blood vessels, tissue edema, improper location or dislocation of prosthesis, and hypovolemia.

acute Pain may be related to physical injury agents [traumatized tissues, surgical intervention, degeneration of joints, muscle spasms], possibly evidenced by verbal reports of pain, guarding or distraction behavior, self-focused, and changes in vital signs.

risk for Constipation possibly evidenced by decrease in gastrointestinal motility—anesthesia, opiate analgesics; average daily physical activity is less than recommended for gender/age, insufficient fiber or fluid intake, dehydration.

Tourette's syndrome   CH
chronic low Self-Esteem may be related to [inherited disorder], inadequate belonging, inadequate respect from others, possibly evidenced by shame, exaggerated negative feedback about self, hesitancy to try new experiences.

Social Isolation may be related to social behavior incongruent with norms, inability to engage in satisfying personal relationships, possibly evidenced by disabling condition, feeling different from others, withdrawn, history of rejection.

risk for Injury possibly evidenced by adverse side effects of medications, negative response of uneducated individuals.

Toxemia of pregnancy   OB
Refer to Hypertension, gestational

Toxic enterocolitis   PED/MS
Also refer to Colostomy
deficient Fluid Volume may be related to fulminating losses into the bowel, diarrhea, lack of intake evidenced by decreased concentrated urine, dry mucous membranes, poor skin turgor, decreased venous filling, change in mentation.

risk for decreased Cardiac Output possibly evidenced by decreased venous return, altered heart rate and rhythm.

Toxic megacolon   MS
Refer to Toxic enterocolitis

Toxic shock syndrome   MS
Also refer to Sepsis
Hyperthermia may be related to inflammatory process, hypermetabolic state and dehydration, possibly evidenced by increased body temperature; warm, flushed skin; and tachycardia.

deficient Fluid Volume [isotonic] may be related to increased gastric losses (diarrhea, vomiting), fever, hypermetabolic state, and decreased intake, possibly evidenced by dry mucous membranes, increased pulse, hypotension, delayed venous filling, decreased concentrated urine, and hemoconcentration.

acute Pain may be related to biological injury agent—inflammatory process, effects of circulating toxins, possibly evidenced by verbal reports of pain, guarding or distraction behavior, self-focused, and changes in vital signs.

impaired Skin/Tissue Integrity may be related to [effects of circulating toxins and dehydration], possibly evidenced by alteration in skin integrity (desquamating rash), redness, and [inflammation of mucous membranes].

Traction   MS
Also refer to Casts; Fractures
acute Pain may be related to physical injury agent—direct trauma to tissue and bone, muscle spasms, movement of bone fragments, edema, injury to soft

tissue], possibly evidenced by verbal reports of pain, guarding or distraction behavior, self-focused, alteration in muscle tone, and changes in vital signs.

impaired physical Mobility may be related to (neuromuscular and skeletal impairment), pain, and therapeutic restrictions of movement, possibly evidenced by limited range of motion, inability to move purposefully in environment, reluctance to attempt movement, and decreased muscle strength and control.

risk for Infection possibly evidenced by (invasive procedure [including insertion of foreign body through skin and bone]), presence of traumatized tissue, and reduced activity with stasis of body fluids.

decreased Diversional Activity Engagement may be related to length of hospitalization or therapeutic intervention and environmental lack of usual activity, possibly evidenced by statements of boredom, restlessness, and irritability.

Transfusion reaction, blood   MS
Also refer to Anaphylaxis
risk for imbalanced Body Temperature possibly evidenced by infusion of cold blood products, systemic response to toxins.

risk for impaired Skin Integrity possibly evidenced by (immunodeficiency).

Transient ischemic attack   CH
ineffective cerebral Tissue Perfusion may be related to interruption of blood flow (e.g., vasospasm), possibly evidenced by altered mental status, behavioral changes, language deficit, change in motor and sensory response.

Anxiety [specify level]/Fear may be related to threat to current status, stressors, (situational crisis), possibly evidenced by apprehensiveness, restlessness, irritability, self-focused.

risk for ineffective Denial possibly evidenced by change in health status requiring change in lifestyle, fear of consequences, lack of motivation.

Transplant, living donor   MS
Also refer to Surgery, general; Nephrectomy
Decisional Conflict may be related to conflicting information sources, conflict with moral obligation, possibly evidenced by vacillating among choices, recognizes undesired consequences of actions being considered, delay in decision making.

[moderate to severe] Anxiety/Fear may be related to (situational crisis), unconscious conflict

about essential beliefs or values, threat to current status or death, possibly evidenced by apprehensiveness, uncertainty, increase in tension, fear, sympathetic stimulation.

Transplantation, recipient   MS
Also refer to Surgery, general; Cardiac surgery
Anxiety [specify level]/Fear may be related to threat of current status, value conflict, (situational crisis), possibly evidenced by increase in tension, apprehensiveness, uncertainty, fear, sympathetic stimulation, insomnia.

risk for Infection possibly evidenced by (chronic illness, medically induced immunosuppression, suppressed inflammatory response, invasive procedures).

(Refer to specific conditions relative to compromise or failure of individual transplanted organ, e.g., Renal failure, acute; Heart failure, chronic; Pancreatitis.)

CH

compromised family Coping may be related to coexisting situations affecting the support person, exhaustion of support person's capacity, family disorganization or role changes, possibly evidenced by assistive behaviors by support person produce unsatisfactory results, protective behavior by support person incongruent with client's abilities/need for autonomy, support person reports preoccupation with own reaction to client's need.

ineffective Protection may be related to treatment regimen/pharmaceutical agents, compromised immune system possibly evidenced by weakness, maladaptive stress response.

readiness for enhanced Health Management possibly evidenced by expresses desire to enhance management of illness/prescribed regimens and management of risk factors.

risk for ineffective Health Management possibly evidenced by difficulty managing complex treatment regimen, navigating complex healthcare systems, (economically disadvantaged.

Transurethral resection of prostate   MS
Refer to Prostatectomy

Traumatic brain injury (TBI)   MS
ineffective cerebral Tissue Perfusion may be related to (brain injury), [interruption of blood flow], possibly evidenced by altered level of consciousness, memory loss, changes in motor or sensory responses, restlessness, changes in vital signs.

risk for decreased intracranial Adaptive Capacity possibly evidenced by brain injuries, systemic hypotension with intracranial hypertension.

risk for ineffective Breathing Pattern possibly evidenced byneuromuscular dysfunction—injury to respiratory center of brain; perception or cognitive impairment, tracheobronchial obstruction.

[disturbed Sensory Perception (specify)] may be related to altered sensory reception, transmission or integration (neurological trauma or deficit), possibly evidenced by disorientation to time, place, person; motor incoordination; altered communication patterns; restlessness or irritability; change in behavior pattern.

risk for Infection possibly evidenced by alteration in skin integrity/traumatized tissues, (invasive procedures, decreased ciliary action), stasis of body fluids, nutritional deficits, (suppressed inflammatory response).

risk for imbalanced Nutrition: less than body requirements possibly evidenced by food intake less than recommended daily allowance, altered ability to ingest food, weakness of muscles required for chewing or swallowing.

CH

impaired physical Mobility may be related to alteration in cognitive functioning, sensory-perceptual impairment, decrease in muscle strength or endurance, possibly evidenced by uncoordinated movement, decrease in range of motion, decrease in fine/gross motor skills.

risk for impaired Memory/chronic Confusion possibly evidenced by head injury, neurological disturbances.

interrupted Family Processes may be related to (situational transition and crisis, shift in health status of a family member), shift in family roles, possibly evidenced by change in family satisfaction, change in stress-reduction behavior, decrease in mutual support, change in communication pattern.

Self-Care deficit (specify) may be related to (neuromuscular or musculoskeletal impairment), weakness, pain, (perceptual disorder, alteration in cognitive functioning), possibly evidenced by inability to perform desired or appropriate activities of daily living.

Trench foot   MS
Refer to Immersion foot

Trichinosis   CH
acute Pain may be related to biological injury agent—parasitic invasion of intestines migrating to muscle tissues, edema of upper eyelids, small localized hemorrhages, and development of urticaria], possibly evidenced by verbal reports of pain, guarding/distraction behavior, restlessness, and changes in vital signs.

deficient Fluid Volume may be related to hypermetabolic state (fever, diaphoresis); excessive gastric losses (vomiting, diarrhea); and decreased intake and difficulty swallowing, possibly evidenced by dry mucous membranes, decreased skin turgor, hypotension, decreased venous filling, decreased concentrated urine, and hemoconcentration.

ineffective Breathing Pattern may be related to myositis of the diaphragm and intercostal muscles, possibly evidenced by resulting changes in respiratory depth, tachypnea, dyspnea, and abnormal arterial blood gases.

deficient Knowledge regarding cause, prevention of condition, therapy needs, and possible complications may be related to lack of information, misinterpretation, possibly evidenced by statements of concern, questions, and misconceptions.

Tricuspid insufficiency   CH
Refer to Valvular heart disease

Tricuspid stenosis   CH
Refer to Valvular heart disease

Tubal pregnancy   OB
Refer to Ectopic pregnancy (tubal)

Tuberculosis (pulmonary)   CH
risk for Infection [spread/reactivation] possibly evidenced by status of body fluids (secretions), inadequate vaccination, (decrease in ciliary action, immunosuppression, chronic illness), insufficient knowledge to avoid exposure to pathogens [inadequate therapeutic intervention].

ineffective Airway Clearance may be related to (infection), excessive mucus, retained secretions, possibly evidenced by alteration in respiratory rate/pattern, excessive sputum, ineffective cough, adventitious breath sounds, and dyspnea.

risk for impaired Gas Exchange possibly evidenced by ventilation-perfusion imbalance—[decrease in effective lung surface; atelectasis; destruction of alveolar-capillary membrane].

Activity Intolerance may be related to imbalance between oxygen supply and demand, possibly evidenced by reports of fatigue, weakness, and exertional dyspnea.

*imbalanced Nutrition: less than body require-
ments* may be related to insufficient dietary intake,
(economically disadvantaged), possibly evidenced by
[weight loss], insufficient interest in food, or alteration
in taste sensation, and insufficient muscle tone.

risk for ineffective Health Management possibly evidenced by complexity of therapeutic regimen,
economic difficulties, family patterns of healthcare,
perceived seriousness or benefits (especially during
remission), side effects of therapy.

TURP   MS
Refer to Prostatectomy

Twin-twin transfusion syndrome   OB
decreased Cardiac Output may be related to altered
preload (hypovolemia, anemia) to donor fetus, possibly
evidenced by oliguria, oligohydramnios.

excess Fluid Volume may be related to excess
fluid intake (shunting of circulation) to recipient fetus,
possibly evidenced by polyuria, polyhydramnios.

[risk for disproportionate Growth] possibly evidenced multiple gestation with imbalanced circulation
and nutrition to both fetuses.

Tympanoplasty   MS
Refer to Stapedectomy

Typhoid fever   MS
Also refer to Sepsis
risk for Infection [spread] possibly evidenced by inadequate knowledge to avoid exposure to pathogen (food
or water, fecally contaminated objects).

risk for deficient Fluid Volume possibly evidenced by gastric irritation, ulcers.

*imbalanced Nutrition: less than body require-
ments* possibly evidenced by insufficient dietary intake,
(inability to ingest or digest foods, or absorb nutrients);
possibly evidenced by insufficient interest in food,
food intake less than recommended daily allowance,
abdominal pain, [weight loss].

Typhus   CH/MS
Hyperthermia may be related to generalized inflammatory process (vasculitis), possibly evidenced by
increased body temperature, warm flushed skin, and
tachycardia.

ineffective Tissue Perfusion (specify) may be
related to reduction or interruption of blood flow—
generalized vasculitis or thrombi formation, possibly
evidenced by reports of headache, abdominal pain,

changes in mentation, and areas of peripheral ulceration or necrosis.

Ulcer, decubitus   CH/MS
impaired Skin/Tissue Integrity may be related to excretions, secretions, pressure over bony prominence, alteration in fluid volume, inadequate nutrition, [impaired
physical mobility][and sensory impairments] evidenced by [tissue damage or destruction].

acute Pain may be related to physical agent—
tissue trauma, inflammation, infection, dressing
changes/débridement, possibly evidenced by verbal
reports, distraction behaviors, and self-focus.

risk for Infection possibly evidenced by malnutrition, alteration in skin/tissue integrity, and associated conditions of chronic illness, immunosuppression
[immobility, increased environmental exposure].

Ulcer, peptic (acute)   MS/CH
risk for Shock possibly evidenced by hypovolemia,
hypotension.

acute Pain may be related to physical agent—
caustic irritation and destruction of gastric or duodenal
tissues, reflex muscle spasms in stomach wall possibly
evidenced by verbal reports of pain, distraction behavior, self-focused, and changes in vital signs.

*deficient Knowledge regarding condition, ther-
apy, self-care needs, and potential complications* may
be related to lack of information or recall, misinterpretation, possibly evidenced by statements of concern,
questions, misconceptions; inaccurate follow-through
of instructions; and development of preventable complications or recurrence of condition.

Ulcer, pressure   CH/MS
Refer to Ulcer, decubitus

Ulcer, venous stasis   CH
Also refer to Venous insufficiency
impaired Skin/Tissue Integrity may be related to
(impaired [venous] circulation, alteration in sensation), possibly evidenced by destruction of skin layers,
invasion of body structures.

ineffective peripheral Tissue Perfusion may be
related to interruption of venous flow—small-vessel
vasoconstrictive reflex, possibly evidenced by skin
discoloration, edema formation, altered sensation,
delayed healing.

Ulnar neuropathy   CH
Refer to Cubital tunnel syndrome

Unconsciousness   **MS**
Refer to Coma

Upper GI bleeding   **MS**
Refer to Gastritis, acute or chronic; Ulcer, peptic

Urinary diversion   **MS/CH**
risk for impaired Skin Integrity possibly evidenced by excreations—character and flow of urine from stoma, chemical injury agent—reaction to adhesive product, and improperly fitting appliance.

disturbed Body Image may be related to alteration in self-perception; and psychosocial factors—disease process and associated treatment regimen, possibly evidenced by verbalization of change in body image, fear of reaction of others, negative feelings about body, not touching or looking at stoma, refusal to participate in care.

acute Pain may be related to physical injury agents (disruption of skin and tissues, presence of incisions and drains); biological factors—activity of disease process; and psychological factors—fear, anxiety, possibly evidenced by verbal reports of pain, self-focused, guarding or distraction behavior, restlessness, and autonomic responses—changes in vital signs.

impaired urinary Elimination may be related to surgical diversion, tissue trauma, and postoperative edema, possibly evidenced by loss of continence, changes in amount and character of urine, and urinary retention.

Urinary tract infection   **CH**
Refer to Cystitis

Urolithiasis   **MS/CH**
Refer to Calculi, urinary

Uterine bleeding, dysfunctional   **GYN/MS**
Anxiety [specify level] may be related to threat to change in status and unknown etiology, possibly evidenced by apprehensiveness, uncertainty, fear, expressed concerns, and self-focused.

Activity Intolerance may be related to imbalance between oxygen supply and demand (anemia), possibly evidenced by reports of fatigue, weakness.

Uterine myomas (also called fibroids)   **GYN**
Also refer to Anemia
acute Pain/impaired Comfort may be related to physical agent—growth, size, and location of tumors, possibly evidenced by reports of pressure, cramping, guarding behavior, irritability.

impaired urinary Elimination may be related to uterine pressure on bladder, possibly evidenced by frequent voiding, urinary urgency.

risk for deficient Fluid Volume possibly evidenced by excessive or chronic blood loss.

Uterus, rupture of, in pregnancy   **OB**
risk for Shock possibly evidenced by hypovolemia, hypotension.

acute Pain may be related to physical agent—tissue trauma and irritation of accumulating blood, possibly evidenced by verbal reports of pain, guarding or distraction behavior, self-focused, and autonomic responses—changes in vital signs.

Anxiety [specify level] may be related to threat of death of self/fetus, interpersonal contagion, physiological response—release of catecholamines, possibly evidenced by fearful or scared affect, sympathetic stimulation, fear, and expressed concerns.

UTI   **CH**
Refer to Cystitis

Vaginal hysterectomy   **MS**
Refer to Hysterectomy

Vaginismus   **GYN/PSY**
acute Pain may be related to biological or psychological injury agent [when something is entering the vagina (such as object or penis)], possibly evidenced by verbal reports of pain, expressive or distraction behavior, positioning to relieve pain, and self-focused.

Sexual dysfunction may be related to physical or psychological alteration in function (severe spasms of vaginal muscles), possibly evidenced by verbalization of problem, inability to achieve desired satisfaction, and alteration in relationship with SO.

Vaginitis   **GYN/CH**
impaired Tissue Integrity may be related to irritation or inflammation and mechanical trauma (scratching) of sensitive tissues, possibly evidenced by damaged or destroyed tissue, presence of lesions.

acute Pain may be related to biological agent inflammation/tissue trauma; chemical injury agent [e.g., bacterial, viral, fungal, chemicals in soaps, sprays, or clothing], possibly evidenced by verbal reports of pain, distraction behavior, and self-focused.

deficient Knowledge regarding hygienic needs, therapy, and sexual behaviors or transmission of organisms may be related to lack of information, misinterpretation, possibly evidenced by statements of concern, questions, and misconceptions.

Vaginosis, bacterial GYN
risk for impaired *Tissue Integrity* possibly evidenced by (alteration in sensation-vulvar or vaginal irritation, itching).

risk for *[secondary] Infection* possibly evidenced by prescribed antibiotic therapy, insufficient knowledge to avoid exposure to pathogens.

Valvular heart disease MS
decreased *Cardiac Output* may be related to alteration in preload, increased arterial pressure and venous congestion, increased afterload, changes in electrical conduction, possibly evidenced by variations in hemodynamic parameters, dysrhythmias and electrocardiogram changes, dyspnea, adventitious breath sounds, cyanosis or pallor, jugular vein distention, fatigue.

Activity Intolerance may be related to imbalance between oxygen supply and demand (decreased or fixed cardiac output), possibly evidenced by reports of fatigue, generalized weakness, abnormal heart rate and blood pressure in response to activity, exertional discomfort or dyspnea.

Anxiety may be related to threat to change in current status (chronicity of disease), physiological effects, situational crisis (changes in lifestyle, hospitalization), possibly evidenced by expressed concerns, increased tension, apprehension, uncertainty, sympathetic stimulation, insomnia.

risk for excess *Fluid Volume* possibly evidenced by increased sodium and water retention, changes in glomerular filtration.

risk for ineffective *Tissue Perfusion (specify)* possibly evidenced by interruption of arterial-venous flow (systemic emboli), venous thrombosis (venous stasis, decreased activity).

VAP MS/CH
Refer to Ventilator assist/dependence; Bronchopneumonia

Varices, esophageal MS
Also refer to Ulcer, peptic (acute)
risk for *Bleeding/deficient Fluid Volume* possibly evidenced by (impaired liver function), [presence of varices, reduced intake, and gastric losses—vomiting; vascular loss].

Anxiety [specify level]/Fear may be related to change in current status and threat of death], possibly evidenced by increase in tension, apprehensiveness, sympathetic stimulation, restlessness, self-focused and expressed concerns.

Varicose veins CH
chronic *Pain* may be related to venous insufficiency and stasis, possibly evidenced by verbal reports.

disturbed *Body Image* may be related to change in structure (presence of enlarged, discolored tortuous superficial leg veins), possibly evidenced by hiding affected parts and negative feelings about body.

risk for impaired *Skin/Tissue Integrity* may be related to (impaired circulation, [venous stasis, and edema formation]).

Varicose veins ligation/stripping MS
risk for ineffective peripheral *Tissue Perfusion* possibly evidenced by localized edema, vascular irritation, inadequate venous return, dressings.

impaired *Skin Integrity* may be related to [surgical procedure, pressure dressings, tissue edema, vascular engorgement], possibly evidenced by [incisions, development of complications (e.g., ulcerations)].

Varicose veins sclerotherapy MS
risk for impaired *Skin Integrity* possibly evidenced by risk factors of [extravasation of sclerosing agent].

risk for ineffective *Health Management* possibly evidenced by perceived seriousness or benefit, required lifestyle and activity changes, postprocedure dressings.

Variola MS
Refer to Smallpox

Vasculitis CH
Refer to Polyarteritis nodosa; Temporal arteritis

Vasectomy CH/MS
acute *Pain/impaired Comfort* may be related to physical injury agent [surgical manipulation of delicate tissues, edema/hematoma formation], possibly evidenced by verbal reports, guarding behavior, irritability.

deficient *Knowledge regarding self-care and future expectations (issues of reproduction, safety/sexually transmitted diseases)* may be related to information misinterpretation, lack of recall, possibly evidenced by verbalizations, misconceptions, inaccurate follow-through of instructions.

Venereal disease CH
Refer to Sexually transmitted infection

Venous insufficiency   CH

Also refer to Stasis dermatitis; Ulcer, venous stasis

chronic *Pain/impaired Comfort* may be related to altered venous circulation, edema formation, possibly evidenced by reports of aching, fullness, tiredness of lower extremities with activity.

risk for risk-prone Health Behavior possibly evidenced by health status requiring change in lifestyle, lack of motivation to change behaviors.

risk for ineffective Health Management possibly evidenced by economic difficulties, perceived seriousness or benefit, social support deficit.

Ventilator assist/dependence   MS/CH

ineffective Breathing Pattern/impaired spontaneous Ventilation may be related to neuromuscular dysfunction, respiratory muscle fatigue, spinal cord injury, hypoventilation syndrome, possibly evidenced by dyspnea, increased work of breathing/use of accessory muscles, reduced vital capacity and total lung volume, changes in respiratory rate, decreased Po_2/Sao_2, increased Pco_2.

ineffective Airway Clearance may be related to artificial airway in trachea, inability to or ineffective cough, possibly evidenced by changes in rate and depth of respirations, abnormal breath sounds, anxiety, restlessness, cyanosis.

impaired verbal Communication may be related to physical barrier (artificial airway), neuromuscular weakness or paralysis, possibly evidenced by inability to speak.

Fear/Anxiety [specify] may be related to threat of death or dependency on machine, change in health status or role functioning, possibly evidenced by hypervigilance, restlessness, fearfulness, apprehension, expressed concerns, insomnia, negative self-talk.

risk for impaired oral Mucous Membrane possibly evidenced by inability to swallow oral fluids, decreased salivation, ineffective oral hygiene, presence of endotracheal tube in mouth.

risk for imbalanced Nutrition: less than body requirements possibly evidenced by inability to ingest nutrients, increased metabolic demands.

risk for dysfunctional Ventilatory Weaning Response possibly evidenced by limited or insufficient energy stores, sleep disturbance, pain or discomfort, perceived inability to wean, decreased motivation, inadequate support or adverse environment, history of ventilator dependence greater than 1 week or unsuccessful weaning attempts.

Ventricular fibrillation   MS

Also refer to Dysrhythmia, cardiac

decreased Cardiac Output may be related to altered electrical conduction and reduced myocardial contractility, possibly evidenced by absence of measurable cardiac output, loss of consciousness, no palpable pulses.

Ventricular tachycardia   MS

Also refer to Dysrhythmia, cardiac

risk for decreased Cardiac Output possibly evidenced by alteration in heart rhythm, altered contractility.

Vertigo   CH

[disturbed kinesthetic Sensory Perception] may be related to altered status of sensory organ (middle or inner ear), altered sensory integration, possibly evidenced by visual distortions, altered sense of balance, falls.

risk for Falls possibly evidenced by presence of postural hypotension, acute illness, medications, substance abuse.

West Nile Fever   CH/MS

Hyperthermia may be related to infectious process, possibly evidenced by elevated body temperature, skin flushed and warm to touch, tachycardia, increased respiratory rate.

acute Pain may be related to biological injury agent [virus, circulating toxins] possibly evidenced by reports of headache, myalgia, eye pain, abdominal discomfort.

risk for deficient Fluid Volume possibly evidenced by hypermetabolic state, decreased intake, anorexia, nausea, losses from normal routes (vomiting, diarrhea).

risk for impaired Skin Integrity possibly evidenced by hyperthermia (circulating toxins) and associated conditions of alteration in fluid volume and skin turgor.

Whooping cough   PED

Refer to Pertussis

Wilms' tumor   PED

Also refer to Cancer; Chemotherapy

Anxiety [specify level]/Fear may be related to stressors (e.g., change in environment and interaction patterns with family members and threat of death), possibly evidenced by fearful/scared affect, distress, crying, insomnia, and sympathetic stimulation.

risk for Injury possibly evidenced by nature of tumor (vascular, mushy with very thin covering) with increased danger of metastasis when manipulated.

interrupted Family Processes may be related to situational crisis of life-threatening illness, possibly evidenced by a family system that has difficulty meeting physical, emotional, and spiritual needs of its members, and inability to deal with traumatic experience effectively.

decreased Diversional Activity Engagement may be related to environmental lack of age-appropriate activity (including activity restrictions) and length of hospitalization or treatment, possibly evidenced by restlessness, crying, lethargy, and acting-out behavior.

Withdrawal, drugs/alcohol   CH/MS
Refer to Alcohol intoxication, acute; Drug overdose, acute (depressants); Drug withdrawal

Wound, gunshot   MS
(Depends on site and speed/character of bullet.)
risk for Bleeding/deficient Fluid Volume possibly evidenced by (trauma), [vascular losses, restricted oral intake].

acute Pain may be related to physical injury agent [causing destruction of tissue (including organ and musculoskeletal), surgical repair, and therapeutic interventions] possibly evidenced by verbal reports, guarding or distraction behaviors, self-focus, and changes in vital signs.

impaired Tissue Integrity may be related to [mechanical factors—yaw of projectile and muzzle blast], possibly evidenced by damaged or destroyed tissue.

risk for Infection possibly evidenced by alteration in skin/tissue integrity and associated conditions of [increased environmental exposure] invasive procedures, and decreased hemoglobin.

CH

risk for Post-Trauma Syndrome possibly evidenced by risk factors of nature of incident (catastrophic accident, assault, suicide attempt) and possibly injury or death of other(s) involved.

Zollinger-Ellison syndrome   MS/CH
Also refer to Ulcer, peptic
Diarrhea may be related to intestinal irritation—hypersecretion of gastric acid, possibly evidenced by at least three loose liquid stools per day, abdominal pain, change in bowel sounds.

risk for impaired Skin/Tissue Integrity possibly evidenced by excreations, [esophageal regurgitation].

acute/chronic Pain may be related to physical agent (acidic irritation of esophageal mucosa [GERD]), muscle spasm, possibly evidenced by reports of heartburn, distraction behaviors.

risk for ineffective Health Management possibly evidenced by length of therapy, economic difficulties, perceived susceptibility.

APPENDIX A

NANDA-I's Taxonomy II

The 13 domains and their classes are as follows:

Domain 1 Health Promotion: The awareness of well-being or normality of function and the strategies used to maintain control of and enhance that well-being or normality of function

Class 1 Health Awareness: Recognition of normal function and well-being

Class 2 Health Management: Identifying, controlling, performing, and integrating activities to maintain health and well-being

Domain 2 Nutrition: The activities of taking in, assimilating, and using nutrients for the purposes of tissue maintenance, tissue repair, and the production of energy

Class 1 Ingestion: Taking food or nutrients into the body

Class 2 Digestion: The physical and chemical activities that convert foodstuffs into substances suitable for absorption and assimilation

Class 3 Absorption: The act of taking up nutrients through body tissues

Class 4 Metabolism: The chemical and physical processes occurring in living organisms and cells for the development and use of protoplasm, the production of waste and energy, with the release of energy for all vital processes

Class 5 Hydration: The taking in and absorption of fluids and electrolytes

Domain 3 Elimination and Exchange: Secretion and excretion of waste products from the body

Class 1 Urinary Function: The process of secretion, reabsorption, and excretion of urine

Class 2 Gastrointestinal Function: The process of absorption and excretion of the end products of digestion

Class 3 Integumentary Function: The process of secretion and excretion through the skin

Class 4 Respiratory Function: The process of exchange of gases and removal of the end products of metabolism

Domain 4 Activity/Rest: The production, conservation, expenditure, or balance of energy resources

Class 1 Sleep/Rest: Slumber, repose, ease, relaxation, or inactivity

Class 2 Activity/Exercise: Moving parts of the body (mobility), doing work, or performing actions often (but not always) against resistance

Class 3 Energy Balance: A dynamic state of harmony between intake and expenditure of resources

Class 4 Cardiovascular/Pulmonary Responses: Cardiopulmonary mechanisms that support activity/rest

Class 5 Self-Care: Ability to perform activities to care for one's body and bodily functions

Domain 5 Perception/Cognition: The human processing system including attention, orientation, sensation, perception, cognition, and communication

Class 1 Attention: Mental readiness to notice or observe

Class 2 Orientation: Awareness of time, place, and person

Class 3 Sensation/Perception: Receiving information through the senses of touch, taste, smell, vision, hearing, and kinesthesia and the comprehension of sensory data resulting in naming, associating, and/or pattern recognition

Class 4 Cognition: Use of memory, learning, thinking, problem-solving, abstraction, judgment, insight, intellectual capacity, calculation, and language

Class 5 Communication: Sending and receiving verbal and nonverbal information

Domain 6 Self-Perception: Awareness about the self

Class 1 Self-Concept: The perception(s) about the total self

Class 2 Self-Esteem: Assessment of one's own worth, capability, significance, and success

Class 3 Body Image: A mental image of one's own body

Domain 7 Role Relationships: The positive and negative connections or associations between people or groups of people and the means by which those connections are demonstrated

Class 1 Caregiving Roles: Socially expected behavior patterns by people providing care who are not healthcare professionals

Class 2 Family Relationships: Associations of people who are biologically related or related by choice

Class 3 Role Performance: Quality of functioning in socially expected behavior patterns

Domain 8 Sexuality: Sexual identity, sexual function, and reproduction

Class 1 Sexual Identity: The state of being a specific person in regard to sexuality and/or gender

Class 2 Sexual Function: The capacity or ability to participate in sexual activities

Class 3 Reproduction: Any process by which human beings are produced

Domain 9 Coping/Stress Tolerance: Contending with life events/life processes

Class 1 Post-trauma Responses: Reactions occurring after physical or psychological trauma

Class 2 Coping Responses: The process of managing environmental stress

Class 3 Neurobehavioral Stress: Behavioral responses reflecting nerve and brain function

Domain 10 Life Principles: Principles underlying conduct, thought, and behavior about acts, customs, or institutions viewed as being true or having intrinsic worth

Class 1 Values: The identification and ranking of preferred modes of conduct or end states

Class 2 Beliefs: Opinions, expectations, or judgments about acts, customs, or institutions viewed as being true or having intrinsic worth

Class 3 Value/Belief/Action Congruence: The correspondence or balance achieved among values, beliefs, and actions

Domain 11 Safety/Protection: Freedom from danger, physical injury, or immune system damage; preservation from loss; and protection of safety and security

Class 1 Infection: Host responses following pathogenic invasion

Class 2 Physical Injury: Bodily harm or hurt

Class 3 Violence: The exertion of excessive force or power so as to cause injury or abuse

Class 4 Environmental Hazards: Sources of danger in the surroundings

Class 5 Defensive Processes: The processes by which the self protects itself from the non-self

Class 6 Thermoregulation: The physiological process of regulating heat and energy within the body for purposes of protecting the organism

Domain 12 Comfort: Sense of mental, physical, or social well-being or ease

Class 1 Physical Comfort: Sense of well-being or ease and/or freedom from pain

Class 2 Environmental Comfort: Sense of well-being or ease in/with one's environment

Class 3 Social Comfort: Sense of well-being or ease with one's social situation

Domain 13 Growth/Development: Age-appropriate increases in physical dimensions, maturation of organ systems, and/or progression through the developmental milestones

Class 1 Growth: Increases in physical dimensions or maturity of organ systems

Class 2 Development: Progression or regression through a sequence of recognized milestones in life

APPENDIX B

Definitions of Taxonomy II Axes

AXIS 1 FOCUS OF THE DIAGNOSIS: The principal element or the fundamental and essential part, the root, of the diagnostic concept

AXIS 2 SUBJECT OF THE DIAGNOSIS: The subject of the diagnosis. Values are:

Individual: A single human being distinct from others, a person

Caregiver: A family member or helper who regularly looks after a child or sick, elderly, or disabled person

Family: Two or more people having continuous or sustained relationships, perceiving reciprocal obligations, sensing common meaning, and sharing certain obligations toward others; related by blood and/or choice

Group: A number of people with shared characteristics

Community: A group of people living in the same locale under the same governance; e.g., neighborhoods and cities

When the unit of care is not explicitly stated, it becomes the individual by default

AXIS 3 JUDGMENT: A descriptor or modifier that limits or specifies the meaning of the focus of the diagnosis. Values are:

Complicated: Consisting of many interconnecting parts or elements; intricate; involving many different and confusing aspects

Compromised: Made vulnerable or to function less effectively

Decreased: Smaller or fewer in size, amount, intensity, or degree

Defensive: Used or intended to defend or protect

Deficient/Deficit: Not having enough of a specified quality or ingredient; insufficient or inadequate

Delayed: Late, slow, or postponed

Deprivation: Lack or denial of something considered to be a necessity

Disabled: Limited in movements, senses, or activities

Disorganized: Not properly planned or controlled; scattered or inefficient

Disproportionate: Too large or too small in comparison with something else (norm)

Disturbed: Having had its normal pattern or function disrupted

Dysfunctional: Not operating normally or properly; unable to deal adequately with social norms

Emancipated: Free from legal, social, or political restrictions; liberated

Effective: Successful in producing a desired or intended result

Enhanced: Intensify, increase, or further improve the quality, value, or extent

Excess: An amount of something that is more than necessary, permitted, or desirable

Failure: The action or state of not functioning; lack of success

Frail: Weak and delicate; physically or mentally infirm through old age

Functional: Relating to the way in which something works or operates; of or having a specific activity, purpose, or task

Imbalanced: Lack of proportion or relation between corresponding things

Impaired: Weakened or damaged (something, especially a faculty or function)

Ineffective: Not producing any significant or desired effect

Insufficient: Not enough, inadequate, incapable, incompetent

Interrupted: A stop in continuous progress (of an activity or process); to break the continuity of something

Labile: Liable to change; easily altered; of or characterized by emotions which are easily aroused, freely expressed, and tend to alter quickly and spontaneously

Low: Below average in amount, extent, or intensity; small

Non-: expressing negation or absence

Organized: Arranged or structured in a systematic way; efficient

Overload: Too great a burden

Perceived: Become aware or conscious (of something); come to realize or understand

Readiness for: Willingness to do something; state of being fully prepared for something

Risk for: Situation involving exposure to danger, possibility that something unpleasant or unwelcome will happen

Risk-prone: Likely or liable to suffer from, do, or experience something unpleasant or regrettable

Sedentary: (A way of life) characterized by much sitting and little physical exercise

Situational: Related to or dependant on a set of circumstances or state of affairs; relating to the location and surroundings of a place

Unstable: Prone to change, fail; not firmly established; likely to give way; not stable

AXIS 4 LOCATION: Describes the parts/regions of the body and/or their related functions—all tissues, organs, anatomical sites or structures. Values are:

Auditory	*Corneal*
Bladder	*Dentition*
Body	*Eye*
Bowel	*Gastrointestinal*
Breast	
Cardiac	*Genital*
Cardiopulmonary	*Gustatory*
Cardiovascular	*Intracranial*
Cerebral	*Kinesthetic*

Liver	*Skin*
Mouth	*Tactile*
Mucous membranes	*Tissue*
Neurovascular	*Urinary*
Olfactory	*Urinary tract*
Oral	*Vascular*
Peripheral	*Venous*
Peripheral vascular	*Visual*
Renal	

AXIS 5 AGE: The age of the person who is the subject of the diagnosis. Values are:

Fetus: Unborn human more than 8 weeks after conception, until birth

Neonate: Person <28 days of age

Infant: Person ≥28 days and <1 year of age

Child: Person aged 1 to 9 years, inclusive

Adolescent: Person aged 10 to 19 years, inclusive

Adult: Person older than 19 years of age unless national law defines a person as being an adult at an earlier age

Older adult: A person ≥65 years of age

AXIS 6 TIME: The duration of the focus of the diagnosis. Values are:

Acute: Lasting <3 months

Chronic: Lasting ≥3 months

Continuous: Uninterrupted, going on without stop

Intermittent: Stopping or starting again at intervals, periodic, cyclic

AXIS 7 STATUS OF THE DIAGNOSIS: The actuality or potentiality of the problem/health promotion opportunity/syndrome or to the categorization of the diagnosis as a health promotion diagnosis. Values are:

Problem-Focused: Undesirable human response to health conditions/life process that exists in the current moment (includes syndrome diagnoses)

Health Promotion: Motivation and desire to increase well-being and to actualize human health potential that exists in the current moment (Pender, Murdaugh, & Parsons, 2006)

Risk: Susceptibility for developing in the future an undesirable human response to health conditions/life processes (includes syndrome diagnoses)

Pender, N. J., Murdaugh, C. L., & Parsons, M. A. (2006). *Health Principles in Nursing Practice.* 5th ed. Upper Saddle River, NJ: Pearson Prentice-Hall.

Permission from NANDA International. (2018). *NANDA-I Nursing Diagnoses: Definitions & Classification 2018–2020.* New York: Thieme.

APPENDIX C

NANDA-I Nursing Diagnoses Organized According to Maslow's Hierarchy of Needs

SELF-ACTUALIZATION

Coping, readiness for enhanced
Coping, readiness for enhanced community
Coping, readiness for enhanced family
Decision-Making, readiness for enhanced
Development, risk for delayed
Emancipated Decision-Making, impaired
Emancipated Decision-Making, readiness for enhanced

Emancipated Decision-Making, risk for impaired
Health Literacy, readiness for enhanced
Hope, readiness for enhanced
Knowledge, readiness for enhanced
Power, readiness for enhanced
Religiosity, readiness for enhanced
Self-Concept, readiness for enhanced
Spiritual Well-Being, readiness for enhanced

SELF-ESTEEM

Body Image, disturbed
Coping, defensive
Coping, ineffective
Decisional Conflict
Denial, ineffective
Diversional Activity Engagement, decreased
Emotional Control, labile
Human Dignity, risk for compromised
Hopelessness
Impulse Control, ineffective
Moral Distress
Mood Regulation, impaired
Obesity
Overweight
Overweight, risk for
Personal Identity, disturbed

Post-Trauma Syndrome
Post-Trauma Syndrome, risk for
Powerlessness
Powerlessness, risk for
Rape-Trauma Syndrome
Resilience, impaired
Resilience, risk for impaired
Self-Esteem, chronic low
Self-Esteem, situational low
Self-Esteem, risk for chronic low
Self-Esteem, risk for situational low
Self-Mutilation
Self-Mutilation, risk for
Suicide, risk for
Violence, risk for other-directed
Violence, risk for self-directed

LOVE AND BELONGING

Attachment, risk for impaired
Communication, readiness for enhanced

Coping, compromised family
Coping, disabled family

Development, risk for delayed
Family Processes, dysfunctional
Family Processes, interrupted
Family Processes, readiness for enhanced
Immigration Transition, risk for complicated
Loneliness, risk for
Parenting, impaired
Parenting, readiness for enhanced
Parenting, risk for impaired
Religiosity, impaired
Religiosity, risk for impaired

Relocation Stress Syndrome
Relocation Stress Syndrome, risk for
Role Conflict, parental
Role Performance, ineffective
Sexual Dysfunction
Social Interaction, impaired
Social Isolation
Sorrow, chronic
Spiritual Distress
Spiritual Distress, risk for

SAFETY AND SECURITY

Acute Substance Withdrawal Syndrome
Acute Substance Withdrawal Syndrome, risk for
Adverse Reaction to Iodinated Contrast Media, risk for
Allergy Reaction, risk for
Anxiety
Autonomic Dysreflexia
Autonomic Dysreflexia, risk for
Behavior, readiness for enhanced organized infant
Communication, impaired verbal
Confusion, acute
Confusion, chronic
Confusion, risk for acute
Contamination
Contamination, risk for
Coping, ineffective community
Death Anxiety
Disuse Syndrome, risk for
Dry Eye, risk for
Dry Mouth, risk for
Energy Field, imbalanced
Falls, risk for
Fear
Female Genital Mutilation, risk for
Grieving
Grieving, complicated
Grieving, risk for complicated
Health Behavior, risk-prone
Health Maintenance, ineffective
Health Management, ineffective
Health Management, ineffective family
Health Management, readiness for enhanced
Home Maintenance, impaired
Hyperbilirubinemia, neonatal
Hyperbilirubinemia, risk for neonatal

Infection, risk for
Injury, risk for
Injury, risk for corneal
Injury, risk for urinary tract
Knowledge, deficient (specify)
Latex Allergy Reaction
Latex Allergy Reaction, risk for
Lifestyle, sedentary
Maternal-Fetal Dyad, risk for disturbed
Memory, impaired
Mobility, impaired bed
Mobility, impaired wheelchair
Neonatal Abstinence Syndrome
Neurovascular Dysfunction, risk for peripheral
Occupational Injury, risk for
Perioperative Positioning Injury, risk for
Poisoning, risk for
Protection, ineffective
Role Strain, caregiver
Role Strain, risk for caregiver
Self-Neglect
Sitting, impaired
Standing, impaired
Stress Overload
Sudden Infant Death, risk for
Surgical Site Infection, risk for
Thermal Injury, risk for
Transfer Ability, impaired
Trauma, risk for physical
Trauma, risk for vascular
Unilateral Neglect
Thromboembolism, risk for venous
Walking, impaired
Wandering [specify sporadic or continuous]

Activity Intolerance [specify level]
Activity Intolerance, risk for
Adaptive Capacity, decreased intracranial
Airway Clearance, ineffective
Aspiration, risk for
Behavior, disorganized infant
Behavior, risk for disorganized infant
Bleeding, risk for
Blood Glucose Level, risk for unstable
Blood Pressure, risk for unstable
Breast Milk Production, insufficient
Breastfeeding, ineffective
Breastfeeding, interrupted
Breastfeeding, readiness for enhanced
Breathing Pattern, ineffective
Cardiac Output, decreased
Cardiac Output, risk for decreased
Childbearing Process, ineffective
Childbearing Process, risk for ineffective
Comfort, impaired
Comfort, readiness for enhanced
Constipation
Constipation, chronic functional
Constipation, perceived
Constipation, risk for
Constipation, risk for chronic functional
Dentition, impaired
Diarrhea
Eating Dynamics, ineffective adolescent
Eating Dynamics, ineffective child
Eating Dynamics, ineffective infant
Electrolyte Imbalance, risk for
Elimination, impaired urinary
Frail Elderly Syndrome
Frail Elderly Syndrome, risk for
Fatigue
Feeding Pattern, ineffective infant
Fluid Volume, deficient
Fluid Volume, excess
Fluid Volume, risk for deficient
Fluid Volume, risk for imbalanced
Gas Exchange, impaired
Gastrointestinal Motility, dysfunctional
Gastrointestinal Motility, risk for dysfunctional
Hyperthermia
Hypothermia
Hypothermia, risk for
Hypothermia, risk for perioperative

Incontinence, bowel
Incontinence, functional urinary
Incontinence, overflow urinary
Incontinence, reflex urinary
Incontinence, stress urinary
Incontinence, urge urinary
Incontinence, risk for urge urinary
Insomnia
Liver Function, risk for impaired
Metabolic Imbalance Syndrome, risk for
Mobility, impaired physical
Mucous Membrane, impaired oral
Mucous Membrane, risk for impaired oral
Nausea
Nutrition: less than body requirements, imbalanced
Nutrition, readiness for enhanced
Pain, acute
Pain, chronic
Pain, labor
Pain Syndrome, chronic
Pressure Ulcer, risk for
Retention, urinary [acute/chronic]
Self-Care, readiness for enhanced
Self-Care Deficit (specify): bathing, dressing, feeding, toileting
[Sensory Perception, disturbed (specify: visual, auditory, kinesthetic, gustatory, tactile, olfactory)]
Sexuality Pattern, ineffective
Skin Integrity, impaired
Skin Integrity, risk for impaired
Sleep, readiness for enhanced
Sleep Deprivation
Sleep Pattern, disturbed
Suffocation, risk for
Surgical Recovery, delayed
Surgical Recovery, risk for delayed
Swallowing, impaired
Thermoregulation, ineffective
Thermoregulation, risk for ineffective
Tissue Integrity, impaired
Tissue Integrity, risk for impaired
Tissue Perfusion, ineffective peripheral
Tissue Perfusion, risk for decreased cardiac
Tissue Perfusion, risk for ineffective cerebral
Tissue Perfusion, risk for ineffective peripheral
Ventilation, impaired spontaneous
Ventilatory Weaning Response, dysfunctional

DOENGES & MOORHOUSE'S DIAGNOSTIC DIVISION INDEX

Doenges & Moorhouse's Diagnostic Division Index

---

in multiple organ dysfunction, 1031
NIC linkages, 903
NOC linkages, 903
nursing priorities, 904–906
in peripheral vascular disease, 1042
in pressure ulcer or sore, 1049
in puerperal sepsis, 1059
in Raynaud's disease, 1053
in reflex sympathetic dystrophy, 1053
in thrombophlebitis, 1067
in venous stasis ulcer, 1071
peripheral, risk for, 915–918
in amputation, 966
definition of, 915
documentation focus, 917–918
in electrical injury, 1000
in femoral popliteal bypass, 1003
in gastroplasty, 1006
NIC linkages, 916
in nicotine abuse, 1036
NOC linkages, 915
nursing priorities, 916–917
in total joint replacement, 1068
in varicose veins ligation/stripping, 1073
in pheochromocytoma, 1043
in polyarteritis nodosa, 1045
in polycythemia vera, 1045
risk for
in abdominal aortic aneurysm and repair, 971
in endocarditis, 1001
in lumbar laminectomy, 1024
in metabolic syndrome, 1030
in newborn, 1034
in valvular heart disease, 1073
in scleroderma, 1058
in shock, 1060
in sickle cell anemia, 968
in typhus, 1071
uteroplacental
in postmaturity pregnancy, 1049
risk for, in cardiac conditions, prenatal, 980
in ventricular aneurysm, 968
TMJ syndrome. See Temporomandibular joint syndrome
Toileting, self-care deficit for. See Self-care deficit: bathing, dressing, feeding, toileting
Tonsillectomy. See Adenoidectomy
Tonsillitis, 1067–1068
Total joint replacement, 1068
Tourette's syndrome, 1068
Toxemia of pregnancy. See Hypertension, gestational
Toxic enterocolitis, 1068

Toxic megacolon. See Toxic enterocolitis
Toxic shock syndrome, 1068
Traction, 1068–1069
Transfer ability, impaired, 918–921
definition of, 918
documentation focus, 921
NIC linkages, 919
NOC linkages, 919
nursing priorities, 919–920
in paraplegia, 1040
Transfusion reaction, blood, 1069
Transient ischemic attack (TIA), 1069
Transplant, living donor, 1069
Transplantation, recipient, 1069
Transurethral resection of prostate. See Prostatectomy
Trauma
in Alzheimer's disease, 966
head/neck, risk for, in thyroidectomy, 1067
physical, risk for, 921–927
in cataract, 981
in Cushing's syndrome, 990
definition of, 921
in dementia, 992
in diabetes mellitus, intrapartum, 994
documentation focus, 926
in Down syndrome, 997
in drug overdose, 998
in electrical injury, 1000
in encephalitis, 1001
in fractures, 1004
in hemothorax, 1012
in heroin abuse, 1013
in hyperparathyroidism, 1015
in lead poisoning, 1024
in LSD intoxication, 1026
in meningitis, 1029
in narcolepsy, 1033
NIC linkages, 923
NOC linkages, 922
in nonketotic hyperglycemic-hyperosmolar coma, 1036
nursing priorities, 923–926
in PCP intoxication, 1041
in peritoneal dialysis, 995
in quadriplegia, 1052
in rabies, 1052
in Rett's syndrome, 1056
in Reye's syndrome, 1056
risk for
in brain abscess, 961
in carbon monoxide poisoning, 980
in lumbar laminectomy, 1024
in osteoporosis, 1037
in physical abuse, 961
in seizure disorder, 1059
in sick sinus syndrome, 1061
in stapedectomy, 1063

vascular, risk for, 927–930
definition of, 927
documentation focus, 930
NIC linkages, 928
NOC linkages, 927
nursing priorities, 928–930
Traumatic brain injury (TBI), 1069–1070
Trench foot. See Immersion foot
Trichinosis, 1070
Tricuspid insufficiency. See Valvular heart disease
Tricuspid stenosis. See Valvular heart disease
Tubal pregnancy. See Ectopic pregnancy
Tuberculosis, 1070–1071
TURP. See Prostatectomy
Twin-twin transfusion syndrome, 1071
Tympanoplasty. See Stapedectomy
Typhoid fever, 1071
Typhus, 1071

Ulcer
decubitus, 1071
peptic, 1071
pressure. See Ulcer, decubitus
venous stasis, 1071
Ulnar neuropathy. See Cubital tunnel syndrome
Unconsciousness. See Coma
Unified Medical Language System Metathesaurus, 9
Unilateral neglect, 931–935
definition of, 931
documentation focus, 934
NIC linkages, 932
NOC linkages, 931
nursing priorities, 932–934
risk for, in cerebrovascular accident, 982
Upper GI bleeding. See Gastritis; Ulcer, peptic
Urinary diversion, 1072
Urinary elimination
impaired, 291–295
in bladder cancer, 976
in calculi, urinary, 979
in circumcision, 984
in cystitis, 990
definition of, 291
documentation focus, 294–295
in enuresis, 1002
in hyperparathyroidism, 1015
in hysterectomy, 1018
in intrapartum hypertension, 1016
in labor, 1022
NIC linkages, 291
NOC linkages, 291
nursing priorities, 292–294
in paraplegia, 1040